ADVANCED RECONSTRUCTION

Shoulder 2

Arthroscopy, Arthroplasty, and Fracture Management

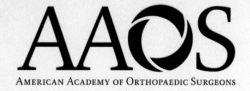

AAOS

AMERICAN ACADEMY OF ORTHOPAEDIC SURGEONS

Video Access

Your purchase of *Advanced Reconstruction: Shoulder 2. Arthroscopy, Arthroplasty, and Fracture Management* includes online access to streaming videos referenced in select chapters throughout the book. Purchasers interested in institutional access to these videos should contact AAOS Licensing at connect@aaos.org or call AAOS Customer Service at 1-800-626-6726. Dial 1-847-823-7186 outside of the U.S. and Canada.

Initial Registration

- Go to www.aaos.org/ARShoulder/video and follow the instructions to redeem your code and gain video access for this title.

Your access code:

For Technical Support

- Email customerservice@aaos.org or call 1-800-626-6726.

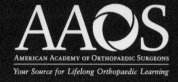

AMERICAN ACADEMY OF ORTHOPAEDIC SURGEONS
Your Source for Lifelong Orthopaedic Learning

ADVANCED RECONSTRUCTION

Shoulder 2

Arthroscopy, Arthroplasty, and Fracture Management

Edited by

Jeffrey S. Abrams, MD
Clinical Professor
Department of Surgery
Seton Hall University
Orange, New Jersey
Attending Surgeon
Department of Surgery
University Medical Center of Princeton
Princeton, New Jersey

Robert H. Bell, MD
Crystal Clinic Orthopaedic Center
Akron, Ohio

John M. Tokish, MD
Clinical Professor
University of South Carolina School of Medicine Greenville
Greenville, South Carolina
Adjunct Professor, Department of Bioengineering
Professor, School of Health Research
Clemson University
Clemson, South Carolina
Associate Director, Sports Medicine Fellowship
Steadman Hawkins Clinic of the Carolinas
Greenville, South Carolina

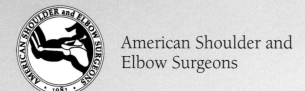

American Shoulder and
Elbow Surgeons

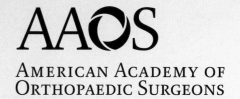

AMERICAN ACADEMY OF
ORTHOPAEDIC SURGEONS

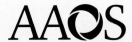

The material presented in *Advanced Reconstruction: Shoulder 2* has been made available by the American Academy of Orthopaedic Surgeons for educational purposes only. This material is not intended to present the only, or necessarily best, methods or procedures for the medical situations discussed, but rather is intended to represent an approach, view, statement, or opinion of the author(s) or producer(s), which may be helpful to others who face similar situations.

Some drugs or medical devices demonstrated in Academy courses or described in Academy print or electronic publications have not been cleared by the Food and Drug Administration (FDA) or have been cleared for specific uses only. The FDA has stated that it is the responsibility of the physician to determine the FDA clearance status of each drug or device he or she wishes to use in clinical practice.

Furthermore, any statements about commercial products are solely the opinion(s) of the author(s) and do not represent an Academy endorsement or evaluation of these products. These statements may not be used in advertising or for any commercial purpose.

Library of Congress Control Number: 2016937873

Published 2016 by the
American Academy of Orthopaedic Surgeons
9400 West Higgins Road
Rosemont, IL 60018

Copyright 2016
by the American Academy of Orthopaedic Surgeons

ISBN 978-1-62552-544-4
Printed in the USA

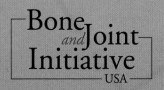

Acknowledgments

Advanced Reconstruction: Shoulder 2
Editorial Board

Jeffrey S. Abrams, MD

Robert H. Bell, MD

John M. Tokish, MD

American Shoulder and Elbow Surgeons
Executive Committee, 2015-2016

Jesse B. Jupiter, MD
President

Felix H. Savoie III, MD
President-Elect

Anthony A. Romeo, MD
Vice President

C. Craig Satterlee, MD
Secretary/Treasurer

William J. Mallon, MD
Immediate Past President

Robert H. Bell, MD
Past President

John E. (Jed) Kuhn, MD
Member-at-Large

Joseph A. Abboud, MD
Member-at-Large

Explore the full portfolio of AAOS educational programs and publications across the orthopaedic spectrum for every stage of an orthopaedic surgeon's career, at www.aaos.org. The AAOS, in partnership with Jones & Bartlett Learning, also offers a comprehensive collection of educational and training resources for emergency medical providers, from first responders to critical care transport paramedics. Learn more at www.aaos.org/ems.

Contributors

Joseph A. Abboud, MD
Orthopaedic Surgeon and Associate Professor
Department of Shoulder and Elbow Surgery
Rothman Institute
Philadelphia, Pennsylvania

Jeffrey S. Abrams, MD
Clinical Professor
Department of Surgery
Seton Hall University
Orange, New Jersey
Attending Surgeon
Department of Surgery
University Medical Center of Princeton
Princeton, New Jersey

Christopher S. Ahmad, MD
Professor of Orthopedic Surgery
Columbia Orthopedics
Columbia University Medical Center
New York, New York

Michael H. Amini, MD
Shoulder and Elbow Fellow
Orthopaedic and Rheumatologic Institute
Cleveland Clinic
Cleveland, Ohio

Jeffrey O. Anglen, MD
Professor
Department of Orthopaedics
Indiana University
Indianapolis, Indiana

Cameron Michael Anley, MD
Fellow
Arthroscopic Reconstruction
University of British Columbia
Vancouver, British Columbia, Canada

John M. Apostolakos, BS
Department of Orthopaedic Surgery
University of Connecticut Health Center
Farmington, Connecticut

Robert Arciero, MD
Professor
Department of Orthopaedics
University of Connecticut
Farmington, Connecticut

Luke S. Austin, MD
Assistant Professor of Orthopaedic Surgery
Rothman Institute
Philadelphia, Pennsylvania

Frank R. Avilucea, MD
Orthopaedic Trauma Fellow
Vanderbilt Medical Center
Nashville, Tennessee

Jeffrey Backes, MD
Orthopaedic Surgeon
Department of Orthopaedic Surgery
Greenville Health System
Greenville, South Carolina

Jonathan D. Barlow, MD, MS
Assistant Professor, Shoulder and Elbow Surgery
Department of Sports Medicine
Ohio State University
Columbus, Ohio

Carl J. Basamania, MD
Orthopaedic Surgeon
Department of Orthopedic Surgery
The Polyclinic
Department of Orthopedic Surgery
Swedish Orthopedic Institute
Seattle, Washington

Robert H. Bell, MD
Crystal Clinic Orthopaedic Center
Akron, Ohio

Jared C. Bentley, MD
Orthopaedic Surgeon
Steadman Hawkins Clinic of the Carolinas
Greenville Health System
Greenville, South Carolina

Randa Berdusco, MD, MSc, FRCS
Orthopaedic Surgeon
Department of Orthopaedic Surgery
Pan Am Clinic
Winnipeg, Manitoba, Canada

Kamal I. Bohsali, MD, FACS
Jacksonville Orthopaedic Institute
Orthopaedic Surgeon, Shoulder and Elbow Reconstruction
Department of Orthopaedics
Baptist Beaches Medical Center
Jacksonville Beach, Florida

James P. Bradley, MD
Clinical Professor, Orthopaedic Surgery
Burke and Bradley Orthopedics
University of Pittsburgh Medical Center
Pittsburgh, Pennsylvania

Stephen S. Burkhart, MD
Orthopaedic Surgeon
The San Antonio Orthopaedic Group
San Antonio, Texas

Wayne Z. Burkhead, Jr, MD
Orthopedic Surgeon
The Shoulder Service
W.B. Carrell Memorial Clinic
Dallas, Texas

Robert T. Burks, MD
Professor of Orthopaedic Surgery
University of Utah
Salt Lake City, Utah

Ryan M. Carr, MD
Orthopaedic Fellow
Department of Orthopaedics
Cleveland Shoulder Institute
Beachwood, Ohio

Danielle Casagrande, MD
Orthopaedic Surgical Fellow
Department of Orthopaedics
Shoulder, Elbow, and Hand Clinic
San Francisco, California

Peter N. Chalmers, MD
Chief Resident
Department of Orthopedic Surgery
Midwest Orthopaedics at Rush
Rush University Medical Center
Chicago, Illinois

John J. Christoforetti, MD
Assistant Professor, Orthopedic Surgery
Sports Medicine Division
Drexel University College of Medicine
Allegheny Health Network
Pittsburgh, Pennsylvania

Frank A. Cordasco, MD, MS
Attending Orthopaedic Surgeon
Department of Orthopaedic Surgery
Hospital for Special Surgery
Weill Cornell Medical College
New York, New York

Mark P. Cote, DPT, MSCTR
Sports Medicine Clinical Outcomes Facilitator
Department of Orthopaedic Surgery
University of Connecticut Health Center
Farmington, Connecticut

Lynn A. Crosby, MD
Professor and Director of Shoulder Surgery
Department of Orthopaedic Surgery
Medical College of Georgia
Georgia Regents University
Augusta, Georgia

S. David Daniels, BS
Research Assistant
Department of Orthopedic Surgery
Brigham and Women's Hospital
Boston, Massachusetts

Omkar H. Dave, MD
Physician
Department of Orthopaedics
Mississippi Sports Medicine and Orthopaedic Center
Jackson, Mississippi

David M. Dines, MD
Attending Orthopedic Surgeon
Sports Medicine and Shoulder Service
Hospital for Special Surgery
New York, New York

Joshua S. Dines, MD
Attending Orthopedic Surgeon
Sports Medicine and Shoulder Service
Hospital for Special Surgery
New York, New York

Jessica DiVenere, BS
Research Assistant 1
Department of Orthopaedic Surgery
University of Connecticut Health Center
Farmington, Connecticut

Thomas R. Duquin, MD
Assistant Professor
Department of Orthopaedic Surgery
University at Buffalo
Buffalo, New York

Kenneth A. Egol, MD
Professor and Vice Chair
Department of Orthopaedic Surgery
NYU Hospital for Joint Diseases
NYU Langone Medical Center
New York, New York

Neal S. ElAttrache, MD
Kerlan-Jobe Orthopaedic Clinic
Los Angeles, California

Bassem T. Elhassan, MD
Consultant
Department of Orthopedic Surgery
Mayo Clinic
Rochester, Minnesota

Gregory A. Erickson, MD
Orthopaedic Surgeon
OrthoWest
Omaha, Nebraska

Larry D. Field, MD
Physician
Department of Orthopaedics
Mississippi Sports Medicine and Orthopaedic Center
Jackson, Mississippi

Leslie A. Fink Barnes, MD
Fellow
Department of Orthopaedic Surgery
Mount Sinai School of Medicine
New York, New York

Kelly Fitzpatrick, DO
Orthopaedic Surgeon
Department of Orthopaedics
Blanchfield Army Community Hospital
Fort Campbell, Kentucky

Evan L. Flatow, MD
Professor, Orthopaedic Surgery
Mount Sinai School of Medicine
President, Roosevelt Hospital
New York, New York

Janice Flocken, BA, MS
Research Assistant
Cleveland Shoulder Institute
University Hospitals of Cleveland
Beachwood, Ohio

Salvatore J. Frangiamore, MD, MS
Department of Orthopaedic Surgery
Cleveland Clinic
Cleveland, Ohio

Mark A. Frankle, MD
Chief of Shoulder and Elbow Surgery
Florida Orthopaedic Institute
Tampa, Florida

Matthew Furey, MD, MSc, FRCSC
Trauma and Upper Extremity Fellow
St. Michael's Hospital
University of Toronto
Toronto, Ontario, Canada

E'Stephan J. Garcia, MD
Orthopaedic Surgeon
Department of Orthopaedic Surgery
Keller Army Community Hospital
West Point, New York

Grant E. Garrigues, MD
Associate Professor
Shoulder and Elbow Surgery
Department of Orthopaedic Surgery
Duke University Medical Center
Durham, North Carolina

Mark H. Getelman, MD
Southern California Orthopedic Institute
Van Nuys, California

Blake P. Gillette, MD
Sports Medicine Fellow
Department of Orthopedic Surgery
Southern California Orthopedic Institute
Van Nuys, California

Reuben Gobezie, MD
Director, Cleveland Shoulder Institute
University Hospitals of Cleveland
Cleveland, Ohio

Brian Grawe, MD
Assistant Professor
Department of Orthopaedics and Sports Medicine
University of Cincinnati
Cincinnati, Ohio

Andrew Green, MD
Chief, Division of Shoulder and Elbow Surgery
Associate Professor
Department of Orthopaedic Surgery
University Orthopedics
Warren Alpert Medical School
Brown University
Providence, Rhode Island

Joshua A. Greenspoon, BSc
Visiting Research Scholar
Center for Outcomes-Based Orthopaedic Research
Steadman Philippon Research Institute
Vail, Colorado

Adam D. Hall, MD
Upper Extremity Surgeon
Fort Wayne Orthopedics
Fort Wayne, Indiana

Samuel Harmsen, MD
Physician
The San Francisco Shoulder, Elbow, and Hand Clinic
San Francisco, California

Robert U. Hartzler, MD, MS
Orthopaedic Surgeon
The San Antonio Orthopaedic Group
San Antonio, Texas

Richard J. Hawkins, MD
Orthopaedic Surgeon
Steadman Hawkins Clinic of the Carolinas
Greenville Health System
Greenville, South Carolina

Laurence D. Higgins, MD
Chief of Sports Medicine
Department of Orthopedic Surgery
Brigham and Women's Hospital
Boston, Massachusetts

Michael M. Hussey, MD
Shoulder and Elbow Specialist
Arkansas Specialty Orthopaedics
Little Rock, Arkansas

Joseph P. Iannotti, MD, PhD
Maynard Madden Professor and Chair
Orthopaedic and Rheumatologic Institute
Cleveland Clinic
Cleveland, Ohio

Akshay Jain, MD
Research Fellow
Department of Orthopaedic Surgery
Rush University Medical Center
Chicago, Illinois

Charles M. Jobin, MD
Assistant Professor
Department of Orthopedic Surgery
Columbia University Medical Center
New York, New York

Jesse B. Jupiter, MD
Hansjorg Wyss AO Professor of Orthopedic Surgery
Harvard Medical School
Department of Orthopaedic Surgery
Massachusetts General Hospital
Boston, Massachusetts

Michael J. Kissenberth, MD
Orthopedic Surgeon
Steadman Hawkins Clinic of the Carolinas
Greenville Health System
Greenville, South Carolina

Michael Knesek, MD
Sports Medicine and Shoulder Fellow
Department of Orthopaedic Surgery
Northwestern Memorial Hospital
Chicago, Illinois

Jia-Wei Kevin Ko, MD
Shoulder & Elbow Fellow
Department of Shoulder and Elbow Surgery
Rothman Institute
Philadelphia, Pennsylvania

Jason L. Koh, MD
Chairman
Department of Orthopaedic Surgery
NorthShore University HealthSystem
Evanston, Illinois

Sanjit R. Konda, MD
Assistant Professor
Department of Orthopaedic Surgery
NYU Hospital for Joint Diseases
NYU Langone Medical Center
New York, New York

John E. Kuhn, MD, MS
Kenneth D. Schermerhorn Professor of Orthopaedics
Department of Sports Medicine and Rehabilitation
Vanderbilt University Medical Center
Nashville, Tennessee

Marc R. Labbé, MD
Clinical Associate Professor
Department of Orthopedic Surgery
Baylor College of Medicine
Houston, Texas
University of Texas Medical Branch
Galveston, Texas

Mark D. Lazarus, MD
Associate Professor
Department of Orthopaedic Surgery
Rothman Institute
Sidney Kimmel Medical College
Thomas Jefferson University
Philadelphia, Pennsylvania

Ian K.Y. Lo, MD, FRCSC
Department of Surgery
University of Calgary
Calgary, Alberta, Canada

Adam J. Lorenzetti, MD
Orthopedic Surgeon
Department of Orthopaedic Surgery
Florida Orthopaedic Institute
Tampa, Florida

Peter B. MacDonald, MD, FRCSC
Professor and Head
Section of Orthopaedics
University of Manitoba
Winnipeg, Manitoba, Canada

William J. Mallon, MD
Triangle Orthopaedic Associates
Durham, North Carolina

Guido Marra, MD
Professor of Orthopaedic Surgery
Department of Orthopaedic Surgery
Northwestern University
Chicago, Illinois

Augustus D. Mazzocca, MS, MD
Chair, Department of Orthopaedic Surgery
Director, New England Musculoskeletal Institute
University of Connecticut Health Center
Farmington, Connecticut

Michael McKee, MD, FRCSC
Professor
Division of Orthopaedic Surgery, Faculty of Medicine
University of Toronto
Toronto, Ontario, Canada

Chris R. Mellano, MD
Orthopedic Surgeon
Beach Cities Orthopedics and Sports Medicine
Manhattan Beach, California

Bruce S. Miller, MD, MS
Associate Professor
Department of Orthopaedic Surgery
University of Michigan
Ann Arbor, Michigan

Peter J. Millett, MD, MSc
Director of Shoulder Service
Steadman Clinic
Steadman Philippon Research Institute
Vail, Colorado

Anthony Miniaci, MD, FRCSC
Attending Physician
Cleveland Clinic Orthopaedic and Rheumatologic Institute
Cleveland Clinic Foundation
Cleveland, Ohio

Brent Mollon, MD, FRCSC
Clinical Fellow, Shoulder and Elbow
Department of Orthopaedics
NYU Hospital for Joint Diseases
NYU School of Medicine
NYU Langone Medical Center
New York, New York

Brian H. Mullis, MD
Chief of Orthopaedic Trauma Service
Eskenazi Health
Indiana School of Medicine
Indianapolis, Indiana

Jeffrey S. Noble, MD
Associate Professor of Orthopaedic Surgery
Crystal Clinic Orthopaedic Center
Akron, Ohio

William T. Obremskey, MD, MPH, MMHC
Chief of Orthopaedic Trauma
Vanderbilt Medical Center
Nashville, Tennessee

Michael J. O'Brien, MD
Assistant Professor
Department of Orthopaedics
Tulane University School of Medicine
New Orleans, Louisiana

Yohei Ono, MD, PhD
Shoulder Fellow
Department of Surgery
University of Calgary
Calgary, Alberta, Canada

Michael B. O'Sullivan, MD
Department of Orthopaedic Surgery
University of Connecticut Health Center
Farmington, Connecticut

Brett D. Owens, MD
Chief of Orthopaedic Surgery
Keller Army Hospital
West Point, New York

Stephen A. Parada, MD
Shoulder and Sports Medicine Surgeon
Department of Orthopaedics
Eisenhower Army Medical Center
Fort Gordon, Georgia

Maxwell C. Park, MD
Partner Physician
Department of Orthopaedic Surgery
Kaiser Permanente
Woodland Hills, California

E. Scott Paxton, MD
Assistant Professor
Department of Orthopaedic Surgery
Warren Alpert Medical School
Brown University
Providence, Rhode Island

Maximilian Petri, MD
Orthopaedic Surgeon and Research Fellow
Steadman Clinic
Steadman Philippon Research Institute
Vail, Colorado

Roger G. Pollock, MD
Assistant Professor of Clinical Orthopaedic Surgery
Columbia University
New York, New York

Matthew T. Provencher, MD, CDR, MC, USNR
Chief, Department of Sports Medicine
Massachusetts General Hospital
Boston, Massachusetts

William D. Regan, MD, FRCSC
Department of Orthopedics
UBC Hospital
Vancouver, British Columbia, Canada

Eric T. Ricchetti, MD
Staff, Orthopaedic and Rheumatologic Institute
Cleveland Clinic
Cleveland, Ohio

Anthony A. Romeo, MD
Orthopaedic Surgeon
Department of Orthopedics
Midwest Orthopaedics at Rush
Chicago, Illinois

Matthew D. Saltzman, MD
Assistant Professor
Department of Orthopaedic Surgery
Northwestern University
Chicago, Illinois

George Sánchez, BS
Research Coordinator
Department of Sports Medicine and Surgery
Massachusetts General Hospital
Boston, Massachusetts

Joaquin Sanchez-Sotelo, MD, PhD
Consultant and Professor of Orthopedics
Department of Orthopedic Surgery
Mayo Clinic
Rochester, Minnesota

Felix H. Savoie III, MD
Professor and Vice Chairman
Department of Orthopaedics
Tulane University School of Medicine
New Orleans, Louisiana

Mark A. Schrumpf, MD
Attending Surgeon
San Francisco Shoulder, Elbow and Hand Clinic
California Pacific Medical Center
San Francisco, California

Benjamin S. Shaffer, MD
Associate Professor
Department of Orthopaedics
Johns Hopkins Sibley Memorial Medical Center
Washington, District of Columbia

Yousef Shishani, MD
Research Fellow
Cleveland Shoulder Institute
University Hospitals of Cleveland
Beachwood, Ohio

Monica Shoji, BA
Department of Orthopaedic Surgery
University of Connecticut Health Center
Farmington, Connecticut

Amit Sood, MD
Fellow
Department of Orthopaedic Surgery
Massachusetts General Hospital
Harvard Medical School
Shoulder and Elbow Fellow
Department of Orthopedic Surgery
Brigham and Women's Hospital
Boston, Massachusetts

John W. Sperling, MD, MBA
Professor of Orthopedic Surgery
Mayo Clinic
Rochester, Minnesota

Scott P. Steinmann, MD
Consultant
Department of Orthopedic Surgery
Mayo Clinic
Rochester, Minnesota

Brent Stephens, MD
Department of Orthopaedic Surgery
Florida Orthopaedic Institute
Tampa, Florida

Geoffrey P. Stone, MD
Orthopaedic Surgeon
Department of Shoulder and Elbow Surgery
Florida Orthopaedic Institute
Tampa, Florida

Philipp N. Streubel, MD
Assistant Professor
Department of Orthopaedic Surgery
University of Nebraska Medical Center
Omaha, Nebraska

Fotios P. Tjoumakaris, MD
Associate Professor
Department of Orthopaedic Surgery
Jefferson Medical College
Philadelphia, Pennsylvania

John M. Tokish, MD
Clinical Professor
University of South Carolina School of Medicine Greenville
Greenville, South Carolina
Adjunct Professor, Department of Bioengineering
Professor, School of Health Research
Clemson University
Clemson, South Carolina
Associate Director, Sports Medicine Fellowship
Steadman Hawkins Clinic of the Carolinas
Greenville, South Carolina

Nikhil N. Verma, MD
Assistant Professor
Department of Orthopaedic Surgery
Rush University Medical Center
Chicago, Illinois

Mandeep S. Virk, MD
Clinical Fellow, Orthopaedic Surgeon
Department of Orthopedics
Midwest Orthopaedics at Rush
Rush University Medical Center
Chicago, Illinois

George Christian Vorys, MD
Fellow
Department of Sports Medicine
Massachusetts General Hospital
Boston, Massachusetts

Jon J.P. Warner, MD
Chief, Shoulder Service
Department of Orthopedics
Massachusetts General Hospital
Harvard Medical School
Boston, Massachusetts

Russell F. Warren, MD
Professor, Orthopedics
Department of Sports Medicine
Hospital for Special Surgery
New York, New York

K. Durham Weeks, MD
Orthopedic Surgery
Sports Medicine Service
OrthoCarolina
Charlotte, North Carolina

Ian G. Wilkofsky, MD
Orthopedic Surgeon
Shoulder Service
W.B. Carrell Memorial Clinic
Dallas, Texas

Gerald R. Williams, Jr, MD
John M. Fenlin, Jr., MD Professor of Shoulder and Elbow
    Surgery
Department of Orthopaedic Surgery
Rothman Institute
Sidney Kimmel Medical College
Thomas Jefferson University
Philadelphia, Pennsylvania

Joseph B. Wilson, MD
Department of Sports Medicine and Shoulder Reconstruction
Triangle Orthopaedics
Raleigh, North Carolina

Michael A. Wirth, MD
Professor and Charles A. Rockwood Chair, Orthopaedics
Department of Orthopaedics
University of Texas Health Sciences Center at San Antonio
San Antonio, Texas

Justin S. Yang, MD
Orthopaedic Sports Medicine Fellow
Department of Orthopaedics
University of Connecticut
Farmington, Connecticut

Seung Jin Yi, MD
Sports Fellow
Department of Orthopaedic Surgery
University of Chicago
Chicago, Illinois

Joseph D. Zuckerman, MD
Professor and Chairman
Department of Orthopaedic Surgery
NYU Hospital for Joint Diseases
NYU School of Medicine
NYU Langone Medical Center
New York, New York

Foreword

It is a privilege and an honor to write the foreword for this comprehensive shoulder textbook, *Advanced Reconstruction: Shoulder 2: Arthroscopy, Arthroplasty, and Fracture Management*. It is an honor because the three editors for the book, Dr. Jeffrey Abrams, Dr. Rob Bell, and Dr. John (JT) Tokish have been three of the best fellows that I have ever had the privilege of training. This publication is a combined effort of the American Shoulder and Elbow Surgeons (ASES) and the American Academy of Orthopaedic Surgeons (AAOS). You will see from the table of contents that an international roster of authors contributed their expertise; many authors are members of ASES.

The chapter design for this edition is unique in that it begins with a case presentation, followed by a discussion of indications for treatment, patient assessment, and a bulleted presentation of the surgical technique steps. Several chapters feature associated videos. The bibliographies reflect advances in the field. This carefully structured and organized, well-written, and expertly illustrated publication, along with the associated videos, presents comprehensive and up-to-date information on shoulder reconstruction.

It is with great personal pride that I watch Drs. Abrams, Bell, and Tokish spearhead this publication.

On a sadder note, in 2015 we lost one of our authors, Dr. Benjamin Shaffer. He wrote Chapter 27, "Arthroscopic Distal Clavicle Resection: Optimizing Technique." Dr. Shaffer passed away at the young age of 57. He was an active member of all of our societies, including ASES, Arthroscopy Association of North America, AAOS, and American Orthopaedic Society for Sports Medicine, and was a champion for shoulder education. During his career, he was team physician for the Georgetown Hoyas, the Washington Nationals, and the Washington Capitals. He will be missed greatly by Jill, his loving wife of 20 years, his daughter Emma, his son Noah, and all of us.

Richard J. Hawkins, MD
Orthopaedic Surgeon
Steadman Hawkins Clinic of the Carolinas
Greenville Health System
Greenville, South Carolina

Preface

Advanced Reconstruction: Shoulder 2: Arthroscopy, Arthroplasty, and Fracture Management, follows on the success of the first edition published more than 9 years ago. Case-based physician education that can be directly applied to clinical pathology is the new learning model. Currently, physician meetings include clinical panels and debates in which accepted and new theories in managing symptomatic shoulders are presented. Following that learning model, this expanded publication presents common and complex shoulder maladies with a unique modernized approach that includes case-based presentations, detailed descriptions of surgical technique, and video to illustrate repair and reconstruction techniques.

The table of contents covers 61 topics, including sports, trauma, and degenerative and neurovascular deficits. Each chapter was authored by an expert on the topic and begins with an illustrative case scenario, including noteworthy aspects of patient history, physical examination findings, and preferred imaging to best illustrate the pathoanatomy. Multiple treatment options ranging from nonsurgical to arthroscopic and open surgical approaches are compared and contrasted, and authors present their justification for their preferred treatment method. In addition to the illustrated, detailed descriptions of safe and efficient surgical approaches, authors present pearls and pitfalls; 26 chapters have associated video. The balanced approach to presenting multiple techniques further enhances the reader's knowledge and informs surgical planning and patient care, with the goal of reducing the risk of complications during and after treatment.

Advanced Reconstruction: Shoulder 2: Arthroscopy, Arthroplasty, and Fracture Management is a landmark textbook providing the reader with clinical pearls, a discussion of the controversies on best approaches to manage common and complex shoulder problems, time-tested and cutting-edge surgical techniques, and an up-to-date bibliography for researching topics of interest. The American Shoulder and Elbow Surgeons (ASES) joined forces with the American Academy of Orthopaedic Surgeons (AAOS) to create this state-of-the-art reference that can be immediately applied to clinical evaluation and decision making and that can serve as a resource for surgical planning. The AAOS staff has been invaluable in the production of this important work. Laura Goetz, Managing Editor, and Rachel Winokur, Editorial Coordinator, provided hands-on assistance, joining Lisa Claxton Moore, Senior Manager, Book Program, and Elizabeth Durham, Instructional Designer, to organize the chapter collections, provide instruction to authors, and facilitate seamless interaction with the three editors. Katie Hovany, Digital Media Specialist, collaborated with authors on polishing their video submissions. The editors thank the contributing ASES authors, the AAOS staff, and everyone who helped to create this educational resource.

Jeffrey S. Abrams, MD
Robert H. Bell, MD
John M. Tokish, MD
Editors

Table of Contents

Video Index

Video 31.1 Arthroscopic Capsular Release: Keys to Safe and Effective Restoration of Motion. Bruce S. Miller, MD, MS (2 min)

 Video 32.1 Arthroscopic Management of Glenohumeral Osteoarthritis: Nonarthroplasty Options for Joint Preservation. Maximilian Petri, MD; Joshua A. Greenspoon, BSc; Peter J. Millett, MD, MSc (7 min)

 Video 36.1 Uncomplicated Total Shoulder Arthroplasty. Joseph D. Zuckerman, MD; Brent Mollon, MD, FRCSC; William E. Ryan, Jr, BS (9 min)

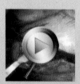 **Video 37.1** The Difficult Glenoid in Total Shoulder Arthroplasty: Reaming and Bone Grafting Techniques to Ensure Long-Term Stability. David M. Dines, MD; Joshua S. Dines, MD (8 min)

 Video 38.1 Cuff Tear Arthropathy Reverse Shoulder Arthroplasty: Steps to Get it Right. Richard J. Hawkins, MD; Jeffrey R. Backes, MD; Jared C. Bentley, MD; Michael J. Kissenberth, MD (15 min)

 Video 41.1 Revision Total Shoulder Arthroplasty to Reverse Total Shoulder Arthroplasty. Reuben Gobezie, MD; Yousef Shishani, MD (9 min)

 Video 45.1 Proximal Humerus Intramedullary Nail Technique. Brian H. Mullis, MD; Jeffrey O. Anglen, MD (15 min)

 Video 46.1 Fracture Platform Prosthesis. Michael A. Wirth, MD; Kamal I. Bohsali, MD, FACS (13 min)

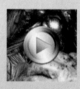 **Video 47.1** Reverse Shoulder Arthroplasty for Acute Proximal Humerus Fractures. Michael M. Hussey, MD; Brent Stephens, MD; Mark A. Frankle, MD (4 min)

 Video 60.1 Scapulothoracic Fusion for Facioscapulohumeral Muscular Dystrophy. Anthony A. Romeo, MD (39 min)

Solid Foundations for Successful Shoulder Surgery
Jeffrey S. Abrams, MD

Chapter 1

The Beach-Chair and Lateral Decubitus Positions: Key Surgical Principles

Seung Jin Yi, MD

Jason L. Koh, MD

 ## Introduction

Two positions commonly used in arthroscopic shoulder procedures are the lateral decubitus position and the beach-chair position. The lateral decubitus position was first described for shoulder arthroscopy in 1984. The beach-chair position was introduced in 1988 in an effort to decrease the number of neuropathies seen with the lateral decubitus position. The choice of position is typically based on the surgeon's training and comfort with the position, the risk of complications, the ease of conversion to an open procedure if needed, and the access to the shoulder afforded by the position. Advantages and disadvantages of each position are listed in **Table 1**.

 ## Indications

Advocates of the lateral decubitus position claim that it allows better visualization of the joint and the subacromial space. Traction of the arm is accomplished with the use of a pulley on a boom without the need for an assistant to pull traction. The traction pulls the humeral head down and away from the acromion, allowing ample room to work in the subacromial space. Balanced suspension traction places the glenoid parallel to the floor and provides equal access to the posterior and anterior glenoid margins and inferior pouch. The traction also increases the work space around the limited inferior and posterior quadrants of the glenohumeral joint. For this reason, some surgeons who mainly use the beach-chair position prefer the lateral decubitus position when performing surgical procedures to address instability.

Proponents of the beach-chair position claim that it allows increased visualization of the joint with a lower risk of nerve injuries. In a cadaver study, the musculocutaneous and axillary nerves were found to be closer to the anteroinferior portal in the lateral decubitus position than in the beach-chair position. The upright, anatomic position makes orientation to the anatomic structures and teaching easier. Because the entire extremity can be positioned during the surgical procedure, the beach-chair position allows the surgeon to move the arm to improve access to different parts of the joint, which is particularly important during rotator cuff repair. The beach-chair position is preferable when conversion from an arthroscopic to an open procedure may be required because there is no need to reposition and redrape the patient. The neutral position of the cervical spine in the beach-chair position can be maintained during an intraoperative change of procedures. Some shoulder surgeons prefer the beach-chair position simply because the same setup is used for other shoulder procedures, and the use of a consistent position minimizes confusion and variability for the support staff. In addition, some surgeons prefer the beach-chair position because it facilitates the use of regional rather than general anesthesia.

 ## Controversies and Alternative Approaches

Many variations of these positions are available, and surgeon preference dictates which is used. The arthroscopic portal skin incisions may be slightly different with the two position options. Surgeons using the lateral decubitus position prefer different angles and

Dr. Koh or an immediate family member serves as a paid consultant to Aesculap/B. Braun Medical, Aperion Biologics, and Arthrex; has stock or stock options held in Aperion Biologics; and serves as a board member, owner, officer, or committee member of the American Orthopaedic Society for Sports Medicine, the Arthroscopy Association of North America, the Illinois Association of Orthopaedic Surgeons, and the Patellofemoral Foundation. Neither Dr. Yi nor any immediate family member has received anything of value from or has stock or stock options held in a commercial company or institution related directly or indirectly to the subject of this chapter.

Table 1 Advantages and Disadvantages of the Lateral Decubitus and Beach-Chair Positions

Factor	Lateral Decubitus Position	Beach-Chair Position
Advantages	Traction increases space in joint and subacromial space	Upright, anatomic position
	Traction accentuates labral tears	Ease of examination under anesthesia
	Surgical table/patient's head not in the way of posterior and superior shoulder	Arm not hanging in the way of anterior portal
	Cautery bubbles move laterally out of view	No need to reposition or redrape to convert to open procedure
	No increased risk of hypotension/bradycardia; better cerebral perfusion	Can use regional anesthesia
		Mobility of operated arm
Disadvantages	Nonanatomic orientation	Potential mechanical blocks to use of arthroscope in posterior or superior portals
	Must reach around arm for anterior portal	Increased risk of hypotension/bradycardia causing cardiovascular complications
	Must reposition and redrape to convert to open procedure	Cautery bubbles obscure view in subacromial space
	Patients do not tolerate regional anesthesia	Fluid can fog arthroscope
	Traction can cause neurovascular and soft-tissue injury	Theoretically increased risk of air embolus
	Increased risk of injury to axillary and musculocutaneous nerves when placing anteroinferior portal	Expensive equipment if using beach-chair attachment with or without mechanical arm holder

Adapted with permission from Peruto CM, Ciccotti MG, Cohen SB: Shoulder arthroscopy positioning: Lateral decubitus versus beach chair. *Arthroscopy* 2009;25(8):891-896.

amounts of traction. Some surgeons prefer to have the shoulder in a so-called lazy lateral position (in which the operated shoulder is allowed to fall back 20°), with the glenoid parallel to the floor. Several commercially available arm holders have been developed for use with the lateral decubitus position. Some surgeons prefer to have the patient rotated 180° in the operating room such that the anesthesia device is at the foot of the table and sedation is monitored remotely. This position allows the surgeon to work easily near the patient's head, with good access to both sides of the joint.

In the beach-chair position, the angle of inclination can vary from 45° to 90°. To support the operated arm, a mechanical arm holder (such as Trimano [Arthrex], Spider2 limb positioner [Smith & Nephew] or McConnell arm holder [McConnell Orthopedic Manufacturing]) or a simple padded Mayo stand can be used. The beach-chair position can be achieved with the use of commercial table attachments, breakaway surgical tables, or a beanbag on a standard surgical table. Most surgeons turn the table approximately 45° away from the anesthesia device to give surgeons and assistants adequate room to work behind the shoulder without interfering with the anesthesia setup.

Results

No scientific evidence suggests that either position is superior to the other.

No studies have proved that one position is better than the other in terms of technique or outcomes. Successful results in both positions have been clinically proved. Both positions have risks specific to the position, and it is difficult to determine which position is safer overall.

Technical Keys to Success

Lateral Decubitus Position

- The patient is placed on top of a beanbag on the surgical table.
- General anesthesia is administered through endotracheal intubation.
- A draw sheet is used to turn the patient onto the nonoperated side so that the operated side is up.
- In the Gross-Fitzgibbons modification of the lateral decubitus position, the table is tilted 20° to 30° to align the glenoid parallel to the floor. Many surgeons have adapted this technique by using the lazy lateral position previously described.
- An axillary roll is placed between the table and the axilla of the nonoperated side to prevent compression of the brachial plexus.
- The legs and stress points are well padded.
- The arm is placed in traction in 45° of flexion and 60° of abduction by using a 10-lb sandbag attached to a boom (**Figure 1**).
- The surgical table is turned approximately 45° away from the anesthesia device to allow the surgeon and assistant sufficient room to work near the patient's head.
- The patient is draped with a combination of sterile U-drapes and sheets.
- During the procedure, a bump made of rolled sterile towels wrapped in cohesive elastic wrap can be placed under the axilla to

facilitate lateral distraction of the glenohumeral joint.
- A second traction strap or an assistant can also pull the arm laterally to distract the joint.
- The arm can be translated anteriorly or posteriorly to allow the surgeon to work on the posterior or anterior labral surface.
- Depending on the traction setup, the arm may be rotated externally and internally to help expose different parts of the humeral head for anchor placement.
- The degree of abduction for inferior access to the pouch can vary. Abduction is more common with the lateral decubitus position than with the beach-chair position.

Beach-Chair Position

- The patient is positioned on a surgical table designed for the beach-chair position with a back attachment that allows the surgeon to secure the patient's head, neck, and torso for greater access to the posterior shoulder.
- If regional anesthesia is desired, it is administered before patient positioning. If general anesthesia is preferred, it can be administered with the patient lying supine.
- A particular concern with the beach-chair position is the maintenance of adequate cerebral oxygenation in patients who are under general anesthesia and are unable to perform usual autoregulation. The maintenance of systolic blood pressure at 20% of baseline or the use of regional anesthesia and sedation rather than general anesthesia can help avoid this complication. An inclined rather than vertical position can decrease the so-called watershed effect of decreased cerebral blood flow to critical areas of the brain. If general anesthesia is used, the authors of this chapter recommend hypercapnia (Pa$_{CO_2}$ of

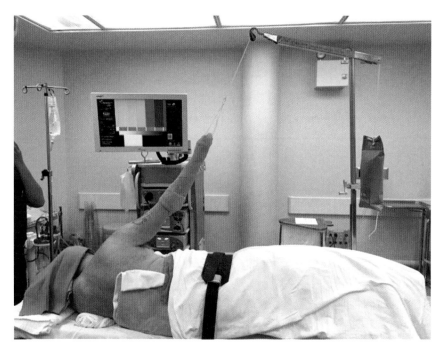

Figure 1 Photograph shows the lateral decubitus position with the use of a traction device.

39 to 42 mm Hg), which improves cerebral oxygenation.
- The head and neck are maintained in neutral rotation.
- The patient is typically placed in a 10° to 15° Trendelenburg position, with 45° to 60° of hip flexion and 30° of knee flexion.
- The pressure points are well padded.
- The patient is draped with a combination of sterile U-drapes and sheets.
- The arm is placed into a padded Mayo stand or a commercially available arm holder (**Figure 2**).
- At this time, some surgeons inject a diluted solution of epinephrine into the subacromial space to improve visualization later in the procedure. During the procedure, lactated Ringer solution augmented with epinephrine can be used as arthroscopy fluid to decrease bleeding and improve visualization.
- During the procedure, the humerus

can be repositioned by an assistant or with the use of a dynamic arm holder to take advantage of the free draping of the arm. Forward flexing and externally rotating the arm can facilitate débridement of articular-sided partial tears of the rotator cuff and exposure of the lesser tuberosity attachment of the subscapularis. External rotation of the arm can accommodate examination of the posterior labrum from the posterior portal by relaxing the posterior capsule and allowing the arthroscope to pull back farther while being maintained in the joint. Pushing the elbow up can allow a better view of the inferior pouch.
- If fog-resistant arthroscopic equipment is not available, fogging of the arthroscope during the procedure can be avoided by placing the arthroscope in a limited uphill position and using rubber caps to limit the effluence of fluid down the arthroscope.

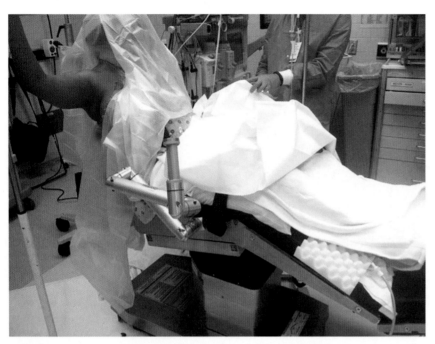

Figure 2 Photograph shows the beach-chair position with the use of a commercially available arm holder (Trimano [Arthrex]).

 Avoiding Pitfalls

In either approach, the shoulder should be examined with the patient supine on the surgical table before positioning because this method ensures the most accurate examination. The ease of stabilizing the scapula makes examination under anesthesia easier in the beach-chair position. To facilitate the examination when using the lateral decubitus position, range of motion and stability should be checked before the patient is prepped and draped.

In the lateral position, injury of the brachial plexus and neurapraxia are the main concerns resulting from the use of persistent traction on the arm to improve visualization. Traction has been shown to cause decreased limb perfusion in some studies. An incidence of nerve injury of up to 10% has been reported with the arm in traction. In one study, 45° of forward flexion with either 90° or 0° of abduction was found to maximize visibility and minimize strain. Regardless of arm position, traction should be limited to no more than 15 to 20 lb.

Reports of neurovascular complications associated with the beach-chair position have included devastating neurologic events, such as stroke and spinal cord injuries, resulting in permanent blindness, coma, and death. These complications could be related to either neck positioning or relative cerebral deoxygenation. Many ischemic events are related to errors in interpretation of blood pressure. The blood pressure cuff should be placed at the level of the heart rather than on the calf to ensure accuracy. However, hypoxic injury has been reported when relative normotension was maintained. Some adverse outcomes were related to a severely hyperflexed position of the neck. To prevent rare catastrophic outcomes, such as spinal cord infarction and mid-cervical quadriplegia, the patient's neck must be maintained in neutral alignment with no flexion. In one study, the rate of cerebral desaturation events was statistically significantly greater in patients undergoing shoulder arthroscopy in the beach-chair position with general anesthesia compared with those undergoing the procedure in the lateral decubitus position with general anesthesia (80.3% and zero, respectively). Concerns of cerebral oxygenation in the beach-chair position can be addressed by using regional anesthesia and sedation, which has been found to have a lower rate of cerebral deoxygenation events compared with general anesthesia (zero and 56.7%, respectively). As noted previously, if general anesthesia is used, hypercapnia ($Paco_2$ of 39 to 42 mm Hg) has been found to improve cerebral oxygenation.

Despite these potential problems, the lateral decubitus and beach-chair positions have been widely used and are regarded as safe. For most procedures, the optimal position is ultimately determined on the basis of surgeon comfort and clinical experience.

Bibliography

Andrews JR, Carson WG Jr, Ortega K: Arthroscopy of the shoulder: Technique and normal anatomy. *Am J Sports Med* 1984;12(1):1-7.

Costouros JG, Clavert P, Warner JJ: Trans-cuff portal for arthroscopic posterior capsulorrhaphy. *Arthroscopy* 2006;22(10):1138.e1-1138.e5.

Cullen DJ, Kirby RRS: Beach chair position may decrease cerebral perfusion: Catastrophic outcomes have occurred. *Anesthesia Patient Safety Foundation Newsletter* 2007;22(2):25-27.

Gelber PE, Reina F, Caceres E, Monllau JC: A comparison of risk between the lateral decubitus and the beach-chair position when establishing an anteroinferior shoulder portal: A cadaveric study. *Arthroscopy* 2007;23(5):522-528.

Gross RM, Fitzgibbons TC: Shoulder arthroscopy: A modified approach. *Arthroscopy* 1985;1(3):156-159.

Hennrikus WL, Mapes RC, Bratton MW, Lapoint JM: Lateral traction during shoulder arthroscopy: Its effect on tissue perfusion measured by pulse oximetry. *Am J Sports Med* 1995;23(4):444-446.

Klein AH, France JC, Mutschler TA, Fu FH: Measurement of brachial plexus strain in arthroscopy of the shoulder. *Arthroscopy* 1987;3(1):45-52.

Koga T, Miyao M, Sato M, et al: Pituitary apoplexy during general anesthesia in beach chair position for shoulder joint arthroplasty. *J Anesth* 2010;24(3):476-478.

Koh JL, Levin SD, Chehab EL, Murphy GS: Cerebral oxygenation in the beach chair position: A prospective study on the effect of general anesthesia compared with regional anesthesia and sedation. *J Shoulder Elbow Surg* 2013;22(10):1325-1331.

Murphy GS, Szokol JW, Avram MJ, et al: Effect of ventilation on cerebral oxygenation in patients undergoing surgery in the beach chair position: A randomized controlled trial. *Br J Anaesth* 2014;113(4):618-627.

Murphy GS, Szokol JW, Marymont JH, et al: Cerebral oxygen desaturation events assessed by near-infrared spectroscopy during shoulder arthroscopy in the beach chair and lateral decubitus positions. *Anesth Analg* 2010;111(2):496-505.

Papadonikolakis A, Wiesler ER, Olympio MA, Poehling GG: Avoiding catastrophic complications of stroke and death related to shoulder surgery in the sitting position. *Arthroscopy* 2008;24(4):481-482.

Paxton ES, Backus J, Keener J, Brophy RH: Shoulder arthroscopy: Basic principles of positioning, anesthesia, and portal anatomy. *J Am Acad Orthop Surg* 2013;21(6):332-342.

Peruto CM, Ciccotti MG, Cohen SB: Shoulder arthroscopy positioning: Lateral decubitus versus beach chair. *Arthroscopy* 2009;25(8):891-896.

Phillips BB: Arthroscopy of the upper extremity, in Canale ST, Beaty JH, eds: *Campbell's Operative Orthopaedics*, ed 11. Philadelphia, PA, Mosby Elsevier, 2008, pp 2923-2926.

Pohl A, Cullen DJ: Cerebral ischemia during shoulder surgery in the upright position: A case series. *J Clin Anesth* 2005;17(6):463-469.

Rains DD, Rooke GA, Wahl CJ: Pathomechanisms and complications related to patient positioning and anesthesia during shoulder arthroscopy. *Arthroscopy* 2011;27(4):532-541.

Skyhar MJ, Altchek DW, Warren RF, Wickiewicz TL, O'Brien SJ: Shoulder arthroscopy with the patient in the beach-chair position. *Arthroscopy* 1988;4(4):256-259.

Terry MA, Altchek DW: Diagnostic shoulder arthroscopy technique: Beach chair position, in Tibone JE, Savoie FH III, Shaffer BS, eds: *Shoulder Arthroscopy.* New York, NY, Springer-Verlag, 2003, pp 9-15.

Tibone JE: Diagnostic shoulder arthroscopy in the lateral decubitus position, in Tibone JE, Savoie FH III, Shaffer BS, eds: *Shoulder Arthroscopy.* New York, NY, Springer-Verlag, 2003, pp 3-8.

Warren RF, Morgan C: Shoulder positioning: Beach chair vs. lateral decubitus. Point/counterpoint. *Arthroscopy Association of North America Newsletter* 2008;March:4-5.

Introduction

Arthroscopic portals are small skin incisions created with a surgical blade for transcutaneous passage of arthroscopic instruments. The use of shoulder arthroscopy solely for diagnosis is limited in modern orthopaedics, and currently, surgeons routinely perform complex procedures arthroscopically. When performing arthroscopic procedures, the surgeon must navigate around bony obstructions and vital neurovascular structures to view and manipulate deep tissues of the shoulder. In addition, the need to perform mobile assessments of the limb with the arthroscope placed deep within the joint as well as the demand for manipulative examination of deep soft tissues compounds the importance of proper positioning and establishment of portals. Considerable educational, laboratory, and surgical observation hours are necessary for mastery of shoulder arthroscopy.

Case Presentation

A 63-year-old woman presents with a 6-month history of unpredictable acute, sharp pains in the left shoulder that are associated with locking. These episodes of pain have occurred at least daily for the past 3 weeks. She has no other resting pain, night pain, or motion-related pain. Physical examination reveals good overall health and only subtle loss of active and passive glenohumeral motion on the affected side. All provocative tests are negative. Radiographs demonstrate moderate glenohumeral osteoarthritis with a loose osteochondral body in the inferior axillary pouch, and MRI confirms these diagnoses.

Because of the mechanical nature of the patient's symptoms, the patient's relatively good function and moderate degree of osteoarthritis, and the potential morbidity of open exposure, an arthroscopic procedure is performed. The goal of the procedure is to identify and remove the large, loose osseous body from the arthritic shoulder with minimal damage to the surrounding soft tissues.

A standard posterior viewing portal allows access of the arthroscope to the glenohumeral joint. The skin incision is located overlying the midlevel of the glenohumeral joint and 1 cm lateral to the joint. The intermediate path is through the posterior deltoid and the infraspinatus muscle, and the deep window is at the midlevel of the posterior shoulder capsule. The loose body is identified in the axillary pouch with the use of a standard 30° arthroscopic lens, after which a 70° arthroscopic lens is used via the same portal to view the loose body from the superior glenoid, thereby separating the inflow direction from the loose body.

With the use of a slightly oversized anterior skin portal with an intermediate path avoiding the coracoacromial arch and a deep window through the rotator interval, a large, closed cannula is used to access the glenohumeral joint for containment of the loose body. After the cannula is established, a grasper is inserted to access the large, loose body in the anterior axillary pouch and remove the specimen en bloc (**Figure 1**).

Indications

The arthroscopic approach has multiple indications in the surgical management of shoulder pathology. Specific procedural indications are beyond the scope of this chapter. However, the systematic approach described later will be of use to any surgeon contemplating portal selection in well-indicated surgical cases.

Dr. Christoforetti or an immediate family member has received royalties from, is a member of a speakers' bureau or has made paid presentations on behalf of, and serves as a paid consultant to Arthrex and Breg; has received research or institutional support from Arthrex; and serves as a board member, owner, officer, or committee member of the International Society for Hip Arthroscopy.

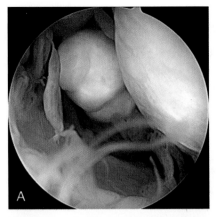 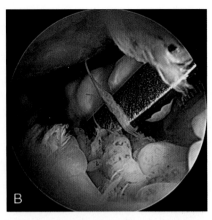

Figure 1   Arthroscopic images of a loose body in an axillary pouch as viewed from the posterior portal using a 70° arthroscopic lens with the camera tip positioned at the 12-o'clock position on the glenoid (**A**). This positioning allows free access of the grasper from the anterior portal (rotator interval) for en bloc removal of the loose body (**B**).

Controversies and Alternative Approaches

Exposure and Angles of Approach

The authors of recent studies of portal placement continue to challenge established standards as demands for closer replication of benchmark open techniques grow. In anterior capsulolabral reconstruction procedures, the placement of suture anchors on the anterior-inferior glenoid from an accessory posterior (7-o'clock; posterolateral) portal has been introduced as an alternative to the standard anterior and anterior-inferior portals. New portals have been recommended for access to the subdeltoid space, the retrocoracoid space, and the suprascapular and infrascapular fossae in an attempt to optimize working angles.

The 70° arthroscopic lens has gained popularity as well. Although the 30° lens is the standard lens for most arthroscopic shoulder procedures, the more highly angled 70° lens offers certain advantages. As illustrated in the case presented in this chapter, the inflow direction, which often runs along the sheath of the arthroscope, diverges from the field of view. This setup avoids the tendency of the fluid inflow to drive loose materials away from the arthroscope and out of view. The view with the 70° lens is much closer to a 90° periscope-style view than it is to a straight-ahead view; therefore, a blind spot exists directly at the tip of the arthroscope. This blind spot allows use of the lens tip itself for deep retraction of tissues without blocking the aperture for viewing. Challenges associated with the 70° lens include the risk of iatrogenic scuffing of cartilage with the tip of the lens in the blind spot as well as the fact that it allows the surgeon to view structures that, nonetheless, cannot be easily accessed to perform procedures. An example of this difficulty of access to the viewed area occurs when the 70° lens is placed through the posterior portal and directed medially over the anterior glenoid rim, thereby bringing the subcoracoid space and anterior glenoid neck into view. The standard anterior portal may not allow safe access this far medially because of the presence of the conjoint tendon and neurovascular structures. In response to this challenge, an accessory anteromedial portal has been developed to allow the surgeon to complete advanced procedures in this space. Specific discussion of alternative portals is provided later in this chapter.

Advantages of the 70° lens in specific procedures are shown in **Table 1**.

Outside-in Versus Inside-out Technique

A technical distinction exists concerning the methods of establishing subsequent portals after the initial blind portal is established. The results of published preclinical studies suggest that these methods create different deep pathways and entail different risks. Surgeons who use skin landmarks, awareness of the desired deep-tissue entry point, and tactile feedback to create portals from the skin to the deep area of interest use the outside-in method. In the visualized outside-in technique, a palpated landmark and arthroscopic view of internal structures are used to guide a spinal needle into position for optimal angle selection followed by portal placement. Conversely, in the inside-out technique, an established portal is used to guide a switching stick from deep space outward, resulting in tented skin that guides placement of the incision for the new portal. Particularly for anterior portals, the inside-out technique has been both advocated for increasing portal access and criticized for increasing proximity to neurovascular structures as a result of the limitations created by the established portal. The outside-in technique may require more advanced triangulation skill and be subject to variability related to surface landmarks, surgical experience, and tactile dexterity. Finally, a growing trend inspired by hip arthroscopy favors the Seldinger technique, or the passage of instruments such as anchors or deep retractors over a guidewire for precision and accuracy of placement. Use of this technique results in greater precision with the outside-in method compared with the method of spinal needle localization followed by complete removal of the needle and insertion of a separate device at the same angle. All recent publications reviewed for this work advocate outside-in techniques. The author of this

Table 1 Advantages of the 70° Arthroscope in Shoulder Procedures

Procedure	Advantages
Anterior glenohumeral stabilization	Provides superior visualization of a medially displaced anterior labroligamentous periosteal sleeve avulsion lesion from the posterior portal
	Allows full mobilization of the capsulolabral complex without the instrument crowding that occurs when the camera and working instruments are placed in dual anterior portals
Coracoclavicular ligament reconstruction	Allows for visualization of the coracoid process from the posterior portal, enabling dissection and graft passage around the coracoid through working anterolateral and anterior portals without instrument crowding
Distal clavicle excision	Provides an excellent view of the entire acromioclavicular joint and distal clavicle from a posterior portal, often obviating the need to shift the arthroscope to an anterolateral or anterior position to confirm adequate resection
Rotator cuff repair	Particularly useful for subscapularis and leading-edge supraspinatus tears
	The entire tear pattern can be visualized from the posterior portal, allowing for unencumbered suture passage and management through anterolateral and anterior portals
Subdeltoid shoulder arthroscopy	Useful in this compartment for arthroscopic biceps tenodesis or transfer procedures, proximal humerus fracture fixation, pectoralis tendon repair, and arthroscopically assisted hardware removal

Adapted with permission from Bedi A, Dines J, Dines DM, et al: Use of the 70° arthroscope for improved visualization with common arthroscopic procedures. *Arthroscopy* 2010;26(12):1684-1696.

chapter prefers to identify the postero-lateral corner of the acromion, place an outside-in posterior portal, and then use spinal needle localization to establish subsequent portals.

Cannula Use

A disposable cannula is often placed in the established skin portal. The cannula may have a variety of internal and external design features (fully or partially threaded exterior, diameter of aperture, diameter of outer dimension, inflow/outflow valves, rigid or flexible plastic design, fixed or variable length, clear or opaque material, open or closed external aperture, single-use or reusable obturators). Advantages of cannula use include preservation of a single three-dimensional portal tract to the deep tissues, which facilitates easy insertion and removal of the arthroscope and instruments; containment of fluid flow, which allows for maintenance of internal pressure for visualization and hemostasis; decreased risk of tissue entrapment in sutures (bridge formation); and the ability to use advanced techniques in which the end, side, or other areas of the cannula itself are used to

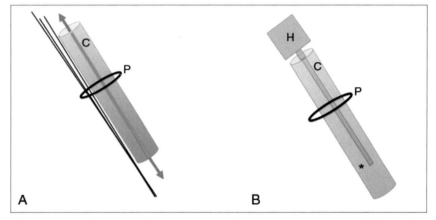

Figure 2 **A,** Illustration depicts passage of an arthroscopic cannula (C) through a skin portal (P) and the creation of working spaces inside the cannula (green arrow) and outside the cannula but inside the portal (black lines). The space outside the cannula is frequently used in shoulder arthroscopy for suture management. **B,** Illustration depicts passage of an arthroscopic cannula (C) through a skin portal (P) and attempted passage of an arthroscopic instrument with appropriate size at the shaft and working end but an oversized handle (H) that blocks the exit from the cannula. The asterisk marks the end of the instrument inside the cannula.

pin, organize, or retract soft tissues or sutures. In addition, the placement of a cannula within a portal tract establishes two working spaces within the portal: inside the cannula and outside the cannula (**Figure 2, A**). The space outside the cannula can be used for storing sutures that have been passed through to deeper structures while new sutures or anchors are passed through the cannula, thereby enabling multifunctional use of a single skin incision.

Drawbacks of cannula use can include cost; crowding of deep-tissue spaces with rigid cannula ends (such as occurs during arthroscopic Bankart

Table 2 Posterior Shoulder Arthroscopy Portals: Anatomic Considerations

Portal Name	Portal Landmarks	Nearest Structures at Risk (Relation to Portal; Distance From Portal Pathway)
Soft spot (posterior)[a,b]	1.5 cm inferior and 2 cm medial to the postero-lateral acromion	Suprascapular artery/nerve (medial; 29 mm)
		Axillary nerve (inferior; 30-49 mm)
Posterior central[a]	2 cm medial and 3 cm inferior to the postero-lateral acromion	Suprascapular artery/nerve (medial; 2.9 cm)
Posterolateral[a]	2 cm below the lateral edge of the acromion in the prolongation of its posterior edge	Axillary nerve/tendinous infraspinatus (inferior/deep lateral; 56 mm)
Posteroinferior (7-o'clock)[b,c]	4 cm lateral to the posterolateral corner of the acromion (following the direction of the posterior clavicle laterally)	Axillary nerve and posterior circumflex humeral artery (inferior; 30-40 mm)
		Suprascapular nerve and artery (medial; 28 mm)
Axillary pouch[b]	2-3 cm inferior to the posterolateral corner of the acromion and 2 cm lateral to the posterior central portal	Axillary nerve and posterior circumflex humeral artery (inferior; no data available)
		Suprascapular nerve and artery (medial; no data available)

[a] Data from Meyer M, Graveleau N, Hardy P, Landreau P: Anatomic risks of shoulder arthroscopy portals: Anatomic cadaveric study of 12 portals. *Arthroscopy* 2007;23(5):529-536.

[b] Data from Paxton ES, Backus J, Keener J, Brophy RH: Shoulder arthroscopy: Basic principles of positioning, anesthesia, and portal anatomy. *J Am Acad Orthop Surg* 2013;21(6):332-342.

[c] Data from Cvetanovich GL, McCormick F, Erickson BJ, et al: The posterolateral portal: Optimizing anchor placement and labral repair at the inferior glenoid. *Arthrosc Tech* 2013;2(3):e201-e204.

reconstruction, which requires two anterior rotator interval portals, each with cannulas); mismatch of the internal diameter of the cannula and the dimensions of the required arthroscopic instruments, which prevents smooth instrument passage; increased soft-tissue swelling because of the containment of arthroscopy fluid flow; and, when the length of the cannula exceeds the length of the arthroscope, elimination of use of the cannula-occupied portal for viewing. Frequently, the handle, shaft, or working-end dimensions of arthroscopic instruments pose a challenge in attempts to navigate the anatomic or cannula-created boundaries of portal pathways (**Figure 2, B**). For example, use of a 90-mm cannula requires use of an instrument with a shaft longer than 90 mm.

Technical Keys to Success

The exposure for shoulder arthroscopy in any position typically begins with establishment of an initial viewing portal. On the basis of surface landmark palpation, typically focusing on the coracoacromial arch and clavicle, the soft spot of the posterior glenohumeral joint, and preoperative imaging, the surgeon passes a blunt-tipped obturator and arthroscope sheath into position. Anterior and lateral portals as well as accessory posterior portals complement the initially established diagnostic posterior portal.

Although rare, complications related to portal establishment have been reported. The major nerves and blood vessels at risk include the axillary nerve, the cephalic vein, the suprascapular nerve and artery, the nerve to the subscapularis, and, during procedures requiring exposure medial to the coracoid base, the brachial artery, the subclavian vein, and the brachial plexus. The tendon insertional fibers of the rotator cuff, the muscles and intramuscular veins of the rotator cuff, and the deltoid can also be injured during portal creation or repeat access. The best available data on portal anatomy are presented in **Tables** 2 through 5. However, distance measurements from portals to vital structures are always estimates because individual patient anatomy, limb position, and the method of portal creation affect these values. These variables are important to consider when selecting the size and location of arthroscopic portals.

Portal Placement
POSTERIOR

Posterior portals (**Table 2**) allow visualization and access to the entire joint as well as the subacromial space with a standard 30° arthroscopic lens. However, the authors of recent studies caution that posterosuperior pathology within the joint at the rotator cuff insertion may be underappreciated from the posterior viewing portals, and those authors support the use of multiple positions of the arthroscope to ensure thorough diagnosis. Preoperative assessment of the relationship of the glenohumeral joint to the posterolateral corner of the acromion is necessary. Surface palpation of this landmark guides portal placement, and anatomic variation may result in the need to deviate from published guidelines on distance.

Surgeons must consider the intent of the posterior portals when selecting the portal type and location. Posterior portals intended for viewing of the joint tend to be more medially located to allow for visualization of anterolateral joint structures without damage to the articular humerus. Posterior portals intended to facilitate posterior anchor placement must be placed laterally and either superiorly or inferiorly to allow access to the corresponding region of the glenoid. Posterior portals that are intended to assist primarily in rotator cuff repair or anterior shoulder procedures may be placed more laterally and proximally.

ANTERIOR

The working anterior portal is typically the second portal established during an arthroscopic procedure. Outside-in and inside-out techniques are both acceptable methods of creating the initial or subsequent anterior portals. Typically, the rotator interval serves as the deep entry point for anterior portals. The skin entry point and therefore the angle of approach to the rotator interval vary according to the intended use of the portal. For standard diagnostic arthroscopy, an anterior central portal consists of a skin incision lateral to the point overlying the coracoid and relatively direct entry to the rotator interval. Anterior portals created for the placement of glenoid anchors or manipulation of the subscapularis tendon are positioned more laterally on the skin.

Regardless of the purpose or method of establishing an anterior portal, awareness of the proximity of vital structures is critical (**Table 3**). The cephalic vein is the most commonly encountered neurovascular structure. In addition, the surgeon must avoid the dense fibers of the coracoacromial arch below the deltoid fascia. Entrapment of the portal in

Table 3 Anterior Shoulder Arthroscopy Portals: Anatomic Considerations

Portal Name	Portal Landmarks	Nearest Structures at Risk (Distance)
Anterior superior[a]	Start: midway between the coracoid and the acromion Deep: rotator interval anterior to biceps	Cephalic vein (39 mm) Axillary artery (53 mm) Axillary nerve (54 mm)
Anterior central[a]	Start: skin point lateral to the coracoid Deep: central rotator interval area	Cephalic vein (17 mm) Axillary nerve (31 mm) Axillary artery (33 mm)
Anterior inferior (inside-out)[a]	Start: through posterior soft spot portal; exits through anterior rotator interval and then inferior to coracoid tip	Cephalic vein (17 mm) Axillary nerve (40 mm) Axillary artery (42 mm)
Anterior inferior (outside-in)[b]	Start: lateral to coracoid Deep: just above the lateral half of the subscapularis tendon	Cephalic vein (18 mm) Musculocutaneous nerve (36 mm) Lateral cord (37 mm) Axillary nerve (44 mm) Axillary artery (46 mm)
5-o'clock (inside-out)[a]	Start: through the posterior soft spot portal; exits at the leading edge of the anterior inferior glenohumeral ligament	Cephalic vein (17 mm) Axillary artery (13 mm) Axillary nerve (15 mm)
5-o'clock (outside-in)[b]	Start: 1 cm below the anterior inferior portal Deep: through the subscapularis tendon	Cephalic vein (10 mm) Musculocutaneous nerve (28 mm) Lateral cord (35 mm) Axillary nerve (33 mm) Axillary artery (38 mm)

[a] Data from Meyer M, Graveleau N, Hardy P, Landreau P: Anatomic risks of shoulder arthroscopy portals: Anatomic cadaveric study of 12 portals. *Arthroscopy* 2007;23(5):529-536.

[b] Data from Lo IK, Lind CC, Burkhart SS: Glenohumeral arthroscopy portals established using an outside-in technique: Neurovascular anatomy at risk. *Arthroscopy* 2004;20(6):596-602.

the lateral edge of the coracoacromial ligament or in the dense clavipectoral fascia may limit mobility of the portal. Recently, some experts have advocated arthroscopic exploration or even portal placement medial to the coracoid process. Because of the increased risk of these maneuvers, extreme caution should be used by any surgeon attempting these advanced techniques.

Advances in arthroscopic access to the anterior shoulder for management of coracoclavicular disorders, procedures in the biceps groove area, repair of the pectoralis major insertion, and subscapularis repair have alerted surgeons

to new possibilities. The subdeltoid space exists between the deep deltoid and the clavipectoral fascia; this space is bounded medially by the coracobrachialis and distally by the deltoid insertion and pectoralis insertion. With preservation of the deep deltoid fascia, anterior portals can be placed in the skin areas overlying this region provided a safe distance from the axillary nerve is maintained.

LATERAL

Surface palpation of the region between the posterolateral corner of the acromion and the anterolateral corner of

Table 4 Lateral Shoulder Arthroscopy Portals: Anatomic Considerations[a]

Portal Name	Portal Landmarks	Nearest Structures at Risk (Relation to Portal; Distance From Portal Pathway)
Superolateral	Start: lateral to the acromion on a line drawn from the acromion to the coracoid Deep: rotator interval overlying the biceps tendon	Axillary nerve (lateral; 58 mm)
Port of Wilmington (posterosuperolateral)	Start: 1 cm anterior and 1 cm lateral to the posterolateral corner of the acromion Deep: transmuscular through the infraspinatus angled to the posterosuperior glenoid	Axillary nerve (lateral; 55 mm)
Trans–rotator cuff	Start: 1 cm posterior and 2 cm lateral to the posterolateral corner of the acromion Deep: transmuscular through the infraspinatus angled to the posterosuperior glenoid	Axillary nerve (lateral; 53 mm)
Lateral anterior	Start: 2 cm below the lateral edge of the acromion in the prolongation of its anterior edge Deep: subacromial space	Axillary nerve (lateral; 70 mm)
Lateral posterior	Start: 2 cm below the lateral edge of the acromion in the prolongation of its posterior edge Deep: subacromial space	Axillary nerve (lateral; 56 mm)

[a] Data from Meyer M, Graveleau N, Hardy P, Landreau P: Anatomic risks of shoulder arthroscopy portals: Anatomic cadaveric study of 12 portals. *Arthroscopy* 2007;23(5):529-536.

Table 5 Superior Shoulder Arthroscopy Portals: Anatomic Considerations[a]

Portal Name	Portal Landmarks	Nearest Structures at Risk (Distance From Portal Pathway)
Neviaser	Start: superior soft spot surrounded by the clavicle anteriorly, the acromion laterally, and the scapular spine posteriorly Deep: transmuscular through the supraspinatus muscle angled to the posterosuperior glenoid	SSN and suprascapular artery (30 mm)
SSN (G)	Start: 7 cm medial to the lateral acromion (2 cm medial to the Neviaser portal) Deep: through the trapezius to a point just medial to the conoid ligament at the coracoid	SSN and suprascapular artery (directly under pathway)

SSN = suprascapular nerve.

[a] Data from Meyer M, Graveleau N, Hardy P, Landreau P: Anatomic risks of shoulder arthroscopy portals: Anatomic cadaveric study of 12 portals. *Arthroscopy* 2007;23(5):529-536.

the acromion along the lateral contour of the shoulder reveals a large and relatively safe zone for lateral portal placement (**Table 4**). The area 4 to 6 cm from the acromial edge anteriorly, laterally, and posterolaterally is the most likely intramuscular (deltoid) location of the axillary nerve and should be avoided. Superiorly placed lateral portals begin immediately lateral to the acromial edge and may traverse the common deltoid origin superficially. Use of these portals for superior glenoid anchor placement may result in inadvertent damage to the insertional tendon fibers of the rotator cuff. Lateral portals placed farther away from the edge of the acromion may be dangerously close to the axillary nerve. Viewing of the subacromial space through a posterosuperolateral portal (Port of Wilmington) is a common approach in rotator cuff repair procedures and posterosuperior glenoid labrum anchor placement, whereas anterosuperolateral portals are used for viewing in subscapularis repair, anterior capsulolabral reconstruction, biceps tenodesis, and other advanced anterior tissue procedures. Regardless of the functional purpose of a lateral portal, preservation of the deep deltoid fascia is critical and is best accomplished by adhering to the technical strategies discussed previously and by avoiding acromioplasty before procedures that require visualization within the subdeltoid space.

SUPERIOR

Portals located over the acromioclavicular joint, suprascapular notch, and spinoglenoid notch allow the surgeon to work in the suprascapular fossa and coracoclavicular space (**Table 5**). Superomedial structures include the spinal accessory nerve, the brachial plexus, and the suprascapular nerve. Portal placement at the juncture of the posterior acromioclavicular joint and the medial border of the acromion at the scapular spine (Neviaser portal) has proved to be safe. Less commonly, a supraclavicular portal placed more medially or an anterosuperomedial portal is used in coracoclavicular ligament reconstruction.

Portal Techniques for Specific Procedures

ROTATOR CUFF REPAIR

Many techniques exist for arthroscopic repair of acute or chronic injury to the rotator cuff tendons. These procedures begin with the creation of standard posterior and anterior glenohumeral and subacromial working portals and incorporate lateral portals for assessment and management of tissue and placement of anchors. Although a standard portal strategy may not exist, some common challenges to portal placement can be identified on the basis of the specific pathology. Partial tears of the rotator cuff present different challenges than do large, full-thickness tears.

In patients with partial rotator cuff tears, the main challenge related to portal selection stems from the lack of communication between the subacromial and glenohumeral spaces. As a result, the posterior and anterior working portals that allow visualization of and access to the glenohumeral joint will not allow visualization of instruments placed via lateral portals into the subacromial space. This difficulty can lead to confusion in the selection and placement of anchors, management of sutures, and tying of arthroscopic knots. Limb position and rotation are critical for success in these procedures and may even require intraoperative adjustment to optimize relationships between the deep tissues and the skin portals. A posterior portal allowing access to and visualization of both the subacromial and glenohumeral spaces is necessary. Because most partial tears occur toward the posterosuperior footprint of the articular cuff, a slightly medial placement of the standard posterior portal improves access to this area. Use of the anterior portal for viewing facilitates visualization of the posterosuperior articular rotator cuff but may require more central and medial placement of the anterior portal to avoid blockage by the coracoacromial arch. Finally, the use of spinal needles passed from the skin incision past the lateral acromial border and through the partially torn rotator cuff to target the correct location for anchor placement portals allows visualization from the glenohumeral joint. This method facilitates accurate passage of anchors through the rotator cuff tissue and placement within the bone.

In patients with full-thickness tears, the subacromial and glenohumeral spaces are continuous at the site of the tear. This scenario typically allows interaction of the arthroscope and the working instruments in the subacromial space. The smaller the tear size, the more similar the procedure becomes to the partial-thickness tear scenario discussed previously. When a full-thickness tear of the rotator cuff is identified on preoperative imaging and the main surgical goals will be addressed in the subacromial space, the posterior and anterior portals may be moved slightly closer to the acromion and more lateral relative to the joint space. This placement will facilitate visualization within the subacromial space.

INSTABILITY PROCEDURES

Instability procedures focus on correcting conditions of the glenoid labrum or glenohumeral ligament. Challenges to portal selection in these procedures include the threat of damage to articular cartilage, crowding of portal entry sites with cannulas in the anterior or posterior shoulder, the presence of neurovascular structures that limit the angle of approach for suture anchor placement or capsulolabral tissue management, disorientation of the surgeon or assistant resulting from movement of the arthroscope to the anterior viewing position, and the need to manage sutures deep within the shoulder.

When capsulolabral procedures are likely to be required, the standard posterior working portal may be placed more superiorly and laterally to allow for placement of a second posterior portal inferiorly and to facilitate use of the portal for anchor placement. Correspondingly, the standard anterior working portal may be placed more laterally and toward the acromion. This adjustment allows use of the portal in anchor placement superiorly on the glenoid, enables top-down visualization of the anteroinferior glenoid, and leaves room for a second anterior portal to be placed inferiorly. Placement of anchors to the superior and inferior glenoid continues to pose a challenge because the risk of injury to neurovascular and tendon structures in this region is high. The posterolateral (7-o'clock) portal, established 4 cm lateral to the posterolateral acromion in line with the posterior border of the clavicle, allows access to the inferior anterior glenoid.

BICEPS TENDON PROCEDURES

Correction of disorders of the long head of the biceps tendon is a common task of the surgeon who specializes in shoulder arthroscopy. The standard posterior and anterior portals provide adequate visualization and access for biceps tenotomy. Development of the subdeltoid space anteriorly allows localization of the tissue overlying the biceps groove. The falciform ligament of the pectoralis major muscle can be used as a guide for spinal needle localization of the biceps groove. After localization, an accessory distal anterolateral portal may be used to access this area directly. Frequently, the top of the groove can be visualized from the lateral portal with a standard lens or from the posterior portal with a 70° lens.

ACROMIOCLAVICULAR JOINT PROCEDURES

Surgical procedures at the acromioclavicular joint include bone resection at the distal clavicle, reconstruction of the coracoclavicular ligaments, and transfer of coracoid bone to reinforce anterior glenoid bone deficiency (Latarjet procedure). The standard posterior portal affords an adequate subacromial view of the posterior acromioclavicular joint. For advanced reconstructive procedures involving the base of the coracoid, a 70° lens may be placed in the standard posterior glenohumeral portal and directed medially over the anterior glenoid. The lateral portal will provide an end-on view of the distal clavicle.

The standard anterior portal is frequently moved superiorly and medially to lie directly anterior to the acromioclavicular joint, lateral to the coracoid tip and at the superior aspect of the glenoid. This position allows direct access to the plane of the acromioclavicular joint for visualization or resection of the distal clavicle. The space medial to the conoid ligament of the coracoclavicular ligament complex is also a key landmark for decompression of the suprascapular nerve at the suprascapular notch. Through the posterior viewing portal, the medial border of the

conoid is visualized, and a spinal needle is used to localize an accessory and slightly medially placed Neviaser portal for access down onto the transverse scapular ligament for release. In general, the approach to the medial structures of the shoulder girdle is in close proximity to large neurovascular danger zones and should be undertaken only after mastery of more lateral techniques is achieved.

DORSAL SCAPULAR ARTHROSCOPY

The dorsal surface of the scapula, which contains the scapular spine and the spinoglenoid notch, requires attention in the management of dynamic compression of the suprascapular nerve at the spinoglenoid notch. A two-portal approach to this area involves a posterior portal located 4 cm medial to the posterolateral corner of the acromion for instrument access to the spinoglenoid ligament and a second portal placed 4 cm medial to the first. After blunt dissection of the working space, the second portal allows submuscular visualization of the initial portal and the spinoglenoid ligament. Creation of this space through these portals is not part of standard glenohumeral arthroscopy and should be reserved for patients with appropriate preoperative diagnoses.

 Avoiding Pitfalls

Correct patient positioning and draping are critically important for successful portal creation and use in shoulder arthroscopy. The surgeon must have a thorough preoperative understanding of the intended strategies to ensure not only a sterile and accessible skin incision site but also enough sterile, unobstructed working room for instrument and arthroscope handles, cord security and passage, and manipulation of the patient's limbs to keep all safe options available. To ensure safety, the surgeon and the anesthesiology team must meticulously consider the patient's head,

neck, and torso structures that are out of the sterile field.

The portal strategy should focus on patient safety, visual access, and technical access (**Figure 3**). The surgeon must possess a comprehensive understanding of the surgical goals before planning the portals. The viewing capabilities offered by the available lenses in the portals selected and the effect of fluid flow should be taken into account to maximize the probability of success. Coordination of the working portals with the visual zones and fluid flow is necessary.

When planning the procedure, the surgeon must systematically consider the portal pathway in three dimensions. First, the surgeon defines the primary purpose for entering the anatomic area at the deep end of the portal path: visualization, working space, or both. The anatomic layers between the target zone and the skin are then considered. The boundary margins on each tissue plane are defined with consideration of important neurovascular structures, traversing musculoskeletal tissues, and mobility of the limb and tissues. These considerations typically allow for skin portal incision locations within a range of areas that may change for each patient.

Arthroscopic portal pathways will remain accessible in most patients if careful precision is applied during portal creation and subsequent access attempts. The surgeon should avoid using excessive force or blind, sweeping motions during portal establishment or repeat access (**Figure 4**). The basic portal pathway in shoulder arthroscopy is a simple path from the skin incision through to the deep working space. The fascial envelope maintains the tract of the portal automatically if the surgeon takes care to guide a rigid switching stick or obturator without excessive sweeping motions that can disrupt these natural planes. As the arthroscope is moved within the portal or switched to other portals, care should be taken

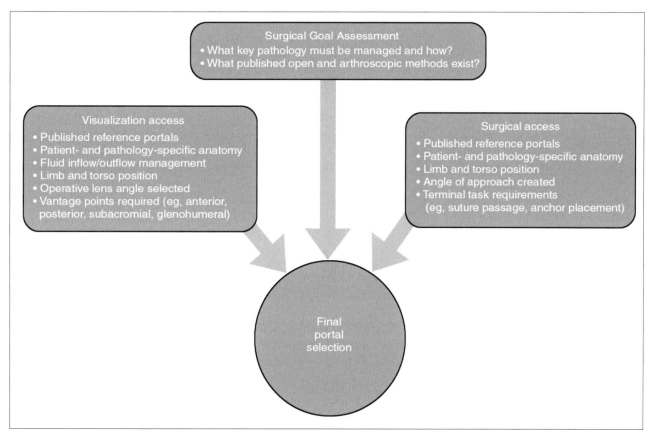

Figure 3   Diagram depicts the strategy for portal selection in shoulder arthroscopy.

to maintain the same pathway to minimize the creation of leakage points for fluid and the obstruction of access by interposed tissue.

Tactile feedback during portal creation and instrument passage should be smooth and consistent with the density of underlying tissues. Portal pathways traverse soft-tissue structures in the shoulder; thus, a sensation that the cannula or instrument will not pass smoothly typically indicates a need for adjustment in angle of approach, portal start location, or both. Slightly increased resistance of tissue to instrument passage is expected at the rotator cuff and capsule, but gentle twisting of the instrument with steady pressure should accomplish the goal. Increased resistance may suggest that a change in location is necessary to avoid injury to the patient.

Within the safe zones for portal establishment, the surgeon should

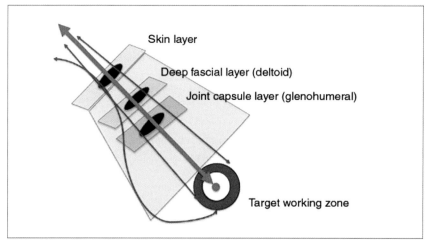

Figure 4   Illustration depicts alignment of established arthroscopy portals in three dimensions. The green arrow indicates the optimal path for instrument passage to preserve the tissue planes. Red arrows demonstrate inaccurate pathways to the target working zone that disrupt the tissue planes.

balance the optimal angle of approach and viewing with the need to establish additional portals or reposition the patient's limb. Multifunctional access through few skin portals is typically possible with a combination of careful planning and the ability to vary the angle of the arthroscopic lens, the entry portal of the arthroscope, and the rotational or spatial position of the limb. In certain patients these techniques may result in suboptimal approach angles for procedural steps or viewing. Surgeons must actively balance the potential for obstruction of access resulting from the creation of additional portals with the need to safely approach and access deeper structures. The use of a spinal needle for percutaneous access to the deep area in question allows surgeons to test the possible portal location, angle,

and fit. The author of this chapter routinely uses this technique when faced with complex procedural steps or variant anatomy. When small spaces result in crowding that cannot be avoided, placing guidewires or switching sticks into portals as placeholders while withdrawing cannulas out of the deep space increases working room and allows for easy reestablishment of portals that are not in use.

Each surgeon must understand the limitations of arthroscopy in general and his or her own skill and facility with the procedure to be performed. Comfort

with the open surgical procedure is requisite to any attempt at an arthroscopic approach. Even with modern advancements in equipment and surgical technique, limitations of the arthroscopic method must be respected. Having the necessary sterile equipment and surgical skill to convert an arthroscopic procedure to an open technique is imperative. Although the surgeon must make every effort to plan the arthroscopic approach and predict which patients can be safely treated arthroscopically, achieving the correction of pathology must remain the primary goal of surgical management.

 Bibliography

Bedi A, Dines J, Dines DM, et al: Use of the 70° arthroscope for improved visualization with common arthroscopic procedures. *Arthroscopy* 2010;26(12):1684-1696.

Bhatia DN, de Beer JF, Dutoit DF: An anatomic study of inferior glenohumeral recess portals: Comparative anatomy at risk. *Arthroscopy* 2008;24(5):506-513.

Burkhead WZ Jr, Scheinberg RR, Box G: Surgical anatomy of the axillary nerve. *J Shoulder Elbow Surg* 1992;1(1):31-36.

Cvetanovich GL, McCormick F, Erickson BJ, et al: The posterolateral portal: Optimizing anchor placement and labral repair at the inferior glenoid. *Arthrosc Tech* 2013;2(3):e201-e204.

Davidson PA, Rivenburgh DW: The 7-o'clock posteroinferior portal for shoulder arthroscopy. *Am J Sports Med* 2002;30(5):693-696.

Dwyer T, Petrera M, White LM, et al: Trans-subscapularis portal versus low-anterior portal for low anchor placement on the inferior glenoid fossa: A cadaveric shoulder study with computed tomographic analysis. *Arthroscopy* 2015;31(2):209-214.

Frank RM, Mall NA, Gupta D, et al: Inferior suture anchor placement during arthroscopic Bankart repair: Influence of portal placement and curved drill guide. *Am J Sports Med* 2014;42(5):1182-1189.

Gelber PE, Reina F, Caceres E, Monllau JC: A comparison of risk between the lateral decubitus and the beach-chair position when establishing an anteroinferior shoulder portal: A cadaveric study. *Arthroscopy* 2007;23(5):522-528.

Han Y, Shin JH, Seok CW, Lee CH, Kim SH: Is posterior delamination in arthroscopic rotator cuff repair hidden to the posterior viewing portal? *Arthroscopy* 2013;29(11):1740-1747.

Hoenecke H, Fronek J: The posterior-medial portal. *Arthroscopy* 2006;22(2):232.e1-232.e3.

Lo IK, Lind CC, Burkhart SS: Glenohumeral arthroscopy portals established using an outside-in technique: Neurovascular anatomy at risk. *Arthroscopy* 2004;20(6):596-602.

Meyer M, Graveleau N, Hardy P, Landreau P: Anatomic risks of shoulder arthroscopy portals: Anatomic cadaveric study of 12 portals. *Arthroscopy* 2007;23(5):529-536.

Morgan RT, Henn RF III, Paryavi E, Dreese J: Injury to the suprascapular nerve during superior labrum anterior and posterior repair: Is a rotator interval portal safer than an anterosuperior portal? *Arthroscopy* 2014;30(11):1418-1423.

Nord KD, Mauck BM: The new subclavian portal and modified Neviaser portal for arthroscopic rotator cuff repair. *Arthroscopy* 2003;19(9):1030-1034.

Oh JH, Kim SH, Lee HK, Jo KH, Bae KJ: Trans-rotator cuff portal is safe for arthroscopic superior labral anterior and posterior lesion repair: Clinical and radiological analysis of 58 SLAP lesions. *Am J Sports Med* 2008;36(10):1913-1921.

Paxton ES, Backus J, Keener J, Brophy RH: Shoulder arthroscopy: Basic principles of positioning, anesthesia, and portal anatomy. *J Am Acad Orthop Surg* 2013;21(6):332-342.

Pearsall AW IV, Holovacs TF, Speer KP: The low anterior five-o'clock portal during arthroscopic shoulder surgery performed in the beach-chair position. *Am J Sports Med* 1999;27(5):571-574.

Romeo AA, Mazzocca AD, Tauro JC: Arthroscopic biceps tenodesis. *Arthroscopy* 2004;20(2):206-213.

Totlis T, Natsis K, Pantelidis P, Paraskevas G, Iosifidis M, Kyriakidis A: Reliability of the posterolateral corner of the acromion as a landmark for the posterior arthroscopic portal of the shoulder. *J Shoulder Elbow Surg* 2014;23(9):1403-1408.

Uno A, Bain GI, Mehta JA: Arthroscopic relationship of the axillary nerve to the shoulder joint capsule: An anatomic study. *J Shoulder Elbow Surg* 1999;8(3):226-230.

Woolf SK, Guttmann D, Karch MM, Graham RD II, Reid JB III, Lubowitz JH: The superior-medial shoulder arthroscopy portal is safe. *Arthroscopy* 2007;23(3):247-250.

Chapter 3

The Deltopectoral Approach: Options for Management of the Subscapularis Tendon

Justin S. Yang, MD

Robert Arciero, MD

Case Presentation

A 33-year-old man presents with chronic, recurrent shoulder instability after sustaining a traumatic anterior shoulder dislocation 10 years earlier. Since that injury, the patient has experienced progressively increasing episodes of recurrent instability, resulting in an inability to perform activities of daily living without dislocating his shoulder. No substantial improvement has been achieved with physical therapy that includes strengthening of the rotator cuff and periscapular muscles. The patient has not had any previous surgical treatment. Advanced imaging shows a glenoid in the shape of an inverted pear and approximately 25% bone loss on the anterior glenoid (**Figure 1**). Based on the amount of glenoid bone loss, bone block transfer of the coracoid process is identified as the best treatment option.

Indications

Most open procedures performed to address anterior instability are done through the deltopectoral interval. At the superficial level, the deltopectoral interval uses an internervous plane that offers maximal exposure with the least harm to muscles, vasculature, and nerves. As the approach deepens past the clavipectoral fascia, however, the anteroinferior glenoid is obscured by the subscapularis tendon, which crosses the field transversely to insert on the lesser tuberosity. To perform the bone block transfer, the dissection must be carried deep to the subscapularis tendon. The surgeon must decide how to manage the subscapularis tendon to expose the anterior glenoid defect. The goal is to balance good exposure with preservation of the integrity of the subscapularis tendon and the lesser tuberosity (**Figure 2**). The options, which are presented here

along a continuum from the technique that provides maximal exposure to the technique that best maintains subscapularis integrity, are as follows: complete subscapularis tenotomy (longitudinal, L-shaped, or T-shaped), subscapularis tendon peel, lesser tuberosity osteotomy, partial subscapularis tenotomy, subscapularis transverse (horizontal) split, and subscapularis tendon retraction (superiorly, inferiorly, or both).

The authors of this chapter prefer the subscapularis split technique for anterior glenoid-based procedures because it allows for adequate exposure without compromising the integrity of the subscapularis tendon. Surgeon comfort with any of these procedures is an important factor in determining how to manage the subscapularis tendon.

Controversies and Alternative Approaches

Subscapularis Tenotomy

Several variations of subscapularis tenotomy have been described. In each variation, the vertical limb is started 1 to 1.5 cm medial to the lesser tuberosity so as to leave a healthy cuff of tissue to be used in the tenotomy repair

Dr. Arciero or an immediate family member is a member of a speakers' bureau or has made paid presentations on behalf of Arthrex and Mitek Sports Medicine; serves as a paid consultant to Biomet, Mitek Sports Medicine, and Soft Tissue Regeneration; has stock or stock options held in Soft Tissue Regeneration; has received research or institutional support from Arthrex; and serves as a board member, owner, officer, or committee member of the American Orthopaedic Society for Sports Medicine. Neither Dr. Yang nor any immediate family member has received anything of value from or has stock or stock options held in a commercial company or institution related directly or indirectly to the subject of this chapter.

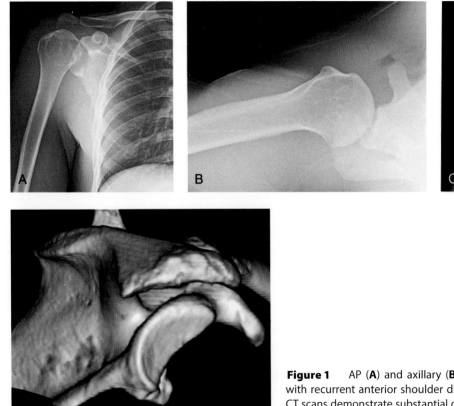

Figure 1 AP (**A**) and axillary (**B**) radiographs from a 33-year-old man with recurrent anterior shoulder dislocation. **C** and **D,** Three-dimensional CT scans demonstrate substantial glenoid bone loss with an inverted pear appearance.

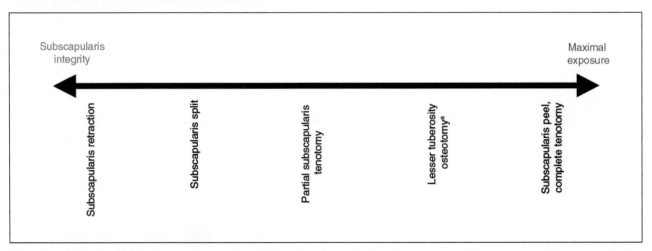

Figure 2 Diagram shows the continuum of surgical options from the least disruptive to subscapularis integrity (subscapularis retraction) to the most disruptive (maximal exposure [subscapularis peel, complete tenotomy]). ª Subscapularis integrity is defined by the entire subscapular complex, including the lesser tuberosity.

(**Figure 3, A**). In patients with degenerative fraying of the subscapularis tendon insertion such that a healthy cuff is not available, care should be taken to repair the tenotomized subscapularis directly to the lesser tuberosity. With the arm in neutral to slight external rotation, the tenotomy is begun at the rotator interval and extended through the tendon to the inferior border of the subscapularis tendon (**Figure 3, B** and **C**). Typically, the circumflex vessels can be spared. By dissecting medially approximately 1 cm from the vertical incision in the tendon just proximal

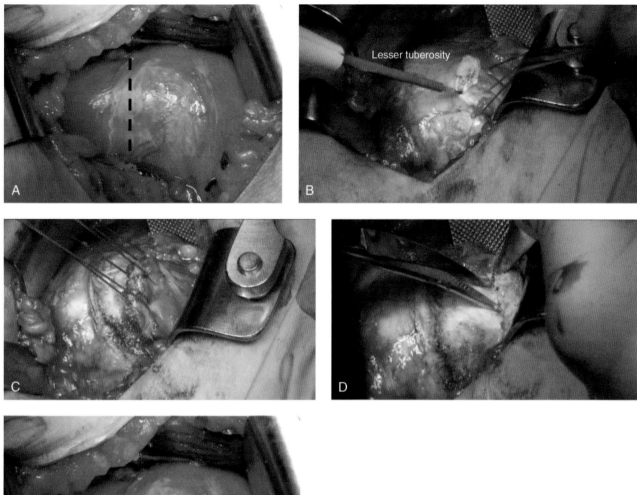

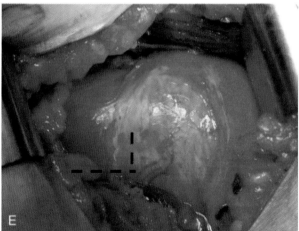

Figure 3 Intraoperative photographs show the steps of full tenotomy that can be performed while avoiding the anterior circumflex vessels. **A,** The vertical portion of the tenotomy is denoted by the dashed line. **B,** The tenotomy is started at the rotator interval. This patient does not exhibit degenerative fraying. **C,** The tenotomy is carried distally to the circumflex vessel. **D,** The tendon is carefully separated from the underlying capsule. **E,** A planned partial L-shaped tenotomy is indicated by the dashed lines.

to the anterior circumflex vessels, it is possible to develop a plane separating the muscle from the capsule. The tendon can be separated from the capsule and the tendon released, with dissection from inferior to superior (**Figure 3, D**). The anterior circumflex vessels occasionally may be sacrificed because they do not provide the predominant blood supply to the proximal humerus. The capsule can be incised either with

the tendon or separately depending on the surgical procedure performed. Anatomic repair of the tenotomy should be done meticulously with nonabsorbable No. 2 high tensile strength braided suture.

The senior author (R.A.) has described a technique using a partial L-shaped tenotomy for exposure in patients with humeral avulsion of the inferior glenohumeral ligament. The

vertical tenotomy is limited to the lower third of the tendon, thereby preserving the anterior circumflex vessels, and then is extended horizontally to create an L-shaped partial tenotomy (**Figure 3, E**). This technique affords better exposure of the inferior capsule than does an isolated subscapularis split. With partial tenotomy, it may be possible to leave some proprioceptive fibers intact.

Video 3.1 Subscapularis Tenotomy in the Deltopectoral Approach. Justin S. Yang, MD; Robert Arciero, MD (5 min)

Historically, complete subscapularis tenotomy has been the preferred technique for arthroplasty because healing rates as high as 90% have been reported. Complete subscapularis tenotomy offers the best exposure of both the glenoid and the humeral head. Other benefits of this technique include its simplicity, its ability to maintain the integrity of the humeral cortex, and its ability to balance soft-tissue tension with medialization of the subscapularis tendon insertion. The weakness of complete subscapularis tenotomy is that the integrity of the subscapularis tendon cannot be maintained. Violation of the integrity of the subscapularis tendon can lead to decreased strength, range of motion, and outcome scores and to fatty degeneration of the muscle belly. In addition, the reported healing rates of tenotomy have been called into question because most studies are based on physical findings, such as the lift-off, belly press, and bear hug tests, which do not correlate well with ultrasound findings. With the use of ultrasound, healing rates of tenotomy as low as 50% have been reported. However, some authors have pointed out that in patients who have undergone arthroplasty, pain and functional scores do not correlate with subscapularis tendon healing.

Subscapularis Tendon Peel

An alternative to subscapularis tenotomy is subscapularis peel, in which the tendon is taken down subperiosteally from its origin on the lesser tuberosity. This technique may be particularly useful in cases in which lengthening of the subscapularis tendon may be necessary, such as in patients with chronic degenerative tendon laxity or in whom increased glenohumeral offset after arthroplasty must be accommodated. To repair the subscapularis tendon, bone tunnels are created from the neck of the humerus to the lesser tuberosity. If arthroplasty is being performed, then the suture can be wrapped around the prosthesis for better fixation in poor-quality bone. Suture anchors can also be used. The strong bone of the medial bicipital groove is ideal for the placement of repair sutures. Meticulous care must be taken while passing and tying sutures to reduce the tendon to bone.

Increasing biologic evidence has shown that tendon-to-bone healing occurs more slowly and less reliably than tendon-to-tendon healing. This finding may be because healing between non-homogeneous tissues is slower than healing of homogeneous tissue. Biomechanically, a subscapularis peel has been shown to have the lowest fatigue load-to-failure rates and the highest complete failure rates compared with osteotomy of the lesser tuberosity (bone-to-bone interface) and complete subscapularis tenotomy (tendon-to-tendon interface). The authors of a 2014 study found subscapularis peel to be clinically inferior to lesser tuberosity osteotomy based on Disabilities of the Arm, Shoulder, and Hand scores and Constant scores. They also found the subscapularis tendon to be abnormal on postoperative ultrasound in 13% of patients treated with subscapularis peel, whereas no patients treated with osteotomy had an abnormal subscapularis tendon. Thus, subscapularis tenotomy or lesser tuberosity osteotomy is preferred when access to the glenohumeral joint necessitates complete takedown of the subscapularis tendon.

Lesser Tuberosity Osteotomy

Lesser tuberosity osteotomy allows access to the glenohumeral joint and preserves its insertion on the lesser tuberosity. Lesser tuberosity osteotomy is used most commonly as an alternative to subscapularis tenotomy in patients undergoing arthroplasty. Exposure is the key to performing a safe and adequate osteotomy. The superior and inferior borders of both the subscapularis tendon and the lesser tuberosity are identified. The rotator interval along with any remaining bursa is dissected so that the subscapularis tendon can be palpated and visualized anterior to posterior, along with the mass of the lesser tuberosity. The biceps tendon should be either tenotomized or retracted laterally. The bicipital and subdeltoid bursae should be freed from the bicipital groove so that the starting point of the osteotomy can be visualized. The anterior humeral circumflex vessels should be ligated and the patient's arm placed in internal rotation and adduction. The osteotomy can be done using an osteotome or a saw, starting at the medial aspect of the bicipital groove and parallel to the subscapularis tendon. The osteotomy should exit at the transition point of the lesser tuberosity and the humeral head cartilage (**Figure 4**). The goal is to remove a wafer of bone approximately 3 to 4 cm long and 5 to 10 mm thick. Authors have reported using a thinner, fleck osteotomy with no difference in function, healing, or biomechanical strength compared with standard, thicker osteotomy. Traction sutures are then placed around the piece of bone at the bone-tendon junction.

In repair of the lesser tuberosity and subscapularis tendon, heavy, nonabsorbable braided sutures are passed around the lesser tuberosity and through the subscapularis tendon at the bone-tendon junction. The heavy needles are then passed through the medial aspect of the bicipital groove. Three or four sutures are typically needed, so spacing should be planned. The lesser tuberosity is reduced anatomically, creating bone-to-bone contact, and is secured by tying the transosseous sutures. In addition, the sutures may be wrapped around the humeral stem to improve biomechanical fixation. A small plate may be used for cortical bone augmentation to improve

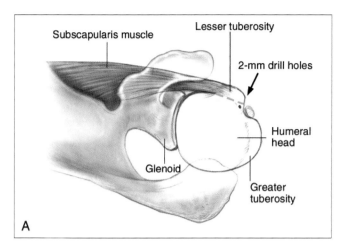
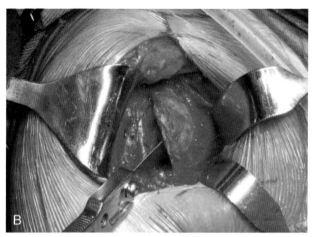

Figure 4   **A,** Illustration depicts the axial view of the lesser tuberosity osteotomy. The dashed blue line at the lesser tuberosity depicts the intended plane of the osteotomy. Drill holes are made in the bicipital groove for later fixation. **B,** Intraoperative photograph shows the osteotomized tuberosity in a right shoulder. (Reproduced with permission from Gerber C, Pennington SD, Yian EH, et al: Lesser tuberosity osteotomy for total shoulder arthroplasty. *J Bone Joint Surg Am* 2006;88[1 suppl 2]:170-177.)

suture pullout strength and to permit safe, active rehabilitation.

Numerous arthroplasty studies have compared lesser tuberosity osteotomy with tenotomy. Biomechanically, the lesser tuberosity osteotomy seems to result in less gap formation and stronger resistance to cyclic load, although ultimate failure load seems to be similar between lesser tuberosity osteotomy and tenotomy. Long-term clinical comparative studies are lacking because of the novelty of the procedure. In midterm results, lesser tuberosity osteotomy had better clinical outcome scores, less subscapularis tendon pathology on ultrasound, high rates of osteotomy healing (as high as 100%), and better belly press strength. The advantage of lesser tuberosity osteotomy is that healing can be monitored reliably on radiographs; however, if the osteotomy site cannot be visualized, CT should be done at 6 months to rule out nonunion. Despite these advantages, lesser tuberosity osteotomy is limited by the inability to medialize the insertion to adjust subscapularis tension, risk of intraoperative fracture, and loss of stem fixation. In addition, osteotomy should be used with caution in patients undergoing nonarthroplasty

procedures because of the risk of damaging the articular cartilage.

Subscapularis Tendon Retraction

For limited indications, the glenohumeral joint may be accessed by retracting the subscapularis tendon inferiorly (through the rotator interval) and/or retracting the subscapularis tendon superiorly along the inferior border. This technique is described in studies published in 2009 and 2013; specialized retractors and reamers are used to visualize and work around a relatively small area. Long-term results of this technique are not available, but short-term results show fast recovery of motion and strength, with the added benefit that full active and passive motion can begin immediately after the procedure. The authors of one study expressed concerns regarding visualization of inferior osteophytes and nonanatomic humeral neck osteotomies. Other researchers have used the space just inferior to the subscapularis tendon to repair a humeral avulsion of the glenohumeral ligament. This technique, which involved ligating the anterior humeral circumflex vessels and retracting the subscapularis tendon

superiorly, is limited to repair of the anterior and middle band of the inferior glenohumeral ligament.

■ Results

In a sequential sectional study of 10 cadaver specimens, researchers measured the area of glenoid and humeral head exposure afforded by the subscapularis split technique compared with partial or complete tenotomy. The glenoid exposure with the subscapularis split technique (2 cm²) did not differ significantly compared with the exposure with a partial (L-shaped) tenotomy (2.2 cm²) or a full (T-shaped) tenotomy (2.4 cm²). However, the subscapularis split afforded only 3.2 cm² of humeral head exposure, whereas the partial and full tenotomies allowed substantially more access to the humeral head (8.1 and 11 cm², respectively). Thus, the authors of that study recommended subscapularis split for glenoid-only procedures because a subscapularis tenotomy offers no added advantage in exposure. Additionally, they recommended a partial or complete tenotomy for combined glenoid and humeral procedures.

Functionally, subscapularis split has been shown to be superior to subscapularis tenotomy for surgical management of instability. In a study of 102 young patients (mean age, 26.8 years) undergoing the Latarjet procedure, the results of partial (L-shaped) tenotomy were compared with the results of subscapularis split (69 and 37 patients, respectively). Patients treated with tenotomy had lower Walch-Duplay scores, lower lift-off strength, and greater loss of internal rotation. At average 7-year follow-up, higher fatty subscapularis muscle belly degeneration was noted on CT from patients treated with tenotomy. In a similar study of 376 patients undergoing the Bristow-Latarjet procedure, those treated with the subscapularis split technique had a decreased incidence of positive belly press and lift-off tests, as well as higher strength scores for internal rotation with the arms at the side. These comparative studies were retrospective and nonrandomized, however. Although the preoperative parameters of the two treatment groups were similar, the selection criteria are not outlined in the studies. Another study of the subscapularis split technique for the Latarjet procedure also showed favorable results. In this prospective study of 15 patients who underwent a Latarjet procedure with the subscapularis split technique, no difference in preoperative and postoperative quantified belly press strength was found.

The literature on subscapularis tendon management is summarized in **Tables 1** and **2**.

Technical Keys to Success: Subscapularis Split

- The patient is placed in the standard beach-chair position, which allows for optimal exposure of the subscapularis tendon, subsequent retractor placement, and protection of neurovascular structures.
- The standard deltopectoral approach is used and the vein is retracted laterally, after which the deltoid and pectoralis major muscles are retracted, typically with a self-retaining retractor.
- The coracoid is identified along with the conjoined tendon and the coracoacromial ligament.
- The clavipectoral fascia is incised just lateral to the fleshy fibers of the short head of the biceps muscle to minimize bleeding (**Figure 5**).
- The self-retaining retractor is then placed one level deeper, retracting the conjoint muscles medially and the deltoid laterally to visualize the subscapularis tendon (**Figure 6**).
- Scarring from previous surgery may exist at the deltopectoral interval; internal and external rotation of the arm helps to define the underlying subscapularis tendon. Although a self-retaining retractor aids exposure, prolonged use should be avoided because it may put the musculocutaneous nerve at risk for injury.
- The superior and inferior borders of the subscapularis tendon are defined, with attention given to the surrounding neurovascular structures.
- The anterior circumflex vessels mark the inferior aspect of the subscapularis tendon; the axillary nerve can be palpated immediately inferior to this point (**Figure 7**).
- A horizontal split in line with the subscapularis tendon fibers is made between the junction of the superior two-thirds and inferior one-third of the subscapularis tendon insertion (**Figure 7**). Anatomically, this split divides the tendinous portions of the subscapularis insertion from the muscular portions. However, this proportion is not an anatomic constant; thus, visualizing both portions may be the best way to determine where to split the fibers. In the coronal plane, the split typically starts 1.5 cm medial to the lesser tuberosity and extends another 1.5 to 2 cm medially.
- The axillary nerve is palpated before the split is initiated to make sure that the nerve is not at risk. Care must be taken not to penetrate the glenohumeral capsule. Identifying the plane between the two structures is easier medially near the myotendinous junction. Blunt dissection with a finger, a Cobb elevator, or a moist sponge can help define the planes between the subscapularis tendon and capsule and permit the muscle to be teased or pushed off the capsule. The authors of this chapter prefer to start more medial because the tissue plane can be difficult to identify more laterally. If the plane is started too far laterally, a needle-tip Bovie cautery device can be used to help identify the tissue plane.
- Traction sutures are placed superior and inferior to the split to assist in tendon mobilization and glenohumeral visualization. Alternatively, self-retaining retractors can be used.
- At the end of the procedure, the split subscapularis tendon is repaired with absorbable suture; however, some authors have suggested that a pure horizontal split does not need to be repaired.
- Additional exposure can be created by connecting the transverse incision to a vertical (T- or L-shaped) tenotomy in the subscapularis tendon. However, doing so compromises the integrity of the subscapularis tendon and creates a potential site of failure.

Table 1 Results of Subscapularis Tendon Management Techniques (2005-2009)

Authors	Journal (Year)	Technique	Outcomes[a]	Failure Rate[b]	Comments
Gerber et al	*J Bone Joint Surg Am* (2005)	Osteotomy	100% union rate 25% of shoulders had a positive lift-off test, 11% had a positive belly press test, and 55% had increased fatty infiltration postoperatively as noted on CT	0	Case series of 36 patients (39 shoulders) treated with arthroplasty Mean age, 57 yr
Maynou et al	*J Bone Joint Surg Br* (2005)	Subscapularis split or L-shaped tenotomy	Lower lift-off strength and decreased internal rotation after tenotomy compared with the contralateral limb Lower outcome scores and more fatty atrophy after tenotomy at avg 7-yr follow-up Subscapularis atrophy was noted on CT	NR	Retrospective cohort study of 102 patients treated with the Latarjet procedure Mean age, 27 yr
Ponce et al	*J Bone Joint Surg Am* (2005)	Peel, tenotomy, or osteotomy (biomechanical testing); osteotomy (clinical results)	Osteotomy demonstrated the least gap formation with cyclic loading and the highest ultimate load to failure in biomechanical testing 5 patients had a positive lift-off or belly press test postoperatively (none preoperatively)	1.3% (1 subscapularis nonunion/ rupture)	Biomechanical testing on 27 cadavers and a case series of 76 patients Mean age, 61.7 yr
Armstrong et al	*J Shoulder Elbow Surg* (2006)	Complete tenotomy	Poor sensitivity (23%) of belly press test in assessing subscapularis tendon integrity Subscapularis tendon rupture did not correlate well with ASES shoulder scores	13% (subscapularis rupture)	Case series of 23 patients treated with arthroplasty Mean age, 70 yr Ultrasound was used to evaluate subscapularis tendon integrity
Scheibel et al	*Am J Sports Med* (2006)	L-shaped tenotomy	High rate of positive belly press sign in primary and revision patients (53% and 91%, respectively) Marked atrophy and fatty infiltration found on MRI, particularly in the upper part of the subscapularis muscle	No complete tendon ruptures	Retrospective cohort study of 25 patients treated with primary or revision anterior stabilization Mean age, 35 yr
Qureshi et al	*J Shoulder Elbow Surg* (2008)	Osteotomy	100% union rate 17% of patients had positive lift-off test, and 12% of patients had positive belly press test postoperatively	0	Case series of 28 patients treated with arthroplasty Mean age, 66 yr
Caplan et al	*J Shoulder Elbow Surg* (2009)	Complete tenotomy	All patients had a negative belly press test, and 9% of patients had a positive lift-off test	NR	Case series of 43 patients treated with arthroplasty Mean age, 65 yr
Krishnan et al	*J Shoulder Elbow Surg* (2009)	Tenotomy, fleck versus standard osteotomy (biomechanical testing); osteotomy (case series)	97% union rate Cadaver study: ultimate load to failure was higher after osteotomy, and earlier gap formation with cyclic loading was noted after tenotomy Case series: 14% of patients had a positive belly press test, and 18% had a positive lift-off test (all were normal preoperatively)	3% (3 nonunions)	Biomechanical testing on 15 cadavers and a case series of 100 patients

ASES = American Shoulder and Elbow Surgeons shoulder outcome, NR = not reported.
[a] Ability to tuck in shirt behind the back is used synonymously with lift-off test in some studies.
[b] Failure rate is defined as the subscapularis tendon rupture rate (by imaging).

Table 2 Results of Subscapularis Tendon Management Techniques (2010-2014)

Authors	Journal (Year)	Technique	Outcomes[a]	Failure Rate[b]	Comments
Elkousy et al	*Orthopedics* (2010)	Subscapularis split	No difference in preoperative versus postoperative isometric belly press strength at 6 mo No difference compared with age-matched normative values	No ruptures	Case series of 15 patients treated with the Latarjet procedure Mean age, 23 yr
Jackson et al	*J Shoulder Elbow Surg* (2010)	Complete tenotomy	High rate of subscapularis rupture noted on ultrasound Lower DASH score in patients with rupture Poor sensitivity (43%) of combined belly press and lift-off test in detecting ruptures	47% subscapularis rupture	Case series of 15 patients treated with arthroplasty Mean age, 67 yr
Scalise et al	*J Bone Joint Surg Am* (2010)	Tenotomy or osteotomy	100% union rate with osteotomy Better Penn Shoulder Score and less tendon pathology on ultrasound in the osteotomy group; equivalent range of motion and strength	Subscapularis tendon pathology after tenotomy in 47% (7 of 15 shoulders) Subscapularis pathology with osteotomy in 10% (2 shoulders)	Retrospective cohort study of 34 patients (35 shoulders) treated with arthroplasty Mean age, 67 yr
Jandhyala et al	*J Shoulder Elbow Surg* (2011)	Complete tenotomy or osteotomy	100% union rate after osteotomy Higher rate of positive belly press tests in the tenotomy group Equivalent range of motion and lift-off test results between groups	None after osteotomy Rupture rate for tenotomy not studied	Retrospective cohort study of 36 patients treated with arthroplasty Mean age, 67 yr
Paladini et al	*J Shoulder Elbow Surg* (2012)	Subscapularis split or L-shaped tenotomy	Higher rates of positive belly press and lift-off tests after tenotomy Better isometric strength in internal rotation after subscapularis split	NR	Retrospective cohort study of 376 patients treated with the Bristow-Latarjet procedure Mean age, 27 yr
Bellamy et al	*J Shoulder Elbow Surg* (2014)	Subscapularis split, L- or T-shaped tenotomy	Glenoid exposure did not change significantly among the three techniques Exposure of the humeral head was best with complete T-shaped tenotomy	N/A	Cadaver study (10 shoulders)

DASH = Disabilities of the Arm, Shoulder and Hand; N/A = not applicable; NR = not reported; WOOS = Western Ontario Osteoarthritis of the Shoulder.

[a] Ability to tuck in shirt behind the back is used synonymously with lift-off test in some studies.

[b] Failure rate is defined as the subscapularis tendon rupture rate (by imaging).

Table 2 Results of Subscapularis Tendon Management Techniques (2010-2014) (*continued*)

Authors	Journal (Year)	Technique	Outcomes[a]	Failure Rate[b]	Comments
Buckley et al	*J Shoulder Elbow Surg* (2014)	Subscapularis peel or osteotomy	Lower WOOS score and higher rate of abnormal ultrasound findings after subscapularis peel Equivalent DASH scores	6.3% of patients (2 of 32) in the peel group had an abnormal subscapularis tendon; none in the osteotomy group 1 of 28 patients had fibrous union of osteotomy (3.6%)	Retrospective cohort study of 50 patients treated with arthroplasty Mean age, 68 yr
Fishman et al	*J Shoulder Elbow Surg* (2014)	Complete tenotomy, fleck osteotomy, or standard osteotomy	Tenotomy repair showed increased gap formation with increasing cyclic loading No difference between the two types of osteotomy Similar ultimate failure strength with all three techniques	N/A	Cadaver study (20 shoulders)

DASH = Disabilities of the Arm, Shoulder and Hand; N/A = not applicable; NR = not reported; WOOS = Western Ontario Osteoarthritis of the Shoulder.
[a] Ability to tuck in shirt behind the back is used synonymously with lift-off test in some studies.
[b] Failure rate is defined as the subscapularis tendon rupture rate (by imaging).

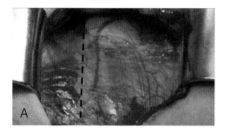 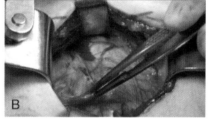

Figure 5 **A,** Intraoperative photograph shows the incision (dashed line) of the clavipectoral fascia lateral to the conjoined tendon in a right shoulder. **B,** Care should be taken when incising the fascia because the conjoined tendon has an associated muscle belly, which may bleed if the incision is made too medial.

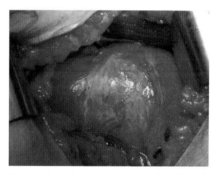

Figure 6 Intraoperative photograph of a left shoulder shows the exposure of the subscapularis tendon with retraction of the conjoined tendon medially. Note the anterior circumflex vessels inferiorly.

 Rehabilitation

In general, the primary surgical procedure should dictate the rehabilitation regimen. For example, after procedures performed to manage instability, 4 to 6 weeks of immobilization is recommended. The timing of the return of subscapularis tendon function after subscapularis tenotomy, measured by the positive results of the lift-off or belly press test, averages 8 to 10 weeks but can take up to 20 weeks. Thus, the protocol should be tailored to each patient, based on progression and symptoms.

The recommendations in **Tables 3** and **4** are based on the subscapularis tendon management technique only and should be modified on the basis of the primary surgical procedure.

 Avoiding Pitfalls

A good surgical technique balances exposure, protection of neurovascular structures, and minimal damage to surrounding soft tissue and bone.

The axillary nerve branches from the posterior cord of the brachial plexus posterior to the axillary artery. It crosses anterior to the subscapularis muscle and exits inferior to that muscle. It then dives posteriorly through the quadrilateral space. Care must be taken to identify or palpate the axillary nerve and to ensure it is free of tension throughout the procedure.

The anterior humeral circumflex artery, accompanied by two veins, lies inferior to the subscapularis tendon. Historically, this artery was thought to contribute a substantial blood supply to

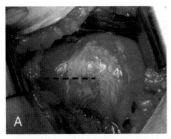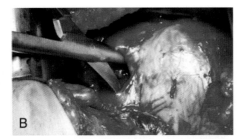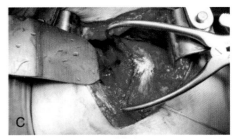

Figure 7 Intraoperative photographs show a left shoulder. **A,** The subscapularis split is shown, with the dashed line signifying the junction between the upper two-thirds and lower one-third of the insertion. **B** and **C,** The split is demonstrated. Note the preservation of the anterior circumflex vessels with this technique.

Table 3 Rehabilitation Protocol After Subscapularis Split or Lesser Tuberosity Osteotomy

Postoperative Week	Range of Motion	Strengthening	Return to Play	Comments/Emphasis
0-2	Full active and passive in all planes	None	None	Emphasis on restoring full range of motion
2-6	Full active and passive in all planes	Gentle deltoid, scapular, and rotator cuff strengthening	None	—
6-12	Full active and passive in all planes	Full strengthening in all planes	Can start gradual return-to-play exercises	Emphasis on strengthening
12-24	Full active and passive in all planes	Full strengthening in all planes	Goal of full return to play	—

Table 4 Rehabilitation Protocol After Subscapularis Tenotomy

Postoperative Week	Range of Motion	Strengthening	Return to Play	Comments/Emphasis
0-2	Full active and passive; however, no external rotation beyond neutral	None	None	—
2-6	Full active and passive; however, no external rotation beyond neutral	Gentle scapular and deltoid strengthening	None	—
6-12	Full active and passive	Progressive rotator cuff strengthening Limit internal rotation strengthening based on symptoms	Can start gradual return-to-play exercises	Emphasis on restoring full range of motion
12-24	Full active and passive	Full strengthening in all planes	Goal of full return to play	Emphasis on strengthening

the humeral head, and efforts were made to preserve it in the nonarthroplasty setting. However, recent literature has shown that the posterior humeral circumflex artery provides the dominant blood supply to the humeral head. No cases of osteonecrosis following isolated surgical ligation of the anterior humeral circumflex artery have been reported. The vessels can typically be saved if an isolated transverse subscapularis split is performed; however, if additional exposure is needed inferiorly, the vessels can be sacrificed.

Although the horizontal split of the subscapularis tendon is made between the junction of the superior two-thirds and inferior one-third of the subscapularis tendon insertion, visualization of both portions may be the best way to determine where to split the fibers. Care must be taken to palpate or visualize the axillary nerve as the split is carried medially.

▮ Bibliography

Arciero RA, Mazzocca AD: Mini-open repair technique of HAGL (humeral avulsion of the glenohumeral ligament) lesion. *Arthroscopy* 2005;21(9):1152.e1-1152.e4.

Armstrong A, Lashgari C, Teefey S, Menendez J, Yamaguchi K, Galatz LM: Ultrasound evaluation and clinical correlation of subscapularis repair after total shoulder arthroplasty. *J Shoulder Elbow Surg* 2006;15(5):541-548.

Bellamy JL, Johnson AE, Beltran MJ, Hsu JR; Skeletal Trauma Research Consortium STReC: Quantification of the exposure of the glenohumeral joint from the minimally invasive to more invasive subscapularis approach to the anterior shoulder: A cadaveric study. *J Shoulder Elbow Surg* 2014;23(6):895-901.

Bhatia DN, DeBeer JF, van Rooyen KS: The "subscapularis-sparing" approach: A new mini-open technique to repair a humeral avulsion of the glenohumeral ligament lesion. *Arthroscopy* 2009;25(6):686-690.

Buckley T, Miller R, Nicandri G, Lewis R, Voloshin I: Analysis of subscapularis integrity and function after lesser tuberosity osteotomy versus subscapularis tenotomy in total shoulder arthroplasty using ultrasound and validated clinical outcome measures. *J Shoulder Elbow Surg* 2014;23(9):1309-1317.

Budge MD, Nolan EM, Wiater JM: Lesser tuberosity osteotomy versus subscapularis tenotomy: Technique and rationale. *Operative Techniques in Orthopaedics* 2011;21(1):39-43.

Caplan JL, Whitfield B, Neviaser RJ: Subscapularis function after primary tendon to tendon repair in patients after replacement arthroplasty of the shoulder. *J Shoulder Elbow Surg* 2009;18(2):193-196, discussion 197-198.

DeFranco MJ, Higgins LD, Warner JJ: Subscapularis management in open shoulder surgery. *J Am Acad Orthop Surg* 2010;18(12):707-717.

Elkousy H, Gartsman GM, Labriola J, O'Connor DP, Edwards TB: Subscapularis function following the Latarjet coracoid transfer for recurrent anterior shoulder instability. *Orthopedics* 2010;33(11):802.

Fishman MP, Budge MD, Moravek JE Jr, et al: Biomechanical testing of small versus large lesser tuberosity osteotomies: Effect on gap formation and ultimate failure load. *J Shoulder Elbow Surg* 2014;23(4):470-476.

Gerber C, Yian EH, Pfirrmann CA, Zumstein MA, Werner CM: Subscapularis muscle function and structure after total shoulder replacement with lesser tuberosity osteotomy and repair. *J Bone Joint Surg Am* 2005;87(8):1739-1745.

Habermeyer P, Magosch P, Lichtenberg S: Recentering the humeral head for glenoid deficiency in total shoulder arthroplasty. *Clin Orthop Relat Res* 2007;(457):124-132.

Hettrich CM, Boraiah S, Dyke JP, Neviaser A, Helfet DL, Lorich DG: Quantitative assessment of the vascularity of the proximal part of the humerus. *J Bone Joint Surg Am* 2010;92(4):943-948.

Hinton MA, Parker AW, Drez D Jr, Altcheck D: An anatomic study of the subscapularis tendon and myotendinous junction. *J Shoulder Elbow Surg* 1994;3(4):224-229.

Jackson JD, Cil A, Smith J, Steinmann SP: Integrity and function of the subscapularis after total shoulder arthroplasty. *J Shoulder Elbow Surg* 2010;19(7):1085-1090.

Jandhyala S, Unnithan A, Hughes S, Hong T: Subscapularis tenotomy versus lesser tuberosity osteotomy during total shoulder replacement: A comparison of patient outcomes. *J Shoulder Elbow Surg* 2011;20(7):1102-1107.

Jobe FW: Unstable shoulders in the athlete. *Instr Course Lect* 1985;34:228-231.

Krishnan SG, Stewart DG, Reineck JR, Lin KC, Buzzell JE, Burkhead WZ: Subscapularis repair after shoulder arthroplasty: Biomechanical and clinical validation of a novel technique. *J Shoulder Elbow Surg* 2009;18(2):184-192, discussion 197-198.

Lafosse L, Schnaser E, Haag M, Gobezie R: Primary total shoulder arthroplasty performed entirely thru the rotator interval: Technique and minimum two-year outcomes. *J Shoulder Elbow Surg* 2009;18(6):864-873.

Lui P, Zhang P, Chan K, Qin L: Biology and augmentation of tendon-bone insertion repair. *J Orthop Surg Res* 2010;5:59.

Maynou C, Cassagnaud X, Mestdagh H: Function of subscapularis after surgical treatment for recurrent instability of the shoulder using a bone-block procedure. *J Bone Joint Surg Br* 2005;87(8):1096-1101.

Miller SL, Hazrati Y, Klepps S, Chiang A, Flatow EL: Loss of subscapularis function after total shoulder replacement: A seldom recognized problem. *J Shoulder Elbow Surg* 2003;12(1):29-34.

Paladini P, Merolla G, De Santis E, Campi F, Porcellini G: Long-term subscapularis strength assessment after Bristow-Latarjet procedure: Isometric study. *J Shoulder Elbow Surg* 2012;21(1):42-47.

Ponce BA, Ahluwalia RS, Mazzocca AD, Gobezie RG, Warner JJ, Millett PJ: Biomechanical and clinical evaluation of a novel lesser tuberosity repair technique in total shoulder arthroplasty. *J Bone Joint Surg Am* 2005;87(suppl 2):1-8.

Qureshi S, Hsiao A, Klug RA, Lee E, Braman J, Flatow EL: Subscapularis function after total shoulder replacement: Results with lesser tuberosity osteotomy. *J Shoulder Elbow Surg* 2008;17(1):68-72.

Scalise JJ, Ciccone J, Iannotti JP: Clinical, radiographic, and ultrasonographic comparison of subscapularis tenotomy and lesser tuberosity osteotomy for total shoulder arthroplasty. *J Bone Joint Surg Am* 2010;92(7):1627-1634.

Scheibel M, Tsynman A, Magosch P, Schroeder RJ, Habermeyer P: Postoperative subscapularis muscle insufficiency after primary and revision open shoulder stabilization. *Am J Sports Med* 2006;34(10):1586-1593.

Simovitch R, Fullick R, Zuckerman JD: Use of the subscapularis preserving technique in anatomic total shoulder arthroplasty. *Bull Hosp Jt Dis (2013)* 2013;71(suppl 2):94-100.

Slabaugh MA, Bents RT, Tokish JM: Timing of return of subscapularis function in open capsular shift patients. *J Shoulder Elbow Surg* 2007;16(5):544-547.

Small KM, Siegel EJ, Miller LR, Higgins LD: Imaging characteristics of lesser tuberosity osteotomy after total shoulder replacement: A study of 220 patients. *J Shoulder Elbow Surg* 2014;23(9):1318-1326.

Van den Berghe GR, Nguyen B, Patil S, et al: A biomechanical evaluation of three surgical techniques for subscapularis repair. *J Shoulder Elbow Surg* 2008;17(1):156-161.

Video Reference

Yang JS, Arciero R: Video. Subscapularis Tenotomy in the Deltopectoral Approach. Los Angeles, CA, 2015.

Chapter 4
Open Posterior Approach for the Management of Posterior Shoulder Instability

Robert H. Bell, MD

Jeffrey S. Noble, MD

 Introduction

Shoulder instability is the single most common shoulder disorder affecting young athletes, with an incidence higher than that of rotator cuff tears, arthritis, and fractures. However, the treatment for instability remains somewhat unclear in many patients, especially those with anterior instability combined with bone loss and those with posterior instability. Posterior instability, which occurs in less than 10% of patients, is problematic for the patient and can be difficult to treat.

Techniques to manage posterior instability have changed across time, beginning with biceps transfers and moving to anterior capsulorrhaphy, rotational osteotomies, and, more recently, arthroscopic approaches. Ligamentous laxity and patient volition are now understood to contribute to failure. In addition, surgeons have learned to successfully apply knowledge gained from anterior reconstruction techniques

to better address posterior instability with well-designed and -performed capsulorrhaphies.

 Case Presentation

A 21-year-old man presents with chronic, recurrent instability of the right shoulder 1 year after sustaining a traumatic, season-ending shoulder injury during a swimming competition. The patient reports that as he performed his final turn in the 100-yard butterfly race, he grabbed the wall of the pool with his arms fully extended forward and his hands placed together, adducted at the wrist, and in an internally rotated position. During the turn, the patient felt a pop and immediate pain, along with a sensation of his shoulder giving way and coming out. The patient subsequently underwent two arthroscopic posterior capsulolabral repairs, after which he experienced decreased pain but had a residual sensation of looseness in his

shoulder. No substantial improvement was achieved with a 3-month course of physical therapy, which included an exercise program to strengthen the periscapular musculature. The patient continues to report posterior shoulder pain, occasional crepitus, and the sensation of the shoulder slipping out the back (especially with the provocative position of forward elevation, abduction, and internal rotation). The symptoms interfere with the patient's activities of daily living, such as dressing, getting out of bed, rolling over, and performing overhead motions.

During the physical examination, the patient has a full range of motion, ligamentous laxity with hyperextension of the elbows and knees, pain along the glenohumeral joint line, and a subtly audible and palpable click. In addition, he can reproduce his subluxation with selected muscular contraction and arm position (forward elevation, adduction, and internal rotation). Mild scapular winging is noted. Positive results are noted on the modified load and shift test posteriorly, the jerk test, and the pivot shift test of the shoulder. Further examination reveals a grade 2+ sulcus sign; however, the patient does not correlate that maneuver with a sensation of inferior instability. A displaced capsulolabral complex and a redundant

Dr. Bell or an immediate family member has received royalties from DePuy Synthes and Ortho-Helix; is a member of a speakers' bureau or has made paid presentations on behalf of and serves as a paid consultant to ArthroCare; serves as an unpaid consultant to ExacTech; has stock or stock options held in Cayenne Medical and OrthoHelix; and serves as a board member, owner, officer, or committee member of the American Shoulder and Elbow Surgeons and the Orthopaedic Learning Center. Dr. Noble or an immediate family member is a member of a speakers' bureau or has made paid presentations on behalf of and serves as a paid consultant to Stryker.

patulous posterior capsule are seen on MRI. Glenoid version is within normal limits. The patient is diagnosed with an episode of traumatic posterior instability and as having signs and symptoms of recurrent posterior subluxation of the shoulder. Based on the clinical findings, the open posterior approach is identified as the best treatment option.

Indications

Unidirectional recurrent posterior subluxation is a common condition in overhead athletes. Posterior instability can be traumatic and sport specific, as in a contact sport in which the patient recalls a specific episode that initiated his or her symptoms. Posterior instability also can be the result of repetitive microtrauma with resultant posterior capsular laxity.

Although unidirectional and bidirectional posterior subluxation of the shoulder are less common than anterior instability, such posterior subluxation often occurs in athletes. Most patients are successfully treated nonsurgically. Initial management consists of physical therapy to strengthen the internal and external rotators as well as the periscapular musculature. A standard upper extremity exercise program is prescribed. Overhead athletes are treated with 3 to 6 months of high-intensity, supervised rehabilitation. If symptoms are not relieved with nonsurgical management, reconstruction can be considered. The ideal indications for open surgical reconstruction in athletes are instability episodes that interfere with participation in competitive sports and, especially, activities of daily living.

Because of advances in instrumentation, reduced morbidity, and high success rates, most surgeons believe that posterior subluxation of the shoulder is best managed arthroscopically. However, arthroscopy may not be possible in cases of revision surgery or in patients

with associated bony and soft-tissue deficiencies. Such patients may be best treated using an open approach to reconstruction.

Controversies and Alternative Approaches

The open posterior approach described in this chapter is indicated for a patient with prior failed arthroscopic stabilizations; ongoing symptoms of posterior instability; and no associated bony glenoid bone loss, excessive retroversion, or a strong voluntary component to instability. The surgical goal is to address bidirectional instability (that is, posterior and inferior), which should be distinguished from the more global pattern seen in patients with multidirectional instability. However, the posterior approach can be performed on patients with bony deficiencies of the shoulder who need a posterior bone block or glenoid osteotomy. These procedures are considered salvage procedures. Posterior bone block and glenoid osteotomy should be used only with strict indications and performed only by those surgeons who have extensive knowledge of the techniques.

Patients who have undergone prior attempts at stabilization or who have ligamentous laxity are candidates for a posterior-inferior capsular shift. With this approach, volume and capsular redundancy are addressed, and any additional pathology (including detachment of the labrum) is easily repaired. In patients who exhibit associated soft-tissue or bony issues not amenable to a standard posterior capsulorrhaphy, other options include posterior bone block, glenoid osteotomy, and infraspinatus tenodesis. These are considered salvage procedures; they are rarely used and should be performed only by those surgeons who have an extensive knowledge of the technique.

Results

Published results from current and/or important studies on posterior instability management are summarized in **Table 1**.

Video 4.1 Infraspinatus - Capsular Reconstruction for Posterior Instability. Richard J. Hawkins, MD (5 min)

Technical Keys to Success

Positioning

- The patient is placed in the lateral decubitus position.
- The patient is stabilized using a full-length, inflatable beanbag device. All potential pressure points are identified and padded, and the head is secured in neutral alignment.
- A large axillary roll is placed beneath the unaffected axilla. The entire surgical arm and shoulder are draped free with fluid-impervious drapes to block out the axilla.
- The head of the table is elevated slightly, and the patient's torso is rolled anteriorly to achieve the optimal position for posterior shoulder exposure.
- A general anesthetic is applied, and it may be augmented with preoperative placement of an intrascalene block for postoperative pain control. Anesthesia personnel and equipment are positioned superior to the patient and well out of the surgical field to allow easy access to the posterior and anterior shoulder.
- Arthroscopic assessment of the intra-articular structures and glenohumeral articulation can be performed before reconstruction. If arthroscopic evaluation is planned, then a sterilized arm traction device can be applied to the arm

Table 1 Results of the Open Approach for the Management of Posterior Shoulder Instability

Authors	Journal (Year)	Technique	Outcomes	Failure Rate (%)	Comments
Neer and Foster	*J Bone Joint Surg Am* (1980)	Humeral based T-capsular shift	Of 32 patients, 18 had anterior instability and 15 had posterior instability (1 patient underwent a combined anterior/posterior approach)	0	Osteoarthritis in 1 patient Follow-up >5 yr (44%)
Fronek et al	*J Bone Joint Surg Am* (1989)	Open medially based posterior shift alone (6 patients) and with bone block (5 patients)	10 of 11 patients had no further instability, but only 3 returned to their preinjury level of sports	9	1 superficial infection Mean follow-up, 5 yr
Bigliani et al	*J Bone Joint Surg Am* (1995)	Open posterior-inferior capsular shift	28 of 35 shoulders (80%) exhibited a successful result (good or excellent)	11	6 of the 7 shoulders with unsatisfactory results had undergone previous attempts at stabilization Mean follow-up, 5 yr
Fuchs et al	*J Bone Joint Surg Am* (2000)	Open posterior-inferior capsular shift	Of 26 shoulders, 8 (31%) still had discomfort and 5 (21%) necessitated a change in profession	23	1 patient had subcoracoid impingement Mean follow-up, 7.6 yr
Misamore and Facibene	*J Shoulder Elbow Surg* (2000)	Open posterior-inferior capsular shift	13 of 14 patients achieved good to excellent results (Rowe scores)	7	13 patients returned to unrestricted sports without recurrence of pain and instability Mean follow-up, 3.7 yr
Choi and Ogilvie-Harris	*Br J Sports Med* (2002)	Posterior-inferior capsular shift, with the infraspinatus divided and retracted	Achieved posterior stability in 11 of 16 athletic patients with multidirectional instability (69%)	12	1 patient experienced recurrent dislocation 75% of patients returned to sports Mean follow-up, 3.5 yr
Shin et al	*Bull Hosp Jt Dis* (2005)	Open posterior capsulorrhaphy with infraspinatus split	Of the 17 patients treated, results were excellent in 8, good in 5, fair in 2, and poor in 2	12	Patients rated the overall function of the treated shoulder as 81% that of the unaffected shoulder Mean follow-up, 3.9 yr
Wolf et al	*J Shoulder Elbow Surg* (2005)	Open posterior capsular shift	Significantly poorer satisfaction and outcome scores were seen in patients with chondral defect and age >37 yr at the time of surgery	19	44 shoulders in 41 patients Mean follow-up, 8 yr

while prepping the patient. However, the posterior approach and its dissection is made more difficult by the extravasation of even small amounts of fluid. Thus, the authors of this chapter prefer to assess the structures intra-articularly by using physical examination and a preoperative MRI.

Incision

- A longitudinal incision is made in the posterior axillary fold beginning at 0.2 cm medial to the posterolateral corner of the acromion and extending distally, following the course of the posterior axillary fold.
- The skin flaps are developed, exposing the underlying deltoid muscle.

- The deltoid muscle is split bluntly along the line of its fibers from the acromial spine distally, and a self-retaining retractor is placed. The surgeon must take care to avoid the axillary nerve, which lies inferior to the teres minor muscle.

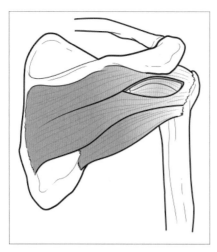

Figure 1 Illustration shows a posterior split of the bipennate infraspinatus, revealing the underlying posterior capsule.

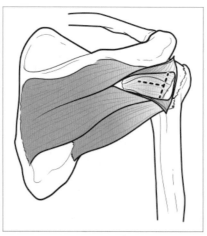

Figure 2 Illustration shows further exposure of the underlying posterior capsule during the infraspinatus split. The tendinous insertion is sharply undermined and elevated laterally, similar to flipping up the collar of a shirt, but some tendinous insertion is left intact. The dashed lines indicate the course of the capsulotomy along the margin of the articular surface.

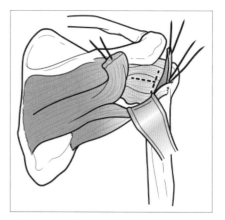

Figure 3 Illustration shows the surgical site after the deltoid muscle fibers have been split. A self-retaining retractor is placed for exposure. With traction sutures applied, the infraspinatus tendon is released vertically by making a vertical incision laterally, leaving enough of the infraspinatus tendon laterally to reattach during closure. The mobilized and released tendon is retracted medially. The dashed lines indicate the course of the capsulotomy along the margin of the articular surface.

Infraspinatus Split

- The underlying infraspinatus muscle, which has a bipennate structure, is visualized and either split or released. The least traumatic approach is to split the infraspinatus muscle horizontally in line with the raphe between the superior and inferior muscle bodies (**Figure 1**).
- Careful sharp, blunt dissection is performed to develop the plane deep to the infraspinatus and the underlying posterior capsule. If the infraspinatus split is used but further capsular exposure is required, then the lateral infraspinatus insertion can be partially released and its corners flipped up like a shirt collar (**Figure 2**).
- A small self-retaining retractor may be placed in this interval for exposure. Alternatively, a tenotomy can be performed 1 cm medial to the humeral insertion of the tendon.
- Traction sutures are applied, and gentle dissection is used to elevate the infraspinatus from the underlying posterior capsule in a fashion similar to the manner in which the subscapularis is evaluated in anterior approaches to the shoulder (**Figure 3**).

Posterior Capsulorrhaphy

- The decision to perform posterior capsulorrhaphy is based on patient laxity and tissue quality. If posterior capsulorrhaphy is to be performed, then the arm is held in neutral rotation, and a vertical capsulotomy is made 1 cm from its humeral insertion (**Figure 4**).
- The traction sutures are applied at the mid portion of the capsule.
- The horizontal limb of the capsulotomy is developed beginning laterally at the vertical limb and working medially to the glenoid labrum to create a T-shaped capsulotomy (**Figure 5**). The surgeon must take care to avoid injury to the axillary nerve, which lies at the inferior extent of the wound.
- The authors of this chapter prefer to use the humeral based, T-shaped capsulotomy because the capsular flaps can be easily tensioned and a larger volume of capsular redundancy can be addressed if desired.
- The posterior labrum is inspected

and any detachment repaired before completing the capsular shift procedure.
- The inferior flap of the posterior capsule is carefully mobilized inferiorly past the 6-o'clock position of the glenoid, extending along the inferior aspect of the humeral head. This step is critical to address posterior-inferior capsular redundancy.
- A high-speed burr is used to decorticate the nonarticular portion of the humeral metaphysis in preparation for repair of capsular mobilization (**Figure 6**).
- With the arm held in 45° of abduction and 20° of external rotation, the inferior flap is brought superiorly and laterally and then sutured to the humeral capsular remnant.
- In a similar fashion, the superior capsular flap is shifted inferiorly over the inferior flap and sutured (**Figure 7**).

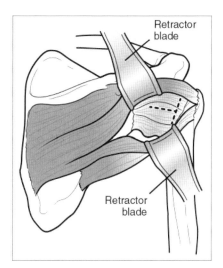

Figure 4 Illustration shows the underlying capsule exposed as a single layer. A vertical capsulotomy is performed first, starting on the humeral side. The dashed lines indicate the course of the initial capsulotomy along the margin of the articular surface.

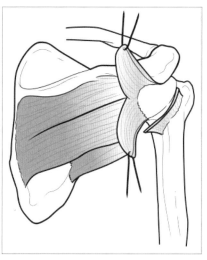

Figure 5 Illustration shows the placement of traction stitches after the capsule is released laterally on the humeral side. The superior and inferior leaflets are produced by dividing the posterior capsule medially toward the glenoid.

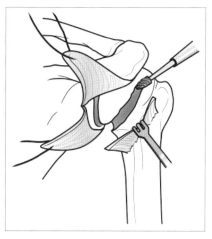

Figure 6 Illustration shows the capsular flaps fully elevated past the 6-o'clock position and exposure of the metaphyseal area just medial to the capsular insertion. The nonarticular portion of the humeral metaphysis is decorticated by using a high-speed burr to enhance healing.

Wound Closure

- The horizontal portion of the T-shaped capsulorrhaphy is closed with nonabsorbable sutures.
- The infraspinatus split is allowed to reapproximate, and its fascia is closed with similar suture. If the infraspinatus was tenotomized, then it is anatomically sutured back to the tendinous stump.
- Routine wound closure is performed, and the arm is placed in a postoperative orthosis that incorporates 20° of external rotation and 20° of abduction. Either a commercially available, prefabricated orthosis or a fiberglass shoulder spica cast may be used for immobilization.

Rehabilitation

The postoperative rehabilitation protocol is summarized in **Table 2**. The immediate postoperative management of the patient is extremely important. It is critical to protect the repair during the first month, especially if

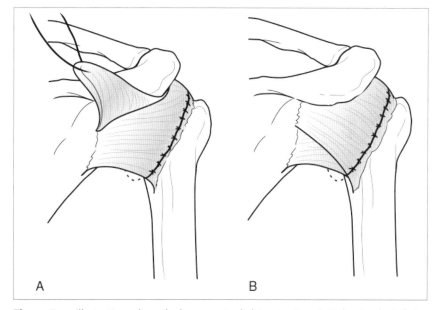

Figure 7 Illustrations show the humerus in slight extension. **A,** To begin, the inferior capsule is shifted superiorly with the arm positioned in 45° of abduction. **B,** In a similar fashion, the superior capsule is then subsequently shifted inferiorly, thus reducing capsular volume and inferior capsular redundancy.

the infraspinatus has been taken down from its tendinous insertion. Most patients are fitted with a commercially available abduction shoulder orthosis that incorporates 20° of abduction and 20° of external rotation. However, the patient who is unable or unwilling to comply with orthosis use can be placed

Table 2 Rehabilitation Protocol After the Open Approach for the Management of Posterior Shoulder Instability

Postoperative Week	Range of Motion	Strengthening	Return to Play
0-4	Gentle elbow and wrist motion Assisted external rotation to 45° to 50° FE in the scapular plane is added as tolerated by the patient	None	None
4-8	Active FE and ER are begun IR to the abdomen and extension of the arm to the trochanter also is slowly incorporated	Gentle periscapular resistive exercises are added	None
8-12	Continued stretching to achieve full FE and ER; if IR is limited, more aggressive stretching in this plane is allowed	Gentle, progressive resistance maneuvers in all planes of motion	None
≥12	Nearly full FE and ER should be achieved, with only mild limitation of IR Sport-specific motion exercises are begun	Sport-specific strengthening is begun	Timing is dependent on the patient and the specific sport, with the goal of returning to play by 6 mo postoperatively

ER = external rotation, FE = forward elevation, IR = internal rotation.

in a shoulder spica cast; this cast is removed 4 weeks postoperatively. Patients who are immobilized with an orthosis are allowed to remove the device twice daily to work on gentle elbow and wrist motion and assisted external rotation to 45° to 50°. Forward elevation in the scapular plane is added as tolerated by the patient. None of these maneuvers should put the repair at risk.

At 4 to 8 weeks postoperatively, a formal physical therapy program is instituted to foster restoration of motion. Forward elevation and external rotation often return quickly. However, internal rotation posterior to the coronal plane can be more troublesome and uncomfortable and is one of the last motions the patient will recover. Internal rotation posterior to the coronal plane must be gradually regained in a controlled, progressive fashion under the direction of a physical therapist. The goal of therapy is to achieve nearly full active forward elevation and external rotation by 6 to 8 weeks postoperatively and internal rotation to the lower lumbar spine by 2 months postoperatively. It is important that the patient understands that it

may take 3 to 4 months before ultimate internal rotation is achieved.

At 2 months postoperatively, strengthening exercises are instituted using gentle, progressive resistance maneuvers in all planes of motion. Strict attention is given to external rotation so as not to overstress the infraspinatus and the posterior capsulorrhaphy.

At 3 months postoperatively, the patient should achieve nearly full forward elevation and external rotation, with only mild limitations of internal rotation. At this time, sport-specific motion and strengthening exercises are added. Return to sport is somewhat dependent on the individual and his or her sport. Swimmers are allowed to return to the pool at 4 months postoperatively but are counseled to avoid wall contact. Football linemen are allowed to engage in full contact, including pass blocking, at 5 to 6 months postoperatively. Athletes who participate in racquet and overhead throwing sports are placed in a regressive exercise program at 3 months, with the goal of returning to competition by 6 months postoperatively.

 Avoiding Pitfalls

Diagnosis

The surgeon should be alert for the rare patient who pathologically and voluntarily dislocates his or her shoulder for secondary gain. Failure to identify such patients is usually accompanied by failure of the procedure. The patient who voluntarily dislocates his or her shoulder for secondary gain should not be confused with the patient who has learned the provocative position of his or her instability through arm position and voluntary muscle control. This patient often can reproduce the instability in the office but is not seeking secondary gain.

Excessive glenohumeral retroversion or glenoid rim deficiency is rarely encountered but should be ruled out before surgical intervention. In patients with either diagnosis, soft-tissue reconstruction alone is insufficient to correct the condition, and the surgeon must be prepared to address glenoid version and bone loss accordingly. Appropriate preoperative imaging, including three-dimensional CT and MRI, provides the data necessary to quantify the loss and plan corrective measures. A glenoid osteotomy or glenoid augmentation may be performed in combination with a posterior-inferior capsular procedure.

Patients who were previously treated with thermal capsulorrhaphy may have experienced failure of subsequent treatments because of the extensive scarring, loss of the posterior capsular restraints, and, in severe cases, total loss of the posterior capsule. The surgeon must carefully manage such patients; preoperative studies may be indicated to assess tissue deficiency.

Exposure

Exposure may be difficult in individuals who have a large body habitus, are well muscled, and have a considerable amount of posterior deltoid musculature. In these situations, the deltoid muscle cannot be split more distally without risking injury to the axillary nerve. Alternatively, the deltoid can be detached from the posterolateral corner of the acromion. The repair can be accomplished in one of two ways, by either leaving a small tendinous attachment for later repair or taking down the subperiosteal envelope of the deltoid off the acromial spine and placing small drill holes in the scapular spine for later repair (**Figure 8**).

After the deltoid muscle has been split and the self-retaining retractor placed, the infraspinatus is identified for capsular exposure. The infraspinatus is characterized by its bipennate structure with a small, central, fatty raphe

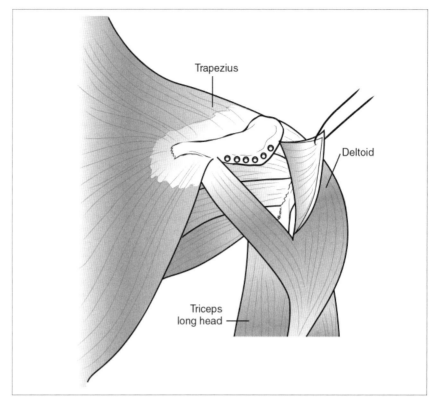

Figure 8   Illustration shows the posterior deltoid muscle fibers split bluntly. The exposure can be further expanded by detaching the lateral portion of the deltoid muscle toward the posterolateral aspect of the acromion, by either leaving a small tendinous stump or using drill holes through the posterior acromion in individuals who have a large deltoid muscle.

dividing its two heads. The ability to identify the appearance and the orientation of the infraspinatus muscle is critical to ensure that the appropriate interval is entered. The infraspinatus can be further characterized based on the direction of its muscle fibers. The muscle fiber of the teres minor, which is located inferior to the infraspinatus,

has a more oblique orientation than that of the infraspinatus. Dissection inferior to the teres minor muscle can jeopardize the axillary nerve before its arborization. In addition, large vessels of the posterior humeral circumflex artery and vein accompany the axillary nerve and are placed at risk with dissection and retraction in this area.

 ## Bibliography

Bell RH, Noble JS: An appreciation of posterior instability of the shoulder. *Clin Sports Med* 1991;10(4):887-899.

Bigliani LU, Pollock RG, McIlveen SJ, Endrizzi DP, Flatow EL: Shift of the posteroinferior aspect of the capsule for recurrent posterior glenohumeral instability. *J Bone Joint Surg Am* 1995;77(7):1011-1020.

Choi CH, Ogilvie-Harris DJ: Inferior capsular shift operation for multidirectional instability of the shoulder in players of contact sports. *Br J Sports Med* 2002;36(4):290-294.

Fronek J, Warren RF, Bowen M: Posterior subluxation of the glenohumeral joint. *J Bone Joint Surg Am* 1989;71(2):205-216.

Fuchs B, Jost B, Gerber C: Posterior-inferior capsular shift for the treatment of recurrent, voluntary posterior subluxation of the shoulder. *J Bone Joint Surg Am* 2000;82(1):16-25.

Hernandez A, Drez D: Operative treatment of posterior shoulder dislocations by posterior glenoidplasty, capsulorrhaphy, and infraspinatus advancement. *Am J Sports Med* 1986;14(3):187-191.

Misamore GW, Facibene WA: Posterior capsulorrhaphy for the treatment of traumatic recurrent posterior subluxations of the shoulder in athletes. *J Shoulder Elbow Surg* 2000;9(5):403-408.

Neer CS II, Foster CR: Inferior capsular shift for involuntary inferior and multidirectional instability of the shoulder: A preliminary report. *J Bone Joint Surg Am* 1980;62(6):897-908.

Pollock RG, Bigliani LU: Recurrent posterior shoulder instability: Diagnosis and treatment. *Clin Orthop Relat Res* 1993;291:85-96.

Shaffer BS, Conway J, Jobe FW, Kvitne RS, Tibone JE: Infraspinatus muscle-splitting incision in posterior shoulder surgery: An anatomic and electromyographic study. *Am J Sports Med* 1994;22(1):113-120.

Shin RD, Polatsch DB, Rokito AS, Zuckerman JD: Posterior capsulorrhaphy for treatment of recurrent posterior glenohumeral instability. *Bull Hosp Jt Dis* 2005;63(1-2):9-12.

Wirth MA, Butters KP, Rockwood CA Jr: The posterior deltoid-splitting approach to the shoulder. *Clin Orthop Relat Res* 1993;(296):92-98.

Wolf BR, Strickland S, Williams RJ, Allen AA, Altchek DW, Warren RF: Open posterior stabilization for recurrent posterior glenohumeral instability. *J Shoulder Elbow Surg* 2005;14(2):157-164.

 Video Reference

Hawkins RJ: Video. *Infraspinatus - Capsular Reconstruction for Posterior Instability.* Copyright Richard J. Hawkins, MD, Greenville, SC, 2015.

Chapter 5

The Anterosuperior Approach to the Shoulder: Indications, Advantages, and Pitfalls

Grant E. Garrigues, MD

Luke S. Austin, MD

Gerald R. Williams, Jr, MD

 ## Introduction

The anterosuperior approaches to the shoulder involve splitting of the deltoid. The main advantages of these approaches are direct access to the posterosuperior rotator cuff and greater tuberosities for management of fractures and rotator cuff pathology. When these approaches are used in reverse total shoulder arthroplasty (RTSA), the procedure is performed through the preexisting rotator cuff defect without disrupting the subscapularis. In addition, an anterosuperior approach gives an excellent view of the glenoid face.

For management of rotator cuff tears, a deltoid-splitting approach with rotation of the humerus can provide exposure of the rotator cuff. Splitting the deltoid muscle without detaching the deltoid from the acromion is referred to as the mini-open rotator cuff approach. The split can be extended over the acromion

with subperiosteal dissection of the anterior deltoid off the acromion. The approach that involves detaching a portion of the deltoid from the acromion is known as the open rotator cuff exposure. The dissection can be carried through the acromioclavicular (AC) joint capsule and the AC joint resected to improve access for larger tears. Although humeral rotation allows access to a substantial amount of the rotator cuff with these approaches, variations may be used for the management of specific tears. For retracted posterior tears, some authors have advocated shifting the deltoid split posteriorly. Massive anteroposterior tears can be managed with two incisions: a deltoid-splitting approach for the posterosuperior tear and a deltopectoral approach for the subscapularis.

For shoulder arthroplasty, the anterosuperior approach that first gained popularity involved subperiosteal release of the anterior head of the deltoid from the

acromion, and the RTSA technique presented in this chapter is based on that method. Although some authors have performed anatomic total shoulder arthroplasty (TSA) through a deltoid split using the rotator interval for glenoid access, most anatomic TSA procedures are performed through a deltopectoral approach with a variety of methods used for division and repair of the subscapularis. However, in patients with a massive rotator cuff tear or cuff tear arthropathy without arthritis, the RTSA prosthesis can be implanted through the rotator cuff defect without disrupting the remaining, intact portions of the rotator cuff. A transacromial approach for RTSA has been described but is no longer widely used.

Anterosuperior approaches can be used for the management of fractures. Humeral intramedullary nails can be inserted through a deltoid split or through a deltoid split extended to detach some of the anterior deltoid. However, newer small-diameter, straight nails are designed to be inserted more medially through the rotator cuff and the articular surface. This smaller, more medial trajectory has allowed insertion through the AC joint and through the Neviaser portal medial to the acromion. The axillary nerve was previously considered the limit of the deltoid split, limiting the

Dr. Garrigues or an immediate family member is a member of a speakers' bureau or has made paid presentations on behalf of and serves as a paid consultant to DePuy Synthes and Tornier; has received research or institutional support from Arthrex, Tornier, and Zimmer; and has received nonincome support (such as equipment or services), commercially derived honoraria, or other non–research-related funding (such as paid travel) from DJO and Zimmer. Dr. Austin or an immediate family member serves as a paid consultant to Tornier and has received research or institutional support from Zimmer. Dr. Williams or an immediate family member has received royalties from CoorsTek Medical and DePuy Synthes; serves as a paid consultant to DePuy Synthes; has stock or stock options held in Cross Current Corporation, FORCE Therapeutics, for[MD], InVivo Therapeutics, and Oberd; and has received research or institutional support from DePuy Synthes, Synthasome, and Tornier.

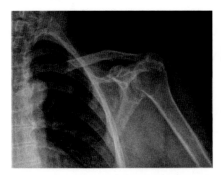

Figure 1 AP radiograph of a left shoulder demonstrates a decreased acromiohumeral interval and humeral head osteophytes consistent with rotator cuff tear arthropathy.

surgeon's ability to achieve safe fixation of locking plates in the humeral shaft. Within the past decade, investigations into the anterolateral approach have shown that splitting the deltoid distal to the axillary nerve can be done safely because only one nerve branch crosses from the middle head to the anterior head across the anterior raphe. This approach provides access to posterior fracture fragments and direct visualization of the lateral cortex for plate application, and cadaver studies have shown minimal disruption of the blood supply to the articular surface. The anterolateral approach continues to be studied to determine whether it offers improved functional results and whether rates of osteonecrosis are better than those of the deltopectoral approach.

Case Presentation

A 75-year-old, right-hand–dominant woman reports pain and difficulty raising her left arm. She reports no prior fracture, dislocation, or surgical treatment involving her shoulders. Initial treatment consists of a course of NSAIDs, acetaminophen, and a corticosteroid injection, none of which yields lasting alleviation of pain or improved strength. The patient is referred to a shoulder specialist for further evaluation.

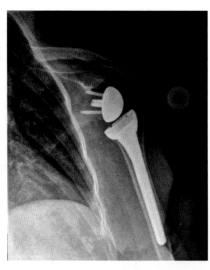

Figure 2 Postoperative AP radiograph demonstrates reverse shoulder arthroplasty. Note the low position of the baseplate on the glenoid and the absence of superior tilt.

Physical examination reveals signs of a massive rotator cuff tear, including reduced active forward elevation of 80° (passive, 150°) and a 5° lag with resisted external rotation with the arm at the side (active, 40°; passive, 45°). The patient is able to actively externally rotate her shoulder at 90° of abduction (negative hornblower sign). The examination is also notable for a Popeye sign; a normal cervical spine; and normal neurologic findings, including intact deltoid function.

A decreased acromiohumeral interval and moderate glenohumeral osteoarthritis consistent with rotator cuff tear arthropathy are noted on radiographs (**Figure 1**). MRI findings are consistent with the physical examination and radiographs, demonstrating a massive, retracted rotator cuff tear with fatty atrophy of the supraspinatus and infraspinatus muscles.

After a thorough discussion of the risks and benefits of surgical treatment, the patient elects to undergo RTSA. The anterosuperior approach described in this chapter is used, allowing the surgeon to implant the RTSA prosthesis

through a deltoid split and through the preexisting rotator cuff defect without division of any remaining intact cuff (**Figure 2**).

The patient starts active, overhead activities at 6 weeks. By 3 months postoperatively, she exhibits 155° of pain-free active forward elevation.

Indications

Anterosuperior approaches have been used in the management of a variety of shoulder pathologies, including rotator cuff tears, pathology of the long head of the biceps tendon, and conditions requiring acromioplasty or AC joint resection. These approaches have been used for fracture fixation with intramedullary nailing or, when the approach is extended past the axillary nerve in a deltoid-splitting anterolateral approach, with proximal humerus locking plates. Anterosuperior approaches have also been used in arthroplasty, hemiarthroplasty, and total RTSA for fracture management. The anterosuperior approach is particularly straightforward in RTSA for fracture management because fragmentation of the proximal humerus facilitates glenoid exposure, and the deltoid split facilitates manipulation of the posterior greater tuberosity fragment. Anterosuperior approaches, including a specialized approach for anatomic arthroplasty through the rotator interval, can be used in arthroplasty for the management of arthritis and, most commonly, in RTSA for the management of rotator cuff tear arthropathy. An anterosuperior approach has even been described for revision shoulder arthroplasty; however, a second incision for access to the humeral shaft may be required.

The authors of this chapter use arthroscopic techniques or the deltopectoral approach for most of their shoulder procedures. However, the anterosuperior approach has been helpful in the management of proximal humerus fractures with intramedullary nailing because a deltoid-splitting approach facilitates access to the entry point on the humeral head and preserves the vascularity of the fracture site. The anterosuperior approach has also been helpful in RTSA for the management of rotator cuff tear arthropathy or massive rotator cuff tear without arthritis, as long as the patient has none of the contraindications noted in the following section.

 ## Contraindications

When exposure of the proximal medial humerus or the humeral shaft is required, the authors of this chapter prefer the deltopectoral approach, which is an extensile exposure within internervous planes. Specific contraindications to the anterosuperior approach include the presence of a substantial medial humeral osteophyte (minimal osteophytes are acceptable), passive external rotation less than 30°, and fixed proximal humeral migration that cannot be reduced under anesthesia (sulcus sign maneuver under anesthesia). Prior open surgical treatment may also be a contraindication. These criteria include most revision cases. In the practice of the senior author (G.R.W.), approximately 10% of patients treated with RTSA satisfy these criteria and undergo the procedure through this approach. The authors of this chapter recommend avoiding the anterosuperior approach when performing RTSA in patients with morbid obesity because that condition may limit the amount of adduction required for placement of the humeral stem.

 ## Controversies and Results

The optimal approach for RTSA is the subject of debate. The most commonly used surgical approaches for RTSA are the anterosuperior and deltopectoral exposures. Although each has its advantages and disadvantages, surgeon training and comfort with the particular approach, a factor likely underestimated in the available nonrandomized studies comparing these techniques, may be the most important variable. The available studies are summarized in **Table 1**.

The deltopectoral approach has several advantages relevant to RTSA, including dissection through the superficial shoulder-girdle musculature through an extensile, atraumatic, internervous, and intermuscular plane between the deltoid and pectoralis major muscles. In addition, the ability to access the medial portion of the humeral head and the medial humeral metaphysis can be helpful for removal of medial osteophytes and release of the humeral insertion of the glenohumeral capsule. The extensile nature of the exposure facilitates revision surgery by eliminating the need for a second incision to access the humeral shaft. Perhaps most importantly, the RTSA prosthesis is primarily powered by the deltoid, and a deltopectoral approach preserves the deltoid origin and muscle belly. Although the deltopectoral approach is internervous, axillary nerve injury during anatomic arthroplasty has been reported to be more common with the deltopectoral approach than with an anterosuperior approach.

Proponents of the anterosuperior approach for RTSA, however, note that the rate of deltoid dehiscence with the anterosuperior approach is extremely low (occurring in 2 of 1,099 patients in one review). In addition, deltoid dehiscence has been reported after the use of the deltopectoral approach for RTSA in patients who have previously undergone open rotator cuff repair. The authors of that study posited that the use of an anterosuperior approach for RTSA allows assessment and possible repair or reinforcement of any prior deltoid division. Surprisingly, neurapraxia of the axillary nerve to the anterior deltoid is infrequent with the anterosuperior approach. In fact, a higher incidence of nerve injury has been reported with the deltopectoral approach than with the anterosuperior approach for anatomic arthroplasty. Evaluation of this complication in patients undergoing RTSA has shown a statistically equivalent rate of axillary nerve palsy between the two approaches.

The advantages of the anterosuperior approach for RTSA are the ability to work through the massive rotator cuff defect and the quality of the en face glenoid exposure. Although the superficial shoulder muscular envelope is divided, the deep layer, consisting of the remaining rotator cuff and the subscapularis, is left undisturbed. The role of the subscapularis muscle in providing stability and function after RTSA is debated even in studies of the deltopectoral approach; however, in several studies subscapularis dysfunction has been found to be associated with a greater risk of instability. Although not all variations of the anterosuperior approach preserve the subscapularis muscle, an anterosuperior approach that preserves the subscapularis theoretically would preserve the compressive, stabilizing effect of the anterior force couple. This factor may explain why the anterosuperior approach has a reported lower rate of dislocation than the deltopectoral approach in both primary RTSA (zero to 1% and 2% to 9%, respectively) and revision RTSA (zero and 6% to 14%, respectively).

The potential stability imparted by the anterior soft tissues in a subscapularis-sparing anterosuperior approach may reduce the need to lengthen the arm to achieve a stable articulation, thereby potentially reducing the incidence of plexopathy and acromial stress fractures from overlengthening. This scenario may explain the lower incidence of acromial stress fractures with the anterosuperior approach than with the deltopectoral approach in one multicenter study (2.2%

Table 1 Results of Reverse Shoulder Arthroplasty

Author(s)	Source (Year)	Technique (No. of Shoulders)	Outcomes[a]	Failure Rate (%)	Comments
Delloye et al	*Rev Chir Orthop Reparatrice Appar Mot* (2002)	Revision RTSA: AS (4)	No instability Complications: glenosphere unscrewing in 1 shoulder and baseplate loosening with notching in 2 shoulders Improvement was noted in Constant-Murley score, pain, and ROM	75	Mean patient age, 73 yr Mean follow-up, 81 mo
Frankle et al	*J Bone Joint Surg Am* (2005)	Primary RTSA: DP (60)	Significant improvement noted for all measures ($P < 0.0001$): ASES score, VAS pain and function, FF, and abduction 5 patients with baseplate failure were revised to RTSA and 2 with deep infection were revised to hemiarthroplasty No scapular notching	13.3	Mean patient age, 71 yr Mean follow-up, 33 mo
Werner et al	*J Bone Joint Surg Am* (2005)	Primary RTSA: DP (17); revision RTSA: DP (41)	Instability in 5.4% of primary RTSA patients and 14.3% of revision RTSA patients Complications: 2 deep infections, 4 baseplate loosenings, 1 repeated instability, 4 acromial stress fractures, 12 hematomas Improvement was noted in Constant-Murley score, subjective shoulder evaluation, pain, and ROM	Primary RTSA: 0 Revision RTSA: 14.6	Mean patient age, 68 yr Mean follow-up, 38 mo
Boileau et al	*J Shoulder Elbow Surg* (2006)	Primary RTSA: DP (21); revision RTSA: DP (19)	Instability in 4.8% of primary RTSA patients and 10.5% of revision RTSA patients Complications: 1 glenoid fracture, 2 periprosthetic humerus fractures, 2 acromial stress fractures, 1 axillary nerve palsy, and 3 dislocations Scapular notching occurred in 68% 78% of patients were satisfied or very satisfied Rate of no or slight pain in 67% Improvement was noted in Constant-Murley score, ASES, pain, and ROM	22.2	Mean patient age, 72 yr Mean follow-up, 40 mo
Nové-Josserand	*Reverse Shoulder Arthroplasty: Nice Shoulder Course* (2006)	Primary RTSA: DP (92) and AS (37); revision RTSA: DP (84) and AS (5)	Primary RTSA: instability in 9.0% of DP group, none in AS group Revision RTSA: instability in 10.7% of DP group, none in AS group Improvement was noted in Constant-Murley score and pain	NR	Mean follow-up after primary RTSA, 49 mo Mean follow-up after revision RTSA, 44 mo
Simovitch et al	*J Bone Joint Surg Am* (2007)	Primary RTSA: DP (77)	Scapular notching in 44% Study evaluated Constant-Murley score, subjective shoulder value, pain, active flexion/abduction/internal/external rotation, strength, and radiographic findings Placement of the glenosphere low on the glenoid was associated with decreased rates of notching Notching was associated with lower Constant-Murley scores, lower subjective shoulder value, decreased active flexion, and decreased active abduction	NR	Mean age, 71 yr Mean follow-up, 44 mo

AS = anterosuperior approach, ASES = American Shoulder and Elbow Surgeons shoulder outcome, DP = deltopectoral approach, ER = external rotation, FF = forward flexion, NR = not reported, ROM = range of motion, RTSA = reverse total shoulder arthroplasty, SST = Simple Shoulder Test, VAS = visual analog scale.

[a] All data are mean values unless otherwise noted.

Table 1 Results of Reverse Shoulder Arthroplasty *(continued)*

Author(s)	Source (Year)	Technique (No. of Shoulders)	Outcomes[a]	Failure Rate (%)	Comments
Cuff et al	*J Bone Joint Surg Br* (2008)	Revision RTSA: DP (22)	Instability in 5.9% All infections cleared with one- or two-stage conversion to RTSA Complications: 1 baseplate loosening, 2 polyethylene dissociations, 1 periprosthetic fracture, 1 humeral loosening, 2 heterotopic ossifications, 1 radial nerve palsy, 3 hematomas Improvement was noted on ASES score, VAS pain score, and ROM	NR	Mean patient age, 67 yr Mean follow-up, 43 mo
Chacon et al	*J Bone Joint Surg Am* (2009)	Revision RTSA: DP (25)	Instability in 8.0% Complications: 1 periprosthetic fracture, 1 dislocation, 1 recurrent instability, and 1 acromial stress fracture Improvement was noted in ASES score, SST, pain, FF, abduction, and internal rotation	4	Mean patient age NR Mean follow-up, 30 mo
Holcomb et al	*J Shoulder Elbow Surg* (2009)	Revision RTSA: DP (14)	Instability in 7.1% Complications: 1 hematoma, 2 recurrent baseplate failures, 1 dislocation Improvement was noted in ASES score, pain, FF, and abduction	14 (2 patients)	Mean patient age, 70.6 yr Mean follow-up, 33 mo
Lévigne et al	*Clin Orthop Relat Res* (2011)	Primary RTSA: DP (254) and AS (207)	Scapular notching in 56% of DP group and 86% of AS group Notching increased in incidence and severity over time. Notching was associated with decreased strength and anterior elevation but was not associated with a change in Constant-Murley score or pain.	NR	Mean follow-up, 51 mo
Molé et al	*Clin Orthop Relat Res* (2011)	Primary RTSA: AS (227) and DP (300)	Instability in 5.1% of DP group and 0.8% of AS group Scapular notching in 63% of DP group and 74% of AS group Glenoid loosening in 2.3% of DP group and 6.6% of AS group Acromial stress fracture in 5.6% of DP group and 2.2% of AS group Final Constant-Murley scores: 62.5 (DP), 62.2 (AS) Final pain scores: 12.5 (DP), 12.7 (AS) Final anterior active elevation: 127° (DP), 132° (AS)	NR	Large, multicenter study Mean patient age NR Mean follow-up after DP, 43 mo Mean follow-up after AS, 59 mo
Gillespie et al	*Orthop Clin North Am* (2015)	Primary RTSA: DP (31) and AS (62)	Instability in 3.0% of DP group, none in AS group Scapular notching in 100% of DP group and 88% of AS group	NR	Mean follow-up, 37 mo Study compared radiographic parameters

AS = anterosuperior approach, ASES = American Shoulder and Elbow Surgeons shoulder outcome, DP = deltopectoral approach, ER = external rotation, FF = forward flexion, NR = not reported, ROM = range of motion, RTSA = reverse total shoulder arthroplasty, SST = Simple Shoulder Test, VAS = visual analog scale.
[a] All data are mean values unless otherwise noted.

and 5.6%, respectively). It is unclear whether the deltoid tension is truly less with an anterosuperior approach than with a deltopectoral approach for RTSA, but a different multicenter study comparing the two approaches showed that patients who underwent RTSA through an anterosuperior approach had a more generous humeral cut (presumably to facilitate glenoid access) that was only partially corrected with thicker polyethylene inserts, resulting in slightly decreased lengthening, on average, in the patients treated with the anterosuperior approach.

The largest study comparing the results of anterosuperior and deltopectoral approaches is a multicenter French study of 527 patients undergoing primary RTSA for massive rotator cuff tears or rotator cuff tear arthropathy. In this large series, the anterosuperior approach resulted in a lower rate of instability (0.8%, compared with 5.1% with the deltopectoral approach), which is consistent with the published results of noncomparative studies. In addition, the rate of acromial stress fracture was also lower (2.2% with anterosuperior approach and 5.6% with the deltopectoral approach), as discussed previously. However, scapular notching and glenoid baseplate loosening occurred more frequently with the anterosuperior approach than with the deltopectoral approach (74% and 63%, respectively, for scapular notching; 6.6% and 2.3%, respectively, for glenoid baseplate loosening). These complications may be attributable to the longer average follow-up in patients treated with the anterosuperior approach but also could be the result of an association between baseplate tilt and the anterosuperior approach. Similarly, in a large cohort of patients undergoing RTSA (461 shoulders) that included both anterosuperior and deltopectoral approaches, notching was more common in patients who underwent RTSA via an anterosuperior approach (86% and 56%, respectively). The authors of the study concluded that the anterosuperior approach tended to make it more difficult to avoid high positioning of the glenoid baseplate and superior tilt and that implant malposition led to scapular notching and glenoid baseplate loosening. The need to retract the proximal humerus inferiorly instead of posteriorly to access the glenoid for preparation and component implantation may explain why the anterosuperior approach is more prone to implantation of the glenoid component in superior tilt.

A recent review of deltopectoral and subscapularis-sparing anterosuperior approaches included 93 patients with average 22-month follow-up. The deltopectoral approach was used in 31 patients and the anterosuperior approach

in 62. In contrast to previous studies, that review demonstrated the baseplate position low on the glenoid and an equivalent incidence of notching. As in previous studies, the authors of that review found a slight tendency toward superior baseplate tilt with the anterosuperior approach (6°, with a range of 10° inferior to 23° superior; and 1° inferior, with a range of 20° inferior to 24° superior, respectively [*P* < 0.005]). The relative contraindications listed previously were used to ensure that the patients were selected appropriately for an anterosuperior approach. Interestingly, the authors of that review found slight valgus position of the humeral stem of 2° in patients treated with the anterosuperior approach and posited that this result may be attributable to the hindrances of this exposure. Because the humeral socket-shaft angle has been shown to correlate with notching, slight approach-specific variation on the humeral implant side may affect notching and glenosphere loosening as much as positioning of the glenosphere does.

Choosing the proper procedure for the indication may be an important factor in achieving acceptable outcomes. In a recent systematic review, successful results were demonstrated with the anterosuperior approach for RTSA in the management of acute proximal humerus fractures, although no specific approach was found to be superior for this indication. In patients with proximal humerus fracture, the surgeon's ability to attain proper baseplate tilt is aided by the lack of intact proximal humeral bone that, if present, could hinder correct positioning of the implant. Superior tilt of the baseplate is likely to occur with the anterosuperior approach because the soft-tissue and bony anatomy make positioning the baseplate low and without superior tilt a challenge. The authors of this chapter recommend using the patient selection algorithm discussed previously to determine the suitability of this approach for patients

with rotator cuff tear arthropathy or massive rotator cuff tears. In addition, patients with proximal humerus fractures may be treated successfully with the anterosuperior approach because the fragmented proximal humerus facilitates glenoid exposure. However, the surgeon's experience with the particular approach may be the most critical factor, regardless of the approach chosen.

Technical Keys to Success

The anterosuperior approach for total RTSA is described below.

Video 5.1 Reverse Shoulder Arthroplasty Through the Anterosuperior Approach. Luke S. Austin, MD; Grant E. Garrigues, MD; Gerald R. Williams, Jr, MD (8 min)

Setup

- The patient is examined under anesthesia before draping to confirm that none of the previously described contraindications is present. In particular, the surgeon must confirm that external rotation is greater than 30° and superior subluxation is reducible with the sulcus maneuver. These criteria confirm that the humerus can be retracted sufficiently. If mobility is insufficient on this preoperative examination under anesthesia, a standard deltopectoral approach is used.
- The patient is placed in the Fowler or modified beach-chair position with the head of the bed elevated 60° and the patient's head tilted slightly away (**Figure 3**).

Instruments/Equipment/ Implants Required

- No specific shoulder instruments are required for the anterosuperior

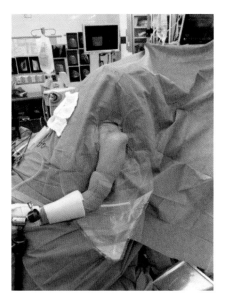

Figure 3 Photograph shows patient positioning for reverse total shoulder arthroplasty through an anterosuperior approach. The patient is in the Fowler or modified beach-chair position with the head of the bed elevated 60°, the head tilted slightly away, and the arm draped free in an arm holder.

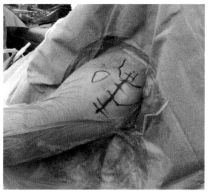

Figure 4 Intraoperative photograph demonstrates the superficial anatomy and planned surgical excision to the anterosuperior approach to reverse total shoulder arthroplasty.

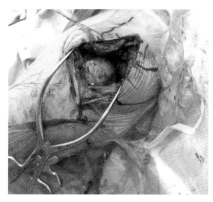

Figure 5 Intraoperative photograph demonstrates release of the anterior deltoid, the coracoacromial ligament, and the anterior portion of the acromioclavicular joint capsule with subperiosteal dissection.

approach. The authors of this chapter use the same shoulder instrument tray that is used for open shoulder procedures performed through the deltopectoral approach.

- The glenoid drill guides, drills, reamers, trial implants and liners, and final implants are the same as those used in the deltopectoral approach. A reversed, double-pronged retractor is often useful because it can be placed directly inferiorly on the glenoid to accomplish inferior humeral retraction.
- Most implant systems do not have specific humeral cutting guides for an anterosuperior approach. Although guides may be used, a freehand cut, perhaps using a humeral trial implant as a guide, may be more practical in the anterosuperior approach.

Procedure

- A 7-cm incision is made at the junction of the anterior and middle thirds of the clavicle (in the anteroposterior dimension) beginning 1 cm medial to the AC joint and extending along the anterior acromion and toward the deltoid insertion.
- Some surgeons favor an incision in the Langer lines for better cosmesis. However, the authors of this chapter have found that an incision in the long axis of the clavicle allows better access to both the AC joint and the glenoid. An incision in the Langer lines that is medial enough to allow exposure of the distal clavicle will often make glenoid access challenging (**Figure 4**).
- Wide, full-thickness subcutaneous flaps are developed at the level of the deltotrapezial fascia.
- Starting 1 cm medial to the AC joint, the anterior third of the AC joint capsule, the anterior deltoid origin, the roof of the subacromial bursa, and the coracoacromial ligament are released in a single layer using electrocautery for subperiosteal dissection (**Figure 5**).
- The subperiosteal dissection is continued laterally over the superior surface of the acromion to the point where the anterior raphe meets the anterolateral corner of the acromion.
- Patients with rotator cuff tear arthropathy will typically have an anterior acromial spur that projects anterior to the clavicle. If this spur is present, approximately 1 cm of the deltotrapezial fascia as well as the coracoacromial ligament should be released in continuity with the anterior head of the deltoid. Maintaining a good periosteal/fascial sleeve for deltoid repair is critical.
- The release of the anterior head is continued down the anterior raphe for 4 cm.
- The axillary nerve can be palpated immediately distal to the inferior reflection of the subdeltoid bursa, approximately 5 to 6 cm distal to the acromion. A stay suture may be placed at the inferior margin of the deltoid split to guard against inadvertent extension of the split and potential axillary neurapraxia.
- Acromioplasty is performed with the use of an oscillating saw or a medium-sized rongeur. The acromion should not be shortened beyond the anterior margin of the clavicle because excessive

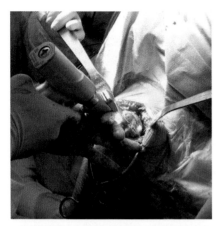

Figure 6 Intraoperative photograph demonstrates the humeral head osteotomy, which facilitates glenoid exposure.

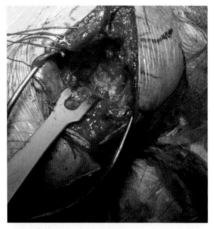

Figure 7 Intraoperative photograph demonstrates excellent glenoid exposure after release of the glenoid capsule. A double-pronged retractor straddles the lateral scapular pillar.

shortening may interfere with secure repair of the deltoid.

- The superior, rolled border of the subscapularis is identified, and any remaining cuff or bursal tissue between this insertion and the infraspinatus muscle are removed. The subscapularis muscle is not released or divided.
- A blunt Hohmann retractor is placed inside the joint at the anterior articular margin to protect the subscapularis muscle.
- If the long head of the biceps tendon is present, tenotomy may be performed, or the tendon may be sewn to the upper border of the pectoralis major tendon. The intra-articular portion of the tendon is excised.
- The sulcus where the medial edge of the supraspinatus footprint meets the articular margin is often effaced by lateral osteophytes. However, that location defines the starting point for the humeral head osteotomy. Guides may be used, or a freehand cut can be made by visualizing 135° (that is, halfway between a horizontal and a vertical cut) and then cutting at 20° shallower for a 155° cut if a Grammont-type prosthesis is used

(**Figure 6**). Alternatively, a trial implant or a broach may be used as a template. Retroversion should be 0° to 20°, depending on the surgeon's preference.

- The humeral bone is cut to the edge of the remaining, intact rotator cuff to preserve any stabilizing effect of the intact rotator cuff and facilitate glenoid exposure.
- The authors of this chapter prefer to start with preparation of the glenoid to better preserve the integrity of the proximal humeral bone.
- To begin the glenoid exposure, inferior traction is placed on the arm, and the inferior capsule is released from the labrum.
- A double-pronged retractor is inserted with the tines of the retractor on either side of the lateral scapular pillar to retract the humerus inferiorly (**Figure 7**).
- A blunt, self-retaining double-pronged Gelpi retractor may be placed within the joint to provide anterior and posterior retraction of the capsule, deltoid, and remaining rotator cuff muscles.
- The capsule is released from the labrum circumferentially, and the labrum is excised.

- Instead of using the double-pronged Gelpi retractor, blunt Hohmann retractors may be placed through the capsulotomy on the anterior and posterior margins of the glenoid. However, the presence of anterior and posterior retractors may tighten the soft-tissue envelope and interfere with the ability of the surgeon to displace the humerus inferiorly. Therefore, the double-pronged Gelpi retractor may be a better choice.
- The glenoid pin guide is used to ensure inferior placement of the glenosphere, and the guide pin is inserted. Care must be taken to prepare for positioning of the baseplate without superior tilt.
- Central reaming is done to prepare for the baseplate, and then a peripheral reamer is used superiorly to ensure that the glenosphere will seat fully. Care must be taken not to overream, especially in patients with poor bone quality. Hand reaming is also acceptable.
- The baseplate is inserted, screw holes are drilled, and screws are inserted.
- The glenosphere is inserted and affixed. In most patients, the glenosphere is preselected on the basis of patient size. However, all systems have trial implants available for use in case of uncertainty.
- To prepare the humerus for the humeral implant, the double-pronged Gelpi retractor is used to retract the deltoid. The humerus is delivered into the wound by adducting, externally rotating, and extending the patient's arm and applying an upward force on the elbow (**Figure 8**). This maneuver places the humeral epiphysis anterior to the acromion.
- A plastic Darrach retractor is placed medial to the humerus to protect the glenosphere. Blunt Hohmann retractors are placed anteromedially and posterolaterally.

- The humeral shaft is reamed distally. Some implant systems include an epiphyseal reaming guide with accompanying reamers; the use of these reamers is particularly important if noncemented fixation is planned.
- The trial humeral implant and trial liners are inserted to ensure appropriate tension and stability.
- If cemented fixation is planned, a cement restrictor is placed and the humeral canal is filled with cement.
- The implant and the appropriate polyethylene spacer are inserted, and the joint is reduced (**Figure 2**).

Wound Closure

- A suction drain is placed, exiting the joint posteriorly at the approximate location of a standard arthroscopic posterior portal. Typically, the drain is removed on postoperative day 2.
- The deltoid is closed with heavy, No. 2 nonabsorbable braided suture.
- A figure-of-8 suture is placed through the AC joint capsule.
- Two more sutures are placed in a pants-over-vest fashion down through the anterior deltoid, up through the bone of the anterior acromion, and back up through the anterior deltoid.
- A final suture is placed in figure-of-8 fashion at the anterolateral corner of the acromion through the short, tendinous portion of the deltoid origin.
- The entire deltoid split is oversewn with a running No. 0 absorbable braided suture from medial to the AC joint to the distal part of the split for a watertight seal.

Rehabilitation

The rehabilitation protocol is summarized in **Table 2**. The patient is placed in a sling postoperatively. At 2 weeks, the patient may remove the sling and start light activities of daily living with his or her elbow near the side. The patient should not lift more than 2 lb with the operated arm. At 6 weeks, active overhead reaching, lifting, and pulling is encouraged. The patient is taught so-called wall-walking exercises. Driving is permitted when the patient can safely control the car with both hands. Structured physical therapy is not generally used unless the patient exhibits undue stiffness 6 weeks postoperatively. If stiffness is observed, physical therapy or home use of an overhead pulley is recommended.

Avoiding Pitfalls

The axillary nerve is at risk during surgical procedures because it runs inferior to the glenoid and the anterior circumflex branch travels along the deep side of the deltoid. The anterior circumflex branch is specifically of concern in deltoid-splitting exposures. Nerve injury can be avoided by avoiding extension of the deltoid split across this branch. Excessive traction of this branch should also be avoided. A stay suture can be helpful to avoid inadvertent extension of the deltoid split.

The safe distance to which the deltoid can be split distally from the acromion before the axillary nerve is encountered has been identified as 3.8 cm and frequently is identified as 4 to 5 cm. A ratio of one fifth of the patient's arm length has been shown to predict the position anteriorly, and the authors of one study found the axillary nerve to be 1 cm closer to the acromion in women than in men. More recently, the distance has been shown to be 6.7 cm, with humeral rotation or forward flexion having no substantial effect on the distance, and abduction beyond 60° resulting in a slight decrease in the distance. If the dissection must be carried distally, such as to allow placement of a proximal

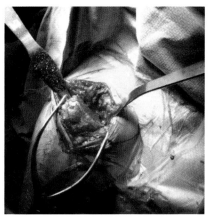

Figure 8 Intraoperative photograph demonstrates preparation for the humeral implant. The exposure of the humerus is aided by adduction, external rotation, and extension of the patient's arm, in combination with an upward force on the humerus applied through the elbow.

humerus locking plate through an anterolateral approach, the axillary nerve can be isolated and protected because only the main motor trunk crosses the anterior deltoid raphe. The axillary nerve runs immediately distal to the inferior reflection of the subdeltoid bursa. After splitting the deltoid proximally, the surgeon can place a finger inside the deltoid split and palpate the inferior reflection of the bursa as a readily identifiable landmark.

Given the importance of the deltoid muscle in shoulder function, secure healing of the deltoid is imperative after any anterosuperior approach. The anterior head of the deltoid originates on the lateral clavicle, with fibers running essentially parallel to the anterior acromion to their insertion on the lateral humerus. For this reason, many authors recommend splitting the deltoid along the anterior raphe to the anterolateral corner of the acromion. This method allows minimal disruption of muscle fibers, and the split can be easily extended onto the acromion to convert a mini-open approach to an open approach by releasing the anterior deltoid. To avoid deltoid rupture, it is critically

Table 2 Rehabilitation Protocol After Reverse Total Shoulder Arthroplasty Through an Anterosuperior Approach

Postoperative Week	Range of Motion	Strengthening	Return to Play	Comments/Emphasis
0-2	—	—	—	Sling immobilization
2-6	Light ADLs begun with the elbow near the side	—	—	Remove sling at 2 wk Avoid lifting >2 lb
6-12	Wall-walking exercises and active overhead reaching, lifting, and pulling are begun at 6 wk	Anti-gravity motion and light resistance bands	Driving permitted when the patient is able to control the car with both hands	Structured physical therapy at the discretion of the treating surgeon. It may not be required if patient exhibits stiffness at 6-wk follow-up and can do a simple home exercise program.
12-24	Daily stretching is recommended	ADLs	Reverse total shoulder arthroplasty is not designed for athletes. However, golf, tennis, and select other low-impact sports may be permitted at the discretion of the surgeon beginning between 3 and 6 mo postoperatively.	Daily stretching is recommended to maintain range of motion

ADLs = activities of daily living.

important to perform meticulous pants-over-vest closure of the anterior deltoid through bone tunnels and to avoid overtensioning.

Finally, to avoid glenoid baseplate malposition, proper patient selection and surgeon comfort with the approach are important. The surgeon should study the relevant anatomy and perform cadaver dissections and open rotator cuff repairs before attempting RTSA via an anterosuperior approach.

Bibliography

Boileau P, Watkinson D, Hatzidakis AM, Hovorka I: The Grammont reverse shoulder prosthesis: Results in cuff tear arthritis, fracture sequelae, and revision arthroplasty. *J Shoulder Elbow Surg* 2006;15(5):527-540.

Brorson S, Rasmussen JV, Olsen BS, Frich LH, Jensen SL, Hróbjartsson A: Reverse shoulder arthroplasty in acute fractures of the proximal humerus: A systematic review. *Int J Shoulder Surg* 2013;7(2):70-78.

Burkhead WZ Jr, Scheinberg RR, Box G: Surgical anatomy of the axillary nerve. *J Shoulder Elbow Surg* 1992;1(1):31-36.

Chacon A, Virani N, Shannon R, Levy JC, Pupello D, Frankle M: Revision arthroplasty with use of a reverse shoulder prosthesis-allograft composite. *J Bone Joint Surg Am* 2009;91(1):119-127.

Cheung S, Fitzpatrick M, Lee TQ: Effects of shoulder position on axillary nerve positions during the split lateral deltoid approach. *J Shoulder Elbow Surg* 2009;18(5):748-755.

Chou YC, Tseng IC, Chiang CW, Wu CC: Shoulder hemiarthroplasty for proximal humeral fractures: Comparisons between the deltopectoral and anterolateral deltoid-splitting approaches. *J Shoulder Elbow Surg* 2013;22(8):e1-e7.

Clark JC, Ritchie J, Song FS, et al: Complication rates, dislocation, pain, and postoperative range of motion after reverse shoulder arthroplasty in patients with and without repair of the subscapularis. *J Shoulder Elbow Surg* 2012;21(1):36-41.

Codman EA: *The Shoulder: Rupture of the Supraspinatus Tendon and Other Lesions in or About the Subacromial Bursa.* Boston, MA, Thomas Todd, 1934.

Cordasco FA, Bigliani LU: The rotator cuff: Large and massive tears. Technique of open repair. *Orthop Clin North Am* 1997;28(2):179-193.

Cuff DJ, Virani NA, Levy J, et al: The treatment of deep shoulder infection and glenohumeral instability with debridement, reverse shoulder arthroplasty and postoperative antibiotics. *J Bone Joint Surg Br* 2008;90(3):336-342.

Delloye C, Joris D, Colette A, Eudier A, Dubuc JE: Mechanical complications of total shoulder inverted prosthesis [French]. *Rev Chir Orthop Reparatrice Appar Mot* 2002;88(4):410-414.

Edwards TB, Williams MD, Labriola JE, Elkousy HA, Gartsman GM, O'Connor DP: Subscapularis insufficiency and the risk of shoulder dislocation after reverse shoulder arthroplasty. *J Shoulder Elbow Surg* 2009;18(6):892-896.

Frankle M, Siegal S, Pupello D, Saleem A, Mighell M, Vasey M: The Reverse Shoulder Prosthesis for glenohumeral arthritis associated with severe rotator cuff deficiency: A minimum two-year follow-up study of sixty patients. *J Bone Joint Surg Am* 2005;87(8):1697-1705.

Gardner MJ, Boraiah S, Helfet DL, Lorich DG: The anterolateral acromial approach for fractures of the proximal humerus. *J Orthop Trauma* 2008;22(2):132-137.

Gardner MJ, Griffith MH, Dines JS, Briggs SM, Weiland AJ, Lorich DG: The extended anterolateral acromial approach allows minimally invasive access to the proximal humerus. *Clin Orthop Relat Res* 2005;(434):123-129.

Gardner MJ, Voos JE, Wanich T, Helfet DL, Lorich DG: Vascular implications of minimally invasive plating of proximal humerus fractures. *J Orthop Trauma* 2006;20(9):602-607.

Gillespie RJ, Garrigues GE, Chang ES, Namdari S, Williams GR Jr: Surgical exposure for reverse total shoulder arthroplasty: Differences in approaches and outcomes. *Orthop Clin North Am* 2015;46(1):49-56.

Gupta AK, Hug K, Berkoff DJ, et al: Dermal tissue allograft for the repair of massive irreparable rotator cuff tears. *Am J Sports Med* 2012;40(1):141-147.

Hatzidakis AM, Shevlin MJ, Fenton DL, Curran-Everett D, Nowinski RJ, Fehringer EV: Angular-stable locked intramedullary nailing of two-part surgical neck fractures of the proximal part of the humerus: A multicenter retrospective observational study. *J Bone Joint Surg Am* 2011;93(23):2172-2179.

Hepp P, Theopold J, Voigt C, Engel T, Josten C, Lill H: The surgical approach for locking plate osteosynthesis of displaced proximal humeral fractures influences the functional outcome. *J Shoulder Elbow Surg* 2008;17(1):21-28.

Holcomb JO, Cuff D, Petersen SA, Pupello DR, Frankle MA: Revision reverse shoulder arthroplasty for glenoid baseplate failure after primary reverse shoulder arthroplasty. *J Shoulder Elbow Surg* 2009;18(5):717-723.

Iannotti JP, Codsi MJ, Lafosse L, Flatow EL: Management of rotator cuff disease: Intact and repairable cuff, in Iannotti JP, Williams GR Jr, eds: *Disorders of the Shoulder: Diagnosis and Management.* Philadelphia, PA, Lippincott Williams & Wilkins, 2007, pp 53-100.

Kempton LB, Balasubramaniam M, Ankerson E, Wiater JM: A radiographic analysis of the effects of prosthesis design on scapular notching following reverse total shoulder arthroplasty. *J Shoulder Elbow Surg* 2011;20(4):571-576.

Knierim AE, Bollinger AJ, Wirth MA, Fehringer EV: Short, locked humeral nailing via Neviaser portal: An anatomic study. *J Orthop Trauma* 2013;27(2):63-67.

Lädermann A, Lubbeke A, Collin P, Edwards TB, Sirveaux F, Walch G: Influence of surgical approach on functional outcome in reverse shoulder arthroplasty. *Orthop Traumatol Surg Res* 2011;97(6):579-582.

Lafosse L, Schnaser E, Haag M, Gobezie R: Primary total shoulder arthroplasty performed entirely thru the rotator interval: Technique and minimum two-year outcomes. *J Shoulder Elbow Surg* 2009;18(6):864-873.

Laver L, Garrigues GE: Avoiding superior tilt in reverse shoulder arthroplasty: A review of the literature and technical recommendations. *J Shoulder Elbow Surg* 2014;23(10):1582-1590.

Lévigne C, Garret J, Boileau P, Alami G, Favard L, Walch G: Scapular notching in reverse shoulder arthroplasty: Is it important to avoid it and how? *Clin Orthop Relat Res* 2011;469(9):2512-2520.

Lynch NM, Cofield RH, Silbert PL, Hermann RC: Neurologic complications after total shoulder arthroplasty. *J Shoulder Elbow Surg* 1996;5(1):53-61.

MacKenzie DB: The antero-superior exposure for total shoulder replacement. *Orthop Trauma* 1993;2:71-77.

Molé D, Wein F, Dézaly C, Valenti P, Sirveaux F: Surgical technique: The anterosuperior approach for reverse shoulder arthroplasty. *Clin Orthop Relat Res* 2011;469(9):2461-2468.

Neer CS II: Replacement arthroplasty for glenohumeral osteoarthritis. *J Bone Joint Surg Am* 1974;56(1):1-13.

Neviaser AS, Hettrich CM, Dines JS, Lorich DG: Rate of avascular necrosis following proximal humerus fractures treated with a lateral locking plate and endosteal implant. *Arch Orthop Trauma Surg* 2011;131(12):1617-1622.

Neviaser TJ, Neviaser RJ, Neviaser JS, Neviaser JS: The four-in-one arthroplasty for the painful arc syndrome. *Clin Orthop Relat Res* 1982;(163):107-112.

Nové-Josserand L: Instability of the reverse prosthesis, in Walch G, Boileau P, Molé D, Favard L, Lévigne C, Sirveaux F, eds: *Reverse Shoulder Arthroplasty: Nice Shoulder Course.* Montpellier, France, Sauramps Medical, 2006, pp 247-260.

Simovitch RW, Zumstein MA, Lohri E, Helmy N, Gerber C: Predictors of scapular notching in patients managed with the Delta III reverse total shoulder replacement. *J Bone Joint Surg Am* 2007;89(3):588-600.

Stecco C, Gagliano G, Lancerotto L, et al: Surgical anatomy of the axillary nerve and its implication in the transdeltoid approaches to the shoulder. *J Shoulder Elbow Surg* 2010;19(8):1166-1174.

Trappey GJ IV, O'Connor DP, Edwards TB: What are the instability and infection rates after reverse shoulder arthroplasty? *Clin Orthop Relat Res* 2011;469(9):2505-2511.

Warner JJ, Higgins L, Parsons IM IV, Dowdy P: Diagnosis and treatment of anterosuperior rotator cuff tears. *J Shoulder Elbow Surg* 2001;10(1):37-46.

Werner CM, Steinmann PA, Gilbart M, Gerber C: Treatment of painful pseudoparesis due to irreparable rotator cuff dysfunction with the Delta III reverse-ball-and-socket total shoulder prosthesis. *J Bone Joint Surg Am* 2005;87(7):1476-1486.

Whatley AN, Fowler RL, Warner JJ, Higgins LD: Postoperative rupture of the anterolateral deltoid muscle following reverse total shoulder arthroplasty in patients who have undergone open rotator cuff repair. *J Shoulder Elbow Surg* 2011;20(1):114-122.

Young SW, Everts NM, Ball CM, Astley TM, Poon PC: The SMR reverse shoulder prosthesis in the treatment of cuff-deficient shoulder conditions. *J Shoulder Elbow Surg* 2009;18(4):622-626.

 Video Reference

Austin LS, Garrigues GE, Williams GR Jr: Video. *Reverse Shoulder Arthroplasty Through the Anterosuperior Approach.* Durham, NC, 2015.

Chapter 6

Arthroscopic Bankart Repair for Management of Uncomplicated Anterior Instability

Brett D. Owens, MD

E'Stephan J. Garcia, MD

 ## Introduction

Shoulder instability is common in young athletes. The focus in the literature has historically been on dislocation; however, subluxation has recently been shown to account for 85% of instability events and to result in substantial pathologic changes. Although the natural history of subluxation is less well understood, research on first-time anterior dislocation suggests that young athletes experience recurrence at a high rate. Early surgical stabilization has been repeatedly shown to decrease recurrence and improve patient-reported outcome measures.

A clear association between progressive pathologic changes and subsequent instability events has been demonstrated in the literature. In one series of patients undergoing arthroscopic stabilization, statistically significantly more glenoid and humeral bone loss was found in patients with recurrent instability than in patients with primary dislocation. In a similar study, a lower recurrence rate was shown among patients treated within 6 months of the initial dislocation. A higher number of preoperative instability events is associated with the presence of an anterior labroligamentous periosteal sleeve avulsion lesion rather than with the classic Bankart lesion. These findings underscore the importance of early stabilization of initial dislocation and suggest that early stabilization minimizes the risk of bone and soft-tissue lesions that can make arthroscopic stabilization technically challenging and result in poorer clinical outcomes.

 ## Case Presentation

A 20-year-old male collegiate football player experienced recurrent anterior subluxation of the right (dominant) shoulder during a fall football season. He was treated with a motion-limiting brace during the season and never experienced a complete dislocation requiring manual reduction. Similar instability of the contralateral shoulder during the previous season was managed successfully with arthroscopic stabilization. The patient now seeks similar treatment to manage the current instability. Physical examination demonstrates full range of motion and no neurovascular pathology. Results are normal on examination of the rotator cuff and biceps. Scapulothoracic motion is excellent, and no evidence of ligamentous laxity is observed. The patient has positive apprehension and relocation test results. The load-and-shift test is limited by patient guarding, but a grade 2 anterior translation that reproduced the patient's symptoms is noted. Plain radiographs demonstrate a concentrically reduced glenohumeral joint with no evidence of bony injury (**Figure 1**). Because the patient reported no clear recent injury, MRI with intra-articular dye injection was performed. Magnetic resonance arthrography demonstrated a Bankart lesion with minimal displacement and a small glenolabral articular disruption lesion (**Figure 2**). No evidence of a humeral avulsion of the glenohumeral ligament or a substantial Hill-Sachs lesion was observed.

 ## Indications

Anterior shoulder instability is common in young, active individuals. Nonsurgical management is a viable

Dr. Owens or an immediate family member serves as a paid consultant to Mitek Sports Medicine and the Musculoskeletal Transplant Foundation; has received nonincome support (such as equipment or services), commercially derived honoraria, or other non–research-related funding (such as paid travel) from SLACK; and serves as a board member, owner, officer, or committee member of the American Orthopaedic Society for Sports Medicine. Neither Dr. Garcia nor any immediate family member has received anything of value from or has stock or stock options held in a commercial company or institution related directly or indirectly to the subject of this chapter.

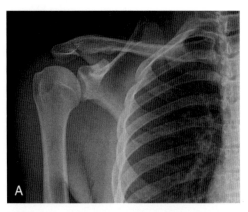
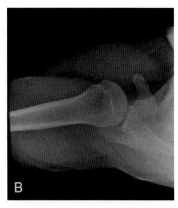

Figure 1 AP (**A**) and axillary (**B**) radiographs demonstrate the right shoulder of a 20-year-old male football player who experienced traumatic anterior subluxation during football season. No evidence of glenoid or humeral bone lesions is present.

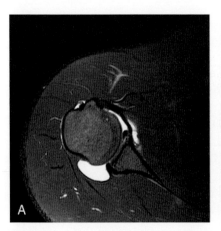
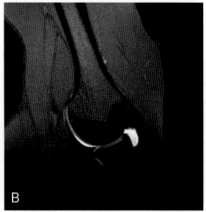

Figure 2 Magnetic resonance arthrograms of the same patient described in Figure 1. **A,** Axial view demonstrates an anteroinferior labral avulsion (Bankart lesion) and a small glenolabral articular disruption lesion. **B,** Abduction and external rotation slice demonstrates a minimally displaced Bankart lesion.

Controversies and Alternative Approaches

Several techniques have been described for the management of anterior shoulder instability. The most commonly used techniques are arthroscopic and open Bankart repairs using suture anchors. Arthroscopic repair is becoming the technique of choice. The key to both procedures is appropriate tensioning of the anteroinferior capsule and glenohumeral ligament complex. Age, activity level, and participation in contact or overhead sports can substantially increase the risk of failure of arthroscopic stabilization. The instability severity index score (ISIS) is used to identify patients who may be at increased risk for failure of arthroscopic treatment. The researchers who developed this score identified patient age younger than 20 years, competitive sport participation, contact sport participation, shoulder hyperlaxity, Hill-Sachs lesion visible on external rotation radiograph, and loss of normal inferior glenoid contour observed on AP radiograph as statistically significantly increasing the rate of failure. They recommended open stabilization in these high-risk patients. Although the validity of the ISIS as a decision-making tool is being evaluated, it is definitely a useful adjunct to patient risk stratification. In patients with a high ISIS, the surgeon should at least consider open procedures such as Bankart repair or Latarjet coracoid transfer because these options may provide more reliable outcomes in this subset of patients with instability.

The question of open versus arthroscopic stabilization has been investigated in many studies; however, the controversy continues. Three high-quality randomized controlled trials examined this question, with mixed results. In one study, researchers randomized 60 patients to undergo either open or arthroscopic repair and reported no

option, but the risk of recurrent instability increases with younger patient age and increased activity level. Nonsurgical management consists of rest and rehabilitation focusing on periscapular muscular stabilization and rotator cuff strengthening. Midseason athletes may return to sport within 1 to 2 weeks depending on the sport and the position played; however, recurrence can be expected in two-thirds of these patients. Surgical intervention should be considered in young, active patients with acute anterior shoulder instability and in patients with recurrent instability. Patients with acute instability after a dislocation should be evaluated for bony or other ligamentous injuries because the presence of these injuries influences the surgical management. Patients with recurrent instability should be evaluated for glenoid bone loss. Bony defects can be noted on MRI but are often best measured using CT. The authors of this chapter prefer routine initial use of MRI, with CT reserved for patients with suspicious bone loss. If bone loss is present, glenoid augmentation should be considered because outcomes after soft-tissue stabilization are less reliable in these patients. Patients without evidence of large bony lesions or bone loss are candidates for arthroscopic stabilization.

Table 1 Results of Arthroscopic Bankart Repair

Authors	Journal (Year)	No. of Patients (Shoulders)	Mean Follow-up (mo)	Outcomes[a]	Failure Rate (%)[b]
Cole et al	*J Bone Joint Surg Am* (2000)	37	54	ASES score, 87 Rowe score, 83 46% returned to activity	0
Kandziora et al	*Arthroscopy* (2000)	55	38.4	Rowe score, 84.6 83.6% returned to activity	16.4
Karlsson et al	*Am J Sports Med* (2001)	60	28	Rowe score, 93 Constant score, 91	11.7
Bottoni et al	*Am J Sports Med* (2002)	9	36	ASES score, 91.9 Rowe score, 92.3 Constant score, 33.3 91% returned to activity	11.1
Kim et al	*Arthroscopy* (2002)	58 (59)	33	Rowe score, 92.7 UCLA score, 33.1 Outcomes based on 59 shoulders	3.4
Kim et al	*J Bone Joint Surg Am* (2003)	167	44	ASES score, 91.9 Rowe score, 92.3 UCLA score, 33.3 91% returned to activity	0.6
Fabbriciani et al	*Arthroscopy* (2004)	30	24	Constant score, 89.5	0
Mazzocca et al	*Am J Sports Med* (2005)	18	37	ASES score, 89.5 Rowe score, 93.6 100% returned to activity	11.1
Boileau et al	*J Bone Joint Surg Am* (2006)	91	36	Rowe score, 77.8 75% returned to activity	6.6
Carreira et al	*Am J Sports Med* (2006)	69	46	ASES score, 95 Rowe score, 97	5.8
Cho et al	*Arthroscopy* (2006)	29	62.1	Constant score, 88.9 65.5% returned to activity	13.8

ASES = American Shoulder and Elbow Surgeons shoulder outcome, UCLA = University of California–Los Angeles Shoulder Rating Scale.

[a] Values are based on number of patients unless otherwise indicated.

[b] Failure is defined as recurrent dislocation.

recurrent instability and similar Constant and Rowe scores at 2-year follow-up, with greater range of motion in the arthroscopic group. The authors of a different study randomized 64 military patients to receive either open or arthroscopic repair and found similar outcome scores, similar failure rates (two open, one arthroscopic), and motion loss in the open group. The authors of a recent randomized trial of 196 patients found no differences in Western Ontario Shoulder Instability Index or American Shoulder and Elbow Surgeons scores at 2 years but a significantly higher failure rate in the arthroscopic group compared with the open group (23% and 11%, respectively). The literature is mixed, but it is important to note that although arthroscopic Bankart repair can have outcomes equivalent to those of open Bankart repair in general, further consideration of open repair is warranted in patients at high risk for failure.

Results

The outcomes of arthroscopic anterior stabilization have been reported in several studies (**Table 1**). The reported rates of recurrent instability after arthroscopic stabilization range from zero to 19.4%. In all the studies listed in **Table 1**, follow-up was at least 2 years, and a high rate of return to activity and excellent outcomes were reported. However, the measures of subjective outcome

Table 1 Results of Arthroscopic Bankart Repair (*continued*)

Authors	Journal (Year)	No. of Patients (Shoulders)	Mean Follow-up (mo)	Outcomes[a]	Failure Rate (%)[b]
Marquardt et al	*Arthroscopy* (2006)	27 (54)	44.4	ASES score, 91.8 Rowe score, 92.1 Constant score, 92.7 85.7% returned to activity Outcomes based on 54 shoulders	5.7
Rhee et al	*Am J Sports Med* (2006)	16	72	Rowe score, 35.4 83.6% returned to activity	18.8
Tan et al	*Arthroscopy* (2006)	124	31	85% returned to activity	5.6
Thal et al	*Arthroscopy* (2007)	72	24	ASES score, 96 UCLA score, 96	6.9
Castagna et al	*Am J Sports Med* (2010)	30 (31)	130.8	Rowe score, 80.1 UCLA score, 32.1 71% returned to activity Outcomes based on 31 shoulders	19.4
Voos et al	*Am J Sports Med* (2010)	73	33	ASES score, 94.9	9.6

ASES = American Shoulder and Elbow Surgeons shoulder outcome, UCLA = University of California–Los Angeles Shoulder Rating Scale.

[a] Values are based on number of patients unless otherwise indicated.

[b] Failure is defined as recurrent dislocation.

used are variable. Few longer term studies are available.

Video 6.1 Uncomplicated Anterior Instability: The "Simple" Arthroscopic Bankart Repair. Brett D. Owens, MD; E'Stephan Garcia, MD (6 min)

Technical Keys to Success

Setup/Exposure

- Arthroscopic anterior stabilization can be performed with the patient in the lateral decubitus position or the beach-chair position. The authors of this chapter prefer the beach-chair position for the following reasons: ease of orientation of both the surgical team and trainees; ease of concomitant shoulder procedures, such as rotator cuff repair; ease of conversion to open surgery, such as the Latarjet procedure; and improved ability to assess the glenohumeral joint through complete range of motion. When choosing the position, the surgeon should take into account all aspects of the repair, including concomitant posterior labral repair/plication or rotator cuff repair.
- With the patient in the beach-chair position, an interscalene block with sedation can be used, providing excellent pain relief and relaxation both intraoperatively and postoperatively. With the patient in the lateral decubitus position, general anesthesia is usually administered with a laryngeal mask airway or intubation.
- The arm and entire shoulder girdle are draped free to ensure circumferential access to the shoulder (**Figure 3**).

Instruments/Equipment/Implants Required

- A 30° and a 70° arthroscope are used.
- Two 7- or 8-mm cannulas are used.
- An arthroscopic periosteal elevator is used.
- A 3.5-mm mechanical shaver is used.
- A suture-shuttling device of the surgeon's choice is used.
- An anchor of the surgeon's choice is used.
- If knot tying is required, an arthroscopic knot pusher is required.

Procedure

- The patient is examined under anesthesia to quantify the severity of anterior, inferior, and posterior translation, and the findings are compared with those from the clinical examination, preoperative imaging, and examination of the contralateral side under anesthesia.

- The bony anatomy and all portal locations are drawn on the patient's skin (**Figure 4**).
- A posterior portal is created 2 cm distal and 1 cm medial to the posterolateral border of the acromion, and the arthroscope is introduced into the glenohumeral joint.
- A low anterior portal is created with the use of the needle-localization technique to ensure appropriate placement. This anterior portal allows inferior access to the axillary pouch and permits the surgeon to reach the 5:30 or 6:30 clock-face position on the glenoid rim for placement of the inferiormost anchor at a low angle to minimize risk of breaching the posterior cortex.
- The skin incision is typically located distal to the lateral edge of the coracoid in the area of a standard deltopectoral approach. The needle is inserted into the capsule and is directed superiorly over the superior edge of the subscapularis tendon (**Figure 5**).
- An 8.25-mm arthroscopic cannula is placed into the glenohumeral joint (**Figure 6**).
- A standard diagnostic arthroscopy is performed. Special attention is given to the humeral attachment of the glenohumeral ligaments. Even in patients with a Bankart lesion, the presence of a floating anterior band of the inferior glenohumeral ligament is possible.
- The anterosuperior portal is created, again with the use of a spinal needle for localization. The portal enters the glenohumeral joint lateral to the biceps tendon in the rotator interval. This portal allows the surgeon to work either anterior or posterior to the biceps tendon to facilitate both repair preparation and concomitant procedures (**Figure 7**).
- The lesion is evaluated with the arthroscope in the anterosuperior

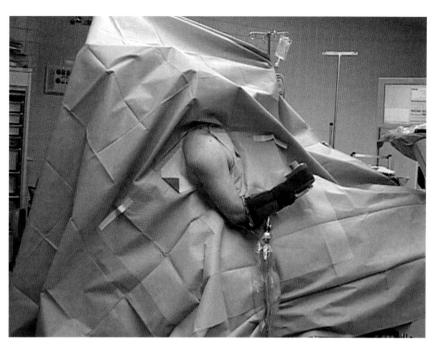

Figure 3 Intraoperative photograph shows a patient in the beach-chair position with the surgical arm draped free and supported with an arm positioner.

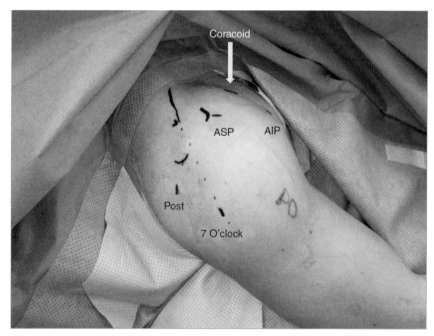

Figure 4 Photograph shows the bony anatomy and portal locations drawn on a patient's skin. The posterior portal (Post) is placed 2 cm inferior and 1 cm medial to the posterolateral border of the acromion. The anteroinferior portal (AIP) is created lateral to the coracoid, along the line of a standard incision for open Bankart repair, typically 6 cm inferior to the anterior acromion; this portal is placed using needle localization. The anterosuperior portal (ASP) is placed just distal to the anterolateral corner of the acromion. The 7-o'clock (accessory posterolateral) portal is placed approximately 4 cm distal to the posterolateral corner of the acromion, typically along a line extending from the posterior border of the clavicle. (Copyright Brett D. Owens, MD, West Point, NY.)

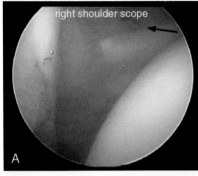 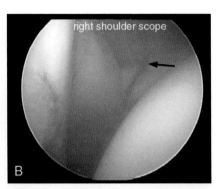

Figure 5 Arthroscopic views of a right shoulder from the posterior portal demonstrate creation of the anteroinferior portal pathway with the use of spinal needle localization (arrow). Low placement of the anteroinferior portal ensures that the needle crests just over the subscapularis tendon (**A**) and is able to translate inferiorly (**B**) to easily reach the 5:30 clock-face position to facilitate proper inferior anchor placement.

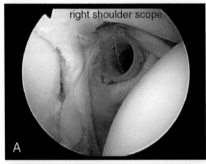 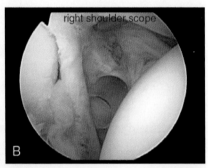

Figure 6 Arthroscopic views of a right shoulder from the posterior portal. **A,** Anteroinferior portal placement with an 8.25-mm cannula cresting just over the subscapularis tendon. **B,** This anteroinferior portal allows access to the inferior glenoid for anchor placement.

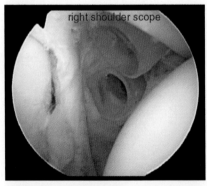 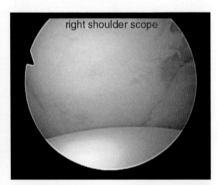

Figure 7 Arthroscopic view of a right shoulder from the posterior portal demonstrates placement of the anterosuperior portal with an 8.25-mm cannula placed lateral to the biceps tendon.

Figure 8 Arthroscopic view of a right shoulder from the anterosuperior portal demonstrates the so-called 50-yard-line view of the lesion.

portal (**Figure 8**). This view is referred to as the 50-yard-line view and allows visualization of medialized anterior labroligamentous periosteal sleeve avulsion lesions as well as an improved vantage point to view the posterior labrum and evaluate for a humeral avulsion of the glenohumeral ligament lesion.

- An arthroscopic load-and-shift test can be performed and correlated to the examination under anesthesia and the clinical data to finalize the treatment plan.
- An arthroscopic periosteal elevator is used to free the labrum and capsule from the glenoid face (**Figure 9**). The anteroinferior capsule and ligament complex should be fully mobilized from the glenoid neck such that the muscle fibers of the subscapularis can be visualized.
- After the soft tissue has been sufficiently mobilized, the anterior glenoid is prepared. Soft tissue is gently débrided using a mechanical shaver, and the anterior glenoid neck and rim is decorticated to facilitate soft-tissue healing. Articular cartilage that could inhibit visualization may be gently removed at the rim.
- A suture-shuttling device (angled 25° toward the ipsilateral side for anterior work) is used to shuttle a suture-passing wire through the anteroinferior soft tissue. Either a pleat of capsule should be grabbed before the labrum is captured or a large amount of capsule should be grabbed in a single pass along with the labrum. Working from inferior to superior will allow progressive tensioning of the anterior soft tissues. The first suture should be passed through the tissue as low as possible (approximately the 6-o'clock position) so that a suture shuttle can be placed at the 5:30 clock-face position (right shoulder).
- The soft tissues are grabbed lower and fixed in a superior and lateral position (anteroinferior capsular shift). An arthroscopic grasper can be used to aid with this step (**Figure 10**).
- A drill-sleeve cannula is used to guide drilling and placement of

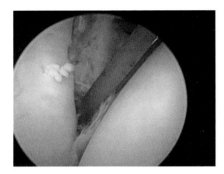

Figure 9 Arthroscopic view of a right shoulder from the posterior portal demonstrates the use of an arthroscopic periosteal elevator to free the labrum and capsule from the glenoid face.

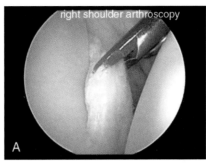

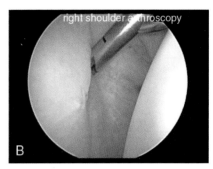

Figure 10 Arthroscopic views of a right shoulder from the posterior portal demonstrate suture shuttling facilitated with the use of a grasping instrument brought through the anterosuperior portal. **A,** The labrum and capsule are pulled laterally and superiorly during shuttling to achieve a low position; however, this method may limit visualization of the anteroinferior capsule, as in this example. **B,** The grasped tissue is medialized to improve visualization of the capsule and the inferior glenohumeral ligament to ensure appropriate placement of the shuttling device. After the shuttling device has penetrated the capsule, the tissue can be moved superiorly and laterally.

suture anchors into the glenoid. Anchors are placed a few millimeters onto the glenoid face. This placement will aid in appropriate lateralization of the labrum and capsule. In the right shoulder, the first anchor is generally placed at the 5:30 clock-face position. In the left shoulder, the first anchor is placed at the 6:30 clock-face position (**Figure 11**). Subsequent anchors are evenly spaced to provide a balanced repair (**Figure 12**).

Wound Closure

- Subcutaneous closure usually is not necessary for the portals.
- Skin is closed with 3-0 nylon sutures placed in a horizontal mattress, figure-of-8, or interrupted simple pattern.

 Rehabilitation

A sample rehabilitation protocol is presented in **Table 2**. The patient is maintained in a sling for 4 to 6 weeks, during which time range-of-motion exercises under the supervision of a therapist are initiated. The goal is to achieve full motion by 12 weeks postoperatively. Gentle strengthening is allowed at 8 to

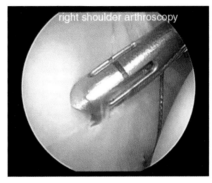

Figure 11 Arthroscopic view of a right shoulder from the posterior portal demonstrates placement of a low anchor at the 5:30 clock-face position. The suture shuttle has already been passed to allow proper planning of the anchor location.

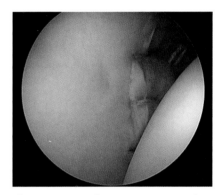

Figure 12 Arthroscopic view of a right shoulder from the posterior portal demonstrates a completed arthroscopic Bankart repair.

10 weeks. Progressive weight training is delayed until 12 weeks postoperatively, when full motion is obtained. Sport-specific training is initiated 4 to 5 months postoperatively, with return to sport allowed at 6 months.

 Avoiding Pitfalls

Excellent outcomes of Bankart reconstruction can be achieved by adhering to some key principles. Patient selection is paramount for obtaining reliable outcomes. In general, shoulder instability

occurs in young, active individuals. With increasing patient age, outcomes of shoulder stabilization become less reliable, and in the experience of the authors of this chapter, postoperative stiffness or loss of range of motion becomes a concern. In addition, each patient should undergo an appropriate and thorough preoperative evaluation. This evaluation should include scrutiny of imaging for concomitant pathology and glenoid or humeral bone defects (such as capsular stretch injury/laxity, glenoid bone loss, Hill-Sachs lesion). Intraoperative keys to success include appropriate tissue mobilization, adequate capsular tightening, appropriate anchor placement,

Table 2 Rehabilitation Protocol After Arthroscopic Bankart Repair

Postoperative Week	ROM	Strengthening/Exercises	Return to Play	Comments/Emphasis
0-2	Flexion of 0°-90° External rotation neutral	Supported modified pendulum exercises Supine assisted shoulder flexion	None	Goal is to protect the surgical repair and avoid shoulder stiffness Full-time use of sling/immobilizer
2-4	Flexion of 0°-110° External rotation to 10°	Gentle isometric internal and external rotation Scapular protraction and retraction	None	Full-time use of sling/immobilizer
4-6	Flexion of 0°-130° External rotation to 20°	Shoulder active-assisted ROM Add lower extremity strengthening	None	Full-time use of sling/immobilizer
6-8	Full flexion and internal rotation External rotation 90% of contralateral side	Upper body cycling Active and active-assisted ROM Shoulder stabilization exercises	None	Goal is to achieve pain-free activities of daily living
8-12	Full flexion and internal and external rotation	Progressive strengthening	Walk-run progression	Goal is to achieve full ROM, increasing strength
12-16	Full ROM	Push-ups at patient's own pace without pain High-repetition, low-weight weight training	No contact or collision sports	—
16-26	Full ROM	Sport-specific training progression	Return to sport at 6 mo	—

ROM = range of motion.

and appropriate concomitant pathology management (such as superior labrum anterior to posterior lesions, posterior labral tear/laxity). Adequate liberation of the anteroinferior soft tissues allows for proximal and lateral translation of the capsuloligamentous tissue with each subsequent suture anchor. Intraoperative stability should be assessed; if appreciable laxity remains, adjunctive procedures can be considered.

Bibliography

Arciero RA, Wheeler JH, Ryan JB, McBride JT: Arthroscopic Bankart repair versus nonoperative treatment for acute, initial anterior shoulder dislocations. *Am J Sports Med* 1994;22(5):589-594.

Balg F, Boileau P: The instability severity index score: A simple pre-operative score to select patients for arthroscopic or open shoulder stabilisation. *J Bone Joint Surg Br* 2007;89(11):1470-1477.

Boileau P, Villalba M, Héry JY, Balg F, Ahrens P, Neyton L: Risk factors for recurrence of shoulder instability after arthroscopic Bankart repair. *J Bone Joint Surg Am* 2006;88(8):1755-1763.

Bottoni CR, Smith EL, Berkowitz MJ, Towle RB, Moore JH: Arthroscopic versus open shoulder stabilization for recurrent anterior instability: A prospective randomized clinical trial. *Am J Sports Med* 2006;34(11):1730-1737.

Bottoni CR, Wilckens JH, DeBerardino TM, et al: A prospective, randomized evaluation of arthroscopic stabilization versus nonoperative treatment in patients with acute, traumatic, first-time shoulder dislocations. *Am J Sports Med* 2002;30(4):576-580.

Burkhart SS, De Beer JF: Traumatic glenohumeral bone defects and their relationship to failure of arthroscopic Bankart repairs: Significance of the inverted-pear glenoid and the humeral engaging Hill-Sachs lesion. *Arthroscopy* 2000;16(7):677-694.

Carreira DS, Mazzocca AD, Oryhon J, Brown FM, Hayden JK, Romeo AA: A prospective outcome evaluation of arthroscopic Bankart repairs: Minimum 2-year follow-up. *Am J Sports Med* 2006;34(5):771-777.

Castagna A, Markopoulos N, Conti M, Delle Rose G, Papadakou E, Garofalo R: Arthroscopic Bankart suture-anchor repair: Radiological and clinical outcome at minimum 10 years of follow-up. *Am J Sports Med* 2010;38(10):2012-2016.

Cho NS, Hwang JC, Rhee YG: Arthroscopic stabilization in anterior shoulder instability: Collision athletes versus noncollision athletes. *Arthroscopy* 2006;22(9):947-953.

Cole BJ, L'Insalata J, Irrgang J, Warner JJ: Comparison of arthroscopic and open anterior shoulder stabilization: A two to six-year follow-up study. *J Bone Joint Surg Am* 2000;82(8):1108-1114.

Dickens JF, Owens BD, Cameron KL, et al: Return to play and recurrent instability after in-season anterior shoulder instability: A prospective multicenter study. *Am J Sports Med* 2014;42(12):2842-2850.

Fabbriciani C, Milano G, Demontis A, Fadda S, Ziranu F, Mulas PD: Arthroscopic versus open treatment of Bankart lesion of the shoulder: A prospective randomized study. *Arthroscopy* 2004;20(5):456-462.

Hovelius L, Eriksson K, Fredin H, et al: Recurrences after initial dislocation of the shoulder: Results of a prospective study of treatment. *J Bone Joint Surg Am* 1983;65(3):343-349.

Jakobsen BW, Johannsen HV, Suder P, Søjbjerg JO: Primary repair versus conservative treatment of first-time traumatic anterior dislocation of the shoulder: A randomized study with 10-year follow-up. *Arthroscopy* 2007;23(2):118-123.

Kandziora F, Jäger A, Bischof F, Herresthal J, Starker M, Mittlmeier T: Arthroscopic labrum refixation for post-traumatic anterior shoulder instability: Suture anchor versus transglenoid fixation technique. *Arthroscopy* 2000;16(4):359-366.

Karlsson J, Magnusson L, Ejerhed L, Hultenheim I, Lundin O, Kartus J: Comparison of open and arthroscopic stabilization for recurrent shoulder dislocation in patients with a Bankart lesion. *Am J Sports Med* 2001;29(5):538-542.

Kim DS, Yoon YS, Yi CH: Prevalence comparison of accompanying lesions between primary and recurrent anterior dislocation in the shoulder. *Am J Sports Med* 2010;38(10):2071-2076.

Kim SH, Ha KI, Cho YB, Ryu BD, Oh I: Arthroscopic anterior stabilization of the shoulder: Two to six-year follow-up. *J Bone Joint Surg Am* 2003;85(8):1511-1518.

Kim SH, Ha KI, Kim SH: Bankart repair in traumatic anterior shoulder instability: Open versus arthroscopic technique. *Arthroscopy* 2002;18(7):755-763.

Kirkley A, Griffin S, Richards C, Miniaci A, Mohtadi N: Prospective randomized clinical trial comparing the effectiveness of immediate arthroscopic stabilization versus immobilization and rehabilitation in first traumatic anterior dislocations of the shoulder. *Arthroscopy* 1999;15(5):507-514.

Marquardt B, Witt KA, Liem D, Steinbeck J, Pötzl W: Arthroscopic Bankart repair in traumatic anterior shoulder instability using a suture anchor technique. *Arthroscopy* 2006;22(9):931-936.

Mazzocca AD, Brown FM Jr, Carreira DS, Hayden J, Romeo AA: Arthroscopic anterior shoulder stabilization of collision and contact athletes. *Am J Sports Med* 2005;33(1):52-60.

Mohtadi NG, Chan DS, Hollinshead RM, et al: A randomized clinical trial comparing open and arthroscopic stabilization for recurrent traumatic anterior shoulder instability: Two-year follow-up with disease-specific quality-of-life outcomes. *J Bone Joint Surg Am* 2014;96(5):353-360.

Owens BD, Agel J, Mountcastle SB, Cameron KL, Nelson BJ: Incidence of glenohumeral instability in collegiate athletics. *Am J Sports Med* 2009;37(9):1750-1754.

Owens BD, Duffey ML, Nelson BJ, DeBerardino TM, Taylor DC, Mountcastle SB: The incidence and characteristics of shoulder instability at the United States Military Academy. *Am J Sports Med* 2007;35(7):1168-1173.

Owens BD, Harrast JJ, Hurwitz SR, Thompson TL, Wolf JM: Surgical trends in Bankart repair: An analysis of data from the American Board of Orthopaedic Surgery certification examination. *Am J Sports Med* 2011;39(9):1865-1869.

Owens BD, Nelson BJ, Duffey ML, et al: Pathoanatomy of first-time, traumatic, anterior glenohumeral subluxation events. *J Bone Joint Surg Am* 2010;92(7):1605-1611.

Ozbaydar M, Elhassan B, Diller D, Massimini D, Higgins LD, Warner JJ: Results of arthroscopic capsulolabral repair: Bankart lesion versus anterior labroligamentous periosteal sleeve avulsion lesion. *Arthroscopy* 2008;24(11):1277-1283.

Porcellini G, Campi F, Pegreffi F, Castagna A, Paladini P: Predisposing factors for recurrent shoulder dislocation after arthroscopic treatment. *J Bone Joint Surg Am* 2009;91(11):2537-2542.

Pulavarti RS, Symes TH, Rangan A: Surgical interventions for anterior shoulder instability in adults. *Cochrane Database Syst Rev* 2009;4:CD005077.

Rhee YG, Ha JH, Cho NS: Anterior shoulder stabilization in collision athletes: Arthroscopic versus open Bankart repair. *Am J Sports Med* 2006;34(6):979-985.

Sachs RA, Lin D, Stone ML, Paxton E, Kuney M: Can the need for future surgery for acute traumatic anterior shoulder dislocation be predicted? *J Bone Joint Surg Am* 2007;89(8):1665-1674.

Tan CK, Guisasola I, Machani B, et al: Arthroscopic stabilization of the shoulder: A prospective randomized study of absorbable versus nonabsorbable suture anchors. *Arthroscopy* 2006;22(7):716-720.

Thal R, Nofziger M, Bridges M, Kim JJ: Arthroscopic Bankart repair using Knotless or BioKnotless suture anchors: 2- to 7-year results. *Arthroscopy* 2007;23(4):367-375.

Voos JE, Livermore RW, Feeley BT, et al, HSS Sports Medicine Service: Prospective evaluation of arthroscopic Bankart repairs for anterior instability. *Am J Sports Med* 2010;38(2):302-307.

Wheeler JH, Ryan JB, Arciero RA, Molinari RN: Arthroscopic versus nonoperative treatment of acute shoulder dislocations in young athletes. *Arthroscopy* 1989;5(3):213-217.

Zhang AL, Montgomery SR, Ngo SS, Hame SL, Wang JC, Gamradt SC: Arthroscopic versus open shoulder stabilization: Current practice patterns in the United States. *Arthroscopy* 2014;30(4):436-443.

 ## Video Reference

Owens BD, Garcia E: Video. *Uncomplicated Anterior Instability: The "Simple" Arthroscopic Bankart Repair.* Providence, RI, 2015.

Chapter 7
Anterior Instability With Moderate Glenoid Bone Loss: The Latarjet Procedure

Stephen S. Burkhart, MD

Robert U. Hartzler, MD, MS

 ## Introduction

Recurrent anterior shoulder instability can be disabling for patients and frustrating for the treating surgeon. Patients who are at high risk for unsuccessful soft-tissue reconstruction, particularly those with substantial glenoid bone loss, can be effectively treated with the Latarjet procedure, which involves transfer of the coracoid process and the attached conjoint tendon to the anterior glenoid. In addition to the stability provided by the coracoid as a so-called bone block, the sling effect of the conjoint and subscapularis tendons and anterior capsular reconstruction contribute to shoulder stabilization. Numerous techniques for coracoid bone transfer have been described in the literature. The chapter authors' preferred techniques, instrumentation, and rehabilitation protocols for the congruent-arc Latarjet procedure are described.

 Video 7.1 Latarjet Surgical Technique. Stephen S. Burkhart, MD; Robert U. Hartzler, MD, MS (8 min)

 ## Case Presentation

A 24-year-old right-hand–dominant man has recurrent anterior instability of the right shoulder that has continued for 6 months. The traumatic initial dislocation occurred during a soccer game, at which time the shoulder was reduced on the field. Despite undergoing physical therapy, the patient has experienced subluxation events several times per week as well as one recurrent dislocation that occurred during sleep. Preoperative radiographs, CT scans, and MRIs are obtained for diagnosis and to calculate glenoid bone loss (**Figure 1**). A shallow Hill-Sachs lesion is noted as well.

Diagnostic arthroscopy reveals two associated lesions (one type II superior labrum anterior to posterior tear and one capsular split [a variant posterior humeral avulsion of the glenohumeral ligament]) that are repaired arthroscopically (**Figure 2**). The patient has an inverted pear–shaped glenoid and 25% bone loss (as calculated intraoperatively using the bare area of the glenoid as a landmark; **Figure 3**). On the basis of this amount of glenoid bone loss, the

decision is made to proceed with the congruent-arc modification of the Latarjet procedure.

The inferior coracoid surface matched the shape of the native glenoid well in this patient, and the congruent-arc modification resulted in an anatomic-appearing reconstruction of the bone-deficient anteroinferior glenoid (**Figure 4, A**). A capsular repair was performed at the glenoid margin to produce an extra-articular graft, per the preference of the authors of this chapter (**Figure 5**). Such repair is not possible in all patients. To create a capsular rim repair, the takedown of the capsule is done medial to the joint line to provide added length (**Figure 6**). Postoperative radiographs demonstrate the typical appearance of the graft and the cannulated screws (**Figure 4, B, C, and D**).

 ## Indications

The case described in this chapter illustrates the value of arthroscopy in patients who have recurrent anterior shoulder instability. In this patient, arthroscopic evaluation showed bone loss to be greater than anticipated based on preoperative imaging. The authors of this chapter consider intraoperative arthroscopic measurement to be the determining factor in deciding whether to

Dr. Burkhart or an immediate family member has received royalties from and serves as a paid consultant to Arthrex. Dr. Hartzler or an immediate family member has received nonincome support (such as equipment or services), commercially derived honoraria, or other non–research-related funding (such as paid travel) from Wolters Kluwer Health–Lippincott Williams & Wilkins.

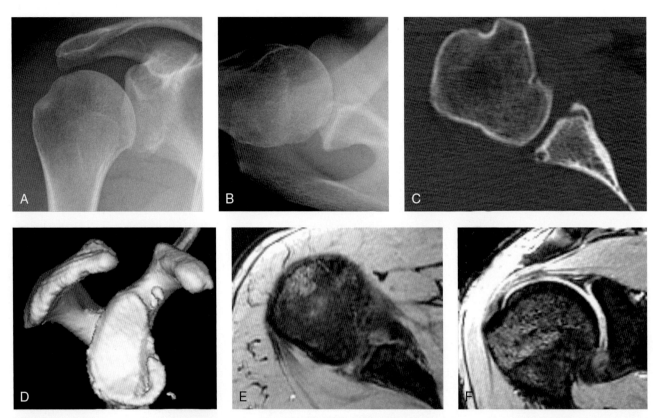

Figure 1   Preoperative Grashey internal rotation (**A**) and axillary lateral (**B**) radiographs demonstrate a shallow Hill-Sachs lesion and substantial anterior glenoid bone loss. CT (**C**) and corresponding three-dimensional CT reconstruction (**D**) were used to calculate bone loss, which was found to be 22% compared with the contralateral uninjured glenoid (not shown). MRIs demonstrate the associated capsulolabral injury anteroinferiorly (**E**) and the superior labral anterior and posterior tear lesion superiorly (**F**).

perform soft-tissue repair or the Latarjet procedure. As shown in the patient described in the case study, associated lesions such as superior labrum anterior to posterior tear and humeral avulsion of the glenohumeral ligament are common and may be repaired arthroscopically before the open Latarjet procedure is performed.

In considering the Latarjet procedure for any patient, the authors of this chapter take into account the quantity and morphology of glenoid and humeral bone loss, the status of the capsule and the subscapularis, and the patient demands on the shoulder. The one unyielding indication for the Latarjet procedure, independent of any other risk factor, is intraoperatively measured glenoid bone loss of 25% or greater.

In 2007, the authors of this chapter described the engaging Hill-Sachs lesion as an indication for the Latarjet procedure. A study published in 2014 presented the glenoid track concept for categorizing bipolar bone lesions (that is, Hill-Sachs lesion and glenoid bone loss), in which Hill-Sachs lesions are classified as either off-track (engaging) or on-track (nonengaging). The authors of this chapter have since performed soft-tissue reconstructions as described in that 2014 study in the treatment of nearly all patients with bipolar bone lesions with mild glenoid bone loss (≤15%). On-track lesions are managed with arthroscopic Bankart repair, and off-track lesions are managed with arthroscopic Bankart repair plus remplissage of the rotator cuff into the Hill-Sachs defect. Therefore, some lesions that the authors of this chapter might have previously treated with the Latarjet procedure for so-called engagement

are treated entirely arthroscopically with soft-tissue procedures.

In patients with bipolar bone lesions with moderate glenoid bone loss (15% to 24%), the authors of this chapter strongly consider the Latarjet procedure if there are other risk factors for recurrent instability. These factors include previous surgery for instability, poor soft-tissue quality, participation in contact sports, and presence of a deep Hill-Sachs lesion. For example, the Latarjet procedure might be recommended to a wrestler who has 20% glenoid bone loss.

Sometimes the Latarjet procedure is indicated solely for the management of deficient soft tissues. For example, failure of a well-performed Bankart repair is indicative of poor-quality capsulolabral tissues; in most patients with such failure, the Latarjet procedure is required. Using the Latarjet procedure, the authors of this chapter have successfully managed irreparable subscapularis tendon loss after failed open instability surgery. Soft-tissue loss after failed thermal capsulorrhaphy is another (if rare) indication for the Latarjet procedure.

Controversies and Alternative Approaches

The Latarjet procedure has been suggested as a routine alternative to soft-tissue repair or reconstruction for the treatment of anterior shoulder instability. In the opinion of the authors of this chapter, a large percentage of patients who have anterior shoulder instability, even when recurrent, can be successfully treated with arthroscopic soft-tissue repairs. Associated morbidity is higher with the Latarjet procedure than with arthroscopic soft-tissue reconstruction. Complications both unique to the Latarjet procedure and occurring at a high rate also have been reported. In the opinion of the authors of this chapter, use of the Latarjet procedure would represent overtreatment in nearly all patients with primary shoulder dislocation and in most patients with recurrent instability without bone loss.

Techniques and results of the Latarjet procedure performed entirely via arthroscopy have been reported in several studies. The rates of complications, reoperations, and graft nonunions have been high at short-term follow-up. The authors of this chapter have found the open Latarjet procedure to be safe and reliable and thus consider the open Latarjet procedure to be the current best treatment for patients who have anterior instability with an appropriate indication for the procedure, as described previously in this chapter.

The authors of this chapter prefer to orient the coracoid graft so that the undersurface (inferior surface) of the coracoid is aligned with the glenoid

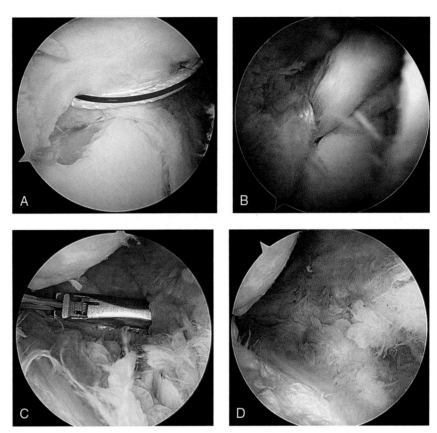

Figure 2   Arthroscopic views. The type II superior labral anterior and posterior tear lesion (**A**) was repaired arthroscopically (**B**) before open Latarjet reconstruction occurred. An unexpected diagnostic finding was a posterior capsular split (**C**) (variant posterior humeral avulsion of the glenohumeral ligament). Routine arthroscopy performed before the open procedure makes it possible to diagnose and repair these associated lesions. **D,** Final appearance of the repaired posterior humeral avulsion of the glenohumeral ligament lesion.

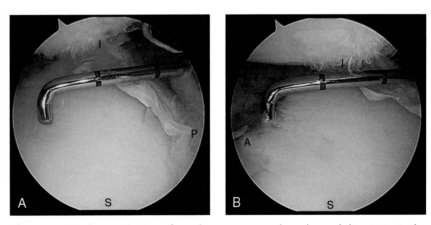

Figure 3   Arthroscopic views from the anterosuperolateral portal demonstrate the taking of measurements used in calculating bone loss (in this patient, 25%). **A,** The width of the posterior half of the glenoid is 12 mm, using the bare area as the center of the glenoid. **B,** The anterior width is 6 mm, which indicates a 6-mm bone loss. The morphology of the glenoid is an inverted pear shape. A = anterior, I = inferior, P = posterior, S = superior.

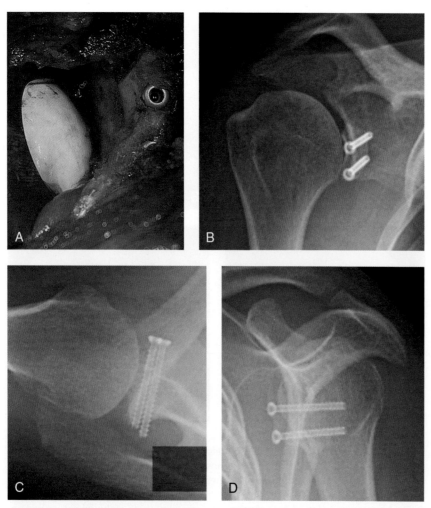

Figure 4 **A,** Intraoperative photograph of a shoulder shows final graft congruency with the glenoid. Final postoperative Grashey (**B**), axillary (**C**), and scapular Y (**D**) radiographs demonstrate the placement of cannulated screws and the appearance of the graft.

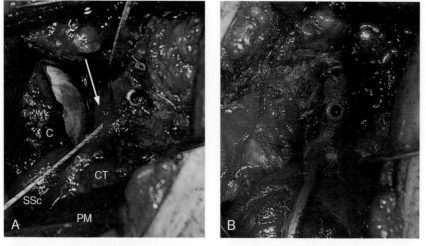

Figure 5 Intraoperative photographs of a shoulder show repair of the capsular flap to the native glenoid (**A**) and the appearance of the repair tied such that the coracoid bone graft is extra-articular (**B**). C = capsule, CT = coracoid tip, PM = pectoralis major muscle, SSc = subscapularis, arrow = placement of suture anchor.

(**Figure 7**). In contrast, in the traditional orientation of the graft, the lateral aspect of the coracoid is aligned with the glenoid articular surface. As illustrated in the case study described in this chapter (**Figure 4, A**), the shape of the undersurface of the coracoid truly is congruent with the anterior glenoid; equal radii of curvature for these surfaces have been demonstrated on CT. Biomechanically, the congruent-arc configuration results in more favorable loading characteristics compared with the traditional orientation, with decreased contact pressure, increased contact area, and increased diameter of the reconstructed glenoid. In some patients of small stature, the coracoid is too thin to accept screws and the graft must be oriented in the traditional manner. Even in such patients, the authors of this chapter do not attach the joint capsule to the stump of the coracoacromial ligament; rather, the joint capsule is attached to the native glenoid so that the graft remains extra-articular.

Some surgeons prefer to approach the anterior glenoid by using a subscapularis split, which obviates any need to protect a tendon repair postoperatively. In contrast, the authors of this chapter prefer to manage the subscapularis by taking down the superior half as a flap separate from the anterior capsule. In this manner, the capsule is then reflected from the glenoid neck from medial to lateral (**Figure 6**). The authors of this chapter believe taking down the upper subscapularis to be a safer and more effective approach. If the subscapularis split is not made in an optimal location, poor glenoid exposure can result. However, discerning the landmarks for an upper subscapularis tendon flap—the rolled upper tendon border, the rotator interval, and the lesser tuberosity—visually and by palpation is straightforward. A subscapularis flap is also more extensile than a subscapularis split. In the experience of the authors of this

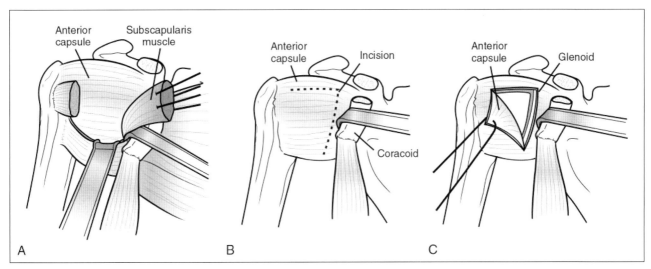

Figure 6 Illustrations depict upper subscapularis tenotomy and capsular flap technique. **A,** A tenotomy through the upper 50% of the subscapularis tendon exposes the joint capsule. **B,** An L-shaped capsular flap is developed from medial to lateral beginning approximately 1 cm medial to the rim of the glenoid. **C,** The flap is retracted to expose the glenohumeral joint, but it will be closed back to the glenoid rim to make the coracoid graft extra-articular.

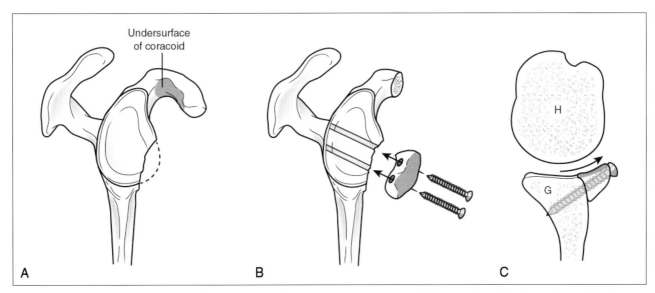

Figure 7 Illustrations depict the graft orientation in the congruent-arc Latarjet technique preferred by the authors of this chapter. En face view of the glenoid (**A**) shows how the undersurface of the coracoid will be oriented and fixed (**B**) to the deficient glenoid to restore the bone defect while maintaining the shape of the articular surface (**C**). G = glenoid, H = humerus.

chapter, strength deficits and problems with healing after subscapularis tenotomy are rare.

 Results

In multiple published studies with mid- to long-term follow-up, the Latarjet procedure has been shown to be durable and effective, with an acceptable rate of complications (**Table 1**).

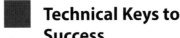 **Technical Keys to Success**

Setup/Exposure

- Before performing open reconstruction, the patient is placed in the lateral decubitus position, and diagnostic arthroscopy is performed through posterior and anterosuperolateral portals.
- Associated pathology that is inaccessible by means of the anterior open approach is repaired, and the arthroscopic portals are closed.
- In preparation for open repair, the patient is placed in the modified

Table 1 Results of the Latarjet Procedure

Authors	Journal (Year)	Number	Outcomes	Failure Rate (%)[a]	Comments
Singer et al	*J Bone Joint Surg Br* (1995)	14 patients	Rowe score was excellent in 5 patients, good in 8, and fair in 1 Mean Constant score, 80	7.1	Mean follow-up, 20.5 yr No graft complications
Allain et al	*J Bone Joint Surg Am* (1998)	58 shoulders	Rowe score was excellent in 37 shoulders, good in 14, fair in 5, and poor in 2 Mean Constant score, 84	1.7	Mean follow-up, 3 yr 7% complication rate
Hovelius et al	*J Shoulder Elbow Surg* (2004)	118 shoul-ders	Mean Rowe score, 89.4 (good) 98% of patients were satisfied with the surgical repair	3.4	Mean follow-up, 15.2 yr 1.7% complication rate
Burkhart et al	*Arthroscopy* (2007)	102 patients	Mean Constant score, 94.4[b] Mean Walch-Duplay score, 91.7[b]	4.9[c]	Mean follow-up, 4.9 yr[b]
Mizuno et al	*J Shoulder Elbow Surg* (2014)	68 shoulders	Mean Rowe score increased from 37.9 to 89.6 Mean subjective shoulder value, 91% 96% of patients were very satisfied or satisfied	5.9	Mean follow-up, 20 yr

[a] Recurrent instability.
[b] For 47 patients personally examined. The other 55 patients were contacted by telephone or letter.
[c] Based on the full cohort of 102 patients.

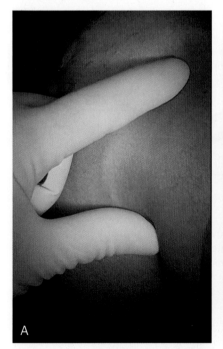
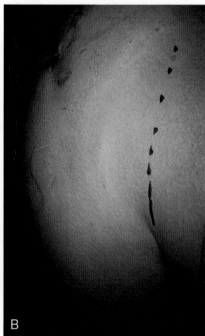

Figure 8 Preoperative photographs show palpation of the coracoid tip and anterior axillary fold by the surgeon (**A**) and the standard incision (dotted line) marked over the deltopectoral groove between these landmarks (**B**).

beach-chair position, with the head elevated approximately 20°.
- A bump is placed under the ipsilateral scapula.

Instruments/Equipment/ Implants Required

- A specific Latarjet instrument set (such as the Glenoid Bone Loss Instrument Set, Arthrex) greatly facilitates performing the procedure versus using freehand instrumentation.
- Both straight and angled microsagittal saw blades (70°).
- Curved and straight osteotomes.
- Specific retractors that should be available include Fukuda, Hohmann, Chandler, Richardson, and anterior and posterior glenoid retractors.

Procedure

- The coracoid tip and anterior axillary fold are palpated (**Figure 8, A**), and the incision is placed between these two landmarks (**Figure 8, B**).

- A deltopectoral approach is used with the cephalic vein mobilized on the medial aspect to be retracted laterally with the deltoid.
- To harvest the coracoid bone, the coracoacromial ligament and pectoralis minor attachments are incised and then elevated from the bone using subperiosteal dissection (**Figure 9, A**).
- The soft tissues are dissected from the bone to an extent that the surgeon's finger can be placed under the coracoid (**Figure 9, B**).
- A 70° oscillating saw is used to osteotomize the coracoid at the base of the coracoclavicular ligaments. Ideally, the graft should include a small spike of bone inferiorly if the maximal length of the graft available is taken (**Figure 10**).
- The conjoint tendon is dissected free from its attachment to the pectoralis minor to increase its excursion. The length of dissection measures approximately 1 cm, and care is taken at this point not to stray too far distally to avoid the musculocutaneous nerve.

- The coracoid is grasped gently with a Kocher clamp.
- A flat-blade microsagittal saw is used to remove the spike and a thin wafer of bone from the medial aspect of the graft (the minor attachment side of the pectoralis; **Figure 10**).

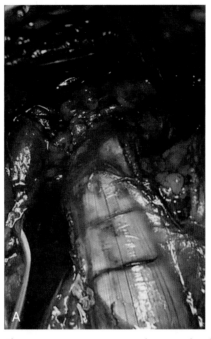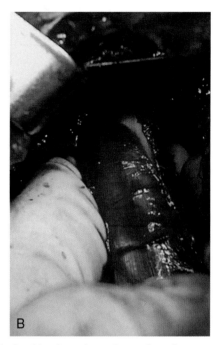

Figure 9 Intraoperative photographs of a shoulder show the end point for soft-tissue dissection off the coracoid. **A,** The characteristic anatomy of the conjoint tendon origin from the coracoid is shown. **B,** Sufficient room exists for an index finger to be placed under the coracoid process.

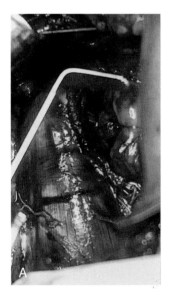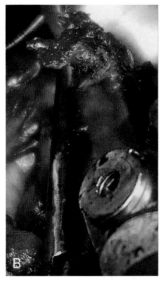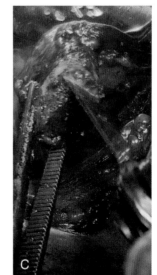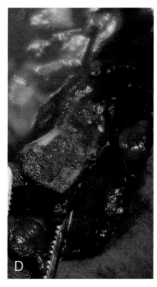

Figure 10 Intraoperative photographs of a shoulder. **A,** A 70° angled saw blade is used to enable harvest of the maximum length of coracoid. **B,** After harvest of the maximum length, removal of a small spike of bone from the inferior surface of the graft using a straight microsagittal saw blade. Decortication of the medial side of the coracoid is with a straight saw blade (**C**) so that a flat surface (**D**) may be compressed against the prepared surface of the glenoid.

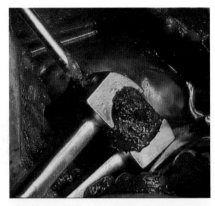

Figure 11 Intraoperative photograph of a shoulder shows a graft clamped in a drill guide with the circular holes on the lateral face of the graft (coracoacromial ligament) and the oblong holes on the medial decorticated face (pectoralis minor) in preparation for drilling gliding holes used to insert lag screws in the congruent-arc Latarjet technique.

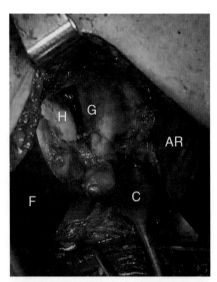

Figure 12 Intraoperative photograph of a shoulder shows the preferred retractor placement for glenoid (G) exposure. AR = anterior glenoid retractor, C = Chandler leverage retractor, F = Fukuda retractor, H = humeral head.

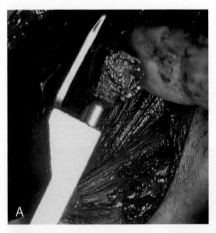

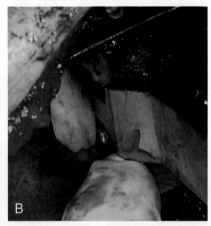

Figure 13 Intraoperative photographs of a shoulder show a parallel drill guide with approximately 2 mm of space positioned between the fin and the coracoid bone (**A**) and the resulting placement of the graft in the ideal position and at the proper angle (**B**).

- The authors of this chapter prefer to use the Glenoid Bone Loss Instrument Set (Arthrex) rather than a freehand technique to prepare the graft.
- The graft is grasped in the coracoid drill guide with the oblong slots on the medial (pectoralis minor) side (**Figure 11**).
- If using the lag screw technique, a retractor is placed medially to protect from plunging, after which two 4-mm gliding holes are drilled in the coracoid.
- The coracoid is tucked into the medial soft tissues while the joint is exposed and prepared.
- The upper one-half of the subscapularis is taken down, beginning 1 cm medial to the lesser tuberosity (**Figure 6, A**).

- An L-shaped capsular flap (**Figure 6, B**) is taken down from medial to lateral. Subperiosteal dissection of the capsular flap is begun approximately 1 cm medial to the glenoid rim; the superior margin of the flap will be through the rotator interval (**Figure 6, B**). A traction stitch placed at the corner of the flap aids in creation of the flap and retraction (**Figure 6, C**).
- Several retractors are placed (**Figure 12**). A Fukuda retractor is positioned behind the glenoid to retract the humeral head laterally. A two-pronged anterior glenoid retractor is placed medially at the glenoid neck. Either a Chandler or a blunt Hohmann retractor is placed under the neck of the coracoid to retract the lower subscapularis. An Army-Navy or other right-angle retractor is often positioned superiorly.
- Meticulous glenoid bone bed preparation for the graft is important to facilitate union. A 70° angled saw blade is used to create a flat, bleeding bone surface centered at the 4:30 clock-face position.
- The ease and accuracy of graft positioning and fixation is greatly aided by the use of commercially available instruments at this point.
- The surgeon should use a parallel drill guide that will leave at least 2 mm of space between the guide and the coracoid process (usually the +6 offset) (**Figure 13, A**). The guide is placed into the 4-mm drill holes in the graft, and the graft is positioned so that it is congruent with the glenoid articular surface (**Figure 13, B**).
- The screws are placed at a 5° to 10° angle from lateral to medial (**Figure 6, C**).
- It is important to place the graft inferiorly on the glenoid, typically centered at approximately the 4:30 clock-face position (right shoulder).

Table 2 Rehabilitation Protocol After the Open Congruent-Arc Latarjet Procedure

Postoperative Week	ROM	Strengthening	Return to Activities	Comments
0-6	Pendulum (Codman) exercises are allowed	None	None	Sutures must be left in place for at least 3 wk postoperatively
6-12	Active-assisted forward elevation, external rotation, and internal rotation are begun	None	Resume light ADLs	The goal of the ROM exercises is to achieve external rotation equal to half that of the opposite shoulder by 12 wk
12-24	Continue active ROM	Rotator cuff strengthening by means of an exercise band is begun	May begin sports-specific rehabilitation except for contact sports or heavy labor	—
>24	—	Return to strengthening in the gym is allowed	Return to contact sports or heavy labor is allowed when bony union is evident radiographically (typically 9-12 mo after surgery)	—

ADLs = activities of daily living, ROM = range of motion.

- Guide pins are placed through the drill guide and advanced until they pass through the posterior cortex.
- In most patients, 34 mm (placed inferior) and 36 mm (placed superior) 3.75-mm cannulated screws can be placed over the guide pins without measuring. These self-drilling, self-tapping screws usually will penetrate the posterior cortex without predrilling the posterior cortex.
- The guide pins are removed before final seating of the screws.
- Two suture anchors are placed into the glenoid just superior and inferior to the graft-glenoid interface. Simple sutures are placed to reattach the capsular flap to the glenoid, leaving the graft extra-articular (**Figure 5**).
- The subscapularis tenotomy is closed with No. 2 nonabsorbable sutures.

Wound Closure
- The wound is irrigated.
- A standard layered skin closure is performed.

Rehabilitation

Some surgeons, especially those who advocate performing a subscapularis split, place few limitations on patients in the immediate postoperative period and allow return to full-contact athletics by 3 months postoperatively. In contrast, the authors of this chapter do not allow patients to engage in active-assisted range-of-motion exercises until 6 weeks postoperatively (**Table 2**). The authors of this chapter do not allow return to competitive athletic activities until union of the graft is seen on an axillary radiograph, which is often between 9 and 12 months postoperatively.

Avoiding Pitfalls

A preoperative CT scan should be obtained to measure glenoid bone loss and ensure that the coracoid has not been compromised by recurrent instability. When osteotomizing the coracoid, it is important to take care that neither the saw blade nor the osteotome exits into the face of the glenoid. Lateral

malpositioning of the graft should be avoided because it has been associated with arthritis at mid- and long-term follow-up. The congruent-arc technique often results in the appearance of slight overhang on a postoperative Grashey view (**Figure 4, B**) because of the extended length and curvature of the undersurface of the coracoid. The angle of the screws should be kept within 10° of the plane of the glenoid (the axial plane). Maintaining such an angle decreases the danger of too-medial exit of the screws, which would damage the suprascapular neurovascular structures. To minimize the risk of shearing off the tip of the guide pins, the authors of this chapter recommend removing the pins before fully seating the cannulated screws.

Bibliography

Allain J, Goutallier D, Glorion C: Long-term results of the Latarjet procedure for the treatment of anterior instability of the shoulder. *J Bone Joint Surg Am* 1998;80(6):841-852.

Armitage MS, Elkinson I, Giles JW, Athwal GS: An anatomic, computed tomographic assessment of the coracoid process with special reference to the congruent-arc Latarjet procedure. *Arthroscopy* 2011;27(11):1485-1489.

Arrigoni P, Huberty D, Brady PC, Weber IC, Burkhart SS: The value of arthroscopy before an open modified Latarjet reconstruction. *Arthroscopy* 2008;24(5):514-519.

Boileau P, Mercier N, Roussanne Y, Thélu CÉ, Old J: Arthroscopic Bankart-Bristow-Latarjet procedure: The development and early results of a safe and reproducible technique. *Arthroscopy* 2010;26(11):1434-1450.

Burkhart SS, De Beer JF, Barth JR, Cresswell T, Roberts C, Richards DP: Results of modified Latarjet reconstruction in patients with anteroinferior instability and significant bone loss. *Arthroscopy* 2007;23(10):1033-1041.

Burkhart SS, DeBeer JF, Tehrany AM, Parten PM: Quantifying glenoid bone loss arthroscopically in shoulder instability. *Arthroscopy* 2002;18(5):488-491.

Butt U, Charalambous CP: Arthroscopic coracoid transfer in the treatment of recurrent shoulder instability: A systematic review of early results. *Arthroscopy* 2013;29(4):774-779.

de Beer J, Burkhart SS, Roberts CP, van Rooyen K, Cresswell T, du Toit DF: The congruent-arc Latarjet. *Techniques in Shoulder & Elbow Surgery* 2009;10(2):62-67.

Di Giacomo G, Itoi E, Burkhart SS: Evolving concept of bipolar bone loss and the Hill-Sachs lesion: From "engaging/non-engaging" lesion to "on-track/off-track" lesion. *Arthroscopy* 2014;30(1):90-98.

Dumont GD, Fogerty S, Rosso C, Lafosse L: The arthroscopic Latarjet procedure for anterior shoulder instability: 5-year minimum follow-up. *Am J Sports Med* 2014;42(11):2560-2566.

Edwards TB, Walch G: The Latarjet procedure for recurrent anterior shoulder instability: Rationale and technique. *Oper Tech Sports Med* 2002;10(1):25-32.

Ghodadra N, Gupta A, Romeo AA, et al: Normalization of glenohumeral articular contact pressures after Latarjet or iliac crest bone-grafting. *J Bone Joint Surg Am* 2010;92(6):1478-1489.

Giles JW, Puskas G, Welsh M, Johnson JA, Athwal GS: Do the traditional and modified Latarjet techniques produce equivalent reconstruction stability and strength? *Am J Sports Med* 2012;40(12):2801-2807.

Griesser MJ, Harris JD, McCoy BW, et al: Complications and re-operations after Bristow-Latarjet shoulder stabilization: A systematic review. *J Shoulder Elbow Surg* 2013;22(2):286-292.

Hovelius L, Sandström B, Sundgren K, Saebö M: One hundred eighteen Bristow-Latarjet repairs for recurrent anterior dislocation of the shoulder prospectively followed for fifteen years: Study I. Clinical results. *J Shoulder Elbow Surg* 2004;13(5):509-516.

Koo SS, Burkhart SS, Ochoa E: Arthroscopic double-pulley remplissage technique for engaging Hill-Sachs lesions in anterior shoulder instability repairs. *Arthroscopy* 2009;25(11):1343-1348.

Advanced Reconstruction: Shoulder 2   *© 2016 American Academy of Orthopaedic Surgeons*

Lädermann A, Denard PJ, Burkhart SS: Injury of the suprascapular nerve during Latarjet procedure: An anatomic study. *Arthroscopy* 2012;28(3):316-321.

Lafosse L, Boyle S: Arthroscopic Latarjet procedure. *J Shoulder Elbow Surg* 2010;19(2 suppl):2-12.

Mizuno N, Denard PJ, Raiss P, Melis B, Walch G: Long-term results of the Latarjet procedure for anterior instability of the shoulder. *J Shoulder Elbow Surg* 2014;23(11):1691-1699.

Shah AA, Butler B, Romanowski J, Goel D, Karadagli D, Warner JJP: Short-term complications of the Latarjet procedure. *J Bone Joint Surg Am* 2012;94(6):495-501.

Singer GC, Kirkland PM, Emery RJ: Coracoid transposition for recurrent anterior instability of the shoulder: A 20-year follow-up study. *J Bone Joint Surg Br* 1995;77(1):73-76.

Walch G, Boileau P: Latarjet-Bristow procedure for recurrent anterior instability. *Techniques in Shoulder & Elbow Surgery* 2000;1(4):256-261.

Yamamoto N, Muraki T, An KN, et al: The stabilizing mechanism of the Latarjet procedure: A cadaveric study. *J Bone Joint Surg Am* 2013;95(15):1390-1397.

Video Reference

Burkhart SS, Hartzler RU: Video. *Latarjet Surgical Technique.* San Antonio, TX, 2015.

Chapter 8

Anterior Instability With Severe Glenoid Bone Loss: Bone Grafting Options and Techniques

Matthew T. Provencher, MD, CDR, MC, USNR

George Christian Vorys, MD

George Sánchez, BS

 ## Introduction

The management of recurrent traumatic anterior shoulder instability remains a controversial and challenging topic. Shoulder instability occurs as a result of multiple, often overlapping factors. One common factor is glenoid bone loss (GBL). Bone loss occurs from recurrent subluxations or dislocations in conjunction with attritional bone loss. Paramount to the success of a surgical stabilization is a thorough understanding of the lesion type in a given patient. Injury to the anterior labrum or attenuation of the capsule is the most common cause of instability and can be addressed with a soft-tissue procedure alone; however, a growing body of evidence suggests that GBL exists more frequently than previously appreciated and is a common cause of recurrent instability if not addressed. It is generally accepted that bony reconstruction of the glenoid is recommended in patients who have substantial bone loss.

When GBL is suspected, CT with three-dimensional reconstructions should be obtained to fully appreciate and quantify the amount of bone loss. A reliable technique for this purpose is the so-called perfect circle measurement. The glenoid is carefully examined in the sagittal en face and oblique views. The inferior two-thirds of the glenoid closely approximates a perfect circle, allowing for accurate measurement of the percentage of anterior bone loss on the sagittal en face view. On the sagittal oblique view, the anterior glenoid should have a sharp contour, whereas anterior bone loss shows a blunted edge.

Traditionally, bone loss resulting from recurrent anterior instability has been studied in isolation, on the humeral side (the Hill-Sachs lesion) or the glenoid side. Recently, it has been shown that shoulder instability in the setting of bone loss is a bipolar issue. The introduction of the glenoid track concept has shed further light on the effects of bone loss resulting from anterior shoulder instability. The glenoid track is defined as the region on the superolateral humeral head articulating with the anterior glenoid in arm positions of abduction and external rotation. A Hill-Sachs lesion inside the glenoid track has little chance for engagement and resulting instability, whereas a lesion outside the track will lead to engagement and, ultimately, cause instability. Biomechanical studies have shown that the glenoid track depends entirely on the width of the glenoid; therefore, GBL leads to a decrease in the size of the glenoid track and a greater likelihood that a Hill-Sachs lesion will engage (**Figure 1**). Reconstruction of the glenoid or the Hill-Sachs lesion with bone graft restores the glenoid track. A clinical study of a series of 205 patients by the senior author of this chapter (M.T.P.) validated that measurements of Hill-Sachs and glenoid deficits taken using the glenoid track concept predict engagement, aiding preoperative planning. Some patients have severe defects on the glenoid and the humeral side, requiring both defects to be addressed at the time of surgery; however, most patients have a clinically insignificant Hill-Sachs lesion after bony glenoid reconstruction.

Dr. Provencher or an immediate family member has received royalties from Arthrex; serves as a paid consultant to or is an employee of Arthrex and the Joint Restoration Foundation; and serves as a board member, owner, officer, or committee member of the American Academy of Orthopaedic Surgeons, the American Orthopaedic Society for Sports Medicine, the American Shoulder and Elbow Surgeons, the Arthroscopy Association of North America, the San Diego Shoulder Institute, the Society of Military Orthopaedic Surgeons, and the International Society of Arthroscopy, Knee Surgery and Orthopaedic Sports Medicine. Neither of the following authors nor any immediate family member has received anything of value from or has stock or stock options held in a commercial company or institution related directly or indirectly to the subject of this chapter: Dr. Vorys and Mr. Sanchez.

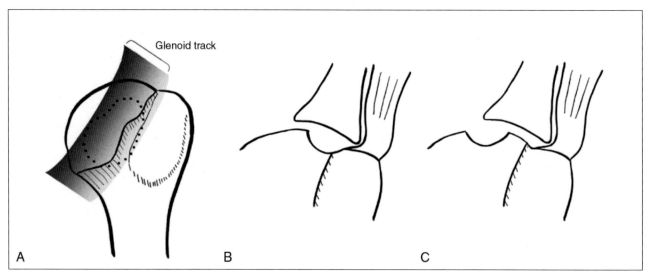

Figure 1   Illustrations depict the glenoid track concept, which is used to take into account both glenoid and humeral head bone loss to determine the risk of instability and engagement. **A,** With the arm in abduction and external rotation, the glenoid is in contact with the lateral articular margin of the humerus. **B,** If a Hill-Sachs lesion lies medial to this zone of contact, it can engage, causing instability. **C,** If the defect is inside the glenoid track, however, it will not engage and will be asymptomatic. (Reproduced from Provencher MT, Frank RM, LeClere LE, et al: The Hill-Sachs lesion: Diagnosis, classification, and management. *J Am Acad Orthop Surg* 2012;20[4]:242-252.)

Many surgical techniques have been described to reconstruct bony loss on the glenoid, including the Bristow procedure, the Latarjet procedure, and the iliac crest autograft technique as well as various allograft options. The Bristow and Latarjet procedures are nonanatomic reconstruction procedures and are effective at restoring stability, but they have been shown to have related complications such as degenerative changes that develop in the glenohumeral joint, hardware failure, and graft resorption. Bone grafting with the coracoid process may also be insufficient or unavailable in patients who have severe bone loss or in revision settings; these conditions would be better addressed with autograft or allograft reconstruction.

 Case Presentation

The patient is a 25-year-old, right-hand–dominant man in an active-duty U.S. Army Special Forces unit who has recurrent traumatic right shoulder instability. He initially sustained a traumatic anterior dislocation, which was reduced in the emergency department and managed nonsurgically in a sling. Recurrent instability subsequently developed during minimal levels of activity, with more than 30 dislocations as well as subluxation events. The patient's instability was so severe that dislocations became frequent during sleep. Plain radiographs demonstrated severe GBL, which was confirmed as involving 40% of the anterior glenoid on sagittal three-dimensional CT. In addition, a small Hill-Sachs lesion was present (**Figure 2**). Given the extensive bone loss and multiple recurrences, a soft-tissue procedure was deemed to be insufficient for the goal of long-term stability of the shoulder. Thus, a bony augmentation procedure was chosen.

Indications

Shoulder instability resulting from injury to the capsulolabral complex without substantial GBL can be managed with open or arthroscopic shoulder stabilization alone. Most surgeons recommend bone grafting to manage GBL greater than 20% to 25%. In patients who have severe GBL, however, the coracoid process may be insufficient for reconstruction of the glenoid. Some studies have suggested that GBL greater than 30% to 40% is a contraindication to the Latarjet procedure. In patients who have severe GBL or in the revision setting (that is, after a failed Latarjet procedure), tricortical iliac crest autograft and fresh distal tibia allograft are viable options.

In biomechanical studies, the distal tibia has been shown to have a radius of curvature almost identical to that of the glenoid. The distal tibia also has a cartilaginous surface that is identical in thickness to that of the glenoid and confers near anatomic articular conformity to the native glenoid (**Figure 3**). A biomechanical study examining the glenohumeral contact area, contact pressure, and peak forces seen in a Latarjet reconstruction or distal tibia allograft reconstruction of a 30% glenoid defect demonstrated substantially higher glenohumeral contact areas and substantially lower peak forces after distal tibia allograft. Distal tibia allograft offers a number of benefits, including a source

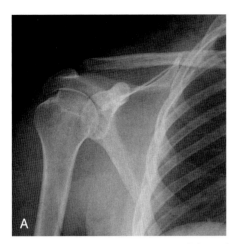
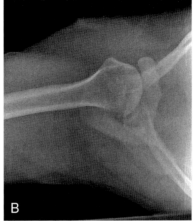
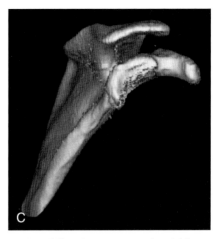

Figure 2 Preoperative images of the right shoulder of a patient with recurrent anterior instability demonstrate glenoid bone loss and a moderate Hill-Sachs lesion. **A,** AP radiograph of the shoulder with the humerus in slight internal rotation demonstrates a Hill-Sachs lesion as well as anterior cortical irregularity of the glenoid, which suggests anterior glenoid bone loss. **B,** Axillary radiograph demonstrates loss of cortical contour of the anterior glenoid, which suggests anterior glenoid bone loss. **C,** Preoperative three-dimensional sagittal CT scan demonstrates approximately 40% to 45% attritional glenoid bone loss of the anterior glenoid.

of articular cartilage, a robust subchondral bone ideal for fixation, lack of donor site morbidity, and considerable availability without the need for size-matched donor grafts. The inner table of the iliac crest also provides a suitable match to the radius of curvature of the glenoid articular surface. Although iliac crest autograft is readily available and theoretically has better healing potential and a lower risk of infection than allograft, autograft has the disadvantage of substantial donor site morbidity.

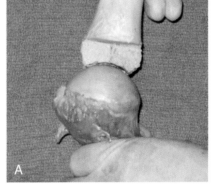
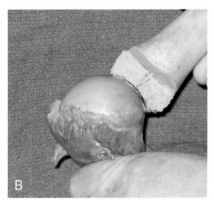

Figure 3 **A** and **B,** Clinical photographs of unmatched cadaver specimens show excellent articular conformity (radius of curvature) between the humeral head and the lateral aspect of the distal tibia along different points of the humeral head.

Controversies and Alternative Approaches

Numerous grafting alternatives have been described for patients who have severe GBL or in the revision setting, including fresh osteochondral glenoid, frozen humeral head, and frozen femoral head, with a paucity of outcomes reported in the literature because of the relative rarity of severe GBL. The literature supports arthroscopic shoulder stabilization in patients in whom the bony fragment can be mobilized and repaired back to its anatomic location. In the setting of attritional bone loss, however, a high rate of recurrent instability with arthroscopic management has been demonstrated in multiple studies. The principles of surgical management are guided by the extent of the combined glenoid and humeral bone defects, surgeon preference, and patient-specific factors such as work or athletic demands and preferences regarding allograft versus autograft.

Results

The results of prominent studies using techniques similar to those described in this chapter are summarized in **Table 1.** Positive outcomes were achieved with each bone augmentation technique studied, including the iliac crest bone autograft, tricortical iliac crest bone graft, and distal tibia allograft procedure. Failure rates were minimal, and return to activity was rapid. In addition, for each procedure, graft incorporation

Table 1 Results of Iliac Crest Autograft and Distal Tibia Allograft to Manage Anterior Instability With Severe Glenoid Bone Loss

Authors	Journal (Year)	Technique (No. of Patients)	Outcomes	Failure Rate (%)	Comments
Haaker et al	*Mil Med* (1993)	Iliac crest autograft (24)	No dislocations 90% patient satisfaction rate	0	Graft incorporation was verified radiographically Follow-up, 6-42 mo
Warner et al	*Am J Sports Med* (2006)	Tricortical iliac crest bone graft (11)	No dislocations All patients returned to their preinjury levels of sport	0	Graft incorporation was verified via three-dimensional CT Follow-up, 4-6 mo
Khazzam et al	*Am J Orthop (Belle Mead NJ)* (2009)	Iliac crest autograft (10)	1 failure from trauma Mean outcomes scores: Constant, 94; ASES, 83; UCLA, 32	10	Outcome scores recorded at mean follow-up of 25 mo
Provencher et al	*Arthroscopy* (2009)	Distal tibia allograft (3)	Return to full activity at 4-6 mo	0	Full incorporation to native glenoid demonstrated on CT Mean follow-up, 4 mo
Provencher et al	*J Bone Joint Surg Am* (2010)	Distal tibia allograft (1)	Return to full duties at 7 mo	0	Follow-up, 16 mo

ASES = American Shoulder and Elbow Surgeons shoulder outcome, UCLA = University of California–Los Angeles Shoulder Rating Scale.

was verified on plain radiographs or three-dimensional CT. However, lack of postoperative morbidity was unique to the distal tibia allograft procedure.

Technical Keys to Success

Tricortical Iliac Crest Autograft for GBL

SETUP

- The procedure is performed under general anesthesia, with regional anesthesia if desired.
- The patient must be anesthetized sufficiently to allow muscle paralysis to relax the shoulder and facilitate exposure.
- The patient is placed in the beach-chair position with the head of the bed elevated to 40°.
- A bump is placed under the contralateral hip to prepare for a contralateral iliac crest bone graft harvest. The iliac crest also is prepared

separately from the surgical field.
- Several blue towels are placed behind the medial border of the scapula to prevent anterior rotation of the glenoid and scapula and to stabilize the area for glenoid preparation and fixation. This position also optimizes the trajectory of the screw fixation of the allograft.
- The surgical arm is placed in a commercially available arm holder or left free on a padded Mayo stand (**Figure 4**).

EXPOSURE

- A deltopectoral approach is used, with an incision extending from the tip of the coracoid process directly inferior to the superior axillary fold for approximately 7 cm. The incision is more medial than the standard incision used in arthroplasty.
- After the deltopectoral interval is identified, the cephalic vein is retracted laterally, and the fascia over the conjoined tendon is identified

and incised with Metzenbaum scissors.
- The lateral aspect of the conjoined tendon is incised just lateral to the muscle belly of the short head of the biceps.
- Retractors are placed under the deltoid as well as underneath the lateral aspect of the conjoined tendon to expose the subscapularis muscle. The glenoid is exposed with a subscapularis split.
- The subscapularis tendon is identified and incised longitudinally at the midpoint. The capsule is separated off the subscapularis medially. In a revision setting, it may be necessary to incise the subscapularis tendon with the capsule.
- After the capsule is identified, it is incised with an inverted L-shaped capsulotomy such that the apex of the "L" is toward the superomedial aspect of the joint capsule. The capsule is elevated as far medially off the glenoid as possible in a

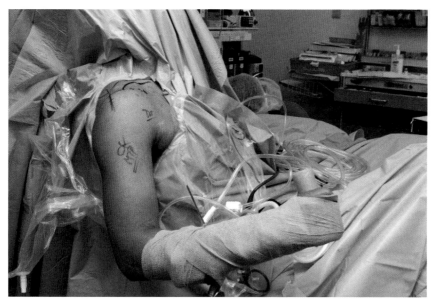

Figure 4 Preoperative photograph shows a patient prepared and draped in the beach-chair position with the head of the bed elevated to 40° in preparation for bone grafting to manage severe glenoid bone loss.

subperiosteal fashion, and the corner of the "L" is tagged with a No. 2 nonabsorbable suture.

- After identifying the anterior glenoid, the amount of GBL is confirmed and compared with that seen during preoperative planning. In general, bone loss of approximately 25% to 30% requires a graft measuring 8 to 9 mm. Every 1.5 mm of bone loss corresponds to approximately 5% of GBL.

- Any remaining labral tissue is preserved carefully and dissected medially, taking care to preserve the axillary nerve. The labrum may be deficient, particularly in a revision setting, and may not be amenable to repair.

- A high-speed burr and/or a hand rasp is used to prepare the native anterior glenoid and create a uniform surface as perpendicular as possible to the articular surface to accommodate graft fixation.

- Attention is turned to the iliac crest autograft harvest.

TRICORTICAL ILIAC CREST AUTOGRAFT HARVEST AND FIXATION

- The anterior superior iliac spine (ASIS) and the iliac crest are identified. The incision is made just posterior to the ASIS and parallel to the iliac crest, taking care to avoid the lateral femoral cutaneous nerve.

- The fascia is incised parallel to the iliac crest, and the soft tissue is dissected off the inner and outer table. A wide, bent Hohmann retractor is useful to expose the inner table.

- The graft is outlined using an oscillating saw to harvest a tricortical iliac crest bone graft measuring approximately 3 cm long and 1.5 cm deep.

- With the help of an assistant, the graft is contoured with the sagittal saw on the back table. The inner concave table of the iliac crest will become the articulating portion of the graft.

- Attention is returned to the glenohumeral joint exposure and defect. The graft is placed into the defect

to confirm the fit and is contoured further if necessary.

- The graft is fixed provisionally with Kirschner wires (K-wires) at a 45° angle to the glenoid.

- Final fixation is achieved with two 3.5 or 4.0 fully threaded noncannulated screws, which are placed as parallel as possible to the glenoid, using a lag technique. Again, the inner table of the graft provides the concave articulating portion of the reconstruction.

- The interface is palpated to confirm a smooth transition and is contoured with a burr if fine adjustments are required.

- The capsulolabral complex then is repaired with No. 2 nonabsorbable sutures that are anchored under the screw heads or suture washers.

- The wound is irrigated, and closure is completed in the standard fashion.

- The subscapularis is reapproximated with a No. 2 nonabsorbable suture in the tendinous portion. The capsule is repaired, making this an interarticular graft.

- Typically, a drain is not required. The arm is placed in an abduction sling.

Alternative Technique: Distal Tibia Allograft for GBL

Video 8.1 Distal Tibial Allograft for Glenoid Bone Loss and Loss of Articular Cartilage. Matthew T. Provencher, MD, CDR, MC, USNR (8 min)

- The patient is placed in the beach-chair position, and the glenoid is exposed as described previously.

- After identifying and confirming the size of the glenoid defect, the surgeon focuses on allograft preparation.

- With the help of an assistant, the fresh distal tibia allograft is prepared on the back table. After the graft is removed from the serum bath, the lateral one-third of the tibial plafond is measured and marked to accommodate the glenoid defect. An assistant stabilizes the graft with two large clamps, and the graft is cut with a 0.5-in thin blade sagittal saw.

- Frequent irrigation is used to prevent thermal necrosis.
- The allograft is cut medially at a 10° to 15° angle to accommodate any changes in glenoid slope and to restore the natural concavity.
- The superior and inferior aspects of the graft are rounded with the sagittal saw to match the native glenoid contour. The graft is 1 cm deep medial to lateral and 22 to 25 mm long superior to inferior, with a 7- to 10-mm anterior-posterior articular surface (**Figure 5**).
- Two 1.6-mm K-wires are placed in the graft at a 45° angle to the articular surface, away from the location of screw fixation (**Figure 6**).
- Before fixation, the graft is copiously irrigated with 3 L of lactated Ringer solution using pulsed lavage.
- The graft is transferred to the native glenoid to assess the fit and the congruity. Final adjustments are made with the sagittal saw as necessary.
- The K-wires are driven into the glenoid for provisional fixation.
- Two 3.5-mm cortical screws are placed in a lag fashion with a washer, as parallel to the glenoid as possible (**Figure 7**).
- The labrum and capsule are repaired with No. 2 nonabsorbable sutures anchored under the washer before final tightening.
- The wound is irrigated, and closure is completed in the standard fashion.
- The subscapularis split is reapproximated with a No. 2 nonabsorbable suture in the tendinous portion.
- Typically, a drain is not required. The arm is placed in an abduction sling.

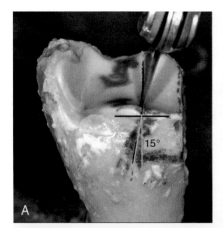
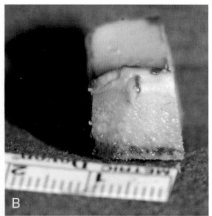
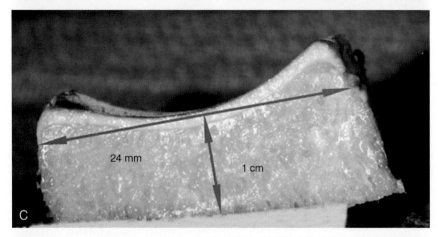

Figure 5   Intraoperative photographs demonstrate distal tibia allograft preparation. **A,** The lateral aspect of the distal tibia is measured and cut for the graft. Note the 15° angle of the sagittal saw on the graft-glenoid interface side of the distal tibia. **B,** The width of the graft is measured based on preoperative CT and intraoperative findings. **C,** The superior-inferior view of the prepared graft is shown. The graft is contoured to a depth of 1 cm and a superior-inferior dimension of 24 mm.

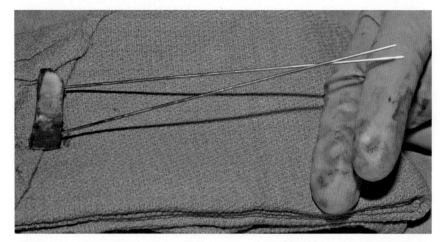

Figure 6   Intraoperative photograph shows provisional fixation of a distal tibia allograft. Two 1.6-mm Kirschner wires are placed away from the final screw fixation sites at a 45° angle to avoid penetration of the articular surface.

Rehabilitation

Postoperatively, the patient begins pendulum and passive range of motion (ROM) exercises in the scapular plane for the first 2 weeks as well as

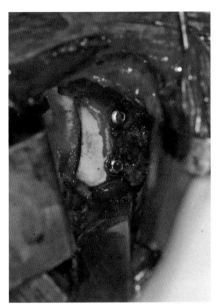

Figure 7 Intraoperative photograph of the anterior glenoid demonstrates two 3.5-mm screws that are used to fix the distal tibia to the anterior glenoid via the lag technique.

scapular strengthening exercises such as low rows (**Table 2**). From postoperative weeks 2 to 4, progressive passive and active-assisted ROM exercises are begun. At 4 weeks postoperatively, active ROM begins, followed by a more extensive strengthening program. Return to sport occurs at 4 to 6 months postoperatively, depending on graft incorporation, functional ROM, and strength. CT is obtained routinely to confirm graft incorporation (**Figures 8** and **9**).

Avoiding Pitfalls

Tricortical Iliac Crest Autograft for GBL

The exposure of the anterior glenoid is optimized with proper patient positioning and the use of towels under the medial border of the scapula. It is important to preserve as much of the capsulolabral tissue as possible during the exposure using a humeral-based, inverted, L-shaped capsulotomy because the tissue, if available, will be repaired to the graft. The K-wires are placed at a 45° angle to the articular surface to achieve

optimal purchase and avoid articular surface penetration. The screws, however, are placed as parallel as possible to the glenoid. To prevent graft rotation, the surgeon should avoid fully tightening the first screw until the second screw is seated. The typical screw length is between 32 and 38 mm.

Distal Tibia Allograft for GBL

It is important to ensure that the graft bed is as perpendicular as possible to the glenoid articular surface to allow for optimal congruity of the graft/articular surface. In general, cutting the allograft medial interface at 10° to 15° best restores the natural concavity of the glenoid. The K-wires are placed at the superior and inferior margins of the graft for provisional fixation. The fully threaded cortical screws are later placed in different locations for final fixation using a lag technique. Washers are used with No. 2 nonabsorbable sutures secured underneath to secure the anterior capsule. Before fixation, the graft is irrigated generously on the back table with 3 L of lactated Ringer solution using pulsed lavage.

Table 2 Rehabilitation Protocol After Bone Augmentation for Severe Glenoid Bone Loss

Postoperative Week	ROM	Strengthening	Return to Play	Comments/ Emphasis
0-2	Pendulum and passive exercises	Scapular (eg, low rows, prone extension, prone rowing exercise, external rotation and internal rotation exercises)	NA	NA
2-4	Progressive passive and active-assisted exercises are begun	Scapular (eg, low rows, prone extension, prone rowing exercise, external rotation and internal rotation exercises)	NA	NA
4-16	At 4 wk, active is begun	Scapular exercises and exercises of other shoulder girdle musculature at approximately 4 mo	NA	NA
16-24	Full ROM exercises and terminal stretching are emphasized	Full strengthening program is begun at 10-20 wk	Begun depending on graft incorporation, functional ROM, and strength	Obtain CT routinely to confirm graft incorporation

NA = not applicable, ROM = range of motion.

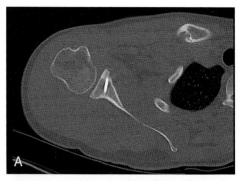 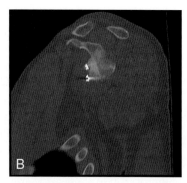 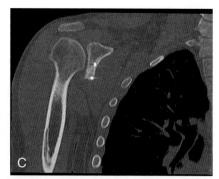

Figure 8   Images obtained 4 months postoperatively demonstrate incorporation of a fresh distal tibia allograft on axillary (**A**) and sagittal (**B**) CT scans and incorporation and bridging of bone with no evidence of lysis on a coronal CT scan (**C**).

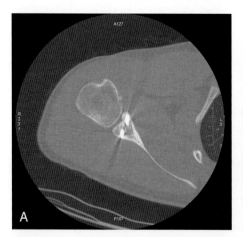 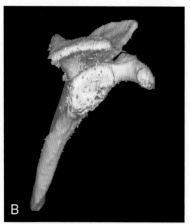

Figure 9   Images of a severe glenoid defect that was treated with tricortical iliac crest bone graft (autograft). Postoperative axial CT scan (**A**) and three-dimensional CT reconstruction (**B**) demonstrate graft incorporation and good hardware position.

 # Bibliography

Arciero RA, Parrino A, Bernhardson AS, et al: The effect of a combined glenoid and Hill-Sachs defect on glenohumeral stability: A biomechanical cadaveric study using 3-dimensional modeling of 142 patients. *Am J Sports Med* 2015;43(6):1422-1429.

Bhatia S, Frank RM, Ghodadra NS, et al: The outcomes and surgical techniques of the latarjet procedure. *Arthroscopy* 2014;30(2):227-235.

Bhatia S, Van Thiel GS, Gupta D, et al: Comparison of glenohumeral contact pressures and contact areas after glenoid reconstruction with latarjet or distal tibial osteochondral allografts. *Am J Sports Med* 2013;41(8):1900-1908.

Bigliani LU, Newton PM, Steinmann SP, Connor PM, McIlveen SJ: Glenoid rim lesions associated with recurrent anterior dislocation of the shoulder. *Am J Sports Med* 1998;26(1):41-45.

Burkhart SS, De Beer JF: Traumatic glenohumeral bone defects and their relationship to failure of arthroscopic Bankart repairs: Significance of the inverted-pear glenoid and the humeral engaging Hill-Sachs lesion. *Arthroscopy* 2000;16(7):677-694.

Griesser MJ, Harris JD, McCoy BW, et al: Complications and re-operations after Bristow-Latarjet shoulder stabilization: A systematic review. *J Shoulder Elbow Surg* 2013;22(2):286-292.

Griffith JF, Antonio GE, Yung PS, et al: Prevalence, pattern, and spectrum of glenoid bone loss in anterior shoulder dislocation: CT analysis of 218 patients. *AJR Am J Roentgenol* 2008;190(5):1247-1254.

Haaker RG, Eickhoff U, Klammer HL: Intraarticular autogenous bone grafting in recurrent shoulder dislocations. *Mil Med* 1993;158(3):164-169.

Huijsmans PE, Haen PS, Kidd M, Dhert WJ, van der Hulst VP, Willems WJ: Quantification of a glenoid defect with three-dimensional computed tomography and magnetic resonance imaging: A cadaveric study. *J Shoulder Elbow Surg* 2007;16(6):803-809.

Huysmans PE, Haen PS, Kidd M, Dhert WJ, Willems JW: The shape of the inferior part of the glenoid: A cadaveric study. *J Shoulder Elbow Surg* 2006;15(6):759-763.

Itoi E, Lee SB, Amrami KK, Wenger DE, An KN: Quantitative assessment of classic anteroinferior bony Bankart lesions by radiography and computed tomography. *Am J Sports Med* 2003;31(1):112-118.

Itoi E, Lee SB, Berglund LJ, Berge LL, An KN: The effect of a glenoid defect on anteroinferior stability of the shoulder after Bankart repair: A cadaveric study. *J Bone Joint Surg Am* 2000;82(1):35-46.

Khazzam M, Kane SM, Smith MJ: Open shoulder stabilization procedure using bone block technique for treatment of chronic glenohumeral instability associated with bony glenoid deficiency. *Am J Orthop (Belle Mead NJ)* 2009;38(7):329-335.

LeClere L, Bernhardson AS, Metzger P, et al: Recent advances in the diagnosis and treatment of glenohumeral bone loss, in Provencher MT, Romeo AA, eds: *Shoulder Instability: A Comprehensive Approach.* Philadelphia, PA, Saunders, 2012, pp 248-258.

Metzger PD, Barlow B, Leonardelli D, Peace W, Solomon DJ, Provencher MT: Clinical application of the "glenoid track" concept for defining humeral head engagement in anterior shoulder instability: A preliminary report. *Orthop J Sports Med* 2013;1(2):2325967113496213.

Mologne TS, Provencher MT, Menzel KA, Vachon TA, Dewing CB: Arthroscopic stabilization in patients with an inverted pear glenoid: Results in patients with bone loss of the anterior glenoid. *Am J Sports Med* 2007;35(8):1276-1283.

Provencher MT, Bhatia S, Ghodadra NS, et al: Recurrent shoulder instability: Current concepts for evaluation and management of glenoid bone loss. *J Bone Joint Surg Am* 2010;92(suppl 2):133-151.

Provencher MT, Ghodadra N, LeClere L, Solomon DJ, Romeo AA: Anatomic osteochondral glenoid reconstruction for recurrent glenohumeral instability with glenoid deficiency using a distal tibia allograft. *Arthroscopy* 2009;25(4):446-452.

Rowe CR, Zarins B, Ciullo JV: Recurrent anterior dislocation of the shoulder after surgical repair: Apparent causes of failure and treatment. *J Bone Joint Surg Am* 1984;66(2):159-168.

Sugaya H, Moriishi J, Dohi M, Kon Y, Tsuchiya A: Glenoid rim morphology in recurrent anterior glenohumeral instability. *J Bone Joint Surg Am* 2003;85(5):878-884.

Warner JJ, Gill TJ, O'Hollerhan JD, Pathare N, Millett PJ: Anatomical glenoid reconstruction for recurrent anterior glenohumeral instability with glenoid deficiency using an autogenous tricortical iliac crest bone graft. *Am J Sports Med* 2006;34(2):205-212.

Yamamoto N, Itoi E, Abe H, et al: Contact between the glenoid and the humeral head in abduction, external rotation, and horizontal extension: A new concept of glenoid track. *J Shoulder Elbow Surg* 2007;16(5):649-656.

 Video Reference

Provencher MT: Video. *Distal Tibial Allograft for Glenoid Bone Loss and Loss of Articular Cartilage.* San Diego, CA, 2015.

Chapter 9

The Open Bankart Procedure for Bone Loss, Revision Surgery, and Soft-Tissue Deficiency

Russell F. Warren, MD

K. Durham Weeks, MD

 Case Presentation

Case 1

A 22-year-old college student who is a rugby player sustained a dislocated shoulder and experienced multiple recurrences. Examination of the shoulder elicits apprehension at 90° of elevation, which is relieved by a relocation test, and a 2+ sulcus sign with anterior apprehension and crepitus with some posterior play. Radiographic evaluation demonstrates a centered humeral head, a small Hill-Sachs lesion, and glenoid bone loss of approximately 15% (**Figure 1**). Glenoid bone loss of approximately 20% and a small Hill-Sachs lesion are noted on CT (**Figure 2**). On MRI, the rotator cuff is shown to be intact, and bone loss and the presence of a Bankart lesion are confirmed.

A surgical approach is discussed with the patient, who elects to undergo arthroscopy followed by an open Bankart repair and capsular shift. The authors of this chapter routinely perform arthroscopy on all shoulders after examination under anesthesia. The examination is critical in determining the degree and direction of the instability.

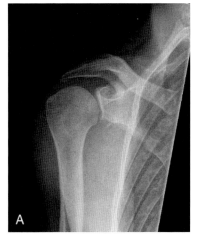 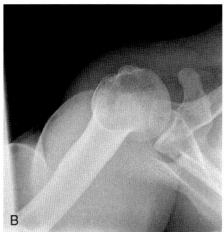

Figure 1   **A,** AP radiograph of the shoulder demonstrates a bony Bankart lesion with a concentric joint. **B,** Axillary radiograph demonstrates a small Hill-Sachs lesion and anterior glenoid bone loss.

Subluxation without bone loss is managed with an arthroscopic repair, but an open procedure is warranted to manage marked laxity and bone loss of 20%. The instability severity index score can aid in identifying patients who may benefit from an open rather than an arthroscopic approach. Successful results without grafting have been reported in patients with less than 20% bone loss; the need for graft in such situations is not definitive. The arthroscopy

preceding the open procedures helps identify posterior injury that might require a repair. In rare instances, if a Hill-Sachs lesion is large, remplissage can be performed before repair.

Case 2

An 18-year-old lacrosse player had undergone radiofrequency capsular shrinkage that had provided stability for 2 years, after which he experienced several more episodes of instability. On stability examination, the patient has apprehension at 90° of elevation and increased translation. His strength is normal. Radiographs demonstrate excellent bone stock, and MRI demonstrates

Dr. Warren or an immediate family member has received royalties from Biomet and has stock or stock options held in Ivy Sports Medicine and OrthoNet. Neither Dr. Weeks nor any immediate family member has received anything of value from or has stock or stock options held in a commercial company or institution related directly or indirectly to the subject of this chapter.

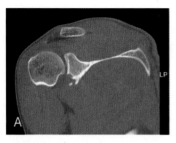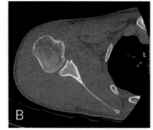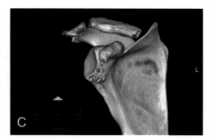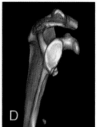

Figure 2   Coronal (**A**) and axial (**B**) CT scans demonstrate anterior glenoid bone loss and a Hill-Sachs lesion. **C** and **D**, Three-dimensional CT reconstructions demonstrate the glenoid injury and the Hill-Sachs lesion.

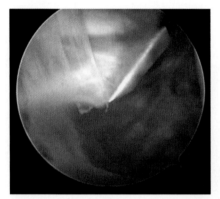

Figure 3   Arthroscopic view of a translucent anterior capsular deficiency resulting from previous radiofrequency ablation.

capsular injury with an intact subscapularis. Surgical options are discussed with the patient, and he elects to undergo arthroscopy (**Figure 3**) followed by an open capsular repair with a human dermal allograft.

 Indications

Open Bankart repair allows the surgeon to address inferior and anterior capsular laxity by means of an open lateral shift on the humeral head down to the 6-o'clock position while advancing the capsule superiorly and laterally, followed by closure of the rotator interval. The Bankart repair is performed in an inside-out manner. This technique is indicated in patients who participate in high-impact sports, for recurrent instability after arthroscopic stabilization, in patients with midsubstance capsular tears and anterior laxity, and for primary repair of bony avulsions. Open surgery is associated with more risks compared with arthroscopic stabilization. The primary concerns after any open procedure for shoulder instability are injury to the subscapularis, loss of external rotation, and increased incidence of osteoarthritis.

 Controversies and Alternative Approaches

Bone Loss

After primary arthroscopic stabilization, an increased failure rate has been noted in patients with glenohumeral bone loss. The amount of bone loss associated with failure is unknown. However, in the past few years, bone grafting has been increasingly used to repair these defects. The authors of this chapter support the use of a Latarjet or Bristow procedure to manage bony defects greater than 25% (approximately 6 mm). However, in many patients with smaller defects, an isolated Bankart repair with or without a capsular shift is sufficient, depending on the degree of capsular laxity. If a substantial Hill-Sachs lesion is present, then arthroscopic remplissage without grafting can be added to the open repair. Advanced imaging, including CT, can help elucidate the amount of bone loss and evaluate for a humeral-side engaging Hill-Sachs lesion.

Revision Surgery

Revision surgery to manage anterior shoulder instability is fraught with problems and failures. The anatomic, surgical, and patient-specific issues that led to failure must be identified. The initial surgical report should be reviewed, if possible. The treating surgeon should discern whether the surgeon who performed the previous procedure or procedures addressed all pathology, note how many anchors were used and where they were placed, consider the current diagnosis, note whether the patient has joint laxity, assess the uninjured shoulder, and inquire about family history of shoulder instability. Radiographs, CT, and MRI are of paramount importance in patient evaluation and determining whether arthroscopic surgery could be successful. Glenoid bone defects of greater than 25% require bone graft; smaller defects are managed with arthroscopy followed by open Bankart repair and a capsular shift.

Capsular Deficiency

Soft-tissue deficiency may present as capsular rupture, damage to the capsule caused by prior radiofrequency ablation, loss or attenuation of the subscapularis, or a combination of these with bone loss. If radiofrequency ablation was used, then the capsule may be deficient. If an open procedure was performed, then the subscapularis may have avulsed and retracted to a variable degree. In either case, anterior shoulder

Table 1 Results of Revision Open Bankart Repair

Author(s)	Journal (Year)	Technique (No. of Patients)	Outcomes	Failure Rate (%)[a]	Comments
Rowe et al	*J Bone Joint Surg Am* (1984)	Revision open Bankart repair (24)	10 excellent, 12 good, 2 poor	8	Mean follow-up, 24 mo 84% of shoulders had a new Bankart lesion at the time of revision
Sisto	*Am J Sports Med* (2007)	Revision open Bankart repair with capsular shift (30)	Significant improvement in Rowe and UCLA scores ($P < 0.05$)	0	Mean follow-up, 46 mo 87% returned to preinjury level of sports activity 13% were unable to return to their preinjury level of sports activity
Cheung et al	*J Shoulder Elbow Surg* (2008)	Revision open Bankart repair with capsular shift (34)	Improvements in Rowe, ASES, and SST scores as well as functional measures; no significant difference in outcomes were found between primary and revision surgery	0	Mean follow-up, 22 yr Clinically important osteoarthritis rarely developed
Cho et al	*Am J Sports Med* (2009)	Revision open Bankart repair (26)	Significant improvement in Rowe and Constant scores ($P < 0.05$)	11.8	Mean follow-up, 42 mo 46.2% returned to preinjury level of sports activity

ASES = American Shoulder and Elbow Surgeons shoulder outcome, SST = Simple Shoulder Test, UCLA = University of California–Los Angeles Shoulder Rating Scale.
[a] Rate of recurrence.

instability may result, necessitating open revision surgery. The authors of this chapter have noted an approximate 80% success rate in revision for traumatic instability; in patients with multidirectional instability of the shoulder, the success rate is approximately 50%. In a patient whose previous open or arthroscopic procedure has failed, arthroscopic technique may be of great value, particularly in older patients or in young athletes or throwers with a labral tear who experience only subluxation. However, in patients with soft-tissue deficiency, an open approach may be more effective.

 Results

Results of select studies on open revision Bankart repair with and without capsular shift are reported in **Table 1**.

 Technical Keys to Success

Case 1

- A deltopectoral incision is made after administration of epinephrine.
- The cephalic vein is identified and laterally retracted.
- The deltoid and pectoralis major muscles are separated from proximal to distal, and the proximal edge of the pectoralis major tendon insertion on the humerus is incised.
- The clavipectoral fascia is identified, and an incision is made along the lateral edge of the short head of the biceps muscle and opened to the coracoacromial ligament and distally. The three sister vessels—two veins and one artery—running along the subscapularis should be identified.

- The subscapularis is exposed, and two sutures are placed medially. Using a periosteal elevator, an opening approximately 1.5 cm long is made proximal to the vasculature in a lateral to medial direction and extended down to the capsule under the muscle between the middle and lower thirds of the capsule (**Figure 4**).
- A Kelly clamp is placed proximally under the muscle but above the capsule up to the rotator interval.
- The subscapularis tendon is cut obliquely down to the clamp, leaving some tendon laterally and medially for a good repair.
- Using a periosteal elevator, the separation of the capsule and muscle is completed. The glenoid neck is palpated medially, and a retractor is inserted deep to the subscapularis muscle.

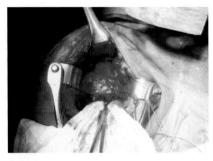

Figure 4 Intraoperative photograph shows the exposed subscapularis muscle through a deltopectoral approach. Medial traction stitches are in place. A curved clamp enters the plane between the capsule and the subscapularis just above the vessels and 1.5 cm medial to the subscapularis insertion onto the lesser tuberosity.

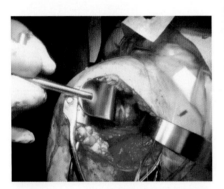

Figure 7 Intraoperative photograph shows medial longitudinal capsulotomy performed in a laterally based manner near the humeral attachment in a patient undergoing a simple capsular shift.

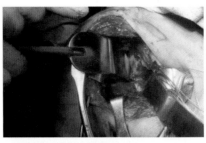

Figure 5 Intraoperative photograph shows the capsule retracted medially and the elevated anteroinferior Bankart component.

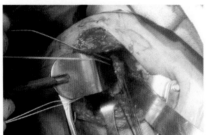

Figure 8 Intraoperative photograph shows three suture anchors placed in the glenoid rim at a 45° angle.

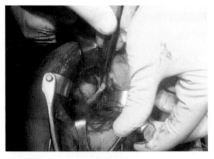

Figure 6 Intraoperative photograph shows lateral capsulotomy prior to shift.

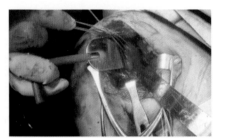

Figure 9 Intraoperative photograph shows sutures from anchors on the glenoid rim passed out through the medial capsulolabral complex, which was then tied down at this site. A superolateral capsular shift is then performed with excision of any redundant capsule from the lateral edge before it is reattached to the humeral side with suture anchors.

- If the repair includes a capsular shift, the patient's arm is placed in external rotation and the capsule is opened laterally from proximal to the 6-o'clock position. If inferior laxity is not present, a standard opening is created medially just off the edge of the glenoid (**Figure 5**). It is important to maintain the patient's arm in external rotation to avoid overtightening the capsule in a medial direction.
- In the patient described in case 1, capsular shift was required to eliminate the sulcus sign and tighten the capsule (**Figure 6**).
- After the capsule is opened, the head

is pushed posteriorly and a Fukuda retractor is inserted to achieve excellent visualization of the glenoid.
- The Bankart lesion is noted (**Figure 7**) and freed from the glenoid. A curet is used to prepare the attachment site of the cartilage defect on the anterior 25% of the glenoid. It may be necessary to advance the labral capsule onto the face of the glenoid to smooth the defect and promote healing if there is cartilage loss on the glenoid.
- Excellent visualization is achieved by placing the retractor deep to the subscapularis medially on the neck of the glenoid and using the Fukuda retractor to position the humeral head.
- Three or four anchors with sutures are placed at a 45° angle on the corner of the glenoid (**Figure 8**).
- The sutures are passed through the medial capsule and tied from the inferior to the superior aspect

to reapproximate the capsule and any remaining labrum (**Figure 9**). The mattress sutures are placed approximately 5 mm apart to avoid tearing the capsule.
- The Fukuda retractor is removed, and the humeral head is released. Pushing the humeral head superiorly and externally rotating the patient's arm allows the surgeon to determine where the capsule should be anchored on the humeral head at the 6-o'clock position.
- Sutures placed in the proximal lateral edge of the capsule aid in determining the correct placement and tension within the capsule. Three or four anchors are placed around the neck deep to the lateral capsule that was incised initially. To prevent

Table 2 Rehabilitation Protocol After Open Bankart Repair

Postoperative Week	Range of Motion	Strengthening	Return to Activities	Comments/Emphasis
0-4	Pendulum exercises	—	—	Sling is used
4-7	—	Patient-initiated active elevation at 4 wk Use of resistance bands is begun at 5-6 wk	—	Sling is discontinued after 4 wk
7-12	Physical therapy is begun at wk 7	Use of light weights in flexion at 7-8 wk	—	By wk 7, elevation to 120°, 20° of ER at the side, and 30° of ER at 90° of abduction should be achieved
12-20	—	Bench press exercise is begun at wk 12, including exercises for the scapula	Contact sports allowed at 16-20 wk	By wk 12, elevation to 170°-180°, 45° of ER at the side, and 90° of ER at 90° of abduction should be achieved The military press and use of dependent weights is not allowed

ER = external rotation.

laxity, sutures are placed sequentially from inferior to superior with an assistant pushing the head proximally while the sutures are tied.

- The superior border of the capsule is reefed to the proximal capsule with the patient's arm in 45° of external rotation. This maneuver closes the rotator interval and prevents overtightening.
- The arm is tested in all planes; it should be quite stable.
- The subscapularis is repaired laterally to the lateral tendon.
- The arm is set in neutral rotation and tendon-to-tendon repair of the subscapularis is performed with No. 5 nonabsorbable braided suture. The repair is made in edge-to-edge fashion; overlapping should be avoided because it leads to contracture.
- Hemostasis is critical to avoid postoperative pain. After the self-retainer is removed, the veins are carefully inspected. A drain is inserted between the deltoid and the pectoralis major, exiting proximally but not through the muscle.
- The wound is closed with monofilament absorbable suture or monofilament nonabsorbable polypropylene suture.

Case 2

- The technique and exposure used on the patient in case 2 are similar to those used in case 1, but insufficient capsule remained for a repair. The technique consists of using a human dermal allograft to replace the capsule in this young athlete. In an older patient, tenodesis of the subscapularis to the glenoid with multiple sutures could be performed.
- To create a new capsule, the human dermal allograft is placed anterior to the glenoid and humeral head to replace the normal capsule.
- Four anchors are placed medially and laterally to attach the membrane to bone. The anchors are placed under tension and pulled proximally, similar to the previously described process of reefing the normal capsule. Sutures are used to attach the anchor to any remaining capsule and close the interval proximally. The humeral head is translated, and

stability is noted with the arm in neutral rotation.

- The subscapularis is reattached laterally with No. 5 nonabsorbable braided suture. If needed, anchors can be added.

 Rehabilitation

The rehabilitation protocol is noted in **Table 2**. A sling is applied to the elbow for proximal support; the sling should have an abdominal strap to help prevent external rotation greater than neutral. Pendulum exercises are started on postoperative day 1. After 4 weeks, the sling is discontinued, and active elevation is initiated by the patient. At week 7, the patient begins physical therapy and increases motion. Typically, 90° has been achieved by the start of week 5, with external rotation of 0°. By week 7, the patient should have 120° of elevation, 20° of external rotation at the side, and 30° of external rotation at 90° of abduction. By week 12, the patient should have elevation to 170° to 180°, external rotation to 45° at the side, and external rotation to 90° at 90° of abduction.

The strengthening program consists of use of a resistance band at weeks 5 and 6 and light weights in flexion by weeks 7 and 8. Bench press exercise is initiated at week 12, with exercises for the scapula. The military press is avoided, as is the use of dependent weights. Activities such as contact sports are started approximately 4 to 5 months postoperatively.

Avoiding Pitfalls

A high rate of failure has been reported after primary arthroscopic stabilization in patients with bone loss. Recently, grafting is more frequently used in the management of bone defects smaller than 25%. Although the senior author of this chapter (R.F.W.) agrees that defects greater than 20% to 25% are best managed with a Latarjet or Bristow procedure, smaller defects may be sufficiently managed with isolated open Bankart repair with a capsular shift (depending on the degree of capsular laxity). If a substantial Hill-Sachs lesion is present, a remplissage can be added to the open repair without grafting.

Bibliography

Balg F, Boileau P: The instability severity index score: A simple pre-operative score to select patients for arthroscopic or open shoulder stabilisation. *J Bone Joint Surg Br* 2007;89(11):1470-1477.

Burkhart SS, De Beer JF: Traumatic glenohumeral bone defects and their relationship to failure of arthroscopic Bankart repairs: Significance of the inverted-pear glenoid and the humeral engaging Hill-Sachs lesion. *Arthroscopy* 2000;16(7):677-694.

Cheung EV, Sperling JW, Hattrup SJ, Cofield RH: Long-term outcome of anterior stabilization of the shoulder. *J Shoulder Elbow Surg* 2008;17(2):265-270.

Cho NS, Yi JW, Lee BG, Rhee YG: Revision open Bankart surgery after arthroscopic repair for traumatic anterior shoulder instability. *Am J Sports Med* 2009;37(11):2158-2164.

Pagnani MJ: Open capsular repair without bone block for recurrent anterior shoulder instability in patients with and without bony defects of the glenoid and/or humeral head. *Am J Sports Med* 2008;36(9):1805-1812.

Rowe CR, Zarins B, Ciullo JV: Recurrent anterior dislocation of the shoulder after surgical repair: Apparent causes of failure and treatment. *J Bone Joint Surg Am* 1984;66(2):159-168.

Sisto DJ: Revision of failed arthroscopic Bankart repairs. *Am J Sports Med* 2007;35(4):537-541.

Zabinski SJ, Callaway GH, Cohen S, Warren RF: Revision shoulder stabilization: 2- to 10-year results. *J Shoulder Elbow Surg* 1999;8(1):58-65.

Chapter 10

Arthroscopic Management of Anterior Instability in Patients With Moderate Humeral Bone Loss: The Remplissage Technique

John M. Tokish, MD

Jeffrey S. Abrams, MD

Introduction

Bone loss is a known associated finding in anterior shoulder instability, but only recently has the role of bone loss in failed arthroscopic stabilization of the shoulder been recognized. In a classic study of glenohumeral bone defects after arthroscopic Bankart repair, the rate of recurrent instability was found to be 10 times greater in patients with bone loss than in patients with no bone loss. The rate of recurrent instability after arthroscopic stabilization in the presence of bone loss was even higher in contact athletes (89%). More recently, a recurrence rate of 75% was noted after arthroscopic Bankart repair in patients with capsular laxity and bone loss greater than 25%. The authors of that study developed an algorithm to estimate the risk of failure after arthroscopic stabilization. Bone loss alone resulted in a 50% failure rate, and when bone loss was combined with young age

or participation in competitive contact sports, the rate of failure increased to 75%.

The amount of bone loss required to proceed with adjunctive treatment has not been determined. In one study in which progressive osteotomies of the glenoid were performed, a 21% glenoid defect was found to decrease the stability of a Bankart repair. The inverted pear appearance of the glenoid has been described as a risk factor for failure of arthroscopic stabilization, and the inverted-pear glenoid has been shown to correspond with bone loss of at least 7.5 mm or 29%.

Although humeral bone loss has been associated with up to 100% of recurrent dislocations, its diagnosis and treatment have been less well reported than those of glenoid bone loss. In one series in which a low overall failure rate was noted after Bankart repair, four of five patients who had recurrent dislocation also had a moderate or severe Hill-Sachs

lesion. In a larger study, patients were evaluated after open revision Bankart repair of a failed arthroscopic procedure. An engaging Hill-Sachs lesion was found in all cases of failure, and the authors of that study concluded that the large Hill-Sachs lesion is a risk factor for failure. Several classifications of the Hill-Sachs lesion have been published (**Table 1**).

Humeral bone loss can be measured qualitatively or quantitatively. Qualitative bone loss is defined as the presence of an engaging Hill-Sachs lesion, in which the humeral head defect displaces over the anterior glenoid in a position of function. In a study published in 2007, researchers quantified the risk of engaging Hill-Sachs lesions by marking the contact area of the glenoid on the humerus throughout the range of motion. The edge of the glenoid track was found to be approximately 18.4 mm medial to the rotator cuff footprint; Hill-Sachs lesions extending beyond this point are at risk for engagement.

Finally, bone loss has been recognized to be a bipolar problem, with both glenoid and humeral bone loss affecting the glenoid track. The authors who proposed this concept described bone loss as either on track or off track, and they proposed that off-track lesions are unsuitable for arthroscopic repair (**Figure 1**). The first author of this chapter (J.M.T.) and colleagues

Dr. Tokish or an immediate family member is a member of a speakers' bureau or has made paid presentations on behalf of Arthrex; serves as a paid consultant to Arthrex, DePuy Synthes, and Mitek Sports Medicine; and serves as a board member, owner, officer, or committee member of the Arthroscopy Association of North America. Dr. Abrams or an immediate family member has received royalties from Smith & Nephew; serves as a paid consultant to ConMed Linvatec, Mitek Sports Medicine, Rotation Medical, and Smith & Nephew; serves as an unpaid consultant to Ingen Technologies and KFx Medical; has stock or stock options held in Cayenne Medical, Ingen Technologies, KFx Medical, Rotation Medical, and Smith & Nephew; and serves as a board member, owner, officer, or committee member of the American Shoulder and Elbow Surgeons and the Arthroscopy Association of North America.

Table 1 Classifications of Hill-Sachs Lesions

Grading System	Imaging	Description
Rowe et al	Axillary radiograph	Mild, 2 cm long × ≤0.3 cm deep; moderate, 2-4 cm long × 0.3-1 cm deep; severe, 4 cm long × ≥1 cm deep
Calandra et al	Direct visualization	Grade I, confined to articular cartilage; grade II, extension into subchondral bone; grade III, large subchondral defect
Franceschi et al	Direct visualization	Grade I, cartilaginous; grade II, bony scuffing; grade III, hatchet fracture
Flatow and Warner	Direct visualization	Clinically insignificant, <20%; variable significance, 20% to 40%; clinically significant, >40%
Hall et al	Notch view radiograph	Percent involvement in 180° articular arc
Richards et al	Axillary MRI	Axillary degrees involved (anterior articular margin, zero degrees)

Reproduced from Provencher MT, Frank RM, LeClere LE, et al: The Hill-Sachs lesion: Diagnosis, classification, and management. *J Am Acad Orthop Surg* 2012;20(4):242-252.

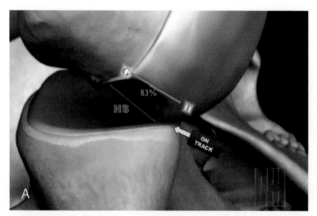
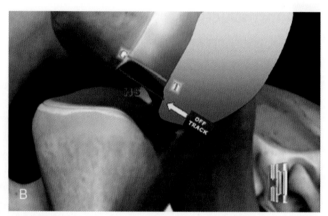

Figure 1   Illustrations depict the glenoid track concept of glenoid bone loss. **A,** The appearance of an on-track Hill-Sachs lesion (HS); the lesion does not engage because minimal glenoid bone loss exists. The glenoid track (G-T) is 83% of the intact glenoid diameter. Bone loss reduces the size of the track, making it more likely to engage. **B,** The additional glenoid bone loss depicted in this illustration results in an off-track engaging Hill-Sachs lesion. (Reproduced with permission from Di Giacomo G, Itoi E, Burkhart SS: Evolving concept of bipolar bone loss and the Hill-Sachs lesion: From "engaging/non-engaging" lesion to "on-track/off-track" lesion. *Arthroscopy* 2014;30[1]:90-98.)

recently indicated anecdotally that track determination is a better predictor of arthroscopic outcome than is glenoid bone loss alone.

Research on the management of substantial Hill-Sachs lesions is ongoing. One option that has gained popularity is transfer of the infraspinatus and posterior capsule directly into the Hill-Sachs defect. Originally described in 1972 as an open procedure, the transfer of the infraspinatus and capsule excludes the defect from the intra-articular aspect of the joint and prevents engagement of the Hill-Sachs lesion with the glenoid. The arthroscopic version of this technique

has gained popularity as an adjunct to arthroscopic Bankart repair in patients with substantial bone loss that precludes isolated labral repair.

■ Case Presentation

A 19-year-old, right-hand–dominant man who plays collegiate lacrosse has a history of 5 anterior dislocations and more than 12 subluxations of his left, nondominant shoulder. He reports that his shoulder has become "easier to pop out" and that he has had one episode of dislocation in his sleep. Several

dislocations have required reduction at a medical facility. He is otherwise healthy. Physical examination reveals substantial anterior apprehension, good symmetric strength in the rotator cuff and periscapular musculature, and no scapular winging. A push-pull test demonstrates posterior instability. The patient has no substantial sulcus sign and does not demonstrate joint hyperlaxity as measured by the Beighton criteria or a Gagey test. Several months of physical therapy have failed, and he has been unable to participate in lacrosse. Radiographs demonstrate a well-reduced shoulder without evidence of glenoid erosion or a substantial Hill-Sachs lesion. MRI reveals anterior and posterior labral pathology with glenoid bone loss and a substantial Hill-Sachs lesion, and CT demonstrates approximately 18% glenoid bone loss. The Hill-Sachs lesion extends 16 mm from the edge of the rotator cuff insertion (**Figure 2**). Measurement reveals a glenoid width of 30 mm and glenoid bone loss of 5.5 mm (**Figure 3**). Thus, the glenoid track (**Table 2**) is calculated as follows:

$$0.83(30 \text{ mm}) - 5.5 \text{ mm} = 19.4 \text{ mm}$$

Because the size of the Hill-Sachs lesion at its greatest dimension (16 mm) is less than the calculated glenoid track (19.4 mm), the patient's bone loss is defined as on track, although it is close to the limit. The patient and his family were counseled about the treatment options. After consideration of his entire clinical situation, he elected to proceed with arthroscopic management of the instability with augmentation of the Hill-Sachs lesion with an arthroscopic remplissage procedure.

 ## Indications

In athletic patients with primarily anterior instability with moderate bone loss and an on-track lesion, several approaches might be taken, ranging from a minimally invasive arthroscopic Bankart repair to a Latarjet bone transfer of the coracoid to the glenoid. Individual patient factors influence the selection of arthroscopic labral repair with remplissage augmentation. Young age, contact athlete status, and competitive sports participation increase the risk of failure after an arthroscopic Bankart repair alone. Furthermore, posterior labral pathology, which can be observed on MRI and in a physical examination with a push-pull test consistent with posterior instability, would be difficult to address with an open anterior procedure.

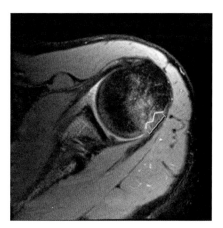

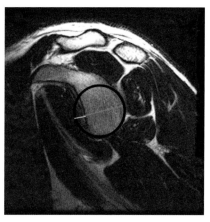

Figure 2 Proton density axial MRI demonstrates a 16-mm-wide Hill-Sachs lesion (highlighted in yellow).

Figure 3 T1-weighted sagittal MRI demonstrates glenoid bone loss. The black circle represents the idealized glenoid circumference; the blue line is the diameter of the idealized glenoid; and the yellow line represents bone loss (5.5 mm, or 18%).

Table 2 Glenoid Track Calculation

Step	Procedure
1	Measure diameter (D) of the inferior glenoid using the perfect circle method.
2	Measure the amount of glenoid bone loss (d).
3	Determine the width of the glenoid track (GT); $GT = 0.83D - d$.
4	Measure the width of the Hill-Sachs lesion (HS).
5	Measure the width of the bone bridge between the rotator cuff and the Hill-Sachs lesion (BB).
6	Determine the Hill-Sachs interval (HSI); $HSI = HS + BB$.
7	If $HSI > GT$, the shoulder is off track; if $HSI < GT$, the shoulder is on track.

Adapted with permission from Di Giacomo G, Itoi E, Burkhart SS: Evolving concept of bipolar bone loss and the Hill-Sachs lesion: From "engaging/non-engaging" lesion to "on-track/off-track" lesion. *Arthroscopy* 2014;30(1):90-98.

The instability severity index score has been described to aid in prediction of failure after arthroscopic stabilization of the shoulder; a score above 6 correlates with an unacceptable failure rate of 70% (**Table 3**). The patient in the case presented in this chapter would receive 2 points for young age (<20 years), 1 point for being a contact athlete, and 2 points for being a competitive athlete, for a total of 5 points before bone loss is even considered.

Based on the amount of glenoid bone loss in this patient (18%) and the substantial Hill-Sachs lesion, an isolated Bankart repair would likely be inadequate to restore stability. Other studies have demonstrated the superiority of remplissage augmentation over isolated Bankart repair, and although rates of return to sport have been modest, an arthroscopic approach allows the surgeon to address both posterior and anterior labral pathology and to augment humeral bone loss using a minimally invasive approach.

Table 3 Instability Severity Index Score

Prognostic Factors	Points
Patient age	
≤20 yr	2
>20 yr	0
Degree of sports participation (preoperative)	
Competitive	2
Recreational or none	0
Type of sport (preoperative)	
Contact or forced overhead	1
Other	0
Shoulder hyperlaxity	
Shoulder hyperlaxity (anterior or inferior)	1
Normal laxity	0
Hill-Sachs lesion on AP radiograph	
Visible in external rotation	2
Not visible in external rotation	0
Glenoid loss of contour on AP radiograph	
Loss of contour	2
No lesion	0
Total	10

Adapted with permission from Balg F, Boileau P: The instability severity index score: A simple pre-operative score to select patients for arthroscopic or open shoulder stabilisation. *J Bone Joint Surg Br* 2007;89(11):1470-1477.

Controversies and Alternative Approaches

Several alternatives to this approach are available. First, an arthroscopic Bankart repair may be sufficient. Bone loss of 20% to 25% is often cited as the level at which an isolated arthroscopic Bankart repair becomes insufficient. According to the criteria used in an early study of bone loss, which demonstrated a low recurrence rate after arthroscopic Bankart repair, the patient in the case presented in this chapter may not have been classified as having an engaging Hill-Sachs lesion, and neither would he have been classified as having an inverted-pear glenoid. Furthermore, some authors have suggested that an isolated arthroscopic Bankart repair may be sufficient

in patients with glenoid bone loss defined as on track. Recent data, however, have questioned the critical level of bone loss at which augmentation should be considered. The authors of a study published in 2015 demonstrated that bone loss greater than 13.5% resulted in lower functional scores, even in patients without subsequent instability events. In a different study, remplissage augmentation of Bankart repair resulted in recurrence rates lower than those of isolated Bankart repair, and several studies have shown successful results of remplissage augmentation in patients with moderate bone loss.

Another option is an open Bankart repair with inferior capsular shift. In a series of patients with anterior instability, more than 80% of whom were contact athletes with Hill-Sachs lesions, this

open approach resulted in a 2% recurrence rate. This study raises the possibility that bone loss may be a risk factor for failure of arthroscopic instability procedures rather than a risk factor for failure of all instability procedures. In the case presented in this chapter, this approach was avoided because the patient demonstrated posterior labral pathology. Addressing posterior instability through an anterior open approach is difficult, whereas bidirectional and circumferential lesions of the glenoid labrum have been successfully addressed with the use of arthroscopic techniques.

The Latarjet procedure is another option that has been successful in patients with substantial bone loss. Return-to-sports rates of 96% to 100% after the Latarjet procedure have been reported in athletes, including contact athletes. Other studies, however, have demonstrated up to a 30% complication rate after the Latarjet procedure; therefore, this procedure may be best reserved for revision situations or patients with more severe bone loss. In the case presented in this chapter, the presence of posterior labral pathology also made the Latarjet procedure a less appropriate option.

Other options, such as grafting of the Hill-Sachs defect, partial prosthetic replacement of the humeral head, and humeral derotational osteotomy, have been attempted. However, results of these procedures have not been reported in large series.

Results

Clinical outcomes of the remplissage technique to address anterior instability are summarized in **Table 4**. Systematic reviews have reported overall recurrence rates of 5.4%. Rowe scores improved from an average of 36 to 88 points, without substantial loss of motion. Other studies have reported small losses of motion, which may be an important consideration in throwing

Table 4 Clinical Results of Remplissage in the Management of Anterior Instability

Authors	Journal (Year)	Technique (No. of Patients)	Outcomes[a]	Failure Rate (%)[b]	Comments
Nourissat et al	*Am J Sports Med* (2011)	Remplissage (15), isolated Bankart repair (17)	No differences in ROM	6	One-third of patients in the remplissage group had postoperative pain
Park et al	*Arthroscopy* (2011)	Remplissage (20)	ASES score, 93 Penn shoulder score, 90 WOSI, 73%	15	Large lesions (>25%)
Zhu et al	*Am J Sports Med* (2011)	Remplissage (49)	ASES score improved from 85 to 96 Constant score improved from 94 to 98 Rowe score improved from 37 to 90	8	MRI demonstrated successful healing
Boileau et al	*J Bone Joint Surg Am* (2012)	Remplissage (47)	90% returned to sport 68% returned to same level of sports participation	2	All imaged patients healed
Franceschi et al	*Am J Sports Med* (2012)	Remplissage (25), isolated Bankart repair (25)	UCLA, Constant, and Rowe scores improved significantly ($P < 0.00001$)	20 (Bankart) 0 (remplissage)	No loss of ROM after remplissage
Park et al	*Am J Sports Med* (2012)	Remplissage (11)	75% to 100% healing of lesions seen on MRI WOSI, 74%	9	4 of 9 patients demonstrated tendinopathy or partial tears
Garcia et al	*Orthopedics* (2013)	Remplissage (20), osteochondral graft substitute (19)	WOSI scores were significantly better after remplissage ($P = 0.016$)	15 (remplissage) 32 (graft)	Results of synthetic grafts were worse than those of remplissage
McCabe et al	*Arthroscopy* (2014)	Remplissage (31)	ASES score improved from 50 to 91	36 (revision) 0 (primary)	Effective as primary procedure High failure rates in revision
Wolf and Arianjam	*J Shoulder Elbow Surg* (2014)	Remplissage (45)	Rowe score, 95 Constant score, 95 WOSI, 110	4.4	Avg follow-up, 58 mo
Merolla et al	*Am J Sports Med* (2015)	Remplissage (61), healthy control subjects (40)	Constant score improved from 62 to 90	2	Largest series in the literature Median follow-up, 40 mo Slight decrease in external rotation in remplissage
Brilakis et al	*Knee Surg Sports Traumatol Arthrosc* (2016)	Remplissage (48)	ASES score improved from 68 to 91 Rowe score improved from 38 to 94	6	71% returned to same level of sports participation

ASES = American Shoulder and Elbow Surgeons shoulder outcome, ROM = range of motion, UCLA = University of California–Los Angeles Shoulder Rating Scale, WOSI = Western Ontario Shoulder Instability Index.
[a] All outcomes are mean values unless otherwise indicated.
[b] Failure is defined as recurrence except where noted.

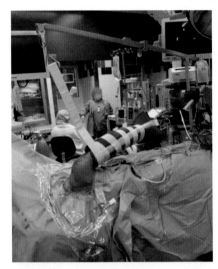

Figure 4   Photograph shows a patient in the lateral decubitus position with traction, which allows an ideal approach for the Bankart procedure.

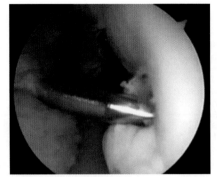

Figure 5   Arthroscopic view of a glenohumeral joint from the posterior portal demonstrates introduction of a narrow switching stick with appropriate trajectory through the capsule to the anterior aspect of the Hill-Sachs defect.

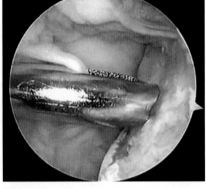

Figure 6   Arthroscopic view of a glenohumeral joint from the posterior portal demonstrates positioning of a drill guide for the posterior anchor at the posterior border of the Hill-Sachs lesion.

athletes; however, this result has not been systematically studied.

 Video 10.1 Double-pulley Remplissage for the Management of Moderate-size Hill-Sachs Lesions. John M. Tokish, MD; Jeffrey S. Abrams, MD (3 min)

Technical Keys to Success

Setup/Exposure
- Remplissage can be performed in either the beach-chair or the lateral decubitus position. However, the lateral decubitus position provides substantial advantages for visualization. The lateral traction afforded by the lateral position can aid in the Bankart repair, and abduction of the arm, which is critical in visualization and performance of the procedure, is far easier to maintain in the lateral position.
- The authors of this chapter perform the remplissage with the arm in approximately 60° of abduction without lateral traction and then

reposition the patient's arm in 20° to 30° of abduction to facilitate the Bankart repair (**Figure 4**). This position allows complete visualization of the rotator cuff insertion and the Hill-Sachs lesion and facilitates approximation of the proper portion of the infraspinatus footprint to the defect itself.

Instruments/Equipment/ Implants Required
- One 8-mm lateral portal cannula is required.
- A small switching stick is used.
- A 3.5-mm drill guide is used.
- Two 3.0 biocomposite suture anchors are used.

Procedure
- Standard posterior, anterosuperior, and midglenoid portals are used to perform the Bankart procedure.
- The arm is placed into abduction, and the lateral traction strap is removed.
- The Hill-Sachs lesion is identified and is biologically prepared with the use of a rasp or shaver until punctate bleeding bone is encountered.
- Remplissage can be performed with one or two additional portals. In

the single-portal technique, the arthroscope remains intra-articular throughout the entire procedure.
- A spinal needle is used to penetrate the skin and enter the joint near the midpoint of the lateral acromial border, approximately 1 to 2 cm lateral to the acromion. Care must be taken to ensure that the spinal needle can easily reach the anterior and posterior limits of the Hill-Sachs defect and that the angle of the spinal needle allows a relatively perpendicular approach to the humeral head.
- After the correct position and trajectory of the spinal needle are determined, a skin incision is made around the spinal needle, the needle is replaced with a switching stick, and the proper angle of approach is confirmed (**Figure 5**).
- An 8-mm arthroscopic cannula is placed through the skin and deltoid down to but not through the infraspinatus. It is not necessary to débride the subacromial space for subsequent suture tying, which is one of the advantages of this technique. The position of this lateral portal is critical. It must be near the midpoint of the remplissage lesion so that the anchors can be directed

to both the posterior and anterior aspects of the Hill-Sachs lesion with sufficient separation between passes through the rotator cuff to allow adequate tissue spanning of the defect. The depth of the portal is critical because it must extend into the subacromial space, just adjacent to the bursal surface of the rotator cuff. This portal placement ensures that the double-pulley construct will have no soft tissue intervening and that the distance between anchors will be appropriate to span but not overconstrain the remplissage.

- After the switching stick has been placed, a drill guide is placed over it and positioned at the posterior aspect of the Hill-Sachs lesion (**Figure 6**).

- The trajectory of the switching stick is critical. The point at which it passes through the rotator cuff will determine the point of fixation between the cuff and the Hill-Sachs lesion. If this point is too medial, it can result in an overaggressive shift and may limit motion. The ideal point of penetration is adjacent to the medial edge of the Hill-Sachs lesion, through the tendinous portion of the infraspinatus.

- With the drill guide held in place, a drill is advanced and is followed by a suture anchor.

- The guide is removed from the cannula, leaving this posterior anchor with sutures exiting through the posterior capsule and infraspinatus tendon (**Figure 7**).

- The same narrow switching stick is reintroduced through the cannula but is redirected anteriorly, and the tissue of the infraspinatus and capsule is indented bluntly until the tip of the switching stick is at the most anterior aspect of the Hill-Sachs defect.

- The switching stick is advanced through the tendon and capsule,

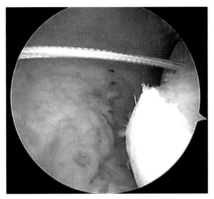

Figure 7   Arthroscopic view of a glenohumeral joint from the posterior portal demonstrates positioning of a posterior anchor and the exit of the suture through the capsule and infraspinatus tendon.

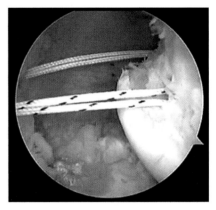

Figure 8   Arthroscopic view of a glenohumeral joint from the posterior portal demonstrates dual anchor placement spanning the Hill-Sachs lesion for double-pulley remplissage.

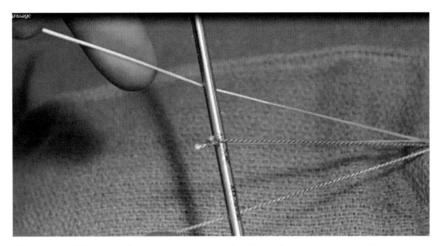

Figure 9   Photograph demonstrates the double-pulley construct used in the remplissage technique. One limb from each suture anchor is tied over a switching stick outside the shoulder. The other two limbs, when tensioned, use the suture anchor eyelets as pulleys and reduce the posterior capsule and infraspinatus into the defect with a mattress suture.

and care is taken to ensure that it can reach the anterior edge of the Hill-Sachs lesion.

- The anchor drilling steps are repeated, and the guide is again removed, leaving one anchor at each of the anterior and posterior borders of the Hill-Sachs lesion, with the sutures exiting with similar spacing through the capsule and tendon (**Figure 8**).

- One limb from each suture anchor is tied over a switching stick outside

the shoulder with a surgeon's knot and three reversed half-hitches on alternating posts, and the excess suture limbs are cut.

- With the use of a double-pulley technique, the opposite limbs of each suture anchor are tensioned (**Figure 9**). This technique delivers the knotted ends down to the top of the infraspinatus and capsule, creating a mattress suture that reduces the tendon into the entire anterior-to-posterior length of the

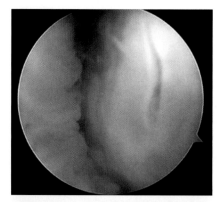

Figure 10 Arthroscopic view of a glenohumeral joint from the posterior portal demonstrates a completed remplissage, which excludes the Hill-Sachs lesion from view.

Hill-Sachs lesion. This reduction can be visualized from the intra-articular side.

- After proper tension has been obtained such that the lesion is excluded from the joint, an arthroscopic sliding knot is tied in the two tension sutures and advanced to secure the double-pulley construct.
- Excess suture length is trimmed, and the remplissage is examined through a gentle range of motion to ensure that it remains reduced. The final construct completely excludes the Hill-Sachs lesion from the joint (**Figure 10**).
- Alternatively, the anchors can be placed through separate percutaneous insertions instead of a single portal. This method may have the advantages of allowing better spacing through the posterior capsule and tendon between the anchors and incorporating a broader area of tendon and capsule into the repair. However, in this technique the subacromial space must be entered and the sutures retrieved into a single cannula for tying, which requires additional subacromial bursal clearance and is slightly less efficient.
- Another alternative is to pass one limb of each suture anchor through a separate stitch through the rotator cuff, more medial than the anchor position. This technique can be accomplished with a spinal needle and suture shuttling techniques. After the anchor is placed, a spinal needle is percutaneously inserted into the joint 1 cm medial to the anchor. With the anterosuperior portal used for viewing, a small-caliber passing suture, such as a polydioxanone suture, is threaded through the spinal needle and retrieved through the posterior cannula. One limb from the suture anchor is likewise grasped through this portal. The two retrieved limbs are tied together, and the subacromial limb of the passing suture is pulled, shuttling the anchor stitch through the capsule and rotator cuff. This step creates a medial-to-lateral mattress stitch. This step is repeated for the second anchor, and the final repair construct has a rectangular footprint instead of a linear one. This method has the advantage of a broader footprint of repair but involves additional steps to pass the sutures and requires retrieval from the subacromial space.

Wound Closure

- All arthroscopic equipment is removed, and the wounds are closed with 3-0 absorbable sutures.
- Dressings are applied to the wound in sterile fashion.
- The arm is placed in a sling with an abduction pillow.

 Rehabilitation

The addition of the remplissage procedure to a Bankart repair changes the postoperative rehabilitation regimen. Because the success of the procedure depends on the healing of the capsule and tendon through the repair sutures, the repair must be protected. Active abduction and external rotation are avoided for 4 to 6 weeks postoperatively. The patient uses a sling with an abduction pillow for 6 weeks at all times except when performing hand, wrist, and elbow exercises and pendulum exercises. Passive elevation to 90° and passive external rotation to 30° are allowed. The restriction on active motion is removed at 6 weeks, and strengthening begins at 12 weeks. Because many patients who undergo this procedure are athletes, the surgeon should work closely with physical therapists and athletic trainers to ensure that the patient progresses through a return-to-sport program of scapular and periscapular strength training with an emphasis on core and dynamic stabilization. The rehabilitation protocol is summarized in **Table 5**.

 Avoiding Pitfalls

Although remplissage can be useful and efficient in the management of instability, several technical pitfalls must be avoided to ensure its success. Before the procedure, care should be taken to ensure that the entire Hill-Sachs lesion can be visualized with working space between the lesion and the edge of the rotator cuff. Visualization is optimized by removal of any lateral traction used to perform the Bankart repair and by placement of the arm into abduction. Rotation can aid in visualization, but the authors of this chapter recommend ensuring that the entirety of the lesion can be visualized without requiring movement of the arm during this portion of the procedure. Typically the surgeon can accomplish the entire procedure while viewing from the anterosuperior portal with a 30° arthroscope and using the posterior portal and lateral subacromial portals as the working portals; however, the surgeon should not hesitate to change to the posterior portal for viewing or to use a 70° arthroscope to obtain

Table 5 Rehabilitation Protocol After Arthroscopic Remplissage

Postoperative Week	ROM	Strengthening	Return to Play	Comments/Emphasis
0-2	Passive pendulums Active hand, wrist, and elbow motion	Hand, wrist, and elbow, ADLs Core strengthening maintained	None	Emphasis on wound healing, protection
2-6	Passive pendulums Active hand, wrist, and elbow motion Passive elevation to 90°, passive external rotation to 30°	Hand, wrist, and elbow, ADLs Scapular engagement: protraction, retraction, elevation, depression Core strengthening maintained	None	ROM in safe positions Reengagement of the scapular muscles is begun early, but with the arm fixed to protect remplissage repair
6-12	Active motion progressed in all planes Restoration of full ROM	Progression from isometric to dynamic exercises Rotator cuff and periscapular strengthening	None	Emphasis on dynamic co-contraction Scapular rhythm and reconnection to core musculature
12-24	Maintenance of full motion	Functional strengthening in multiplanar positions with perturbations	At discretion of therapist/trainer Progression demonstrating dynamic stability, strength, confidence, and endurance	Communication with patient, trainer, coaches, and (if applicable) patient's family critical to determine appropriate return to play

ADLs = activities of daily living, ROM = range of motion.

better visualization of the anterior edge of the Hill-Sachs lesion.

The order of the steps in the procedure can also be critical. Repair of the Bankart lesion can decrease the space available to view the Hill-Sachs lesion, and vice versa. Many authors therefore recommend beginning the procedure by placing the Bankart anchors and sutures but leaving them untied and parked through the midglenoid portal. After the remplissage is performed, the Bankart repair sutures are securely tied. The authors of this chapter have found this method unnecessary in most patients and typically perform the Bankart repair with the arm in lateral traction and relative adduction first and then remove the lateral traction, place the arm into abduction, and perform the remplissage.

Anchor placement can be challenging to visualize, and choosing the appropriate anchor and method of insertion can help to avoid pitfalls. The choice of an anchor that can be inserted through a drill guide allows the surgeon to accomplish the anchor placement step with one pass. After the switching stick has been inserted at the correct point in the capsule and tendon, the surgeon can proceed to anchor placement without reinserting or adjusting the anchor position. Minimizing the number of steps, particularly when they involve passing instruments through the capsule and rotator cuff, results in a more efficient procedure and protects the repair tissue from additional insertional trauma. An additional tip to improve visualization is to pass the drill guide over the switching stick with the switching stick in the joint rather than on the footprint site. Placing the switching stick into the joint allows the drill guide to be inserted well past the capsule, and the switching stick can then be easily repositioned onto the footprint, allowing excellent visualization of the remaining procedure steps.

The site of penetration of the capsule and infraspinatus is a key aspect of the remplissage procedure. To avoid overtensioning the capsule, the sutures should be introduced through the tendon rather than through the muscle. Overtensioning also can occur in patients with very large Hill-Sachs lesions if attempts are made to bring the capsule and tendon to the medial edge of the defect. For these patients, the authors of this chapter recommend placing the suture anchor off the medial edge and into the defect. A biomechanical study of remplissage techniques demonstrated that the results of anchor placement in the valley of the defect were similar to those of placement of anchors on the edge of the defect but that the use of more medialized sutures resulted in increased restriction of range of motion.

Suture management is a key part of the remplissage technique. Because the final knots are tied into the subacromial space, the surgeon must ensure that the space is clear of bursa or soft-tissue bridges before advancing the knots. The safest method is to begin the procedure by clearing bursa from the subacromial space and directly visualizing the infraspinatus to ensure that the path of the sutures is unobstructed. Surgeons who are more familiar with the remplissage technique may prefer to tie the sutures blind, but this method does not eliminate the risk of soft-tissue interposition; therefore, the authors of this chapter recommend routine direct inspection of the bursal side of the repair site. If the surgeon plans to tie the sutures blind, aggressively sweeping a switching stick along the rotator cuff from front to back during establishment of the subacromial portal can help to clear bursa from the eventual path of the suture.

Bibliography

Ahmed I, Ashton F, Robinson CM: Arthroscopic Bankart repair and capsular shift for recurrent anterior shoulder instability: Functional outcomes and identification of risk factors for recurrence. *J Bone Joint Surg Am* 2012;94(14):1308-1315.

Balg F, Boileau P: The instability severity index score: A simple pre-operative score to select patients for arthroscopic or open shoulder stabilisation. *J Bone Joint Surg Br* 2007;89(11):1470-1477.

Beighton P, Horan F: Orthopaedic aspects of the Ehlers-Danlos syndrome. *J Bone Joint Surg Br* 1969;51(3):444-453.

Boileau P, O'Shea K, Vargas P, Pinedo M, Old J, Zumstein M: Anatomical and functional results after arthroscopic Hill-Sachs remplissage. *J Bone Joint Surg Am* 2012;94(7):618-626.

Boileau P, Villalba M, Héry JY, Balg F, Ahrens P, Neyton L: Risk factors for recurrence of shoulder instability after arthroscopic Bankart repair. *J Bone Joint Surg Am* 2006;88(8):1755-1763.

Brilakis E, Mataragas E, Deligeorgis A, Maniatis V, Antonogiannakis E: Midterm outcomes of arthroscopic remplissage for the management of recurrent anterior shoulder instability. *Knee Surg Sports Traumatol Arthrosc* 2016;24(2):593-600.

Burkhart SS, De Beer JF: Traumatic glenohumeral bone defects and their relationship to failure of arthroscopic Bankart repairs: Significance of the inverted-pear glenoid and the humeral engaging Hill-Sachs lesion. *Arthroscopy* 2000;16(7):677-694.

Burkhart SS, De Beer JF, Barth JR, Cresswell T, Roberts C, Richards DP: Results of modified Latarjet reconstruction in patients with anteroinferior instability and significant bone loss. *Arthroscopy* 2007;23(10):1033-1041.

Buza JA III, Iyengar JJ, Anakwenze OA, Ahmad CS, Levine WN: Arthroscopic Hill-Sachs remplissage: A systematic review. *J Bone Joint Surg Am* 2014;96(7):549-555.

Calandra JJ, Baker CL, Uribe J: The incidence of Hill-Sachs lesions in initial anterior shoulder dislocations. *Arthroscopy* 1989;5(4):254-257.

Cerciello S, Edwards TB, Walch G: Chronic anterior glenohumeral instability in soccer players: Results for a series of 28 shoulders treated with the Latarjet procedure. *J Orthop Traumatol* 2012;13(4):197-202.

Cho NS, Hwang JC, Rhee YG: Arthroscopic stabilization in anterior shoulder instability: Collision athletes versus noncollision athletes. *Arthroscopy* 2006;22(9):947-953.

Cho NS, Yi JW, Lee BG, Rhee YG: Revision open Bankart surgery after arthroscopic repair for traumatic anterior shoulder instability. *Am J Sports Med* 2009;37(11):2158-2164.

Connolly JF: Humeral head defects associated with shoulder dislocation: Their diagnostic and surgical significance. *Instr Course Lect* 1972;21:42-54.

Di Giacomo G, Itoi E, Burkhart SS: Evolving concept of bipolar bone loss and the Hill-Sachs lesion: From "engaging/non-engaging" lesion to "on-track/off-track" lesion. *Arthroscopy* 2014;30(1):90-98.

Elkinson I, Giles JW, Boons HW, et al: The shoulder remplissage procedure for Hill-Sachs defects: Does technique matter? *J Shoulder Elbow Surg* 2013;22(6):835-841.

Flatow EL, Warner JI: Instability of the shoulder: Complex problems and failed repairs. Part I: Relevant biomechanics, multidirectional instability, and severe glenoid loss. *Instr Course Lect* 1998;47:97-112.

Flinkkilä T, Hyvönen P, Ohtonen P, Leppilahti J: Arthroscopic Bankart repair: Results and risk factors of recurrence of instability. *Knee Surg Sports Traumatol Arthrosc* 2010;18(12):1752-1758.

Franceschi F, Longo UG, Ruzzini L, Rizzello G, Maffulli N, Denaro V: Arthroscopic salvage of failed arthroscopic Bankart repair: A prospective study with a minimum follow-up of 4 years. *Am J Sports Med* 2008;36(7):1330-1336.

Franceschi F, Papalia R, Rizzello G, et al: Remplissage repair: New frontiers in the prevention of recurrent shoulder instability. A 2-year follow-up comparative study. *Am J Sports Med* 2012;40(11):2462-2469.

Garcia GH, Park MJ, Baldwin K, Fowler J, Kelly JD IV, Tjoumakaris FP: Comparison of arthroscopic osteochondral substitute grafting and remplissage for engaging Hill-Sachs lesions. *Orthopedics* 2013;36(1):e38-e43.

Griesser MJ, Harris JD, McCoy BW, et al: Complications and re-operations after Bristow-Latarjet shoulder stabilization: A systematic review. *J Shoulder Elbow Surg* 2013;22(2):286-292.

Grondin P, Leith J: Case series: Combined large Hill-Sachs and bony Bankart lesions treated by Latarjet and partial humeral head resurfacing. A report of 2 cases. *Can J Surg* 2009;52(3):249-254.

Hall RH, Isaac F, Booth CR: Dislocation of the shoulder with special reference to accompanying small fractures. *J Bone Joint Surg Am* 1959;41(3):489-494.

Itoi E, Lee SB, Berglund LJ, Berge LL, An KN: The effect of a glenoid defect on anteroinferior stability of the shoulder after Bankart repair: A cadaveric study. *J Bone Joint Surg Am* 2000;82(1):35-46.

Kim SH, Ha KI, Jung MW, Lim MS, Kim YM, Park JH: Accelerated rehabilitation after arthroscopic Bankart repair for selected cases: A prospective randomized clinical study. *Arthroscopy* 2003;19(7):722-731.

Koo SS, Burkhart SS, Ochoa E: Arthroscopic double-pulley remplissage technique for engaging Hill-Sachs lesions in anterior shoulder instability repairs. *Arthroscopy* 2009;25(11):1343-1348.

Lo IK, Parten PM, Burkhart SS: The inverted pear glenoid: An indicator of significant glenoid bone loss. *Arthroscopy* 2004;20(2):169-174.

McCabe MP, Weinberg D, Field LD, O'Brien MJ, Hobgood ER, Savoie FH III: Primary versus revision arthroscopic reconstruction with remplissage for shoulder instability with moderate bone loss. *Arthroscopy* 2014;30(4):444-450.

Merolla G, Paladini P, Di Napoli G, Campi F, Porcellini G: Outcomes of arthroscopic Hill-Sachs remplissage and anterior Bankart repair: A retrospective controlled study including ultrasound evaluation of posterior capsulotenodesis and infraspinatus strength assessment. *Am J Sports Med* 2015;43(2):407-414.

Miniaci A, Gish MW: Management of anterior glenohumeral instability associated with large Hill-Sachs defects. *Techniques in Shoulder & Elbow Surgery* 2004;5(3):170-175.

Neyton L, Young A, Dawidziak B, et al: Surgical treatment of anterior instability in rugby union players: Clinical and radiographic results of the Latarjet-Patte procedure with minimum 5-year follow-up. *J Shoulder Elbow Surg* 2012;21(12):1721-1727.

Nourissat G, Kilinc AS, Werther JR, Doursounian L: A prospective, comparative, radiological, and clinical study of the influence of the "remplissage" procedure on shoulder range of motion after stabilization by arthroscopic Bankart repair. *Am J Sports Med* 2011;39(10):2147-2152.

Pagnani MJ: Open capsular repair without bone block for recurrent anterior shoulder instability in patients with and without bony defects of the glenoid and/or humeral head. *Am J Sports Med* 2008;36(9):1805-1812.

Park MJ, Garcia G, Malhotra A, Major N, Tjoumakaris FP, Kelly JD IV: The evaluation of arthroscopic remplissage by high-resolution magnetic resonance imaging. *Am J Sports Med* 2012;40(10):2331-2336.

Park MJ, Tjoumakaris FP, Garcia G, Patel A, Kelly JD IV: Arthroscopic remplissage with Bankart repair for the treatment of glenohumeral instability with Hill-Sachs defects. *Arthroscopy* 2011;27(9):1187-1194.

Provencher MT, Frank RM, Leclere LE, et al: The Hill-Sachs lesion: Diagnosis, classification, and management. *J Am Acad Orthop Surg* 2012;20(4):242-252.

Purchase RJ, Wolf EM, Hobgood ER, Pollock ME, Smalley CC: Hill-Sachs "remplissage": An arthroscopic solution for the engaging Hill-Sachs lesion. *Arthroscopy* 2008;24(6):723-726.

Richards RD, Sartoris DJ, Pathria MN, Resnick D: Hill-Sachs lesion and normal humeral groove: MR imaging features allowing their differentiation. *Radiology* 1994;190(3):665-668.

Rowe CR: Prognosis in dislocations of the shoulder. *J Bone Joint Surg Am* 1956;38(5):957-977.

Rowe CR, Patel D, Southmayd WW: The Bankart procedure: A long-term end-result study. *J Bone Joint Surg Am* 1978;60(1):1-16.

Rowe CR, Zarins B, Ciullo JV: Recurrent anterior dislocation of the shoulder after surgical repair: Apparent causes of failure and treatment. *J Bone Joint Surg Am* 1984;66(2):159-168.

Shah AA, Butler RB, Romanowski J, Goel D, Karadagli D, Warner JJ: Short-term complications of the Latarjet procedure. *J Bone Joint Surg Am* 2012;94(6):495-501.

Shaha JS, Cook JB, Song DJ, et al: Redefining "critical" bone loss in shoulder instability: Functional outcomes worsen with "subcritical" bone loss. *Am J Sports Med* 2015;43(7):1719-1725.

Song DJ, Cook JB, Krul KP, et al: High frequency of posterior and combined shoulder instability in young active patients. *J Shoulder Elbow Surg* 2015;24(2):186-190.

Taylor DC, Arciero RA: Pathologic changes associated with shoulder dislocations: Arthroscopic and physical examination findings in first-time, traumatic anterior dislocations. *Am J Sports Med* 1997;25(3):306-311.

Tokish JM, McBratney CM, Solomon DJ, Leclere L, Dewing CB, Provencher MT: Arthroscopic repair of circumferential lesions of the glenoid labrum. *J Bone Joint Surg Am* 2009;91(12):2795-2802.

Voos JE, Livermore RW, Feeley BT, et al; HSS Sports Medicine Service: Prospective evaluation of arthroscopic Bankart repairs for anterior instability. *Am J Sports Med* 2010;38(2):302-307.

Weber BG, Simpson LA, Hardegger F: Rotational humeral osteotomy for recurrent anterior dislocation of the shoulder associated with a large Hill-Sachs lesion. *J Bone Joint Surg Am* 1984;66(9):1443-1450.

Wolf EM, Arianjam A: Hill-Sachs remplissage, an arthroscopic solution for the engaging Hill-Sachs lesion: 2- to 10-year follow-up and incidence of recurrence. *J Shoulder Elbow Surg* 2014;23(6):814-820.

Yamamoto N, Itoi E, Abe H, et al: Contact between the glenoid and the humeral head in abduction, external rotation, and horizontal extension: A new concept of glenoid track. *J Shoulder Elbow Surg* 2007;16(5):649-656.

Zhu YM, Lu Y, Zhang J, Shen JW, Jiang CY: Arthroscopic Bankart repair combined with remplissage technique for the treatment of anterior shoulder instability with engaging Hill-Sachs lesion: A report of 49 cases with a minimum 2-year follow-up. *Am J Sports Med* 2011;39(8):1640-1647.

 ## Video Reference

Tokish JM, Abrams JS: Video. Double-pulley Remplissage for the Management of Moderate-size Hill-Sachs Lesions. Princeton, NJ, 2015.

Chapter 11

Graft and Prosthetic Options for the Management of Anterior Instability Resulting From Severe Humeral Bone Loss

Salvatore J. Frangiamore, MD, MS

Anthony Miniaci, MD, FRCSC

 ## Introduction

The unique anatomy of the shoulder enables freedom of movement in multiple planes and renders the shoulder one of the most mobile joints in the body; however, the multidirectional range of motion (ROM) of the shoulder also places it at risk of instability and dislocation. The shoulder is the most commonly dislocated joint in the body, with an incidence of dislocation of 23.1 per 100,000 person-years. Young adult men have the highest rate of dislocation. Anterior glenohumeral dislocation is the most common presentation, accounting for more than 95% of all dislocations.

Anterior dislocation results in compression of the anteroinferior glenoid against the posterolateral humeral head, often leading to reciprocal injury on both sides. The Hill-Sachs lesion is an impaction fracture on the posterolateral aspect of the humeral head. Hill-Sachs lesions are estimated to occur in 40%

to 90% of all anterior dislocation events and may occur in up to 100% of patients with recurrent dislocations. Both anteroinferior glenoid bone loss and Hill-Sachs defects alter the contact area in the glenohumeral joint and the function of static shoulder stabilizers, which together may result in recurrent anterior instability. When managing anterior instability, it is critical to address any clinically significant humeral bone loss, because isolated soft-tissue stabilization has a recurrence rate as high as 67% in patients with bone defects.

Anterior glenohumeral dislocation is caused by excessive force placed on the arm while the joint is in abduction and external rotation. In this mechanism of injury, the humeral head translates anteriorly along the glenoid, damaging and possibly tearing soft-tissue structures such as the labrum and capsule. Further anterior translation of the humeral head results in a loss of articular contact and anterior dislocation of the humerus. In

this position, the posterosuperolateral aspect of the humeral head comes into contact with the anterior glenoid rim, causing a Hill-Sachs compression fracture on the humeral head. Because of the substantial loss of stability caused by combined defects in the anterior soft-tissue structures and the humeral head, repeated anterior dislocations are even more likely. Recurrent dislocations cause repeated contact between the Hill-Sachs lesion and hard cortical anterior glenoid bone, resulting in further damage to the humeral head. The defect may be altered by repeated dislocations, a history of seizure or failed reduction, delayed reduction, and a missed diagnosis.

Of further clinical importance is whether a Hill-Sachs lesion is engaging or nonengaging. In a patient with an engaging lesion, the long axis of the humeral head defect is oriented parallel to and contacts the anterior glenoid with the joint in a functional position of 90° of abduction and zero degrees to 135° of external rotation. The disruption within the native glenohumeral articulation during engagement (that is, in contact) is called an articular arc deficit. Larger engaging lesions engage the anterior glenoid at angles less than the traditional 90° of abduction and 90° of external rotation and can cause a sensation of instability. In a patient with a nonengaging lesion, the long axis of the humeral head defect is diagonal to or not parallel

Dr. Miniaci or an immediate family member has received royalties from Arthrosurface and Zimmer; is a member of a speakers' bureau or has made paid presentations on behalf of Arthrosurface, ConMed Linvatec, and Smith & Nephew; serves as a paid consultant to Arthrosurface, ConMed Linvatec, Smith & Nephew, Stryker, and Zimmer; has stock or stock options held in Arthrosurface, DePuy, Medtronic, Stryker, and Zimmer; has received nonincome support (such as equipment or services), commercially derived honoraria, or other non–research-related funding (such as paid travel) from Arthrosurface and Stryker; and serves as a board member, owner, officer, or committee member of the American Orthopaedic Society for Sports Medicine, the American Shoulder and Elbow Surgeons, the Arthroscopy Association of North America, and the International Society of Arthroscopy, Knee Surgery and Orthopaedic Sports Medicine. Neither Dr. Frangiamore nor any immediate family member has received anything of value from or has stock or stock options held in a commercial company or institution related directly or indirectly to the subject of this chapter.

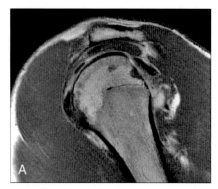
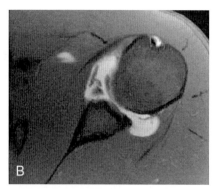

Figure 1   Sagittal (**A**) and axial (**B**) T1-weighted MRIs of a shoulder demonstrate a Hill-Sachs lesion.

to the anterior glenoid when the shoulder is in a functional position. Because a nonengaging lesion passes diagonally across the anterior glenoid, the articular surfaces are in continual contact, and no articular arc deficit is present.

A biomechanical model called the glenoid track concept, which is used to assess the risk of anterior instability, incorporates both glenoid and humeral bone loss. The glenoid track concept is helpful in understanding whether a Hill-Sachs lesion is engaging. The glenoid track is the zone of contact between the glenoid and the humeral head as the shoulder moves through ROM. If a Hill-Sachs lesion stays within the glenoid track (that is, on track) during motion, it has no chance of engaging and overriding the glenoid rim. If the medial margin of a lesion is outside the glenoid track (that is, off track), the risk of the lesion overriding the glenoid rim and engaging is higher. The width of the glenoid track is estimated to be 84% of the width of the glenoid; therefore, glenoid bone loss causes a narrower glenoid track, leading to a higher risk of dislocation.

 Case Presentation

A 21-year-old professional athlete presents for an evaluation of recurrent anterior shoulder instability. His first left glenohumeral dislocation occurred 4 years before. He had two subsequent

dislocations before undergoing an arthroscopic Bankart repair 3 years before. Six months after the soft-tissue stabilization procedure, he experienced a repeat dislocation and has dislocated eight or nine times since. Physical examination reveals apprehension at 45° of abduction and substantial splinting and spasms during external rotation, which is suggestive of rotational humeral head pathology. MRI demonstrates anteroinferior glenoid pathology associated with a Hill-Sachs lesion measuring approximately one-third of the humeral head radius of curvature (**Figure 1**).

Because the patient had an extensive and substantial humeral head defect and evidence of an engaging lesion on physical examination, it was decided that a reconstruction of the glenoid and the humeral head gave the best possibility for long-term success. After discussing all treatment options with the patient, the decision was made to proceed with a humeral head allograft reconstruction, an open Latarjet procedure with glenoid reconstruction, and a Bankart repair with capsular shift. Five months postoperatively, the patient experienced no feelings of instability, achieved full ROM with a 5° loss of external rotation, and had no apprehension in any position. Radiographs demonstrated good hardware positioning, with sclerosis at the interface between the allograft and the native humeral head, which was suggestive of healing (**Figure 2**).

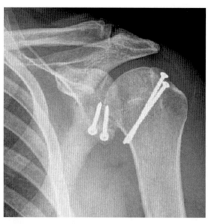

Figure 2   Postoperative AP radiograph of a left shoulder demonstrates the positions of the humeral head allograft and the Latarjet hardware 5 months postoperatively.

 Indications

Indications for addressing the humeral head vary, depending on surgeon preference. In the practice of the senior author of this chapter (A.M.), the approach to anterior instability is determined based on both physical examination findings and advanced imaging. Hill-Sachs lesions that are small (<10% to 15% of the humeral head) or nonengaging do not require surgical management targeted at the humeral head defect. Anterior instability in patients with small Hill-Sachs lesions may be managed by addressing anterior soft-tissue damage alone, including capsulolabral repair and plication and rotator cuff repair if indicated. Many of these procedures are augmented with remplissage. Elderly and low-demand patients also may be better suited for nonsurgical treatment.

Surgical indications for the management of Hill-Sachs lesions guided by level I or II research are lacking; therefore, management is guided by level IV evidence (case series) and level V expert opinion. The management of Hill-Sachs lesions depends on the size and location of a lesion and whether a lesion is engaging.

In one study, glenohumeral stability was found to be substantially decreased when the Hill-Sachs lesion took up 62.5% of the humeral head radius or 30% of diameter. The authors of another study discovered substantially less stability when humeral head lesions involved more than 25% of the humeral head. For certain Hill-Sachs lesions, humeral head management in addition to soft-tissue and glenoid procedures may be necessary. The authors of this chapter propose that humeral head lesions greater than 25% of the humeral head with chronic dislocations or recurrent anterior instability and engaging lesions greater than 20% to 25% of the humeral head should be considered for surgical management to reconstruct the humeral head defect. Surgical options to address Hill-Sachs humeral head defects include nonanatomic and anatomic approaches.

Nonanatomic procedures do not address the Hill-Sachs lesion directly. Instead, they are performed in an attempt to indirectly prevent the lesion from engaging the anterior glenoid. Examples of nonanatomic procedures include the Putti-Platt, Magnuson-Stack, rotational humeral osteotomy or Weber osteotomy, coracoid transfer procedures, and remplissage. The Putti-Platt, Magnuson-Stack, and rotational humeral osteotomy procedures attempt to decrease external rotation to prevent engagement but are associated with an increased risk of glenohumeral osteoarthritis, nonunion, malrotation, and loss of ROM. The Bristow and Latarjet procedures involve coracoid transfers to restore articular arc length but also can lead to osteoarthritis, hardware complications, and nonunion. The remplissage procedure is a tenodesis of the infraspinatus tendon to the defect with suture anchors, which prevents engagement.

For patients who have anterior instability resulting from severe humeral bone loss, treatment options include humeroplasty (that is, disimpaction of the humeral head), osteochondral allograft, and use of prosthetic surface implants. All of these anatomic surgical procedures attempt to imitate the natural shape of the articular surface of the humeral head. Humeroplasty is a relatively novel procedure that directly corrects a Hill-Sachs lesion using a bone tamp or balloon to elevate the depressed defect and fill it with cancellous bone or cement.

The goal of osteochondral allograft reconstruction, whether osteochondral plug transfer or bulk allograft, is to re-create the articular arc of the humeral head. Few case reports and case series exist documenting osteochondral plug transfers. The procedure involves grafting fresh-frozen allograft plugs tangential to the articular surface in the humeral head to restore normal humeral head anatomy. Possible complications include graft resorption and graft failure. In addition, using multiple plugs makes it difficult to achieve a perfect surface. If the grafts have different heights, then these irregularities could create abrasion or even catching during rotational motion. Bulk humeral head allografts are size- and side-matched to a Hill-Sachs lesion to re-create the articular arc and humeral head sphericity. The height of the cadaver model from which an allograft is harvested is the single most accurate indicator of the anatomy and curvature of the cadaveric allograft humeral head. Femoral head osteoarticular allograft or iliac crest autograft tissue also can be used. Ideal candidates for osteochondral allograft reconstruction are young patients without degenerative joint disease. In the experience of the authors of this chapter, this procedure most commonly is performed secondary to other failed soft-tissue stabilization procedures but can be used with primary anterior soft-tissue procedures if a large and engaging Hill-Sachs lesion is discovered preoperatively.

For many years, the senior author of this chapter (A.M.) used irradiated matched humeral head allograft. In the first 20 patients treated, two of the grafts partially resorbed, which required hardware removal but did not result in recurrent instability. A switch was made to using size- and side-matched fresh-frozen grafts, which led to excellent functional results and, to the author's knowledge, no instances of resorption. The increased popularity of this procedure has made it more difficult to find appropriate graft material, with substantial delays in sourcing. Thus, for patients with substantial instability, the authors of this chapter began using metal partial resurfacing implants, which can be matched to the size of the defect and the curvature of the humeral head. Use of these implants has resulted in excellent outcomes with no recurrent instability and no implant-related complications. The authors of this chapter have almost 10 years' experience with this approach.

Fresh-frozen allograft is used in very young patients (younger than 20 years) who do not want a metal implant and are willing to wait for an appropriate allograft. Most of these patients are severely functionally compromised, however, and are not willing to delay surgery. Thus, the authors of this chapter have considerable experience with excellent functional results using metal partial resurfacing even in very young patients.

If surgery is indicated, three-dimensional CT reconstruction is used to prepare a size-matched fresh-frozen cryopreserved humeral head. Alternatively, MRI can help determine the exact location and extent of Hill-Sachs lesions. The allograft ideally should measure within 2 mm of the native humeral head. The contralateral head can be used as a reference if the surgical side anatomy is obscured by the defect. Three-dimensional CT reconstruction images also provide details about the patient's glenoid morphology or bony defects related to instability to ensure articular congruency (**Figure 3**).

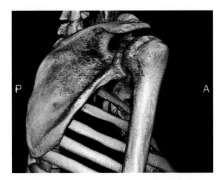

Figure 3 Three-dimensional CT reconstruction of a right shoulder demonstrates a large Hill-Sachs lesion. A = anterior, P = posterior.

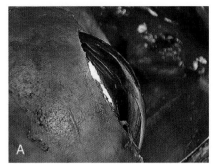
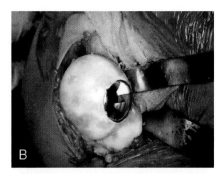

Figure 4 **A** and **B,** Intraoperative photographs of a shoulder show partial humeral resurfacing using the Shoulder HemiCAP System prosthesis (Arthrosurface).

Traditionally, the senior author of this chapter (A.M.) determines the functional impact of a lesion by its position relative to the anterior glenoid with the shoulder in a functional position of abduction and external rotation. The key to identifying humeral head lesions is to use rotational apprehension in positions of 45° or less. Regardless of the relative size of a lesion, if it engages the anterior glenoid at this position, it will continue to engage and disrupt the articular arc unless the humeral head pathology is addressed. The bipolar defects of the humeral head and glenoid rim are assessed with three-dimensional CT, with the patient's arm in external rotation, abduction, and extension in the horizontal plane to assess tracking.

It is much more difficult to determine a treatment plan for patients who have combined lesions. If a humeral lesion is contained within the glenoid track, that is, 84% of the distance measured from the medial margin of the rotator cuff insertion to the middle of the humeral head, it should not engage in the functional arc of motion. Lesions that are either outside the glenoid track or partially contained will limit functional ROM. Although lesions that are perpendicular and nonengaging should not be problematic in theory, lesions that are larger than 30% of the humeral head still can cause instability. The indications for anatomic allograft reconstruction of the

humeral head defect include ongoing symptomatic anterior glenohumeral instability or painful clicking, catching, or popping in a patient with a large engaging Hill-Sachs lesion. Contraindications to surgical management include advanced glenohumeral arthrosis, an existing infection, or unaddressed or irreparable rotator cuff deficiency.

Controversies and Alternative Approaches

In patients with large Hill-Sachs lesions, addressing engaging or off-track lesions to maintain a congruent articular arc can result in fewer episodes of instability and improved outcomes compared with solely addressing the glenoid defect. Humeral head allograft reconstruction offers younger patients a viable option to humeral head arthroplasty, soft-tissue procedures, and other options that have had variable success rates. Another option is humeral head resurfacing, which does not carry the same risk for nonunion, disease transmission, and graft resorption as allograft reconstruction. Potential complications for prosthetic implants include hardware loosening, glenoid wear, and adverse reactions to metal. Partial humeral head resurfacing uses a cobalt-chromium articular component to fill the symptomatic Hill-Sachs lesion. A cobalt-chromium partial humeral head resurfacing implant may

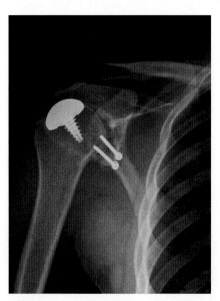

Figure 5 Postoperative AP radiograph of a right shoulder demonstrates the Shoulder HemiCAP System prosthesis (Arthrosurface) next to hardware from a concurrent Latarjet procedure.

be an option for an engaging Hill-Sachs lesion or a reverse Hill-Sachs lesion if a size-matched allograft is unavailable (**Figures 4** and **5**).

Partial humeral head resurfacing is indicated in younger patients who have small- to moderate-size lesions that affect less than 40% of the humeral head, who have normal bone stock, and who do not have osteoporosis. For larger Hill-Sachs lesions that affect more than 40% of the humeral head, partial or complete humeral head resurfacing, hemiarthroplasty, or total shoulder arthroplasty (TSA) is most suitable to re-create the articular arc. Hemiarthroplasty and, in some patients, TSA, are indicated in older patients who have lower activity levels and preexisting glenohumeral osteoarthritis. These implants can facilitate correction of the humeral defect and transition to the adjacent chondral defect with preservation of intact articular cartilage, avoiding failure at the graft-host junction that can occur with osteochondral allograft. Studies of prosthetic options to manage Hill-Sachs lesions are limited, and further work is needed to better define the indications.

Results

The few published studies documenting outcomes for humeroplasty and graft procedures in anterior shoulder instability have relatively small patient populations (**Table 1**). In one small series of patients who were treated with humeroplasty, no instability or complications were noted at 1-year follow-up. Multiple case reports describe the management of anterior instability with humeral head allografts, but a paucity of case series exist. In one published study, most patients who underwent side- and size-matched humeral head allograft reconstruction after previous failed anterior instability repairs were able to return to work, and although seven complications were reported, no patient had recurrent instability. In a series of four patients who underwent humeral head allograft reconstruction, no recurrence of dislocations or subluxations occurred, and there was no radiographic evidence of graft resorption. Patients had losses in ROM, however.

Reports of prosthetic outcomes for anterior instability also are rare. In a report of two patients who were treated with partial humeral head resurfacing to manage anterior instability, neither patient had repeat dislocation at 1-year follow-up, and outcomes scores improved. In a case series of 13 patients who underwent humeral head resurfacing for a Hill-Sachs lesion in anterior instability, none of the patients suffered a repeat dislocation, and 10 patients reported a return to preinjury activity levels.

Few complications were reported in a case series of 10 patients who underwent complete humeral head resurfacing. No signs of implant loosening were found, and outcomes scores improved. In a case series of 11 patients who were treated with either hemiarthroplasty or TSA, outcomes scores improved, although complications were reported and 2 patients required revision surgery. In a separate small series of patients who underwent hemiarthroplasty or TSA, no patients had repeat dislocations and only one complication occurred.

Video 11.1 Osteochondral Allograft Humeral Head Reconstruction for Anterior Shoulder Instability. Anthony Miniaci, MD, FRCSC (5 min)

Technical Keys to Success

- After the patient is intubated and sedated, a proper evaluation of humeral translation on the glenoid is assessed in five directions and three positions of arm rotation to determine the position of instability and the degree of abduction and external rotation at which the instability occurs.
- The examination is repeated in the same fashion after the glenoid pathology is addressed in bipolar defects to confirm engaging, off-track lesions.
- The patient is placed in the beach-chair position with the head of the bed raised 30° to 45° without limitations in glenohumeral or scapular motion.
- The coracoid is identified, and an incision is made in line with the raphe separating the anterior deltoid and the pectoralis to perform a standard deltopectoral approach.
- After the interval between the anterior deltoid and the pectoralis is developed, the arm is externally rotated, and the interval between the clavipectoral fascia and the subscapularis is identified.
- The subscapularis is released in line with the glenohumeral joint off the lesser tuberosity. A small cuff of tendon should remain on the lesser tuberosity for later repair.
- Stay sutures are placed in the subscapularis and retracted medially.
- The superior and inferior borders of the subscapularis must be developed and released so that the humeral head can be exposed adequately posteriorly.
- The arm is rotated maximally externally and flexed to deliver the humeral head for the reconstruction of the posterior defect.
- The interval between the subscapularis muscle and the deep capsule is identified and developed medial to the glenoid.
- A capsulotomy is performed, and pathology in the anteroinferior-capsulolabral complex and glenoid is identified.
- Medial sutures are placed in the capsulolabral junction, and the labrum, which is torn most often, is detached from the glenoid. The labrum will be reattached in the later stages of the procedure after treatment of the humeral head.
- The humeral head lesion is identified and delivered into the incision by maximal external rotation and slight forward flexion. The condition of the surrounding bone and the quality of the neighboring cartilage are assessed for viability to determine the position of the osteotomy cuts (**Figure 6, A**). In many patients, the humeral articular

Table 1 Results of Arthroplasty, Resurfacing, and Grafting in the Management of Anterior Instability in Patients With Severe Humeral Bone Loss

Authors	Journal (Year)	Technique (No. of Patients)	Outcomes	Failure Rate (%)[a]	Comments
Pritchett and Clark	*Clin Orthop Relat Res* (1987)	Hemiarthroplasty (4), TSA (3)	No redislocations Avg Rowe and Zarins score, 70 units (good)	0	1 patient had transient axillary nerve palsy
Miniaci and Gish	*Techniques in Shoulder & Elbow Surgery* (2004)	Humeral head allograft reconstruction (18)	Avg Constant-Murley score, 78.5 Radiographic partial graft collapse in 2 patients Early evidence of osteoarthritis in 3 patients Hardware-related pain that required screw removal 2 yr postoperatively in 2 patients	0	16 patients returned to work, and no patient had recurrent instability Avg follow-up, 50 mo
Matsoukis et al	*J Bone Joint Surg Am* (2006)	Hemiarthroplasty (7), TSA (4)	Mean Constant score improved from 21.1 to 46	14 (hemiarthroplasty) 75 (TSA)	7 complications in 5 patients, requiring 2 reoperations: 3 patients with TSA had anterior dislocations, 2 patients with TSA had glenoid component loosening (requiring 1 patient to undergo revision surgery to remove the glenoid component), 1 patient with hemiarthroplasty had an anterior dislocation, and 1 patient with hemiarthroplasty had bone graft migration requiring screw removal.
Re et al	*Arthroscopy* (2006)	Humeroplasty (4)	All patients had return of full ROM and returned to their preinjury level of function	0	Avg follow-up, 12 mo
Grondin and Leith	*Can J Surg* (2009)	Partial humeral head resurfacing (2)	ASES and WOSI scores improved	0	No redislocation Follow-up, 12 mo
Raiss et al	*Int Orthop* (2009)	Complete humeral head resurfacing (10)	Mean Constant score improved from 20 to 61 No signs of implant loosening	10	1 patient underwent revision to manage redislocation 1 patient developed glenoid erosion and required revision to TSA Mean follow-up, 24 mo
DiPaola et al	*Bull NYU Hosp Jt Dis* (2010)	Humeral head allograft reconstruction (4)	Mean ASES score, 85.3 Mean UCLA score, 28.4 No dislocations, subluxations, or graft resorption	0	Losses in ROM occurred, 1 patient developed reflex sympathetic dystrophy, and 1 patient required revision surgery for removal of a prominent screw Avg follow-up, 28 mo
Frisch et al	ISAKOS Biennial Congress (Abstract; 2013)	Humeral head resurfacing (13) for anterior instability	85% achieved full ROM 77% returned to their pre-injury level of function Significant improvement in MSROS and SF-12 scores	0	Avg follow up, 36.4 mo

ASES = American Shoulder and Elbow Surgeons shoulder outcome, MSROS = musculoskeletal review of systems, ROM = range of motion, SF-12 = Medical Outcomes Study 12-Item Short Form, TSA = total shoulder arthroplasty, UCLA = University of California–Los Angeles Shoulder Rating Scale, WOSI = Western Ontario Shoulder Instability Index.
[a] Recurrent instability.

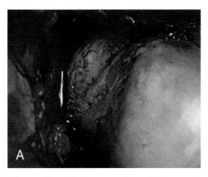 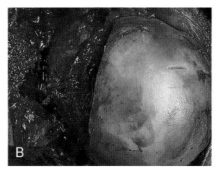 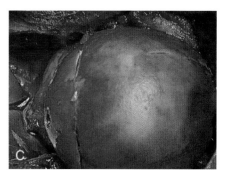

Figure 6 Intraoperative photographs of a shoulder show osteochondral allograft reconstruction to manage a Hill-Sachs lesion. **A,** Humeral head bone loss is shown. **B,** A chevron-type osteotomy encompassing the humeral head defect is shown. **C,** Osteochondral allograft fixation has been performed using a countersunk screw.

surface hangs over the Hill-Sachs defect; this overhang is removed to create a chevron defect to allow easier fit of the allograft (**Figure 6, B**).

- Intraoperative measurements of the machined defect are taken to the nearest millimeter to determine depth, width, and length.
- The matching allograft is sized and cut to fit the humeral head osteotomy site. The matching allograft initially is cut 2 to 3 mm larger in all dimensions and then resized carefully with a microsagittal saw in all three planes until it becomes a perfect size match.
- The allograft is placed into the defect and temporarily secured with Kirschner wires.
- Fully-threaded 3.5-mm cortical screws are placed in a lag fashion to achieve fixation, and the articular congruency is evaluated for any mismatch between the graft and the native humeral head. Step-off must be avoided because it leaves an irregular articulating surface, which will catch or abrade during rotational motion.
- After acceptable positioning is confirmed, definitive screw fixation is achieved by countersinking the screw head to ensure a smooth arc within the functional ROM (**Figure 6, C**). Solid-bore screws are less likely to break compared with a cannulated screw, but any type of

compression screw configuration can be used. Countersinking the screws is crucial so that they do not catch or abrade, especially in patients with small amounts of graft resorption or collapse.

- At this stage of the procedure, if the surgeon chooses to use a partial humeral resurfacing device, the guidewires and instrumentation are used to fill the defect and re-create the curvature of the humeral head.
- After the humeral head is reconstructed, it is reduced and retracted with a Fukuda retractor.
- Remaining glenoid pathology is addressed with a procedure such as a Bankart repair, Latarjet procedure, or bone graft procedure.
- The capsule is closed with the patient's arm in external rotation to avoid overtightening and postoperative loss of motion, specifically external rotation.
- Proper closure is essential to protect the repair and enhance stability.
- If a Latarjet procedure has been performed, inferior subscapularis release must be done to avoid tethering by the conjoined tendon as the conjoined tendon passes underneath the subscapularis. Tethering can result in tightness in external rotation or avulsion of the subscapularis repair if external rotation cannot be achieved intraoperatively.
- The incised subscapularis tendon

is repaired in side-to-side fashion. If there is an insufficient sleeve of tendon for repair, a medial anchor can be placed to augment repair to the humerus (**Figure 1, A**).

- During subscapularis repair as well as capsular closure, it is critical to maintain the arm in external rotation to avoid overtightening and loss of external rotation.
- Before fascial closure, a smooth, uninterrupted range of functional motion should be demonstrated under direct visualization.

Rehabilitation

The affected arm is placed in a sling for comfort postoperatively, and passive ROM is begun immediately postoperatively (**Table 2**). Full forward elevation is encouraged. To protect the subscapularis repair, however, external rotation past 20° and resisted internal rotation are avoided for approximately 6 weeks postoperatively. Terminal stretching and strengthening exercises are begun after this 6-week period. Radiographs of the treated shoulder are obtained at 6 weeks postoperatively and again at 6 months postoperatively to assess for consolidation and incorporation of the graft. CT also is obtained at 6 months postoperatively.

In the experience of the senior author of this chapter (A.M.), some degree of

Table 2 Rehabilitation Protocol After Grafting or Prosthesis Implantation to Manage Anterior Instability in Patients With Severe Humeral Bone Loss

Postoperative Week	ROM	Strengthening	Return to Play	Comments/Emphasis
0-2	Passive ROM is begun immediately postoperatively Full forward elevation is encouraged External rotation past 20° and resisted internal rotation are avoided	None	None	Sling is used for comfort
2-6	External rotation past 20° and resisted internal rotation are avoided	None	None	—
6-12	External rotation past 20° and resisted internal rotation are begun	Terminal stretching and strengthening exercises are begun	—	Radiographs obtained at 6 wk to assess for graft consolidation and incorporation
12-24	—	—	Can return to play at 6 mo if graft shows signs of incorporation and physical therapy has been completed	CT and repeat radiographs obtained to evaluate graft consolidation and incorporation

ROM = range of motion.

graft incorporation is always seen, and partial graft collapse is rare. In addition, neither partial collapse nor delayed incorporation has affected postoperative outcomes, and it is believed that restricting rehabilitation would be more detrimental. Imaging does not guide the rehabilitation protocol. Activity is not restricted in terms of return to sports; however, some athletes choose not to participate in contact sports postoperatively because of the associated risks and their previous disability.

Avoiding Pitfalls

Humeral allograft reconstruction is a technically demanding procedure, and multiple steps must be taken to obtain a successful outcome. If capsulolabral structures are addressed concurrently with a Hill-Sachs lesion, then the anterior capsule and the subscapularis can be left together and elevated as one complex. The authors of this chapter find it simpler to expose the humeral head

and repair the capsulolabral structures separately, however. This technique enables better release of the subscapularis, which makes humeral head exposure easier and facilitates the mobilization and repair of capsulolabral structures. To provide better visualization of the Hill-Sachs defect and allow a greater range of external rotation of the humerus, the interval tissue overlying the tendon of the long head of the biceps should be unroofed. Subscapularis release is key. In making a chevron-type osteotomy to remove damaged humeral cartilage and bone, extra attention should be given to the preparation of surfaces along the base and sides of the recipient site to enable a smooth transition for the best fit of the donor allograft.

When cutting and sizing the allograft humeral head, it is best to err on the side of creating a larger allograft plug that can be adjusted to fit the defect. It is better to cut and size repeatedly than to undercut the graft all at once. Failure to recognize that adjustments in one plane will affect the final size of

the allograft in the other two dimensions will result in a graft that is mismatched to the recipient defect. Little can be done to ensure a perfect fit if the allograft piece is too small, but the surfaces must be aligned perfectly. Steps are not acceptable, because they can catch, abrade, or impinge. During definitive graft fixation, it is imperative that the screw heads be countersunk below the articular cartilage. Prominent screws can cause abrasive wear; in addition, enough of the screw head should be buried so that if the allograft collapses or resorbs, screw wear does not develop. Moving the shoulder through a ROM intraoperatively helps to assess whether any catching or clicking is present from a step between the graft and the humeral head or from a prominent screw.

Acknowledgment

The authors thank Samir Oak, BS, for his significant support in preparing the manuscript and the video.

Bibliography

Bois AJ, Walker RE, Kodali P, Miniaci A: Imaging instability in the athlete: The right modality for the right diagnosis. *Clin Sports Med* 2013;32(4):653-684.

Bollier MJ, Arciero R: Management of glenoid and humeral bone loss. *Sports Med Arthrosc* 2010;18(3):140-148.

Burkhart SS, De Beer JF: Traumatic glenohumeral bone defects and their relationship to failure of arthroscopic Bankart repairs: Significance of the inverted-pear glenoid and the humeral engaging Hill-Sachs lesion. *Arthroscopy* 2000;16(7):677-694.

Cho SH, Cho NS, Rhee YG: Preoperative analysis of the Hill-Sachs lesion in anterior shoulder instability: How to predict engagement of the lesion. *Am J Sports Med* 2011;39(11):2389-2395.

DiPaola MJ, Jazrawi LM, Rokito AS, et al: Management of humeral and glenoid bone loss associated with glenohumeral instability. *Bull NYU Hosp Jt Dis* 2010;68(4):245-250.

Frisch N, Jones MH, Miniaci A: Abstract: Outcome of a partial cap resurfacing implant for humeral head defects in patients with shoulder instability. Presented at the 2013 ISAKOS Biennial Congress, Toronto, Canada, May 12-16, 2013. Available at: https://www.isakos.com/meetings/2013congress/onsite/AbstractView.aspx?EventID=6634. Accessed October 29, 2015.

Gebhart JJ, Miniaci A, Fening SD: Predictive anthropometric measurements for humeral head curvature. *J Shoulder Elbow Surg* 2013;22(6):842-847.

Grondin P, Leith J: Case series: Combined large Hill-Sachs and bony Bankart lesions treated by Latarjet and partial humeral head resurfacing: A report of 2 cases. *Can J Surg* 2009;52(3):249-254.

Kaar SG, Fening SD, Jones MH, Colbrunn RW, Miniaci A: Effect of humeral head defect size on glenohumeral stability: A cadaveric study of simulated Hill-Sachs defects. *Am J Sports Med* 2010;38(3):594-599.

Kodali P, Jones MH, Polster J, Miniaci A, Fening SD: Accuracy of measurement of Hill-Sachs lesions with computed tomography. *J Shoulder Elbow Surg* 2011;20(8):1328-1334.

Leroux T, Wasserstein D, Veillette C, et al: Epidemiology of primary anterior shoulder dislocation requiring closed reduction in Ontario, Canada. *Am J Sports Med* 2014;42(2):442-450.

Matsoukis J, Tabib W, Guiffault P, et al: Primary unconstrained shoulder arthroplasty in patients with a fixed anterior glenohumeral dislocation. *J Bone Joint Surg Am* 2006;88(3):547-552.

Miniaci A, Gish MW: Management of anterior glenohumeral instability associated with large Hill-Sachs defects. *Techniques in Shoulder & Elbow Surgery* 2004;5:170-175.

Najarian R, Fening SD, Jones MH, Miniaci A: Abstract: Engaging versus non-engaging Hill-Sachs defects within the functional shoulder range of motion. Presented at The American Shoulder and Elbow Surgeons (ASES) 2011 Open Meeting/Specialty Day, August 18, 2011. Available at: http://www.jshoulderelbow.org/pb/assets/raw/Health%20Advance/journals/ymse/ASES_2011_Abstracts.pdf. Accessed May 3, 2016.

Patel RM, Amin NH, Lynch TS, Miniaci A: Management of bone loss in glenohumeral instability. *Orthop Clin North Am* 2014;45(4):523-539.

Pritchett JW, Clark JM: Prosthetic replacement for chronic unreduced dislocations of the shoulder. *Clin Orthop Relat Res* 1987;(216):89-93.

Provencher MT, Frank RM, Leclere LE, et al: The Hill-Sachs lesion: Diagnosis, classification, and management. *J Am Acad Orthop Surg* 2012;20(4):242-252.

Raiss P, Aldinger PR, Kasten P, Rickert M, Loew M: Humeral head resurfacing for fixed anterior glenohumeral dislocation. *Int Orthop* 2009;33(2):451-456.

Re P, Gallo RA, Richmond JC: Transhumeral head plasty for large Hill-Sachs lesions. *Arthroscopy* 2006;22(7):798.e1-798.e4.

Rowe CR, Zarins B, Ciullo JV: Recurrent anterior dislocation of the shoulder after surgical repair: Apparent causes of failure and treatment. *J Bone Joint Surg Am* 1984;66(2):159-168.

Sekiya JK, Wickwire AC, Stehle JH, Debski RE: Hill-Sachs defects and repair using osteoarticular allograft transplantation: Biomechanical analysis using a joint compression model. *Am J Sports Med* 2009;37(12):2459-2466.

Skendzel JG, Sekiya JK: Diagnosis and management of humeral head bone loss in shoulder instability. *Am J Sports Med* 2012;40(11):2633-2644.

Walia P, Miniaci A, Jones MH, Fening SD: Theoretical model of the effect of combined glenohumeral bone defects on anterior shoulder instability: A finite element approach. *J Orthop Res* 2013;31(4):601-607.

Yamamoto N, Itoi E, Abe H, et al: Contact between the glenoid and the humeral head in abduction, external rotation, and horizontal extension: A new concept of glenoid track. *J Shoulder Elbow Surg* 2007;16(5):649-656.

 ## Video Reference

Miniaci A: Video. *Osteochondral Allograft Humeral Head Reconstruction for Anterior Shoulder Instability*. Cleveland, OH, 2015.

Chapter 12

Posterior Labral Repair for Management of Uncomplicated Posterior Shoulder Instability

Fotios P. Tjoumakaris, MD

James P. Bradley, MD

Introduction

Posterior instability of the glenohumeral joint was originally thought of in terms of macroinstability, or posterior glenohumeral dislocation. Although posterior dislocation can occur in select patients, it is usually the result of more violent trauma, electrocution, or seizure disorders. Posterior shoulder subluxation with or without labral tearing (that is, microinstability) is the more common but perhaps historically less recognized manifestation of posterior glenohumeral instability. This subluxation may be more challenging to diagnose, with patients often presenting with vague symptoms and subtle findings on physical examination. Sports medicine clinicians are likely to encounter many patients who have posterior shoulder subluxation with or without labral tearing.

Case Presentation

An 18-year-old man presents with the sudden onset of right shoulder pain as a result of a traumatic event on a basketball court several months earlier. He reports that he was coming down from a rebound when he was fouled from behind, which caused him to land on his outstretched arm. He had severe pain in his right shoulder and elbow immediately after the injury; however, during the following week, the pain subsided. After 4 weeks of treatment recommended by his athletic trainer, which consisted of icing, anti-inflammatory medication, and the use of an isometric rotator cuff strengthening program, the patient returned to the basketball court. He finished the basketball season with only mild soreness in his shoulder after practice and games.

Several months later, during baseball season, the patient noted the recurrence of pain in his shoulder and decreased throwing velocity from the shortstop position. He reports anterior and posterior shoulder pain throughout the throwing motion and soreness after competition. He denies any neurovascular issues, such as numbness or tingling radiating into his right upper extremity, but reports feeling his whole arm "go dead" after throwing. Despite rest and continued treatment as recommended by his athletic trainer, the patient continues to experience debilitating symptoms.

The patient is 6 feet 2 inches tall and weighs 205 lb. His blood pressure and pulse are normal. He has no obvious atrophy about the shoulder girdle or the supraspinatus and infraspinatus fossa. His right shoulder demonstrates full range of motion (ROM) symmetric to that of his left shoulder and no evidence of internal rotation deficit. Manual muscle strength testing is normal and symmetric compared with the contralateral shoulder. No tenderness to palpation over the acromioclavicular joint, anterior capsule, and greater tuberosity is exhibited by the patient. Slight tenderness is observed along the posterior capsule and periscapular muscles. Anterior and posterior glide with the patient seated and supine is assigned a grade of 1+ on the load and shift test. Negative results are noted on the apprehension test, the relocation test, and the Neer and Hawkins impingement tests. The jerk test elicits mild pain, but no obvious instability is noted; however, severe sudden posterior pain is elicited with the Kim test. The O'Brien active compression test result is positive, with the patient reporting pain over the posterior joint capsule of the shoulder. Negative results are noted on the sulcus

Dr. Bradley or an immediate family member has received royalties and research or institutional support from Arthrex, and serves as a board member, owner, officer, or committee member of the American Orthopaedic Society for Sports Medicine. Neither Dr. Tjoumakaris nor any immediate family member has received anything of value from or has stock or stock options held in a commercial company or institution related directly or indirectly to the subject of this chapter.

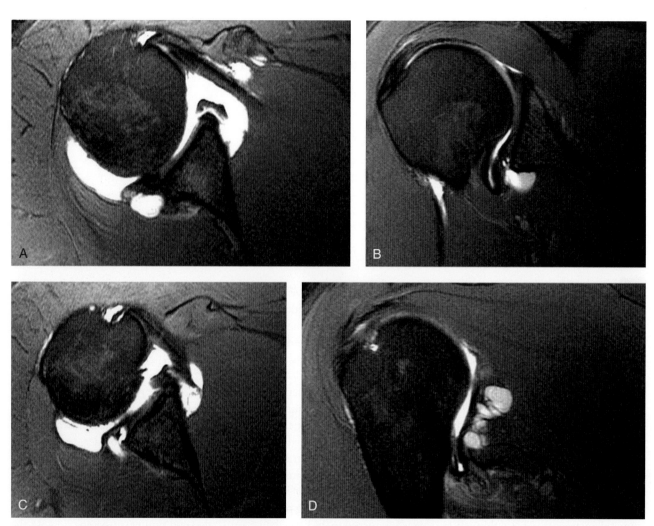

Figure 1   Axial (**A**) and coronal (**B**) T2-weighted magnetic resonance arthrograms demonstrate a posterior ganglion and a cordlike middle glenohumeral ligament. Axial (**C**) and coronal (**D**) T2-weighted magnetic resonance arthrograms demonstrate a posterior labral tear with a moderately sized posterior paralabral cyst.

sign and the global laxity assessment (knee, elbow, metacarpophalangeal joint hyperextension).

AP, scapular Y, and axillary right shoulder radiographs are normal, with no evidence of fracture, dislocation, or degenerative changes or deficiency of the humeral head or glenoid. Magnetic resonance arthrography demonstrates a posterior labral tear without evidence of increased glenoid retroversion or osseous deficiency (**Figure 1**). A loculated paralabral cyst is noted, but no atrophy of the supraspinatus or infraspinatus muscles that would indicate compression of the suprascapular nerve is found.

In patients with posterior labral tearing, imaging may demonstrate labral fraying; posterior glenoid erosion or remodeling; a Kim lesion (that is, concealed incomplete detachment of the posterior labrum); increased glenoid or chondrolabral retroversion; and/or associated pathology of the rotator cuff, biceps anchor, and superior labrum (with paralabral cyst formation).

The diagnosis in this patient was an episode of traumatic posterior instability and signs and symptoms of recurrent posterior subluxation of the right shoulder. Because of the size of the labral tear and the lack of response to extended

nonsurgical treatment, the patient underwent arthroscopy of the right shoulder with posterior labral repair without capsular plication. The patient used a sling for 6 weeks postoperatively and began passive ROM exercises on postoperative day 10. On discontinuation of the sling, active-assisted ROM exercises were begun, with progression to strengthening after 10 weeks. A throwing program was begun at 6 months, and the patient returned to basketball at 9 months. Baseball was resumed nearly 1 year postoperatively. Two years after the surgical repair, the patient was engaged in collegiate athletics. He reported full ROM, the ability to play at his previous level of competition, and no pain.

Indications

Patients are considered candidates for surgery when pain and disability have not been alleviated by nonsurgical means. Nonsurgical management of posterior shoulder instability primarily consists of physical therapy aimed at restoring balance to the glenohumeral joint through scapular and rotator cuff stretching and strengthening. Any patient with an internal rotation contracture is prescribed a posterior capsular stretching program. Despite physical therapy, nonsurgical treatment is unsuccessful in many patients with posterior instability of the shoulder. Surgery is indicated when the symptoms interfere with activities of daily living or restrict a patient's ability to engage in athletics. Patients with posterior instability resulting from a traumatic event, such as electrocution, seizure, or frank dislocation, may require an urgent intervention, such as closed reduction or acute stabilization. An open approach may be needed for patients with an osseous deficiency, such as glenoid hypoplasia, reverse Hill-Sachs lesions, or reverse bony Bankart lesions. Patients who are not willing or able to comply with postoperative restrictions and participate in a lengthy postoperative rehabilitation program also are not considered good surgical candidates.

Controversies and Alternative Approaches

Arthroscopic management of posterior shoulder instability has advanced substantially in the past two decades. Despite considerable initial debate on whether an open or arthroscopic technique should be used for repair

of posterior labral tears, the results of arthroscopic repair have surpassed those of open repair. However, whether an arthroscopic or open approach is best for patients with evidence of increased glenoid or chondrolabral retroversion or substantial bone defects caused by recurrent posterior dislocation remains controversial. Glenoid osteotomy, humeral derotational osteotomy, or allograft reconstruction may be appropriate for patients with substantial bone defects or deformity that could place them at higher risk for failure with an arthroscopic technique. In patients requiring revision surgery, arthroscopic treatment may be possible, depending on the quality of the remaining labral and capsular tissue. The advantages of arthroscopy include decreased morbidity without the need for deltoid detachment or exposure; improved ROM without scarring of the deltoid; the ability to address concomitant pathology, such as rotator cuff tear, impingement syndrome, superior labrum anterior to posterior lesions, loose body removal, biceps treatment, or panlabral pathology; and decreased perioperative morbidity. Controversy has emerged on the necessity of closing the rotator interval in patients with unidirectional posterior instability. Although some studies have advocated closure of the rotator interval during labral repair, the authors of this chapter do not routinely close the rotator interval because of concerns for postoperative stiffness, particularly in athletic patients who use throwing or overhead motions.

Results

The results of arthroscopic posterior labral repair for the treatment of instability have been excellent, with multiple studies reporting recurrence rates less than 10%. In addition, studies of contact athletes have reported low recurrence rates (<8%), with recurrences primarily

in patients who sustained traumatic events in the postoperative period. Because of the successful results of arthroscopic treatment and the poor outcomes of open surgical treatment (for example, an aggregate failure rate of 23% with open capsular shift), most surgeons use an arthroscopic technique for posterior labral repair and stabilization. The results of prominent studies that used a technique similar to that described in this chapter are summarized in **Table 1**.

Technical Keys to Success

Successful surgical treatment begins with proper patient selection and surgical planning. A thorough history and physical examination that corroborates magnetic resonance arthrography findings is key to achieving the best outcome. Several steps can facilitate a stress-free surgical workflow. First, the lateral decubitus position allows unfettered access to the posterior capsule and labrum without the need for an assistant to provide shoulder distraction. Placing the arm in slight traction (10 to 15 lb) with 20° to 30° of forward flexion and 45° of abduction can facilitate access to the posterior glenoid. Second, protection of the labrum during labral preparation is important because the posterior labrum and capsule can be patulous and easily injured iatrogenically. If a motorized shaver or burr is used, it is important to protect the labrum by débriding the undersurface of the labrum and not the external tissue because débridement of the external tissue could compromise labral integrity. Third, anchor placement is improved with proper placement of the posterior portal. Two-portal repair is possible if the posterior portal is positioned slightly lateral and inferior to the location of a standard posterior shoulder arthroscopy portal. This posterior portal position allows for a tangential

Table 1 Results of Arthroscopic Posterior Labral Repair

Authors	Journal (Year)	No. of Patients	Mean Follow-up (mo)	Outcomes Measures	Failure Rate (%)	Comments
Kim et al	*J Bone Joint Surg Am* (2003)	27	39	ASES, Rowe, and UCLA scores	4	>90% good to excellent results
Williams et al	*Am J Sports Med* (2003)	27	61	L'Insalata Shoulder Rating Questionnaire, SF-36	8	Traumatic etiology in all patients
Bottoni et al	*Am J Sports Med* (2005)	19	34	SANE, Rowe score, SST, WOSI	10	Outcomes were better after arthroscopy than after open repair
Savoie et al	*Arthroscopy* (2008)	131	28	Neer-Foster rating scale	3	—
Bahk et al	*Arthroscopy* (2010)	29	66	ASES score, UCLA score, SST, WOSI	3.4	85% of patients returned to sports
Pennington et al	*Arthroscopy* (2010)	28	24	ASES, UCLA, and Rowe scores	7[a]	All patients in the study were athletes
Lenart et al	*Arthroscopy* (2012)	34	36	ASES, SST, VAS	6	—
Bradley et al	*Am J Sports Med* (2013)	183	36	ASES	10[a]	Suture anchor repairs demonstrated superior outcomes
Wooten et al	*J Pediatr Orthop* (2015)	22	63	ASES, Marx activity score	8	Younger patients (≤18 yr)

ASES = American Shoulder and Elbow Surgeons shoulder outcomes, SANE = Single Assessment Numeric Evaluation, SF-36 = Medical Outcomes Study 36-Item Short Form, SST = Simple Shoulder Test, UCLA = University of California–Los Angeles Shoulder Rating Scale, VAS = visual analog scale, WOSI = Western Ontario Shoulder Instability Index.

[a] Defined as failure to return to sport.

drilling angle (>30°) to the glenoid that will help avoid injury to the articular cartilage during anchor placement. If an accessory posterior portal is required for placement of anchors, this portal is typically created slightly lateral (approximately 2 cm) to the standard posterior viewing portal. Finally, the repair technique should be tailored to the specific pathology and needs of the patient. Capsular plication may be needed in patients with multidirectional instability or in athletes who participate in contact sports, whereas overhead-throwing athletes may require only labral restoration to regain high-velocity throwing.

The video cited in this chapter demonstrates arthroscopic posterior labral repair for uncomplicated posterior shoulder instability. The arthroscope in the video is in the anterior viewing portal, and the patient is in the lateral decubitus position.

Video 12.1 Uncomplicated Posterior Shoulder Instability/Labral Repair. Fotios P. Tjoumakaris, MD; James P. Bradley, MD (2 min)

Surgical Technique

- Arthroscopic posterior labral repair can be performed with the patient placed in either the lateral decubitus or the beach-chair position. The authors of this chapter prefer the lateral decubitus position (**Figure 2**) because it allows for easy access to the posterior glenohumeral joint.

- Typically, two portals are used (one anterior and one posterior); however, it may be necessary to place the inferior anchor (6- to 7-o'clock position) through an accessory inferior lateral portal.

- The location of the posterior portal is critical for optimization of the technique, and it should be located more lateral and inferior

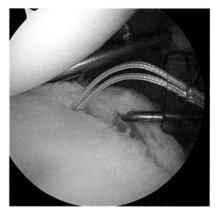

Figure 3 Arthroscopic view from the anterior portal, which provides a panoramic view of the posterior glenoid, labrum, and capsule, with adequate space for working.

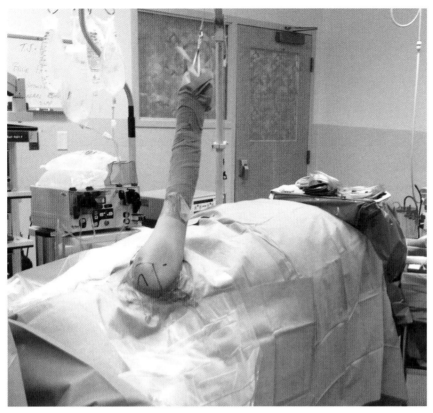

Figure 2 Photograph shows the surgical setup for repair of posterior shoulder instability. The patient is in the lateral decubitus position, with the right shoulder placed in slight forward flexion and abduction with 15 lb of traction applied.

(1 cm in each direction) than the portal typically used for shoulder arthroscopy. Labral preparation and anchor placement can be performed through this portal without the need for further violation of the posterior capsule.

- After the arthroscope is inserted, a comprehensive diagnostic arthroscopy is performed.
- The anterior portal is created in the rotator interval, 1 cm lateral to the coracoid process, with the use of an outside-in technique and a spinal needle.
- The articular cartilage, rotator cuff, biceps anchor, and anterior and superior labrum are inspected and probed to evaluate for concomitant pathology.
- After the diagnostic arthroscopy is completed, attention is turned

to the posterior labrum. Working cannulas (preferably measuring 8.25 mm, although 7-mm cannulas can be used in smaller shoulders) are placed into both portals, and the scope is placed into the anterior portal to obtain a panoramic view of the posterior labrum (**Figure 3**).

- The extent of damage to the posterior structures can range from a partial-thickness rotator cuff tear with labral fraying to complete detachment of the posterior labrum with glenoid remodeling and bone loss.
- Capsular tears, loose bodies, and subtle Kim lesions may be present and can be recognized from the preoperative MRI.
- The labrum is prepared with a periosteal elevator to remove any adhesions or scar tissue, the

presence of which typically causes the labrum to heal in a medialized fashion along the glenoid. In some patients, the elevator may be inserted through the anterior portal and viewed posteriorly because this angle allows for excellent elevation without the risk for damage to the posterior labrum. This is often done in patients in whom the posterior viewing portal is not 45° tangential to the glenoid and manipulation of the elevator through the posterior portal could cause cleavage or tearing of the labrum during labral manipulation.

- An angled rasp or motorized shaver can be used to decorticate the glenoid rim and abrade the undersurface of the labrum to create a vascular environment for healing.
- During labral preparation, preservation of the labral tissue is paramount to prevent damage to the labrum or posterior capsule that could compromise the surgical result.
- Paralabral cysts can be decompressed during labral preparation; however, decompression is not necessary to allow for resorption of the cyst and resolution of neurologic symptoms associated with the suprascapular nerve resulting from

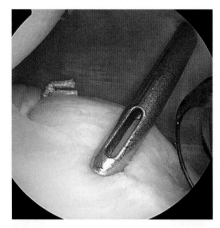

Figure 4 Arthroscopic image viewed from the anterior portal toward the posterior labrum. An accessory posterior and inferior portal has been made to assist with inferior anchor placement with a trajectory of 45° to the glenoid rim. This approach can help prevent iatrogenic injury to the articular cartilage during anchor placement.

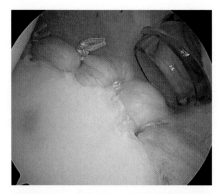

Figure 7 Arthroscopic view from the anterior portal demonstrates four anchors placed on the posterior glenoid rim. Above the equator of the glenoid, knotless anchors are used (white sutures in this image) to reduce knot impingement during overhead motion.

compression at the spinoglenoid notch.

- The labrum is repaired back to the glenoid rim by placing suture anchors along the rim of the glenoid from inferior to superior.
- In patients who require plication, the capsule can be shifted during labral repair to further

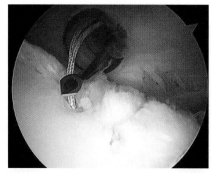

Figure 5 Arthroscopic view from the anterior portal demonstrates the use of a suture-passing device to shuttle the suture around the labrum for labral repair.

reduce pathologic translation of the humerus.

- The authors of this chapter typically use 2.4-mm biocomposite anchors with a single-loaded No. 2 braided composite suture.
- During anchor placement, the drilling angle to the posterior glenoid must be such that the drill guide will not slide along the glenoid face and cause injury to the articular cartilage.
- An accessory portal can be established if the existing posterior portal does not allow for adequate placement of suture anchors along the glenoid rim (**Figure 4**).
- The inferior anchor is placed at the most inferior portion of the posterior labral tear.
- A suture-passing device is used to shuttle the posterior suture through the capsulolabral complex (**Figure 5**). A No. 0 polydioxanone suture can be used as the suture shuttle for this purpose (**Figure 6**).
- In a single-portal technique, the suture shuttle and suture to be passed are grabbed simultaneously and brought out through the posterior cannula.
- After the suture shuttle knot has been tied for passage of the non-absorbable suture, firm tension is maintained on the opposite limb of the polydioxanone suture to enable

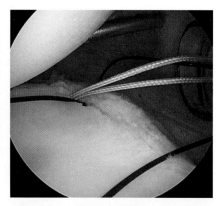

Figure 6 Arthroscopic view from the anterior portal demonstrates the polydioxanone suture that is used as a suture shuttle and passed through the posterior labrum to achieve labral repair.

easy passage of suture and avoid knot entanglement. The shuttled braided composite suture is then used as the post during knot tying, and a sliding, locking knot is used to repair the labrum back to the glenoid rim.

- Additional suture anchors are placed sequentially and superiorly along the glenoid rim until adequate repair of the labrum is achieved (**Figure 7**).
- The authors of this chapter have recently begun using a knotless 2.9-mm suture anchor above the equator of the glenoid, as shown in the video cited in this chapter. Use of knotless technology above the equator of the glenoid eliminates irritation to the biceps muscle and rotator cuff that is caused by knots; such irritation can occur during overhead activity.
- After the labrum and capsule are repaired, an arthroscopic awl is used to penetrate the bare area of the humerus to allow for egress of stem cells to augment the healing response.
- The posterior cannula is slightly backed out beyond the capsule, and the posterior capsule is closed. Closure of the posterior capsule

is accomplished by passing a polydioxanone suture through the capsule, just lateral to the portal,

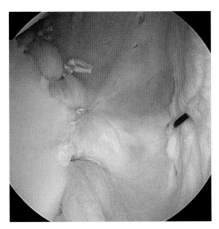

Figure 8 Arthroscopic view from the anterior portal demonstrates the final repair, with closure and suture of the posterior portal in an extracapsular fashion.

and retrieving the suture on the medial side with a penetrating suture grasper. The capsule can be plicated by varying the distance at which the suture is retrieved.

- The polydioxanone suture is tied over the capsule in a blind fashion, completing the surgical procedure (**Figure 8**).

Rehabilitation

After the surgical procedure, the arm is placed in a sling with an abduction pillow, which prevents excessive internal rotation. The authors of this chapter use a cryotherapy device during postoperative week 1 to reduce swelling and control pain. Patients are instructed to begin a home exercise program the day

after the surgical procedure for active ROM of the elbow, wrist, and hand (**Table 2**). After the first postoperative visit (approximately 7 to 10 days), an outpatient physical therapy program is begun. Passive forward flexion and abduction in the scapular plane to 90° is usually initiated in the first week postoperatively, with full passive ROM achieved by 6 weeks postoperatively. After 6 weeks postoperatively, use of the sling is discontinued, and active-assisted ROM exercises are begun, with progression to full active motion as tolerated. Two to 3 months postoperatively, strengthening of the deltoid, rotator cuff, and periscapular muscles is begun.

After the patient has achieved nearly 80% strength in the shoulder (measured by isokinetic strength testing), a sport-specific rehabilitation program is

Table 2 Rehabilitation Protocol After Simple Posterior Labral Repair

Postoperative Week	ROM	Strengthening	Return to Play	Comments/Emphasis
0-2	Home exercise program for active ROM of the elbow, wrist, and hand is begun on postoperative day 1 Passive forward flexion and abduction in the scapular plane to 90° is usually initiated in postoperative week 1	None	N/A	The arm is placed in a sling with an abduction pillow Cryotherapy is used during postoperative week 1 to reduce swelling and control pain Outpatient physical therapy is begun at 7-10 d
2-6	Outpatient physical therapy is initiated, and passive ROM is begun in all planes; internal rotation past the midline is not allowed	None	N/A	Care is taken to avoid excessive stretching of the posterior capsule Limiting internal rotation and cross-body adduction to 50% of normal is critical during this phase
6-12	Active-assisted ROM is begun Progression to full active ROM as tolerated Slight posterior capsule stretching is begun	Strengthening of the deltoid, rotator cuff, and periscapular muscles is begun at 2-3 mo	N/A	Use of the sling is discontinued at 6 wk
12-24	Full ROM should be restored during this phase	Continue with strengthening of the deltoid, rotator cuff, and scapular muscles	N/A	Sport-specific rehabilitation is begun after the patient has achieved 80% strength in the shoulder, typically at 4-6 mo postoperatively Return to sports at 6 mo is typical Return to throwing may not occur until 9-12 mo in overhead throwing athletes

N/A = not applicable, ROM = range of motion.

begun (typically 4 to 6 months post-operatively). Most athletes return to competitive sports by 6 to 9 months after surgery, depending on the results of stability and functional testing. Throwing athletes typically require a longer time before returning to competition compared with other athletic patients. A throwing program is begun at 6 months postoperatively and progresses until nearly full-speed pitching is achieved without soreness. Most throwing athletes return to competition 9 to 12 months postoperatively.

 Avoiding Pitfalls

Experience is key to avoiding the most common complications of posterior labral repair. Surgeons should use the anchors and suture-passing devices with which they are most familiar and experienced. A variety of commercially available products are offered, any of which can be used to achieve a successful posterior labral repair. Similarly, any arthroscopic knot-tying technique can be used; however, the surgeon should have proficiency in using the chosen knot. The authors of this chapter prefer a Weston knot with three half hitches for suture tying because a locking, sliding knot helps avoid knot slippage and because the Weston knot in particular has a relatively low profile. The knots should be tied with the suture limb traversing the labrum as the post to pull the labrum to the glenoid rim. In addition, care should be taken to tie the knot over the labrum and/or posterior capsule to prevent engagement of the knot in the joint during active shoulder motion. Although double-loaded suture anchors can be used to achieve the desired result, using this technique increases the number of knots in the joint and could cause further rotator cuff irritation and scar tissue. Cadaver laboratories and courses are available for surgeons who want to incorporate posterior labral repair into their practice.

 Bibliography

Bahk MS, Karzel RP, Snyder SJ: Arthroscopic posterior stabilization and anterior capsular plication for recurrent posterior glenohumeral instability. *Arthroscopy* 2010;26(9):1172-1180.

Bottoni CR, Franks BR, Moore JH, DeBerardino TM, Taylor DC, Arciero RA: Operative stabilization of posterior shoulder instability. *Am J Sports Med* 2005;33(7):996-1002.

Bradley JP, McClincy MP, Arner JW, Tejwani SG: Arthroscopic capsulolabral reconstruction for posterior instability of the shoulder: A prospective study of 200 shoulders. *Am J Sports Med* 2013;41(9):2005-2014.

Bradley JP, Tejwani SG: Arthroscopic management of posterior instability. *Orthop Clin North Am* 2010;41(3):339-356.

Kim DS, Park HK, Park JH, Yoon WS: Ganglion cyst of the spinoglenoid notch: Comparison between SLAP repair alone and SLAP repair with cyst decompression. *J Shoulder Elbow Surg* 2012;21(11):1456-1463.

Kim SH, Ha KI, Park JH, et al: Arthroscopic posterior labral repair and capsular shift for traumatic unidirectional recurrent posterior subluxation of the shoulder. *J Bone Joint Surg Am* 2003;85(8):1479-1487.

Kim SH, Ha KI, Yoo JC, Noh KC: Kim's lesion: An incomplete and concealed avulsion of the posteroinferior labrum in posterior or multidirectional posteroinferior instability of the shoulder. *Arthroscopy* 2004;20(7):712-720.

Lenart BA, Sherman SL, Mall NA, Gochanour E, Twigg SL, Nicholson GP: Arthroscopic repair for posterior shoulder instability. *Arthroscopy* 2012;28(10):1337-1343.

Misamore GW, Sallay PI, Didelot W: A longitudinal study of patients with multidirectional instability of the shoulder with seven- to ten-year follow-up. *J Shoulder Elbow Surg* 2005;14(5):466-470.

Pennington WT, Sytsma MA, Gibbons DJ, et al: Arthroscopic posterior labral repair in athletes: Outcome analysis at 2-year follow-up. *Arthroscopy* 2010;26(9):1162-1171.

Provencher MT, Mologne TS, Romeo AA, Bradley JP: The use of rotator interval closure in the arthroscopic treatment of posterior shoulder instability [comment on Savoie FH III, Holt MS, Field LD, Ramsey JR: Arthroscopic management of posterior instability: Evolution of technique and results. Arthroscopy 2008;24(4):389-396]. *Arthroscopy* 2009;25(1):109-110, author reply 110-111.

Savoie FH III, Holt MS, Field LD, Ramsey JR: Arthroscopic management of posterior instability: Evolution of technique and results. *Arthroscopy* 2008;24(4):389-396.

Shah N, Tung GA: Imaging signs of posterior glenohumeral instability. *AJR Am J Roentgenol* 2009;192(3):730-735.

Tjoumakaris FP, Bradley JP: The rationale for an arthroscopic approach to shoulder stabilization. *Arthroscopy* 2011;27(10):1422-1433.

Weber SC, Caspari RB: A biochemical evaluation of the restraints to posterior shoulder dislocation. *Arthroscopy* 1989;5(2):115-121.

Williams RJ III, Strickland S, Cohen M, Altchek DW, Warren RF: Arthroscopic repair for traumatic posterior shoulder instability. *Am J Sports Med* 2003;31(2):203-209.

Wooten CJ, Krych AJ, Schleck CD, Hudgens JL, May JH, Dahm DL: Arthroscopic capsulolabral reconstruction for posterior shoulder instability in patients 18 years old or younger. *J Pediatr Orthop* 2015;35(5):462-466.

Video Reference

Tjoumakaris FP, Bradley JP: Video. *Uncomplicated Posterior Shoulder Instability/Labral Repair.* Ocean View, NJ, 2015.

Chapter 13

Shoulder Arthroplasty for the Management of Chronic Glenohumeral Dislocation

E. Scott Paxton, MD

Andrew Green, MD

 ## Introduction

Chronic locked dislocations of the glenohumeral joint are challenging for patients and surgeons. Although the glenohumeral joint is the most commonly dislocated major joint in the body, chronic locked dislocations are uncommon in active individuals. Most acute dislocations are anterior, readily recognized and diagnosed, and successfully managed with early closed reduction. Acute posterior glenohumeral dislocations are much less common, reportedly accounting for less than 3% of dislocations; however, acute posterior glenohumeral dislocations are more frequently missed at the initial presentation and often result in chronic locked dislocation, reportedly in 50% to 80% of patients. The mean age of patients treated with shoulder arthroplasty for chronic posterior dislocation is approximately 53 years, whereas the mean age of patients treated for chronic anterior dislocation is approximately 68 years.

Chronic dislocations must be clearly differentiated from recurrent dislocations. The specific definition of chronic dislocation is debatable. Any dislocation that is not recognized on initial presentation can be considered chronic; closed reduction is unlikely to be possible in any dislocation that goes unrecognized for more than 3 or 4 weeks. Despite repeated warnings in the literature about the incidence of missed dislocations, chronic dislocations remain a problem and often go undiscovered until an average of 2 years after injury. In many patients, missed dislocation is the result of inadequate initial patient evaluation and imaging.

 ## Patient Evaluation

History
It is essential to obtain an accurate history of the mechanism of injury for any patient with a history of traumatic shoulder injury and functional limitation. A patient without a history of recent injury may have a glenohumeral dislocation that is not acute. This presentation is not uncommon in elderly patients with altered mental status. A history of seizure or electrocution should elicit suspicion for posterior dislocation because 50% of posterior dislocations have been reported to be a result of these mechanisms. Patients who awaken from sleep with a shoulder dislocation should be thoroughly evaluated for a seizure disorder. Because alcohol withdrawal can result in seizure, a history of alcoholism also may be associated with chronic unrecognized dislocation. Patients with polytrauma should be thoroughly examined to rule out glenohumeral dislocation. In patients with persistent absence of glenohumeral rotation after a shoulder injury, appropriate imaging is needed to rule out a chronic locked dislocation.

Particular attention should be given to a patient's level of function. Some patients with chronic locked glenohumeral dislocation are relatively pain free despite limited shoulder motion. In some elderly patients with low function, in patients with severe cognitive limitations, and in patients with severe medical comorbidities, acceptance of functional limitation may be preferable to surgical treatment.

Dr. Green or an immediate family member has received royalties from and serves as a paid consultant to Tornier; is a member of a speakers' bureau or has made paid presentations on behalf of DJO; has stock or stock options held in IlluminOss Medical and Pfizer; has received research or institutional support from DJO and DePuy Synthes; has received nonincome support (such as equipment or services), commercially derived honoraria, or other non–research-related funding (such as paid travel) from Arthrex and Smith & Nephew; and serves as a board member, owner, officer, or committee member of the American Academy of Orthopaedic Surgeons and the American Shoulder and Elbow Surgeons. Neither Dr. Paxton nor any immediate family member has received anything of value from or has stock or stock options held in a commercial company or institution related directly or indirectly to the subject of this chapter.

Physical Examination

A careful and thorough physical examination is necessary. Patients with posterior dislocation may have a flattened anterior shoulder, a prominent coracoid, and posterior prominence of the humeral head, whereas patients with anterior dislocation may have a sulcus under the acromion and anterior prominence of the shoulder. However, deformity may not be visible in patients who are overweight or obese. Limited shoulder elevation and rotation are classic findings in patients with chronic locked dislocation. Patients with posterior dislocation cannot externally rotate their hand from their abdomen, whereas patients with locked anterior dislocation may not be able to internally rotate their hand to their abdomen. Some patients with chronic anterior dislocation may have glenohumeral rotation in the presence of an associated fracture of the anterior glenoid rim. In both anterior and posterior locked dislocations, patients usually exhibit substantial limitations in both active and passive shoulder elevation.

The initial evaluation should include a detailed neurovascular examination. With anterior and inferior dislocations, the humeral head presses against the distal aspects of the brachial plexus, the axillary and musculocutaneous nerves, and the adjacent vascular structures. Fractures and fracture-dislocations of the proximal humerus are reported to be associated with neurologic injury in up to 50% of patients. The status of the deltoid muscle can usually be evaluated; however, assessment of rotator cuff strength may be difficult or impossible in patients who do not have glenohumeral rotation. The vascular structures are at particular risk in patients who sustain high-energy trauma as well as in older patients who may have rigid atherosclerotic vessels. In some patients with proximal vascular injuries, the extensive collateral circulation around the shoulder girdle can provide sufficient distal perfusion of the forearm and hand as well as obscure more obvious signs of vascular injury that would be expected in the setting of true ischemia of the upper limb. Any patient with questionable vascular status should be further evaluated using Doppler ultrasonography or arteriography.

Imaging

The initial plain radiographic evaluation of any patient with a traumatic injury of the shoulder girdle should include the trauma series (true AP, axillary lateral, and scapular Y views). Failure to obtain adequate and complete plain radiographs may result in a missed glenohumeral dislocation. Far too often, the initial evaluation includes only AP internal and external rotation views of the shoulder girdle without orthogonal imaging of the glenohumeral joint, resulting in a missed dislocation. Most anterior glenohumeral dislocations are readily apparent on AP radiographs because the humeral head displaces in an anterior and inferior direction. However, an anterior glenoid fracture may be missed in the initial evaluation; lack of diagnosis and treatment may lead to redislocation of the humeral head, especially in older patients.

In patients with posterior dislocation, the humeral head displaces directly posterior, which typically results in overlap of the humeral head on the glenoid on the standard AP shoulder view. Internal rotation of the humerus results in the so-called lightbulb sign because the contours of the tuberosities are lost, which is suggestive of a posterior dislocation. On true AP plain radiographs (Grashey view), any overlap of the humeral head on the glenoid suggests posterior dislocation. Orthogonal imaging with axillary lateral and scapular Y views provides additional information about the position of the humeral head and is required to make the diagnosis. Although several modified axial views are available, CT is the best imaging method to rule out posterior dislocation. In patients with chronic dislocation, plain radiographs may demonstrate osteopenia and heterotopic ossification as well as erosive changes of the glenoid or humerus secondary to either the initial injury or the attempted motion of the dislocated joint over a prolonged period.

In patients with chronic dislocation, CT is essential to fully evaluate the anatomy of the humeral head and glenoid. CT should be obtained with imaging planes perpendicular to the plane of the scapula. Three-dimensional reconstruction can be particularly helpful to better define bony defects. The quality of the rotator cuff muscles also can be assessed with CT. In most patients, MRI is not essential for evaluation but can be used to assess the rotator cuff tendons and muscles. Although rotator cuff tears are unlikely in patients younger than 40 years, older or elderly patients are more likely to have either an associated acute traumatic or a degenerative preexisting tear of the rotator cuff.

The extent of bony defects of the glenoid and humeral head can be determined on CT. An en face CT scan of the glenoid can be used to determine the amount of glenoid bone loss. Axial images of the humeral head can be used to measure the size and location of the damaged articular segment, defined as a reverse Hill-Sachs defect (**Figure 1**).

 Case Presentations

Case 1: Chronic Posterior Glenohumeral Dislocation With a Large Humeral Head Defect and an Intact Glenoid

A 45-year-old, right-hand–dominant man presents with a history of having awakened with right shoulder bruising and pain and with a diagnosis of a right proximal humerus fracture. He reports that 2 months later he awoke with left shoulder pain and the diagnosis was a left proximal humerus fracture. One

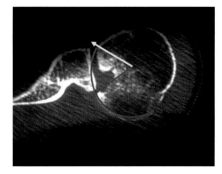

Figure 1 Axial CT scan demonstrates the measurement of the percentage of humeral head articular segment injury in a patient with posterior glenohumeral dislocation. The red arrow indicates the posterior margin of the defect, the red arc indicates the total arc of the articular surface, and the yellow arrow indicates the anterior margin of the defect. (Reproduced from Green A: Chronic posterior dislocation: Open reduction and tendon-bone transfers, in Zuckerman JD, ed: *Advanced Reconstruction: Shoulder.* Rosemont, IL, American Academy of Orthopaedic Surgeons, 2007, pp 111-119.)

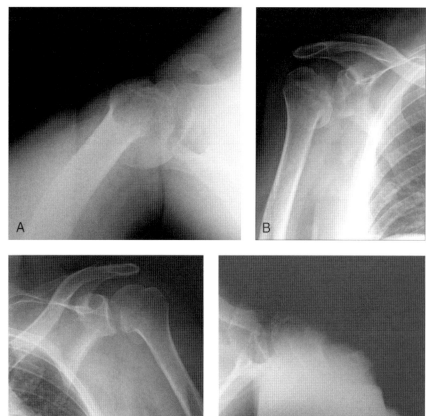

Figure 2 AP (**A**) and axillary (**B**) radiographs of the right shoulder and AP (**C**) and axillary (**D**) radiographs of the left shoulder demonstrate bilateral posterior glenohumeral dislocations resulting from seizure.

month later, he presented to the clinic with bilateral shoulder pain and limited range of motion (ROM). Bilateral posterior fracture-dislocations and a large anterior humeral head defect of the right shoulder were noted on radiographs and CT (**Figures 2** and **3**). Neurologic evaluation revealed no obvious evidence of seizure activity. Humeral head arthroplasty was performed 6 months after the initial right shoulder injury. The anterior humeral head defect was composed of approximately 40% of the articular segment, and the glenoid cartilage was intact. The subscapularis peel technique was used to expose the glenohumeral joint, and anatomic humeral head arthroplasty was performed using a press-fit humeral implant. One year postoperatively, the right shoulder was pain free, and shoulder motion was 125° of active forward elevation, 15° of active external rotation, and internal rotation to L3, with normal strength on manual muscle testing (**Figure 4**).

Case 2: Chronic Anterior Glenohumeral Dislocation and a Large Glenoid Defect

A 71-year-old, right-hand–dominant, morbidly obese woman who uses a wheelchair reports shoulder pain and limited ROM 8 months after sustaining an injury after a fall. Locked anterior dislocation is noted on imaging, with nearly 40% humeral head bone loss and 40% glenoid bone loss (**Figure 5**). At 9 months after injury, the patient is treated with humeral head arthroplasty, glenoid bone grafting using the humeral head, and Achilles tendon allograft reconstruction of the deficient anterior capsule and subscapularis (**Figures 6** and **7**). The upper 50% of

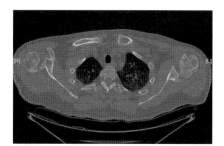

Figure 3 Axial CT scan demonstrates evidence of bilateral posterior glenohumeral dislocations. A humeral head defect of 40% to 50% is visible in the right shoulder.

the pectoralis major tendon is released to facilitate reduction, and the press-fit humeral implant is placed in slightly

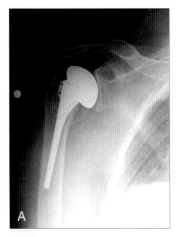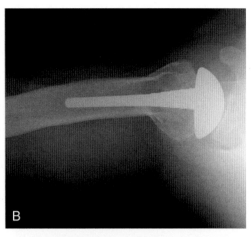

Figure 4   Postoperative true AP (**A**) and axillary (**B**) radiographs of the right shoulder of a patient who underwent humeral head arthroplasty.

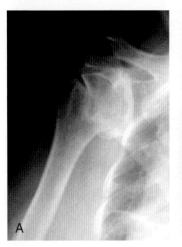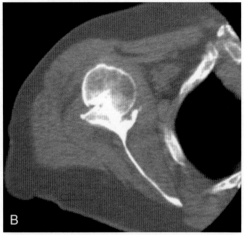

Figure 5   Preoperative AP radiograph (**A**) and axial CT scan (**B**) of a right shoulder demonstrate locked anterior dislocation with substantial humeral and glenoid bone loss.

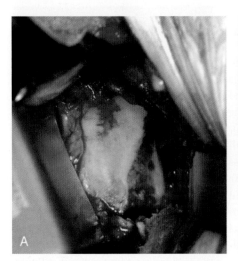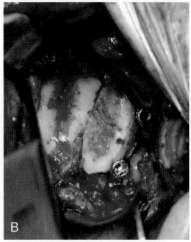

Figure 6   Intraoperative photographs show an anterior glenoid defect of nearly 50% (**A**) and reconstruction of the anterior glenoid using a segment of the humeral head and fixation with two 4.5-mm cortical screws (**B**).

greater than normal retroversion. At 9 months postoperatively, the patient exhibits 70° of active forward elevation and 20° of active external rotation, with good strength and no recurrent instability (**Figure 8**).

Case 3: Chronic Posterior Glenohumeral Dislocation

An 88-year-old, right-hand–dominant man is seen in the clinic with bilateral shoulder injuries 2 weeks after experiencing a grand mal seizure. The patient has a three-part proximal humerus fracture of the left shoulder that is managed nonsurgically and a locked posterior dislocation of the right shoulder (**Figures 9** and **10**). The patient is medically evaluated and cleared for surgical treatment, and the surgical procedure is performed 6 weeks after the injury (**Figure 11**). The glenohumeral joint is opened using the subscapularis peel technique. Because the glenoid articular cartilage is damaged, anatomic total shoulder arthroplasty (TSA) is performed. The subscapularis repair allows nearly full ROM. At 5 months postoperatively, the patient has minimal pain in the right shoulder and has active forward elevation to 90° and active external rotation to 10°.

Case 4: Chronic Anterior Glenohumeral Dislocation With a Large Glenoid Bone Defect

A 79-year-old, right-hand–dominant, obese woman reports shoulder pain 4 months after sustaining a shoulder injury. Limited shoulder ROM with intact neurovascular status is noted on physical examination. Plain radiographs demonstrate anterior-inferior glenohumeral dislocation (**Figure 12**). Because of the patient's age, obesity, and chronic glenohumeral dislocation, nonsurgical treatment is initially attempted. The patient, who had been high functioning and independent before the injury, returns for reevaluation because she is unable to tolerate the pain and dysfunction,

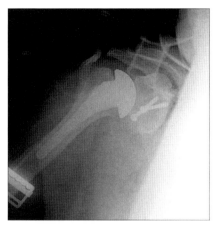

Figure 7 True AP radiograph obtained immediately postoperatively demonstrates anatomic humeral head arthroplasty and reconstruction of the anterior glenoid.

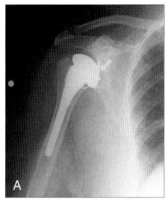
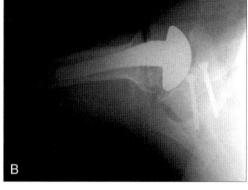

Figure 8 True AP (**A**) and axillary lateral (**B**) radiographs demonstrate anatomic reduction and graft healing 9 months after humeral head arthroplasty, glenoid bone graft, and Achilles tendon allograft reconstruction of the deficient anterior capsule and the subscapularis.

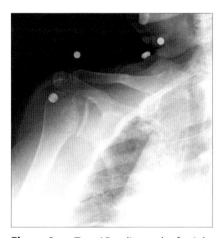

Figure 9 True AP radiograph of a right shoulder demonstrates posterior shoulder dislocation with a large (50%) anterior humeral head defect.

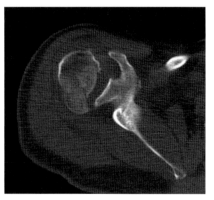

Figure 10 Axial CT scan of a right shoulder demonstrates a locked posterior dislocation with a 50% humeral head defect.

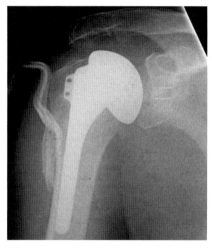

Figure 11 AP radiograph obtained immediately after anatomic total shoulder arthroplasty demonstrates a keeled glenoid component and a noncemented humeral component.

and she requests surgical reconstruction. CT demonstrates a defect of approximately 30% of the anterior glenoid and a defect of approximately 50% of the posterior humeral head (**Figure 13**). A massive rotator cuff tear including the subscapularis, supraspinatus, and infraspinatus tendons is discovered intraoperatively. The patient is treated with reverse TSA and reconstruction of the anterior glenoid using humeral head autograft (**Figure 14**). The patient reports good results 2 months postoperatively.

 Indications

In patients with chronic glenohumeral dislocation, the primary indications for arthroplasty are pain and upper extremity dysfunction that substantially affect a patient's quality of life in the presence of bony deficiency of the humeral head, the glenoid, or both, with or without glenohumeral arthritis. The status of the rotator cuff also is considered because it is often scarred, immobile, or torn, especially in older patients. The presence

of rotator cuff deficiency strongly influences the type of surgery selected. Some elderly patients are not good candidates for surgical treatment because of the presence of severe medical comorbidities or limited functional goals. Patients with mental or psychological disabilities may not be appropriate candidates for complex reconstructive surgical procedures. Even in some younger patients, long-standing chronic dislocation may be a contraindication to surgical treatment, especially if a patient has minimal

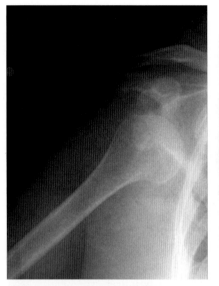

Figure 12 True AP radiograph of a right shoulder demonstrates a chronic locked anterior dislocation.

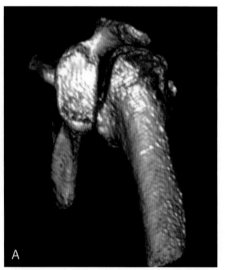

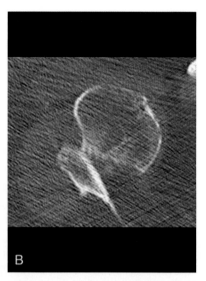

Figure 13 Three-dimensional CT reconstruction (**A**) and axial CT scan (**B**) of a right shoulder demonstrate a chronic anterior dislocation with an anterior glenoid defect of approximately 30% and a posterior humeral head defect of approximately 50%.

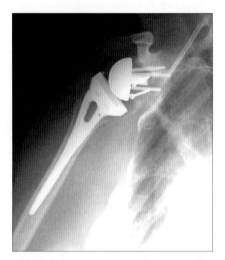

Figure 14 True AP radiograph of a right shoulder obtained 2 months after reverse total shoulder arthroplasty and anterior glenoid bone grafting demonstrates graft incorporation.

pain and is able to tolerate the impairment and disability. Active infection and uncontrolled seizure activity are contraindications to arthroplasty. Chronic brachial plexus or axillary nerve injury with loss of deltoid function, especially with rotator cuff dysfunction, is usually a contraindication to reconstructive arthroplasty.

Historically, arthroplasty was considered for the management of humeral articular segment defects greater than 40% in patients with locked posterior dislocations. In some patients, lesser defects can be managed with humeral allograft or lesser tuberosity transfer procedures without arthroplasty. The length of time from dislocation also must be taken into account because of the development of osteopenia in the humeral head, cartilage degeneration, and rotator cuff scarring that can occur over time. Six months has been suggested as the duration at which prosthetic arthroplasty is preferred to alternatives such as open reduction with or without allograft reconstruction of the humeral head. Nevertheless, in physiologically older patients, arthroplasty is generally considered earlier because long-term implant survivorship is of less concern.

Although the extent of glenoid bone loss that should be considered acceptable in patients with chronic glenohumeral dislocation has not been specifically studied, recommendations gleaned from the literature on the management of recurrent anterior glenohumeral dislocations suggest that

reconstruction is necessary in patients with glenoid deficiency greater than 25%. Because the glenoid bone loss in these patients is often associated with articular cartilage damage that will be reconstructed with anatomic or reverse TSA, the size and design of the glenoid implant will determine whether graft is needed. Although anatomic arthroplasty can be performed with glenoid bone grafting, relatively little has been published on the use of this technique in patients with chronic dislocation, and data on the long-term outcomes of posterior glenoid bone grafting for glenohumeral osteoarthritis are limited. However, anatomic arthroplasty can be considered in younger patients to avoid reverse TSA. Reverse TSA can be performed with glenoid bone grafting by using longer central fixation (such as extended pegs, threaded post baseplate) of the baseplate to the native scapula to enhance the overall glenoid fixation and to protect the graft during incorporation.

If the shoulder remains unstable after nonprosthetic reconstruction, prosthetic arthroplasty is required. The type of prosthetic arthroplasty required (anatomic or reverse) depends on several factors, including patient age, chronicity of injury, rotator cuff and capsular contracture, and the extent of glenoid bone loss.

Anatomic Arthroplasty

Anatomic arthroplasty is indicated for patients in whom the capsular contracture and rotator cuff can be adequately mobilized so that the glenohumeral joint volume and soft-tissue envelope are sufficient to fit the implants and allow functional shoulder motion. This scenario is more likely in patients with acute rather than chronic dislocation. Regardless of the direction of the dislocation, the subscapularis tendon is almost always contracted. In patients with chronic anterior dislocation, contracture of the pectoralis major muscle is not uncommon, and release of the upper portion or, occasionally, even the entire pectoralis major tendon may be necessary.

The authors of this chapter prefer to perform a lesser tuberosity osteotomy to expose the glenohumeral joint when performing anatomic shoulder arthroplasty. However, if subscapularis mobility is a concern, a subscapularis tendon peel is a better option. In most patients, the subscapularis can be mobilized by releasing the capsule, coracohumeral ligament, rotator cuff interval, and subcoracoid adhesions to regain motion and permit repair. Alternatively, a coronal Z-plasty of the subscapularis tendon can be performed by separating the subscapularis tendon from the anterior capsule, releasing the subscapularis on the humeral side and releasing the anterior capsule from the glenoid side. The anterior capsule and the subscapularis tendon are repaired end-to-end, allowing for greater external rotation without tension on the subscapularis repair. If the subscapularis cannot be repaired, reverse TSA should be considered. Although younger age is generally considered a contraindication to reverse TSA, this procedure may be preferable to a stiff anatomic arthroplasty in younger patients. In younger patients, a compromise between implant longevity and functional outcome may be required.

In patients with posterior dislocation, the posterior capsule can be redundant, and plication may be required to prevent posterior instability. The posterior capsular redundancy can be corrected with plication sutures with or without suture anchors in the posterior glenoid, with the goal of allowing 50% posterior translation of the humeral head with spontaneous reduction.

Humeral implant positioning is an important consideration. Previous suggestions have included altering the version of the humeral implant to account for the direction of glenohumeral dislocation, with increased anteversion for posterior dislocation and increased retroversion for anterior dislocation. However, data supporting this recommendation are limited, and most surgeons prefer to position the humeral head to re-create the patient's native version. Most current anatomic arthroplasty designs include offset humeral heads that facilitate optimal positioning of the humeral head.

Glenoid bone defects can be managed with a variety of techniques. For larger defects managed with anatomic TSA, bone grafting is required to restore glenohumeral stability and support a glenoid implant. The authors of this chapter recommend that in patients with chronic dislocation, the glenoid component of an anatomic total shoulder prosthesis be completely supported by native glenoid bone; if support from the native glenoid bone cannot be achieved, bone grafting or reverse TSA should be considered. If humeral head arthroplasty is performed in the presence of a glenoid defect, the authors' experience with the management of recurrent anterior glenohumeral dislocations suggests that reconstruction is required in the setting of glenoid deficiency greater than 20% to 25%. In patients with chronic dislocation, extreme caution should be taken if considering anatomic humeral head arthroplasty in the presence of any glenoid defect because of the risk for instability. Typically, the humeral head is an excellent source of autogenous graft to manage glenoid bone defects. Screw fixation to the native scapula is preferred to improve the stability of the graft and to facilitate healing.

Glenohumeral stability and ROM should be assessed before and after repair of the subscapularis tendon. The limits of external rotation depend on the degree of preoperative subscapularis contracture. Motion limitation and capsular tightness are more common than instability in patients with chronic glenohumeral dislocation.

Reverse Arthroplasty

Until the advent of contemporary reverse TSA, anatomic arthroplasty was the only option for arthroplasty in the management of chronic glenohumeral dislocation. Reverse arthroplasty provides advantages over anatomic arthroplasty by obviating the need for a functioning rotator cuff to achieve active shoulder elevation and by providing a constrained and stable fulcrum for glenohumeral stability and motion. In many patients with chronic glenohumeral dislocation, the outcome of anatomic arthroplasty is not ideal because rotator cuff function and glenohumeral stability are compromised. The general considerations for surgical preparation, patient positioning, and surgical approach for anatomic arthroplasty also apply to reverse TSA.

Complete, unimpeded exposure of the glenoid is necessary to fully evaluate the glenoid and scapular anatomy, appropriately position the reamers, and implant the glenoid baseplate. To achieve such exposure, soft-tissue release is performed to enable posterior retraction of the proximal humerus, and retractors are used around the glenoid (**Figure 15**).

Manipulation of implant version in

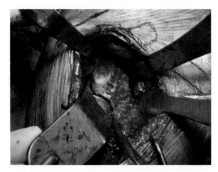

Figure 15 Intraoperative photograph of a right shoulder shows the complete exposure of the glenoid necessary for the assessment of defects and the appropriate instrumentation and implant positioning required for successful shoulder arthroplasty.

reverse TSA is frequently discussed but not entirely understood. The available arc of motion is limited by the geometry of the implants and by impingement of the humeral socket on the scapula. Some surgeons recommend less retroversion or neutral positioning of the humeral implant if greater internal rotation is desired; however, this technique may lead to earlier posterior impingement with external rotation. The effect of humeral version also depends on the glenosphere and humeral designs. Designs with lateralized glenoids and lower-angle humeral sockets may have greater arcs of rotation and a decreased risk for scapular notching. The authors of this chapter prefer to place the humeral implant in the patient's native version unless the native version is excessive in either direction.

Fixation of the glenoid implant depends on bone quality. The baseplate should be completely supported with bone; therefore, the need for bone graft depends on the size of the baseplate and the extent of bone deficiency. In recent studies, values of 80% and 50% have been suggested as the acceptable amount of native bone support before bone grafting is needed. An exact number is unknown, but the authors of this chapter prefer to have nearly complete native

support for the baseplate. To achieve this recommended level of support, it may be necessary to perform reaming medially to gain more native support. However, if reaming would result in substantial medialization of the glenosphere, the surgeon can select from one of three options. Reaming can be progressed until more than 50% native bone support is available, and the deficit can be reconstructed with a structural bone graft. Alternatively, if sufficient bone support to permit complete reaming is available, the glenosphere can be lateralized by selecting an appropriate implant design or by using bone graft. If bone graft is used behind a glenoid baseplate, the central post must be long enough to achieve fixation to the native scapula. Eccentric baseplate or glenosphere designs also may facilitate optimal fixation and positioning.

Glenohumeral stability is a major concern in patients treated with reverse TSA for a chronic locked dislocation. The stability of reverse TSA depends on the status of the remaining rotator cuff, the tension of the deltoid and other muscle groups, and the constrained glenohumeral articulation. The desired ideal tension is difficult to quantify. The authors of this chapter prefer to maintain enough tension to prevent easy intraoperative dislocation. This amount of tension usually corresponds with an implant combination that does not easily reduce. An easy reduction indicates that the joint may not be sufficiently stable. In addition, implant impingement is important in postoperative stability. Many patients have substantial scar tissue around the glenoid periphery, which can increase the likelihood of impingement and result in dislocation of the humeral implant. Healed, malunited fracture fragments and heterotopic ossification also can promote instability. Therefore, it is imperative to remove impinging bone or soft tissue and to check the stability of the implant in multiple positions, including maximum

adduction to assess for substantial gapping of the components superiorly if they are impinging inferiorly. Stability may be improved with the use of humeral inserts that either lengthen or lateralize the humerus or with the use of a larger glenosphere with or without a constrained humeral socket insert.

 ## Controversies and Alternative Approaches

The main controversy in patients with chronic glenohumeral dislocation involves the decision to perform arthroplasty rather than other reconstructive procedures. In patients with posterior dislocation, the native joint can be salvaged if the humeral head defect is less than 40%. Options include transfer of the subscapularis tendon into the defect, transfer of the lesser tuberosity into the defect (McLaughlin procedure), plication or tenodesis of the subscapularis into the defect, allograft reconstruction of the defect, or partial head resurfacing. In younger patients, osteochondral allograft or autograft may be performed. If the condition is managed early enough, it may be possible to tamp out the head defect and support the articular surface with cancellous graft, rafting screws, or synthetic bone void filler. Another controversy relates to the use of reverse TSA in younger patients. However, recent studies have reported promising outcomes after reverse TSA in patients younger than 65 years. Resection arthroplasty and arthrodesis are rarely indicated.

 ## Results

The outcomes of anatomic arthroplasty for chronic glenohumeral dislocation vary (**Table 1**). Although published data are limited, the experience of the authors of this chapter suggests that

Table 1 Results of Anatomic Arthroplasty for Chronic Glenohumeral Dislocation[a]

Authors	Journal (Year)	Technique (No. of Patients)	Outcomes
Rowe and Zarins	*J Bone Joint Surg Am* (1982)	TSA (7)	Rowe and Zarins criteria:[b] 1 good (score, 75) and 1 fair (score, 60)
Hawkins et al	*J Bone Joint Surg Am* (1987)	HHA (9), TSA (6)	HHA: 6 good; 3 failures (2 were referrals) were converted to TSA TSA: 5 good; 1 failure (posterior dislocation) occurred
Pritchett and Clark	*Clin Orthop Relat Res* (1987)	Anterior dislocation: TSA (2), HHA (2) Posterior dislocation: HHA (2), TSA (1)	Anterior dislocation: 2 fair, 2 good Posterior dislocation, Rowe and Zarins criteria:[b] HHA: 1 patient improved from a score of 55 to 70; 1 patient improved from a score of 55 to 80 TSA: 1 patient improved from a score of 55 to 85
Flatow et al	*J Shoulder Elbow Surg* (1993)	Anterior dislocation: TSA (8), HHA (1)	4 excellent, 4 satisfactory, 1 unsatisfactory
Cheng et al	*J Shoulder Elbow Surg* (1997)	TSA (7)	VAS pain score improved from 7.7 to 3.5 External rotation improved from −4° to 11.4° Forward flexion improved from 76° to 109° Internal rotation improved from S2 to T10 ASES score improved from 20.1 to 55.6
Checchia et al	*J Shoulder Elbow Surg* (1998)	HHA (8), TSA (5)	UCLA score HHA: mean score of 25.6 (range, 7-35) 3 excellent, 2 good, 1 fair, 2 poor TSA: mean score of 17 (range, 3-30) 1 good, 1 fair, 3 poor
Boileau et al	*J Shoulder Elbow Surg* (2001)	HHA (8), TSA (1)	Pain (Constant score) was 11.5 on a 15-point scale Forward elevation improved from 57° to 114° External rotation improved from −2° to 42°
Sperling et al	*J Shoulder Elbow Surg* (2004)	HHA (6), TSA (6)	VAS pain score improved from 4.6 to 2.7 External rotation improved from −13° to 28° Abduction improved from 82° to 96° Internal rotation improved from sacrum to L4 HHA: 4 satisfactory, 2 unsatisfactory (both revised) TSA: 1 excellent, 2 satisfactory, 3 unsatisfactory (1 revised)
Gavriilidis et al	*Int Orthop* (2010)	HHA (10), RTSA (2)	Mean Constant score, 59.4 (normative age- and sex-related Constant score, 67.1) Flexion improved from 84.2° to 125° Abduction improved from 55.4° to 95.8° External rotation improved from −6.7° to 36.7° 1 revision at 36 mo (polyethylene insert exchange; original was metal backed) Humeral head migration: 1 mild, 1 severe
Schliemann et al	*Arch Orthop Trauma Surg* (2011)	HHA (1), RTSA (1)	Avg Constant score, 51 Avg Rowe score, 56

ASES = American Shoulder and Elbow Surgeons shoulder outcome, HHA = humeral head arthroplasty, RTSA = reverse total shoulder arthroplasty, TSA = total shoulder arthroplasty, UCLA = University of California–Los Angeles Shoulder Rating Scale, VAS = visual analog scale.

[a] All dislocations are posterior except as noted.

[b] Score out of a total of 100 units.

Table 1 Results of Anatomic Arthroplasty for Chronic Glenohumeral Dislocation[a] (*continued*)

Authors	Journal (Year)	Technique (No. of Patients)	Outcomes
Wooten et al	*J Bone Joint Surg Am* (2014)	HHA (18), TSA (14)	Pain score decreased from 4 to 3 (5-point scale)
			Median external rotation improved from 21.5° to 50° (*P* < 0.001)
			HHA: 4 excellent, 8 satisfactory, 6 unsatisfactory
			TSA: 7 satisfactory, 7 unsatisfactory
			HHA: 6 revisions (1 removal at 2 mo for infection; 1 removal related to instability and Parkinson disease; 2 revisions to TSA with posterior capsule plication for instability, at 2 and 11 mo; 2 revisions to TSA for pain and glenoid wear at 3 and 10 yr)
			TSA: 3 revisions (1 removal at 7 mo for infection; 1 revision for humeral fracture nonunion; 1 revision to HHA for metal-backed glenoid loosening at 14 yr)

ASES = American Shoulder and Elbow Surgeons shoulder outcome, HHA = humeral head arthroplasty, RTSA = reverse total shoulder arthroplasty, TSA = total shoulder arthroplasty, UCLA = University of California–Los Angeles Shoulder Rating Scale, VAS = visual analog scale.

[a] All dislocations are posterior except as noted.

[b] Score out of a total of 100 units.

several factors affect outcomes, including the chronicity of the injury, the status of the rotator cuff, the severity of the soft-tissue contracture, and the motivation of the patient. Most patients experience improvement in the level of pain and function. However, persistent limited ROM and associated limited function are common.

Published experience with reverse TSA for chronic glenohumeral dislocation is limited (**Table 2**). The outcomes of posttraumatic reverse TSA are generally inferior to those of reverse TSA for the management of rotator cuff tear arthropathy; therefore, the results of this procedure for the management of chronic glenohumeral dislocation may be similarly limited.

Technical Keys to Success

Anatomic Arthroplasty

- Preoperative planning with plain radiography and CT is necessary to assess the extent and location of humeral and glenoid bone defects.
- An interscalene nerve block and general anesthesia are administered. Endotracheal anesthesia should be used if complete paralysis is necessary.
- Perioperative antibiotics are administered.
- The patient's skin is scrubbed and rinsed, and an alcohol-based prep solution is applied.
- An iodine-impregnated drape is placed on the shoulder.
- The patient is placed in the beach-chair position for ease of fluoroscopic imaging intraoperatively. The surgeon should confirm that the humerus can be positioned vertically to gain access to the humeral intramedullary canal.
- No attempt at closed reduction should be made.
- The arm is placed in a sterile arm positioner.
- A deltopectoral approach is used, with the cephalic vein retracted laterally.
- A variety of humeral implants, including press-fit, cemented, long-stem, and short-stem implants, as well as resurfacing of the humeral heads may be used. The most important consideration is the ability to restore the articular anatomy of the humeral head and achieve adequate soft-tissue balance.
- The authors of this chapter prefer to use noncemented, short-stem humeral implants for both anatomic and reverse arthroplasty. However, in patients with poor humeral bone quality, cement fixation may be required.
- Humeral resurfacing is technically challenging and requires adequate humeral head bone stock.
- The conjoined tendon and coracoid are identified as landmarks. Care must be taken to remain lateral to the conjoined tendon.
- The clavipectoral fascia is incised.
- Subdeltoid and subacromial adhesions are released.
- The long head of the biceps tendon is sutured to the pectoralis major tendon with nonabsorbable sutures. The tendon of the long head of the biceps is released proximally.
- The upper 2 cm of the pectoralis major tendon may be released as needed for humeral retraction and to counter anterior force in patients

Table 2 Results of Reverse Total Shoulder Arthroplasty (RTSA) for Chronic Glenohumeral Dislocation[a]

Authors	Journal (Year)	Indication for RTSA	No. of Patients	Mean Patient Age in Years (Range)	Mean Follow-up in Years (Range)	Results
Cuff et al	J Bone Joint Surg Am (2012)	Rotator cuff deficiency	94 (96 shoulders)	70.4 (51.7-88.0)	5.2 (5.0-6.4)	Avg ASES score improved from 32 to 75 Avg elevation improved from 64° to 144° Avg ER improved from 15° to 51° 5 revisions: 3 for instability, 1 for humeral and baseplate loosening, 1 for allograft resorption
Werner et al	J Shoulder Elbow Surg (2014)	Chronic anterior dislocation (combined with glenoid bone grafting)	21	71 (50-85)	4.9 (2-10)	Mean Constant score improved from 5.7 to 57.2 Mean elevation improved from 35° to 128° Mean ER improved from 2.4° to 8.4° 2 revisions for baseplate loosening 19 grafts healed completely
Ross et al	J Shoulder Elbow Surg (2015)	Acute 3- and 4-part fractures in the elderly	28 (29 shoulders)	79 (67-90)	4.6 (2.1-8.9)	Mean ASES score, 89.3 Mean Constant score, 70.9 Avg elevation, 130° Avg ER, 30° No revisions

ASES = American Shoulder and Elbow Surgeons shoulder outcome, ER = external rotation.

[a] Representative results for rotator cuff–deficient shoulder (rotator cuff tear arthropathy and chronic massive rotator cuff tear) and acute proximal humerus fractures are provided for comparison.

with chronic anterior dislocation.
- The axillary nerve and artery are palpated.
- Glenohumeral arthrotomy is performed.
- Lesser tuberosity osteotomy may be performed if mild contracture is present. In patients with moderate to severe contracture, a subscapularis peel should be performed.
- The humeral neck capsule is released inferiorly past the 6-o'clock position.
- The rotator cuff is evaluated for integrity and quality.
- In patients with chronic posterior dislocation, a Darrach elevator is used across the glenoid to lever the humeral head off the back of the glenoid (**Figure 16**). A bone hook is used to pull the humeral head away from the glenoid laterally. Reduction is achieved by externally rotating the humeral head. An in situ cut of the humeral head may be required.
- In patients with anterior dislocation, reduction can be achieved with the use of a bone hook on the humeral neck.
- An anatomic cut of the humeral neck is performed.
- The humerus is prepared for the implant.
- The humerus is retracted posteriorly with a Fukuda retractor (or similar) to expose the glenoid.
- The glenoid cartilage is assessed.
- The glenoid is prepared for an anatomic implant in standard fashion. Capsular release is performed to expose the glenoid and enhance shoulder motion. In patients with chronic posterior instability, release of the posterior capsule may not be required.
- A trial reduction is performed to assess the stability of the implant and ROM.
- Subscapularis tension and suitability for repair are assessed. If the subscapularis repair would be too tight, the surgeon should consider abandoning the procedure and performing humeral head arthroplasty with no glenoid component (in physiologically younger patients) or

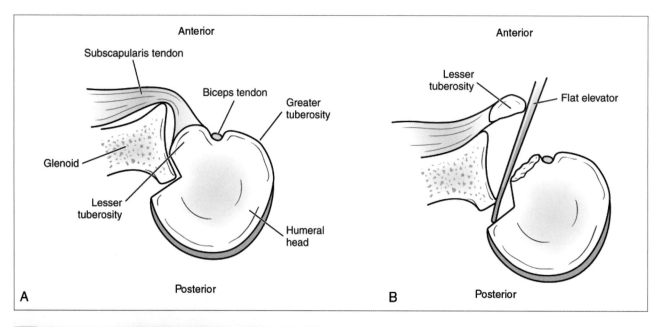

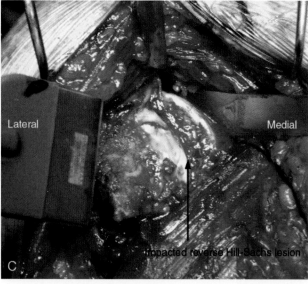

Figure 16 **A,** Illustration depicts open reduction of a chronic posterior glenohumeral dislocation. **B,** Illustration depicts lesser tuberosity osteotomy. A wide, flat elevator is placed between the posterior glenoid rim and the dislocated humeral head to lever the head away from the glenoid rim and facilitate reduction. **C,** Intraoperative photograph shows an elevator placed between the posterior glenoid rim and the dislocated humeral head. (Reproduced from Green A: Chronic posterior dislocation: Open reduction and tendon-bone transfers, in Zuckerman JD, ed: *Advanced Reconstruction: Shoulder*. Rosemont, IL, American Academy of Orthopaedic Surgeons, 2007, p 111-119.)

reverse TSA (in older patients).

- The final humeral implants are placed.
- The subscapularis repair is secured with high-strength transosseous sutures. If the anterior humeral bone is weak, sutures are placed around the neck of the humeral implant.
- Glenohumeral stability and motion are assessed.
- The patient's arm is placed in a sling for immobilization. A position of external rotation should be considered in patients with chronic posterior dislocation.

Reverse TSA

- The preoperative planning, patient positioning and preparation, and surgical approach up to the humeral exposure are the same as those described for anatomic arthroplasty.
- A superior deltoid-splitting approach may be used; however, the authors of this chapter prefer the deltopectoral approach.
- A humeral osteotomy is performed, extending from the upper aspect of the greater tuberosity to the medial aspect of the humeral head. The angle of the cut depends on the specific implant system that will be used.
- The humerus can be prepared for the implant at this time or after the glenoid preparation is completed.
- Exposure of the glenoid is the same as that for anatomic TSA.
- The glenoid implant should be placed in the neutral position or in slight (<10°) inferior tilt to avoid superior tilt.

Table 3 Rehabilitation Protocol After Total Shoulder Arthroplasty

Postoperative Week	Range of Motion	Strengthening	Return to Play	Comments/Emphasis
0-2	None	None	None	Sling immobilization
2-6	None	None	None	Sling immobilization
6-12	Passive, self-assisted stretching	None	Light activity permitted (no lifting >5 lb)	Discontinue sling at 6 wk
12-24	Full	Resistive strengthening at 12 wk depending on progress and radiographic findings	Resume activity at 12 wk Avoid impact activities and heavy lifting	Patients who had prolonged chronic dislocation may require longer rehabilitation

- If a bony defect that requires grafting is encountered, the baseplate center post or screw must be fixed into native scapular bone at the base of the glenoid vault.
- In some patients, it may be necessary to place the baseplate in slightly altered version to gain adequate purchase.
- Solid, structural bone grafting of a glenoid defect is preferred. Usually, the humeral head can be used as graft material. The graft can be either fixed to the native intact scapula with screws or incorporated into the baseplate fixation.
- If the baseplate cannot be adequately supported with the combination of native bone and bone grafting, a two-stage procedure should be considered to achieve graft healing before implant placement.
- The baseplate, peripheral screws, and glenosphere are implanted according to the technique specified by the manufacturer of the implant. If a screw-in baseplate is used, the graft must be stabilized so that it does not rotate after the baseplate is implanted.
- The humerus is prepared as required for the implant that will be used. The authors of this chapter prefer to use press-fit fixation if possible.

- A trial reduction is performed to assess implant stability.
- The authors of this chapter recommend repairing the subscapularis if possible, provided that the repair does not limit external rotation or elevation.
- Postoperatively, the patient's arm is immobilized in a sling with a small abduction cushion. Use of a closed suction drain is recommended to decrease the likelihood of postoperative hematoma.

 Rehabilitation

Rehabilitation after arthroplasty to manage chronic glenohumeral dislocation has not been specifically studied. The authors of this chapter prefer abduction sling immobilization for 6 weeks. The suggested rehabilitation protocol is summarized in **Table 3**.

After anatomic arthroplasty, ROM is usually initiated the day after surgery. If posterior instability is a concern, an external rotation immobilizer should be used, internal rotation should be delayed, and elevation should be in or posterior to the scapular plane. If the arthroplasty is thought to be stable, pendulum circumduction ROM; self-assisted supine passive forward elevation and external rotation; and motion

of the elbow, hand, and wrist are initiated on postoperative day 1. After reverse arthroplasty, pendulum circumduction motion exercises are initiated on postoperative day 1. Active-assisted ROM is initiated after 6 weeks.

After either anatomic or reverse arthroplasty, the sling is usually discontinued 6 weeks postoperatively, at which time active use of the shoulder is permitted. Passive self-assisted stretching is continued until patients reach a plateau in their motion recovery. Patients are allowed to use the arm for light activities (lifting restricted to <5 lb). Patients may begin resistive strengthening at 12 weeks postoperatively depending on their progress and radiographic findings. At this time, patients are allowed to resume activities; however, impact activities and heavy lifting should be avoided. For patients with prolonged chronic dislocation, rehabilitation time may be considerable because of long-standing muscle inactivity.

 Avoiding Pitfalls

Common pitfalls in shoulder arthroplasty include neurovascular injury, iatrogenic fracture, overstuffing of the glenohumeral joint, weak subscapularis repair, instability, and failure of the glenoid baseplate. To avoid these pitfalls, proper patient selection, thorough preoperative planning, and technical expertise are necessary. Matching the correct procedure to the correct patient is key to success. A patient who lacks a functioning rotator cuff will typically achieve better functional results with reverse arthroplasty than with anatomic arthroplasty. The surgeon must be aware of any preoperative vascular disturbances (radial pulse asymmetry) in the affected arm, which may indicate a previous vascular injury that could increase the risk for complications. In patients with long-standing anterior dislocation, the axillary artery and the brachial plexus can become scarred to the humerus. Meticulous and careful dissection is imperative. The axillary nerve should be palpated and protected because careful release of the capsule is required in these patients.

Scarring and osteopenia increase the risk for intraoperative fracture of the humerus. Adequate capsular releases are required to facilitate safe exposure of the humerus and glenoid. Careful retractor placement and force can facilitate exposure and prevent iatrogenic fracture.

Overstuffing of the glenohumeral joint in anatomic arthroplasty results in limited ROM and excessive tension on the subscapularis repair. Adequate soft-tissue releases and mobilization as well as appropriate implant selection can help achieve the soft-tissue laxity and balance that is required to avoid overstuffing of the glenohumeral joint.

To avoid failure of the anatomic arthroplasty, the subscapularis repair must be strong and protected. If the subscapularis repair would be too tight, reverse TSA should be considered.

Glenohumeral stability depends on achieving appropriate balance between the soft tissues and the implant. If stability is difficult to achieve with anatomic arthroplasty, reverse TSA should be considered.

Failure of the glenoid baseplate is a considerable concern. Appropriate placement, avoidance of superior tilt, adequate fixation into native bone, and the use of peripheral locking screws help decrease the risk for this complication.

Bibliography

Boileau P, Trojani C, Walch G, Krishnan SG, Romeo A, Sinnerton R: Shoulder arthroplasty for the treatment of the sequelae of fractures of the proximal humerus. *J Shoulder Elbow Surg* 2001;10(4):299-308.

Checchia SL, Santos PD, Miyazaki AN: Surgical treatment of acute and chronic posterior fracture-dislocation of the shoulder. *J Shoulder Elbow Surg* 1998;7(1):53-65.

Cheng SL, Mackay MB, Richards RR: Treatment of locked posterior fracture-dislocations of the shoulder by total shoulder arthroplasty. *J Shoulder Elbow Surg* 1997;6(1):11-17.

Cuff D, Clark R, Pupello D, Frankle M: Reverse shoulder arthroplasty for the treatment of rotator cuff deficiency: A concise follow-up, at a minimum of five years, of a previous report. *J Bone Joint Surg Am* 2012;94(21):1996-2000.

Cuff D, Pupello D, Virani N, Levy J, Frankle M: Reverse shoulder arthroplasty for the treatment of rotator cuff deficiency. *J Bone Joint Surg Am* 2008;90(6):1244-1251.

Flatow EL, Miller SR, Neer CS II: Chronic anterior dislocation of the shoulder. *J Shoulder Elbow Surg* 1993;2(1):2-10.

Gavriilidis I, Magosch P, Lichtenberg S, Habermeyer P, Kircher J: Chronic locked posterior shoulder dislocation with severe head involvement. *Int Orthop* 2010;34(1):79-84.

Hawkins RJ, Neer CS II, Pianta RM, Mendoza FX: Locked posterior dislocation of the shoulder. *J Bone Joint Surg Am* 1987;69(1):9-18.

Pritchett JW, Clark JM: Prosthetic replacement for chronic unreduced dislocations of the shoulder. *Clin Orthop Relat Res* 1987;(216):89-93.

Ross M, Hope B, Stokes A, Peters SE, McLeod I, Duke PF: Reverse shoulder arthroplasty for the treatment of three-part and four-part proximal humeral fractures in the elderly. *J Shoulder Elbow Surg* 2015;24(2):215-222.

Rowe CR, Zarins B: Chronic unreduced dislocations of the shoulder. *J Bone Joint Surg Am* 1982;64(4):494-505.

Schliemann B, Muder D, Gessmann J, Schildhauer TA, Seybold D: Locked posterior shoulder dislocation: Treatment options and clinical outcomes. *Arch Orthop Trauma Surg* 2011;131(8):1127-1134.

Sperling JW, Pring M, Antuna SA, Cofield RH: Shoulder arthroplasty for locked posterior dislocation of the shoulder. *J Shoulder Elbow Surg* 2004;13(5):522-527.

Werner BS, Böhm D, Abdelkawi A, Gohlke F: Glenoid bone grafting in reverse shoulder arthroplasty for long-standing anterior shoulder dislocation. *J Shoulder Elbow Surg* 2014;23(11):1655-1661.

Wooten C, Klika B, Schleck CD, Harmsen WS, Sperling JW, Cofield RH: Anatomic shoulder arthroplasty as treatment for locked posterior dislocation of the shoulder. *J Bone Joint Surg Am* 2014;96(3):e19.

Chapter 14

Arthroscopic Techniques to Minimize Recurrence of Multidirectional Instability

Omkar H. Dave, MD

Larry D. Field, MD

 ## Introduction

Multidirectional instability (MDI) is shoulder instability in more than one direction, one of which is inferior. Patients with MDI usually do not have a history of traumatic injury. The term was first coined in 1980 to describe instability in the anterior, posterior, and inferior planes in a cohort of patients, most of whom were successfully treated with open inferior capsular shift. Nevertheless, MDI can be challenging to diagnose and treat. Most patients are treated nonsurgically with physical therapy, but arthroscopic suture capsulorrhaphy with or without closure of the rotator interval can be an option when nonsurgical management is unsuccessful.

In all patients with MDI, a preoperative clinical assessment that includes a careful history and a thorough physical examination should be performed to identify the predominant direction of the instability. If either anteroinferior or posteroinferior instability is identified, this finding affects the order of the arthroscopic capsulorrhaphy procedure. The authors of this chapter prefer to pass all inferior capsular sutures before any sutures are tied, and the capsulorrhaphy sutures in the direction of predominant instability are tied first. For example, if the instability is primarily anteroinferior, the posteroinferior sutures should be passed first and left untied until after the anteroinferior sutures have been passed and tied. In this way, the surgeon can more reliably and fully access all aspects of the inferior capsule than would be possible if some sutures were tied before all sutures were passed.

 ## Case Presentation

A 19-year-old woman who is a collegiate volleyball player has a 3-year history of intermittent and slowly progressive dull pain in her dominant shoulder. She describes recurrent subluxations occurring during activities including but not limited to volleyball participation. She also has transient tingling in the arm, especially during strenuous and/or overhead activities. She denies popping or clicking in the shoulder. She has no history of shoulder dislocation or any personal or family history of connective tissue disorders such as Marfan syndrome or Ehlers-Danlos syndrome. She reports no previous surgical procedures on either shoulder.

Inspection of the shoulder girdle reveals no skin changes, scars, glenohumeral joint effusion, or muscular atrophy. The scapula is slightly protracted. Palpation of the shoulder and shoulder girdle does not elicit tenderness. Range of motion of the shoulder, including flexion, abduction, and internal and external rotation with the arm both adducted and abducted, is full and symmetric with the contralateral shoulder, with no crepitus. Muscle strength is full and equal bilaterally. A sulcus sign test is performed by applying an inferiorly directed pull on the arm while the shoulder is in an adducted position. The test result is positive when the inferior translation of the humeral head leaves a sulcus, or a hollow appearance, between the lateral acromion and the superior aspect of the humeral head. The patient's sulcus sign is 1+ on both shoulders as

Dr. Field or an immediate family member is a member of a speakers' bureau or has made paid presentations on behalf of Smith & Nephew; serves as a paid consultant to Mitek Sports Medicine and Smith & Nephew; has received research or institutional support from Arthrex, Mitek Sports Medicine, and Smith & Nephew; has received nonincome support (such as equipment or services), commercially derived honoraria, or other non–research-related funding (such as paid travel) from Elsevier, Thieme, and Wolters Kluwer Health; and serves as a board member, owner, officer, or committee member of the American Academy of Orthopaedic Surgeons, the American Orthopaedic Society for Sports Medicine, the American Shoulder and Elbow Surgeons, and the Arthroscopy Association of North America. Neither Dr. Dave nor any immediate family member has received anything of value from or has stock or stock options held in a commercial company or institution related directly or indirectly to the subject of this chapter.

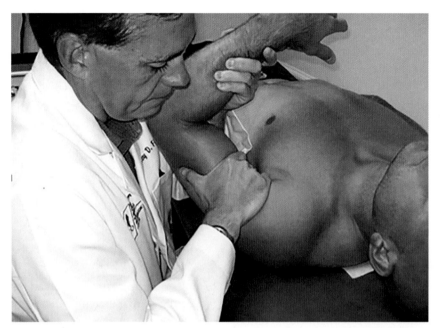

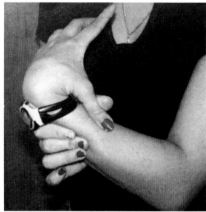

Figure 2 Clinical photograph shows a positive thumb-to-forearm test result, which is common in patients with multidirectional instability.

Figure 1 Clinical photograph shows performance of the load-and-shift test. The patient is placed in the supine position, with the elbow in 90° of flexion. The shoulder is translated anteriorly while axial load is applied, and the degree of humeral head translation is assessed.

confirmed by the presence of less than 1 cm of distance between the inferior margin of the acromion and the humeral head.

The results of the anterior apprehension test, performed while the patient is supine, are also positive because of the patient's obvious and expressed apprehension when the arm is positioned in 90° of abduction and maximum external rotation. The patient's apprehension is even more pronounced when an anteriorly directed force is applied to the shoulder while the shoulder is in an abducted and externally rotated position. The apprehension is relieved when a posteriorly directed force is applied to the anterior humeral head while maintaining the same position of the arm; this finding represents a positive Jobe relocation test result. The load-and-shift test is also performed with the patient in the supine position (**Figure 1**). In this test, humeral head translation is assessed and graded with the elbow positioned in approximately 90° of flexion while the examiner stabilizes the

forearm with one hand and uses the other hand to apply an anterior and posterior force while the glenohumeral joint is axially loaded. If the humeral head can be translated to the edge of the glenoid, the result is graded as 1+. If the humeral head can be subluxated over the glenoid rim with spontaneous reduction, the grade is 2+. If the shoulder can be dislocated without a spontaneous reduction, the grade is 3+. In this patient, this test reveals 1+ increased anterior and no increased posterior humeral head translations compared with the contralateral shoulder. Examination of rotator cuff strength causes mild shoulder pain but no weakness compared with the contralateral shoulder. Finally, the patient has positive thumb-to-forearm test results, suggesting generalized hyperlaxity (**Figure 2**). Results of complete cervical, neurologic, and vascular examinations of both upper extremities are within normal limits.

Standard AP, axillary lateral, and scapular Y radiographic views demonstrate no deformities or bony

deficiencies of the glenoid or humeral head. Joint spaces are maintained. MRI with intra-articular contrast demonstrates increased capsular volume and a large axillary fold, but no labral tears or capsular disruptions such as humeral avulsion of the glenohumeral ligament. The rotator cuff and all other shoulder structures are normal in appearance.

Because nonsurgical treatment is successful in most patients with MDI, the patient undergoes a structured nonsurgical treatment course for 6 months. This program consists of formal physical therapy, focusing first on proper scapular control using bracing, taping, and an isometric exercise program. Subsequently, a strengthening exercise program focusing on the scapular stabilizers, deltoid, and rotator cuff muscles is incorporated into the therapy schedule. Despite excellent compliance, the patient continues to have persistent shoulder pain and episodes of subluxation that preclude her from participating in overhead activities, including volleyball. This young, athletic individual is substantially limited by the instability symptoms despite an appropriately conducted and overseen rehabilitation program that was continued for more than 6 months. Physical examination continues to suggest MDI. Although imaging studies revealed no labral tear, MRI with intra-articular contrast material demonstrates increased capsular volume. Arthroscopic capsulorrhaphy is therefore performed.

Indications

Patients with MDI are candidates for surgical intervention only after extensive nonsurgical treatment has proved to be inadequate in improving their symptoms. The motivated, compliant patient must complete an extended trial of appropriate physical therapy (overseen by knowledgeable medical staff) before surgical intervention is considered. Typically, surgery is discussed with a patient only after he or she has completed at least 6 months of organized physical therapy with no substantial improvement in symptoms.

Contraindications

Patients with generalized joint hypermobility resulting from connective tissue disorders such as Ehlers-Danlos syndrome are poor surgical candidates. Patients with Ehlers-Danlos syndrome typically have joint hypermobility and laxity, dystrophic scarring, hyperextensible skin, and connective tissue fragility. Patients with hypermobility-type Ehlers-Danlos syndrome generally have a greater-than-average range of motion and are more prone to joint instability because of altered vibratory perception and proprioception.

Voluntary dislocation is a relative contraindication to surgical management. These patients may achieve secondary gain from the instability and may attempt to redislocate the shoulder after surgical stabilization. Because these patients will likely have chronically poor results, surgical treatment should be avoided.

Controversies and Alternative Approaches

The landmark study on open capsulorrhaphy for the management of MDI was published in 1980. Patients who underwent the inferior capsular shift procedure described in that study had a 97% rate of satisfactory outcomes, with full strength, full return to activity, and no substantial postoperative pain or recurrent instability. Similarly successful results after open surgical treatment of MDI have been reported in several other studies. Capsulorrhaphy involving a glenoid-side shift rather than a humeral-side shift, along with a combined open Bankart procedure, has also been described with excellent results. Although studies comparing open capsulorrhaphy with arthroscopic capsulorrhaphy are lacking, both basic science and clinical results have shown the approaches to be equally effective. Several other controversies persist, including the value of rotator interval closure, use of sutures only or suture anchors, number of sutures used, and use of absorbable versus nonabsorbable sutures.

Capsulorrhaphy for the management of MDI can be performed with the patient in either the beach-chair position or the lateral decubitus position (**Figure 3**). The authors of this chapter prefer the lateral decubitus position because it provides improved access to the inferior capsule. In addition, recent clinical evidence suggests lower recurrence rates among patients undergoing arthroscopic stabilization in the lateral decubitus position. The advantages and disadvantages of each position are shown in **Table 1**.

Results

The literature describing outcomes of arthroscopic management of shoulder MDI is scarce (**Table 2**). Most of the

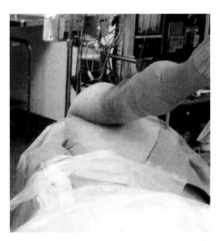

Figure 3 Intraoperative photograph shows the lateral decubitus position. This patient position provides improved access to the inferior capsule during capsulorrhaphy.

published studies demonstrate successful outcomes.

A technique for arthroscopic stabilization of MDI was first described in a 1993 study of 10 patients who were followed for 1 to 3 years. According to the Neer criteria, all patients exhibited satisfactory results, and the average postoperative Bankart score was 90. Two patients required revision surgery for the management of symptomatic sutures. The authors of another study used the transglenoid suture technique in 25 patients with minimum 2-year follow-up and reported 88% satisfactory results according to the Neer criteria.

In a study of a technique involving multiple sutures in the anterior and posterior capsule, researchers reported 95% good to excellent results in 19 patients, with 89% of patients returning to their former level of competition. Another study likewise reported good or excellent results in 94% of 47 patients treated with a pancapsular plication technique; 85% of patients in that study resumed their previous activity levels.

In a study of 40 patients with MDI treated using arthroscopic capsular

Table 1 Advantages and Disadvantages of the Beach-Chair and Lateral Decubitus Positions in Arthroscopic Management of Multidirectional Instability

Position	Advantages	Disadvantages
Lateral decubitus	Efficient setup	Nonanatomic orientation
	Less fatigue because most of the procedure is done with the surgeon's arms at the side	Need for repositioning and redraping for conversion to open procedures
	Better access to the inferior glenoid and the inferior capsule	Less ability to rotate the shoulder due to constraints of the traction device
	Increased joint space through lateralization and labral tears, sometimes accentuated by traction	More difficult anesthesia airway management
	Ease of performing instability repairs	Arm-holding device and balanced suspension device required
	Excellent visualization of subacromial space as a result of maintained traction	Risk of traction-related injury
	Lateral flotation of arthroscopic bubbles within the subacromial space (subdeltoid space) out of the field of view	Increased risk of axillary and musculocutaneous nerve damage during anteroinferior portal placement
	Decreased risk of cerebral hypoperfusion	General anesthesia is typically required because regional anesthesia is not well tolerated
Beach-chair	Anatomic orientation	Possible increased fatigue because the surgeon's arms are abducted at the glenohumeral joint for most of the procedure
	Ease of setup	
	Ease of conversion to open procedures	Decreased visualization of the posteroinferior and anteroinferior aspects of the joint
	No additional required equipment, although specific beach-chair attachments are often used	Difficulty providing balanced suspension without an assistant or a specialized shoulder-holding device
	Excellent visualization of the subacromial space	Increased risk of cerebral hypoperfusion
	Optimal rotational control of the shoulder, which is especially helpful for positioning during closure of the rotator interval	Potential for obscured visualization of the subacromial space because of arthroscopic bubbles

Adapted with permission from Frank RM, Saccomanno MF, McDonald LS, Moric M, Romeo AA, Provencher MT: Outcomes of arthroscopic anterior shoulder instability in the beach chair versus lateral decubitus position: A systematic review and meta-regression analysis. *Arthroscopy* 2014;30(10):1349-1365.

plication with 2- to 5-year follow-up, 86% of patients ultimately returned to sport. A study of 13 patients with MDI and 270° labral tears had an 84% satisfaction rate and recurrent instability in 15% of patients after minimum follow-up of 2 years. In a study of nine young overhead athletes with MDI, seven patients had good or excellent results and returned to sports. In a study of a laser-assisted technique with suture plication of the rotator interval, 26 of 27 shoulders remained stable at 2-year follow-up, and 86% of patients returned to their previous level of sport.

Technical Keys to Success: Arthroscopic Capsulorrhaphy

Setup/Exposure
- An interscalene block is administered, followed by the induction of general anesthesia.
- The procedure can be performed with the patient in either the beach-chair position or the lateral decubitus position.
- If the lateral decubitus position will be used, the patient should be examined carefully under anesthesia before positioning. Translations of both shoulders in the anterior,

posterior, and inferior directions should be assessed and compared.
- The patient is supported with the use of a deflatable bean bag.
- The patient's body is tilted 30° posteriorly to position the glenoid parallel to the floor.
- The area around the patient's head is cleared to provide easy access to both the anterior and posterior shoulder.
- The dependent leg is well padded to protect the common peroneal nerve.
- The affected extremity is positioned in 70° of abduction, 10° of forward flexion, and neutral external rotation, and 10 lb (4.5 kg) of balanced suspension is applied (**Figure 3**).

Table 2 Results of Arthroscopic Management of Multidirectional Instability

Authors	Journal (Year)	Technique (No. of Patients)	Outcomes	Comments
Duncan and Savoie	*Arthroscopy* (1993)	Arthroscopic stabilization (10)	All patients had satisfactory results (Neer criteria) Avg Bankart score, 90	Follow-up, 1-3 yr 2 patients required revision surgery for symptomatic sutures
McIntyre et al	*Arthroscopy* (1997)	Multiple-suture technique in the anterior and posterior capsules (19)	95% good or excellent results (Tibone and Bradley outcome scale)	89% of patients returned to their former level of competition
Treacy et al	*J Shoulder Elbow Surg* (1999)	Transglenoid suture technique (25)	88% satisfactory results (Neer criteria)	Minimum follow-up, 2 yr
Gartsman et al	*Arthroscopy* (2001)	Pancapsular plication (47)	Rowe scores were good or excellent in 94% of patients	85% of patients returned to previous activity levels
Lyons et al	*Arthroscopy* (2001)	Laser-assisted technique with suture plication of the rotator interval (27)	96% were stable and asymptomatic, 86% returned to sports	26 of 27 shoulders remained stable at 2-yr follow-up
Alpert et al	*Arthroscopy* (2008)	Arthroscopic stabilization with labral repair (13)	84% satisfaction	Patients had multidirectional instability and 270° labral tears 15% of patients had recurrent instability Minimum follow-up, 2 yr
Baker et al	*Am J Sports Med* (2009)	Arthroscopic capsular plication (40)	91% full or satisfactory range of motion 98% normal or slightly decreased strength 86% return to sports with little or no limitation	Follow-up, 2-5 yr
Voigt et al	*Open Orthop J* (2009)	Arthroscopic capsular plication (9)	7 patients had good or excellent results	7 patients returned to sports

Instruments/Equipment/Implants Required

- Either an arthroscopic pump or a gravity system may be used for fluid inflow. If a pump is used, the flow must be kept low to avoid excessive soft-tissue swelling. The authors of this chapter prefer to use gravity inflow with four 5-L bags of lactated Ringer fluid.
- A standard 4.0-mm arthroscope with a 30° lens is typically used. A 70° lens should also be available.
- A 4.5-mm full-radius shaver should be available to débride the capsule and the glenoid labrum without damaging the surrounding soft tissues.
- A 7-mm translucent, threaded cannula and a 5-mm threaded cannula

with a sharp trocar are required for instrument passage. The threaded design helps to prevent the cannula from backing out of the glenohumeral joint, and the translucent body allows visualization of the sutures and knots through the cannula itself. The sharp trocar facilitates insertion through the interval tissue.
- Small-diameter glenoid labrum anchors should be available for use in the event that an unexpected labral tear is identified.
- Several nonabsorbable, braided free sutures are typically used to perform the capsulorrhaphy.
- A suture-passing device is necessary for suture passage through the capsule and/or labrum.

Procedure

PORTAL PLACEMENT AND DIAGNOSTIC ARTHROSCOPY

- A skin marker is used to outline the posterior and lateral borders of the acromion as well as the coracoid process.
- The posterior arthroscopic portal is established first. This portal should be located slightly more lateral than the standard posterior portal, bringing the portal closer to the humeral head and thereby allowing improved access to the posterior glenoid labrum and capsule.
- The arthroscope is introduced through the posterior portal.
- Diagnostic arthroscopy is performed. The surgeon should observe the amount of overall

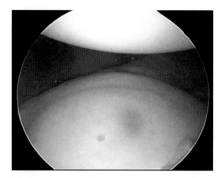

Figure 4 Arthroscopic view from the anterosuperior portal demonstrates a positive drive-through sign, in which the arthroscope can easily pass between the humeral head (top) and the glenoid (bottom).

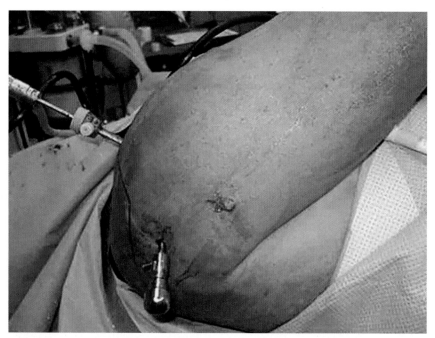

Figure 5 Intraoperative photograph shows the arthroscopic portals typically used for suture capsulorrhaphy in patients with multidirectional instability, as viewed from posterior with the patient's head to the left of the image. Anterosuperiorly, a plastic cannula is used primarily for viewing with the arthroscope but can also be used for labral preparation and suture management as necessary. A metal cannula is in the standard posterior portal. The accessory posterolateral portal, indicated in this photograph by the spinal needle with a green cap, lies distal and lateral to the position of the standard posterior portal. This posterolateral portal is created under direct arthroscopic visualization and is necessary for effective access to the inferior capsule. This portal provides the proper trajectory for posterior anchor placement when anchors are used and allows the surgeon to more easily access the posteroinferior capsule for capsular shift and plication.

capsular volume, the biceps anchor, the attachment of glenohumeral ligaments, and the status of the anterior, inferior, and posterior labrum as well as the rotator cuff. The patulousness of the capsule and the status of the rotator interval should also be examined (**Figure 4**). In many patients with MDI, the posterior capsule is thin, and the infraspinatus muscle may be visible through it. Care must therefore be taken to avoid damage to the posterior capsular tissue.

- The first of two anterior portals is established. A spinal needle is placed just lateral and 1 cm proximal to the coracoid process from outside in through the rotator interval tissue. After verifying proper placement of the spinal needle inferiorly within the rotator interval and immediately adjacent and superior to the subscapularis tendon, a small skin incision is made.
- A switching stick is introduced into the joint through this anterior portal. To ensure adequate access to the inferior capsule, the switching stick is used to gently palpate the anterior-inferior glenoid and then is directed into the anteroinferior capsular pouch.
- A large 7-mm cannula is placed

over the switching stick and gently twisted through the skin incision into the joint.
- The switching stick is removed.
- Anterior fluid inflow is established by removing the inflow tubing from the scope and connecting it to the anterior cannula.
- The second anterior portal is established superior to the first (**Figure 5**). A spinal needle is introduced approximately 1 cm lateral and proximal to the anterior portal into the joint, through the rotator interval. A small skin incision is made at this level, and a 5-mm cannula is introduced adjacent to the larger cannula and just posterior to the biceps tendon such that the biceps tendon is flanked

on either side by the two cannulas.
- The arthroscope can be placed into either of the anterior portals for visualization. The anterosuperior portal allows excellent top-down visualization of the entire anterior and posterior labrum and capsule.
- In patients with primarily anteroinferior instability, the arthroscope is placed into the anterosuperior portal, and the posterior portal is used as the initial working portal. In addition, depending on the surgeon's ability to adequately access the posteroinferior capsule through the posterior portal, an accessory (posterior instability) portal may be created at the 5-o'clock position. This portal, which is typically located approximately 2 cm lateral

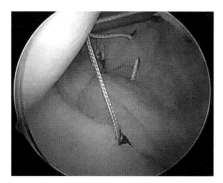

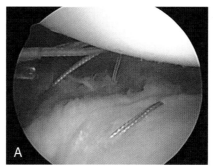

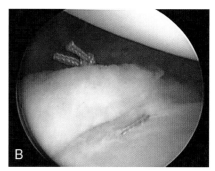

Figure 6 Arthroscopic view from an anterosuperior portal demonstrates the use of suture anchors in posterior capsulorrhaphy. The capsular limb of the anchor suture has been passed inferior and lateral to its respective anchor. The sutures have been tied, resulting in superior shift of the capsule; the redundant capsule has been plicated to form a labral bumper. Anchor placement and suture tying proceeded from inferior to superior.

Figure 7 Arthroscopic views from the anterior portal demonstrate plication of the inferior capsule to the intact glenoid labrum. **A,** A permanent, nonabsorbable braided suture has been passed across the labrum in a horizontal mattress fashion but has not yet been tied. **B,** The appearance of effective capsular plication after suture tying.

and 2 cm inferior to the standard posterior portal, greatly improves access to the inferior capsule for suture passage.

SUTURE PASSAGE AND CAPSULAR PLICATION

- After portal placement and careful diagnostic assessment, the entire shoulder capsule is stimulated anteriorly, posteriorly, and inferiorly with the use of an arthroscopic synovial rasp to create a reactive, bleeding surface that will enhance soft-tissue healing. Alternatively, a full-radius shaver without teeth can be used without suction.

- Sutures are passed beginning posteroinferiorly. A No. 1 absorbable polydioxanone suture is loaded onto an arthroscopic suture passer. The first suture is the most inferior of the plication sutures.

- The suture passer is used to pierce the capsule at the 6-o'clock position, approximately 1 cm inferior to the labrum.

- The suture passer is rotated to advance the capsule superiorly.

- The capsule is lifted proximally toward the inferior labrum to draw the capsule up and away from the axillary nerve. Regardless which suture-passing device is used for this step, it is critically important to limit penetration inferiorly through the capsule to minimize the risk of damage to the axillary nerve.

- After the inferior capsular tissue is captured, the suture passer is advanced under the labrum, exiting at the labral-chondral junction (**Figure 6**).

- The polydioxanone suture is shuttled out of the suture passer and into the joint.

- A grasper is used to retrieve the intra-articular end of the shuttled polydioxanone suture through the anterolateral cannula.

- The capsular plication can be accomplished with the polydioxanone suture or with a shuttled nonabsorbable braided suture. If the surgeon chooses to use a nonabsorbable suture, the polydioxanone suture is simply tied around the tail of the nonabsorbable suture outside the anterolateral portal. The polydioxanone suture tail is pulled out of the posterior portal, shuttling the nonabsorbable suture through the capsulolabral complex in a retrograde fashion. Both ends of the nonabsorbable suture are brought

out through the posterior cannula.

- Either a simple or mattress suture construct is used to perform the capsulorrhaphy (**Figure 7**). Typically, two to four posteroinferior sutures are sufficient to eliminate capsular redundancy. As noted previously, in a patient with primarily anteroinferior instability, the posteroinferior sutures should not be tied until after the anterior sutures have been passed and tied.

- After all posterior plication sutures have been passed through the posteroinferior capsule, the anteroinferior capsule is plicated in a similar manner.

- The anterior capsule is abraded to create a reactive surface as described previously, if this step has not already been accomplished.

- As in the posterior capsular plication, the first anterior suture is placed most inferiorly. Subsequent anterior sutures are passed through the capsule progressively more superiorly as needed to achieve adequate reduction of capsular volume and ligamentous retensioning.

- Two to four sutures are typically required for adequate anterior capsular plication.

- After the posterior and anterior capsular plication sutures have been placed, they are tied sequentially, beginning with the anterior plication sutures. Any sutures passed using a simple suture limb construct should always use the capsular suture limb as the post limb. Using the capsular suture limb instead of the labral suture limb serves to position the knot away from the labrum and articular surfaces, thus preventing knot impingement and potential articular cartilage damage.

- If the labral tissue is poorly defined and/or is insufficient to support the capsulorrhaphy, suture anchors are used much as they would be if labral detachments were present. These anchors are placed along the glenoid rim inferiorly, posteriorly, and anteriorly as necessary. The sutures are then passed and tied as described previously.

ROTATOR INTERVAL CLOSURE
- Closure of the rotator interval may be performed as a supplemental procedure at the surgeon's discretion, depending on the degree of instability determined preoperatively, the soft-tissue quality determined intraoperatively, and the surgeon's ability to securely and adequately stabilize the shoulder using the suture capsulorrhaphy technique.
- Closure of the rotator interval, if performed, should include both the inner and the outer layers of the rotator interval.
- A braided suture is delivered into the joint through the anterosuperior cannula and is grasped with a retrograde suture retriever inserted through the inferiorly placed anterior cannula.
- The suture retriever is used to grasp the end of the free suture and is backed out of the glenohumeral joint along with the anterior portal cannula through which it was inserted. However, the cannula is backed out only to a point that is immediately adjacent and anterior

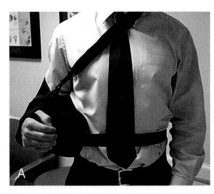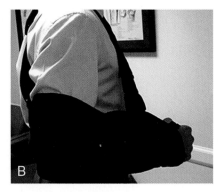

Figure 8 Photographs demonstrate the sling position from the front (**A**) and lateral (**B**) views.

to the rotator interval capsular tissue.
- The suture retriever is blindly redirected back into the glenohumeral joint through the rotator interval tissue at its most superior extent such that the suture completely spans the rotator interval from superior to inferior and incorporates both the inner and outer layers of the rotator interval tissue.
- The redelivered end of the free suture is retrieved through the anterosuperior portal. In this way, one suture has been successfully passed around and across the entire rotator interval, and both limbs of the suture are within the anterosuperior portal.
- The arm is removed from balanced suspension and placed in approximately 60° of abduction and approximately 45° of external rotation.
- While the arm is held in this position, the rotator interval suture is tied.
- Depending on the size of the rotator interval, more than one suture may be passed around the rotator interval and tied in this way.

Wound Closure
- The wound is closed with an absorbable subcutaneous stitch.
- Thin adhesive strips are used on large portal sites.

- The patient's arm is immobilized in an abduction brace or gunslinger brace (**Figure 8**).

Rehabilitation

The rehabilitation protocol is summarized in **Table 3**. Patients are typically kept in a shoulder immobilizer with the surgical arm in approximately neutral rotation for 4 to 6 weeks after the procedure. The patient participates in gentle elbow, wrist, and hand range-of-motion exercises during the initial 6-week postoperative phase. Active and active-assisted shoulder range-of-motion exercises are generally initiated between 6 and 12 weeks postoperatively, with an emphasis on proper scapular positioning. Neuromuscular proprioception and rotator cuff strengthening are not usually begun until 3 months postoperatively. Clinical end point examination should be used to determine healing of capsular reconstruction during this phase. Sport-specific conditioning is begun at 4 months, and return to sports is generally allowed anytime from 6 to 12 months postoperatively.

Avoiding Pitfalls

Proper diagnosis of MDI is the keystone to success. Careful and thorough assessment is critical because patients

Table 3 Rehabilitation Protocol After Arthroscopic Capsulorrhaphy to Manage Multidirectional Instability

Postoperative Week	ROM	Strengthening	Return to Play	Comments/Emphasis
0-6	Immobilization in an abduction brace or gunslinger brace Gentle elbow, wrist, and hand ROM exercise program	—	—	Stiffness is uncommon; overzealous early rehabilitation can increase the risk of recurrent instability
6-12	Active and active-assisted ROM No aggressive passive ROM	—	—	Emphasis on correct scapular position Early static scapular bracing or taping may be needed for short periods in patients with scapular protraction
12-16	Proprioceptive neuromuscular facilitation exercises Plyometrics	Rotator cuff strengthening	—	Continue maintenance of correct scapular posture Clinical end point examination should be used to determine healing of capsular reconstruction
16-52	Integrated rehabilitation following the Kibler protocol from 4-8 mo	Rotator cuff strengthening	Return to sports at 6-12 mo depending primarily on shoulder tracking patterns and position	Sport-specific conditioning from 4-8 mo

ROM = range of motion.

commonly report pain without a clear history of instability. Careful preoperative evaluation is necessary to determine whether the direction of instability is predominantly anteroinferior or posteroinferior; this information is used to direct the sequence of suture passage and tying intraoperatively. The surgeon should determine the magnitude and direction of instability by performing a careful examination of both shoulders with the patient under anesthesia.

The use of an outside-in technique to establish portals can help to ensure access to all areas of the shoulder. To improve access to the posterior labrum and capsule, the posterior portal should be placed slightly more lateral than a standard posterior portal. Failure to optimize portal placement may limit access to the inferior capsule. If a pump is used for fluid inflow, the flow must be kept low to avoid excessive swelling about the shoulder, which can limit access to the inferior capsule. To avoid injury to the axillary nerve, the surgeon should visualize the penetration of devices across the inferior capsule and limit the depth of penetration to the amount necessary to capture the capsule.

The goal of arthroscopic capsulorrhaphy is to obtain a stable glenohumeral joint by balancing the anterior and posterior capsular plication. If the patient's labrum is inadequate to support the stabilization, anchors may be used to secure the shifted tissues. In patients with thin and patulous capsular tissue, the surgeon should liberally use additional sutures as necessary to add structural support to the capsulorrhaphy. The procedure should be tailored to the individual patient to address the pathology identified arthroscopically. In selected patients, the procedure may include closure of the rotator interval incorporating the coracohumeral ligament and the superior and middle glenohumeral ligaments. When a simple suture construct is used for knot tying, the suture limb that passes through the capsule should be used as the post limb. This method avoids the placement of knots adjacent to the articular surface.

Bibliography

Alpert JM, Verma N, Wysocki R, Yanke AB, Romeo AA: Arthroscopic treatment of multidirectional shoulder instability with minimum 270 degrees labral repair: minimum 2-year follow-up. *Arthroscopy* 2008;24(6):704-711.

Altchek DW, Warren RF, Skyhar MJ, Ortiz G: T-plasty modification of the Bankart procedure for multidirectional instability of the anterior and inferior types. *J Bone Joint Surg Am* 1991;73(1):105-112.

Bak K, Spring BJ, Henderson JP: Inferior capsular shift procedure in athletes with multidirectional instability based on isolated capsular and ligamentous redundancy. *Am J Sports Med* 2000;28(4):466-471.

Baker CL III, Mascarenhas R, Kline AJ, Chhabra A, Pombo MW, Bradley JP: Arthroscopic treatment of multidirectional shoulder instability in athletes: A retrospective analysis of 2- to 5-year clinical outcomes. *Am J Sports Med* 2009;37(9):1712-1720.

Brems JJ, Bergfeld J: Multidirectional shoulder instability. *Orthop Trans* 1991;15:84.

Burkhead WZ Jr, Rockwood CA Jr: Treatment of instability of the shoulder with an exercise program. *J Bone Joint Surg Am* 1992;74(6):890-896.

Duncan R, Savoie FH III: Arthroscopic inferior capsular shift for multidirectional instability of the shoulder: A preliminary report. *Arthroscopy* 1993;9(1):24-27.

Frank RM, Saccomanno MF, McDonald LS, Moric M, Romeo AA, Provencher MT: Outcomes of arthroscopic anterior shoulder instability in the beach chair versus lateral decubitus position: A systematic review and meta-regression analysis. *Arthroscopy* 2014;30(10):1349-1365.

Gartsman GM, Roddey TS, Hammerman SM: Arthroscopic treatment of multidirectional glenohumeral instability: 2- to 5-year follow-up. *Arthroscopy* 2001;17(3):236-243.

Kibler WB: Rehabilitation of the shoulder, in Kibler WB, Herring SA, Press JM, eds: *Functional Rehabilitation of Sports and Musculoskeletal Injuries*. Gaithersburg, MD, Aspen Publishers, 1998, pp 149-170.

Lebar RD, Alexander AH: Multidirectional shoulder instability. Clinical results of inferior capsular shift in an active-duty population. *Am J Sports Med* 1992;20(2):193-198.

Lyons TR, Griffith PL, Savoie FH III, Field LD: Laser-assisted capsulorrhaphy for multidirectional instability of the shoulder. *Arthroscopy* 2001;17(1):25-30.

Marberry TA: Experience with the Neer inferior capsular shift for multidirectional instability. *Orthop Trans* 1988;15:747.

McIntyre LF, Caspari RB, Savoie FH III: The arthroscopic treatment of multidirectional shoulder instability: Two-year results of a multiple suture technique. *Arthroscopy* 1997;13(4):418-425.

Misamore GW, Sallay PI, Didelot W: A longitudinal study of patients with multidirectional instability of the shoulder with seven- to ten-year follow-up. *J Shoulder Elbow Surg* 2005;14(5):466-470.

Neer CS II: Involuntary inferior and multidirectional instability of the shoulder: Etiology, recognition, and treatment. *Instr Course Lect* 1985;34:232-238.

Neer CS II, Foster CR: Inferior capsular shift for involuntary inferior and multidirectional instability of the shoulder: A preliminary report. *J Bone Joint Surg Am* 1980;62(6):897-908.

Treacy SH, Savoie FH III, Field LD: Arthroscopic treatment of multidirectional instability. *J Shoulder Elbow Surg* 1999;8(4):345-350.

Voigt C, Schulz AP, Lill H: Arthroscopic treatment of multidirectional glenohumeral instability in young overhead athletes. *Open Orthop J* 2009;3:107-114.

Chapter 15

Multidirectional Instability: Open Surgical Revision in Patients With Soft-Tissue Deficiency or Collagen Disorders

Roger G. Pollock, MD

Peter B. MacDonald, MD, FRCSC

 ## Introduction

Multidirectional instability (MDI) is defined as symptomatic glenohumeral instability in the anterior, posterior, and inferior directions. It consists of anteroinferior dislocation with posterior subluxation, posteroinferior dislocation with anterior subluxation, or dislocation in all three directions. In normal shoulders, passive manipulation can result in a wide range of translation because laxity varies widely. In patients with MDI, symptoms result from excessive translation of the humeral head on the glenoid with use of the arm. The definition of MDI does not refer to the amount of native laxity in the shoulder but to the occurrence of symptoms when subluxation or dislocation occurs in multiple directions.

Factors that can contribute to the development of MDI include excessive inherent ligamentous laxity, repetitive microtrauma to the shoulder over a period of years, and at least one episode of major trauma. Many patients with MDI have generalized ligamentous laxity and fit the classic stereotype of patients with this diagnosis: atraumatic and bilateral instability as well as hyperextensibility in other joints. This group includes patients with collagen disorders, such as Ehlers-Danlos syndrome or Marfan syndrome. However, many patients with MDI do not have ligamentous laxity in all joints, but only so-called loose shoulders. They are frequently athletes who repetitively stress the shoulder capsule with activities such as throwing, gymnastics, or swimming. These patients' overhead sports activities are thought to have stretched the shoulder ligaments. Even in patients at risk for MDI, a frank instability event may occur only after substantial trauma to the shoulder.

MDI can therefore result from a combination of etiologic factors. Limiting the diagnosis of MDI to patients with atraumatic instability and generalized ligamentous laxity would omit a substantial group of patients. In a clinical population, patients with overlapping factors contributing to the instability are precisely those in whom the instability may be underdiagnosed and incorrectly managed with a surgical repair that fails to address the multidirectional nature of the instability.

Reasons for Failed Surgical Instability Repair in Patients With MDI

The most common reason for failure of surgical repair in patients with MDI is recurrent instability of the shoulder. Historically, unidirectional dislocation was managed with procedures such as the Putti-Platt and Magnuson-Stack repairs, which tightened the anterior side of the shoulder joint and are inadequate to address MDI. Although these procedures are no longer performed, unidirectional tightening can still occur in inadequate capsulorrhaphy procedures (open or arthroscopic) in which only the anterior capsule is shifted and tightened, leaving the inferior capsular volume unaddressed. Asymmetric unidirectional tightening can allow persistent subluxation in the untouched inferior capsular pouch and/or subluxation in the opposite direction, resulting in altered glenohumeral joint mechanics and even leading to the early development of glenohumeral arthritis.

Other intraoperative technical factors can contribute to the recurrence of instability after primary repair. Ligamentous avulsion from the glenoid insertion (that is, a Bankart lesion) can occasionally be present, especially in patients with an episode of trauma contributing to the development of MDI. Failure to repair a Bankart lesion and to re-anchor the

Dr. Pollock or an immediate family member has stock or stock options held in Merck and Pfizer. Dr. MacDonald or an immediate family member has received research or institutional support from Arthrex, Conmed Linvatec, and Össur and serves as a board member, owner, officer, or committee member of the American Shoulder and Elbow Surgeons.

capsule and labrum to the glenoid rim prevents proper anteroinferior capsular tensioning and can allow persistent subluxation or dislocation. Similarly, repair of a Bankart lesion too far medially rather than to the anatomic insertion site on the glenoid rim (immediately adjacent to the articular cartilage) can allow residual laxity and contribute to recurrent instability.

Management of MDI with thermal capsular shrinkage, using either laser or radiofrequency devices, has yielded relatively poor outcomes, resulting in high recurrence rates, persistent pain in some patients, and capsular damage, which can make revision surgery problematic. In one study, 9 of 19 patients who underwent thermal capsulorrhaphy with the use of a monopolar radiofrequency device had recurrent instability at a mean 9-month follow-up. Four patients also had neurapraxic injuries to the axillary nerve, although symptoms resolved within 9 months. At the time of revision surgery, the capsular tissue was found to be abnormal in seven patients (thickened and difficult to mobilize in four patients and thin and friable in three patients, requiring an allograft procedure in one patient). A different group of authors reported an unsatisfactory outcome in 22 of 53 patients in an MDI subgroup (42%). Nine patients later underwent open revision procedures in which the capsular tissue was found to be thin and attenuated, enabling plication. Other authors have reported similar high failure rates of thermal capsulorrhaphy in patients with MDI (28% in one study and 59% in another study). Severe glenohumeral chondrolysis has been reported after the use of thermal capsulorrhaphy to manage shoulder instability.

Errors in postoperative rehabilitation can result in recurrence of instability after surgical repair of MDI. After an open capsulorrhaphy procedure, aggressive early stretching exercises, especially in external rotation, can cause pull-off of

the subscapularis or the repaired capsular flaps, resulting in recurrent instability and shoulder weakness with use of the arm in certain planes. Aggressive restoration of full motion after a capsulorrhaphy procedure for MDI can stretch the repaired capsule and lead to recurrent instability. In contrast to patients with unidirectional instability who may experience a stiff shoulder after instability repair, patients with MDI and natural capsular laxity are much less likely to have a stiff shoulder after a well-performed capsulorrhaphy procedure. Particularly in patients with an atraumatic etiology of the instability, the shoulder is much more likely to become loose again than permanently stiff. Advancing stretching and resistive exercises too quickly as well as allowing a return to high-demand activities, such as overhead sports, too early may result in recurrence of the instability.

Unsatisfactory outcomes after surgical repair of MDI can result from other factors as well. Asymmetric capsular tightening can produce stiffness in the plane that was overtightened, which usually results in restriction of external rotation, especially with the arm at the side. This restricted external rotation, in turn, may cause altered joint kinematics and contact patterns, resulting in pain, chondral damage over time, and, in some patients, early development of glenohumeral osteoarthritis. Loose, migrating, or prominent intra-articular hardware from previous instability surgery may cause pain and result in chondral injury. Chondrolysis of the glenohumeral joint, which occurs in some patients after thermal capsulorrhaphy procedures, results in a stiff and painful shoulder. This diagnosis is confirmed by loss of joint space on plain radiographs and abnormal cartilage signal on MRI.

An incorrect initial diagnosis also can result in an unsatisfactory outcome of instability repair. A patient with normal shoulder laxity may receive an

incorrect diagnosis of instability and may undergo an inappropriate capsular tightening. Acromioclavicular joint pathology or bicipital tendon pathology, which may be the actual source of the patient's symptoms, may be missed if an examiner is preoccupied with a loose shoulder. Similarly, mistaking postero-inferior instability for anteroinferior instability may lead a surgeon to perform capsular tightening that exacerbates instability on the opposite side of the joint.

Among patients in whom standard nonsurgical management of MDI was unsuccessful, those who have Ehlers-Danlos syndrome often present the most challenging scenario. In these patients, abnormalities of collagen makeup can lead to early stretching and failure of conventional surgical procedures, including capsular shift, open or arthroscopic capsular plication, and thermal modification with radiofrequency devices. After failure of these procedures, other methods of stabilization, including the use of allograft tissue, can be attempted. The use of allograft tissue is based on the theory that shoulder stability can be achieved despite the intrinsic collagen abnormality, at least until prolonged remodeling of the allograft tissue takes place. Surgeons often are reluctant to attempt additional surgical procedures in patients with Ehlers-Danlos syndrome, and persistent pain and instability can result in a poor quality of life, leading to a sense of desperation and even clinical depression. Because these patients typically have bilateral disease, the authors of this chapter believe that allograft reconstruction, even if successful for only 3 to 5 years, is preferable to fusion, which can result in extremely poor function and preclude salvage procedures. Most patients who are given the option prefer allograft to arthrodesis.

In patients with voluntary instability that is intentional or willful, an instability repair will almost always result in a poor outcome. In these patients, shoulder instability may be a manifestation of an underlying emotional or psychiatric problem. These patients often will have undergone multiple failed attempts at stabilization. If this type of voluntary instability is suspected, then the patient should be referred for psychological evaluation so that the underlying emotional pathology can be addressed. In this subgroup of patients with voluntary instability, further surgical revision procedures should be avoided.

Diagnosis After Failed Surgical Management of MDI

A careful history and physical examination is essential in diagnosing MDI of the shoulder. Details about the onset of symptoms, such as whether the symptoms began with an episode of major trauma, recurrent or repetitive microtrauma, or no trauma are helpful in making the diagnosis. Knowing the position of the arm at the time of the initial event helps establish the predominant direction of the instability. Information about the extent or degree of the instability (locked dislocation versus transient or self-reduced subluxation) is helpful in classifying the disorder.

Especially in patients who have undergone prior surgical procedures, it is important to obtain information about previous treatment. Prior surgical reports are useful in assessing the pathology encountered and procedures performed. The type and position of postoperative immobilization, the length of immobilization, the specific timing and nature of the rehabilitation program, and the timing of return to sports activities may yield insight into the reasons for failure of the prior repair. After the history of instability events and prior surgical treatment has been established, present symptoms should be investigated. Patients may have pain only with episodes of instability or in certain arm positions, although some patients with MDI may experience a

constant ache in the shoulder. The location of pain and information about the arm position or activity that evokes pain can help establish the directional components of the instability. Patients with MDI will often experience symptoms with extremes of combined abduction, external rotation, and extension (anterior component); combined flexion, adduction, and internal rotation (posterior component); and weighted activities with the arm at the side (inferior component). Furthermore, patients with inferior subluxation may report numbness and a "dead arm" sensation when carrying heavy objects, such as suitcases, with the arm at the side. Patients with glenohumeral instability often report a sensation of slippage or subluxation in addition to pain. Functional loss or disability can vary widely, ranging from an inability to perform even routine activities of daily living because of pain or apprehension to interference with only high-demand overhead activities, such as throwing or swimming. The frequency and severity of symptoms must be considered in deciding whether revision surgery is indicated.

The issue of voluntary control over instability also must be addressed in taking a patient's history. As noted previously, surgery to address instability will fail in patients with underlying psychiatric or emotional problems who use the ability to voluntarily dislocate the shoulder as a means of getting attention. However, not all voluntary instability is of this type. Some patients are able to demonstrate instability (especially posterior subluxation) by placing the arm in the provocative position. Typically, these patients report that this positional type of voluntary instability developed after multiple episodes of instability. This subgroup of patients who are capable of voluntary dislocation typically responds favorably to surgical treatment. Serial office examinations and observation of a patient's interaction with other family members during these visits can help

determine whether orthopaedic treatment or psychological treatment is most appropriate in each patient.

Physical examination of patients with MDI frequently reveals signs of generalized ligamentous laxity: elbow hyperextension, the ability to appose the thumb to the forearm, metacarpophalangeal joint hyperextension, and hypermobility of the patella. Some patients also may have hypermobility of the acromioclavicular and sternoclavicular joints. The hallmark of inferior instability and MDI is the sulcus sign. The sulcus sign should be tested with the arm at the side and again with the shoulder abducted to 90°. Patients with MDI may have positive findings with provocative stress testing, including the anterior apprehension and posterior stress tests, the relocation maneuver, and the anterior and posterior drawer tests. These translations should be measured in the symptomatic and asymptomatic shoulders and correlated with a patient's symptoms to make the diagnosis.

Determining the primary direction of instability on physical examination can be difficult. If a patient guards because of pain, provocative tests may not yield meaningful information. Care also must be taken to distinguish between a maneuver that produces a subluxation and one that reduces a subluxated humeral head. Using the coracoid process and posterolateral corner of the acromion as landmarks can assist in making such determinations. Because the examination of painful or heavily muscled shoulders can be difficult, multiple examinations in sequential office visits can be useful in assessing patients with suspected shoulder instability.

Plain radiographs of patients with MDI are usually normal but occasionally demonstrate humeral head defects or glenoid lesions, such as bony rim avulsions, reactive changes, or erosion from multiple instability events. If a patient has undergone a prior asymmetric tightening procedure, the axillary radiograph may demonstrate a fixed humeral subluxation in the opposite direction. Loss of the glenohumeral joint space is seen in patients with secondary osteoarthritis and in the rare patient with chondrolysis. Occasionally, CT scans or CT arthrograms are obtained, especially if axillary radiographs suggest glenoid deficiency or dysplasia. In patients who have undergone a prior attempt at stabilization, MRI can provide helpful data concerning labral healing or detachment and subscapularis healing. Electromyography can be helpful in patients with prominent neurologic symptoms, especially in postoperative situations in which the history and physical examination suggest injury to the axillary or musculocutaneous nerves.

Case Presentation

A 25-year-old man has moderately severe Ehlers-Danlos syndrome affecting mainly his shoulders but also his ankles (previous bilateral subtalar arthrodesis) and knees (bilateral patellofemoral instability). His history includes three previous failed attempts at stabilization on each side. In each shoulder, two arthroscopic procedures (one radiofrequency heat probe and one arthroscopic plication) and one open inferior capsular shift were performed. After each previous shoulder procedure, the patient experienced short-term stability followed by recurrence of symptoms after 6 to 8 months. Previous courses of physical therapy and shoulder girdle muscle strengthening and retraining failed. Symptoms include anteroinferior instability and voluntary subluxation on contraction of the anterior deltoid or the pectoralis major. Because the instability episodes are unwanted and the patient attempts to avoid painful subluxation of the shoulder, the instability is judged not to be willful.

Clinical examination reveals signs of generalized ligamentous hyperlaxity in every joint tested. Evidence of hypertrophic scarring is observed in the anterior shoulder along the lines of the previous deltopectoral incisions. The patient's shoulders sit in an anteroinferior subluxated position and are passively reducible with a superior and posterior translation. In addition to a grade III sulcus sign, the patient has grade 3 anterior translation on the load-and-shift test and grade 2 posterior translation. The patient is not symptomatic with posterior load-and-shift testing but is very symptomatic with anterior and inferior translation. The patient is neurovascularly intact and has good deltoid function. After a discussion of the surgical treatment options, the patient elects to proceed with open anteroinferior stabilization and capsular shifting with Achilles tendon allograft augmentation.

Indications

Nonsurgical Treatment

The initial management of MDI is nonsurgical, combining activity modification (avoidance of provocative activities) and a prolonged exercise program. The goal of the exercise program is to strengthen the deltoid and rotator cuff muscles below the horizontal level and address the scapular stabilizers. In one study, researchers found that 29 of 33 shoulders with involuntary, atraumatic multidirectional subluxation had good or excellent results with nonsurgical management (88%). However, in a long-term outcome study of patients treated nonsurgically with rehabilitative exercises for atraumatic MDI, only 17 of 57 patients had satisfactory stability and Rowe scores at 7- to 10-year follow-up, and only 20 patients had good or excellent self-reported results (30% and 35%, respectively).

In patients with prior failed instability surgery for MDI, initial nonsurgical

treatment with an exercise program is often appropriate. The exercise program may help sufficiently reduce instability symptoms to avoid further surgical treatment. Frequent monitoring during the nonsurgical treatment period will enable a surgeon to assess a patient's motivation and ability to cooperate with postoperative restrictions and rehabilitation protocols. In some patients, however, nonsurgical treatment will be less useful. Earlier surgical revision should be considered if radiographs reveal hardware penetration or migration in the joint that risks damage to the articular cartilage, or if radiographs demonstrate fixed subluxation of the humeral head after an asymmetric capsular tightening.

Surgical Treatment

Inferior capsular shift is the most widely used surgical repair for MDI. In the original Neer and Foster repair, the capsule is detached near the lateral insertion on the humeral neck and shifted in a superolateral direction, reducing the capsular redundancy and decreasing the capsular volume on all three sides of the joint. The capsule is overlapped or reinforced on the side of the approach and is tensioned on all three sides of the joint to reestablish soft-tissue balance. This procedure directly addresses the primary pathology in MDI, which is believed to be a loose, redundant capsule. Although the original procedure was an open capsulorrhaphy, an arthroscopic capsular shift also has been described.

Inferior capsular shift is a lateral or humeral-side capsulorrhaphy. Because the joint capsule is funnel-shaped with a wider insertion on the lateral side compared with the medial side, the lateral approach is preferred in the management of MDI because it allows for a greater amount of the capsule to be shifted a greater distance than would be possible in the medial approach. The cleft in the capsule between the superior glenohumeral ligament (SGHL) and middle glenohumeral ligament (MGHL), which is often enlarged in shoulders with MDI, is closed during the procedure. The entire superior flap (consisting of the SGHL and the MGHL) is then repaired in cruciate fashion over the previously shifted inferior flap. If the ligament-labral complex is observed to be detached from the glenoid rim, the labrum is repaired back to the glenoid rim, with sutures passed through bony tunnels or suture anchors before the capsule is shifted. Although labral detachments or Bankart lesions are uncommon in patients with MDI, they can be found in patients in whom major trauma has contributed to instability. Although bone deficiency is rare in patients with MDI, the lateral approach allows for incorporation of a bone graft to augment the glenoid if needed. Specifically, a coracoid transfer is used if a deficiency is anterior, and a scapular or iliac graft is used if a deficiency is posterior.

In the classic inferior capsular shift, the side of the surgical approach depends on the direction of the greatest instability. If a shoulder dislocates anteriorly and inferiorly and only subluxates posteriorly, or if it dislocates in all three directions, an anterior approach is used. If a shoulder dislocates posteriorly and inferiorly and only subluxates anteriorly, a posterior approach is preferred. The primary direction of instability is determined based on preoperative symptoms and the physical examination and is confirmed intraoperatively via careful examination under anesthesia. The findings of the examination under anesthesia rarely differ substantially from preoperative findings; therefore, the side of the approach rarely needs to be changed intraoperatively.

Controversies and Alternative Approaches

In appropriately selected patients, open repair of MDI with an inferior capsular shift has yielded excellent results as a primary repair. In a revision setting, in which a patient may have varying degrees of soft-tissue contracture, soft-tissue deficiency, and even early glenohumeral arthritis, surgical results are more variable and overall less satisfactory. In less symptomatic patients, nonsurgical treatment with an exercise program and avoidance of provocative activities may be the best option. In more symptomatic patients who have not responded to nonsurgical treatment, do not engage in willful voluntary dislocation of their shoulders, and have undergone limited prior surgical instability procedures (preferably one prior repair), a revision procedure using an inferior capsular shift (augmented in rare instances with allograft material for tissue deficiency) may help restore stability and decrease symptoms. Multiple revision attempts are less likely to produce the satisfactory results that surgeons and patients have come to expect with modern instability repairs.

Failed instability procedures remain a surgical challenge, especially in patients with hyperlaxity associated with Ehlers-Danlos syndrome. Affected patients may have instability associated with symptomatic translations in the anterior, posterior, and inferior directions. The small amount of information available in the literature suggests that allograft reconstruction provides relief of symptoms and improved function at short- to intermediate-term follow-up. One case report suggests that simultaneous anterior and posterior allograft stabilization may help completely address symptomatic instability in all directions, but the exact indications for this technique remain unclear. Other options, including bone block procedures, have higher complication rates and offer nonanatomic solutions to this complex problem. In the experience of the second author of this chapter (P.B.M.), allograft stabilization can be repeated after clinical failure.

Results

In the original report on inferior capsular shift for the management of MDI, successful results were reported in 31 of 32 shoulders with at least 1-year follow-up. No recurrent instability was found in the 11 shoulders in which the capsular shift was performed as a revision procedure. In a study of inferior capsular shift using an anterior approach for the management of MDI in 43 shoulders, 39 shoulders had no further instability (91%), and only 1 of the 19 shoulders with prior instability repair became unstable again. In a study of 49 shoulders, inferior capsular shift resulted in stability in 47 shoulders at a mean 5-year follow-up (96%); however, the study included only patients in whom capsular shift represented a primary instability repair. The authors of a different study reported stability in 22 of 25 patients who underwent arthroscopic capsular shift (88%). None of the patients in this series had undergone prior surgical procedures to address instability. In a study of patients with Ehlers-Danlos syndrome or hyperlaxity disorders who required allograft reconstruction after failed prior surgical treatment, midterm results indicated a 45% stability rate at 3.8 years postoperatively. The authors of this study advocated the use of the technique as a salvage procedure.

Other authors have reported less promising results of revision surgery in patients with MDI. In a report on the management of complications of a failed Bristow procedure, researchers reported good or excellent results in 8 of 13 patients. In that study, four of the five patients who had a fair or poor result had MDI. In a different study of revision shoulder stabilization in 44 shoulders, only 9 of the 21 shoulders with MDI (43%) had good or excellent results despite multiple revision procedures. Four of those patients ultimately underwent glenohumeral fusion. These authors

Table 1 Results of Surgical Treatment With Allograft in Patients With Ehlers-Danlos Syndrome or Hyperlaxity-Associated Shoulder Instability

Authors	Journal (Year)	Technique (No. of Patients)	Outcomes	Failure Rate (%)	Comment
MacDonald et al	*Techniques in Shoulder & Elbow Surgery* (2008)	Achilles allograft augmentation (8)	High failure rates reported in this difficult population	69 (avg follow-up, 22 mo)	16 shoulders Mean follow-up, 2.3 yr
Chaudhury et al	*J Shoulder Elbow Surg* (2012)	Bilateral anterior and posterior glenohumeral stabilization using Achilles allograft augmentation (1)	Anterior and posterior stability was achieved	0	Case report of a patient with Ehlers-Danlos syndrome Follow-up, 3 yr
Dewing et al	*Arthroscopy* (2012)	Allograft tibialis (15)	High failure rates in a difficult population	55	20 shoulders Only 5 patients had Ehlers-Danlos syndrome Mean follow-up, 3.8 yr

concluded that revision surgery in patients with MDI has highly unpredictable results and that these patients might be best treated with nonsurgical management and counseling with regard to realistic goals. In a different study of revision stabilization surgery, researchers concluded that poor results of revision instability repairs were associated with atraumatic causes of failure, voluntary dislocation, and multiple prior stabilization attempts. Finally, in a study of 10 patients who had undergone at least three previous stabilizations, the authors performed a procedure that they termed the kitchen sink operation, which involved a humerally based capsular shift, a Nicola biceps tenodesis, and coracohumeral ligament and rotator interval augmentation (using Achilles tendon allograft or a synthetic ligament augmentation device in 7 of the 10 patients). Although nine patients had successful reduction of instability, one-half of those patients continued to have unremitting pain.

Table 1 summarizes the results of surgical treatment with allograft augmentation or reconstruction in patients with Ehlers-Danlos syndrome or hyperlaxity-associated shoulder instability.

 # Technical Keys to Success

Anterior Approach
SETUP/EXPOSURE
- The patient is placed in the modified beach-chair position with the upper portion of the surgical table flexed 20° to 30°.
- A concealed axillary incision measuring approximately 6 to 8 cm is made. The incision begins several centimeters inferior to the tip of the coracoid and continues in an anterior axillary skin fold to the inferior border of the pectoralis major muscle.
- In patients undergoing revision procedures, the prior incision is used unless it is poorly located.

PROCEDURE
- The subcutaneous layer is widely undermined, and the deltopectoral interval is developed.
- The cephalic vein is retracted laterally with the deltoid.
- An incision is made in the clavipectoral fascia lateral to the origin of the coracobrachialis and the short head of the biceps.

- The coracobrachialis and the short head of the biceps are retracted with care in a medial direction.
- In patients undergoing revision, particularly if a patient has undergone prior open instability surgery, abundant scarring may be present between the coracobrachialis and short head of the biceps and the underlying subscapularis. Care is taken to dissect between these layers and identify the axillary nerve on the anteroinferior aspect of the subscapularis.
- Although the axillary nerve does not need to be mobilized or retracted, it must be located and protected during subscapularis and capsular dissection.
- The superior and inferior borders of the subscapularis are identified.
- If the anterior circumflex humeral vessels at the inferior border of the subscapularis were not coagulated during a previous repair, they are coagulated.
- An incision is made in the subscapularis tendon 1 cm medial to its insertion on the lesser tuberosity, starting at the rotator interval and proceeding to the

inferior border of the tendon.

- Blunt and sharp dissection is used to carefully develop the plane between the subscapularis tendon and the underlying capsular ligaments until the dissection extends medial to the glenoid rim.
- The tendon is tagged with nonabsorbable sutures for later repair.
- Care must be taken to avoid perforating the capsule.
- Dissection is continued inferiorly, with care taken to identify and protect the axillary nerve.
- The muscular portion of the subscapularis is separated from the capsule with blunt dissection.
- Complete separation of the capsule from the subscapularis tendon and muscle will prevent tethering of the capsule during its shift.
- The joint capsule is incised laterally at a point 0.5 cm medial to the subscapularis tenotomy. This dissection begins near the capsular cleft between the SGHL and the MGHL and continues inferiorly along the humeral neck.
- A cuff of tissue should be left laterally on the humeral neck so that the capsular flaps can be repaired to it later.
- Care must be taken to ensure inferolateral dissection along the humeral neck to avoid cutting the inferior pouch, which would prevent use of the flaps for a capsular shift and would risk damage to the axillary nerve.
- Dissection is continued inferiorly (and even posteroinferiorly) as necessary to reduce the redundant inferior pouch and allow the freed capsule to be shifted.
- The ability to shift the capsule can be tested by pulling on the traction sutures in the capsule. If an index finger placed in the pouch can be extruded by this maneuver, then the dissection is sufficient (**Figure 1**). Inferior dissection past the

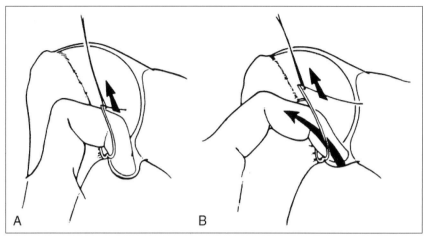

Figure 1   Illustrations of a shoulder show the use of an index finger inserted in the inferior capsular pouch (**A**) to assess the extent of capsular dissection. Dissection proceeds inferiorly until the point at which an upward pull on the capsular traction sutures (short arrows) can extrude the index finger from the pouch (**B,** curved arrow). (Reproduced with permission from Pollock RG, Owens JM, Flatow EL, Bigliani LU: Operative results of the inferior capsular shift procedure for multidirectional instability of the shoulder. *J Bone Joint Surg Am* 2000;82[7]:919-928.)

6-o'clock position on the humeral neck is typically necessary.

- After capsular dissection and mobilization is complete, the humeral head is retracted with a ring retractor to allow for inspection of the anteroinferior labral insertion.
- If the glenohumeral ligaments are avulsed from the glenoid, they are reattached to the glenoid rim with nonabsorbable No. 1 braided nylon sutures passed through osseous tunnels or suture anchors.
- A T-shaped split is made in the capsule almost to its labral insertion, directly superior to the inferior glenohumeral ligament (IGHL).
- The patient's arm is placed in 20° of abduction and 25° to 30° of external rotation.
- The inferior flap (that is, the IGHL) is pulled superolaterally to reduce the capsular pouch and is repaired to the remaining portion of the lateral capsule (**Figure 2, A**).
- The cleft between the SGHL and the MGHL is closed. In a cruciate fashion, this superior flap is shifted

inferolaterally over the inferior flap to reinforce the capsule anteriorly (**Figure 2, B**).

- In rare instances of capsular deficiency, allograft material can be used to augment the repair or substitute for missing tissue.
- The subscapularis tendon is repaired at the tenotomy site with nonabsorbable No. 2 braided nylon sutures.

WOUND CLOSURE

- The deltopectoral interval is closed.
- The skin is closed with subcuticular suture.

Posterior Approach
SETUP/EXPOSURE

- The patient is placed in the lateral decubitus position, with the affected shoulder up.
- A skin incision directed obliquely 60° from the scapular spine is made, beginning at the posterolateral corner of the acromion and extending approximately 10 cm distally.

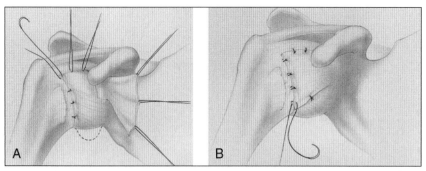

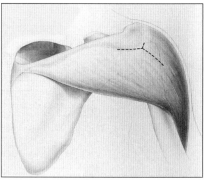

Figure 2 **A,** Illustration of a shoulder shows shift of the inferior capsular flap (the inferior glenohumeral ligament) in a superolateral direction and the suturing of this flap to the lateral capsular tissue. **B,** Illustration of a shoulder shows closure of the capsular cleft between the superior and middle glenohumeral ligaments and the inferolateral shift of the entire superior flap over the inferior flap in a cruciate fashion. (Reproduced with permission from Pollock RG, Owens JM, Flatow EL, Bigliani LU: Operative results of the inferior capsular shift procedure for multidirectional instability of the shoulder. *J Bone Joint Surg Am* 2000;82[7]:919-928.)

Figure 3 Illustration of a shoulder shows incision splitting of the deltoid 4 to 5 cm along a posterolateral raphe and detaching the deltoid 3 to 4 cm from the scapular spine. (Reproduced with permission from Pollock RG, Owens JM, Flatow EL, Bigliani LU: Operative results of the inferior capsular shift procedure for multidirectional instability of the shoulder. *J Bone Joint Surg Am* 2000;82[7]:919-928.)

PROCEDURE

- The subcutaneous layer is widely undermined.
- The deltoid is split 4 to 5 cm along a posterolateral raphe and is detached 3 to 4 cm from the scapular spine, leaving a cuff of tissue for later repair (**Figure 3**).
- The infraspinatus is identified and distinguished from the supraspinatus superiorly and the teres minor inferiorly.
- Palpation of the smaller tubercle, onto which the teres minor inserts, can help identify the correct interval to develop.
- The infraspinatus is separated from the posterior capsule with sharp and blunt dissection, continuing medially past the glenoid rim and laterally to the insertion on the greater tuberosity.
- A vertical incision is made in the infraspinatus, leaving a stump of tissue laterally for later tendon repair.
- An incision is made from superior to inferior in the capsule 1 cm medial to its insertion on the humerus, leaving a cuff of tissue laterally for later repair.
- Blunt dissection is performed in the plane between the teres minor

and the capsule, with care taken to identify and protect the axillary nerve.

- Dissection of the capsule around the humeral neck is continued inferiorly as needed to reduce the posteroinferior capsular redundancy. Dissection past the 6-o'clock position on the humeral neck is typically required. Progressive extension and internal rotation of the arm will enable better exposure of the capsule in this region.
- As described previously in the anterior approach, an index finger can be placed into the pouch to assess the adequacy of the capsular release and mobilization. If pulling on the traction sutures in the capsule extrudes the finger, the mobilization is sufficient to allow for appropriate reduction in capsular volume with the capsular shift.
- Before the flaps are shifted, the medial capsular insertion is assessed. If detachment is observed, the insertion is repaired to the glenoid rim with transosseous sutures or suture anchors.
- A T-shaped split is made in the capsule at the midglenoid region

to create a superior flap and an inferior flap.

- The shoulder is placed in 5° to 10° of external rotation, 10° to 15° of abduction, and neutral flexion-extension.
- The superior flap is shifted in an inferolateral direction and is repaired to the cuff of capsular tissue on the lateral aspect of the humeral neck (**Figure 4, A**).
- The inferior flap is shifted superolaterally to reduce the inferior pouch and reinforce the posterior capsule (**Figure 4, B**).
- If the tissue is deficient and unsuitable for suturing, allograft tissue can be incorporated into the repair.

WOUND CLOSURE

- The infraspinatus is repaired with No. 2 nonabsorbable braided sutures.
- The deltoid is reattached to the scapular spine and the posterolateral split in the deltoid is repaired with nonabsorbable braided sutures.
- The skin incision is closed with subcuticular suture.

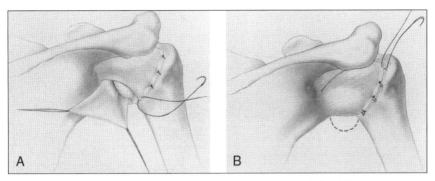

Figure 4 **A,** Illustration of a shoulder shows inferolateral shift of the superior capsular flap and reattachment of this flap to the cuff of tissue on the lateral aspect of the humeral neck. **B,** Illustration of a shoulder shows superolateral shift of the inferior flap to reduce the inferior capsular pouch and repair of the inferior flap in a cruciate fashion over the superior flap. (Reproduced with permission from Pollock RG, Owens JM, Flatow EL, Bigliani LU: Operative results of the inferior capsular shift procedure for multidirectional instability of the shoulder. *J Bone Joint Surg Am* 2000;82[7]:919-928.)

Allograft Procedure in Patients With Ehlers-Danlos Syndrome

SETUP/EXPOSURE

- The patient is placed in the beach-chair position, which facilitates free draping of the affected limb.
- A deltopectoral incision is used, and the hypertrophic scar is excised.
- The cephalic vein is retracted laterally.
- In patients undergoing revision, dissection may be difficult.
- The conjoint tendon is mobilized and retracted medially.
- The deltoid and pectoralis major are retracted with a self-retaining shoulder retraction system.

PROCEDURE

- The insertion of the subscapularis on the lesser tuberosity as well as the biceps groove are identified.
- Approximately 1.5 cm medial to the insert of the subscapularis on the lesser tuberosity, a longitudinal incision is made through the subscapularis and the capsule, and the joint is entered.
- The capsule layer is teased off the overlying subscapularis to establish two distinct layers.
- Dissection is carried down to the anterior labrum and glenoid.

- An incision is made in the labrum, and the underlying extra-articular anterior glenoid is exposed, creating a bed measuring 3 cm from medial to lateral and 2 cm from superior to inferior to accept the glenoid graft.
- Four suture anchors are placed in a perimeter configuration to accept the Achilles tendon allograft.
- High-strength sutures are placed from the anchors through drill holes in the graft such that the graft lies over the anterior glenoid. The sutures are tied, securing the graft (**Figure 5**).
- The soft-tissue portion of the graft is split to create a Y-shaped configuration that is used to reinforce the MGHL and the IGHL. With the patient's arm in 30° of abduction and 30° of external rotation, the graft limbs are attached under some tension to suture anchors that are placed in the corresponding ligament insertion points on the lateral humerus (**Figure 6**).
- To supplement the stabilization provided by the allograft repair, a Neer and Foster inferior capsular shift is performed with supplemental suturing into the allograft tissue.
- Alternatively, the second author

of this chapter (P.B.M.) has used human dermal allograft instead of Achilles tendon allograft in a similar fashion with similar results. The dermal allograft is laid in a sheet-like fashion on top of the inferior capsular shift tissue to reinforce it and provide additional integrity to the anterior capsule.

WOUND CLOSURE

- The subscapularis is repaired anatomically with the same sutures that were used for the inferior capsular shift and the attachment of the allograft to the lateral humerus.
- Care is taken to close the rotator interval.
- The deltopectoral interval, subcutaneous tissue, and skin are closed in layers.

 Rehabilitation

After surgical management of MDI, stiffness is less common compared with recurrence of instability. Therefore, especially in revision patients with poor tissue quality, the rehabilitation protocol should err on the conservative side to prevent tendon pull-off and capsular stretching. The rehabilitation protocol varies depending on the surgical procedure performed.

Anterior Approach

The rehabilitation protocol for the anterior approach is summarized in **Table 2**. The arm is typically protected in a sling for 6 weeks postoperatively. Passive range-of-motion exercises are begun at 10 to 14 days postoperatively and are gradually progressed. External rotation is limited to less than 30° for 6 weeks postoperatively. Frequent monitoring is necessary because patients who regain motion too quickly risk stretching the repair. In these patients, the protocol should be adjusted. Although isometric exercises are begun at 3 weeks postoperatively, most resistive exercises are deferred to 6 weeks postoperatively, and resisted internal rotation is deferred for 12 weeks postoperatively to protect the subscapularis repair. Return to sports should not occur before 6 months postoperatively and is usually deferred until 9 to 12 months postoperatively for high-demand overhead activities such as throwing or swimming. In patients in whom substantial posterior instability required surgical dissection of the posteroinferior capsule, a postoperative brace is used for 6 weeks postoperatively to position the arm in neutral rotation, which protects the capsular repair. In these patients, the postoperative rehabilitation guidelines described previously are individualized to each patient.

Posterior Approach

The rehabilitation protocol for the posterior approach is summarized in **Table 3**. The arm is immobilized in a brace with slight abduction and neutral rotation to protect the capsular repair and the infraspinatus for 6 weeks postoperatively. Range-of-motion exercises, focusing on elevation in the scapular plane and external rotation, are usually begun at 6 weeks postoperatively. Terminal flexion and internal rotation should be avoided for 3 months postoperatively. Isometric exercises are begun at 6 weeks postoperatively. Resisted external rotation should be deferred for 12 weeks postoperatively to protect the infraspinatus repair. Sports activity is restricted for 9 to 12 months postoperatively.

Allograft Procedure in Patients With Ehlers-Danlos Syndrome

The rehabilitation protocol for the allograft procedure in patients with Ehlers-Danlos syndrome is summarized in **Table 4**. The arm is immobilized in

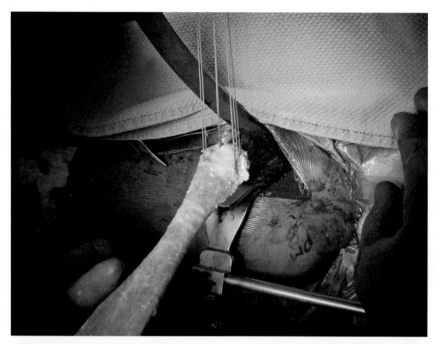

Figure 5   Intraoperative photograph of a shoulder shows placement of the Achilles tendon allograft through suture anchors onto an anterior glenoid bed. Five holes in the graft are connected to anchors on the anterior glenoid. The medial direction is on the right side of the photograph.

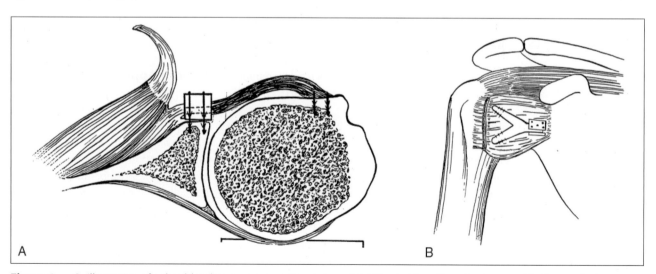

Figure 6   **A,** Illustration of a shoulder shows a cross-sectional view of Achilles tendon allograft placement in the surgical management of multidirectional instability. Arrows indicate anchor placement sites. **B,** Illustration of a shoulder shows an anterior view of the Y-shaped graft placement.

Table 2 Rehabilitation Protocol After Capsular Shift in the Anterior Approach for the Management of Multidirectional Instability

Postoperative Week	ROM	Strengthening	Return to Play	Comments/Emphasis
0-2	Passive ROM is begun at 10 to 14 d and is gradually progressed External rotation is limited to <30°	None	None	The arm is protected in a sling[a]
2-6	External rotation is limited to <30°	Isometric exercises are begun at wk 3	None	The arm is protected in a sling[a]
6-12	Gradual return to full ROM	Resistive exercises are begun at wk 6	None	Sling use is discontinued at 6 wk
12-52	Full ROM achieved	Resisted internal rotation is not allowed until wk 12 to protect the subscapularis repair	Return to sports is allowed beginning at 6 mo High-demand overhead activities are not allowed until 9 to 12 mo	—

ROM = range of motion.

[a] In patients treated with surgical dissection of the posteroinferior capsule to address substantial posterior instability, a brace is used for 6 weeks postoperatively and the rehabilitation protocol is adjusted accordingly.

Table 3 Rehabilitation Protocol After Capsular Shift in the Posterior Approach for the Management of Multidirectional Instability

Postoperative Week	Range of Motion	Strengthening	Return to Play	Comments/Emphasis
0-2	None	None	None	Immobilization in a brace with slight abduction and neutral rotation
2-6	Passive external rotation to 30° in a brace	None	None	Immobilization in a brace with slight abduction and neutral rotation
6-12	Exercises focusing on elevation in the scapular plane and external rotation are begun at 6 wk	Isometric exercises are begun at 6 wk	None	Brace use is discontinued at 6 wk
12-52	Terminal flexion and internal rotation is allowed at 3 mo	Resisted external rotation is begun at 12 wk	Return to sports is allowed at 9 to 12 mo	—

an abduction brace in 30° of abduction and 30° of external rotation postoperatively. Immobilization continues for 8 weeks postoperatively, at which time a slowly progressive rehabilitation protocol begins.

 Avoiding Pitfalls

Accurate diagnosis is the first step in ensuring a successful procedure. The surgeon should first determine whether instability is the problem. The predominant direction of instability should then be determined, and voluntary dislocation should be ruled out. The surgeon should evaluate whether the patient's symptoms are substantial enough to warrant revision surgery.

If using the anterior approach, then the surgeon should take care to identify and protect the axillary nerve. The subscapularis should be separated from the capsule. When releasing the capsule, the surgeon should take care to remain laterally on the humeral neck to avoid transecting the axillary pouch. The capsular release must be sufficient to reduce the inferior pouch. If a Bankart lesion is present, it should be repaired. The superior cleft between the SGHL and the MGHL must be closed. In patients with severe deficiency of the anterior tissues, the use of allograft should be considered.

Table 4 Rehabilitation Protocol After Allograft Procedure in the Management of Multidirectional Instability

Postoperative Week	Range of Motion	Strengthening	Return to Play	Comments/Emphasis
0-2	None	None	None	The arm is immobilized in an abduction brace in 30° of abduction and 30° of external rotation
2-6	None	None	None	Immobilization in the brace is continued
6-12	Slow, progressive rehabilitation is begun at wk 8	None	None	Immobilization in the brace is discontinued at wk 8
12-52	—	Progressive strengthening	None	Limited goals in this patient population; usually, no involvement in sports

If using the posterior approach, then the surgeon should take care to stay above the teres minor to avoid damage to the axillary nerve. Medial dissection should be performed with care to avoid injury to the suprascapular nerve. The capsular release must be sufficient to reduce the capsular pouch. Careful repair of the infraspinatus is necessary. Postoperative positioning in internal rotation should be avoided.

Postoperatively, rapid recovery of motion should be avoided to prevent stretching of the repair. Resistive exercises should be delayed until the tendon has healed. Return to sports should be delayed until 6 to 12 months postoperatively.

 Bibliography

Bigliani LU, Pollock RG, McIlveen SJ, Endrizzi DP, Flatow EL: Shift of the posteroinferior aspect of the capsule for recurrent posterior glenohumeral instability. *J Bone Joint Surg Am* 1995;77(7):1011-1020.

Burkhead WZ Jr, Rockwood CA Jr: Treatment of instability of the shoulder with an exercise program. *J Bone Joint Surg Am* 1992;74(6):890-896.

Chaudhury S, Gasinu S, Rodeo SA: Bilateral anterior and posterior glenohumeral stabilization using Achilles tendon allograft augmentation in a patient with Ehlers-Danlos syndrome. *J Shoulder Elbow Surg* 2012;21(6):e1-e5.

Ciccone WJ II, Weinstein DM, Elias JJ: Glenohumeral chondrolysis following thermal capsulorrhaphy. *Orthopedics* 2007;30(2):158-160.

Cooper RA, Brems JJ: The inferior capsular-shift procedure for multidirectional instability of the shoulder. *J Bone Joint Surg Am* 1992;74(10):1516-1521.

D'Alessandro DF, Bradley JP, Fleischli JE, Connor PM: Prospective evaluation of thermal capsulorrhaphy for shoulder instability: Indications and results, two- to five-year follow-up. *Am J Sports Med* 2004;32(1):21-33.

Dewing CB, Horan MP, Millett PJ: Two-year outcomes of open shoulder anterior capsular reconstruction for instability from severe capsular deficiency. *Arthroscopy* 2012;28(1):43-51.

Fronek J, Warren RF, Bowen M: Posterior subluxation of the glenohumeral joint. *J Bone Joint Surg Am* 1989;71(2):205-216.

Good CR, Shindle MK, Kelly BT, Wanich T, Warren RF: Glenohumeral chondrolysis after shoulder arthroscopy with thermal capsulorrhaphy. *Arthroscopy* 2007;23(7):797.e1-797.e5.

Hawkins RJ, Krishnan SG, Karas SG, Noonan TJ, Horan MP: Electrothermal arthroscopic shoulder capsulorrhaphy: A minimum 2-year follow-up. *Am J Sports Med* 2007;35(9):1484-1488.

Krishnan SG, Hawkins RJ, Horan MP, Dean M, Kim YK: A soft tissue attempt to stabilize the multiply operated glenohumeral joint with multidirectional instability. *Clin Orthop Relat Res* 2004;(429):256-261.

Levine WN, Arroyo JS, Pollock RG, Flatow EL, Bigliani LU: Open revision stabilization surgery for recurrent anterior glenohumeral instability. *Am J Sports Med* 2000;28(2):156-160.

MacDonald P, Mascarenhas R, McRae S, Leiter J: Achilles allograft stabilization of the shoulder in refractory multidirectional glenohumeral instability. *Techniques in Shoulder & Elbow Surgery* 2008;9(2):60-65.

Miniaci A, McBirnie J: Thermal capsular shrinkage for treatment of multidirectional instability of the shoulder. *J Bone Joint Surg Am* 2003;85(12):2283-2287.

Misamore GW, Sallay PI, Didelot W: A longitudinal study of patients with multidirectional instability of the shoulder with seven- to ten-year follow-up. *J Shoulder Elbow Surg* 2005;14(5):466-470.

Mohtadi NG, Kirkley A, Hollinshead RM, et al; Joint Orthopaedic Initiative for National Trials of the Shoulder-Canada: Electrothermal arthroscopic capsulorrhaphy: Old technology, new evidence. A multicenter randomized clinical trial. *J Shoulder Elbow Surg* 2014;23(8):1171-1180.

Neer CS II: Involuntary inferior and multidirectional instability of the shoulder: Etiology, recognition, and treatment. *Instr Course Lect* 1985;34:232-238.

Neer CS II, Foster CR: Inferior capsular shift for involuntary inferior and multidirectional instability of the shoulder: A preliminary report. *J Bone Joint Surg Am* 1980;62(6):897-908.

Pollock RG, Bigliani LU: Glenohumeral instability: Evaluation and treatment. *J Am Acad Orthop Surg* 1993;1(1):24-32.

Pollock RG, Owens JM, Flatow EL, Bigliani LU: Operative results of the inferior capsular shift procedure for multidirectional instability of the shoulder. *J Bone Joint Surg Am* 2000;82(7):919-928.

Rowe CR, Pierce DS, Clark JG: Voluntary dislocation of the shoulder: A preliminary report on a clinical, electromyographic, and psychiatric study of twenty-six patients. *J Bone Joint Surg Am* 1973;55(3):445-460.

Treacy SH, Savoie FH III, Field LD: Arthroscopic treatment of multidirectional instability. *J Shoulder Elbow Surg* 1999;8(4):345-350.

Toth AP, Warren RF, Petrigliano FA, et al: Thermal shrinkage for shoulder instability. *HSS J* 2011;7(2):108-114.

Wirth MA, Groh GI, Rockwood CA Jr: Capsulorrhaphy through an anterior approach for the treatment of atraumatic posterior glenohumeral instability with multidirectional laxity of the shoulder. *J Bone Joint Surg Am* 1998;80(11):1570-1578.

Young DC, Rockwood CA Jr: Complications of a failed Bristow procedure and their management. *J Bone Joint Surg Am* 1991;73(7):969-981.

Zabinski SJ, Callaway GH, Cohen S, Warren RF: Revision shoulder stabilization: 2- to 10-year results. *J Shoulder Elbow Surg* 1999;8(1):58-65.

Chapter 16

Revision Procedures to Manage Soft-Tissue Deficiency: The Role of Muscle Transfer and Grafting

Jonathan D. Barlow, MD, MS

Mark D. Lazarus, MD

 ## Introduction

Nonsurgical management and arthroscopic or open capsulolabral repair restore full function in most patients with recurrent shoulder instability. Additional or alternative procedures are needed to manage more severe pathology. Humeral and glenoid bone loss may be amenable to bone grafting procedures or muscle and soft-tissue transfer or grafting procedures.

In most patients with mild anterior soft-tissue deficiency, coracoid transfer, with its inherent bony and dynamic stabilization properties, is an adequate option for addressing traumatic anteroinferior instability. Some authors advocate primary Latarjet procedures in patients with hyperlaxity and other risk factors for recurrence, even in the absence of substantial glenoid bone loss. In patients with more severe soft-tissue deficiency, including patients with severe multidirectional and inferior instability (many of whom have undergone one or more failed procedures to manage instability), allograft capsular reconstruction and biceps suspension procedures may be indicated.

Subscapularis pathology is extremely common in patients with failed open instability procedures. When subscapularis repair is impossible, pectoralis major transfer is a viable option to improve pain and function.

 ## Case Presentation

A 32-year-old, right-hand–dominant woman who works as a truck driver reports ongoing right shoulder pain and instability. Four years previously, she was injured in a motor vehicle collision while driving her truck and underwent arthroscopic labral repair shortly after the injury. Despite the repair, the patient continued to experience pain and instability. She returned to the same surgeon and underwent a procedure reported to be a capsular shift. She was told at the time of the procedure that the labral repair was intact but the soft tissues were loose. The postoperative course was again complicated by recurrent instability, which began as soon as the brace was removed. Several rounds of physical therapy focusing on scapular stabilization and rotator cuff strengthening did

not lead to resolution of her symptoms. The patient has no other known medical history, no congenital collagen or other genetic disorders, and no other joint subluxation, dislocation, or pain.

The patient's main concerns are instability and pain. She experiences a sensation of posterior dislocation of the shoulder as well as inferior instability. She reports that the shoulder feels unsupported. Physical examination demonstrates clinically evident inferior subluxation. The deltoid is intact and strong. External rotation strength is normal. The patient exhibits dramatic pain and apprehension with sulcus testing. Her sulcus sign persists in external rotation. She has a dramatically positive jerk test, with crepitus on reduction. Her anterior load-and-shift test results in subluxation with spontaneous reduction. She has excellent scapular control with no scapular winging and an intact neurovascular examination distally. Preoperative radiographs demonstrate severe inferior instability (**Figure 1**).

Because of the failure of nonsurgical management and the patient's continued severe pain and disability, the decision is made to proceed with surgical intervention. With the patient under anesthesia, gross posterior dislocation of the shoulder is possible. The patient has 75% inferior subluxation resulting from gravity alone, which does not reduce with external rotation. Anterior

Dr. Lazarus or an immediate family member has received royalties from, is a member of a speakers' bureau or has made paid presentations on behalf of, serves as a paid consultant to, has stock or stock options held in, and has received research or institutional support from Tornier. Neither Dr. Barlow nor any immediate family member has received anything of value from or has stock or stock options held in a commercial company or institution related directly or indirectly to the subject of this chapter.

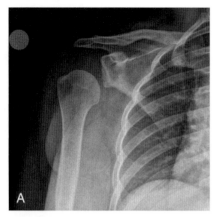 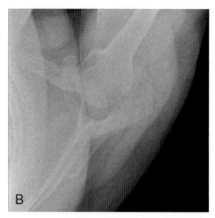

Figure 1 **A,** Grashey radiograph of the right shoulder demonstrates severe inferior instability. **B,** Axillary radiograph of the right shoulder demonstrates an instability pattern that is predominantly inferior rather than anterior or posterior.

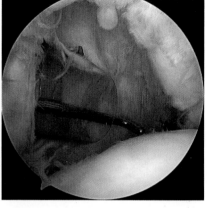

Figure 2 Arthroscopic view of the right shoulder from the anterosuperior portal demonstrates an extremely patulous posteroinferior capsule (indicated by the probe).

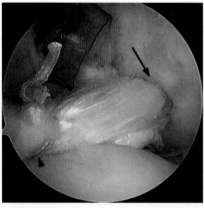 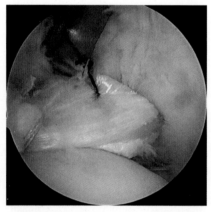

Figure 3 Arthroscopic view from the anterosuperior portal demonstrates allograft reconstruction. With the patient's arm in neutral rotation, the graft is tied to the glenoid (arrow) and to the humeral head (arrowhead).

Figure 4 Arthroscopic view from the anterosuperior portal demonstrates placement of polydioxanone sutures between the reconstructed ligament and the native capsule.

subluxation occurs with stress, but gross dislocation does not.

Arthroscopic portals are placed in the standard fashion for labral procedures, and the joint is inspected. Some arthrosis of the superior aspect of the glenoid is observed. The patient has a normal sublabral foramen, with severely deficient anteroinferior and posteroinferior labral tissue. Three loose sutures are observed in the posteroinferior labrum, with anchors intact to the glenoid but no tissue attached, and one anteroinferior anchor is similar. The subscapularis and rotator

cuff are intact and normal. The biceps tendon is normal.

An anterosuperior viewing portal is established and used for the remainder of the procedure. The posteroinferior labral repair is inspected, and the sutures are removed. The capsule is extremely patulous, with the rotator cuff musculature visible through the capsular tissue (**Figure 2**). For this reason, allograft capsular reconstruction is chosen. The posterior capsular length is measured intra-articularly with a suture, and a semitendinosus allograft is reconstituted and cut to length. Two

3.0-mm double-loaded biocomposite suture anchors are placed in the posteroinferior glenoid, and the remaining posteroinferior capsule is shifted to these anchors, in an inferior-to-superior direction. The suture from one of the placed anchors is retrieved through a cannula and passed through the center of the allograft tendon. The allograft is introduced through the cannula and tied to the glenoid anchor. The suture from the second glenoid anchor is retrieved, passed through the allograft on the glenoid side, and tied, thereby stabilizing the glenoid side of the allograft.

The humerus is placed in neutral rotation, and one 3.0-mm double-loaded biocomposite suture anchor is placed in the anatomic neck, passed through the lateral allograft tissue, and tied. This step is repeated with another superior suture anchor in the anatomic neck to create a robust posteroinferior capsular reconstruction (**Figure 3**). Three size 0 polydioxanone sutures are sequentially passed between the native capsule and the allograft tendon and tied (**Figure 4**).

Attention is focused on the anteroinferior capsule. Because examination demonstrates a reasonably healthy appearance of the anteroinferior capsule and no gross anterior instability, antero-inferior capsular shift without allograft reconstruction is chosen. Three biocomposite anchors are placed, and a superior capsular shift is completed, resulting in a robust repair.

The arthroscope is placed posteriorly to gain a better view of the rotator interval. A working portal is created just superior to the subscapularis. A 3.0-mm double-loaded anchor is placed just anterior to the biceps insertion. The sutures from this anchor are passed through the labrum and laterally through the rotator interval, capturing the middle and superior glenohumeral ligaments and shifting them superiorly and medially to the glenoid rim. This step is repeated with a second double-loaded anchor. At this point, the humerus is well reduced in the glenoid. Because of the patient's severe shoulder instability and the patulous nature of her capsule, an arthroscopic biceps suspension procedure is chosen.

The arm is placed in slight abduction and neutral rotation. A biceps tenodesis anchor is placed to reduce and secure the biceps tendon into the proximal humerus while leaving its glenoid origin intact (**Figure 5**). This technique creates an excellent biceps suspension, with appropriate tension on the biceps tendon at neutral rotation (**Figure 6**). A sulcus test is performed gently with the arm in the neutral position, and the biceps is taut with no sulcus sign.

The patient is placed into a sling postoperatively. Use of the sling is continued with no exercises until 6 weeks postoperatively, with removal only for hygiene and dressing. At 6 weeks, the patient begins performing gentle activities of daily living. Examination demonstrates a firm end point at 0° of external rotation and no sulcus sign. The patient begins scapular stabilization and gentle rotator cuff strengthening exercises at this time. She is instructed to avoid lifting more than 20 lb with the surgical arm and to avoid stretching of the

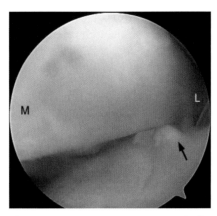

Figure 5 Arthroscopic view of the right shoulder from the posterior portal demonstrates tenodesis of the biceps tendon high in the bicipital groove. The anchor is visible in the bottom right of the picture (arrow). L = lateral, M = medial.

shoulder as a lifetime restriction. She has dramatic improvement in pain and function postoperatively.

Controversies and Alternative Approaches

The classic indication for coracoid transfer is anteroinferior glenoid bone loss, but this procedure has increasingly been used in patients at risk for recurrent instability, including those with humeral-sided bone loss, contact athletes, and patients with anterior soft-tissue deficiency. Preclinical data indicate that in addition to the bony reconstruction enabled by a coracoid transfer, the sling effect resulting from the soft tissue of the conjoined tendon provides a dynamic restraint to anteroinferior instability. In most patients, coracoid transfer should be considered before the following options.

Limited data are available regarding alternative treatment options for patients with severe capsular insufficiency. Although allograft capsular reconstruction has a high rate of failure, few viable alternatives exist. In addition, a capsular reconstruction attempt is often the last

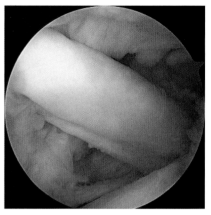

Figure 6 Arthroscopic view of the right shoulder from the posterior portal demonstrates the biceps after biceps suspension. The glenoid attachment was left intact, and tenodesis of the biceps to the proximal bicipital groove was performed, neither of which is visible in this image.

option before glenohumeral arthrodesis. Although arthrodesis can provide excellent pain relief and is durable, functional outcomes are limited. Many patients, after discussion of the risks, benefits, and alternatives of attempted capsular reconstruction compared with glenohumeral arthrodesis, will select one more attempt at joint salvage despite knowledge of the failure rate.

Capsular Reconstruction

Indications
A small subset of patients will require alternatives to the classic instability procedures (arthroscopic or open labral repair, coracoid transfer, bone grafting, remplissage). These patients often have histories similar to the case presentation in this chapter. Many have a long history of instability, often multidirectional. Often the initial episode is atraumatic. Many have had previous failed reconstructive surgical procedures. Finally, many have hyperlaxity or other soft-tissue deficiency.

Treatment of these patients can be particularly challenging. First, patients with baseline soft-tissue deficiency and multiple previous reconstructive shoulder procedures often have profound soft-tissue loss. This soft-tissue loss may result in a patulous or even absent capsule. Second, the multidirectional nature of the instability makes bony reconstruction less effective. Finally, the instability seen in these patients does not always follow standard patterns. The patient in the case presentation demonstrates severe inferior instability, which is common in this group of patients, rare in the typical instability population, and nonexistent in patients with traumatic anterior instability. Because of these considerations, alternative techniques have been developed to address these complex problems. The two main categories of capsular reconstruction for severe soft-tissue deficiency are allograft capsular reconstruction and biceps suspension.

Allograft capsular reconstruction can be done arthroscopically or with an open approach. The typical indication for this procedure is severe soft-tissue loss. Most of these patients will have undergone one or more failed instability procedures. Although magnetic resonance arthrography can indicate somewhat the thickness and quality of the capsular tissue before reconstruction, examination of the tissue is the only true method to assess the quality of the capsular tissue. In many patients, as in the case presented in this chapter, the capsule is extremely thin, and a capsular shift or labral repair will have little chance of success. In these patients with soft-tissue deficiency, allograft capsular reconstruction is a viable option.

Several capsular reconstruction techniques have been described in the literature. The most common is reconstruction of the rotator interval, middle glenohumeral ligament, and anteroinferior glenohumeral ligament with allograft or autograft tissue. Several case reports have documented acceptable results of this procedure. The largest series, with the longest follow-up, demonstrated successful results in most patients but a high rate of recurrent instability (30%). At 3.8-year follow-up, however, 64% of patients were satisfied. This technique has been described with different graft choices and technique variations.

Open Allograft
TECHNICAL KEYS TO SUCCESS
- The authors of this chapter prefer the following technique for open anterior capsular reconstruction. This technique is similar to others described in the literature.
- The patient is placed in the beach-chair position.
- A standard deltopectoral incision is made, and dissection is carried to the subscapularis.
- The subscapularis is divided just medial to its insertion on the lesser tuberosity.
- In most patients, no usable capsule is present on the deep surface of the subscapularis, so the subscapularis tendon and capsule are divided as a unit.
- Usually, the capsule is still present inferiorly, so the inferior capsule can be shifted superiorly to tighten the inferior glenohumeral ligament (IGHL).
- A semitendinosus allograft is prepared.
- The anterior glenoid rim is decorticated, and the midsubstance of the graft is laid on the rim and sutured in place with the use of either transosseous tunnels or anchors. This step recreates the anterior labrum and corrects any labral insufficiency.
- The inferior limb of the graft is brought laterally to the normal insertion site of the anterosuperior band of the IGHL and is secured to the humeral head with a screw-in anchor. The graft is secured with the arm in 45° of abduction and 45° of external rotation.
- In similar fashion, the upper limb of the graft is brought laterally and secured to reconstruct the middle glenohumeral ligament. The graft is tightened with the arm in 25° of abduction and external rotation.
- The two graft ends can also be sutured to each other for added tightening.
- In the rare patient with isolated posterior instability and capsular insufficiency, a similar technique may be used through an intratendinous split between the infraspinatus and teres minor.
- In patients with recurrent anterior and posterior instability with capsular deficiency, combined anterior and posterior approaches may be required.
- The subscapularis is meticulously repaired with permanent sutures, and standard closure of the deltopectoral approach is completed.

REHABILITATION
A sling is applied postoperatively. Use of the sling is continued with no exercises until 6 weeks postoperatively, with removal only for hygiene and dressing. At 6 weeks, the patient begins performing gentle activities of daily living. Active stretching in external rotation and abduction/external rotation is discouraged. At this time, the patient begins scapular stabilization and gentle rotator cuff strengthening exercises and is instructed to avoid lifting more than 20 lb with the surgical arm and to avoid stretching of the shoulder. The lifting and stretching restrictions are lifelong. A rehabilitation protocol is noted in **Table 1**.

AVOIDING PITFALLS
The surgeon must understand the patient's direction or directions of instability and focus the repair or reconstruction on the involved structures. The patient's remaining capsule (usually inferior) should be used to assist in

Table 1 Rehabilitation Protocol After Open Capsular Reconstruction

Postoperative Week	Range of Motion	Strengthening	Return to Play	Comments/Emphasis
0-6	None	None	None	Sling is worn at all times, except for hygiene and dressing
≥6	Gentle activities of daily living are begun No active stretching in external rotation or abduction/ external rotation	Scapular stabilization and gentle rotator cuff strengthening exercises are begun	None	Sling use is discontinued Lifting >20 lb is prohibited (lifetime restriction) Stretching of the shoulder is not allowed (lifetime restriction)

the reconstruction. The reconstruction should re-create the true anatomic insertions of the anterosuperior band of the IGHL and the middle glenohumeral ligament. When each portion of the graft is tightened, careful attention to arm positioning is necessary. A meticulous subscapularis closure is critical to avoid postoperative subscapularis failure.

Arthroscopic Allograft

Although open capsular reconstruction allows reconstruction of the anterior capsule, many of these patients have multidirectional instability. As in the case presented in this chapter, posterior instability may be prominent. Because of this posterior instability, an isolated anterior reconstruction will be ineffective in addressing all of the pathology. In these patients, an arthroscopic approach may allow the surgeon to avoid combined anterior and posterior approaches. The ability to manage all joint pathologies concomitantly makes this technique valuable. In addition, an arthroscopic approach is highly preferred for posterior capsular work because visualization and graft placement through an open posterior approach can be problematic.

TECHNICAL KEYS TO SUCCESS
- The patient is placed in the beach-chair position.
- Portal placement is critical to enable successful reconstruction. A high posterolateral portal is made, and the joint space is visualized.
- A standard comprehensive diagnostic examination is completed. Special attention is focused on the posteroinferior and anteroinferior capsular tissue.
- After the diagnostic examination, an anterior portal is established just superior to the subscapularis, aiming slightly toward the glenoid, so that anchors can be placed through this portal if necessary.
- A shaver is introduced into this portal, and any labral degeneration or loose bodies are removed.
- An anterosuperior viewing portal is established from outside in. A spinal needle is introduced just anterior and lateral to the anterolateral acromion. This needle should enter the joint high in the rotator interval, midway between the humeral head and glenoid, and should be placed to allow easy access in front of and behind the biceps tendon.
- A small metal cannula is introduced, and the arthroscope is transferred to this portal. This portal will allow excellent visualization of the anteroinferior labrum, the anterior capsule, the posterior labrum, and the posterior capsule.
- The following procedure is a posterior capsular allograft

reconstruction; however, the steps are similar for an anterior capsular reconstruction.
- The high posterolateral portal is changed to a working portal.
- With the use of a percutaneous technique, a low posteroinferior 3.0-mm double-loaded biocomposite anchor is placed. A spinal needle is used to localize the position of the skin incision, which is typically lateral to the lateral edge of the acromion and inferior to the high posterolateral initial viewing portal. Using the needle to assess trajectory is helpful to ensure that it will be possible to place anchors. A small stab incision is made adjacent to the needle, and the drill guide with trocar can be introduced in line with the needle into the joint in the appropriate position.
- With the use of a suture hook, one limb is passed through the posteroinferior capsule, creating a posterior and superior shift of the native capsule.
- The suture is tied in place. The second suture is saved for later ligament reconstruction.
- One or two more anchors are placed in a similar manner, creating a standard posterior labral repair with capsular shift. The second suture from each anchor is retained.
- Tendon allograft (typically

semitendinosus or gracilis tendon) is thawed and prepared for reconstruction.

- With the patient's arm in neutral rotation, the distance between the glenoid neck and the bare area of the humeral head is measured with the use of a polydioxanone suture. This measurement is used to estimate the length of allograft tendon that will be required.
- The tendon is folded in half and trimmed to the appropriate length. The folded edge will be placed at the glenoid insertion, and the cut ends will be placed at the humeral insertion.
- Beginning with the most superior glenoid anchor, the sutures are retrieved through the posterior cannula. These sutures are passed in a mattress fashion through the folded edge of the allograft tendon.
- The allograft tendon is passed into the joint through the cannula. The sutures are used to direct the folded surface to the glenoid neck.
- The suture is tied, reducing the allograft tissue to the glenoid neck.
- The sutures from the remaining anchors are retrieved. These sutures are passed through the allograft tissue in the typical manner, reducing the remaining glenoid portion of the allograft to the glenoid rim.
- The patient's arm is placed in the neutral position, and a 3.0-mm double-loaded biocomposite anchor is placed percutaneously into the anatomic neck of the humerus.
- One of these sutures is retrieved and passed through the humeral side of the allograft tendon.
- This suture is tied in place, reducing the lateral portion of the graft to the humeral neck.
- This method is repeated with one or two more anchors to create the desired posterior capsular reconstruction. In most patients, size 0 polydioxanone sutures are

shuttled through the allograft tissue and into the native posterior capsule to imbricate these tissues.
- The wounds are closed with interrupted nylon sutures, and a sling is applied.

REHABILITATION

Rehabilitation is similar to that previously described for the open capsular reconstruction. The authors discourage active stretching because it may predispose the patient to recurrent instability.

AVOIDING PITFALLS

Portal placement is vital to the success of this procedure. The anterosuperior viewing portal should allow easy access in front of and behind the biceps tendon and should be located approximately midway between the cuff insertion and the glenoid. The high posterolateral viewing portal should enter the capsule laterally, allowing anchor placement through this portal as well as access to the anterior glenoid for anterior work. If the posterolateral viewing portal is too medial, it will not allow an appropriate viewing angle for diagnostic arthroscopy and will limit access to the glenoid for anchor placement. The surgeon should take care to keep the posterolateral portal in a high and lateral position.

Systematic suture management is critical. Careful attention should be given to arm position when sutures are passed and tied through the capsule. When working in the posterior shoulder, the surgeon should take care to keep the patient's arm in neutral or internal rotation to avoid overtightening the posterior structures because overtightening can lead to early failure or severe stiffness.

Although arthroscopic posterior capsular reconstruction can be technically challenging, open posterior capsular reconstruction is also technically demanding. In patients who require procedures in more than one area of the shoulder, the surgeon should strongly consider using an arthroscopic approach that will

allow comprehensive treatment instead of using multiple (front and back) open approaches.

Biceps Suspension Procedures

Indications

In patients with recurrent inferior instability with capsular deficiency, anterior or posterior capsular reconstruction will not restore stability. In these patients, as in the case presented in this chapter, a biceps suspension procedure may be used to supplement the reconstruction. The most common indication for this procedure is painful inferior subluxation after multiple unsuccessful shoulder reconstructions. Many of these patients will have a dramatic sulcus sign that does not reduce with external rotation. This sign should alert the clinician to the presence of severe rotator interval attrition. Rotator interval closure is beneficial in these patients. The authors of this chapter recommend rotator interval closure (incorporating anchors to the anterosuperior glenoid) for patients with an inferior instability pattern and a sulcus sign that does not reduce with external rotation. This indication for rotator interval closure is especially true in the revision setting. However, in many patients the interval tissue is deficient and may only partially correct the inferior translation. In these situations, the biceps suspension procedure, which has been successful in patients with neuromuscular disorders, may provide a belt-and-suspenders approach. Results of an open biceps suspension technique were recently published, but data are insufficient to recommend it based on that article alone.

Technical Keys to Success

- The standard arthroscopic approach is used as described previously. Anteroinferior and posteroinferior capsular reconstruction is completed as

Table 2 Results of Allograft Capsular Augmentation Procedures

Authors	Journal (Year)	Technique	Outcomes[a]	Failure Rate (%)	Comments
Iannotti et al	*J Shoulder Elbow Surg* (2002)	Open folded iliotibial band allograft (7 shoulders)	No instability ASES score improved from 30 to 55 External rotation decreased from 72° to 35°	0	All revision operations (mean, 2.2 operations) All maintained physiologic ROM
Warner et al	*J Bone Joint Surg Am* (2002)	Open hamstring autograft (2 patients) or biceps tendon autograft (1 patient)	Only qualitative outcomes were reported	No recurrent instability	Small case study
Alcid et al	*J Shoulder Elbow Surg* (2007)	Open hamstring autograft or allograft tibialis anterior allograft (15 shoulders)	ASES score, 73 Satisfaction was 7.9 on a 10-point scale 13 patients were satisfied Forward flexion decreased 10° External rotation decreased 22° Internal rotation decreased by 4 spinal levels	33 (continued subluxation)	Minimum follow-up, 2 yr 2 shoulders were revised to total shoulder arthroplasty because of arthrosis
Dewing et al	*Arthroscopy* (2012)	Open Achilles allograft anterior capsular reconstruction in 20 shoulders (2 patients with autograft)	Stability achieved in 70% of shoulders ASES score was 84 for stable shoulders	30 (recurrent instability) 15 (required revision for pain)	64% of shoulders had a satisfactory result Largest and longest term study

ASES = American Shoulder and Elbow Surgeons shoulder outcome, ROM = range of motion.

[a] Mean values unless otherwise noted.

described previously (**Table 2**).

- The arthroscope is placed in the high posterolateral portal for improved visualization of the rotator interval. This tissue is often patulous and deficient in these patients.
- The authors of this chapter prefer to repair and shift available interval tissue to a glenoid anchor before performing the biceps suspension procedure.
- The arm is placed in the neutral position, and a 3.0-mm double-loaded anchor is placed just anterior to the biceps insertion into the glenoid. This anchor is passed deep to the labrum and incorporates the labrum in the repair.
- With the use of a hooked suture passer, suture limbs are passed through the interval tissue, shifting the tissue superiorly and medially. A double-loaded anchor allows two passes through the tissue.
- Attention is turned to the biceps suspension procedure. Reduction of the glenohumeral joint is visually confirmed.
- If inferior subluxation persists, support under the elbow or increased support with a pneumatic arm holder should be used to reduce the joint.
- The arm is held in neutral rotation.
- The most superior aspect of the bicipital groove is visualized, and the biceps tendon is retracted posteriorly.
- The authors of this chapter prefer to use a forked biceps tenodesis anchor for the reconstruction.
- A guide pin is placed into the top of the groove, and the appropriate drill is used to make a unicortical drill hole in the bicipital groove. The authors of this chapter typically make an 8.5-mm drill hole for an 8.0- × 19.5-mm tenodesis screw. Using a forked tenodesis screw allows the surgeon to fix the tendon to the hole without cutting the proximal or distal biceps tendon.
- The pin and drill are removed, and the biceps is allowed to reduce over the drill hole.
- The biceps tendon is reduced into the drill hole with the forked end

Table 3 Rehabilitation Protocol After Biceps Suspension Procedures

Postoperative Week	Range of Motion	Strengthening	Return to Play	Comments/Emphasis
0-2	None	None	None	Sling is worn at all times
2-6	None	None	None	Sling is worn at all times
6-12	No stretching	Scapular stabilization, rotator cuff isometrics	None	Sling use is discontinued
12-24	No stretching	As tolerated	None (lifetime limit of 10 lb in operated arm)	Stretching of the shoulder is prohibited (lifetime restriction)

of the anchor, and the anchor is screwed into place. This method creates a stable construct and provides excellent reinforcement of the rotator interval.

- The wounds are closed with interrupted nylon sutures, and a sling is applied.

Rehabilitation

These patients, who are in true salvage situations, are counseled preoperatively that the arm will have a permanent external rotation limit of 0°. The rehabilitation protocol is summarized in **Table 3**.

Avoiding Pitfalls

Visualization via the posterior portal, occasionally with a 70° arthroscope, provides an excellent view of the superior bicipital groove in the location of the biceps tenodesis. The use of a pneumatic arm holder or a padded Mayo stand allows superior support of the arm during the repair.

The surgeon should ensure that the glenohumeral joint is reduced, has no inferior subluxation, and is in neutral rotation before the bicipital anchor is secured. Because this procedure does not involve transection of the biceps in the joint, as is typical with biceps tenodesis, the biceps may be under additional tension during anchor placement. Flexing the elbow may decrease the tension on the biceps tendon and enable easier introduction of the anchor.

 Management of Subscapularis Insufficiency

Indications

Although techniques to manage capsular deficiency are available as described, a subset of patients will have demonstrable subscapularis insufficiency after instability procedures. This finding is especially true of older open stabilization procedures. In one series, 30% of patients had subscapularis insufficiency after open Bankart repair. In that series, subscapularis insufficiency was correlated with worse outcomes. In many patients with subscapularis insufficiency, open or arthroscopic subscapularis repair may be sufficient to restore function. In some patients with long-standing deficiency, however, extensive subscapularis tearing with retraction and fatty atrophy may make subscapularis repair impossible. In these patients, pectoralis major transfer may improve pain and function and provide additional anterior stability. Several case reports have demonstrated satisfactory results of pectoralis major transfer, with the best results seen in patients with isolated subscapularis deficiency (such as after instability procedures).

Controversies and Alternative Approaches

The lack of controversy about the importance of the subscapularis in the unstable shoulder has led to ongoing research into the best way to manage the subscapularis during Bankart repair. Arthroscopic Bankart repair has become a mainstay in the management of primary shoulder instability and does not necessitate incision of the subscapularis. However, a role still exists for open Bankart repair in the management of instability, with some authors using a subscapularis split to reduce the risk of postoperative subscapularis deficiency. Other authors advocate careful repair of the tenotomy. Irrespective of the technique used, protection or repair of the subscapularis is vital. Finally, some controversy exists regarding the relative roles of subscapularis repair and pectoralis major transfer in the management of subscapularis deficiency.

Technical Keys to Success

- When performing pectoralis major transfer, the authors of this chapter prefer to pass the transfer in the subcoracoid position (**Table 4**).
- The patient is placed in the beach-chair position.
- A standard deltopectoral approach is used. The two heads of the pectoralis major are identified and isolated. The sternal head is located deep to the clavicular head.
- The interval between the two heads is developed. This interval is best identified on the medial and inferior surface of the pectoralis major.

Table 4 Results of Split Pectoralis Major Transfer

Authors	Journal (Year)	Technique	Outcomes[a]	Failure Rate (%)	Comments
Resch et al	*J Bone Joint Surg Am* (2000)	Transfer of the superior one-third to one-half of the pectoralis major under the conjoined tendon	Pain improved from 1.7 to 9.6 on a 15-point scale (higher score indicates less pain) No poor outcomes SANE score improved from 20 to 63 Constant score improved from 27 to 67	25 (fair final outcome)	All 4 unstable shoulders became stable 12 patients treated Mean patient age, 65 yr
Jost et al	*J Bone Joint Surg Am* (2003)	Transfer of the entire pectoralis major over the conjoined tendon	Constant score improved from 47 to 70 SANE score improved from 23 to 55	16 (dissatisfied)	Results were more successful in patients with isolated subscapularis tears than in patients with associated tears 28 patients (30 transfers)
Elhassan et al	*J Bone Joint Surg Br* (2008)	Transfer of the sternal head over the conjoined tendon behind the clavicular head	Pain improved in 7 patients Constant score improved from 28 to 50 Subjective shoulder score improved in 7 patients	36	The 11 patients treated had undergone previous failed procedures to manage shoulder instability
Lederer et al	*J Shoulder Elbow Surg* (2011)	Transfer under the conjoined tendon, some with cuff of bone	Constant score improved from 39 to 63 Muscle and tendons intact in 80% on MRI	13 (ruptured tendon on MRI)	Rerupture may decrease with a cuff of bone left on the harvested tendon 54 shoulders
Nelson et al	*J Shoulder Elbow Surg* (2014)	Meta-analysis	Outcome measures included American Shoulder and Elbow Surgeons shoulder outcome score, visual analog scale, and Constant score	NR	168 patients Patients with isolated subscapularis tears had the best outcomes Reliable improvement in pain and function with transfer
Valenti et al	*Int Orthop* (2015)	Transfer of the clavicular head or sternal head	Constant score improved from 36 to 69	20 (dissatisfied)	Similar improvement was noted with clavicular transfer and sternocostal transfer 15 patients treated

NR = not reported, SANE = Single Assessment Numeric Evaluation.

[a] Mean values unless otherwise noted.

- The two heads are isolated from each other, and dissection is performed to the insertion.
- With the long head of the biceps tendon protected, the sternal head of the pectoralis major is released from the humerus, preserving its entire length.
- With the use of two No. 2 permanent braided sutures, Krackow sutures are placed along the superior and inferior borders of the tendon so that four limbs exit the lateral aspect of the tendon (**Figure 7, A**).
- The lateral border of the conjoined tendon is visualized, and the clavipectoral fascia is divided up to but not through the coracoacromial ligament.
- Dissection of the medial conjoined tendon is performed under loupe magnification. The musculocutaneous nerve must be identified and protected. The authors of this chapter prefer to begin dissection proximally, working distally to identify the nerve. Although the location of the nerve in relation to the tip of the coracoid varies, it is typically

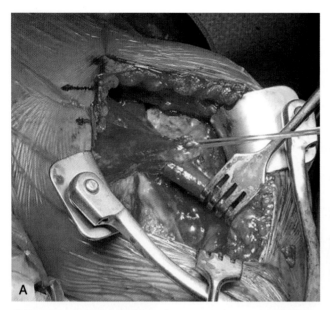 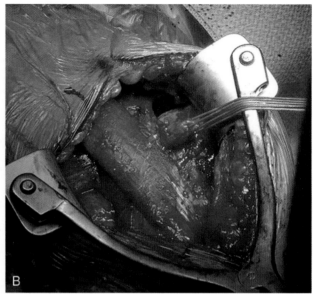

Figure 7 **A,** Intraoperative photograph shows transfer of the sternal head of the pectoralis major in a left shoulder. The clavicular head is being retracted by the rake retractor. The sternal head has been released off the humerus and has been tagged with four sutures. **B,** Intraoperative photograph shows passage of the transfer through a generous tunnel under the coracoid. The transferred muscle has excellent mobility, which will allow it to easily reach the greater tuberosity for reattachment.

Table 5 Rehabilitation Protocol After Split Pectoralis Transfer

Postoperative Week	Range of Motion	Strengthening	Return to Play	Comments/Emphasis
0-4	None	None	None	Sling is worn at all times
4-8	Active-assisted (no external rotation limit)	None	None	—
8-12	No limit	Rotator cuff and scapular strengthening	None	—
12-24	No limit	No limit	Yes, if able	—

located approximately 5 cm distal. Use of a handheld nerve stimulator can be beneficial in patients with distorted anatomy or scar tissue.

- A generous tunnel is created under the conjoined tendon.
- The sternal head of the pectoralis major is transferred under the strap muscles, deep to the conjoined tendon and superficial to the musculocutaneous nerve (**Figure 7, B**).
- Three transosseous tunnels are created in the greater tuberosity, beginning medially at the biceps groove and ending in the greater tuberosity.

- The previously passed sutures in the pectoralis major tendon are passed in a horizontal mattress pattern through the bone tunnels and securely tied.
- The deltopectoral interval is closed in layers.

Rehabilitation

The patient is fitted with a standard sling, to be worn for 4 weeks (**Table 5**). At 4 weeks postoperatively, the patient begins a program of active-assisted range of motion. Because the pectoralis major transfer has sufficient length to permit full range of motion, no external

rotation limit is necessary. At 2 months postoperatively, the patient begins formal physical therapy, focusing on rotator cuff and scapular strengthening as well as transfer training (that is, isometric adduction during active forward flexion). At 4 months, plyometric and endurance training begins. Because the transfer is in phase, biofeedback training typically is not required.

Avoiding Pitfalls

Identifying and separating the two heads of the pectoralis major is critical and is best done medially and inferiorly on the muscle belly. The musculocutaneous nerve must be visualized and freed from the proximal aspect of the conjoined tendon to create an adequate tunnel under the conjoined tendon. Careful identification and dissection of the musculocutaneous nerve is required to allow a large enough tunnel for the graft to pass. Using loupe magnification allows safer and easier dissection of this nerve.

Arthroscopic Bankart repair spares the subscapularis tendon, decreasing the need for pectoralis major transfer. In primary instability procedures, consideration of an arthroscopic approach that spares the subscapularis tendon is warranted.

Bibliography

Alcid JG, Powell SE, Tibone JE: Revision anterior capsular shoulder stabilization using hamstring tendon autograft and tibialis tendon allograft reinforcement: Minimum two-year follow-up. *J Shoulder Elbow Surg* 2007;16(3):268-272.

Braun S, Horan MP, Millett PJ: Open reconstruction of the anterior glenohumeral capsulolabral structures with tendon allograft in chronic shoulder instability. *Oper Orthop Traumatol* 2011;23(1):29-36.

Chechik O, Maman E, Dolkart O, Khashan M, Shabtai L, Mozes G: Arthroscopic rotator interval closure in shoulder instability repair: A retrospective study. *J Shoulder Elbow Surg* 2010;19(7):1056-1062.

Dewing CB, Horan MP, Millett PJ: Two-year outcomes of open shoulder anterior capsular reconstruction for instability from severe capsular deficiency. *Arthroscopy* 2012;28(1):43-51.

Elhassan B, Ozbaydar M, Massimini D, Diller D, Higgins L, Warner JJ: Transfer of pectoralis major for the treatment of irreparable tears of subscapularis: Does it work? *J Bone Joint Surg Br* 2008;90(8):1059-1065.

Giles JW, Boons HW, Elkinson I, et al: Does the dynamic sling effect of the Latarjet procedure improve shoulder stability? A biomechanical evaluation. *J Shoulder Elbow Surg* 2013;22(6):821-827.

Iannotti JP, Antoniou J, Williams GR, Ramsey ML: Iliotibial band reconstruction for treatment of glenohumeral instability associated with irreparable capsular deficiency. *J Shoulder Elbow Surg* 2002;11(6):618-623.

Jost B, Puskas GJ, Lustenberger A, Gerber C: Outcome of pectoralis major transfer for the treatment of irreparable subscapularis tears. *J Bone Joint Surg Am* 2003;85(10):1944-1951.

Lazarus MD, Sidles JA, Harryman DT II, Matsen FA III: Effect of a chondral-labral defect on glenoid concavity and glenohumeral stability: A cadaveric model. *J Bone Joint Surg Am* 1996;78(1):94-102.

Lederer S, Auffarth A, Bogner R, et al: Magnetic resonance imaging-controlled results of the pectoralis major tendon transfer for irreparable anterosuperior rotator cuff tears performed with standard and modified fixation techniques. *J Shoulder Elbow Surg* 2011;20(7):1155-1162.

Namdari S, Keenan MA: Outcomes of the biceps suspension procedure for painful inferior glenohumeral subluxation in hemiplegic patients. *J Bone Joint Surg Am* 2010;92(15):2589-2597.

Nelson GN, Namdari S, Galatz L, Keener JD: Pectoralis major tendon transfer for irreparable subscapularis tears. *J Shoulder Elbow Surg* 2014;23(6):909-918.

Resch H, Povacz P, Ritter E, Matschi W: Transfer of the pectoralis major muscle for the treatment of irreparable rupture of the subscapularis tendon. *J Bone Joint Surg Am* 2000;82(3):372-382.

Valenti P, Boughebri O, Moraiti C, et al: Transfer of the clavicular or sternocostal portion of the pectoralis major muscle for irreparable tears of the subscapularis: Technique and clinical results. *Int Orthop* 2015;39(3):477-483.

Warner JJ, Venegas AA, Lehtinen JT, Macy JJ: Management of capsular deficiency of the shoulder: A report of three cases. *J Bone Joint Surg Am* 2002;84(9):1668-1671.

Yamamoto N, Muraki T, An KN, et al: The stabilizing mechanism of the Latarjet procedure: A cadaveric study. *J Bone Joint Surg Am* 2013;95(15):1390-1397.

Chapter 17

Superior Labrum Anterior to Posterior (SLAP) Repair

Mark H. Getelman, MD

Blake P. Gillette, MD

◼ Introduction

Since its initial description in overhead athletes in 1985 and its subsequent naming—superior labrum anterior to posterior (SLAP) lesion—in an arthroscopic series published in 1990, superior labral tear remains a diagnostic challenge, even after conducting a detailed history and physical examination with the use of modern imaging modalities. Asymptomatic, natural degeneration of the superior labrum is common with increasing age and is different from traumatic, symptomatic SLAP tears. Symptomatic injuries to the superior labrum occur rarely, with a reported incidence of 3% to 6%.

Knowledge of the normal appearance and the anatomic variations of the superior labrum, biceps anchor, and middle glenohumeral ligament is essential to avoid overdiagnosis of SLAP lesions and labral tears, which may lead to inappropriate management. The normal superior labrum is more mobile compared with the inferior labrum and can attach directly to the glenoid margin; it also may be meniscoid in appearance. Furthermore, 73% of normal shoulders have a sublabral recess that is present most

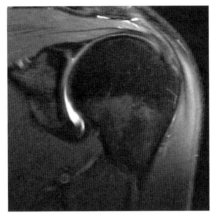

Figure 1 Proton density gadolinium-enhanced coronal magnetic resonance arthrogram of a shoulder demonstrates a normal sublabral recess that was originally interpreted as a possible superior labrum anterior to posterior tear. (Courtesy of Southern California Orthopedic Institute, Van Nuys, CA.)

commonly at the 12 o'clock position. In such patients, the glenoid articular cartilage extends medially over the superior glenoid rim (**Figures 1** and **2**). The long head of the biceps origin also may have great variability, inserting anywhere between 11 and 1 o'clock; it arises directly at the midpoint of the glenoid in only 37% of shoulders. In 55% of shoulders, it originates posterior to the midline.

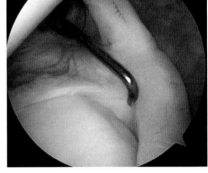

Figure 2 Arthroscopic image of a shoulder from the posterior portal shows a normal superior sublabral recess. No fraying or tearing is present, and the glenoid cartilage extends medially. (Courtesy of Mark H. Getelman, MD, Van Nuys, CA.)

The anatomy in the anterosuperior quadrant of the glenoid anterior to the biceps anchor is the most variable anatomy of the shoulder, and three distinct, normal variations exist. In the first variation, a sublabral foramen with a cord-like middle glenohumeral ligament (MGHL) attaches directly to the anterosuperior labral tissue. This is the most common variant, occurring in 9% of all shoulders (**Figure 3, A**). The second variation is an isolated sublabral foramen, occurring in 3% of shoulders (**Figure 3, B**). The third variant is the Buford complex, which appears in 1.9% of shoulders and has three components: the complete absence of an anterosuperior labrum in the anterosuperior glenoid quadrant and an MGHL that is cord-like

Dr. Getelman or an immediate family member is a member of a speakers' bureau or has made paid presentations on behalf of and serves as a paid consultant to Mitek Sports Medicine, and serves as a board member, owner, officer, or committee member of the Arthroscopy Association of North America. Neither Dr. Gillette nor any immediate family member has received anything of value from or has stock or stock options held in a commercial company or institution related directly or indirectly to the subject of this chapter.

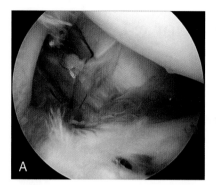 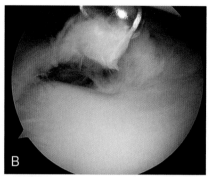 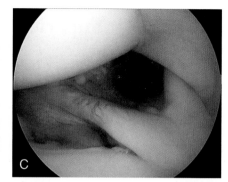

Figure 3   Arthroscopic images of a shoulder show three normal variations in the anatomy of the anterosuperior quadrant of the glenoid anterior to the biceps anchor: sublabral foramen with a cord-like middle glenohumeral ligament (**A**), isolated sublabral foramen in the anterosuperior region of the labrum (**B**), and the Buford complex (**C**). (Courtesy of Mark H. Getelman, MD, Van Nuys, CA.)

and that attaches directly to the base of the biceps tendon (**Figure 3, C**).

Even with the knowledge of the common variants, intraoperative recognition can be difficult, because the MGHL can have great variability and often may demonstrate a frayed appearance as it inserts anterior to the glenoid. It is extremely important to differentiate these entities from a pathologic SLAP tear, because inadvertent "repair" will likely cause postoperative pain and stiffness, limited external rotation, and a poor outcome. In contrast, the posterosuperior labrum consistently is confluent with the glenoid cartilage without a recess or foramen. In general, if the labrum in this region is easily displaced, with associated fraying or tearing, it is likely to be pathologic.

In 1990, SLAP lesions were classified into four distinct types. This classification was followed in 1995 by an analysis of 140 patients with superior labrum injuries to determine the overall incidence in the authors' practice (5.9%), and the frequency of the specific types (**Figure 4**).

Type I SLAP lesions have an incidence of 21%. They display degenerative fraying of the labrum, but the biceps anchor is firmly attached to the glenoid. Type I lesions occur as part of the natural aging process and are most common in patients who are middle-aged or older. They are unlikely

to be a substantial source of clinical symptoms.

Type II SLAP lesions, with an incidence of 55%, have a substantial detachment or tearing of the biceps/labral anchor from the glenoid margin and arthroscopically displace more than 5 mm with retraction by a probe. Often, localized hemorrhagic injection or fraying and associated synovitis are present. Type II lesions are the most common; they require repair and are the main focus of this discussion.

Type III SLAP tears have a 9% occurrence rate and exhibit a bucket-handle longitudinal tear of the superior labrum. The biceps tendon is normal, however, and is firmly attached to the intact labrum and supraglenoid tubercle. Débridement of the displaced superior labrum typically is sufficient.

Type IV SLAP lesions, with an incidence of 10%, have a complex longitudinal bucket-handle tear of the superior labrum with extension of the tear into the biceps tendon. These tears require débridement and repair, or more frequently, strong consideration for concurrent biceps tenodesis, depending on the overall quality of the biceps and a patient's characteristics. Additions to this classification system to include anterior or posterior shoulder instability injury patterns have been described, but they are beyond the scope of this discussion, which

focuses on the management of type II lesions.

Type II lesions may have multiple mechanisms of injury, including traction, forceful rotation, a fall onto an outstretched arm, and a fall directly onto the shoulder. Three subgroups have been described, varying by the predominance of the tear: anterior, posterior, or combined anterior and posterior. SLAP tears with predominantly posterior extension are more likely to occur in younger overhead athletes via a frequently encountered mechanism of injury referred to as the peel-back mechanism. Intraoperatively, labral stability can be assessed dynamically by removing the arm from traction, placing it into the throwing position with abduction to 90°, and increasing external rotation. An unstable labrum will fall medially off the superior glenoid and peel back along the glenoid neck with full cocking of the arm. Concomitant partial articular-side rotator cuff tears may be visualized at the point of contact between the cuff and the posterosuperior glenoid.

Despite advances in MRI techniques and heightened clinical awareness, SLAP lesions remain a diagnostic challenge. However, with a thorough understanding of the anatomic variations, a detailed history of trauma or diagnosis in a throwing or overhead athlete, a careful physical examination with provocative biceps testing, and good quality MRI

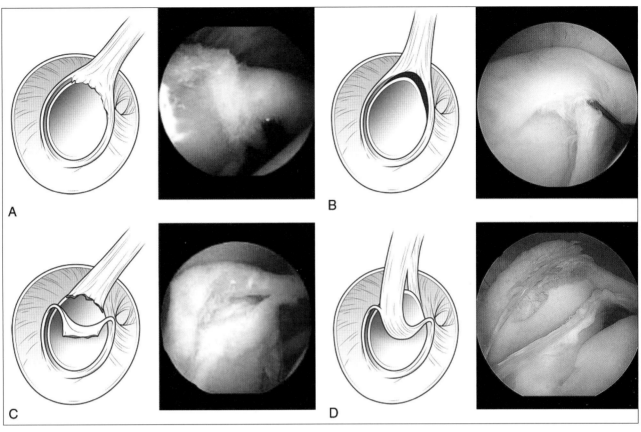

Figure 4   Images show the different types of superior labrum anterior to posterior tears. **A,** Type I tears demonstrate fraying of the superior labrum with an intact biceps anchor. **B,** Type II tears are characterized by a detached superior labrum and biceps anchor. Type III (**C**) and type IV (**D**) tears are bucket-handle tears of the superior labrum. In type III tears, the biceps anchor is intact, whereas type IV tears extend into the biceps tendon and only part of the biceps anchor remains intact. (Reproduced from Werner BC, Brockmeier SF, Miller MD: Etiology, diagnosis, and management of failed SLAP repair. *J Am Acad Orthop Surg* 2014;22[9]:554-565.)

with or without contrast, the surgeon can be more confident in the diagnosis of a symptomatic SLAP tear. Ultimately, after nonsurgical measures have failed and other shoulder pathology has been ruled out, arthroscopy should be considered and remains the standard for the accurate diagnosis and management of SLAP tears.

 Case Presentation

A 32-year-old man presents with 6 months of shoulder pain after a traumatic fall onto his dominant shoulder during a recreational flag football game. He was evaluated initially by his primary care physician, who treated him

with rest, NSAIDs, and a subacromial injection that provided incomplete, transient relief. He completed a course of physical therapy with no substantial improvement in his symptoms. He currently reports substantial weakness and moderate pain in the throwing position or with any prolonged overhead activity.

On physical examination, the patient has full range of motion (ROM), no specific tenderness to palpation, and normal rotator cuff strength. He does not have anterior or posterior instability, but positive results are elicited for the Neer impingement sign and on the Speed and O'Brien tests. Radiographs do not demonstrate a Hill-Sachs lesion or glenohumeral arthritis, but they do demonstrate a Bigliani type 2 acromial

arch. Nonsurgical management was unsuccessful, and gadolinium-enhanced magnetic resonance arthrogram demonstrates increased signal intensity beneath the superior labrum, with ragged lateral extension and a paralabral cyst measuring 1.5 cm that sits adjacent to the posterosuperior labrum (**Figure 5**). After detailed discussion of these findings, the patient elected to proceed with surgical treatment.

Indications

The most common indications for the single-anchor, double-suture repair technique include a patient younger than 35 years with an isolated, traumatic

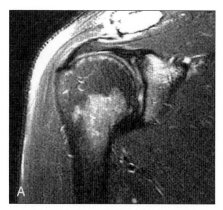 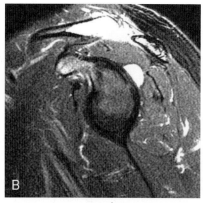

Figure 5   Coronal (**A**) and sagittal (**B**) T2-weighted MRIs of a shoulder demonstrate a superior labrum anterior to posterior tear with lateral extension and a posterosuperior paralabral cyst, respectively. (Courtesy of Southern California Orthopedic Institute, Van Nuys, CA.)

type II SLAP lesion with detachment and unstable tearing of the superior labrum and biceps anchor without coexisting rotator cuff pathology or biceps tendon injury. This approach is used based on the experience of the authors of this chapter and the current body of evidence-based literature.

Historically, before the development of modern anchors and repair techniques, SLAP lesions were managed primarily with simple débridement. Healing was inconsistent, with a reported failure rate of 40% and results that deteriorated over time. Based on the high failure rates associated with débridement alone, many repair techniques were attempted, including staples, transosseous sutures, and absorbable polyglycolic acid tacks and screws. These techniques resulted in some improvement over débridement alone, but complications occurred and occasionally required additional surgery to remove hardware or loose bioabsorbable fragments. Ultimately, suture anchor repair became the standard of care, and most surgical reviews published since 2007 have used suture anchor techniques.

In the management of isolated type II SLAP tears, one double-loaded anchor has been shown to be biomechanically equivalent to two single-loaded anchor repairs. Studies have shown that the anchor-bone interface is an unlikely location for failure; construct failure is most likely to occur at the suture-labral interface. Moreover, a study published in 2013 showed that repair contact pressures were most consistently localized directly beneath the biceps anchor in a single-anchor, double-suture configuration. In a double-anchor repair, contact pressure was seen only under the anchor points with limited contact pressure directly beneath the biceps anchor. From an economic standpoint, the benefits of reducing implant costs with a single-anchor rather than a double-anchor repair cannot be overlooked. Tears with extension beyond the biceps base may require additional anchors, however, and the use of additional anchors depends on the extent of labral tearing and the anatomic location of the tear. Patient age and activity level must be considered carefully in determining appropriate treatment.

Controversies, Alternative Approaches, and Results

Although one study has indicated a substantial increase in SLAP repairs since 2002 and a community incidence reported to be greater than that of historical series, the incidence of isolated SLAP lesion repair declined from 69% to 45% from 2002 to 2011. Several studies indicate that a high percentage of patients have less than excellent outcomes after repair (**Table 1**). As a result of these findings, a recent trend exists toward narrowing the indications for type II SLAP repair and recommending instead that a biceps tenodesis be performed more routinely, especially in older patients.

In a prospective study published in 2009 comparing repair of isolated type II SLAP tears with either two suture anchors or arthroscopic biceps tenodesis, better results were achieved with tenodesis, with an 80% satisfaction rate and 87% of athletes returning to previous levels of athletic participation compared with a 40% satisfaction rate and a 20% return to sports rate in patients treated with SLAP repair. The mean age of patients treated with SLAP repair was 37, a mean of 15 years younger compared with the patients treated with biceps tenodesis. In a study published in 2012, outcome scores after type II SLAP repair tended to be lower and less predictable compared with those of tenodesis in patients older than 35 years. Moreover, the authors of that study noted a trend toward a 3-month longer recovery time for patients who underwent labral repair. The difference was not statistically significant. In a recent large prospective study of military personnel who had isolated type II SLAP lesions, 37% of the repairs failed, and the revision rate was 28%. In patients older than 36 years, the relative risk of failure was 3.5. In contrast, a study published in 2010 showed no clinical difference in outcomes for patients who were treated with type II SLAP repairs regardless whether they were younger or older than 40 years at the time of treatment. The authors of a study published in 2014 performed isolated type II SLAP repairs only in

Table 1 Clinical Results of Repair of Isolated Type II Superior Labrum Anterior to Posterior (SLAP) Lesions

Authors	Journal (Year)	Technique (No. of Patients)	Outcomes	Failure Rate (%)	Comments
Kim et al	*J Bone Joint Surg Am* (2002)	1 single-loaded, metal suture anchor through ASP (34)	UCLA score was good to excellent in 32 patients	6	91% of patients regained preinjury level of shoulder function, but only 41% had no limitations postoperatively 23 patients were collegiate or professional athletes Mean age, 26 yr Mean follow-up, 33 mo
Ide et al	*Am J Sports Med* (2005)	≥2 single-loaded, bioabsorbable suture anchors through the TRCP[a] (40)	Modified Rowe score was good to excellent in 36 patients	10	All patients treated were overhead athletes 75% of patients returned to their preoperative level of competition 63% of baseball players returned to their preoperative level of competition Among baseball players, the return-to-sport rate was higher in patients with overuse injury than with traumatic injury 75% of all patients had partial articular-side rotator cuff tear Mean age, 24 yr Mean follow-up, 41 mo
Enad et al	*J Shoulder Elbow Surg* (2007)	≥2 single-loaded, bioabsorbable anchors through ASP; if posterior extension of tear, then TRCP (portal of Wilmington) (27)	UCLA score was good to excellent in 24 patients Mean ASES score, 86.9	11	All patients were in the military, and 96% returned to full duty 67% of patients had concomitant shoulder pathology that was treated at the time of SLAP repair: PRCT in 4, chondrosis of the humeral head or glenoid in 6, and subacromial impingement in 8 Mean age, 32 yr Mean follow-up, 30.5 mo
Yung et al	*Knee Surg Sports Traumatol Arthrosc* (2008)	Multiple single-loaded knotless through ASP; if posterior extension of tear, then TRCP (portal of Wilmington) (16)	UCLA score was good to excellent in 12 patients	25	Mean age, 24 yr Mean follow-up, 28 mo
Boileau et al	*Am J Sports Med* (2009)	2 single-loaded bioabsorbable anchors (10)	4 patients were satisfied Mean Constant score, 83	60	10 patients underwent SLAP repair 2 patients returned to their previous level of sports participation 4 patients with failed SLAP repair later underwent biceps tenodesis Mean age, 37 yr Mean follow-up, 35 mo

ASES = American Shoulder and Elbow Society shoulder outcome, ASP = anterior-superior portal, KJOC = Kerlan-Jobe Orthopedic Clinic Shoulder and Elbow, NR = not reported, PRCT = partial rotator cuff tear, SF-12 = Medical Outcomes Study 12-Item Short Form, TRCP = trans-rotator cuff portal, UCLA = University of California–Los Angeles Shoulder Rating Scale.

[a] Used as primary lateral portal.

Table 1 Clinical Results of Repair of Isolated Type II Superior Labrum Anterior to Posterior (SLAP) Lesions (*continued*)

Authors	Journal (Year)	Technique (No. of Patients)	Outcomes	Failure Rate (%)	Comments
Brock-meier et al	*J Bone Joint Surg Am* (2009)	≥2 single-loaded, metal or bioab-sorbable anchors through ASP; if posterior exten-sion of tear, then TRCP (portal of Wilmington) (47)	Subjective outcome was good to excellent in 41 patients Median patient-reported satisfaction, 9 (10-point scale) Median L'Insalata score, 93 Median ASES score, 97	15	25 of the 34 athletes treated returned to their preinjury level of competition 7 of the 11 baseball players treated returned to their preinjury level of competition 11 of the 12 athletes who reported a discrete traumatic event returned to their preinjury level of competition 24 patients had a PRCT Mean age, 36 yr Avg follow-up, 32.4 mo
Alpert et al	*Am J Sports Med* (2010)	2 single-loaded anchors posterior to biceps from ASP (52)	Of the 21 patients aged <40 yr, the mean ASES score was 93, and 20 were satisfied or completely satisfied Of the 31 patients aged >40 yr, the mean ASES score was 86, and 26 were satisfied or completely satisfied No significant difference in SF-12, simple shoulder test, or ASES scores	14 (age < 40 yr) 10 (age > 40 yr)	Failure was defined by patient unwillingness to undergo the same procedure again Mean follow-up, 28 mo
Neuman et al	*Am J Sports Med* (2011)	Mean 2.7 single-loaded bioab-sorbable anchors TRCP lateral to midpoint of acro-mion[a] (30)	Mean ASES score, 87.9 Mean overall KJOC score, 73.6 Overall satisfaction rate, 93.3%	7	All patients were overhead ath-letes Athletes perceived that they re-turned to approximately 84% of their preinjury function at mean return-to-play time of 11.7 mo KJOC score was significantly lower in baseball players ($P = 0.006$) Mean age, 24 yr Avg follow-up, 42 mo
Silber-berg et al	*Arthroscopy* (2011)	Group 1: 1 double-loaded, bioab-sorbable anchor with vertical stitch through ASP (15) Group 2: 1 single-loaded bioab-sorbable anchor with horizontal suture through ASP (17)	Group 1: Mean ASES score, 91.9; good to excellent satisfaction in 87% Group 2: Mean ASES score, 95.8; good to excellent satisfaction in 94%	Group 1: 13 Group 2: 6	Prospective, double-blind, ran-domized controlled trial 13 patients in group 1 and 16 patients in group 2 returned to their preinjury level of work activities No significant difference between treatment groups Mean ages: group 1, 29 yr; group 2, 28 yr Mean follow-up, 37 mo

ASES = American Shoulder and Elbow Society shoulder outcome, ASP = anterior-superior portal, KJOC = Kerlan-Jobe Orthopedic Clinic Shoulder and Elbow, NR = not reported, PRCT = partial rotator cuff tear, SF-12 = Medical Outcomes Study 12-Item Short Form, TRCP = trans-rotator cuff portal, UCLA = University of California–Los Angeles Shoulder Rating Scale.

[a] Used as primary lateral portal.

Table 1 Clinical Results of Repair of Isolated Type II Superior Labrum Anterior to Posterior (SLAP) Lesions (*continued*)

Authors	Journal (Year)	Technique (No. of Patients)	Outcomes	Failure Rate (%)	Comments
Denard et al	*Arthroscopy* (2012)	Multiple (mean, 1.9) double-loaded anchors; if posterior extension of tear, then TRCP (portal of Wilmington) (55)	UCLA score was good to excellent in 48 patients Good to excellent UCLA scores achieved in 81% of patients ≥40 yr and in 97% of patients aged <40 yr Good to excellent UCLA scores achieved in 65% of patients who filed a workers' compensation claim, compared with 95% in patients who did not have such a claim (*P* = 0.009)	13	82% of all patients returned to normal sport or activities 88% of overhead athletes returned to normal activities Mean age, 39.7 yr 23 patients aged <40 yr 32 patients aged ≥40 yr No significant difference in outcomes based on patient age Mean follow-up, 77 mo
Park et al	*Am J Sports Med* (2013)	1 double-loaded bioabsorbable anchor (5) Multiple (mean, 3.4) single-loaded metal anchors (18)	Mean ASES score, 87.1 Mean subjective feeling of recovery, 76%	NR	24 elite overhead athletes treated 50% of all overhead athletes returned to play, but only 38% of baseball players returned to play Labral re-tear in 2 patients who failed to return to play (found on postoperative CT arthrogram) Mean age, 23 yr Mean follow-up, 45.8 mo
Provencher et al	*Am J Sports Med* (2013)	1 or 2 single-loaded anchors using a trans-rotator cuff percutaneous technique[a] (179)	Mean ASES score, 88 Mean single assessment numeric evaluation score, 85	37	Prospective study of 179 patients Relative risk of failure of 3.45 in patients aged >36 yr Overall revision rate, 28% Failure was defined as the need for revision surgery, an ASES score <70, and inability to return to sports and/or work 16 of 66 patients separated from the military after treatment failure Mean age, 32 yr Mean follow-up, 40 mo
Ek et al	*J Shoulder Elbow Surg* (2014)	1 double-loaded anchor centered or placed posterior to the biceps anchor TRCP[a] (10)	Mean ASES score, 93.5 Mean subjective shoulder value, 84%	10	6 patients returned to their preinjury level of sports participation 9 patients were satisfied Mean age, 31 yr Mean follow-up, 35 mo

ASES = American Shoulder and Elbow Society shoulder outcome, ASP = anterior-superior portal, KJOC = Kerlan-Jobe Orthopedic Clinic Shoulder and Elbow, NR = not reported, PRCT = partial rotator cuff tear, SF-12 = Medical Outcomes Study 12-Item Short Form, TRCP = trans-rotator cuff portal, UCLA = University of California–Los Angeles Shoulder Rating Scale.

[a] Used as primary lateral portal.

patients younger than 35 years who were active and had healthy-appearing labral tissue. Patients who did not meet these criteria were treated with biceps tenodesis. At follow-up of more than 2 years, no statistical difference was observed in functional outcome, patient satisfaction, or return to play between the treatment groups.

The evidence suggests that repair of type II SLAP lesions remains a viable treatment option for certain patients with superior labral detachments and that it can result in a successful outcome. It is imperative, however, that the surgeon adheres to the surgical principles and techniques described in this chapter and select appropriate patients to achieve a successful repair.

Biomechanical studies have been conducted on specific approaches and techniques for type II SLAP repair, including the number of anchors used, anchor position, and suture configuration. The authors of a cadaver model study published in 2008 found no difference between two types of suture anchor constructs—two posterior sutures versus one anterior suture and one posterior suture—in type II SLAP lesions loaded to failure via a posterior peel-back mechanism. The authors of a study published in 2004 found no difference in mean load to ultimate failure between double-anchor constructs using simple vertical or horizontal mattress sutures. In a different biomechanical model, three common suture anchor configurations were compared: single-anchor simple sutures placed anterior to the biceps, double-anchor simple sutures placed anterior and posterior to the biceps, and single-anchor horizontal mattress sutures placed medial to the biceps. The mean load-to-strain failure was greatest in cadaver model shoulders fixed with a single anchor with a mattress suture. The authors of that study concluded that a single suture anchor with a mattress suture through the biceps anchor was biomechanically advantageous over one

or two suture anchors with a simple suture. Double-suture constructs provided intermediate load-to-strain failure. The literature comparing emerging knotless anchors with standard suture anchors is limited. One study showed equivalent ultimate load to failure; however, a second study found knotless anchors to be weaker in load and in the number of cycles to 2-mm gapping but similar in ultimate load to failure. When considering newly developing technology or techniques, the authors of this chapter recommend a cautious approach, particularly for surgeons whose experience has been predictable and reproducible for many years with the single-anchor, double-suture technique.

The anterosuperior portal (ASP) is not used universally. Some surgeons have indicated that a transtendinous or trans–rotator cuff approach is safe because they believe that it offers improved access to the posterosuperior labrum, which is particularly important in throwing athletes with posterior extension of the tear. In a 2008 study of 58 patients treated with a trans–rotator cuff approach, 6 patients had partial articular-side rotator cuff tears at 1-year follow-up. In four of these six patients, however, these tears had been observed preoperatively, and no worsening of the rotator cuff damage was reported. In a study from 2002 in which a similar transtendinous approach through the supraspinatus or infraspinatus tendon was performed (depending on the patient's anatomy), a 71% good or excellent satisfaction rate and a 52% rate of return to preinjury level of sports was noted among 31 patients who were followed for a minimum of 2 years after SLAP repair. None of the patients with poorer outcomes had symptoms indicative of rotator cuff pathology; the eight patients from this group who underwent postoperative MRI did not show evidence of rotator cuff tearing. Other studies have indicated that substantial damage to the rotator cuff can occur with the

transtendinous approach. The authors of a recent case series of six referred patients identified full-thickness rotator cuff tears that they thought were created iatrogenically, resulting from improper transtendinous portal placement during the initial SLAP repair. All six patients required subsequent rotator cuff repairs, and three also required concurrent revision SLAP repair. The authors of that case series emphasized that, if using a transtendinous portal, the surgeon must ensure that the trans–rotator cuff portal entry occurs medial to the musculotendinous junction of the rotator cuff.

 Video 17.1 Type 2 SLAP Repair. Mark Getelman, MD; Blake Gillette, MD (10 min)

Technical Keys to Success

- The patient is placed in the lateral decubitus position.
- A standard posterior portal is created 1 cm inferior and medial to the posterolateral corner of the acromion at the soft spot.
- A 30° arthroscope is inserted posteriorly, and an ASP is created. The position of the ASP is localized using a spinal needle inserted just off the anterolateral corner of the acromion. It is critical that the needle enters the joint along the superior edge of the rotator interval directly behind the biceps tendon. Orientation of the needle should simulate the trajectory of a drill guide and should allow access to the superior glenoid neck for anchor placement (**Figure 6, A**).
- A small skin incision is made in line with the axilla, and a clear plastic 5.5-mm cannula is placed into the joint, avoiding iatrogenic injury to the anterior edge of the supraspinatus tendon.

- An anterior mid-glenoid (AMG) portal is created similarly with spinal needle localization through the inferior rotator interval directly superior to the subscapularis tendon, maintaining as much distance as possible between the two cannulas to prevent interval crowding.

- A standard 15-point diagnostic examination is performed.

- Using a probe introduced through the AMG portal, the biceps anchor is examined. In patients with pathologic type II SLAP lesions, the biceps anchor insertion exhibits substantial fraying of the undersurface of the labrum (**Figure 6, B**). When the biceps tendon is probed with superiorly directed force, the labrum arches away from the glenoid and displaces 5 to 6 mm. In **Figure 6, C**, the tear extends posteriorly, and a posterosuperior paralabral cyst is visualized adjacent to the tear.

- The patient's arm is removed from traction and placed into the throwing position while viewing the superior labrum from the posterior portal to simulate a peel-back mechanism. The dynamic examination is demonstrated in the video that accompanies this chapter. In that patient, mild displacement of the labrum is evident with the arm in the throwing position, but no damage to the undersurface of the rotator cuff is seen.

- Cysts are commonly associated with labral tears in the posterosuperior glenoid region, and they are readily identified by MRI. If a cyst is large and accessible, it is the opinion of the authors of this chapter that it should be decompressed at the time of labral repair.

- As the biceps anchor and superior labrum are débrided, the cyst may be visualized inferior to the superior labrum. If the cyst is not visualized, a probe may be used to

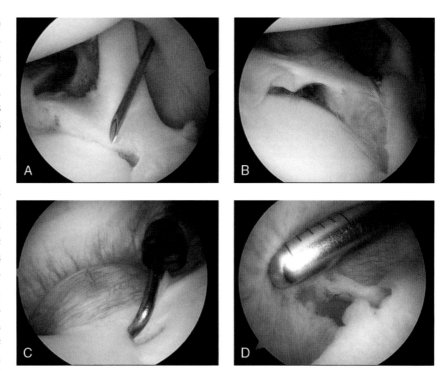

Figure 6   Arthroscopic images of a left shoulder show portal placement during arthroscopic repair of an isolated type II superior labrum anterior to posterior (SLAP) lesion using a single-anchor, double-suture technique. **A,** View from the posterior portal shows proper needle trajectory for the placement of the anterosuperior portal. **B,** The superior labrum is displaced more than 5 mm with substantial tearing of the undersurface. The normal anterosuperior sublabral foramen also is visualized. Views from the anterior portal show a posterosuperior paralabral cyst from the posterior extension of the SLAP tear (**C**) and the posterosuperior paralabral cyst being unroofed or "marsupialized" with a shaver (**D**). (Courtesy of Mark H. Getelman, MD, Van Nuys, CA.)

palpate the area peripheral to the labrum, and the cyst may be decompressed through the tear or by creating a separate capsulotomy.

- A blush of synovial fluid often is visualized as the probe or shaver enters the cyst.

- If no visible evidence is present that the cyst has been decompressed, then further investigation and management may be necessary.

- Viewing from the ASP, the posterior superior capsule is opened using a shaver or radiofrequency device, allowing the cyst to be unroofed or "marsupialized" (**Figure 6, D**).

- Cyst-wall excision can be performed safely within 1.5 cm of the glenoid rim, because the infraspinatus branch of the suprascapular nerve

typically is located approximately 1.8 to 2.1 cm from the glenoid rim, adjacent to the scapular spine. Cyst recurrence is unlikely after decompression and subsequent repair of the labrum.

- The superior labral tear is repaired next. For most type II SLAP lesions, a single-anchor, double-suture technique is performed. In patients with posterior tears, however, an additional double-loaded suture anchor is used in the posterosuperior quadrant to address the posterior extension and the cyst formation.

- The labral edge is débrided gently from anterior to posterior as described previously, and the superior glenoid rim is decorticated slightly with a 4-mm motorized shaver and

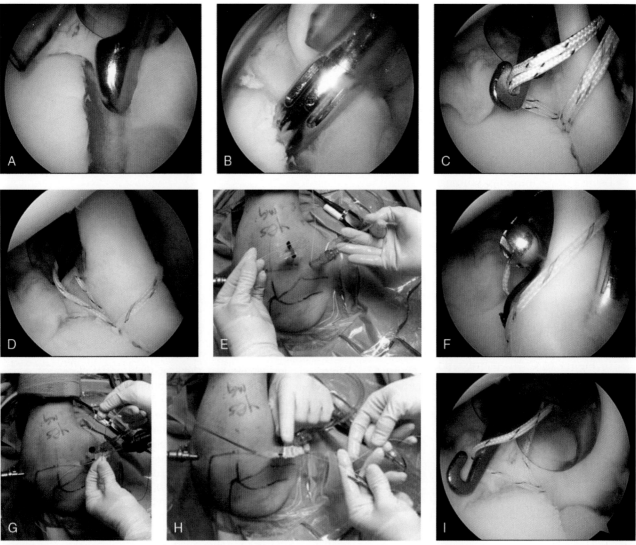

Figure 7   Images of a shoulder show arthroscopic repair of a type II superior labrum anterior to posterior lesion. Arthroscopic images are viewed from the posterior portal. **A,** The prepared superior glenoid is ready for anchor placement. **B,** The correct angle for anchor placement through the anterior-superior portal (ASP) is shown. **C,** The most anterior suture pair is retrieved out the anterior mid glenoid (AMG) with a crochet hook. These sutures are placed outside the cannula. **D,** The black-and-white anterior sutures lie outside the AMG cannula, and one strand from the blue-and-white posterior sutures is pulled into the cannula while its partner remains in the ASP cannula. **E,** Intraoperative photograph shows the cannulas and the suture position. **F,** The shuttle is passed through the superior labrum posterior to the biceps anchor. **G,** Intraoperative photograph shows the shuttling monofilament tied to one limb of the posterior suture from the AMG portal. **H,** Intraoperative photograph shows the posterior sutures in the ASP cannula in preparation for knot tying. **I,** One strand of the anterior pair of sutures is pulled into the AMG portal from the ASP. (Courtesy of Mark H. Getelman, MD, Van Nuys, CA.)

rasp or curet (**Figure 7, A**).
- After the labrum and bone have been prepared, the suture anchor is ready for insertion.
- Suture anchor selection is a personal choice, but small (<3.5-mm), double-loaded anchors made of biocomposite material or the newer all-suture soft anchors

typically are recommended.
- Through the ASP cannula positioned posterior to the biceps, a drill guide for a double-loaded, soft suture anchor is inserted and placed at the anatomic center of the biceps tubercle just medial to the edge of the articular cartilage (**Figure 7, B**). The guide is positioned at

an angle of 45° to the glenoid surface and is aimed toward the center of the glenoid.
- The pilot hole is created, and the soft anchor is inserted and set by pulling on the sutures to ensure secure placement.
- Attention is then directed toward suture passing.

- The most anterior suture limbs are retrieved with a crochet hook through the AMG portal and then stored outside the cannula with a switching stick (**Figure 7, C**).
- The posterior suture limb that is closest to the labrum is retrieved with the crochet hook in the AMG portal in preparation for passing (**Figure 7, D** and **E**).
- A suture-shuttling angled hook is inserted through the ASP (which is positioned posterior to the biceps tendon) and passed through the superior labrum posterior to the biceps tendon, exiting at the base of the superior labrum adjacent to the anchor.
- The suture shuttle or a No. 1 monofilament suture is advanced into the joint and retrieved with a grasper through the AMG portal (**Figure 7, F** and **G**).
- The monofilament suture is tied to the stored suture limb and carried back through the superior labrum, creating a simple vertical stitch.
- At this point, both posterior suture limbs are in the ASP cannula and are ready for knot tying (**Figure 7, H**).
- The suture limb that passed through the labrum serves as the post suture.
- A locking sliding knot is tied and advanced intra-articularly, ensuring that the knot remains superior and medial to the biceps anchor to avoid damage to the humeral head cartilage.
- The knot is backed up with alternating half hitches while reversing the post to maintain knot security. It is important to not over-tension the labrum and to avoid using too much force when tying the knots. Appropriate tension will just indent the labral tissue.
- Attention is directed to suture passing for the anterior sutures.
- One of the stored sutures outside

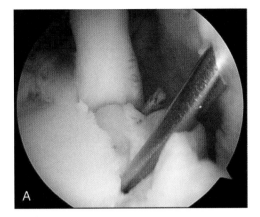
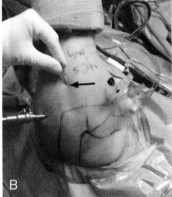
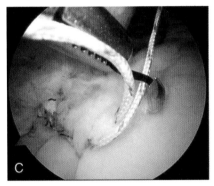
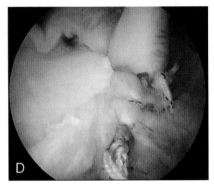

Figure 8 Images of a shoulder show surgical repair of the posterior extension of a superior labrum anterior to posterior (SLAP) tear. **A,** Arthroscopic image from the posterior portal shows the needle position for the transtendinous portal of Wilmington that is used to place an additional anchor in the posterosuperior region. The portal lies medial to the musculotendinous junction of the infraspinatus. **B,** Intraoperative photograph shows the position of the transtendinous portal of Wilmington (arrow). **C,** Arthroscopic image from the anterosuperior portal shows the shuttle passed through the posterosuperior labrum from the posterior portal. **D,** Arthroscopic image from the posterior portal shows the final SLAP repair, which consists of two soft anchors and four double-loaded sutures. (Courtesy of Mark H. Getelman, MD, Van Nuys, CA.)

the AMG portal is placed back into the cannula. This step can be accomplished most easily by retrieving the suture to be passed first into the ASP and then into the AMG portal with a crochet hook to avoid any fraying to the suture that may occur by directly retrieving the suture into the AMG portal (**Figure 7, I**).
- The shuttling steps are performed again, this time passing the shuttling device just anterior to the biceps anchor.
- The suture is tied via the ASP, taking care to ensure knot and loop security.

- To treat patients who have posterior extension of the tear and an associated cyst, a percutaneous transtendinous portal of Wilmington is used to access the posterior glenoid and repair the labrum.
- Needle localization is visualized directly with the arthroscope.
- Typically, the portal of Wilmington is located 1 cm lateral and 1 cm inferior to the posterolateral corner of the acromion (**Figure 8, A** and **B**). This portal is used only for the small-diameter drill guide and for anchor placement to minimize iatrogenic rotator cuff injury.
- After the anchor has been inserted,

Table 2 Rehabilitation Protocol After the Repair of Superior Labrum Anterior to Posterior Lesions

Postoperative Week	Range of Motion	Strengthening	Return to Play	Comment/Emphasis
0-3	Scapular, cervical	None	None	—
3-6	Shoulder (passive, active assisted)	None	None	No forceful passive abduction–external rotation
6-12	Shoulder (active)	Rotator cuff, scapular stabilizers	None	No biceps strengthening
12-24	Full	Biceps resistance	Light sports	Collision sports are not allowed before 6 mo Return to overhead or throwing sports may not be possible until >6 mo

the arthroscope is moved to the ASP for viewing, and the angled hook shuttle device is introduced from the posterior portal to facilitate access to the labrum. Similar shuttling steps are performed via the standard cannulas (**Figure 8, C**).

- The SLAP repair is inspected by probing the biceps anchor and the superior labrum to assess appropriate tension and stability (**Figure 8, D**).
- In a patient who had a demonstrable peel-back lesion, the SLAP repair should correct it, thereby restoring superior labral stability and eliminating any remaining peel-back with the arm in the throwing position.

Rehabilitation

Scarring may occur with portal placement in the rotator interval; thus, the patient's arm is placed postoperatively in neutral to 15° of external rotation while in the sling to prevent internal rotation contracture and to minimize stiffness. Patients are instructed to begin immediate elbow, wrist, and hand ROM exercises, and scapular motion is allowed. For the first 3 weeks postoperatively, the sling should be worn at all times except

during ROM exercises and showering. The rehabilitation protocol is shown in **Table 2**. It is important to maintain the duration guidelines proposed and to not progress the patient too quickly. The physician and therapist must take into consideration an individual patient's healing rate, the extent of surgery, and the subjective and objective findings before advancing to each subsequent phase of rehabilitation. For throwing athletes, a progressive throwing program should begin only after the patient obtains full, pain-free ROM and full strength.

Avoiding Pitfalls

If concomitant pathology, such as rotator cuff tearing or biceps tendon damage, is present and the patient is older than 40 years, biceps tenodesis should be strongly considered for definitive management. Several technical points are vital to a properly positioned and secure SLAP repair. The ASP must be localized with a spinal needle to attain the optimal position for the cannula and subsequent anchor pathway. Ensuring that the drill guide passes posterior to the biceps, sits medial to the glenoid articular surface, is angled 45° to the superior glenoid rim, and aims toward the center of the glenoid helps avoid

entering the spinoglenoid notch and potentially damaging the suprascapular nerve. It is important to maintain proper drill orientation, and the drilling step must be well visualized. If the angle is too steep or too posterior, anchor malpositioning or skiving can occur and may cause injury to the suprascapular nerve in the spinoglenoid notch. When metal or biocomposite anchors are used, the anchor must be seated well below the bone surface to avoid any anchor prominence that could abrade the humeral head cartilage. Posterior and anterior suture limbs must be passed separately through the superior labrum in a simple vertical stitch configuration, with the post and knot maintained superior and medial to avoid potential humeral head abrasion. When the sutures are tied, the appropriate amount of tension should be placed to just indent the tissues. Overtightening of the biceps anchor creates nonphysiologic torsion or translation of the superior labrum and may lead to a poor outcome. To prevent recurrence of paralabral cysts, they can be decompressed and unroofed, or marsupialized, on the capsular side of the labrum, and secure biceps anchor fixation must be achieved. To avoid internal rotation contracture, a neutral rotation or even a 15° external rotation sling must be used postoperatively.

Bibliography

Alpert JM, Wuerz TH, O'Donnell TF, Carroll KM, Brucker NN, Gill TJ: The effect of age on the outcomes of arthroscopic repair of type II superior labral anterior and posterior lesions. *Am J Sports Med* 2010;38(11):2299-2303.

Altchek DW, Warren RF, Wickiewicz TL, Ortiz G: Arthroscopic labral debridement: A three-year follow-up study. *Am J Sports Med* 1992;20(6):702-706.

Andrews JR, Carson WG Jr, McLeod WD: Glenoid labrum tears related to the long head of the biceps. *Am J Sports Med* 1985;13(5):337-341.

Baldini T, Snyder RL, Peacher G, Bach J, McCarty E: Strength of single- versus double-anchor repair of type II SLAP lesions: A cadaveric study. *Arthroscopy* 2009;25(11):1257-1260.

Barber A, Field LD, Ryu R: Biceps tendon and superior labrum injuries: Decision-marking. *J Bone Joint Surg Am* 2007;89(8):1844-1855.

Bigliani LU, Dalsey RM, McCann PD, April EW: An anatomical study of the suprascapular nerve. *Arthroscopy* 1990;6(4):301-305.

Boileau P, Parratte S, Chuinard C, Roussanne Y, Shia D, Bicknell R: Arthroscopic treatment of isolated type II SLAP lesions: Biceps tenodesis as an alternative to reinsertion. *Am J Sports Med* 2009;37(5):929-936.

Brockmeier SF, Voos JE, Williams RJ III, et al; Hospital for Special Surgery Sports Medicine and Shoulder Service: Outcomes after arthroscopic repair of type-II SLAP lesions. *J Bone Joint Surg Am* 2009;91(7):1595-1603.

Cooper DE, Arnoczky SP, O'Brien SJ, Warren RF, DiCarlo E, Allen AA: Anatomy, histology, and vascularity of the glenoid labrum: An anatomical study. *J Bone Joint Surg Am* 1992;74(1):46-52.

Cordasco FA, Steinmann S, Flatow EL, Bigliani LU: Arthroscopic treatment of glenoid labral tears. *Am J Sports Med* 1993;21(3):425-431.

Denard PJ, Lädermann A, Burkhart SS: Long-term outcome after arthroscopic repair of type II SLAP lesions: Results according to age and workers' compensation status. *Arthroscopy* 2012;28(4):451-457.

Denard PJ, Lädermann A, Parsley BK, Burkhart SS: Arthroscopic biceps tenodesis compared with repair of isolated type II SLAP lesions in patients older than 35 years. *Orthopedics* 2014;37(3):e292-e297.

DePalma AF: *Surgery of the Shoulder,* ed 3. Philadelphia, PA, JB Lippincott, 1983, p 58.

DiRaimondo CA, Alexander JW, Noble PC, Lowe WR, Lintner DM: A biomechanical comparison of repair techniques for type II SLAP lesions. *Am J Sports Med* 2004;32(3):727-733.

Domb BG, Ehteshami JR, Shindle MK, et al: Biomechanical comparison of 3 suture anchor configurations for repair of type II SLAP lesions. *Arthroscopy* 2007;23(2):135-140.

Ek ET, Shi LL, Tompson JD, Freehill MT, Warner JJ: Surgical treatment of isolated type II superior labrum anterior-posterior (SLAP) lesions: Repair versus biceps tenodesis. *J Shoulder Elbow Surg* 2014;23(7):1059-1065.

Enad JG, Gaines RJ, White SM, Kurtz CA: Arthroscopic superior labrum anterior-posterior repair in military patients. *J Shoulder Elbow Surg* 2007;16(3):300-305.

Handelberg F, Willems S, Shahabpour M, Huskin JP, Kuta J: SLAP lesions: A retrospective multicenter study. *Arthroscopy* 1998;14(8):856-862.

Ide J, Maeda S, Takagi K: Sports activity after arthroscopic superior labral repair using suture anchors in overhead-throwing athletes. *Am J Sports Med* 2005;33(4):507-514.

Jin W, Ryu KN, Kwon SH, Rhee YG, Yang DM: MR arthrography in the differential diagnosis of type II superior labral anteroposterior lesion and sublabral recess. *AJR Am J Roentgenol* 2006;187(4):887-893.

Kim SH, Ha KI, Kim SH, Choi HJ: Results of arthroscopic treatment of superior labral lesions. *J Bone Joint Surg Am* 2002;84(6):981-985.

Kim SJ, Kim SH, Lee SK, Lee JH, Chun YM: Footprint contact restoration between the biceps-labrum complex and the glenoid rim in SLAP repair: A comparative cadaveric study using pressure-sensitive film. *Arthroscopy* 2013;29(6):1005-1011.

Maffet MW, Gartsman GM, Moseley B: Superior labrum-biceps tendon complex lesions of the shoulder. *Am J Sports Med* 1995;23(1):93-98.

Morgan CD, Burkhart SS, Palmeri M, Gillespie M: Type II SLAP lesions: Three subtypes and their relationships to superior instability and rotator cuff tears. *Arthroscopy* 1998;14(6):553-565.

Morgan RJ, Kuremsky MA, Peindl RD, Fleischli JE: A biomechanical comparison of two suture anchor configurations for the repair of type II SLAP lesions subjected to a peel-back mechanism of failure. *Arthroscopy* 2008;24(4):383-388.

Nam EK, Snyder SJ: The diagnosis and treatment of superior labrum, anterior and posterior (SLAP) lesions. *Am J Sports Med* 2003;31(5):798-810.

Neuman BJ, Boisvert CB, Reiter B, Lawson K, Ciccotti MG, Cohen SB: Results of arthroscopic repair of type II superior labral anterior posterior lesions in overhead athletes: Assessment of return to preinjury playing level and satisfaction. *Am J Sports Med* 2011;39(9):1883-1888.

O'Brien SJ, Allen AA, Coleman SH, Drakos MC: The trans-rotator cuff approach to SLAP lesions: Technical aspects for repair and a clinical follow-up of 31 patients at a minimum of 2 years. *Arthroscopy* 2002;18(4):372-377.

Oh JH, Kim SH, Lee HK, Jo KH, Bae KJ: Trans-rotator cuff portal is safe for arthroscopic superior labral anterior and posterior lesion repair: Clinical and radiological analysis of 58 SLAP lesions. *Am J Sports Med* 2008;36(10):1913-1921.

Onyekwelu I, Khatib O, Zuckerman JD, Rokito AS, Kwon YW: The rising incidence of arthroscopic superior labrum anterior and posterior (SLAP) repairs. *J Shoulder Elbow Surg* 2012;21(6):728-731.

Park JY, Chung SW, Jeon SH, Lee JG, Oh KS: Clinical and radiological outcomes of type 2 superior labral anterior posterior repairs in elite overhead athletes. *Am J Sports Med* 2013;41(6):1372-1379.

Patterson BM, Creighton RA, Spang JT, Roberson JR, Kamath GV: Surgical trends in the treatment of superior labrum anterior and posterior lesions of the shoulder: Analysis of data from The American Board of Orthopaedic Surgery Certification Examination Database. *Am J Sports Med* 2014;42(8):1904-1910.

Provencher MT, McCormick F, Dewing C, McIntire S, Solomon D: A prospective analysis of 179 type 2 superior labrum anterior and posterior repairs: Outcomes and factors associated with success and failure. *Am J Sports Med* 2013;41(4):880-886.

Rao AG, Kim TK, Chronopoulos E, McFarland EG: Anatomical variants in the anterosuperior aspect of the glenoid labrum: A statistical analysis of seventy-three cases. *J Bone Joint Surg Am* 2003;85(4):653-659.

Silberberg JM, Moya-Angeler J, Martín E, Leyes M, Forriol F: Vertical versus horizontal suture configuration for the repair of isolated type II SLAP lesion through a single anterior portal: A randomized controlled trial. *Arthroscopy* 2011;27(12):1605-1613.

Sileo MJ, Lee SJ, Kremenic IJ, et al: Biomechanical comparison of a knotless suture anchor with standard suture anchor in the repair of type II SLAP tears. *Arthroscopy* 2009;25(4):348-354.

Smith DK, Chopp TM, Aufdemorte TB, Witkowski EG, Jones RC: Sublabral recess of the superior glenoid labrum: Study of cadavers with conventional nonenhanced MR imaging, MR arthrography, anatomic dissection, and limited histologic examination. *Radiology* 1996;201(1):251-256.

Snyder SJ, Banas MP, Karzel RP: An analysis of 140 injuries to the superior glenoid labrum. *J Shoulder Elbow Surg* 1995;4(4):243-248.

Snyder SJ, Karzel RP, Del Pizzo W, Ferkel RD, Friedman MJ: SLAP lesions of the shoulder. *Arthroscopy* 1990;6(4):274-279.

Stephenson DR, Hurt JH, Mair SD: Rotator cuff injury as a complication of portal placement for superior labrum anterior-posterior repair. *J Shoulder Elbow Surg* 2012;21(10):1316-1321.

Uggen C, Wei A, Glousman RE, et al: Biomechanical comparison of knotless anchor repair versus simple suture repair for type II SLAP lesions. *Arthroscopy* 2009;25(10):1085-1092.

Vangsness CT Jr, Jorgenson SS, Watson T, Johnson DL: The origin of the long head of the biceps from the scapula and glenoid labrum: An anatomical study of 100 shoulders. *J Bone Joint Surg Br* 1994;76(6):951-954.

Vogel LA, Moen TC, Macaulay AA, et al: Superior labrum anterior-to-posterior repair incidence: A longitudinal investigation of community and academic databases. *J Shoulder Elbow Surg* 2014;23(6):e119-e126.

Warner JP, Krushell RJ, Masquelet A, Gerber C: Anatomy and relationships of the suprascapular nerve: Anatomical constraints to mobilization of the supraspinatus and infraspinatus muscles in the management of massive rotator-cuff tears. *J Bone Joint Surg Am* 1992;74(1):36-45.

Weber SC, Martin DF, Seiler JG III, Harrast JJ: Superior labrum anterior and posterior lesions of the shoulder: Incidence rates, complications, and outcomes as reported by American Board of Orthopedic Surgery. Part II candidates. *Am J Sports Med* 2012;40(7):1538-1543.

Williams MM, Snyder SJ, Buford D Jr: The Buford complex: The "cord-like" middle glenohumeral ligament and absent anterosuperior labrum complex. A normal anatomic capsulolabral variant. *Arthroscopy* 1994;10(3):241-247.

Yoo JC, Ahn JH, Lee SH, et al: A biomechanical comparison of repair techniques in posterior type II superior labral anterior and posterior (SLAP) lesions. *J Shoulder Elbow Surg* 2008;17(1):144-149.

Yung PS, Fong DT, Kong MF, et al: Arthroscopic repair of isolated type II superior labrum anterior-posterior lesion. *Knee Surg Sports Traumatol Arthrosc* 2008;16(12):1151-1157.

Video Reference

Getelman M, Gillette B: Video. *Type 2 SLAP Repair.* Van Nuys, CA, 2015

Chapter 18

Biceps Tenodesis: Arthroscopic Considerations and Fixation Options

Gregory A. Erickson, MD

Robert T. Burks, MD

 ## Introduction

Pathology related to the long head of the biceps tendon, including tendinitis, partial tearing, biceps instability, and superior labrum anterior to posterior (SLAP) tears, is a common cause of shoulder pain. These disorders can often be managed nonsurgically with activity modifications, NSAIDs, physical therapy, and/or corticosteroid injections into the glenohumeral joint or into the sheath of the long head of the biceps tendon. However, when symptoms are not relieved with nonsurgical management, surgery is often required. Surgical management options for pathology related to the long head of the biceps tendon include biceps tenotomy, arthroscopic biceps tenodesis, and open subpectoral biceps tenodesis. Proximal arthroscopic biceps tenodesis techniques and fixation options are discussed herein.

 ## Case Presentation

A 43-year-old man presents with a 1-year history of recurrent, persistent pain in the left shoulder. Two years earlier, he had undergone arthroscopic SLAP repair. He now localizes his pain to the deep, anterior shoulder and states that it is aggravated by activities that involve reaching overhead or behind his back. He had previously undergone nonsurgical treatment that included activity modification, NSAIDs, and physical therapy without marked improvement in his symptoms. He reports having experienced temporary, near-complete pain relief after an ultrasound-guided corticosteroid injection into the glenohumeral joint.

Physical examination reveals full shoulder range of motion and strength with tenderness to palpation over the long head of the biceps tendon. Positive

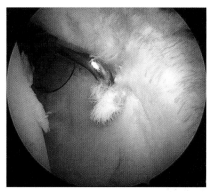

Figure 1 Arthroscopic view of the left shoulder from the posterior portal demonstrates failed repair of a superior labrum anterior to posterior lesion.

results are elicited on the Speed, Yergason, O'Brien, and crank tests. Radiographs of the shoulder are unremarkable, and MRI demonstrates a tear of the superior labrum and increased fluid around the long head of the biceps tendon. After discussion of nonsurgical and surgical treatment options, the patient elects to proceed with surgery.

Left shoulder arthroscopy revealed a failed SLAP repair (**Figure 1**). Because of the patient's age and preoperative symptoms, the decision was made to proceed with arthroscopic biceps tenodesis with interference screw fixation.

After diagnostic arthroscopy was performed, an 18-gauge spinal needle

Dr. Burks or an immediate family member has received royalties from and serves as an unpaid consultant to Arthrex; is a member of a speakers' bureau or has made paid presentations on behalf of Mitek Sports Medicine; serves as a paid consultant to Mitek Sports Medicine and VirtaMed; has received research or institutional support from DePuy Synthes; and serves as a board member, owner, officer, or committee member of the American Shoulder and Elbow Surgeons and the Arthroscopy Association of North America. Neither Dr. Erickson nor any immediate family member has received anything of value from or has stock or stock options held in a commercial company or institution related directly or indirectly to the subject of this chapter.

was placed percutaneously into the glenohumeral joint through the bicipital groove. At this anterolateral location, a No. 11 blade was used to create a portal and open the rotator interval. A cannula was introduced, and two locking sutures were placed into the biceps tendon. A loose suture from the previous SLAP repair was removed, and a tenotomy of the biceps was performed at its insertion into the superior labrum (**Figure 2**). The biceps tendon was exteriorized out the anterolateral incision (**Figure 3**), and a No. 2 braided composite suture whipstitch was placed into the tendon. A cannula was reintroduced into the anterolateral portal, and a guide pin for

the interference screw was placed into the bicipital groove distally. The guide pin was overdrilled with a 6.5-mm drill bit to a depth of 20 mm. After the guide pin was removed, the hole was cleaned with electrocautery and smoothed with a shaver (**Figure 4, A**). The sutures from the biceps tendon were passed into a 7-mm biocomposite suture anchor. The biceps tendon was advanced into the hole (**Figure 4, B**) and secured into position with the screw (**Figure 4, C**).

The patient followed the prescribed postoperative rehabilitation protocol and progressed as expected. By 10 weeks postoperatively, he was pain free and was cleared to begin biceps strengthening

exercises. He returned to all activities without recurrence of symptoms.

Indications

Frequently, disorders associated with pathology of the long head of the biceps tendon or biceps anchor can be managed nonsurgically. However, if nonsurgical management fails to relieve symptoms, surgical treatment can be considered.

Indications for surgical management include partial-thickness tendon tears involving more than 25% to 50% of the tendon diameter (**Figure 5**), medial subluxation of the long head of the biceps tendon, or dislocation of the long head of the biceps tendon associated with a tear of the subscapularis tendon or biceps pulley/sling (**Figure 6**). Relative indications for surgery include type IV SLAP tears, symptomatic type II SLAP tears (**Figure 7**), failed SLAP repair, and chronic pain secondary to long head of the biceps tendinitis that has not responded to nonsurgical management.

Controversies and Alternative Approaches

Surgical alternatives to manage symptomatic pathology of the long head

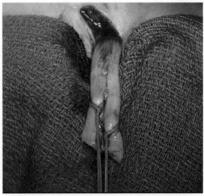

Figure 2 Arthroscopic view of the left shoulder from the posterior portal demonstrates the appearance of a biceps anchor after tenotomy and removal of sutures that had been placed during a previous repair of a superior labrum anterior to posterior lesion.

Figure 3 Intraoperative photograph shows the exteriorized biceps tendon after tenotomy with two looped tag sutures in place before placement of the whipstitch.

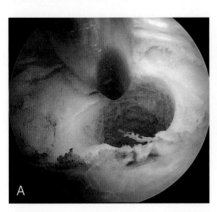
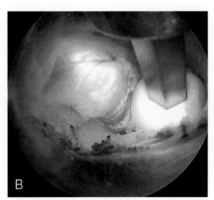
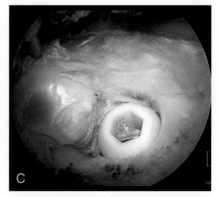

Figure 4 Arthroscopic views of the left shoulder from the lateral portal demonstrate the humeral bone socket with a bevel on the distal cortical rim (**A**), placement of the biceps tenodesis interference screw fixation (**B**), and the completed biceps tenodesis with an interference screw (**C**).

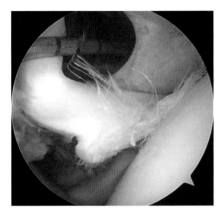

Figure 5 Arthroscopic view of a right shoulder from the posterior portal demonstrates a partial tear of the long head of the biceps tendon.

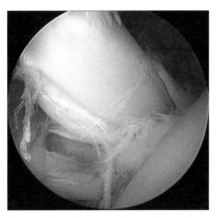

Figure 6 Arthroscopic view of a right shoulder from the posterior portal demonstrates a partial tear of the subscapularis tendon with medial subluxation of the long head of the biceps tendon.

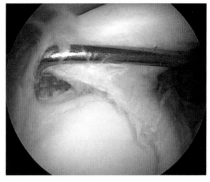

Figure 7 Arthroscopic view of a right shoulder from the posterior portal demonstrates a type II superior labrum anterior to posterior tear.

of the biceps tendon include arthroscopic débridement, arthroscopic tenotomy, and arthroscopic or open subpectoral biceps tenodesis. The preferred surgical treatment remains controversial.

Biceps Tenotomy Versus Biceps Tenodesis

Pathology related to the long head of the biceps tendon is most commonly managed with biceps tenotomy or biceps tenodesis. Biceps tenotomy can be performed relatively simply and quickly, leading to predictable pain relief without the need for substantial postoperative rehabilitation. As a result, patients typically experience a quicker return to activities and a decreased risk for postoperative stiffness.

However, biceps tenotomy has been associated with the development of a cosmetic deformity, muscle cramping, fatigue pain, and a decrease in elbow flexion or supination power. The so-called Popeye deformity is reported to occur in 3% to 70% of patients after biceps tenotomy and can be an unappealing result for patients concerned about the cosmetic appearance of the arm. The potential loss of supination strength may be a concern for patients who work as laborers and may be more important in the dominant arm.

To decrease the possibility of these unwanted outcomes, biceps tenodesis has been recommended over biceps tenotomy because it establishes an appropriate length of the biceps to avoid muscle atrophy, preserves elbow function, and provides better cosmetic results. However, biceps tenodesis has some disadvantages compared with biceps tenotomy. Biceps tenodesis is technically more challenging, requires increased surgical time as well as more substantial postoperative restrictions, and has an added cost of implants for tendon fixation. In addition, it has the potential for pain at the tenodesis site and/or failure of the tenodesis to heal.

Although biceps tenotomy has been associated with a higher incidence of the Popeye deformity, muscle cramping, and fatigue pain, studies comparing biceps tenotomy with biceps tenodesis have not identified statistically significant differences in functional outcomes or patient satisfaction scores. Thus, the decision to perform biceps tenodesis versus biceps tenotomy should take into account patient factors such as age, work, physical activity level, arm dominance, and cosmetic concerns. In general, tenotomy is reserved for patients who are older than 60 years, do not work as laborers, are unlikely to be dissatisfied with cosmetic

changes, or are unwilling or unable to comply with postoperative restrictions. Biceps tenodesis is preferred for younger or active patients, especially those who may be concerned about the cosmetic appearance of the arm.

SLAP Tears: Repair Versus Tenodesis

SLAP tears are commonly managed with arthroscopic repair using suture anchors. However, inconsistent results have been reported after SLAP repair, with good or excellent outcomes ranging from 40% to 94%, and with 22% to 75% of overhead athletes returning to their previous level of play. Furthermore, in studies in which SLAP repair is compared with biceps tenodesis, improved patient satisfaction scores and higher rates of return to previous levels of sports participation are reported in patients who underwent biceps tenodesis. Biceps tenodesis also has been reported to be effective in the management of failed SLAP repairs, with most patients obtaining satisfactory results and returning to previous levels of sports activity.

On the basis of these studies, the indications for SLAP repair are dwindling, and biceps tenodesis is becoming the preferred management method for many SLAP tears. The authors of a 2011 study suggest SLAP repair only for type II SLAP tears in patients younger than

40 years who have a history of acute trauma, physical examination and MRI findings consistent with a SLAP tear, and no arthroscopic evidence of biceps pathology or other relevant pathology. If these criteria are not met, biceps tenodesis is their treatment of choice.

Tenodesis Location

Historically, in arthroscopic biceps tenodesis techniques, the long head of the biceps tendon was secured proximal to the bicipital groove or within the proximal aspect of the bicipital groove. Although these techniques typically result in good outcomes, some patients continue to experience pain localized to the bicipital groove, and high revision rates for proximal arthroscopic tenodesis have been reported. Persistent pain after proximal arthroscopic tenodesis may occur secondary to inflammation of retained tendon in the bicipital groove, which may be eliminated with the use of a more distal tenodesis location.

To eliminate groove pain, some studies have advocated open subpectoral biceps tenodesis over arthroscopic tenodesis. However, the authors of one study described a technique in which biceps tenodesis can be performed arthroscopically distal to the bicipital groove in a suprapectoral location. In a review of 17 patients undergoing arthroscopic biceps tenodesis, 2 of 5 patients who underwent tenodesis in the upper one-half of the bicipital groove had persistent pain at the tenodesis site 12 months after the procedure, whereas none of the 12 patients in the suprapectoral group (tenodesis in the lower groove or humeral shaft) had pain at 12-month follow-up. These results suggest that a more distal tenodesis may decrease the incidence of postoperative pain at the bicipital groove and can still be performed arthroscopically.

The largest series of biceps tenodesis in the literature was published in 2015. This study of 1,083 patients who underwent arthroscopic proximal biceps tenodesis at the articular margin revealed a low overall surgical revision rate (4.1%) as well as a low rate of residual pain and statistically significant improvement in objective shoulder outcome scores. These results are in contrast to those of studies that suggest the bicipital sheath is a substantial source of shoulder pain, which, left unaddressed, is likely to result in persistent shoulder pain and the need for revision surgery. Furthermore, the authors of the 2015 study prefer biceps tenodesis at the articular margin rather than lower in the groove or in the subpectoral position for many reasons, including ease of the procedure, the ability to incorporate the biceps tenodesis construct in the repair of concomitant rotator cuff tears, more reproducible tensioning of the long head of the biceps tendon, and the relative lack of substantial intraoperative or postoperative complications.

Controversy persists regarding the ideal location for biceps tenodesis, and clinical evidence is insufficient to support one location over another. Thus, the choice of proximal, suprapectoral, or subpectoral biceps tenodesis should be guided by the surgeon's preference.

Method of Fixation

Fixation options for arthroscopic biceps tenodesis include soft-tissue fixation, in which the long head of the biceps tendon is sutured to surrounding soft tissues; osseous fixation, in which the tendon is secured to bone with suture anchors; and intraosseous fixation, in which the tendon is secured in a bone tunnel using an interference screw or sutures.

Results of biomechanical studies have been mixed. In some studies, interference screw fixation has been reported to have a higher load to failure compared with suture anchor fixation and to be less resistant to displacement under cyclic loading compared with fixation in a bone tunnel with sutures. In other studies, no statistically significant difference in ultimate load to failure or cyclic displacement has been reported between suture anchor and interference screw fixation. The authors of a 2014 study described an intraosseous suture fixation technique that was superior to interference screw fixation in terms of ultimate failure load.

Results

The clinical outcomes of biceps tenodesis are summarized in **Table 1**. Clinical data are available to support each of the fixation options previously discussed. However, bony fixation has been shown to be superior to soft-tissue fixation in terms of clinical outcome scores and structural integrity of the tenodesis construct. Clinical evidence is insufficient to recommend one form of bony fixation over another.

Technical Keys to Success

Many surgical techniques have been described for arthroscopic biceps tenodesis. These techniques can generally be divided into three categories: soft-tissue fixation, osseous fixation with bone anchors, and intraosseous fixation with an interference screw.

A thorough history and physical examination must be performed preoperatively to diagnose pathology related to the long head of the biceps tendon and to assess for concomitant pathology. Imaging studies, including plain radiographs and MRI, may help confirm the diagnosis and identify associated pathology that may need to be addressed at the time of the surgical procedure.

The setup, positioning, and initial steps of each of the techniques are similar. Each technique can be performed in the beach-chair or lateral decubitus position. For all three techniques, the authors of this chapter prefer the

Table 1 Clinical Outcomes After Biceps Tenodesis

Authors	Journal (Year)	Technique (No. of Patients)	Outcomes	Failure Rate	Comments
Boileau et al	*Arthroscopy* (2002)	Arthroscopic biceps tenodesis with an interference screw (43)	Mean Constant score improved from 43 to 79 Biceps strength on the affected side was 90% of that on the contralateral side (range, 80%-100%)	4.7%	Good clinical results were reported
Elkousy et al	*Orthopedics* (2005)	Percutaneous intra-articular transtendon technique (11)	All patients had postoperative biceps strength equal to that on the contralateral side All patients were satisfied with outcome	0	Use of this technique (soft-tissue tenodesis) resulted in pain relief, an increase in or maintenance of level of strength and function, and no cosmetic deformity
Boileau et al	*Am J Sports Med* (2009)	Arthroscopic biceps tenodesis with an interference screw (15) or SLAP lesion repair (10) for management of type II SLAP lesions	Mean Constant score improved from 59 to 89 after biceps tenodesis and from 65 to 83 after SLAP repair	No revision surgery required for tenodesis group In SLAP repair group, 4 patients (40%) required revision surgery	93% satisfaction rate and 87% return to previous level of sports after biceps tenodesis 40% satisfaction rate and 20% return to previous level of sports after SLAP repair Mean age of tenodesis group was 52 yr (range, 28-64 yr) Mean age of SLAP repair group was 37 yr (range, 19-57 yr) Authors concluded that arthroscopic biceps tenodesis can be an effective alternative for repair of a type II SLAP lesion
Lutton et al	*Clin Orthop Relat Res* (2011)	Arthroscopic biceps tenodesis with an interference screw: upper bicipital groove tenodesis (5) or suprapectoral tenodesis (12)	Mean ASES score improved from 49 to 78 Mean Constant-Murley score improved from 58 to 81	0	Study compared proximal and distal (suprapectoral) arthroscopic biceps tenodesis locations 2 patients treated with upper groove tenodesis had persistent pain at 1-yr follow-up All patients treated with suprapectoral tenodesis were asymptomatic at 1-yr follow-up Authors concluded that a more distal tenodesis location may decrease the incidence of persistent postoperative pain at the bicipital groove

ASES = American Shoulder and Elbow Surgeons shoulder outcome, LHB = long head of the biceps, NR = not reported, ROM = range of motion, SANE = Single Assessment Numeric Evaluation, SLAP = superior labrum anterior to posterior, SST = Simple Shoulder Test, UCLA = University of California–Los Angeles Shoulder Rating Scale, VAS = visual analog scale, VR-36 = Veterans RAND 36-Item Health Survey.

[a] The authors of the study reported their results based on all patients initially treated rather than on the number in each group who completed clinical follow-up.

Table 1 Clinical Outcomes After Biceps Tenodesis (continued)

Authors	Journal (Year)	Technique (No. of Patients)	Outcomes	Failure Rate	Comments
Scheibel et al	Am J Sports Med (2011)	Arthroscopic soft-tissue tenodesis (24) or arthroscopic bony fixation anchor tenodesis (20)	Mean values after soft-tissue tenodesis and after bony fixation tenodesis, respectively: Constant scores, 75 and 78.3 (no significant difference); LHB scores, 80.9 and 91.8 ($P < 0.05$); examiner-dependent evaluation of cosmetic deformity, 8.1 points and 11.2 points ($P < 0.05$) On radiographic evaluation, distalization of the LHB was more common after soft-tissue tenodesis than after bony fixation tenodesis ($P < 0.05$)	NR	Authors recommended bony fixation over soft-tissue fixation because clinical and structural outcomes were better after bony fixation
Werner et al	Am J Sports Med (2014)	Arthroscopic suprapectoral biceps tenodesis with an interference screw (27) or open subpectoral biceps tenodesis with an interference screw (35)[a]	Mean values after arthroscopic tenodesis and after open tenodesis, respectively: Constant-Murley scores, 90.7 and 91.8; ASES scores, 90.1 and 88.4; SANE scores, 87.4 and 86.8; SST scores, 10.4 and 10.6; LHB scores, 91.6 and 93.6; VR-36 scores, 81.0 and 80.1	0	Minimum follow-up of 2 yr No significant differences in clinical outcome measures, ROM, or strength Postoperative stiffness was reported by 3 of 32 patients treated with arthroscopic tenodesis and 3 of 50 patients treated with open tenodesis (9.4% and 6%, respectively) All ROM deficits in both groups resolved with intra-articular corticosteroid injections Authors concluded that both techniques yield excellent clinical and functional results for the management of isolated superior labrum or LHB lesions
Brady et al	Arthroscopy (2015)	Arthroscopic proximal biceps tenodesis with an interference screw (1,083)	Mean VAS pain score (1,083 patients) improved from 6.47 to 1.08 ($P < 0.0001$) Mean UCLA score (928 patients) improved from 14.88 to 30.09 ($P < 0.0001$) Mean SST score (642 patients) improved from 2.72 to 10.21 ($P < 0.0001$)	4.1% overall revision rate (44 of 1,083 patients) 0.4% rate of revision related to biceps tenodesis (4 of 1,083 patients)	No postoperative nerve injuries or humeral fractures Authors concluded that arthroscopic biceps tenodesis performed at the articular margin results in a low surgical revision rate, a low rate of residual pain, and significant improvement in objective outcome scores

ASES = American Shoulder and Elbow Surgeons shoulder outcome, LHB = long head of the biceps, NR = not reported, ROM = range of motion, SANE = Single Assessment Numeric Evaluation, SLAP = superior labrum anterior to posterior, SST = Simple Shoulder Test, UCLA = University of California–Los Angeles Shoulder Rating Scale, VAS = visual analog scale, VR-36 = Veterans RAND 36-Item Health Survey.

[a] The authors of the study reported their results based on all patients initially treated rather than on the number in each group who completed clinical follow-up.

beach-chair position unless a procedure to manage concomitant arthroscopic instability is being performed, in which case the lateral decubitus position is preferred.

Technique 1: Soft-Tissue Fixation

- When the beach-chair position is used, the authors of this chapter typically place the affected arm in a sterile limb holder.
- When the lateral decubitus position is used, the arm should be placed in 30° to 45° of abduction with longitudinal traction. If a technique that requires exteriorization of the tendon will be used, removal of traction and flexion of the elbow may be required to allow for adequate excursion of the tendon.
- After the affected shoulder and upper extremity are positioned, they are prepped and draped in a typical sterile fashion.
- A standard posterior portal is established, after which an anterior portal is created.
- Pump pressure is maintained at 50 mm Hg.
- Diagnostic arthroscopic examination of the glenohumeral joint, including visualization of the intra-articular and proximal extra-articular segments of the long head of the biceps tendon, is performed.
- Pulling the tendon into the joint with a probe can increase visualization of the extra-articular segment.
- Concomitant shoulder pathology, such as a rotator cuff tear, is noted and appropriately managed.
- In this arthroscopic biceps tenodesis technique, described in 2003 and termed the percutaneous intra-articular transtendon technique, the biceps tendon is fixed to the rotator interval tissue.
- An 18-gauge spinal needle is introduced percutaneously near

the anterolateral acromial border through the bicipital groove and into the glenohumeral joint, where it is used to pierce the biceps tendon just proximal to its exit from the glenohumeral joint.
- A No. 1 polydioxanone monofilament suture is shuttled through the spinal needle and retrieved through the anterior portal.
- A second No. 1 polydioxanone monofilament suture is passed percutaneously through the biceps tendon adjacent to the first suture with the use of a spinal needle.
- These two polydioxanone monofilament sutures are then used to pull a No. 2 braided, nonabsorbable suture through the biceps tendon.
- The braided, nonabsorbable suture is tied to one strand of polydioxanone monofilament suture and is pulled from the percutaneous anterolateral puncture wound through the biceps tendon and out the anterior cannula.
- The end of the permanent suture that was pulled out the anterior cannula is then tied to the second polydioxanone monofilament suture and is pulled through the biceps tendon and out the anterolateral puncture wound. This technique creates a mattress suture, which will be used to secure the biceps tendon to the rotator interval.
- Using the same technique, a second No. 2 braided, nonabsorbable suture of different color is passed through the biceps tendon.
- After the biceps tendon is secured with the two nonabsorbable sutures, the biceps tendon is transected proximal to the sutures with the use of arthroscopic scissors, a biter, or electrocautery.
- The remnant biceps anchor stump is débrided down to the superior labrum.
- The arthroscope is then placed into the subacromial space.

- A lateral portal is created, and a subacromial bursectomy is performed to allow for adequate visualization.
- Alternatively, the subacromial bursectomy can be performed before the sutures are passed. Performing the bursectomy first may ease the identification of the sutures in the subacromial space and eliminate the risk of inadvertently cutting the sutures during the bursectomy.
- After the braided, nonabsorbable sutures are identified in the subacromial space, they are pulled out the lateral portal.
- The braided, nonabsorbable sutures are then sequentially tied with the use of standard arthroscopic knot-tying techniques, securing the biceps tendon to the rotator interval.
- The arthroscopic portals are then closed according to the surgeon's preferred method.

Technique 2: Osseous Fixation With Bone Anchors

- The setup, positioning, and initial steps of the technique are similar to those previously described for soft-tissue fixation.
- After diagnostic arthroscopy is performed, an 18-gauge spinal needle is introduced percutaneously near the anterolateral acromial border through the bicipital groove into the glenohumeral joint, where it is used to pierce the biceps tendon.
- One end of a No. 1 polydioxanone or similar suture is then passed through the spinal needle and pulled out the anterior portal to tag the biceps tendon.
- A second tag stitch can be placed if desired.
- After the biceps tendon is secured with the tag sutures, the tendon is transected at its superior labral attachment with the use of arthroscopic scissors, a biter, or electrocautery.

- Alternatively, tendon transection can be delayed until after the tendon has been secured with suture anchors. Delaying the release of the biceps tendon will keep the tendon in its anatomic location, ensuring maintenance of the correct length and tension of the long head of the biceps tendon.
- The arthroscope is moved to the subacromial space, and a lateral portal is created.
- A bursectomy is performed to allow for adequate visualization of the subacromial and anterolateral subdeltoid space.
- A spinal needle or probe is used to localize the biceps tendon at the surgeon's preferred tenodesis location.
- Arthroscopic scissors or electrocautery is used to incise the bicipital sheath, exposing the biceps tendon and bicipital groove.
- The bicipital groove is cleared of soft tissue at the tenodesis site with electrocautery and is lightly decorticated with a motorized shaver or burr.
- A double-loaded suture anchor is inserted at the tenodesis site, and the four suture limbs are passed through the biceps tendon with a suture-passing device, creating two mattress sutures.
- Each suture set is then sequentially tied using standard arthroscopic knot-tying techniques.
- Alternatively, a self-cinching lasso-loop stitch or other locking knot configuration can be used. After fixation of the tendon, the proximal portion of the tendon is excised.
- Knotless suture anchors can be used instead of standard suture anchors.
- When a knotless suture anchor is used, the biceps tendon is tenotomized at its insertion on the superior labrum and is exteriorized through the anterolateral skin

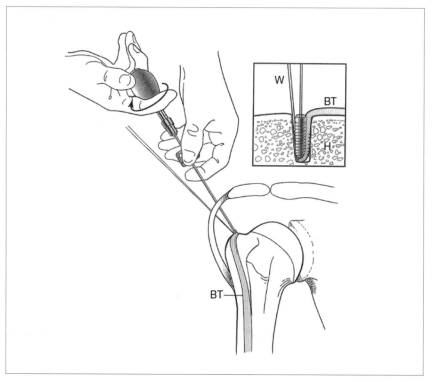

Figure 8   Illustration depicts proximal arthroscopic biceps tenodesis with an interference screw. BT = biceps tendon, H = humerus, W = whipstitch. (Reproduced with permission from Lo IK, Burkhart SS: Arthroscopic biceps tenodesis using a bioabsorbable interference screw. *Arthroscopy* 2004;20[1]:85-95.)

incision. The appropriate length of tendon is excised depending on the chosen tenodesis location, and a No. 2 nonabsorbable suture is whipstitched into the proximal 15 mm of the biceps tendon. A small hole for the anchor is created at the tenodesis site using the appropriate drill or punch, and the knotless suture anchor is loaded with the sutures and inserted into the hole to secure the tendon and complete the tenodesis.

- After the tenodesis is completed, the arthroscopic portals are closed according to the surgeon's preferred method.

Technique 3: Intraosseous Fixation With an Interference Screw

- The setup, positioning, and initial steps of the technique are similar

to those previously described for soft-tissue fixation.

- Several authors have described arthroscopic biceps tenodesis techniques using an interference screw (**Figure 8**).
- In a variation of these techniques, one or two traction sutures are passed through the biceps tendon using a spinal needle as previously described. The biceps tendon is then transected close to its insertion on the superior labrum with the use of arthroscopic scissors, a biter, or electrocautery, and the remnant biceps anchor stump is débrided down to the superior labrum.
- The arthroscope is then moved into the subacromial space, and an anterolateral portal is created approximately 2 to 3 cm anterior and lateral to the anterolateral corner of the acromion.

- A bursectomy is performed to allow for adequate visualization of the subacromial and anterolateral subdeltoid space.
- The traction sutures marking the biceps tendon are then identified in the subacromial space, and arthroscopic scissors or a motorized shaver is used to divide the capsular tissue of the rotator interval, exposing the biceps tendon and bicipital groove.
- The traction sutures and biceps tendon are retrieved through the anterolateral skin incision, and a hemostat is placed on the tendon at the level of the skin to prevent the tendon from retracting. The shoulder and elbow can be flexed to increase the amount of tendon excursion.
- After the tendon is extracted from the anterolateral portal, approximately 20 mm of proximal tendon is excised, depending on the chosen tenodesis location.
- The tenodesis location can be anywhere from the articular margin proximally to below the bicipital groove distally. The choice of tenodesis location will affect how much, if any, of the proximal biceps tendon needs to be excised.
- After the tendon is cut to the appropriate length, a whipstitch of No. 2 braided, nonabsorbable suture is placed on the end of the tendon for a length of approximately 15 mm, and the bulbous end of the tendon is contoured to allow for easy passage into the bone socket.
- After the tendon is sized, the sutures and tendon are allowed to fall back into the subacromial space, and a cannula is placed in the anterolateral portal.
- The tenodesis site is identified and débrided of soft issue using electrocautery to allow for easy visualization.
- The guidewire for the interference screw is inserted into the bicipital groove 10 to 15 mm below the insertion of the supraspinatus or another chosen tenodesis location.
- The bone socket is then created with a 7-, 8-, or 9-mm calibrated reamer depending on the previously measured tendon diameter, and the calibrated reamer is advanced over the guidewire to a depth of 25 mm.
- After the bone socket is created, the guidewire and reamer are removed, and sutures from the biceps tendon are retrieved through the anterolateral portal.
- The screwdriver is assembled and loaded with the appropriate interference screw. Typically, an 8-mm screw is used for an 8-mm bone tunnel.
- One limb of suture is passed through the driver and pulled tightly to secure the end of the tendon against the tip of the driver.
- The tip of the driver and tendon are then seated into the base of the bone socket, and the screw is advanced until it is flush with the cortical bone.
- After the screw has been properly seated, the sutures are retrieved through the anterolateral portal and are tied using standard arthroscopic knot-tying techniques, thus creating a secondary method of fixation.
- The arthroscopic portals are then closed according to the surgeon's preferred method.
- If biceps tenodesis is performed at the articular margin of the humeral head, the entire procedure can be visualized from the intra-articular space. In this variation, an anterolateral portal is created so that it enters the glenohumeral joint through the biceps sheath perpendicular to the biceps tendon. This portal is then used for placement of the interference screw off the articular margin of the humeral head.

Rehabilitation

The rehabilitation protocol for isolated arthroscopic biceps tenodesis is outlined in **Table 2**. Additional restrictions are often required if concomitant procedures, such as rotator cuff repair, are performed.

Avoiding Pitfalls

One of the keys to a successful arthroscopic biceps tenodesis is adequate visualization. When tenodesis is undertaken in an extra-articular location, a thorough bursectomy should be performed with the use of a motorized shaver and electrocautery. When the tenodesis is performed in the lower bicipital groove or suprapectoral location, particular attention must be given to the anterior and lateral gutters. To further aid in visualization of the bicipital groove and open the subdeltoid space, the arm is positioned in 60° of flexion, 30° of external rotation, and 30° of abduction. Shoulder flexion is the key to visualization of the subdeltoid space.

After adequate débridement of the subacromial and subdeltoid space has been performed, the bicipital groove must be identified. This identification can be accomplished by localization of the previously placed traction sutures or by palpation with a spinal needle.

When fixation methods requiring exteriorization of the biceps tendon are used, flexing the elbow and pulling on the tendon with traction sutures can increase tendon excursion. A clamp can then be placed on the tendon at the level of the skin to prevent it from retracting during placement of the whipstitch.

After the site of tenodesis fixation has been selected, electrocautery should be used to clear the soft tissue from the bone and allow visualization of the fixation site. An area approximately 1 cm in diameter should be cleared.

Table 2 Rehabilitation Protocol After Biceps Tenodesis

Postoperative Week	ROM	Strengthening	Return to Play	Comments/Emphasis
0-3	Active ROM of the hand and wrist Active ROM of the gleno-humeral joint (if no rotator cuff repair)	No resisted elbow flexion or forearm supination No lifting	May perform hand functions without biceps resistance (eg, typing)	Full-time sling wear
3-6	ROM of the hand, wrist, and shoulder is continued	No resisted elbow flexion or forearm supination	May return to driving after 5-6 wk	Wean from sling after 5-6 wk
6-10	Active ROM of the elbow is begun ROM of the hand, wrist, and shoulder is continued	Rotator cuff strengthening is begun No resisted elbow flexion or forearm supination	No sports allowed	—
≥10	ROM of the elbow, wrist, hand, and shoulder is continued	Biceps strengthening is begun	Gradual return to sports allowed	—

ROM = range of motion.

When placing bone tunnels or suture anchors, drilling should be perpendicular to the humerus, taking care to ensure placement in a unicortical manner. After drilling is completed, the cortical rim of the tunnel can be gently smoothed with a burr to facilitate passage of the tendon. The authors of this chapter recommend placing a small notch or bevel on the inferior cortical edge of the tunnel. This notch provides a resting place for the tendon, which helps prevent the tendon from wrapping around the interference screw as it is inserted.

One common cause of revision after biceps tenodesis is inadequate restoration of the length-tension relationship of the long head of the biceps tendon. This length-tension relationship is easily maintained with techniques that fix the tendon in its anatomic location, such as soft-tissue tenodesis or suture anchor fixation that is performed before tenotomy.

Restoring the anatomic length-tension relationship of the long head of the biceps tendon can be more challenging with interference screw fixation techniques requiring exteriorization of the tendon. One option is to place the interference screw at the top of the bicipital groove, adjacent to the articular margin of the humeral head. At this location, no resection of the tendon is required because the length of tendon remaining after tenotomy corresponds with the depth of the interference screw socket.

Alternatively, interference screw fixation can be performed in a more distal location with biceps tenodesis systems that do not require exteriorization of the tendon. In this technique, the biceps tendon is stabilized with a spinal needle before tenotomy, and in situ tenodesis is performed.

Bibliography

Boileau P, Krishnan SG, Coste JS, Walch G: Arthroscopic biceps tenodesis: A new technique using bioabsorbable interference screw fixation. *Arthroscopy* 2002;18(9):1002-1012.

Boileau P, Parratte S, Chuinard C, Roussanne Y, Shia D, Bicknell R: Arthroscopic treatment of isolated type II SLAP lesions: Biceps tenodesis as an alternative to reinsertion. *Am J Sports Med* 2009;37(5):929-936.

Brady PC, Narbona P, Adams CR, et al: Arthroscopic proximal biceps tenodesis at the articular margin: Evaluation of outcomes, complications, and revision rate. *Arthroscopy* 2015;31(3):470-476.

Burns JP, Bahk M, Snyder SJ: Superior labral tears: Repair versus biceps tenodesis. *J Shoulder Elbow Surg* 2011; 20(2 suppl):S2-S8.

David TS, Schildhorn JC: Arthroscopic suprapectoral tenodesis of the long head biceps: Reproducing an anatomic length-tension relationship. *Arthrosc Tech* 2012;1(1):e127-e132.

Denard PJ, Dai X, Hanypsiak BT, Burkhart SS: Anatomy of the biceps tendon: Implications for restoring physiological length-tension relation during biceps tenodesis with interference screw fixation. *Arthroscopy* 2012;28(10):1352-1358.

Elkousy HA, Fluhme DJ, O'Connor DP, Rodosky MW: Arthroscopic biceps tenodesis using the percutaneous, intra-articular trans-tendon technique: Preliminary results. *Orthopedics* 2005;28(11):1316-1319.

Gartsman GM, Hammerman SM: Arthroscopic biceps tenodesis: Operative technique. *Arthroscopy* 2000;16(5):550-552.

Lafosse L, Van Raebroeckx A, Brzoska R: A new technique to improve tissue grip: "The lasso-loop stitch." *Arthroscopy* 2006;22(11):1246.e1-1246.e3.

Lo IK, Burkhart SS: Arthroscopic biceps tenodesis using a bioabsorbable interference screw. *Arthroscopy* 2004;20(1):85-95.

Lutton DM, Gruson KI, Harrison AK, Gladstone JN, Flatow EL: Where to tenodese the biceps: Proximal or distal? *Clin Orthop Relat Res* 2011;469(4):1050-1055.

Mazzocca AD, Bicos J, Santangelo S, Romeo AA, Arciero RA: The biomechanical evaluation of four fixation techniques for proximal biceps tenodesis. *Arthroscopy* 2005;21(11):1296-1306.

McCormick F, Nwachukwu BU, Solomon D, et al: The efficacy of biceps tenodesis in the treatment of failed superior labral anterior posterior repairs. *Am J Sports Med* 2014;42(4):820-825.

Nho SJ, Strauss EJ, Lenart BA, et al: Long head of the biceps tendinopathy: Diagnosis and management. *J Am Acad Orthop Surg* 2010;18(11):645-656.

Romeo AA, Mazzocca AD, Tauro JC: Arthroscopic biceps tenodesis. *Arthroscopy* 2004;20(2):206-213.

Sampatacos N, Getelman MH, Henninger HB: Biomechanical comparison of two techniques for arthroscopic suprapectoral biceps tenodesis: Interference screw versus implant-free intraosseous tendon fixation. *J Shoulder Elbow Surg* 2014;23(11):1731-1739.

Sanders B, Lavery KP, Pennington S, Warner JJ: Clinical success of biceps tenodesis with and without release of the transverse humeral ligament. *J Shoulder Elbow Surg* 2012;21(1):66-71.

Scheibel M, Schröder RJ, Chen J, Bartsch M: Arthroscopic soft tissue tenodesis versus bony fixation anchor tenodesis of the long head of the biceps tendon. *Am J Sports Med* 2011;39(5):1046-1052.

Sekiya JK, Elkousy HA, Rodosky MW: Arthroscopic biceps tenodesis using the percutaneous intra-articular trans-tendon technique. *Arthroscopy* 2003;19(10):1137-1141.

Werner BC, Evans CL, Holzgrefe RE, et al: Arthroscopic suprapectoral and open subpectoral biceps tenodesis: A comparison of minimum 2-year clinical outcomes. *Am J Sports Med* 2014;42(11):2583-2590.

Chapter 19

Open Subpectoral Biceps Tenodesis: Surgical Tips to Safely Restore Function and Cosmesis

Mandeep S. Virk, MD

Peter N. Chalmers, MD

Chris R. Mellano, MD

Anthony A. Romeo, MD

 ## Introduction

The anatomy of the long head of the biceps (LHB) is unique. In its proximal part, the LHB tendon is fixed at its site of origin, and after a brief intra-articular course (approximately 3 cm), it is again relatively anchored in the bicipital groove for approximately 3 to 4 cm. This fixation of the proximal part of the LHB at two sites in the setting of extensive mobility of the glenohumeral joint predisposes the LHB tendon to excessive wear and tear stress. Although its functional importance remains the subject of debate, the LHB tendon is well accepted as an important source of anterior shoulder pain. The LHB tendon can be affected by trauma in association with superior labrum anterior to posterior (SLAP) tears or rupture of the LHB, instability associated with subscapularis and supraspinatus tears, intrinsic degeneration, inflammation, and fibrosis or scarring in the rotator interval, which

is often encountered postoperatively or with chronic rotator cuff pathology. Because LHB tendon pathology often occurs concomitantly with other pathology in the shoulder joint, determining the role of the LHB tendon in a patient's pain can be challenging. Clinical tests for LHB pathology are neither sensitive nor specific. Diagnostic injection into the biceps tendon sheath in the bicipital groove can be helpful, but the best corroborative and diagnostic test is arthroscopic examination of the intra-articular and intertubercular portion of the LHB tendon.

Initial management of LHB pathology is nonsurgical and includes activity modification, anti-inflammatory medications, ice, corticosteroid injection, and therapy modalities such as deep friction massage, iontophoresis, and phonophoresis. Continued pain and dysfunction despite a 3-month trial of nonsurgical management is an indication for surgical management.

 ## Case Presentation

A 37-year-old, right-hand–dominant woman who works as a yoga instructor has a long-standing history of atraumatic right anterior shoulder pain. The shoulder pain is exacerbated by certain yoga poses, activities of daily living involving overhead lifting, and swimming. Several rounds of physical therapy, acupuncture, use of an electrical stimulation unit, NSAIDs, and other medications are unsuccessful.

On physical examination, the patient has tenderness to palpation in the bicipital groove region and positive Speed and Yergason test results. Shoulder range of motion, strength testing of the rotator cuff, subacromial impingement signs, and neurovascular examination findings are normal. Plain radiographs do not demonstrate any notable abnormality (**Figure 1, A** through **C**). Magnetic resonance arthrography performed at an outside facility does not demonstrate rotator cuff or superior labrum tears (**Figure 1, D**).

The patient is initially treated with two ultrasonographically guided injections of cortisone and local anesthetic into the bicipital sheath, both of which temporarily provide 100% symptom relief. After a lengthy discussion of

Dr. Romeo or an immediate family member has received royalties from Arthrex; is a member of a speakers' bureau or has made paid presentations on behalf of Arthrex; serves as a paid consultant to Arthrex; has received research or institutional support from Arthrex, DJO, Ōssur, and Smith & Nephew; and serves as a board member, owner, officer, or committee member of the American Orthopaedic Society for Sports Medicine and the American Shoulder and Elbow Surgeons. None of the following authors or any immediate family member has received anything of value from or has stock or stock options held in a commercial company or institution related directly or indirectly to the subject of this chapter: Dr. Virk, Dr. Chalmers, and Dr. Mellano.

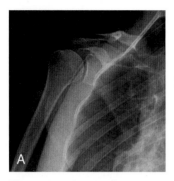 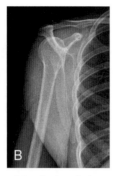 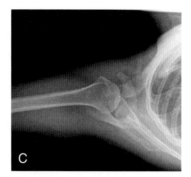 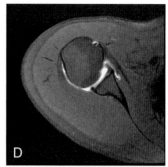

Figure 1   Images from a 37-year-old right-hand–dominant woman who works as a yoga instructor and has a long-standing history of atraumatic right anterior shoulder pain. AP (**A**), scapular Y (**B**), and axillary (**C**) radiographs and an axial T2-weighted magnetic resonance arthrogram (**D**) demonstrate no notable abnormality.

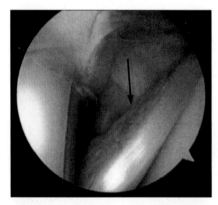

Figure 2   Arthroscopic view of the right shoulder of the same patient described in Figure 1 obtained from the posterior portal demonstrates erythema in the intra-articular and intertubercular part of the long head of the biceps tendon (arrow).

the risks and benefits, the patient undergoes a glenohumeral diagnostic arthroscopy, which demonstrates erythema and inflammatory changes in the intra-articular and intertubercular part of the LHB tendon (**Figure 2**). No superior labrum or subscapularis tears are present. Tenotomy of the LHB tendon is performed intra-articularly and followed by mini-open subpectoral biceps tenodesis. Postoperatively, the patient reports complete relief of her pain and symptoms and is able to return without limitation to her occupation, yoga, and activities of daily living.

Indications

When the pathology is limited to the LHB tendon, mini-open subpectoral biceps tenodesis is indicated in patients following failed nonsurgical management of LHB tendinitis, partial tears of the LHB tendon (>25% to 50%), chronic tendinitis of the LHB tendon or subluxation of the LHB tendon, spontaneous rupture of the LHB tendon with continued pain, and cramping in the arm. Patients with LBH tendon pathology in the presence of other shoulder pathology may require rotator cuff repair or SLAP repair (revision or type IV). Soft-tissue tenodesis or tenotomy of the LHB tendon is also performed as a concomitant procedure through the deltopectoral approach, above the pectoralis major, when performing open reduction and internal fixation of proximal humerus fractures or shoulder arthroplasty.

Controversies and Results

No consensus has been reached on the optimal surgical management of LHB tendon pathology. Substantial debate exists regarding the procedure type (tenotomy versus tenodesis), the anatomic location of tenodesis (suprapectoral versus subpectoral), the type of implant used for tenodesis, and the use

of open versus arthroscopic techniques for LHB tenodesis.

Insufficient high-quality evidence is available in the literature to recommend tenotomy versus tenodesis of the LHB as the ideal strategy for management of LHB pathology. Tenotomy of the LHB relieves pain by preventing traction insult to the inflamed or degenerated biceps tendon. Proponents of LHB tenotomy suggest that it is a simple, safe procedure that consistently relieves pain, allows quicker rehabilitation than does tenodesis, and does not require an additional skin incision. However, clinical studies have demonstrated that patients with LHB tenotomy have higher rates of biceps cramping, Popeye deformity, and weakness in elbow flexion and supination strength testing. Tenodesis provides a new fixation anchor in the proximal humerus for the LHB tendon after tenotomy and thus maintains the length-tension relationship and reduces the risk of Popeye deformity, biceps cramping, muscle weakness, and fatigue (**Table 1**). However, complications such as proximal humerus fracture, infection, loss of fixation, neurovascular injuries, reflex sympathetic dystrophy, and hardware-related complications are rare but known complications associated with LHB tenodesis. A randomized controlled trial comparing LHB tenotomy and tenodesis for lesions of the LHB is under way and is expected

Table 1 Results of Tenodesis of the Long Head of the Biceps Tendon

Authors	Journal (Year)	Technique (No. of Patients)	Outcomes	Failure Rate[a] (%)	Comments
Boileau et al	*Arthroscopy* (2002)	Arthroscopic biceps tenodesis with interference screw (43)	Significant improvement in Constant score (*P* < 0.05)	4.6 (Popeye deformity)	Level IV case series Mean follow-up, 1.4 yr No neurologic or vascular complications 4 patients had temporary reflex sympathetic dystrophy Biceps tenosynovitis (4), prerupture (15), subluxation (11), dislocation (13)
Mazzocca et al	*Am J Sports Med* (2008)	Open subpectoral biceps tenodesis with interference screw (50; 9 lost to follow-up)	Significant improvements in ASES, SST, Constant-Murley, and SANE scores Mean ASES and SST scores were higher in patients without concomitant RCR	2 (Popeye deformity)	Level IV case series Mean follow-up, 2.4 yr Clinical and arthroscopic findings of biceps pathology Concomitant RCR (24), rotator cuff or glenohumeral débridement and SAD (8), SLAP tear repair (1), Bankart repair (1), DCE and SAD (4), glenohumeral débridement and SAD (2)
Millett et al	*BMC Musculoskelet Disord* (2008)	Open subpectoral biceps tenodesis with interference screw (34) or suture anchor (54)	Significant improvements in ASES, VAS, and Constant scores (*P* < 0.0001)	0	Level IV case series Mean follow-up, 1.1 yr 1 patient treated with an interference screw and 4 patients treated with suture anchor had persistent bicipital groove pain Biceps tenosynovitis, partial tear (>50%), biceps tendon subluxation Concomitant RCR (64), SAD (41), capsular reconstruction (8), DCE (12)
Nho et al	*Arthroscopy* (2010)	Open subpectoral biceps tenodesis with interference screw (17; 4 lost to follow-up)	Significant improvements in VAS, ASES, and SST scores (*P* < 0.001)	NR	Level IV case series Mean follow-up, 2.9 yr Biceps instability (subluxation) in setting of rotator cuff tears Concomitant arthroscopic RCR (17)
Nho et al	*J Shoulder Elbow Surg* (2010)	Open subpectoral biceps tenodesis with interference screw (353)	Study of complications found a 2% complication rate (Popeye deformity, 0.57%; deep infection, 0.28%; bicipital pain, 0.57%; musculocutaneous neuropathy, 0.28%; reflex sympathetic dystrophy, 0.28%)	NR	Level IV case series Mean follow-up, 2.3 yr Concomitant RCR, SAD, capsular release, DCE, SLAP tear repair

ASES = American Shoulder and Elbow Surgeons shoulder outcome, DCE = distal clavicle excision, NR = not reported, RCR = rotator cuff repair, SAD = subacromial decompression, SANE = Single Assessment Numerical Evaluation, SLAP = superior labrum anterior to posterior, SST = Simple Shoulder Test, UCLA = University of California–Los Angeles Shoulder Rating Scale, VAS = visual analog scale.

[a] Failure rate is defined as anatomic failure of the tenodesis.

to provide level I evidence to establish clinical guidelines for the management of LHB pathology. The senior author of this chapter (A.A.R.) suggests that older, sedentary patients and those with low functional demands are ideal candidates for LHB tenotomy.

The LHB tenodesis procedure can be performed proximally (in the bicipital groove, soft-tissue tenodesis to the rotator cuff or the conjoint tendon) or distally (in the bicipital groove at the

Table 1 Results of Tenodesis of the Long Head of the Biceps Tendon (*continued*)

Authors	Journal (Year)	Technique (No. of Patients)	Outcomes	Failure Rate[a] (%)	Comments
Lee et al	*J Shoulder Elbow Surg* (2014)	Arthroscopic proximal biceps tenodesis with suture anchor (84)	Significant improvements in ASES, Constant, and VAS scores (*P* < 0.01)	NR	Level IV retrospective case series Mean follow-up, 2.8 yr Complications were Popeye deformity (11 clinical and 15 radiographic) and biceps cramping pain (6) Biceps tears (79.5%), SLAP tears (36.4%), tenosynovitis (4.5%), subluxation (19.3%) Concomitant RCR (96.4%), SAD (75%), calcific material removal (2.3%), microfracture (1.1%), DCE (11.4%)
McCormick et al	*Am J Sports Med* (2014)	Open subpectoral biceps tenodesis with interference screw (46; 4 lost to follow-up)	Significant improvements in ASES, SANE, and Western Ontario Shoulder Instability Index scores (*P* < 0.0001)	NR	Level IV case series Mean follow-up, 3.5 yr 1 patient had musculocutaneous neurapraxia Failed SLAP tear repair
Werner et al	*Am J Sports Med* (2014)	Arthroscopic proximal biceps tenodesis with interference screw (32) Open subpectoral biceps tenodesis with interference screw (50)	No significant difference in outcome scores (ASES, SST, SANE, and Constant-Murley) between open and arthroscopic groups	NR	Level III study Mean follow-up, 3.1 yr 6 patients had postoperative stiffness SLAP tears, partial or complete long head of the biceps tendon tears, tenosynovitis, subluxation
Brady et al	*Arthroscopy* (2015)	Arthroscopic proximal biceps tenodesis with interference screw (1,083)	Significant improvements in UCLA, SST, and pain scores (*P* < 0.0001)	NR	Level IV case series Mean follow-up, 2.6 yr 1 patient required revision for biceps pain 3 patients required revision for Popeye deformity Biceps tendinitis, tears (43%), instability (44.1%), type II SLAP tears (16%) Concomitant RCR (84.5%), SAD (59.1%), acromioplasty (48.3%), coracoplasty (24.5%) capsular release (12.8%), DCE (28.2%)

ASES = American Shoulder and Elbow Surgeons shoulder outcome, DCE = distal clavicle excision, NR = not reported, RCR = rotator cuff repair, SAD = subacromial decompression, SANE = Single Assessment Numerical Evaluation, SLAP = superior labrum anterior to posterior, SST = Simple Shoulder Test, UCLA = University of California–Los Angeles Shoulder Rating Scale, VAS = visual analog scale.

[a] Failure rate is defined as anatomic failure of the tenodesis.

level of the inferior border of the pectoralis major). No high-quality evidence is available to support or recommend one surgical technique over the other. Proponents of distal fixation suggest that removal of the entire LHB tendon allows the surgeon to avoid residual bicipital groove pain originating from the intertubercular part of the LHB tendon, which may be scarred or inflamed.

Several techniques and implants are available for tenodesis of the LHB tendon. Bone tunnels and keyhole techniques anchor the tendon to the bone but do not require the use of implants. Similarly, soft-tissue tenodesis to the short head of the biceps, conjoint tendon, pectoralis major, or rotator cuff does not require an implant for fixation. Alternately, tenodesis of the LHB tendon to bone can be done with the use of an interference screw, a cortical button, or a suture anchor. Both arthroscopic and open techniques have been described with good outcomes. No high-quality evidence is available to recommend one technique over the other. Several controlled laboratory studies have compared the biomechanical properties of various implants for tenodesis of the LHB tendon. These studies have demonstrated that the interference screw offers excellent pullout strength, decreased tendon excursion with cyclic loading, and comparable or superior results in terms of cyclic and maximum load to failure compared with other fixation methods such as suture anchors, unicortical intramedullary buttons, bicortical buttons, or hybrid techniques. However, high-quality clinical outcome data to recommend one method of fixation over the other are not available.

The authors of this chapter prefer mini-open biceps tenodesis because it results in an acceptable cosmetic incision, allows better appreciation of anatomy with minimum dissection through the musculotendinous structures, facilitates reproduction of the length-tension relationship of the LHB tendon with the use of available surrounding landmarks (inferior border of the pectoralis major, musculotendinous junction of the LHB tendon), provides reproducible relief of pain with a low incidence of bicipital groove pain, and is technically less demanding than the arthroscopic techniques.

Video 19.1 Open Biceps Subpectoral Tenodesis: Operative Tips to Safely Restore Function and Cosmesis. Anthony A. Romeo, MD; Mandeep S. Virk, MD (4 min)

Technical Keys to Success

Setup/Exposure
- Before the induction of anesthesia, a preoperative antibiotic is administered.

- Either general or regional anesthesia or both are used, depending on the surgeon's preference and whether LHB tenodesis is being performed as an isolated procedure or as part of a rotator cuff repair or instability repair.
- The skin is infiltrated with local anesthetic and epinephrine before the incision is made and also at the end of the procedure to provide analgesia and maintain hemostasis. A regional (interscalene) block usually does not completely cover this part of the arm.
- Mini-open biceps tenodesis can be performed with the patient in the supine, modified beach-chair, or lateral position.
- When open subpectoral biceps tenodesis is performed for the management of isolated LHB pathology, the patient should be positioned supine with the head and the back of the bed raised to approximately 30°. The arm is usually placed in 30° to 45° of abduction. The authors of this chapter prefer to place the arm on a padded Mayo stand, but the use of an arm positioner is an acceptable alternative.
- When the mini-open subpectoral biceps tenodesis is performed as part of a rotator cuff repair or instability procedure, the beach-chair or lateral position should be modified for the subpectoral biceps tenodesis part of the procedure. If the patient is initially in the beach-chair position, the head end of the bed should be lowered to approximately 30°. If the patient is initially in the lateral position, the surgeon should deflate the beanbag and have the circulating assistant pull the sheet underneath the patient from across the table opposite to the surgeon to bring the patient into a more supine position in a controlled manner.

Procedure
ARTHROSCOPIC EVALUATION AND LHB TENOTOMY
- An examination under anesthesia is performed to assess for signs of restriction of range of motion or abnormal translation.
- Diagnostic arthroscopy of the glenohumeral joint is performed through a standard posterior portal.
- The biceps tendon is initially evaluated with no fluid pressure to avoid compressing the inflamed synovial vessels, which can hinder the surgeon's observation of any inflammation of the tendon where it enters the joint.
- A standard anterior portal is made in the rotator interval using either the inside-out or the outside-in method.
- An arthroscopic probe is used to palpate the insertion of the biceps anchor and assess for any tears or detachment.
- The probe is placed on top of the intra-articular part of the LHB tendon to pull it down and deliver the intertubercular portion of the LHB tendon into the glenohumeral joint; this method allows the surgeon to observe any erythema or structural lesions (**Figure 2**). Findings that indicate a diseased tendon include alteration of the surface architecture in the form of fraying, thickening, or surface irregularity, and partial tears or complete tears of the tendon.
- In addition to the biceps tendon, the supraspinatus and subscapularis tendons are evaluated.
- Tenotomy of the diseased LHB tendon is performed through the anterior portal using an arthroscopic cutting instrument (basket or scissor) or a radiofrequency ablation device. The tenotomy is performed slightly lateral to the superior labrum to avoid cutting into it.
- A stable base is fashioned by

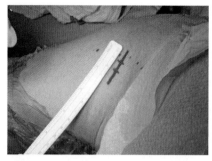

Figure 3 Photograph shows the planned incision for mini-open subpectoral biceps tenodesis. The dashed line indicates the inferior border of the pectoralis major.

débriding the proximal portion of the tendon with a shaver until the tendon stump is confluent with the remaining labral tissue.

MINI-OPEN SUBPECTORAL BICEPS TENODESIS

- The lower border of the pectoralis major muscle is identified as it travels toward the humeral shaft and forms the anterior axillary fold. Placement of the arm in abduction facilitates identification of the lower border of the pectoralis major tendon (**Figure 3**).
- The skin is infiltrated with a mixture of local anesthesia and epinephrine.
- A 3-cm skin incision is made over the humerus along the Langer lines at the junction of the anterior axillary fold and the arm. This incision is typically located approximately at an acute angle to the lower border of the pectoralis major tendon and provides excellent cosmesis. However, the incision can be made closer to the axilla for better cosmesis or can be placed more laterally in patients with compromised axillary hygiene.
- Alternatively, a longitudinal incision can be made over the humerus extending 1 cm above and 2 cm below the lower border of the pectoralis major insertion.

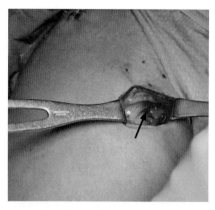

Figure 4 Photograph shows the inferior border of the pectoralis major as visualized during deep dissection (arrow).

- This region contains a substantial amount of adipose tissue. A self-retaining retractor can be placed for improved visualization.
- Hemostasis is achieved with electrocautery.
- The underlying deep fascia is identified and entered with a dissecting scissor to expose the inferior border of the pectoralis major muscle.
- Care should be taken not to create false planes through the substance of the pectoralis major muscle during deep dissection. The pectoralis major muscle runs obliquely in a medial to lateral direction (**Figure 4**). If muscle fibers can be seen running vertically, they are either the deltoid, which indicates that the dissection is too lateral, or the muscles associated with the conjoint tendon, which indicate that the dissection is too medial and distal.
- A band of deep fascia is released laterally to free the inferior border of the pectoralis major muscle laterally and gain extra mobility.
- The conjoint tendon protects the musculocutaneous nerve and the more medial neurovascular bundle. The radial nerve is behind the medial part of the tendon of the latissimus dorsi and teres major almost at the level of the musculocutaneous

nerve. It is critical to use a broad, blunt-tip retractor (Chandler) to avoid penetrating the conjoint or the latissimus dorsi tendon.

RETRIEVAL OF THE LHB TENDON AFTER TENOTOMY

- The LHB tendon is identified in contact with the undersurface of the pectoralis major muscle.
- The pectoralis muscle is retracted superiorly and laterally with an Army-Navy retractor (**Figure 4**). Care should be taken not to place this retractor too deep on the undersurface of the pectoralis major because doing so can trap the LHB tendon and make visualization of the tendon difficult.
- Blunt finger dissection is performed to release the adhesions between the LHB tendon in the bicipital groove.
- After the LHB tendon is freed, it can be retrieved out of the wound with right-angled hemostat forceps or finger dissection (**Figure 5**).
- Occasionally, after spontaneous rupture of the LHB or failure of the tenodesis, the tendon can retract distally and may require a longer and more distal incision for retrieval.

PREPARATION OF THE LHB TENDON

- Approximately 6 to 8 cm of the LHB tendon is delivered out of the wound and débrided of any loose areolar tissue or unhealthy tendon tissue around the musculotendinous junction.
- The authors of this chapter prefer to use a high-strength No. 2 loop suture to run whip stitches through the tendon for a length of approximately 2 cm proximally to the musculotendinous junction (**Figure 6**).
- Alternatively, a No. 2 high-strength nonabsorbable suture can be used to run Krackow stitches in the

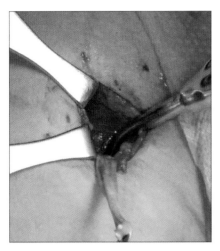

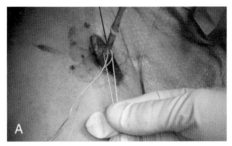

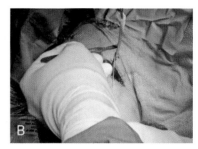

Figure 6 Photographs show preparation of the long head of the biceps tendon after tenotomy. **A,** A high-strength No. 2 loop suture is used to run whip stitches for four to five passes through the tendon for a length of approximately 2 cm proximally to the musculotendinous junction. **B,** The remainder of the long head of the biceps tendon is cut and discarded except for 5 mm proximal to the exit of the suture.

Figure 5 Photograph shows retrieval of the long head of the biceps tendon after tenotomy. The tendon is delivered out of the wound with finger extraction or the use of a right-angled hemostat forceps.

tendon, leaving a tendon stump of 5 mm proximal to the sutures. The free ends of the suture exit 2 cm proximal to the musculotendinous junction (**Figure 7**).

TENODESIS OF THE LHB TENDON
- Multiple techniques and implants are available for tenodesis of the LHB tendon at the subpectoral location. These options include keyhole tenodesis, bone tunnel tenodesis, and tenodesis with an interference screw, a suture anchor, or a cortical button. Tenodesis of the LHB tendon to surrounding soft tissue such as the pectoralis major and conjoint tendon has also been described and is more commonly performed in shoulder arthroplasty procedures.
- The authors of this chapter prefer to use a biceps tenodesis interference screw for fixation of the LHB tendon.
- Anatomic studies have demonstrated that the musculotendinous junction of the LHB tendon is located at the inferior border of the pectoralis major tendon. Therefore, the tenodesis site is selected and marked with an electrocautery

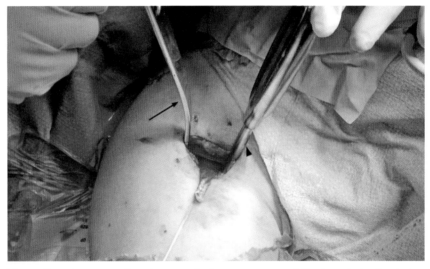

Figure 7 Intraoperative photograph shows exposure of the tenodesis site during deep dissection. A pointed Hohmann retractor (arrow) is placed proximally and laterally under the pectoralis major, and a Chandler retractor (arrowhead) is placed medially to the coracobrachialis and the short head of the biceps muscles.

device in the distal part of the bicipital groove at or slightly proximal to the level of the inferior border of the pectoralis major (**Figure 8, A**). Tenodesis at this site restores the anatomic length-tension relationship of the LHB tendon.
- A guidewire is drilled unicortically at the previously marked site on the bicipital groove of the humerus and placed against the far cortex (**Figure 8, B**).
- The guidewire is overreamed with a cannulated 8-mm drill to a depth of 15 mm. The size of the reamer and the depth of the reaming can be

altered depending on the size of the tendon and patient (**Figure 8, C**).
- The bone debris is removed, and the tunnel is tapped with a cortical tap (**Figure 8, D**).
- One end of the Krackow suture is passed through an interference screw (usually 8 × 12 mm), which is loaded onto a screwdriver using a nitinol wire (**Figure 8, E**).
- The tendon, loaded onto the screw, is pushed into the tunnel, and the screw is advanced until it is flush with the anterior cortex (**Figure 8, F and G**).
- Care must be taken to ensure that

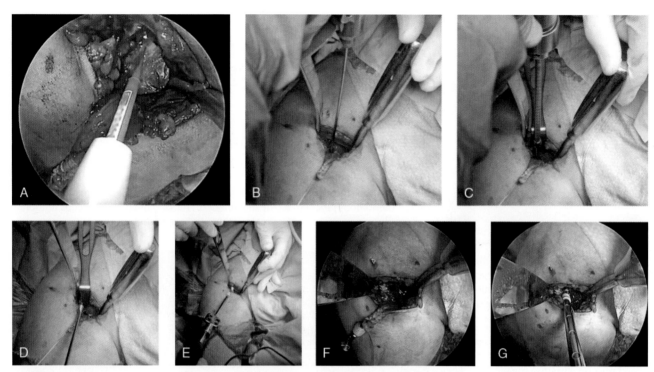

Figure 8   Images demonstrate preparation of the tenodesis site and creation of the bone tunnel. **A,** Image obtained using an arthroscopic camera through the open incision demonstrates marking of the tenodesis site in the bicipital groove at the level of or slightly proximal to the inferior border of the pectoralis major with an electrocautery device. **B,** Photograph shows drilling of a guidewire through the proximal cortex. The guidewire is placed against the opposite endosteum. **C,** Photograph shows passage of a cannulated reamer over the guidewire. **D,** Photograph shows tapping of the bone tunnel with a cortical tap. **E,** Photograph shows insertion of the interference screw with one of the limbs of the No. 2 high-strength nonabsorbable suture threaded through the interference screw. **F** and **G,** Images obtained using an arthroscopic camera through the open incision demonstrate insertion of the screw until it is flush with the cortex (**F**) and tying of the two suture limbs over the screw with square knots (**G**).

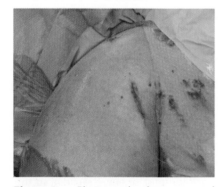

Figure 9   Photograph shows wound closure after open subpectoral biceps tenodesis.

the stump of the tendon is in the tenodesis tunnel before the screw is advanced; otherwise, the screw will not advance.

- Overadvancement of the screw should be avoided to prevent it from dropping into the medullary canal.

- The two ends of the suture are tied together over the screw. This step prevents loss of the screw in case of dislodgment.

- The extra length of the suture is cut, and the wound is irrigated.

Wound Closure

- Because the skin on the medial aspect of the arm and axilla has nociceptive fibers and is sensitive to touch and pressure, the authors of this chapter avoid the use of thin adhesive strips or cutaneous sutures because they can cause considerable discomfort postoperatively.

- The authors of this chapter use a nonabsorbable suture for closure of the deep fascia and absorbable monofilament sutures for subcutaneous and subcuticular closure.

- The incision is covered with a topical skin adhesive glue (**Figure 9**).

Rehabilitation

The rehabilitation protocol following LHB tenodesis is usually determined by the primary procedure (rotator cuff repair, instability repair). The postoperative rehabilitation for isolated LHB tenodesis is aimed at protecting the tenodesis until the tendon-bone repair is able to tolerate normal physiologic loads (**Table 2**). The LHB tendon is stretched when the elbow is extended and the forearm is pronated; therefore, during the first 3 to 4 weeks after LHB tenodesis, patients are required to use

Table 2 Rehabilitation Protocol After Isolated Tenodesis of the Long Head of the Biceps Tendon

Postoperative Week	ROM	Strengthening	Return to Play	Comments/Emphasis
0-6	Active ROM of the hand and wrist from day 1 Therapist-supervised passive ROM of the shoulder from wk 1 Active-assisted ROM of the elbow in all planes (flexion, extension, supination, and pronation) from wk 4 Active-assisted and active ROM of the shoulder and scapular retraction from wk 4	No	No	Immobilization in a shoulder immobilizer until wk 4
6-12	Active ROM of elbow in all planes (no weights) from wk 6	Isometric strengthening of shoulder and scapular muscles is begun at wk 6 Isometric biceps strengthening is begun at wk 8 to 10	No	—
12-24	—	Strengthening of the elbow is begun at wk 12 (start with elastic resistance bands and progress to the use of light weights [1 lb] and advanced strengthening)	Sports-specific rehabilitation is initiated at 3 to 4 mo Return to contact sports is allowed at 6 mo	—

ROM = range of motion.

a sling that keeps the elbow in flexion and the forearm in neutral alignment. Patients are instructed to avoid active elbow flexion, active supination of the forearm, passive stretching of the elbow, and active or passive extension of the shoulder (**Table 2**). At 4 weeks postoperatively, use of the sling is discontinued, and active-assisted followed by active range-of-motion exercises of the elbow are initiated. Submaximal isometric exercises are started at 8 to 10 weeks, and a strengthening protocol is started at 12 weeks. Patients are counseled to avoid lifting heavy objects or doing strengthening exercises with resistance until 12 weeks. Sport-specific rehabilitation is started at 3 to 4 months postoperatively. Return to collision sports is typically allowed at 6 months if all rehabilitation goals have been met.

 Avoiding Pitfalls

Identification of the lower border of the pectoralis major is key to finding the right planes for deeper dissection. To avoid damage to the medial neurovascular structures, deep dissection must be directed toward the humerus and not inferiorly toward the axilla. Staying lateral to the short head of the biceps and close to the humeral shaft prevents inadvertent damage to the musculocutaneous nerve, which runs in the substance of the short head of the biceps at this level. Excessive retraction on the medial side should be avoided for the same reason. Drilling of the humerus for interference screw fixation should be unicortical and at a right angle to the bicipital groove of the humerus. After reaming has been performed over the guidewire, the reamer should be dislodged by hand and not on power. To re-create the normal length-tension relationship of the LHB tendon, the tenodesis site should be at the level of or slightly proximal to the inferior border of the pectoralis major. The tenodesis screw should not be overadvanced and should be flush with the cortex. Overadvancement of the screw can result in loss of the screw in the intramedullary canal.

Bibliography

Amaravathi RS, Pankappilly B, Kany J: Arthroscopic keyhole proximal biceps tenodesis: A technical note. *J Orthop Surg (Hong Kong)* 2011;19(3):379-383.

Bennett WF: Specificity of the Speed's test: Arthroscopic technique for evaluating the biceps tendon at the level of the bicipital groove. *Arthroscopy* 1998;14(8):789-796.

Bicos J: Biomechanics and anatomy of the proximal biceps tendon. *Sports Med Arthrosc* 2008;16(3):111-117.

Boileau P, Baqué F, Valerio L, Ahrens P, Chuinard C, Trojani C: Isolated arthroscopic biceps tenotomy or tenodesis improves symptoms in patients with massive irreparable rotator cuff tears. *J Bone Joint Surg Am* 2007;89(4):747-757.

Boileau P, Krishnan SG, Coste J-S, Walch G: Arthroscopic biceps tenodesis: A new technique using bioabsorbable interference screw fixation. *Arthroscopy* 2002;18(9):1002-1012.

Boileau P, Neyton L: Arthroscopic tenodesis for lesions of the long head of the biceps. *Oper Orthop Traumatol* 2005;17(6):601-623.

Brady PC, Narbona P, Adams CR, et al: Arthroscopic proximal biceps tenodesis at the articular margin: Evaluation of outcomes, complications, and revision rate. *Arthroscopy* 2015;31(3):470-476.

Busconi BB, DeAngelis N, Guerrero PE: The proximal biceps tendon: Tricks and pearls. *Sports Med Arthrosc* 2008;16(3):187-194.

Curtis AS, Snyder SJ: Evaluation and treatment of biceps tendon pathology. *Orthop Clin North Am* 1993;24(1):33-43.

Delle Rose G, Borroni M, Silvestro A, et al: The long head of biceps as a source of pain in active population: Tenotomy or tenodesis? A comparison of 2 case series with isolated lesions. *Musculoskelet Surg* 2012;96(suppl 1):S47-S52.

Elser F, Braun S, Dewing CB, Giphart JE, Millett PJ: Anatomy, function, injuries, and treatment of the long head of the biceps brachii tendon. *Arthroscopy* 2011;27(4):581-592.

Fama G, Edwards TB, Boulahia A, et al: The role of concomitant biceps tenodesis in shoulder arthroplasty for primary osteoarthritis: Results of a multicentric study. *Orthopedics* 2004;27(4):401-405.

Franceschi F, Longo UG, Ruzzini L, Papalia R, Rizzello G, Denaro V: To detach the long head of the biceps tendon after tenodesis or not: Outcome analysis at the 4-year follow-up of two different techniques. *Int Orthop* 2007;31(4):537-545.

Frost A, Zafar MS, Maffulli N: Tenotomy versus tenodesis in the management of pathologic lesions of the tendon of the long head of the biceps brachii. *Am J Sports Med* 2009;37(4):828-833.

Galasso O, Gasparini G, De Benedetto M, Familiari F, Castricini R: Tenotomy versus tenodesis in the treatment of the long head of biceps brachii tendon lesions. *BMC Musculoskelet Disord* 2012;13(1):205.

Gill TJ, McIrvin E, Mair SD, Hawkins RJ: Results of biceps tenotomy for treatment of pathology of the long head of the biceps brachii. *J Shoulder Elbow Surg* 2001;10(3):247-249.

Holtby R, Razmjou H: Accuracy of the Speed's and Yergason's tests in detecting biceps pathology and SLAP lesions: Comparison with arthroscopic findings. *Arthroscopy* 2004;20(3):231-236.

Hsu AR, Ghodadra NS, Provencher MT, Lewis PB, Bach BR: Biceps tenotomy versus tenodesis: A review of clinical outcomes and biomechanical results. *J Shoulder Elbow Surg* 2011;20(2):326-332.

Hussain WM, Reddy D, Atanda A, Jones M, Schickendantz M, Terry MA: The longitudinal anatomy of the long head of the biceps tendon and implications on tenodesis. *Knee Surg Sports Traumatol Arthrosc* 2015;23(5):1518-1523.

Kelly AM, Drakos MC, Fealy S, Taylor SA, O'Brien SJ: Arthroscopic release of the long head of the biceps tendon: Functional outcome and clinical results. *Am J Sports Med* 2005;33(2):208-213.

Khazzam M, George MS, Churchill RS, Kuhn JE: Disorders of the long head of biceps tendon. *J Shoulder Elbow Surg* 2012;21(1):136-145.

Kibler WB, Sciascia AD, Hester P, Dome D, Jacobs C: Clinical utility of traditional and new tests in the diagnosis of biceps tendon injuries and superior labrum anterior and posterior lesions in the shoulder. *Am J Sports Med* 2009;37(9):1840-1847.

Koh KH, Ahn JH, Kim SM, Yoo JC: Treatment of biceps tendon lesions in the setting of rotator cuff tears: Prospective cohort study of tenotomy versus tenodesis. *Am J Sports Med* 2010;38(8):1584-1590.

Lee HI, Shon MS, Koh KH, Lim TK, Heo J, Yoo JC: Clinical and radiologic results of arthroscopic biceps tenodesis with suture anchor in the setting of rotator cuff tear. *J Shoulder Elbow Surg* 2014;23(3):e53-e60.

Lutton DM, Gruson KI, Harrison AK, Gladstone JN, Flatow EL: Where to tenodese the biceps: Proximal or distal? *Clin Orthop Relat Res* 2011;469(4):1050-1055.

Ma H, Van Heest A, Glisson C, Patel S: Musculocutaneous nerve entrapment: An unusual complication after biceps tenodesis. *Am J Sports Med* 2009;37(12):2467-2469.

Mazzocca AD, Bicos J, Santangelo S, Romeo AA, Arciero RA: The biomechanical evaluation of four fixation techniques for proximal biceps tenodesis. *Arthroscopy* 2005;21(11):1296-1306.

Mazzocca AD, Cote MP, Arciero CL, Romeo AA, Arciero RA: Clinical outcomes after subpectoral biceps tenodesis with an interference screw. *Am J Sports Med* 2008;36(10):1922-1929.

Mazzocca AD, Rios CG, Romeo AA, Arciero RA: Subpectoral biceps tenodesis with interference screw fixation. *Arthroscopy* 2005;21(7):896.

McCormick F, Nwachukwu BU, Solomon D, et al: The efficacy of biceps tenodesis in the treatment of failed superior labral anterior posterior repairs. *Am J Sports Med* 2014;42(4):820-825.

Millett PJ, Sanders B, Gobezie R, Braun S, Warner JJ: Interference screw vs. suture anchor fixation for open subpectoral biceps tenodesis: Does it matter? *BMC Musculoskelet Disord* 2008;9(1):121.

Murthi AM, Vosburgh CL, Neviaser TJ: The incidence of pathologic changes of the long head of the biceps tendon. *J Shoulder Elbow Surg* 2000;9(5):382-385.

Nho SJ, Frank RM, Reiff SN, Verma NN, Romeo AA: Arthroscopic repair of anterosuperior rotator cuff tears combined with open biceps tenodesis. *Arthroscopy* 2010;26(12):1667-1674.

Nho SJ, Reiff SN, Verma NN, Slabaugh MA, Mazzocca AD, Romeo AA: Complications associated with subpectoral biceps tenodesis: Low rates of incidence following surgery. *J Shoulder Elbow Surg* 2010;19(5):764-768.

Nho SJ, Strauss EJ, Lenart BA, et al: Long head of the biceps tendinopathy: Diagnosis and management. *J Am Acad Orthop Surg* 2010;18(11):645-656.

Osbahr DC, Diamond AB, Speer KP: The cosmetic appearance of the biceps muscle after long-head tenotomy versus tenodesis. *Arthroscopy* 2002;18(5):483-487.

Ozalay M, Akpinar S, Karaeminogullari O, et al: Mechanical strength of four different biceps tenodesis techniques. *Arthroscopy* 2005;21(8):992-998.

Patzer T, Santo G, Olender GD, Wellmann M, Hurschler C, Schofer MD: Suprapectoral or subpectoral position for biceps tenodesis: Biomechanical comparison of four different techniques in both positions. *J Shoulder Elbow Surg* 2012;21(1):116-125.

Provencher MT, LeClere LE, Romeo AA: Subpectoral biceps tenodesis. *Sports Med Arthrosc* 2008;16(3):170-176.

Richards DP, Burkhart SS: A biomechanical analysis of two biceps tenodesis fixation techniques. *Arthroscopy* 2005;21(7):861-866.

Romeo AA, Mazzocca AD, Tauro JC: Arthroscopic biceps tenodesis. *Arthroscopy* 2004;20(2):206-213.

Sentürk I, Ozalay M, Akpınar S, Leblebici B, Cınar BM, Tuncay C: Clinical and isokinetic comparison between tenotomy and tenodesis in biceps pathologies. *Acta Orthop Traumatol Turc* 2011;45(1):41-46.

Shank JR, Singleton SB, Braun S, et al: A comparison of forearm supination and elbow flexion strength in patients with long head of the biceps tenotomy or tenodesis. *Arthroscopy* 2011;27(1):9-16.

Simmen BR, Bachmann LM, Drerup S, et al: Usefulness of concomitant biceps tenodesis in total shoulder arthroplasty: A prospective cohort study. *J Shoulder Elbow Surg* 2008;17(6):921-924.

Slenker NR, Lawson K, Ciccotti MG, Dodson CC, Cohen SB: Biceps tenotomy versus tenodesis: Clinical outcomes. *Arthroscopy* 2012;28(4):576-582.

Szabó I, Boileau P, Walch G: The proximal biceps as a pain generator and results of tenotomy. *Sports Med Arthrosc* 2008;16(3):180-186.

Walch G, Edwards TB, Boulahia A, Nové-Josserand L, Neyton L, Szabo I: Arthroscopic tenotomy of the long head of the biceps in the treatment of rotator cuff tears: Clinical and radiographic results of 307 cases. *J Shoulder Elbow Surg* 2005;14(3):238-246.

Werner BC, Evans CL, Holzgrefe RE, et al: Arthroscopic suprapectoral and open subpectoral biceps tenodesis: A comparison of minimum 2-year clinical outcomes. *Am J Sports Med* 2014;42(11):2583-2590.

Wittstein JR, Queen R, Abbey A, Toth A, Moorman CT III: Isokinetic strength, endurance, and subjective outcomes after biceps tenotomy versus tenodesis: A postoperative study. *Am J Sports Med* 2011;39(4):857-865.

Video Reference

Romeo AA, Virk MS: Video. *Open Biceps Subpectoral Tenodesis: Operative Tips to Safely Restore Function and Comesis.* Chicago, IL, 2015.

Chapter 20

High-Grade Partial-Thickness Rotator Cuff Tears: Repair In Situ Versus Tear Completion and Repair

Charles M. Jobin, MD

Christopher S. Ahmad, MD

 Introduction

Partial-thickness rotator cuff tears (RCTs) are common pathologic lesions with greater prevalence in older individuals. Factors thought to contribute to the development of partial-thickness RCTs include decreased vascularity, accumulation of microtrauma from intratendinous shear stress, and internal or external impingement. Partial-thickness RCTs are more than twice as likely to be articular sided than bursal sided and commonly occur just posterior to the biceps tendon at the insertion of the rotator cuff cable (**Figure 1**). Partial articular-sided supraspinatus tendon avulsions are commonly called PASTA lesions. In athletes with internal impingement, articular-sided tears occur more posteriorly, at the confluence of the supraspinatus and the infraspinatus at the anterior margin of the bare area. These tears commonly delaminate the infraspinatus tendon into two layers and are referred to as partial articular intratendinous (PAINT) lesions. In the Ellman classification of partial-thickness RCTs, tears are graded on the basis of the thickness (grade 1, <3 mm or <25%; grade 2, 3 to 6 mm or 25% to 50%; grade

3, >6 mm or >50%) and location of the tear (articular, bursal, intratendinous). Tear size greater than 50% carries a higher risk of tear progression, and surgical treatment is indicated in these patients if 3 to 6 months of nonsurgical treatment fails.

Surgical management options for partial-thickness RCTs include tear débridement, in situ transtendon repair, intratendinous repair, and tear completion with repair. Tear etiology, patient-specific factors, favorable biology for cuff healing, and shoulder demands are important factors guiding surgical indications. Repair strategies must take into account patient and tear characteristics, and patients who are throwing athletes should be considered a distinct class. The extent of a partial tear is typically assessed quantitatively after débridement of the diseased tissue to determine the amount and location of exposed footprint and the quality of the remaining intact fibers. True avulsions of the articular-sided supraspinatus fibers are good candidates for in situ transtendon repair, whereas degenerative partial articular-sided tears with tendon attritional loss may be contraindicated for an in situ repair

because of the risk of over tensioning the articular-sided repair. These guidelines are summarized in **Table 1**. In throwing athletes, most partial-thickness RCTs do not require repair unless a laminar tear is present or the size of the tear is substantial (50% to 75% thickness). If repair to bone is performed in a throwing athlete, reattachment of the tendon to the lateral footprint should be attempted because a more medial repair may result in internal impingement at the repair site, which can jeopardize throwing performance.

 Case Presentations

Case 1: Articular-Sided Tear Managed With In Situ Transtendon Repair

A 50-year-old man who works as a laborer reports shoulder pain that is aggravated by overhead activity. A 6-month attempt at nonsurgical management consisting of physical therapy, NSAIDs, and a subacromial corticosteroid injection performed at 3 months is unsuccessful. The workup reveals a high-grade PASTA lesion. Surgical repair is indicated in this patient because of the failure of 6 months of nonsurgical treatment and the patient's high level of activity and relatively young age. Diagnostic arthroscopy reveals tearing of the undersurface of the rotator

Dr. Jobin or an immediate family member is a member of a speakers' bureau or has made paid presentations on behalf of and serves as a paid consultant to Acumed and Tornier. Dr. Ahmad or an immediate family member serves as a paid consultant to Arthrex and has received research or institutional support from Arthrex, Major League Baseball, and Stryker.

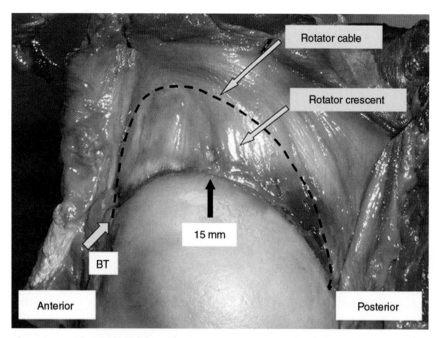

Figure 1 Photograph of a cadaver specimen demonstrates the rotator cuff cable (curved dashed line) and crescent. The rotator cuff cable bridges the anterior and posterior greater tuberosity, off-loading the crescent area and distributing load. BT = biceps tendon. (Adapted with permission from Kim HM, Dahiya N, Teefey SA, et al: Location and initiation of degenerative rotator cuff tears: An analysis of three hundred and sixty shoulders. *J Bone Joint Surg Am* 2010;92[5]:1088-1096.)

cuff (**Figure 2, A**). After débridement of the undersurface of the cuff tear, a tear of 50% of the footprint with 6 mm of exposed footprint is observed (**Figure 2, B**). The remaining bursal-sided cuff fibers appear healthy and intact. The subacromial space is entered and a bursectomy performed. No bursal-sided tear is found. An in situ transtendon repair strategy is therefore chosen, and a 4.5-mm double-loaded anchor is placed at the articular margin (**Figure 2, C**). Sutures are shuttled with the use of a spinal needle and nonabsorbable suture such that the torn articular fibers are grasped with the shuttling needle in a configuration to anatomically reduce the torn articular lamina (**Figure 2, D, E, and F**). Two suture pairs are passed through the torn tendon on the articular side (**Figure 2, F**). The sutures are retrieved and tied in simple mattress fashion in the subacromial space, reducing the torn articular tendon to the footprint (**Figure 2, G**). Intra-articular

visualization confirms anatomic repair of the articular-sided tear (**Figure 2, H**).

Case 2: Bursal-Sided High-Grade Partial Tear Managed With Completion and Repair

A 54-year-old woman who is active in competitive target archery experiences shoulder pain in the arm that draws the bowstring. The pain prevents her from competing. A 6-month course of nonsurgical management consisting of physical therapy, NSAIDs, and a subacromial corticosteroid injection performed at 3 months that alleviates most of her symptoms temporarily, is unsuccessful. The workup reveals a high-grade partial bursal-sided supraspinatus tear (**Figure 3, A**). Surgical repair is indicated in this patient because of the failure of 6 months of nonsurgical treatment and the patient's high level of activity and relatively young age. Diagnostic arthroscopy reveals tendinosis of the undersurface of the supraspinatus

(**Figure 3, B**). The subacromial space is entered, revealing a bursal-sided tear with fraying of the coracoacromial ligament indicative of subacromial impingement (**Figure 3, C**). After débridement of the bursal-sided cuff tear, the footprint is exposed, demonstrating a tear of nearly 90% with 10 mm of exposed footprint (**Figure 3, D**). Intra-articular visualization demonstrates tendinosis and fraying of the few remaining articular fibers, which are sectioned with a shaver. The tear completion technique is chosen because of the poor health of the remaining fibers and the ease of suture passage and cuff repair in a standard full-thickness fashion. The footprint is prepared for full-thickness cuff repair. A medial row anchor is placed, and sutures are passed with a shuttling instrument (**Figure 3, E**). A suture bridge construct with a lateral row anchor is used to compress the repair site and reduce the profile of the knots (**Figure 3, F**).

Case 3: Delaminating Partial-Thickness Articular-Sided Tear in a Throwing Athlete

A 26-year-old competitive baseball pitcher presents with a 2-year history of intermittent shoulder pain that has progressed and is associated with loss of pitching control, reduced velocity, and difficulty warming up. His discomfort is localized to the anterior-superior and posterior-superior shoulder during the late-cocking and acceleration phases of the throwing motion. Pain has progressed to become more intense, limiting the patient's ability to throw at the desired level and recently limiting throwing altogether. He experiences some mechanical clicking with throwing, especially during periods of pain. One year of nonsurgical treatment has failed to relieve the patient's symptoms, and the workup reveals a high-grade partial-thickness articular-sided tear (**Figure 4, A**). Surgical treatment is indicated in this patient because of the failure of

Table 1 Repair of Partial-Thickness Rotator Cuff Tears by Location and Size of Tear

Location of Tear	Percentage of Cuff Torn	Management
Articular-sided tear in patient who is not a throwing athlete	<50%	Débride partial tear and perform subacromial bursectomy; perform acromioplasty only if coracoacromial abrasion is present
	50%-75%, with healthy bursal tendon	Débride pathologic tissue; perform transtendon in situ repair to bone
	>50% with bursal tendon pathology or >75% articular tear	Perform tear completion and repair of full-thickness RCT to footprint
Bursal-sided tear	<50%	Débride partial tear and perform subacromial decompression with bursectomy; perform acromioplasty if coracoacromial abrasion is present
	50%-75%, with healthy articular tendon	Débride pathologic tissue and perform either in situ repair or repair with tear completion if the terminal tendon is deficient
	>50% with articular tendon pathology or >75% articular tear	Perform tear completion and repair of full-thickness RCT to footprint
Articular-sided tear in overhead throwing athlete	<25%	Débride pathologic frayed tissue with or without subacromial bursectomy; perform acromioplasty only if coracoacromial abrasion is present
	25%-75%	Débride pathologic tissue; perform intratendinous repair of PAINT lesion, possible transtendon repair to bone
	≥75% with healthy bursal tendon	Perform intratendinous repair of PAINT lesion, possible transtendon repair to bone
	≥75% with pathologic remaining bursal tendon	Complete and repair tear, favoring fixation at the lateral aspect of the footprint insertion
Intratendinous	<25%	Débride pathologic tissue with or without subacromial bursectomy; perform acromioplasty only if coracoacromial abrasion is present
	25%-75%	Débride pathologic tissue; perform intratendinous repair for PAINT lesion, possible transtendon repair to bone
	≥75% with healthy bursal tendon	Perform intratendinous repair of PAINT lesion, possible transtendon repair to bone
	≥75% with pathologic remaining bursal tendon	Complete and repair tear, favoring fixation at lateral aspect of footprint insertion

PAINT = partial articular intratendinous, RCT = rotator cuff tear.

1 year of nonsurgical treatment with loss of performance and radiographic imaging consistent with the decline in function. Diagnostic arthroscopy reveals a delaminating PAINT lesion with exposed footprint adjacent to the bare area and low-grade fraying of the anterior supraspinatus, which is débrided. The infraspinatus delamination is observed to be mobile and free (**Figure 4, B**). Intratendinous side-to-side repair without repair of the tendon to the bony footprint is chosen because of the internal impingement in this high-level throwing athlete. An intratendinous repair is performed with spinal-needle shuttling of two mattress sutures (**Figure 4, C**). The sutures are tied in the subacromial space (**Figure 4, D**), and intra-articular visualization confirms repair of the laminar tear (**Figure 4, E**).

 Indications

Indications for surgical treatment include failure of a course of nonsurgical management of at least 3 months' duration, including physical therapy, activity modification, NSAIDs, and corticosteroid injections. Surgical indications are based on patient factors, clinical factors, and pathologic factors. Patient factors include age, activity level, occupation, and sports involvement. Clinical factors include severity of pain, response to nonsurgical management, functional deficit, and etiology, whether traumatic or degenerative. Degenerative partial-thickness RCTs in patients older than 65 years with minimal symptoms should be managed nonsurgically. In adults with acute traumatic tears greater than 50% in thickness, early surgical intervention may be beneficial.

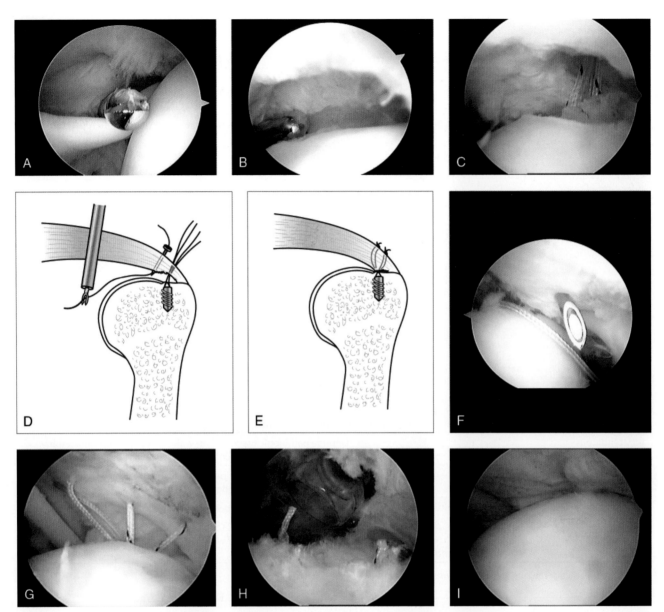

Figure 2   **A,** Arthroscopic view from the posterior portal demonstrates an articular-sided rotator cuff tear. A shaver inserted through the anterior portal is used to débride the partial-thickness tear. **B,** Arthroscopic view from the posterior portal demonstrates an articular-sided tear after débridement. The width of the tear measures 6 mm, or 50% of the footprint. **C,** Arthroscopic view from the posterior portal demonstrates transtendon anchor placement. The anchor is inserted through the bursal cuff tissue into the medial footprint. **D** and **E,** Illustrations depict repair of a partial articular-sided supraspinatus tendon avulsion (PASTA) lesion. **D,** The anchor is inserted through the bursal cuff tissue into the footprint, and a spinal needle is used to shuttle a passing suture through the retracted articular fibers. **E,** The articular lamina tear is differentially reduced to the medial footprint by tensioning and tying the sutures on the bursal surface of the cuff. **F,** Arthroscopic view from the posterior portal demonstrates suture shuttling in transtendon PASTA repair. The articular lamina is differentially reduced to the footprint by means of sutures passed through the articular lamina. **G,** Arthroscopic view from the posterior portal demonstrates transtendon PASTA repair prior to knot tying. The two suture pairs have been shuttled through the retracted articular lamina in preparation for tying in the subacromial space. **H,** Arthroscopic view from the posterior subacromial portal demonstrates the appearance of subacromial knots in transtendon repair. The sutures have been tied, reducing the articular tear to the footprint. **I,** Arthroscopic view from the posterior intra-articular portal demonstrates an articular view of a completed transtendon repair. Secure attachment of the articular tear has been confirmed.

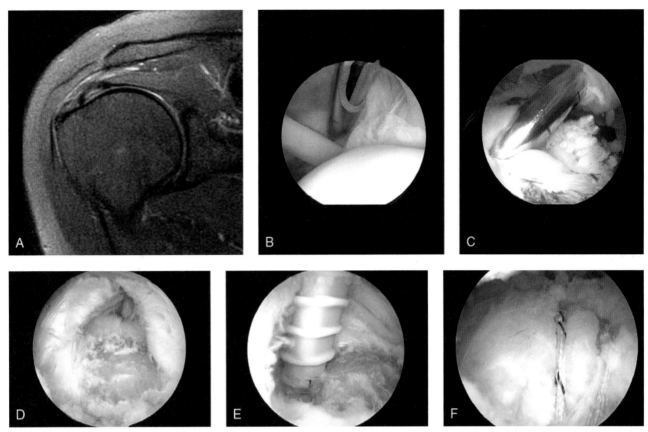

Figure 3   **A,** T2-weighted coronal MRI of a right shoulder demonstrates a partial-thickness, bursal-sided tear of the supraspinatus. **B,** Intra-articular arthroscopic view from the posterior portal demonstrates tendinosis and fraying of the articular fibers. **C,** Subacromial arthroscopic view from the posterior subacromial portal demonstrates a bursal-sided tear with fraying of the coracoacromial ligament. **D,** Arthroscopic view from the lateral subacromial portal demonstrates tear débridement from the subacromial space, which reveals unhealthy articular fibers and a bursal-sided tear of nearly 90% of the footprint. The footprint is abraded to enhance healing and the remaining unhealthy articular fibers resected. **E,** Arthroscopic view from the posterior subacromial portal demonstrates placement of a medial row anchor adjacent to the articular margin. **F,** Arthroscopic view from the lateral subacromial portal demonstrates the final suture bridge construct with compression of the tear and low-profile knots.

Pathologic factors include the tear size, location (bursal, articular, or intratendinous), and associated pathology such as subacromial impingement. The indications for surgical management of partial-thickness RCTs in overhead throwing athletes remains controversial, and repair techniques have been modified to specifically address the unique adaptations of shoulders in throwing athletes.

Controversies and Alternative Approaches

In Situ Transtendon Repair Versus Tear Completion and Repair

Transtendon repair of articular-sided partial-thickness RCTs requires recognition of the retracted articular fibers and differential reduction of the articular retracted fibers relative to the intact bursal fibers. This differential reduction can be performed with shuttling of sutures through the bursal fibers and then through the articular fibers in a more

medial location relative to the bursal suture penetration location to capture the retracted articular lamellae. Cadaver studies of articular-sided tears demonstrate that bursal fiber strain is alleviated when tears of >50% thickness are repaired. Suture anchors that penetrate the intact bursal side of the rotator cuff do not substantially weaken the intact bursal-sided tendon. In light of the biomechanical evidence and early clinical results, the authors of this chapter recommend preserving the integrity of the intact bursal rotator cuff tendon in the absence of substantial tendinosis. A study of progressive

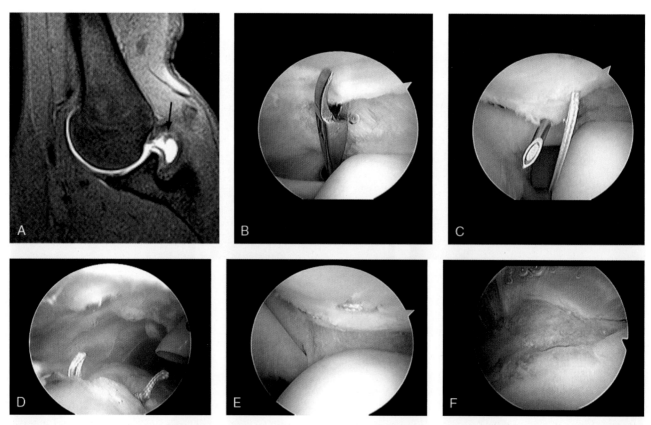

Supraspinatus

Infraspinatus

Horizontal extension into infraspinatus

Figure 4   **A,** T2-weighted coronal MRI in the abduction and external rotation view demonstrates a partial-thickness articular-sided rotator cuff tear (arrow) in a throwing athlete. **B,** Arthroscopic image from the posterior portal shows an intratendinous partial-thickness tear with retraction. The tear is grasped to observe mobility and determine the anatomic repair site. **C,** Arthroscopic image from the posterior portal shows placement of the spinal needle through both laminations of the tear for suture passing. **D,** Arthroscopic image from the posterior portal shows suture tying in the subacromial space from a lateral working portal. Arthroscopic images from the posterior portal show the final intratendinous repair (**E**) and a normal bare area between the lateral and posterior articular margin of the humeral head and the medial and posterior insertion of the rotator cuff (**F**). **G,** Illustration depicts a partial-thickness articular intratendinous lesion.

sectioning of bursal-sided fibers in cadavers demonstrated that when >50% of the bursal tendon is cut, the articular-sided fiber strain increases in a nonlinear and exponential fashion. Takedown tear completion of intact bursal fibers may similarly increase the strain on the repaired articular fibers. Tear completion and single-row repair have been found to have substantial retear rates (approximately 20%) that are greater than those of articular-sided tear takedown repairs. Suture bridge techniques may improve the integrity of the repair because they maximize the pressurized contact area of the footprint and reduce motion compared with standard single-row fixation, thereby increasing the potential for healing between the tendon and the greater tuberosity.

Suture Bridge Construct for Small Tear of the Anterior Rotator Cable

A partial tear of the anterior rotator cuff cable may increase the risk of further tear progression given the increased stress at the attachment of the anterior cable. In these patients, a transtendon repair or tear completion with increased fixation mechanics may be warranted. Double-row or anchor and marginal convergence constructs to counteract the increased forces at the anterior cable have been found to outperform less mechanically robust constructs. In contrast, a partial-thickness articular-sided crescent tear may be more amenable to a single-row transtendon repair given the anterior and posterior biomechanical stability of the intact cable.

Concomitant Acromioplasty

Concomitant acromioplasty during partial-thickness RCT repair is controversial. Theoretical advantages of acromioplasty include reduction of subacromial impingement, release of mesenchymal stem cells from the acromial bone marrow to the healing cuff, and denervation of painful bursal tissue. Successful outcomes have been described with and without acromioplasty. The authors of this chapter recommend acromioplasty in patients with evidence of acromial spurring with fraying of the coracoacromial ligament in bursal-sided tears.

Tear Repair in Throwing Athletes

Differences in anatomy and soft-tissue demands unique to throwing athletes must be considered in the choice of repair strategy. In these patients, repairing partial articular-sided tears to the exposed footprint or to the bare area will limit external rotation and abduction during the late-cocking phase of the throwing motion. This type repair will substantially affect the performance of a throwing athlete and must be avoided.

The footprint of the supraspinatus insertion typically extends approximately 12 to 14 mm in the medial-lateral direction and inserts adjacent to the articular margin. A normal bare area exists between the posterolateral humeral head

articular margin and the infraspinatus rotator cuff insertion (**Figure 4, F**). In throwing athletes, articular-sided tears with internal impingement commonly occur at this bare area (**Figure 4, G**). Therefore, tears with intralaminar extension (PAINT lesions) are commonly managed with intratendinous repair without repair directly to the tuberosity footprint to preserve full motion during throwing. Occasionally, far anterior partial detachments of the rotator cuff are repaired to the bony footprint because repair to this area of the footprint does not result in internal impingement in throwing athletes. In throwing athletes with high-grade, near-complete partial-thickness RCTs that are converted to full-thickness tears, the repair is performed to the lateral aspect of the footprint when possible to allow normal internal impingement during throwing. Repairs must also optimize fixation for accelerated rehabilitation because stiffness in a throwing athlete greatly affects performance and therefore must be avoided.

Results

Outcomes after surgical management of symptomatic partial-thickness RCTs have been reported in many studies, with encouraging results of débridement, intratendinous repair, transtendon repair to bone, and tear completion and repair (**Table 2**). The authors of a systematic review of all types of partial-thickness RCT repair found no evidence to support tear completion versus transtendon repair for tears involving >50% of the tendon because both strategies had favorable outcomes. Tear completion and repair has an 80% to 90% healing rate and more than 90% satisfaction at 1 year postoperatively in most studies. In a study published in 2012, bursal-sided tear completion and single-row repair were found to have substantial retear rates that were greater than those of

articular-sided transtendon repairs (9% and 0%, respectively). Transtendon repair techniques have similarly good outcomes, with 91% of patients feeling satisfied with surgery. Suture bridge techniques may provide improved repair integrity; in one study, no retears were reported following articular-sided tear completion and repair, and a retear rate of 9.5% was reported for bursal-sided tear completion and repair. A study of a modified transtendon repair method with a suture bridge construct demonstrated a satisfaction rate greater than 90% at 1 year postoperatively.

Results of partial-thickness RCT repair have been less successful in overhead throwing athletes than in other patients. Good results of débridement of partial-thickness RCTs in overhead throwing athletes have been reported, with most of these patients returning to competitive pitching (75%); however, only half returned to their previous level of competition. Transtendon repair techniques have had excellent outcomes in most patients, but only 30% of the athletes are able to return to their previous level of competition. In a small series, 89% of baseball players treated with intratendinous repair techniques for laminar-type partial tears were able to return to their previous level of competition or higher.

Technical Keys to Success

In Situ Transtendon Repair
SETUP/EXPOSURE
- The patient is typically placed in the beach-chair position; however, the lateral decubitus position is recommended for throwing athletes because treatment of posterior capsulolabral Bennett lesion often is required and the lesion is more easily accessed with lateral positioning.
- Either general or regional anesthesia is administered.

Table 2 Results of Surgical Management of Partial-Thickness Rotator Cuff Tears

Author(s)	Journal (Year)	Technique (No. of Patients)	Outcomes[a]	Failure Rate (%)	Comments
Ide et al	*Am J Sports Med* (2005)	Transtendon (17)	Results were good or excellent in 16 patients and fair in 1 Of 6 overhead throwing athletes treated, 2 returned to sport at the same level, 3 returned at a lower level, and 1 did not return UCLA shoulder score improved from 17 to 33	5.8	Mean patient age, 42 yr Mean follow-up, 39 mo
Waibl and Buess	*Arthroscopy* (2005)	Transtendon (22)	UCLA shoulder score improved from 17 to 31	9 (clinical)	Mean patient age, 45 yr Mean follow-up, 16 mo
Deutsch	*J Shoulder Elbow Surg* (2007)	Completion to full-thickness RCT (41)	ASES score improved from 42 to 93	2 (clinical)	Mean patient age, 49 yr Mean follow-up, 38 mo Prospective study
Porat et al	*J Shoulder Elbow Surg* (2008)	Completion to full-thickness RCT (51)	No poor results UCLA shoulder score improved from 17 to 31	16 (fair UCLA score)	Mean patient age, 60 yr Mean follow-up, 42 mo Retrospective study
Tauber et al	*Knee Surg Sports Traumatol Arthrosc* (2008)	Transtendon and anchorless transosseous technique (16)	UCLA shoulder score improved from 16 to 33	6 (clinical)	Mean patient age not reported Mean follow-up, 18 mo
Castagna et al	*Am J Sports Med* (2009)	Transtendon (54)	UCLA shoulder score improved from 14 to 33	2 (clinical)	Mean patient age, 56.7 yr Minimum follow-up, 2 yr Better results expected in patients with less retraction, traumatic injury, and of younger age
Kamath et al	*J Bone Joint Surg Am* (2009)	Completion to full-thickness RCT (41)	ASES score improved from 46 to 82	7 (clinical) 12 (ultrasonographic full-thickness retear)	Better healing in younger patients, with a mean age of 51.8 yr in patients with healed repair compared with 62.8 yr in patients with recurrent tear Mean patient age, 53 yr Mean follow-up, 39 mo
Spencer	*Clin Orthop Relat Res* (2010)	Intra-articular (20)	Penn shoulder score improved from 74 to 92	5 (inability to return to sport)	The patients studied were recreational and high school athletes Mean patient age, 41 yr Mean follow-up, 29 mo
Iyengar et al	*Arthroscopy* (2011)	Completion to full-thickness RCT (22)	UCLA shoulder score improved from 19 to 33	18 (full-thickness retear on MRI) 22 (partial retear)	Mean patient age, 57 yr Minimum follow-up, 2 yr 8 patients had a bursal-sided tear

ASES = American Shoulder and Elbow Surgeons, RCT = rotator cuff tear, UCLA = University of California–Los Angeles Shoulder Rating Scale.
[a] All scores are mean values unless otherwise noted.

Table 2 Results of Surgical Management of Partial-Thickness Rotator Cuff Tears (*continued*)

Author(s)	Journal (Year)	Technique (No. of Patients)	Outcomes[a]	Failure Rate (%)	Comments
Seo et al	*Knee Surg Sports Traumatol Arthrosc* (2011)	Transtendon with suture bridge technique (24)	ASES score improved from 38 to 89	8 (clinical)	Mean patient age, 51 yr Final follow-up, 12 mo
Shin	*Arthroscopy* (2012)	Completion to full-thickness RCT (24) or transtendon (24)	ASES score improved from 49 to 86 in the completion group and from 50 to 89 in the transtendon group	Completion group, 8 Transtendon group, 0	Mean age in completion group, 57 yr Mean age in transtendon group, 53 yr Mean follow-up, 31 mo Transtendon repair resulted in slower recovery but better structural integrity Failure was determined on MRI Randomized prospective trial (level II)
Kim et al	*Am J Sports Med* (2014)	Completion to full-thickness RCT (43)	ASES score improved from 47 to 91 (mean final follow-up, 35.5 mo) Radiologic evaluation demonstrated no retear of articular-sided tears (minimum follow-up, 1 yr)	9.5 (retear after bursal-sided repair)	Bursal-side tear in 23 patients (mean age, 48.8 yr) Articular-side tear in 20 patients (mean age, 53.9 yr) Cohort study (level III)
Park et al	*Am J Sports Med* (2015)	Transtendon repair of intra-tendinous tears using suture bridge configuration (33)	ASES score improved from 51 to 91 No retear on MRI Sugaya type 2 healing achieved in 64% of patients and type 3 in 6%	—	Mean patient age, 53.4 yr Mean follow-up, 56 mo Case series (level IV)

ASES = American Shoulder and Elbow Surgeons, RCT = rotator cuff tear, UCLA = University of California–Los Angeles Shoulder Rating Scale.
[a] All scores are mean values unless otherwise noted.

- An examination under anesthesia is performed to evaluate laxity in the anterior, posterior, and inferior directions.
- The arm is positioned such that abduction and forward flexion can be increased as needed intraoperatively. This positioning will allow the surgeon to increase instrument accessibility to the undersurface of the rotator cuff by moving the cuff closer to the anterior working portal.
- Traction also assists in proper positioning by enabling easier access to and instrumentation of the tear.

PROCEDURE

- Portals include an anterior working portal, a lateral working portal, and a standard posterior viewing portal. The anterior working portal is modified and positioned to the superolateral aspect of the rotator interval immediately anterior to the leading edge of the supraspinatus tendon. This position ensures that the surgeon can access the RCT with instruments such as shavers and graspers.
- The arthroscope is inserted into the glenohumeral joint through the posterior portal, and a thorough diagnostic examination is performed

before additional portals are created because further understanding of the complete pathology may affect portal placement.

Video 20.1 PASTA Repair. Christopher S. Ahmad, MD; Charles M. Jobin, MD (5 min)

- The articular surface of the rotator cuff is evaluated from anterior to posterior. The arm may be abducted, adducted, and internally and externally rotated as needed.
- Diagnostic arthroscopy requires visualization from the anterior portal to assess the posterior labrum

and capsule as well as the posterior rotator cuff insertion.

- In throwing athletes, special attention should be given to the undersurface of the rotator cuff at the junction between the supraspinatus and infraspinatus tendons at the anterior margin of the bare area. Tears of the rotator cuff at this location are common, and probing and grasping is performed to evaluate for intratendinous delamination.

- Débridement of the frayed articular surface tear is performed with a small, full-radius resector introduced through the anterior portal. The frayed edges of the rotator cuff are resected down to intact fibers (**Figure 2, A**).

- If a delaminated flap is encountered, a grasper is used to fully assess the flap and its suitability for repair.

- The intact fibers are inspected for substantial tendinosis or lack of integrity.

- The percentage of RCT in the medial to lateral dimension is estimated. This estimation can be made by measuring the exposed bony footprint based on the known diameter of the shaver or probe. The tendon thickness can be assumed to be 12 to 14 mm in the medial to lateral direction, and this value can be used to calculate the percentage of tear (**Figure 2, B**).

- If the tear is low grade, then a simple débridement is performed.

- The arthroscope is introduced in the subacromial space, which is examined carefully for bursitis and evidence of external impingement such as fraying or ossification of the coracoacromial ligament or inflammation of the bursa.

- The edges of the RCT are débrided, and the tear is assessed to determine the amount of footprint exposed.

- If the tear is greater than 50% and

the quality of the bursal lamina tissue is good, then transtendon repair to bone is considered. This technique is most commonly performed for repair of the anterior supraspinatus in patients with minimal retraction.

- The medial aspect of the exposed footprint is débrided and the bone abraded to stimulate healing.

- To allow inspection of the bursal rotator cuff adjacent to the articular surface tear, a marking suture is placed by introducing a spinal needle percutaneously across the tear and delivering a monofilament suture that is retrieved through the anterior cannula.

- After inspection of the subacromial space, a complete bursectomy is performed to ensure uncompromised management of sutures later in the procedure.

- The bursal side of the tendon is inspected for quality, especially at the site of the marking suture.

- After good tissue quality is confirmed, the arthroscope is reintroduced into the glenohumeral joint.

- Double-loaded suture anchors are placed percutaneously through the remaining bursal lamina of the tendon and into the medial footprint (**Figure 2, C**). If the width of the tear is greater than 1.5 cm, two anchors are placed.

- In throwing athletes with obligate internal impingement, several millimeters of bone may be left between the site of the tendon repair and the articular margin of the humeral head to prevent impingement of the repaired tissue.

- After anchors are placed, suture passing is performed. Several types of suture passers can be used. The authors of this chapter prefer an 18-gauge spinal needle, which reduces the risk of trauma to the intact rotator cuff that larger devices can cause (**Figure 2, D, E,** and **F**).

- One suture anchor limb is retrieved out of the anterior working cannula.

- A spinal needle is inserted into the bursal cuff and then into the lamina of the tear on the articular side.

- A monofilament suture passed through the needle is used to shuttle the anchor suture from the anterior cannula. This step is repeated for each suture, with differential passage of sutures through the retracted lamina on the articular side (**Figure 2, G**).

- Additional anchors may be placed for the management of anterior tears.

- The arthroscope is placed in the subacromial space, and the lateral cannula is used to tie the sutures (**Figure 2, H**).

- If compression of the repair site with the creation of low-profile knots is desired, the tied suture limbs can be fixed with a lateral row anchor in a suture bridge construct.

- The repair is inspected from within the glenohumeral joint (**Figure 2, I**).

WOUND CLOSURE

- Arthroscopic portals are closed with simple nylon dermal sutures.

Bursal-Sided High-Grade Partial Tear Completion and Repair
SETUP/EXPOSURE

- The patient is typically placed in the beach-chair position.

- Either general or regional anesthesia is administered.

- An examination under anesthesia is performed to evaluate range of motion and laxity.

- The arm is positioned such that abduction and forward flexion can be increased to allow the instrument accessibility to the undersurface of the rotator cuff by moving the cuff closer to the anterior working portal and improving the working angle to the cuff footprint.

- Gentle traction also assists in proper positioning by enabling easier access to and instrumentation of the tear.

PROCEDURE

- After diagnostic arthroscopy and management of associated pathology, a thorough assessment is performed to determine the presence of articular-sided tears or tendinosis (**Figure 3, B**).
- If tendinosis is found at a potential site of a bursal-sided tear, it can be marked with a monofilament suture inserted through a spinal needle.
- A subacromial bursectomy is performed to expose the bursal side of the cuff. Often in patients with bursal-sided tears, the bursa is absent at the tear site as a result of mechanical subacromial impingement (**Figure 3, C**).
- After the bursal-sided tear is débrided and its size, location, and exposed footprint evaluated, tear completion is performed for tears of greater than 50% to 75% of the medial to lateral footprint and with poor-quality articular tendon tissue (**Figure 3, D**).
- The tear is completed with a sharp, stout blade or shaver until the articular cartilage is reached, and a full-thickness rotator cuff repair is performed. The use of No. 11 blades should be avoided because the tip of the knife blade can easily be broken against the greater tuberosity.
- A stout blade is introduced through the lateral portal and used to release the rotator cuff from its attachment to the greater tuberosity.
- Often, a second lateral portal is needed to visualize the articular margin through the narrow bursal-sided tear, which is frequently far anterior.
- The footprint is abraded with a shaver to facilitate biologic healing. The edges of the rotator cuff are lightly débrided to remove poor-quality tissue in a limited and careful fashion to avoid removing too much tissue.
- Anchors are placed in the footprint percutaneously. If a suture bridge construct is planned, anchors are placed at the articular margin (**Figure 3, E**). Otherwise, a single-row repair may be performed with an anchor in the center of the footprint.
- After anchor placement, standard suture-passing devices are used to pass sutures through the rotator cuff, creating multiple horizontal mattress sutures.
- The sutures are tied. If a suture bridge construct is planned, a lateral row of anchors is placed to complete the construct (**Figure 3, F**).

WOUND CLOSURE

- The arthroscopic portal is closed with simple nylon dermal sutures.

Intratendinous Repair of PAINT Lesion

SETUP/EXPOSURE

- Intratendinous repair of a delaminated articular-sided tear requires careful assessment of the degree of articular footprint exposed, the location of the exposure, and the mobility and extent of the delaminated tear.
- The patient is placed in the lateral decubitus position.
- Portals are established in standard fashion.

PROCEDURE

- Associated pathology is addressed before rotator cuff repair.
- Glenohumeral arthroscopy will reveal degenerated, frayed tearing of the undersurfaces of the supraspinatus and infraspinatus.
- Poor-quality fragmented edges of the tear are removed with a full-radius resector.
- A soft-tissue grasper introduced from the anterior portal can be used to observe the tissue quality and the magnitude and mobility of the lamination (**Figure 4, B**).
- To enhance healing, a shaver or rasp is used to abrade the inside of the lamination, thereby eliminating synovial tissue at the inside edges.
- Before sutures are passed, the subacromial space is inspected and a complete bursectomy is performed to avoid compromised visualization.
- Mattress sutures are placed using the outside-in technique. A spinal needle is inserted lateral to the anterolateral acromion, and the needle is used to insert a passing suture and then shuttle the permanent suture through the anterior portal to capture the cuff delaminated tear (**Figure 4, C**).
- To penetrate the intact bursal lamina, the spinal needle is inserted percutaneously just lateral to the acromion.
- The needle is introduced into the articular lamina at the appropriate location. A soft-tissue grasper can be used to hold the articular lamina in reduction as necessary during needle passage.
- A monofilament suture is passed through the needle and retrieved from the anterior cannula.
- The monofilament suture is tied to a No. 2 nonabsorbable braided suture outside the cannula and shuttled through the tear.
- Another monofilament suture is passed across the RCT and retrieved out of the anterior cannula with the second tail of the braided suture.
- A mattress suture is created by shuttling the second tail of the braided suture through the rotator cuff.
- These steps are repeated to form

Table 3 Rehabilitation Protocol After Partial-Thickness Rotator Cuff Tear Repair

Postoperative Week	ROM	Strengthening	Return to Play	Comments/Emphasis
0-2	None	None	None	Comfort
2-6	Pendulum exercises, passive rotation with the arm at the side	None	None	Protect the repair, prevent severe stiffness
6-12	Obtain full ROM	Active-assisted ROM progressing to active ROM	None	Regain motion, protect repair from excessive force
12-24	—	Strengthening to restore balance, strength, and proprioception	Allowed after 24 wk	Sport-specific training

ROM = range of motion.

additional mattress sutures.

- With the arthroscope in the subacromial space, the sutures are tied through a standard lateral working portal (**Figure 4, D**).
- The arthroscope is moved to the glenohumeral joint to facilitate evaluation of the repair (**Figure 4, E**).

WOUND CLOSURE

- Arthroscopic wound closure is performed with interrupted nylon dermal stitches or with absorbable sutures in the deep dermal layer.

 Rehabilitation

The postoperative rehabilitation protocol after partial-thickness RCT repair is similar to the rehabilitation protocol after repair of small full-thickness tears (**Table 3**). Immediately postoperatively, the patient is placed in an abduction sling with the arm in neutral rotation for pain control and protection of the repair from the mechanical forces of shoulder motion. The sling is worn for 6 weeks except during exercise and bathing.

With the sling off, active flexion and extension of the elbow are performed several times per day. Passive external rotation exercises are allowed immediately postoperatively. Use of the sling is discontinued at 6 weeks, at which time the patient begins overhead stretching with the use of a rope and pulley and internal rotation stretching. Strengthening begins at 10 to 12 weeks postoperatively. A progressive strengthening and sport-specific training program is initiated from 3 to 6 months postoperatively. In overhead throwers, sport-specific therapy is focused on minimizing internal impingement by optimizing throwing mechanics, pectoralis minor stretching, posterior capsular stretching, and scapular dynamics in addition to cuff strengthening. Most patients can return to sports 6 to 9 months postoperatively.

 Avoiding Pitfalls

Paying particular care during a few key steps in PASTA repair can help optimize outcomes. Performing a subacromial bursectomy before intra-articular suture passage prevents difficulty finding the subacromial sutures and accidental cutting of suture with the shaver during subacromial knot-tying. Proper arm position in midrange flexion and abduction helps avoid iatrogenic injury to the superior humeral head cartilage by ensuring a proper working angle of the shaver onto the exposed footprint. Positioning the patient's arm in midrange flexion and abduction also reduces tension on the supraspinatus cuff tissue, thereby creating intra-articular working space for suture management and shuttling. Débridement of the footprint to bleeding cortical bone is important for rotator cuff healing. Identification of the rotator cuff cable and crescent is helpful in identifying the anatomic location for repair. The location of spinal needle passage or suture lasso passage through the articular-sided cuff tissue is the critical step for proper reduction and tensioning of the PASTA repair.

Bibliography

Burkhart SS, Morgan CD, Kibler WB: The disabled throwing shoulder: Spectrum of pathology. Part I: Pathoanatomy and biomechanics. *Arthroscopy* 2003;19(4):404-420.

Castagna A, Delle Rose G, Conti M, Snyder SJ, Borroni M, Garofalo R: Predictive factors of subtle residual shoulder symptoms after transtendinous arthroscopic cuff repair: A clinical study. *Am J Sports Med* 2009;37(1):103-108.

Conway JE: Arthroscopic repair of partial-thickness rotator cuff tears and SLAP lesions in professional baseball players. *Orthop Clin North Am* 2001;32(3):443-456.

Deutsch A: Arthroscopic repair of partial-thickness tears of the rotator cuff. *J Shoulder Elbow Surg* 2007;16(2):193-201.

Ellman H: Diagnosis and treatment of incomplete rotator cuff tears. *Clin Orthop Relat Res* 1990;(254):64-74.

Gonzalez-Lomas G, Kippe MA, Brown GD, et al: In situ transtendon repair outperforms tear completion and repair for partial articular-sided supraspinatus tendon tears. *J Shoulder Elbow Surg* 2008;17(5):722-728.

Ide J, Maeda S, Takagi K: Arthroscopic transtendon repair of partial-thickness articular-side tears of the rotator cuff: Anatomical and clinical study. *Am J Sports Med* 2005;33(11):1672-1679.

Iyengar JJ, Porat S, Burnett KR, Marrero-Perez L, Hernandez VH, Nottage WM: Magnetic resonance imaging tendon integrity assessment after arthroscopic partial-thickness rotator cuff repair. *Arthroscopy* 2011;27(3):306-313.

Kamath G, Galatz LM, Keener JD, Teefey S, Middleton W, Yamaguchi K: Tendon integrity and functional outcome after arthroscopic repair of high-grade partial-thickness supraspinatus tears. *J Bone Joint Surg Am* 2009;91(5):1055-1062.

Kim HM, Dahiya N, Teefey SA, et al: Location and initiation of degenerative rotator cuff tears: An analysis of three hundred and sixty shoulders. *J Bone Joint Surg Am* 2010;92(5):1088-1096.

Kim KC, Shin HD, Cha SM, Park JY: Repair integrity and functional outcome after arthroscopic conversion to a full-thickness rotator cuff tear: Articular- versus bursal-side partial tears. *Am J Sports Med* 2014;42(2):451-456.

Mazzocca AD, Rincon LM, O'Connor RW, et al: Intra-articular partial-thickness rotator cuff tears: Analysis of injured and repaired strain behavior. *Am J Sports Med* 2008;36(1):110-116.

Mesiha MM, Derwin KA, Sibole SC, Erdemir A, McCarron JA: The biomechanical relevance of anterior rotator cuff cable tears in a cadaveric shoulder model. *J Bone Joint Surg Am* 2013;95(20):1817-1824.

Miller SL, Hazrati Y, Cornwall R, et al: Failed surgical management of partial thickness rotator cuff tears. *Orthopedics* 2002;25(11):1255-1257.

Mochizuki T, Sugaya H, Uomizu M, et al: Humeral insertion of the supraspinatus and infraspinatus. New anatomical findings regarding the footprint of the rotator cuff. *J Bone Joint Surg Am* 2008;90(5):962-969.

Nguyen ML, Quigley RJ, Galle SE, et al: Margin convergence anchorage to bone for reconstruction of the anterior attachment of the rotator cable. *Arthroscopy* 2012;28(9):1237-1245.

Park SE, Panchal K, Jeong JJ, et al: Intratendinous rotator cuff tears: Prevalence and clinical and radiological outcomes of arthroscopically confirmed intratendinous tears at midterm follow-up. *Am J Sports Med* 2015;43(2):415-422.

Porat S, Nottage WM, Fouse MN: Repair of partial thickness rotator cuff tears: A retrospective review with minimum two-year follow-up. *J Shoulder Elbow Surg* 2008;17(5):729-731.

Reynolds SB, Dugas JR, Cain EL, McMichael CS, Andrews JR: Débridement of small partial-thickness rotator cuff tears in elite overhead throwers. *Clin Orthop Relat Res* 2008;466(3):614-621.

Seo YJ, Yoo YS, Kim DY, Noh KC, Shetty NS, Lee JH: Trans-tendon arthroscopic repair for partial-thickness articular side tears of the rotator cuff. *Knee Surg Sports Traumatol Arthrosc* 2011;19(10):1755-1759.

Sher JS, Uribe JW, Posada A, Murphy BJ, Zlatkin MB: Abnormal findings on magnetic resonance images of asymptomatic shoulders. *J Bone Joint Surg Am* 1995;77(1):10-15.

Shin SJ: A comparison of 2 repair techniques for partial-thickness articular-sided rotator cuff tears. *Arthroscopy* 2012;28(1):25-33.

Spencer EE Jr: Partial-thickness articular surface rotator cuff tears: An all-inside repair technique. *Clin Orthop Relat Res* 2010;468(6):1514-1520.

Strauss EJ, Salata MJ, Kercher J, et al: The arthroscopic management of partial-thickness rotator cuff tears: A systematic review of the literature. *Arthroscopy* 2011;27(4):568-580.

Tauber M, Koller H, Resch H: Transosseous arthroscopic repair of partial articular-surface supraspinatus tendon tears. *Knee Surg Sports Traumatol Arthrosc* 2008;16(6):608-613.

Waibl B, Buess E: Partial-thickness articular surface supraspinatus tears: A new transtendon suture technique. *Arthroscopy* 2005;21(3):376-381.

Yang S, Park HS, Flores S, et al: Biomechanical analysis of bursal-sided partial thickness rotator cuff tears. *J Shoulder Elbow Surg* 2009;18(3):379-385.

 ## Video Reference

Ahmad CS, Jobin CM: Video. *PASTA Repair*. New York, NY, 2015.

Chapter 21

Managing Simple Full-Thickness Rotator Cuff Tears With Single- or Double-Row Repair Constructs

Maxwell C. Park, MD

Neal S. ElAttrache, MD

 ## Introduction

Simple, typically crescent-shaped, full-thickness rotator cuff tears may be repaired with single- or double-row constructs. The tear must be thoroughly characterized, accounting for tear morphology in relation to the anterior cord of the supraspinatus tendon. Careful assessment of tissue quality and repair tension is critical, particularly in a patient with remnant tissue on the greater tuberosity footprint. The surgeon performing the repair should strive for technical efficiency and biomechanical optimization. Healing and resultant favorable outcomes rely not only on meticulous surgical technique but on patient compliance with the recovery program and its progression in the appropriate time parameters.

 ## Case Presentation

A healthy 60-year-old right-hand–dominant woman who is a golf enthusiast presents with chronic pain (lasting more than 6 months) in her right shoulder. She does not report any specific trauma. Her pain is reproducible with overhead motion and forward-reaching activities. She reports that no substantial improvement was achieved with regular use of ibuprofen or a 3-month course of physical therapy, during which she received two separate corticosteroid injections. On physical examination, the patient has full motor strength that is limited only by pain, and positive results are noted on Neer and Hawkins impingement tests. An MRI of the right shoulder demonstrates a full-thickness tear of the supraspinatus and anterior infraspinatus tendons; however, the anterior cord of the supraspinatus is intact. This latter finding explains the patient's sufficient motor strength during the preoperative examination. Based on clinical and MRI findings, the patient meets indications for arthroscopic rotator cuff repair.

A simple full-thickness, crescent-shaped tear of the supraspinatus and anterior infraspinatus tendons is confirmed intraoperatively (**Figure 1**). The tear is fully reducible to the lateral footprint of the rotator cuff. A medial-pulley transosseous-equivalent (MP-TOE) repair is subsequently performed. The MP-TOE technique achieves supraphysiologic biomechanical results with only two suture passes through the tendon, in contrast to the original transosseous-equivalent (TOE) construct first described in 2005, which required a minimum of four suture passes through the tendon. The medial-pulley technique does not rely on focal spot-weld medial mattress suture configurations (**Figure 2**). The use of tendon-bridging sutures during trial reduction of the tendon can confirm the optimal location of distal-lateral anchor placement (**Figure 3**). The final construct fully restores the anatomy of the rotator cuff footprint (**Figure 4**). In a patient who has involvement of the anterior cord of the supraspinatus, a dedicated anterior anchor can supplement the repair.

 ## Indications

Single- or double-row repair techniques may be used to repair simple, crescent-shaped, full-thickness rotator cuff tears involving the supraspinatus and anterior infraspinatus tendons. The number of rows used depends on the degree of preexisting tendon retraction and tendon tension during trial reduction of the tendon onto the footprint of the rotator cuff. In addition, the integrity of the anterior cord of the supraspinatus must be considered, particularly because of its additional biomechanical role in resisting rotational stress.

Dr. Park or an immediate family member has received royalties and research or institutional support from Arthrex. Dr. ElAttrache or an immediate family member has received royalties and research or institutional support from Arthrex and serves as a board member, owner, officer, or committee member of the American Orthopaedic Society for Sports Medicine.

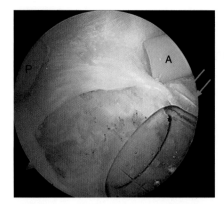

Figure 1 Arthroscopic image of a shoulder from the posterolateral portal demonstrates a simple, crescent-shaped, full-thickness tear of the supraspinatus and anterior infraspinatus tendons. The anterior cord of the supraspinatus (arrows) is intact underneath the blue anterior cannula (A). The clear cannula is at the midlateral position. The posterior cannula (P) is positioned for suture management.

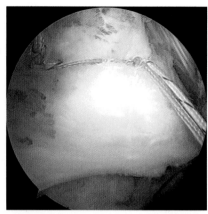

Figure 2 Arthroscopic image of a shoulder from the posterolateral portal demonstrates a broad medial-pulley interimplant mattress suture configuration between knots positioned over the medial anchors located anterior and posterior. Focal spot-weld medial mattress suture configurations are not used, and this resultant broad inter-implant mattress suture configuration has been reported to be biomechanically equivalent but less traumatic to the medial tendon. The knots are not cut, and the sutures are used to secure the tendon over the bony footprint, which is covered in this image. Tendon-bridging sutures compress the tendon, creating a self-reinforcing repair construct.

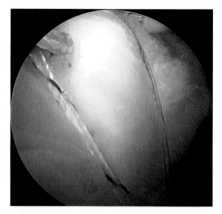

Figure 3 Arthroscopic image of a shoulder from the posterolateral portal demonstrates trial reduction of the posterior suture limbs from each knot to optimally localize the distal-lateral anchor placement.

The single-anchor repair construct may be used to manage relatively small anterior full-thickness tears measuring 10 mm or less in the anterior-posterior dimension. In patients in whom the posterosuperior rotator cuff tendons are mostly intact, placing a row of anchors may be neither necessary nor feasible. In patients whose native rotator cuff footprint is mostly intact, less protection against failure loads is necessary, and a single-anchor repair likely is sufficient. In addition, there is less of a footprint contact area that needs restoring. Because the repair dimension is relatively small, an anchor that occupies the footprint may limit bony surface area for healing. Therefore, a distal-lateral anchor in relation to the footprint may be optimal; an inverted mattress knotless configuration with suture tape can be used in this setting. This construct has been shown to improve tendon repair morphology compared with one in which the anchor occupies the top of the footprint.

Simple crescent-shaped tears that are not fully reducible can be managed with a single-row repair medialized on the native footprint. Single-row repairs with modified suture configurations and triple-loaded anchors have been described. In patients who have tears that are not fully reducible, particularly tears with remnant tissue on the footprint, the amount of tissue loss and degree of inherent tendon retraction make single-row repair the only feasible construct, even if anterior and posterior releases are performed. Insufficient lateral tissue is available to fix or compress with a lateral row, and suture passes tend to be relatively medial near the rotator cable; the cable is normally medial to the footprint and therefore should not be lateralized to the footprint. To address retracted tears that are not fully reducible, bony medialization (up to 10 mm) of the footprint has been shown to be a reasonable and practical option. However, there are limitations to single-row

repair with respect to failure loads, contact area, and self-reinforcement. Biomechanically, for rotator cuff tears with substantial tendon retraction and, thus, substantial chronicity, single-row repair can be sufficient because of the relatively reduced failure loads in the setting of muscle atrophy. As a result, the repair constructs are not under supraphysiologic loading conditions, as in the early postoperative period.

For fully reducible tears in patients who have only moderate tendon retraction and minimal to no tissue loss, double-row repair may be appropriate. Double-row TOE repair has been shown to optimize repair dimensions in simple, full-thickness, crescent-shaped tears that are fully reducible to the lateral footprint and not overtensioned during trial reduction. This repair construct has arguably become the standard by which other repairs are compared. In addition to restoring footprint contact dimensions, other biomechanical advantages of double-row TOE repair over single- and traditional double-row repair include improved failure loads, minimal gap formation, improved anterior cord resistance to rotational stress, decreased fluid extravasation, improved technical efficiency, and improved self-reinforcement effect.

Regardless whether single-row or double-row TOE repair is performed, the indications for the particular technical approach must be considered. Although it is generally understood that the use of more tendon suture passes results in better fixation, biomechanical necessity (healing sufficiency) and increased surgical time must be considered. For example, in patients with single-row repair, the surgeon must determine whether biomechanical advantages exist that may substantially improve healing and therefore patient outcomes with the use of triple-loaded anchors, or whether double-loaded anchors, which are less load-resistant but require less suture management, are sufficient.

These general considerations are the impetus behind the selection of a technically optimized TOE repair construct that uses a medial-pulley inter-implant mattress suture configuration (MP-TOE repair). The MP-TOE repair construct, which requires only two tendon suture passes, has been shown to be biomechanically equivalent to the originally described TOE repair, which uses two separate medial horizontal mattress suture configurations (requiring four tendon suture passes). Medial fixation provides a substantial biomechanical advantage with respect to failure loads and gap resistance. However, medial failure of the rotator cuff repair is a concern with spot-weld mattress suture configurations.

Although some clinical success has been demonstrated with medial knotless bridging constructs, they have been biomechanically outperformed by TOE constructs that use medial knot fixation. The MP-TOE repair does not compromise medial fixation because it provides a broad inter-implant horizontal mattress across the central repair and helps to dissipate the force over a larger tendon surface area. This broad mattress configuration has been shown to provide improved load-sharing capacity and results in less tendon damage

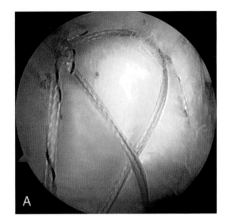 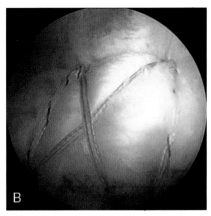

Figure 4 Arthroscopic images of a shoulder viewed from the posterolateral portal (**A**) and the midlateral portal (**B**) demonstrate the final appearance of a broad medial-pulley transosseous-equivalent rotator cuff repair construct.

with failure testing (creating a so-called purse-string effect). In other words, the MP-TOE construct provides the advantages of separate medial spot-weld mattress suture configurations without the potential disadvantages of additional suture management (more than two suture passes), increased surgical times, medial failure tear patterns, and compromised biomechanics that occur with knotless medial fixation.

The unique anatomy of the supraspinatus tendon can affect selection of a specific repair construct, whether single-anchor, single-row, or double-row TOE. The supraspinatus tendon is asymmetric; it is cord-like anteriorly and strap-like posteriorly. In its posterior aspect, the tendon interdigitates with the anterior infraspinatus tendon. This asymmetry creates relatively more stress on the tendon anteriorly, particularly with humeral rotation. Therefore, direct anterior fixation that incorporates the anterior cord (distinct from the anterior cable) may be indicated if the cord is detached from the footprint, because the anterior cord region has been shown to experience more stress and strain with tendon loading compared with the posterior region. In all patients, inserting a dedicated anchor for the anterior supraspinatus region should be considered, if needed.

Controversies and Alternative Approaches

Whether to perform single-row or double-row repair remains controversial. Recent meta-analyses have shown that although double-row repairs result in improved healing, findings on outcome measures are not significantly different from those of single-row repairs. As studies with longer follow-up durations are published, improved healing over time may result in improved outcome measures.

The specific indications for single-row versus double-row repairs have not been fully elucidated. The current indications as outlined previously are based primarily on technical concerns related to tear reducibility and tension with trial reduction of the tendon; a reducible tear with minimal tension may benefit more from a footprint-restoring, double-row TOE technique. When single-row repair techniques are indicated, tears under tension may require either medialization of the repair to the medial native footprint or medialization of the bony footprint itself using a standard burr. However, the presence of repair tension has been shown to be beneficial to the healing environment. Because the optimal amount of repair tension is unknown, controversy persists regarding whether to medialize all repairs (including fully reducible tears) with a single-row construct, which could result in an adverse effect on muscle unit length-tension relationships and the loss of biomechanical advantages seen with TOE constructs.

Biomechanically, tension created by loads that are equal to or below yield loads can demonstrate a relative benefit by means of a self-reinforcement effect. First conceptualized in 2009 for a particular suture tendon-bridging repair construct, self-reinforcement was formally biomechanically characterized, quantified, and validated in 2014. Single-row repair can demonstrate self-reinforcement by creating a "focal loop wedge" effect, in which the focal lateral suture loop (created with simple suture configurations) elongates with tendon loading, resulting in obligatory tendon compression over the footprint deep to the suture loop itself. This compression force increases frictional resistance to failure over the footprint and accounts for the self-reinforcement effect. However, single-row repair, which does not anchor the tendon-bridging suture loop between the medial and distal-lateral anchors, demonstrates a lesser self-reinforcement effect compared with TOE repair. Notably, even with self-reinforcement, loading beyond the yield load with single-row or TOE repairs can create coincidental construct failure with increasing gap formation.

Not only does controversy exist in terms of indications for single- versus double-row repair, but controversy exists regarding whether to perform knotless or medial-knotted repair in double-row constructs. Although knotless repair has demonstrated adequate clinical outcomes, knotted repair has biomechanically outperformed knotless repair. Knotless repair can be technically efficient, but consequences of the lack of knots may include lesser failure loads and decreasing footprint contact with

glenohumeral abduction. However, focal medial knot fixation may overconstrain the construct, inhibit self-reinforcement, and contribute to medial failures. Further studies are needed to elucidate the specific indications for knotless TOE repair over medial-knotted repair.

Alternative approaches can be considered in patients with retracted tears that are not reducible and require medialization. Only a partial repair may be feasible in patients in whom the tension of repair based on trial tendon reduction may be excessive. Tendon transfers can be considered as well. Graft patch augmentation has shown clinical potential for success in patients in whom tendon quality is deficient. In addition, superior capsular reconstruction may be a viable alternative. In a patient with arthropathy, a reverse total shoulder arthroplasty or hemiarthroplasty may be indicated.

Results

Published results from current and important historical studies on rotator cuff tear management are summarized in **Table 1**. Controversy remains regarding the indications for single- and double-row repair. There is no consensus for one type of repair over the other with respect to clinical outcomes; however, double-row repair has demonstrated improved healing rates. The inability to distinguish a statistical difference between single- and double-row outcomes may be related to limited statistical power and follow-up duration.

Video 21.1 Medial-Pulley Transosseous-Equivalent Rotator Cuff Repair With Dedicated Anterior Cord Fixation for the "Simple" Rotator Cuff Tear. Maxwell C. Park, MD (6 min)

Technical Keys to Success

Success depends on optimized arthroscopic portal placement. Needle localization is a simple reproducible method to target portals. The midlateral portal is typically the working portal, and its placement is critical (**Figure 1**). The midlateral portal should be placed as anteriorly as possible (without compromising accessibility to the tear and the footprint) to create separation on the skin in expectation of placing the posterolateral and superior accessory portals. For TOE constructs, the midlateral portal should be placed sufficiently inferior to enable easy distal-lateral anchor placement, but not so inferior or distal that it prevents easy tendon grasping for trial reductions and suture passing.

Typically, particularly if the patient is in the lateral decubitus position, a posterolateral portal is needed to best visualize the entire tear. If the posterolateral portal is placed too posteriorly, then visualization will be compromised. Furthermore, careful attention should be paid to not only the portal placement, but its relationship to other potential portals. The posterolateral portal should be placed close to the midlateral portal, but not so close that it interferes with the midlateral working cannula. Importantly, if a superior accessory portal is to be used for anchor placement along a medial row, then the posterolateral portal should not be too close to the midlateral portal. If the portals are too close, the cannula from the arthroscope, the midlateral cannula, and the punch for the implant could interfere with one another, making the procedure unnecessarily difficult.

Recognition of the rotator cuff tear pattern is essential for successful repair. Trial reduction of the tendon is critical to characterize the tear fully. For simple full-thickness rotator cuff tears, the authors of this chapter believe tendon

Table 1 Results of Single-Row and Double-Row Repair for the Management of Full-Thickness Rotator Cuff Tears

Individual Study Characteristics

Authors (Year)	Intervention	N[a]	Population Differences	Tear Length (sagittal plane)	Mean Follow-Up (months)	Outcomes	Relevant Findings
Gartsman et al (2013)	SR vs DR; re-tear rate	83 (40 SR, 43 DR)	• Included any repairable full-thickness tear • Excluded smokers, steroid users, bilateral cuff repairs, suprascapular nerve decompressions	SR: <2.5 cm DR: <2.5 cm	SR: N/R DR: N/R Mean: 10 (6-12)	Subjective: N/R Objective: N/R Imaging: US	• DR had significantly decreased re-tear rate (7%) compared with SR (25%) (*P* = 0.024)
Carbonel et al (2012)	SR vs DR; clinical outcome and re-tear rate	160 (80 SR, 80 DR)	• Excluded OA, tears >5 cm, Fuchs >4, steroid users	SR 1-3 cm: 51 SR 3-5 cm: 29 DR 1-3 cm: 53 DR 3-5 cm: 27	SR: 24 DR: 24 MRI SR: 24 MRI DR: 24	Subjective: ASES, UCLA, Constant Objective: Physical examination, SSI, ROM in degrees Imaging: MRI	• DR significantly improved over SR in 1- to 3-cm tears with respect to degrees of flexion and abduction, internal rotation SSI and external rotation SSI • DR significantly improved over SR with respect to all measured variables in 3- to 5-cm tears except for Constant score, abduction SSI, and external rotation SSI
Lapner et al (2012)	SR vs DR; clinical outcome and re-tear rate	80 (40 SR, 40 DR)	• Included any full-thickness tear • Excluded SSx <6 months, GFDI >3, ACH distance <7 mm	SR: Mean 1.89 cm DR: Mean 2.38 cm	SR: 24 DR: 24 MRI SR: 24 MRI DR: 24	Subjective: ASES, WORC, Constant Objective: Strength (in kg) Imaging: MRI/US	• DR had significantly decreased re-tear rate • Smaller coronal tear sizes resulted in improved healing rates • Patients with re-tears had larger initial tear sizes • Those with re-tears had significantly decreased strength

AC = acromioclavicular; ACH = acromiohumeral; ASES = American Shoulder and Elbow Surgeons score; DASH = Disability of the Arm, Shoulder and Hand score; DR = double-row; ER = external rotation; FF = forward flexion; GFDI = Global Fatty Degeneration Index; IR = internal rotation; MRA = magnetic resonance arthrography; N/R = not reported; OA = glenohumeral osteoarthritis; ROM = range of motion; SANE = Single Assessment Numeric Evaluation score; SR = single-row; SSI = Shoulder Strength Index; SSx = signs and symptoms; UCLA = University of California–Los Angeles score; US = Ultrasound; VAS = visual analog scale (pain); WORC = Western Ontario Rotator Cuff index.

[a] Number of patients randomized.

Adapted with permission from Millett PJ, Warth RJ, Dornan GJ, Lee JT, Spiegl UJ: Clinical and structural outcomes after arthroscopic single-row versus double-row rotator cuff repair: A systematic review and meta-analysis of level I randomized clinical trials. *J Shoulder Elbow Surg* 2014;23(4):586-597.

Table 1 Results of Single-Row and Double-Row Repair for the Management of Full-Thickness Rotator Cuff Tears (*continued*)

Individual Study Characteristics

Authors (Year)	Intervention	N[a]	Population Differences	Tear Length (sagittal plane)	Mean Follow-Up (months)	Outcomes	Relevant Findings
Koh et al (2011)	SR vs DR; clinical outcome and re-tear rate	71 (37 SR, 34 DR)	• Included OA, smokers • Excluded those without complete footprint coverage on postoperative MRI	SR: Mean 1.72 cm DR: Mean 1.75 cm (all tears 2-4 cm in sagittal oblique or coronal oblique plane)	SR: 31.0 DR: 32.8 MRI SR: 27.4 MRI DR: 27.6	Subjective: ASES, UCLA, VAS Objective: ROM (FF, ER, IR) in degrees Imaging: MRI	• DR showed improvement over SR with respect to internal rotation capacity (approaches statistical significance; $P = 0.053$) • No other clinical or radiographic differences between DR and SR groups reported
Burks et al (2009)	SR vs DR; clinical outcome and re-tear rate	40 (20 SR, 20 DR)	• Excluded smokers, steroid users, U-tears, and workers' compensation • Included OA	SR 1-3 cm: 18 SR >3 cm: 2 DR 1-3 cm: 15 DR >3 cm: 5	SR: 12 DR: 12 MRI SR: 12 MRI DR: 12	Subjective: ASES, UCLA, Constant, SANE, WORC Objective: ROM, strength (IR/ER in N-m) Imaging: MRI	• Differences in clinical or radiographic outcomes between SR and DR
Grasso et al (2009)	SR vs DR; clinical outcome only	80 (40 SR, 40 DR)	• Excluded OA, AC arthritis, workers' compensation, very small or very large tears	SR: Mean 1.56 cm DR: Mean 1.61 cm	SR: N/R DR: N/R Mean: 24.8	Subjective: DASH, WorkDASH, Constant Objective: strength in lb Imaging: N/R	• No differences in clinical outcomes between SR and DR
Franceschi et al (2007)	SR vs DR; clinical outcome and re-tear rate	60 (30 SR, 30 DR)	• Included SSx 3 months, OA • Excluded tendon retraction, SSx instability	SR 3-5 cm: 18 SR >5 cm: 8 DR 3-5 cm: 21 DR >5 cm: 5	SR: N/R DR: N/R Mean: 22.5 MRA: N/R	Subjective: UCLA Objective: FF, ER, IR (degrees) Imaging: MRA	• No differences in clinical or radiographic outcomes between SR and DR

AC = acromioclavicular; ACH = acromiohumeral; ASES = American Shoulder and Elbow Surgeons score; DASH = Disability of the Arm, Shoulder and Hand score; DR = double-row; ER = external rotation; FF = forward flexion; GFDI = Global Fatty Degeneration Index; IR = internal rotation; MRA = magnetic resonance arthrography; N/R = not reported; OA = glenohumeral osteoarthritis; ROM = range of motion; SANE = Single Assessment Numeric Evaluation score; SR = single-row; SSI = Shoulder Strength Index; SSx = signs and symptoms; UCLA = University of California–Los Angeles score; US = Ultrasound; VAS = visual analog scale (pain); WORC = Western Ontario Rotator Cuff index.

[a] Number of patients randomized.

Adapted with permission from Millett PJ, Warth RJ, Dornan GJ, Lee JT, Spiegl UJ: Clinical and structural outcomes after arthroscopic single-row versus double-row rotator cuff repair: A systematic review and meta-analysis of level I randomized clinical trials. *J Shoulder Elbow Surg* 2014;23(4):586-597.

$$\frac{\text{Number of tendon suture passes} \quad + \quad \text{Number of suture limbs} \quad + \quad \text{Number of knots}}{\text{Number of implants used}} \quad = \quad \text{Technical efficiency ratio}$$

Figure 5 Image shows the formula for determining the technical efficiency ratio for any rotator cuff repair construct. When comparing constructs using this ratio, it is most useful to compare the same type of construct (such as single-row to single-row), because different construct types create different footprint characteristics after repair.

reducibility is the essential differentiating factor in determining whether to proceed with a single-row or TOE construct. For tears that are fully reducible even after careful anterior and posterior interval releases have been performed, TOE repair should be considered. For TOE repair to be successful, it must be possible to place medial suture passes at least 10 mm medial to the lateral edge of the tear; otherwise, insufficient lateral tissue will be available for fixation with tendon-bridging sutures; however, suture passes at the level of or medial to the rotator cable should be avoided. Because the rotator cable normally lies medial to the medial footprint, suture passes near this structure would lead to obligatory overtensioning. The risk for overtensioning exists in patients who have residual remnant tissue on the footprint itself (which is equivalent to tissue loss) with or without considerable preexisting tear retraction. Suture passes near the rotator cable may be considered when the bony footprint itself is medialized, for example, during single-row repair.

The anterior cord of the supraspinatus tendon also should be appreciated in relation to the tear. If the anterior cord is detached from the bone in the region posterior to the bicipital groove, then a dedicated anchor for additional fixation should be considered.

Calculation of a technical efficiency ratio is helpful to gauge technical ease for a given repair construct (**Figure 5**). A smaller ratio represents relatively greater efficiency. For example, the originally described TOE repair, which requires four tendon suture passes, four suture

limbs to manage, two medial horizontal mattress knots, and four anchor implants, has a technical efficiency ratio of 2.5:

$$(4+4+2)/4 = 2.5$$

A repair that demonstrates biomechanical superiority but is too technically cumbersome to perform (that is, it has a relatively higher ratio) may not be practical. If, however, a repair is shown to be biomechanically equivalent or superior and is technically easier to perform, then it may be a preferred repair method.

The technically optimized MP-TOE repair construct that was biomechanically tested and validated in 2013 involves a broad medial inter-implant mattress configuration rather than two or more separate and isolated focal mattresses (**Figures 1** through **4**). Because only two tendon suture passes are necessary, the technical efficiency ratio is as follows:

$$(2+4+2)/4 = 2.0$$

This smaller ratio number represents improved efficiency or less difficulty compared with the original TOE repair, which has a ratio of 2.5.

Rehabilitation

A shoulder immobilizer and abduction pillow are applied immediately postoperatively. For single-row and double-row TOE repairs, progressive range of motion exercises only are prescribed for the first 12 weeks postoperatively. Progressive

resistive exercises are initiated after passive range of motion is normalized, but no sooner than 12 weeks postoperatively. Individual clinical responses dictate the pace of rehabilitation progression.

For all rotator cuff repairs, the recovery period is the most important variable related to healing. In many patients, range of motion and pain are improved well before healing is fully optimized at the tendon-footprint interface. Unwillingness or inability to comply with rehabilitation guidelines and timelines increases the risk for tear persistence and recurrent failure. If the repair fails to heal sufficiently before the repaired tendon is exerted, then the risk for predictable failure is increased. Patient-specific rehabilitation (such as for a particular sport) and goal timelines (such as seasonal return-to-play protocols) are important considerations in individualizing patient care.

Avoiding Pitfalls

During diagnostic arthroscopy, appreciation of portal placement to facilitate access as well as characterization of the tear pattern are essential to avoiding pitfalls during rotator cuff repair. With regard to portal placement, for example, if the midlateral working portal is placed too superiorly, then distal-lateral fixation cannot be achieved. If the superior accessory portal is too inferior, then the medial row may not be accessible. Although the shoulder may be adducted intraoperatively, moving the arm back and forth during the procedure is technically suboptimal. Pitfalls related to access can easily be avoided by using a spinal needle to localize the target and confirm instrument trajectory.

Trial reduction is necessary to characterize the tear pattern and identify whether single-row repair or double-row TOE repair should be performed. The tear pattern always dictates the repair strategy. If there are tissue loss and considerable tendon retraction and the tendon reduces to the medial footprint only, then a single-row construct should be used. If a simple tear reduces to the lateral footprint and tissue lateral to the rotator cable is present (≥10 to 15 mm of tissue from the lateral tear edge), then a TOE construct is preferred. Trial reduction helps determine not only appropriate anchor placement but also the correct tendon location for passing sutures. If the anchor is placed correctly but the sutures are not correctly passed through the tendon in relation to the anchor, then dog-ear malreduction will occur.

Regarding anchor placement, it is important to recognize the normal bare area on the greater tuberosity over which the infraspinatus crosses before inserting just laterally on the footprint. For single-row repair, malreduction can occur if this region of the repair is situated at the articular margin, within the normal bare area; if trial reduction reveals relative overtensioning, only a more medial position within the bare area may be feasible. However, for simple rotator cuff tears, particularly posteriorly, it is not uncommon to encounter sufficient mobility and reducibility. For similar reasons, the bare area must be appreciated with TOE constructs as well.

Regardless which construct is used, sutures must be correctly placed in relation to the anchor to avoid malreduction. To optimize placement, with the tendon reduced the surgeon could use a tendon grasper to crimp the tendon above the anchor, thereby leaving a visual mark for later targeting with a suture passer. When more than one anchor is used, care must be taken to pass the sutures from a given anchor through the tendon equidistant to sutures from the other anchor in relation to the anterior-posterior distance between the anchors themselves. Furthermore, it is important to recognize that tendon retraction is not directly medial; the tendons retract posteriorly and medially, in an oblique manner. Typically, in a trial reduction the tendon is pulled laterally and anteriorly; thus, when the tendon is not in the reduced state, sutures can be passed relatively posterior in relation to the anchor from which they came. In the anterior region of the rotator cuff tear at which the anterior cord resides, the reduction maneuver can be less oblique because the target insertion is posterior to the bicipital groove. If the anterior cord of the supraspinatus is involved, dedicated anchor fixation may be preferable.

Medial failure has been well described. Salvage may be challenging because there may be limited or no tissue to receive additional sutures in the revision setting. Therefore, creating a tension-free repair should take priority over complete footprint restoration to minimize the risk of medial failure. For tears that involve considerable tendon retraction or tissue loss, single-row repair with footprint medialization and suture passes near the rotator cable may be necessary. For tears that are readily reducible with at least 10 to 15 mm of tissue preservation medial to the tear edge, TOE repair should be considered. For tears involving the anterior cord, additional fixation involving the cord itself should be considered, regardless whether a single-row or TOE construct is used.

Bibliography

Ahmad CS, Vorys GC, Covey A, Levine WN, Gardner TR, Bigliani LU: Rotator cuff repair fluid extravasation characteristics are influenced by repair technique. *J Shoulder Elbow Surg* 2009;18(6):976-981.

Anderl W, Heuberer PR, Laky B, Kriegleder B, Reihsner R, Eberhardsteiner J: Superiority of bridging techniques with medial fixation on initial strength. *Knee Surg Sports Traumatol Arthrosc* 2012;20(12):2559-2566.

Barber FA, Drew OR: A biomechanical comparison of tendon-bone interface motion and cyclic loading between single-row, triple-loaded cuff repairs and double-row, suture-tape cuff repairs using biocomposite anchors. *Arthroscopy* 2012;28(9):1197-1205.

Boileau P, Brassart N, Watkinson DJ, Carles M, Hatzidakis AM, Krishnan SG: Arthroscopic repair of full-thickness tears of the supraspinatus: Does the tendon really heal? *J Bone Joint Surg Am* 2005;87(6):1229-1240.

Boyer P, Bouthors C, Delcourt T, et al: Arthroscopic double-row cuff repair with suture-bridging: A structural and functional comparison of two techniques. *Knee Surg Sports Traumatol Arthrosc* 2015;23(2):478-486.

Burkhart SS, Adams CR, Burkhart SS, Schoolfield JD: A biomechanical comparison of 2 techniques of footprint reconstruction for rotator cuff repair: The SwiveLock-FiberChain construct versus standard double-row repair. *Arthroscopy* 2009;25(3):274-281.

Burks RT, Crim J, Brown N, Fink B, Greis PE: A prospective randomized clinical trial comparing arthroscopic single- and double-row rotator cuff repair: Magnetic resonance imaging and early clinical evaluation. *Am J Sports Med* 2009;37(4):674-682.

Carbonel I, Martinez AA, Calvo A, Ripalda J, Herrera A: Single-row versus double-row arthroscopic repair in the treatment of rotator cuff tears: A prospective randomized clinical study. *Int Orthop* 2012;36(9):1877-1883.

Cho NS, Yi JW, Lee BG, Rhee YG: Retear patterns after arthroscopic rotator cuff repair: Single-row versus suture bridge technique. *Am J Sports Med* 2010;38(4):664-671.

Franceschi F, Ruzzini L, Longo UG, et al: Equivalent clinical results of arthroscopic single-row and double-row suture anchor repair for rotator cuff tears: A randomized controlled trial. *Am J Sports Med* 2007;35(8):1254-1260.

Gartsman GM, Drake G, Edwards TB, et al: Ultrasound evaluation of arthroscopic full-thickness supraspinatus rotator cuff repair: Single-row versus double-row suture bridge (transosseous equivalent) fixation. Results of a prospective, randomized study. *J Shoulder Elbow Surg* 2013;22(11):1480-1487.

Gates JJ, Gilliland J, McGarry MH, et al: Influence of distinct anatomic subregions of the supraspinatus on humeral rotation. *J Orthop Res* 2010;28(1):12-17.

Gimbel JA, Van Kleunen JP, Lake SP, Williams GR, Soslowsky LJ: The role of repair tension on tendon to bone healing in an animal model of chronic rotator cuff tears. *J Biomech* 2007;40(3):561-568.

Grasso A, Milano G, Salvatore M, Falcone G, Deriu L, Fabbriciani C: Single-row versus double-row arthroscopic rotator cuff repair: A prospective randomized clinical study. *Arthroscopy* 2009;25(1):4-12.

Jost PW, Khair MM, Chen DX, Wright TM, Kelly AM, Rodeo SA: Suture number determines strength of rotator cuff repair. *J Bone Joint Surg Am* 2012;94(14):e100.

Killian ML, Cavinatto L, Galatz LM, Thomopoulos S: The role of mechanobiology in tendon healing. *J Shoulder Elbow Surg* 2012;21(2):228-237.

Kim DH, Elattrache NS, Tibone JE, et al: Biomechanical comparison of a single-row versus double-row suture anchor technique for rotator cuff repair. *Am J Sports Med* 2006;34(3):407-414.

Koh KH, Kang KC, Lim TK, Shon MS, Yoo JC: Prospective randomized clinical trial of single- versus double-row suture anchor repair in 2- to 4-cm rotator cuff tears: Clinical and magnetic resonance imaging results. *Arthroscopy* 2011;27(4):453-462.

Lapner PL, Sabri E, Rakhra K, et al: A multicenter randomized controlled trial comparing single-row with double-row fixation in arthroscopic rotator cuff repair. *J Bone Joint Surg Am* 2012;94(14):1249-1257.

Lorbach O, Kieb M, Raber F, Busch LC, Kohn D, Pape D: Comparable biomechanical results for a modified single-row rotator cuff reconstruction using triple-loaded suture anchors versus a suture-bridging double-row repair. *Arthroscopy* 2012;28(2):178-187.

Mall NA, Lee AS, Chahal J, et al: Transosseous-equivalent rotator cuff repair: A systematic review on the biomechanical importance of tying the medial row. *Arthroscopy* 2013;29(2):377-386.

Mihata T, Lee TQ, Watanabe C, et al: Clinical results of arthroscopic superior capsule reconstruction for irreparable rotator cuff tears. *Arthroscopy* 2013;29(3):459-470.

Millett PJ, Warth RJ: Posterosuperior rotator cuff tears: Classification, pattern recognition, and treatment. *J Am Acad Orthop Surg* 2014;22(8):521-534.

Millett PJ, Warth RJ, Dornan GJ, Lee JT, Spiegl UJ: Clinical and structural outcomes after arthroscopic single-row versus double-row rotator cuff repair: A systematic review and meta-analysis of level I randomized clinical trials. *J Shoulder Elbow Surg* 2014;23(4):586-597.

Minagawa H, Itoi E, Konno N, et al: Humeral attachment of the supraspinatus and infraspinatus tendons: An anatomic study. *Arthroscopy* 1998;14(3):302-306.

Mochizuki T, Sugaya H, Uomizu M, et al: Humeral insertion of the supraspinatus and infraspinatus: New anatomical findings regarding the footprint of the rotator cuff. *J Bone Joint Surg Am* 2008;90(5):962-969.

Mori D, Funakoshi N, Yamashita F: Arthroscopic surgery of irreparable large or massive rotator cuff tears with low-grade fatty degeneration of the infraspinatus: Patch autograft procedure versus partial repair procedure. *Arthroscopy* 2013;29(12):1911-1921.

Nguyen ML, Quigley RJ, Galle SE, et al: Margin convergence anchorage to bone for reconstruction of the anterior attachment of the rotator cable. *Arthroscopy* 2012;28(9):1237-1245.

Park MC: Biomechanical validation of rotator cuff repair techniques and considerations for a "technical efficiency ratio". *Arthroscopy* 2013;29(7):1230-1234.

Park MC, Bui C, Park CJ, Oh JH, Lee TQ: Rotator cuff tendon repair morphology comparing 2 single-anchor repair techniques. *Arthroscopy* 2013;29(7):1149-1156.

Park MC, Elattrache NS, Ahmad CS, Tibone JE: "Transosseous-equivalent" rotator cuff repair technique. *Arthroscopy* 2006;22(12):1360.e1-1360.e5.

Park MC, ElAttrache NS, Tibone JE, Ahmad CS, Jun BJ, Lee TQ: Part I: Footprint contact characteristics for a transosseous-equivalent rotator cuff repair technique compared with a double-row repair technique. *J Shoulder Elbow Surg* 2007;16(4):461-468.

Park MC, Idjadi JA, Elattrache NS, Tibone JE, McGarry MH, Lee TQ: The effect of dynamic external rotation comparing 2 footprint-restoring rotator cuff repair techniques. *Am J Sports Med* 2008;36(5):893-900.

Park MC, Jun BJ, Park CJ, Ahmad CS, ElAttrache NS, Lee TQ: The biomechanical effects of dynamic external rotation on rotator cuff repair compared to testing with the humerus fixed. *Am J Sports Med* 2007;35(11):1931-1939.

Park MC, McGarry MH, Gunzenhauser RC, Benefiel MK, Park CJ, Lee TQ: Does transosseous-equivalent rotator cuff repair biomechanically provide a "self-reinforcement" effect compared with single-row repair? *J Shoulder Elbow Surg* 2014;23(12):1813-1821.

Park MC, Peterson A, Patton J, McGarry MH, Park CJ, Lee TQ: Biomechanical effects of a 2 suture-pass medial inter-implant mattress on transosseous-equivalent rotator cuff repair and considerations for a "technical efficiency ratio". *J Shoulder Elbow Surg* 2014;23(3):361-368.

Park MC, Pirolo JM, Park CJ, McGarry MH, Tibone JE, Lee TQ: The effect of abduction and rotation on footprint contact for single-row, double-row, and modified double-row rotator cuff repair techniques. *Am J Sports Med* 2009;37(8):1599-1608.

Park MC, Tibone JE, ElAttrache NS, Ahmad CS, Jun BJ, Lee TQ: Part II: Biomechanical assessment for a footprint-restoring transosseous-equivalent rotator cuff repair technique compared with a double-row repair technique. *J Shoulder Elbow Surg* 2007;16(4):469-476.

Roh MS, Wang VM, April EW, Pollock RG, Bigliani LU, Flatow EL: Anterior and posterior musculotendinous anatomy of the supraspinatus. *J Shoulder Elbow Surg* 2000;9(5):436-440.

Takeda H, Urata S, Matsuura M, Nakayama A, Yonemitsu H: The influence of medial reattachment of the torn cuff tendon for retracted rotator cuff tears. *J Shoulder Elbow Surg* 2007;16(3):316-320.

Xu C, Zhao J, Li D: Meta-analysis comparing single-row and double-row repair techniques in the arthroscopic treatment of rotator cuff tears. *J Shoulder Elbow Surg* 2014;23(2):182-188.

Yamamoto N, Itoi E, Tuoheti Y, et al: Glenohumeral joint motion after medial shift of the attachment site of the supraspinatus tendon: A cadaveric study. *J Shoulder Elbow Surg* 2007;16(3):373-378.

Yoo JC, Ahn JH, Koh KH, Lim KS: Rotator cuff integrity after arthroscopic repair for large tears with less-than-optimal footprint coverage. *Arthroscopy* 2009;25(10):1093-1100.

 ## Video Reference

Park MC: Video. *Medial-Pulley Transosseus-Equivalent Rotator Cuff Repair With Dedicated Anterior Cord Fixation for the "Simple" Rotator Cuff Repair.* Calabasas, CA, 2015.

Chapter 22

Arthroscopic Repair of Massive Rotator Cuff Tears: Anatomic Considerations, Releases, and Mobilization Techniques

Leslie A. Fink Barnes, MD

Evan L. Flatow, MD

 ## Introduction

A massive rotator cuff tear (RCT) is a tear of two rotator cuff tendons that is sometimes further defined as a combined cuff tear measuring greater than 5 cm in the AP direction. Massive RCTs are particularly disabling because they result in dramatically altered shoulder biomechanics. For example, a single tendon tear, such as complete rupture of the supraspinatus, results in decreased or weakened shoulder elevation, whereas complete loss of the supraspinatus in addition to even partial loss of the infraspinatus may result in a kinematic change during shoulder motion with shifting of the humeral head during attempted shoulder rotation.

Massive RCTs can be repaired arthroscopically as long as appropriate preoperative planning has been done and advanced techniques are used intraoperatively. Muscle quality, patient age, and tendon retraction are crucial determinants of tear reparability. Coexisting factors, such as the presence of arthritis, previous surgery, or nerve injury, should be considered as well.

Physical examination and clinical history are the first steps in determining whether arthroscopic repair of a massive RCT is advisable. Patient age is one of the most important factors related to success. The failure rate is higher in patients older than 60 years than in younger patients. Patient tobacco use is another factor that negatively affects tendon healing. Healed incisions offer information on any previous surgery. Atrophy in the supraspinatus or infraspinatus fossa is a poor prognostic sign indicative of chronicity. Lag signs are useful in predicting the size of the RCT. Restoration of near-full passive range of motion is recommended before rotator cuff repair.

Radiographs and MRIs are obtained in the evaluation of RCTs. Radiographs are helpful in determining acromiohumeral distance. Coronal and sagittal T2-weighted MRIs are helpful in determining the size of the tear, the amount of retraction, and the presence or degree of atrophy of the supraspinatus and infraspinatus tendons. Axial T2-weighted MRIs are helpful for evaluating the subscapularis and very posterior infraspinatus tendon tears. T1-weighted sagittal MRIs obtained just lateral to the medial border of the scapula are useful in assessing fatty infiltration of the rotator cuff muscles, which is an important factor in predicting tendon quality and mobility intraoperatively as well as cuff function after attempted repair. A tear with extensive fatty infiltration is likely to be chronic, and rotator cuff repair may be inadvisable if the degree of fatty infiltration is greater than or equal to the muscle bulk present (Goutallier grade 3 or 4). Ultrasound and CT are warranted only in select cases. For example, in a patient with a pacemaker or other device that prohibits MRI, ultrasound and CT are used in evaluating retraction, atrophy, and fatty infiltration. Electromyography is indicated in patients in whom neuropathy is present or in whom marked atrophy is present on clinical examination and MRI does not demonstrate substantial fatty infiltration.

An RCT may be considered inoperable if the acromiohumeral distance is less than 7 mm (indicating static superior migration of the humeral head) or in the setting of substantial tendon retraction with poor muscle quality, as indicated by advanced fatty infiltration on MRI. Muscle atrophy and fatty infiltration can predict a poor clinical outcome even if the tendon can be restored to the anatomic footprint, and these degenerative

Dr. Flatow or an immediate family member has received royalties from Innomed and Zimmer, serves as an unpaid consultant to Zimmer, and serves as a board member, owner, officer, or committee member of the American Academy of Orthopaedic Surgeons and the Healthcare Association of New York. Neither Dr. Fink Barnes nor any immediate family member has received anything of value from or has stock or stock options held in a commercial company or institution related directly or indirectly to the subject of this chapter.

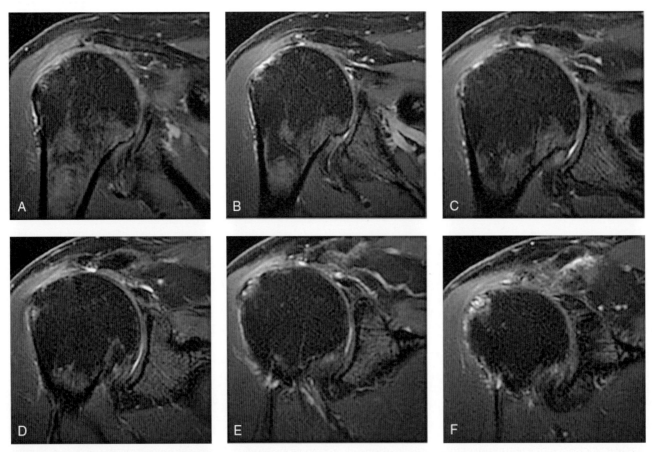

Figure 1 **A-F,** Sequential T2-weighted coronal MRIs of the left shoulder taken at 5-mm increments demonstrate a massive rotator cuff tear with retraction beginning at the leading edge of the supraspinatus and extending posteriorly.

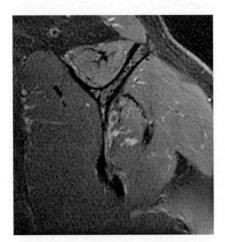

Figure 2 Sagittal T2-weighted MRI demonstrates minimal atrophy of the rotator cuff.

changes do not reverse even after successful surgical repair.

Several studies have shown that repairs of massive RCTs are more prone to failure than are repairs of smaller tears. Outcomes are best after tension-free repair with sufficient tendon-bone fixation. Proper patient selection and surgeon familiarity with advanced arthroscopic surgical techniques are critical factors in achieving successful outcomes after repair of massive RCTs.

Case Presentation

A 55-year-old right-hand–dominant man presents with a 2-month history of left shoulder pain and weakness with overhead activity after a bench press injury. Active range of motion is 170° of forward elevation and 60° of external rotation in the injured shoulder. The patient exhibits grade 4/5 strength with pain on forward elevation (**Figures 1** through **10**).

Indications

In a patient with high functional demands, no arthritis, a normal acromiohumeral interval of greater than 7 mm, and limitations in activities of daily living because of pain or weakness, arthroscopic rotator cuff repair of a massive two-tendon tear is indicated. The authors of this chapter typically reserve arthroscopic repair of massive defects for primary cases, unless the previous arthroscopic repair was very remote.

Patients with long-standing shoulder pain and weakness for more than 1 year are much more likely to have contracted

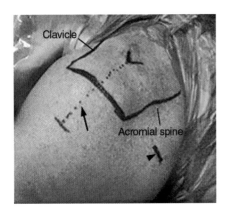

Figure 3 Photograph shows the markings delineating the planned portal sites (dash marks) on the left shoulder of a patient undergoing arthroscopic rotator cuff repair. The patient is in the beach-chair position. The solid lines mark the clavicle anteriorly and the acromion posteriorly and laterally. The dotted line (arrow) indicates the midline of the lateral border of the acromion connecting with the Neviaser point medially. The posterior viewing portal is marked with a dash (arrowhead) approximately 2 cm distal and 1 cm medial to the posterolateral corner of the acromion. The lateral working portal is marked with a dash approximately 3 cm distal to the lateral border of the acromion at the midline.

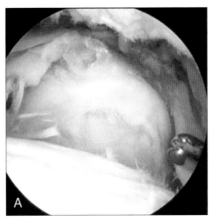 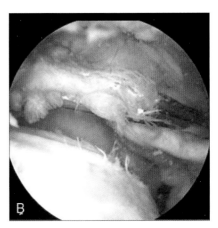

Figure 4 **A,** Arthroscopic view from the lateral portal demonstrates a massive rotator cuff tear that is retracted to the glenoid rim. **B,** Arthroscopic view from the same portal demonstrates use of the grasper to pull the rotator cuff laterally as mobility is assessed for the first time intraoperatively.

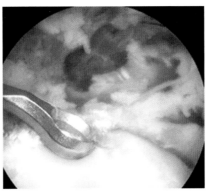

Figure 5 Arthroscopic view from the lateral portal demonstrates preparation of the greater tuberosity with a ring curet. Alternatively, a 4.5-mm shaver can be used.

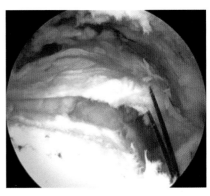

Figure 6 Arthroscopic view from the lateral portal demonstrates placement of a traction stitch, which assists with mobilization and is used to apply gentle tension to the tendon while adhesions are released.

tears with substantial adhesions, making repair more difficult and functional improvement less predictable. Preoperative counseling is advised to set appropriate patient expectations.

Even in the case of recurrent or persistent defects after repair of a massive RCT, patients typically experience predictable improvement in pain postoperatively. This improvement may be the result of the concomitant procedures performed at the time of massive arthroscopic rotator cuff repair, such as subacromial decompression, biceps management, lysis of adhesions, and suprascapular nerve (SSN) release, or it may be the result of rest, physical therapy, and partial maintenance of the cuff repair. Sustained functional gains depend on maintenance of repair integrity.

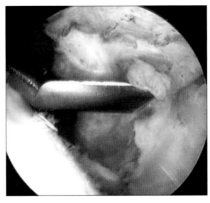

Figure 7 Arthroscopic view from the posterior portal demonstrates capsular release using an arthroscopic elevator inserted through the lateral portal.

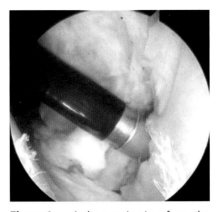

Figure 8 Arthroscopic view from the posterior portal demonstrates electrocautery used for anterior interval release.

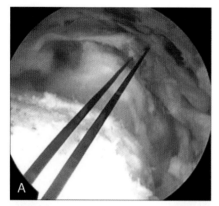
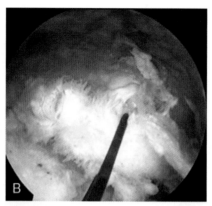
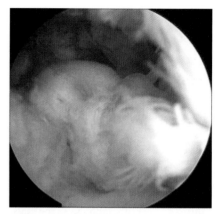

Figure 9   Arthroscopic view from the lateral portal demonstrates the retracted tendon position (**A**) and the mobilization of the tendon to the greater tuberosity after the capsular, bursal, and interval releases were performed (**B**). After adequate releases, the rotator cuff tissue can be mobilized past the articular margin to the medial portion of the rotator footprint on the greater tuberosity.

Figure 10   Arthroscopic view from the posterior portal after anchor placement and suturing, with four simple sutures tied to repair the débrided tendon edge.

Controversies and Alternative Approaches

Nonsurgical treatment, such as physical therapy of the elbow with periscapular muscle strengthening, may be indicated for the asymptomatic patient who has low functional demands and minimal pain and who can perform activities of daily living. The patient with a large RCT but a balanced force couple may have nearly normal shoulder motion with active forward elevation greater than 120°. Relative indications for nonsurgical management in the presence of a massive RCT are previous failed rotator cuff surgery and, in a younger patient (age <60 years), the presence of glenohumeral arthritis. However, the patient who elects nonsurgical treatment should be counseled that if in the future symptoms develop or surgical intervention is desired, then the tear may no longer be reparable. In a patient older than 70 years, the risk of tear progression is mitigated by the potential for future reverse total shoulder arthroplasty. Mini-open approaches with or without biologic or synthetic augmentation may be preferred for revision rotator cuff repair.

In a patient with low functional demands who presents with severe pain but who does not want to undergo immobilization and postoperative rehabilitation, the goals of treatment may be limited to pain relief without rotator cuff repair. Such a patient may be treated nonsurgically with a subacromial injection or surgically with shoulder arthroscopy, biceps tenotomy, removal of a subacromial spur, and débridement of the rotator cuff. In these patients, the coracoacromial ligament should be preserved to help contain superior humeral migration and decentering. Biceps tenotomy alone has been shown to relieve pain in patients with irreparable cuff tears.

In a patient older than 70 years with a massive RCT, arthritis, and poor rotator cuff quality, reverse total shoulder arthroplasty is the treatment of choice. This procedure improves forward elevation; concomitant latissimus dorsi transfer must be performed to improve external rotation. In the presence of axillary nerve palsy or deltoid dysfunction, glenohumeral arthrodesis may be considered.

In young patients with higher functional demands, arthroscopic rotator cuff repair is usually the best treatment option. However, in young patients with irreparable chronic tears or in the presence of superior humeral migration with an acromiohumeral interval less than 7 mm, partial rotator cuff repair with tendon transfers can be considered. In general, partial rotator cuff repair results in only limited temporary improvement. Latissimus dorsi transfers are preferred for addressing posterosuperior cuff deficits, but successful results have been achieved only in the setting of an intact subscapularis. A pectoralis major tendon transfer under the strap muscles can be used to achieve stability in patients with irreparable subscapularis tears and an intact infraspinatus; however, this transfer does not result in increased forward elevation.

Controversies exist regarding concomitant procedures undertaken at the time of arthroscopic repair of massive RCTs. Although release of the SSN has been advocated as a helpful adjunct for pain relief and reversal of muscle atrophy, additional research is needed to determine the role of SSN decompression in the setting of rotator cuff repair. Opinions vary regarding biceps management as well. The authors of this chapter consider biceps tenodesis mainly for younger or very active, muscular patients and prefer biceps tenotomy for older, less active patients. Subacromial decompression is a controversial topic in the published literature. However, the authors of this chapter consider subacromial decompression to be essential for removing external impingement and creating a working space for mobilization of the retracted tendons. If space permits, the rotator cuff repair may be undertaken before decompression to maximize visibility.

 Results

The results of arthroscopic repair of massive RCTs have been mixed (**Table 1**). Generally, high initial success rates for pain relief and functional improvements have been shown. However, high failure rates at midterm follow-up have been reported. Repair technique strongly influences success, and transosseous-equivalent double-row repair in a suture bridge construct has been shown to be the most successful arthroscopic repair technique for massive RCTs. Excessive contact pressures have been shown to impede healing; thus, the surgeon should avoid overtensioning retracted massive RCTs. Adequate mobilization and lysis of adhesions is as crucial in managing massive RCTs as is the repair construct itself.

 Technical Keys to Success

Interval slide techniques may improve shoulder function even if the tear is not completely repairable. Partial repair of the infraspinatus or subscapularis tendons, for example, may rebalance the shoulder forces even if the supraspinatus cannot be repaired. Margin convergence may aid in reinnervating the rotator cuff and buttressing the tendon repair construct.

Tendon mobilization is critical to success because it allows tendon repair. Mobilization allows reduced tension on sutures and anchors and promotes coverage of the anatomic footprint. Tendon gliding is essential and is more important than coverage of the entire anatomic footprint. Tendon releases allow muscle tendon excursion and prevent stiffness. Capsular release can augment bursal-sided releases.

- The authors of this chapter perform rotator cuff repair with the patient under regional anesthesia with sedation and placed in the beach-chair position. The arthroscopy tower is placed on the contralateral side of the patient with the scrub nurse, and the arm is controlled with a pneumatic arm holder.
- The arthroscope is first introduced through a standard posterior viewing portal, after which an anterior portal is established in the rotator interval. Two lateral portals are typically required for repair of massive RCTs. When two lateral portals are used, one serves as the viewing portal and the other as the working portal.
- A 7-mm fully threaded clear cannula is inserted in the working portal.
- After glenohumeral joint débridement and subacromial decompression, attention is turned to the rotator cuff. Assessment of the tear pattern and initial tendon mobility guides the necessary lysis of adhesions and repair strategy.
- Using an arthroscopic elevator or electrocautery through a lateral portal, the capsule and subacromial bursa are elevated off the rotator cuff from the leading edge of the supraspinatus tendon to the scapular spine posteriorly.
- The undersurface of the rotator cuff is lifted off the glenoid in a plane superior and medial to the labrum.
- If the tendon is not sufficiently freed to pass the articular margin

after subacromial lysis of adhesions and the capsular release, then additional releases (slides) are performed. When two tendons have similar retraction, they are mobilized together. For example, if the supraspinatus and subscapularis tendons are both retracted, maintaining their interval connection, that comma-shaped arc of soft tissue (comma sign), will allow each repair to reinforce the other.

- In the setting of differential retraction, an interval release may be considered. For example, if the supraspinatus is retracted but the subscapularis is intact, releasing the anterior rotator interval (anterior interval slide) allows mobilization and realignment of the supraspinatus vis-à-vis the subscapularis. This anterior interval slide consists of release of the supraspinatus tendon from the coracohumeral ligament and the rotator interval tissue to the base of the coracoid (**Figure 11**).
- If part of the rotator cuff is immobile and retracted but another portion has greater excursion, then both anterior and posterior interval slides can be used to mobilize parts of the rotator cuff tendons for reattachment to the greater tuberosity (**Figure 12**).
- In cases of differential mobility, the posterior leaf of the RCT is usually the least retracted. In the posterior interval slide, the supraspinatus tendon is separated from the infraspinatus tendon using electrocautery or arthroscopic scissors. The posterior interval release is directed toward the scapular spine until the surgeon reaches the fat pad that protects the SSN (**Figure 13**).
- The technique of margin convergence can be helpful in managing deep U-shaped tears. With this approach, side-to-side free sutures without an anchor are used to join the anterior and posterior leaves of

Table 1 Results of Arthroscopic Repair of Massive Rotator Cuff Tears

Authors	Journal (Year)	Number	Outcomes[a]	Failure Rate (%)	Comments
Galatz et al	*J Bone Joint Surg Am* (2004)	18 patients	ASES score improved from 48.3 to 79.9 Active FE increased from 92° to 142° Active ER increased from 44.7° to 53.2°	94.4	Recurrent or persistent defect was present in 17 patients on ultrasound Results tended to deteriorate with time All patients stated that they would undergo the procedure again Final follow-up, 24 mo
Bishop et al	*J Shoulder Elbow Surg* (2006)	17 shoulders	ASES score improved from 47 to 73 Constant score improved from 46 to 69 Pain decreased significantly ($P < 0.01$) Strength improvement was not statistically significant	88	The highest failure rate was seen for massive tears (88%) relative to tears <3 cm, which were intact in 84% of cases (16% failure) Final follow-up, 12 mo
Lee et al	*J Shoulder Elbow Surg* (2007)	21 patients	ASES score increased from 41 to 67 Constant score increased from 50 to 68	NR	Pain decreased by half Trend toward improved strength and AROM Mean follow-up, 16.5 mo
Denard, Jiwani et al	*Arthroscopy* (2012)	126 shoulders	FE improved from 132° to 168° VAS pain score improved from 6.3 to 1.3 UCLA score improved from 15.7 to 30.7 ASES score improved from 41.7 to 85.7	NR	Results were best after complete repair and after double-row repair ($P < 0.05$) Single-row and partial repairs were inferior in terms of satisfaction, return to activity, and UCLA functional outcomes No significant difference was seen in ASES score Mean follow-up, 99 mo

AHI = acromiohumeral interval, AROM = active range of motion, ASES = American Shoulder and Elbow Surgeons shoulder outcome, ER = external rotation, FE = forward elevation, NR = not reported, SST = Simple Shoulder Test, UCLA = University of California–Los Angeles Shoulder Rating Scale, VAS = visual analog scale.

[a] All values are means unless otherwise noted.

the tear before tendon-bone reattachment is performed.

- After the rotator cuff tissue has been fully mobilized to a position lateral to the humeral articular surface, repair of the rotator cuff is continued.
- The anatomic footprint is prepared and débrided.
- The patient's arm is positioned in full adduction and then is moved into internal and external rotation to present different portions of the tuberosity. External humeral rotation presents the anterior portion of

the greater tuberosity, whereas internal rotation brings the posterior portion of the tuberosity into view.

- Before anchors are placed percutaneously just lateral to the acromial edge, a spinal needle is inserted to gauge the eventual position of the anchor on the exposed tuberosity. The anchors should be placed at least 5 mm apart.
- The medial row anchors may be placed adjacent to the articular margin.
- Traction stitches often are a helpful

adjunct to keep the tendon edge in proximity of the suture anchors and suture. A No. 2 braided polyester suture with an ultra-high–molecular-weight polyethylene core can be placed at the leading edge and posterior leaf of the tear, then clamped outside the skin with appropriate tension. Alternatively, an assistant can maintain steady lateral traction on the tendon using a tissue grasper.

- Using a spring-needle suture passer, sutures are passed from a

Table 1 Results of Arthroscopic Repair of Massive Rotator Cuff Tears *(continued)*

Authors	Journal (Year)	Number	Outcomes[a]	Failure Rate (%)	Comments
Denard, Lädermann et al	*Arthroscopy* (2012)	39 patients treated with primary repair, 14 with revision repair	***Primary repair*** Active FE improved from 49° to 155° ASES score improved from 37.5 to 84.0 UCLA score improved from 12.7 to 29.4 VAS pain score improved from 5.6 to 1.4 ***Revision*** Active FE improved from 43° to 109° ASES score improved from 40.6 to 56.6 UCLA score improved from 11.8 to 20.6 VAS pain score improved from 5.6 to 2.8	NR	Return to activity was significantly higher after primary care than after revision (80% and 39%, respectively [$P < 0.05$]) Pseudoparalysis was reversed in 90% of primary cases and 43% of revisions ($P < 0.01$) In primary cases, recovery of FE > 90° was associated with a shorter interval before repair and a complete repair ($P < 0.05$) Mean follow-up, 75 mo (primary) and 72 mo (revision)
Chung et al	*Am J Sports Med* (2013)	108 patients	Active FE improved from 165.2° to 175.4° Active ER improved from 65.9° to 70.0° ASES score improved from 55.7 to 83.1 Constant score improved from 47.7 to 71.2 VAS pain score improved from 5.1 to 1.3	39.8	Functional status improved significantly regardless of cuff healing ($P < 0.05$) Fatty infiltration of the infraspinatus muscle and reduced AHI were negative prognostic signs ($P < 0.05$) Mean follow-up, 31.8 ± 15.8 mo
Kim et al	*J Bone Joint Surg Am* (2013)	22 patients treated with posterior slide, 19 with margin convergence	SST score, ASES score, UCLA score, and range of motion improved in both groups ($P < 0.001$ for all) ***Posterior slide*** Active FE improved from 113.9° to 138.6° Active ER improved from 31.4° to 48.4° ASES score improved from 40.3 to 81.5 UCLA score improved from 14.6 to 27.0 ***Margin convergence*** Active FE improved from 115° to 141.1° Active ER improved from 31.8° to 50.8° ASES score improved from 40.3 to 85.6 UCLA score improved from 15.4 to 28.4	91 (retear)	No benefit was seen with the posterior interval slide relative to partial repair via margin convergence Re-tear noted on MRI at 6-mo follow-up Mean follow-up, 24 mo

AHI = acromiohumeral interval, AROM = active range of motion, ASES = American Shoulder and Elbow Surgeons shoulder outcome, ER = external rotation, FE = forward elevation, NR = not reported, SST = Simple Shoulder Test, UCLA = University of California–Los Angeles Shoulder Rating Scale, VAS = visual analog scale.

[a] All values are means unless otherwise noted.

double-loaded anchor through the tendon in a retrograde manner to form a horizontal mattress stitch. The posterior limbs are shuttled out of the posterior portal, and the anterior anchor suture limbs are shuttled out of the anterior portal.

- The posterior anchor and sutures are addressed first. Typically, two double-loaded screw-in bioabsorbable suture anchors are sufficient to span the AP dimension of the RCT.

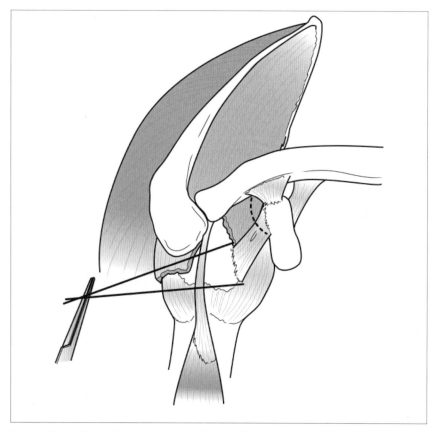

Figure 11 Illustration depicts coracohumeral ligament release (that is, anterior interval slide), which is performed to mobilize a retracted tear of the supraspinatus tendon.

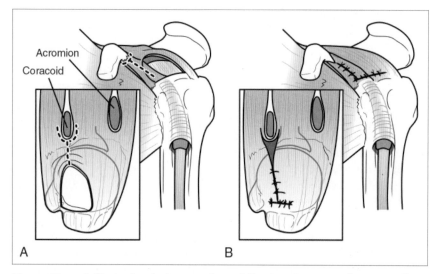

Figure 12 **A,** Illustration depicts anterior mobilization of a retracted rotator cuff tear by releasing the rotator interval. **B,** Illustration depicts repair of the rotator cuff using the anterior interval slide followed by the margin convergence technique.

However, some tears measuring greater than 5 cm may require the insertion of a third anchor posteriorly. The authors of this chapter prefer to tie the medial row of sutures using an alternating half-hitch knot through the lateral cannula.

- After knot-tying, the free suture limbs are threaded through one or two lateral row anchors to create a transosseous-equivalent suture bridge fixation for optimal restoration of the anatomic footprint.
- The lateral row anchors are placed 3 cm distal to the medial row anchors through the lateral working cannula.
- A spot is cleared on the humerus using electrocautery for insertion of the lateral row anchors. The remaining suture tails are cut short after the lateral anchors are secured and appropriate repair tension is confirmed.
- Side-to-side sutures may be used to strengthen the repair of the rotator cuff, as in the case of L-shaped tears or if an interval slide has been performed. In side-to-side repair, suture is passed from the posterior supraspinatus limb anteriorly to the leading edge of the infraspinatus tendon, without the need for an anchor in the humerus. The suture is passed using a spring-needle suture passer, then tied.
- Wound closure is then performed with absorbable buried sutures, and a dressing is applied.
- The arm is placed in a padded shoulder sling with a small abduction pillow unless body habitus provides a sufficient amount of abduction.

Rehabilitation

Delayed motion is the key to rehabilitation after surgery to repair massive RCTs. The risk of re-tear is greater than the risk of stiffness. Greater success is achieved with reoperation to address stiffness (such as a capsular release) than with re-repair of rotator cuff re-tear (**Table 2**).

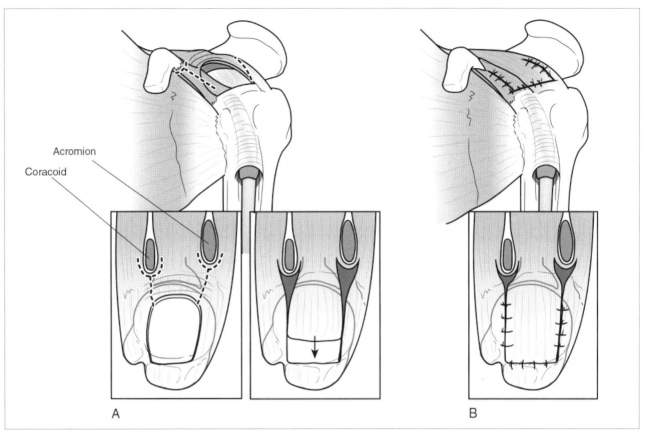

Figure 13   Illustrations depict the double interval slide technique. **A,** The coracohumeral ligament and the rotator interval are released anteriorly, and the interval between the supraspinatus and the infraspinatus is released posteriorly, allowing lateral mobilization of the rotator cuff. **B,** Final appearance of the repair using the double interval slide technique.

 ## Avoiding Pitfalls

The SSN is at risk when performing subacromial lysis of adhesions and during the posterior interval slide technique. The SSN curves tightly around the base of the scapular spine, where it meets the posterior glenoid neck, and the nerve is enveloped in a fat pad approximately 3.5 cm medial to the glenoid rim. The nerve lies approximately 5.3 cm from the articular margin of the rotator cuff footprint and 6 cm from the lateral border of the acromion. The average distance from the posterior rim of the glenoid to the motor branches of the infraspinatus muscle is 2 cm. In addition, the SSN travels across the scapula 3 cm from the supraglenoid tubercle. The average distance from the origin of the long head of

the biceps tendon to the motor branches of the supraspinatus is 2 cm.

It is important not to disrupt the coracoacromial ligament in patients with massive RCTs. This ligament should be elevated as a periosteal sleeve from the anteroinferior acromion if decompression is required in that location. The coracohumeral ligament often requires release from the rotator interval to the base of the coracoid in retracted RCTs to achieve lateral tendon advancement and improved external rotation postoperatively.

The surgeon must take care not to overly tension the repair when mobilizing massive retracted tears. Excursion should be sufficient to cover the humeral head, but the application of undue force must be avoided. If excursion is

not sufficient, repair at the medial border of the anatomic footprint adjacent to the articular surface is preferred over excessive tension on a lateralized repair that would place the construct at high risk for failure. In the setting of differential tension or adhesion, margin convergence followed by partial repair is preferred.

The subscapularis tendon must be thoroughly evaluated because problems related to this tendon are commonly missed. Even partial tears of the upper border of the subscapularis can place tension on the supraspinatus repair. If necessary for visualization, release of the middle glenohumeral ligament should be performed to confirm that the musculotendinous junction of the subscapularis is at the level of the glenoid

Table 2 Rehabilitation Protocol After Arthroscopic Repair of Massive Rotator Cuff Tears

Postoperative Week	ROM	Strengthening	Return to Play	Comments/ Emphasis
0-4	No shoulder ROM allowed Active elbow, wrist, and finger ROM permitted Pendulum exercises (restricted to small arcs) are allowed	None	No	Sling worn at all times No physical therapy Allow rotator cuff healing
4-6	Based on the limits prescribed by the surgeon, PROM and AAROM are begun (forward elevation in scapular plane and external rotation at the side); typically, this consists of forward elevation to 100° and external rotation to the side	None	No	Specific instructions from the surgeon for physical therapy must be followed Some motion is begun
6-12	As symptoms allow, ROM is advanced to full forward elevation, external rotation, and internal rotation Active motion should always be started in the supine position with progression to an upright position	None	No	Full motion should be achieved
12-24	Light strengthening is begun at 3 mo Return to desk job allowed	Light exercises allowed	No	Strengthening is begun
>24	Return to play or heavy labor job allowed	Yes	Yes	Return to full activity

AAROM = active-assisted range of motion, PROM = passive range of motion, ROM = range of motion.

Adapted with permission from Columbia University Shoulder, Elbow, and Sports Medicine Service: *Arthroscopic Massive Rotator Cuff Repair Physical Therapy Protocol*. Available at: http://cses.cumc.columbia.edu/documents/ArthroscopicMassiveRotatorCuffRepair.pdf. Accessed November 10, 2015.

and that the rolled edge is intact. Otherwise, subscapularis repair should be performed before proceeding with repair of the supraspinatus and infraspinatus tendons.

Conversion to an open repair should be considered if visualization becomes impaired or the duration of surgery becomes exceedingly long. Conversion to open repair can be achieved by extending the lateral portals through an open or mini-open deltoid-splitting approach. Care should also be taken to avoid prolonged elevated pump pressure because of the potential for muscle necrosis or compartment syndrome in cases of excessive fluid extravasation. Careful hemostasis with electrocautery and use of epinephrine in the saline solution allow visualization and reduce the need for elevated pump pressure.

Careful rehabilitation is essential after repair of a massive RCT. Early postoperative motion after arthroscopic repair of massive tears is contraindicated. A more conservative approach as described previously yields improved chances of tendon-to-bone healing. The rare problems related to postoperative stiffness can be easily managed with secondary arthroscopic release after the rotator cuff has healed.

Bibliography

Aoki M, Okamura K, Fukushima S, Takahashi T, Ogino T: Transfer of latissimus dorsi for irreparable rotator-cuff tears. *J Bone Joint Surg Br* 1996;78(5):761-766.

Apreleva M, Ozbaydar M, Fitzgibbons PG, Warner JJ: Rotator cuff tears: The effect of the reconstruction method on three-dimensional repair site area. *Arthroscopy* 2002;18(5):519-526.

Bishop J, Klepps S, Lo IK, Bird J, Gladstone JN, Flatow EL: Cuff integrity after arthroscopic versus open rotator cuff repair: A prospective study. *J Shoulder Elbow Surg* 2006;15(3):290-299.

Chung SW, Kim JY, Kim MH, Kim SH, Oh JH: Arthroscopic repair of massive rotator cuff tears: Outcome and analysis of factors associated with healing failure or poor postoperative function. *Am J Sports Med* 2013;41(7):1674-1683.

Collin P, Treseder T, Ladermann A, et al: Neuropathy of the suprascapular nerve and massive rotator cuff tears: A prospective electromyographic study. *J Shoulder Elbow Surg* 2014;23(1):28-34.

Costouros JG, Porramatikul M, Lie DT, Warner JJ: Reversal of suprascapular neuropathy following arthroscopic repair of massive supraspinatus and infraspinatus rotator cuff tears. *Arthroscopy* 2007;23(11):1152-1161.

Denard PJ, Jiwani AZ, Ladermann A, Burkhart SS: Long-term outcome of arthroscopic massive rotator cuff repair: The importance of double-row fixation. *Arthroscopy* 2012;28(7):909-915.

Denard PJ, Ladermann A, Jiwani AZ, Burkhart SS: Functional outcome after arthroscopic repair of massive rotator cuff tears in individuals with pseudoparalysis. *Arthroscopy* 2012;28(9):1214-1219.

Galatz LM, Ball CM, Teefey SA, Middleton WD, Yamaguchi K: The outcome and repair integrity of completely arthroscopically repaired large and massive rotator cuff tears. *J Bone Joint Surg Am* 2004;86(2):219-224.

Gerber C, Fuchs B, Hodler J: The results of repair of massive tears of the rotator cuff. *J Bone Joint Surg Am* 2000;82(4):505-515.

Gerber C, Meyer DC, Schneeberger AG, Hoppeler H, von Rechenberg B: Effect of tendon release and delayed repair on the structure of the muscles of the rotator cuff: An experimental study in sheep. *J Bone Joint Surg Am* 2004;86(9):1973-1982.

Gladstone JN, Bishop JY, Lo IK, Flatow EL: Fatty infiltration and atrophy of the rotator cuff do not improve after rotator cuff repair and correlate with poor functional outcome. *Am J Sports Med* 2007;35(5):719-728.

Goutallier D, Postel JM, Gleyze P, Leguilloux P, Van Driessche S: Influence of cuff muscle fatty degeneration on anatomic and functional outcomes after simple suture of full-thickness tears. *J Shoulder Elbow Surg* 2003;12(6):550-554.

Hertel R, Ballmer FT, Lombert SM, Gerber C: Lag signs in the diagnosis of rotator cuff rupture. *J Shoulder Elbow Surg* 1996;5(4):307-313.

Kim SJ, Kim SH, Lee SK, Seo JW, Chun YM: Arthroscopic repair of massive contracted rotator cuff tears: Aggressive release with anterior and posterior interval slides do not improve cuff healing and integrity. *J Bone Joint Surg Am* 2013;95(16):1482-1488.

Lee E, Bishop JY, Braman JP, Langford J, Gelber J, Flatow EL: Outcomes after arthroscopic rotator cuff repairs. *J Shoulder Elbow Surg* 2007;16(1):1-5.

Lo IK, Burkhart SS: Arthroscopic repair of massive, contracted, immobile rotator cuff tears using single and double interval slides: Technique and preliminary results. *Arthroscopy* 2004;20(1):22-33.

Mallon WJ, Wilson RJ, Basamania CJ: The association of suprascapular neuropathy with massive rotator cuff tears: A preliminary report. *J Shoulder Elbow Surg* 2006;15(4):395-398.

Neer CS II, Satterlee CC, Dalsey RM, Flatow EL: The anatomy and potential effects of contracture of the coracohumeral ligament. *Clin Orthop Relat Res* 1992;(280):182-185.

Nho SJ, Brown BS, Lyman S, Adler RS, Altchek DW, MacGillivray JD: Prospective analysis of arthroscopic rotator cuff repair: Prognostic factors affecting clinical and ultrasound outcome. *J Shoulder Elbow Surg* 2009;18(1):13-20.

Oh JH, Jun BJ, McGarry MH, Lee TQ: Does a critical rotator cuff tear stage exist? A biomechanical study of rotator cuff tear progression in human cadaver shoulders. *J Bone Joint Surg Am* 2011;93(22):2100-2109.

Oh JH, McGarry MH, Jun BJ, et al: Restoration of shoulder biomechanics according to degree of repair completion in a cadaveric model of massive rotator cuff tear: Importance of margin convergence and posterior cuff fixation. *Am J Sports Med* 2012;40(11):2448-2453.

Tauro JC: Arthroscopic repair of large rotator cuff tears using the interval slide technique. *Arthroscopy* 2004;20(1):13-21.

Tingart MJ, Apreleva M, Zurakowski D, Warner JJ: Pullout strength of suture anchors used in rotator cuff repair. *J Bone Joint Surg Am* 2003;85(11):2190-2198.

Vad VB, Southern D, Warren RF, Altchek DW, Dines D: Prevalence of peripheral neurologic injuries in rotator cuff tears with atrophy. *J Shoulder Elbow Surg* 2003;12(4):333-336.

Walch G, Edwards TB, Boulahia A, Nové-Josserand L, Neyton L, Szabo I: Arthroscopic tenotomy of the long head of the biceps in the treatment of rotator cuff tears: Clinical and radiographic results of 307 cases. *J Shoulder Elbow Surg* 2005;14(3):238-246.

Warner JP, Krushell RJ, Masquelet A, Gerber C: Anatomy and relationships of the suprascapular nerve: Anatomical constraints to mobilization of the supraspinatus and infraspinatus muscles in the management of massive rotator-cuff tears. *J Bone Joint Surg Am* 1992;74(1):36-45.

Zanotti RM, Carpenter JE, Blasier RB, Greenfield ML, Adler RS, Bromberg MB: The low incidence of suprascapular nerve injury after primary repair of massive rotator cuff tears. *J Shoulder Elbow Surg* 1997;6(3):258-264.

Chapter 23
Management of Massive Irreparable Rotator Cuff Tears: Muscle Transfer Techniques for Augmentation

Bassem T. Elhassan, MD

 Introduction

Massive irreparable rotator cuff tears (RCTs) can lead to substantial loss of range of motion (ROM) and variable degrees of pain. The loss of the centering force of the rotator cuff results in eccentric loading of the glenoid. Abnormal wear patterns may develop, which can lead to arthritic changes in the shoulder. An anterosuperior RCT usually involves the subscapularis with or without the supraspinatus. With the loss of the subscapularis, the shoulder anterior force couple is lost. With larger tears, the proximal humerus may protrude anterosuperiorly through the anterior cuff defect. The aim of the muscle transfer procedure is to restore the joint mechanics by restoring the force couple across the joint.

In the past few years, several types of muscle transfers, which are often referred to as tendon transfers, have been developed to reconstruct RCTs. The most common transfer for the management of massive irreparable RCTs is transfer of the latissimus dorsi to manage a posterosuperior cuff tear and transfer of the pectoralis major to manage an anterosuperior cuff tear. Additional transfer options include isolated teres major, lower trapezius, and pectoralis minor transfers.

The most commonly reported muscle transfer is the latissimus dorsi transfer. With an intact subscapularis tendon and normal deltoid function, the inferiorly directed force of the latissimus dorsi muscle transfer to the proximal humerus is counterbalanced, which makes this transfer a good option to address the lack of the posterosuperior rotator cuff as an external rotator and humeral head depressor. Despite the major differences in the line of pull, tension, and excursion between the transferred latissimus dorsi and the posterosuperior rotator cuff (supraspinatus and infraspinatus with or without the teres minor) at the conclusion of this transfer, if performed to the level of the proximal insertion of subscapularis tendon along the lateral aspect of the greater tuberosity, the latissimus dorsi takes on the function of abducting and externally rotating the humerus.

The trapezius muscle positions the scapula to support the function of the upper extremity. The upper, middle, and lower parts of the trapezius muscle work together to elevate, retract, and externally rotate the scapula. The trapezius originates from the occiput and spinous processes of C7-T12. The upper trapezius inserts onto the superior aspect of the distal clavicle. The middle and lower trapezius muscle inserts onto the spine of the scapula and extends onto the acromion. The blood supply is derived from the transverse cervical artery. The trapezius muscle is innervated by cranial nerve XI (spinal accessory nerve). Because the origin of the lower trapezius is cranial to the origin of the latissimus dorsi and just medial to the infraspinatus fossa of the scapula, if the lower trapezius is transferred to the greater tuberosity, the line of pull of the muscle fibers mimics that of the infraspinatus (**Figure 1**). Furthermore, the tension and excursion forces of the trapezius are similar to those of the infraspinatus. A biomechanical study demonstrated that a better moment arm of rotation is achieved after transfer of the lower trapezius to the greater tuberosity of the humerus than after transfer of the latissimus dorsi. For these reasons, the author of this chapter prefers transfer of the lower trapezius to the greater tuberosity of the humerus rather than transfer of the latissimus dorsi. The lower trapezius transfer was originally intended to restore shoulder external rotation in patients with shoulder paralysis secondary to brachial plexus injury. Its use was later extended to provide an alternative for the management of irreparable musculotendinous tears of the infraspinatus and

Neither Dr. Elhassan nor any immediate family member has received anything of value from or has stock or stock options held in a commercial company or institution related directly or indirectly to the subject of this chapter.

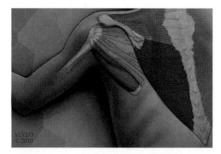

Figure 1 Illustration shows the anatomy of the lower trapezius muscle and its tendinous attachment on the medial spine of the scapula. (Reproduced with permission from the Mayo Foundation for Medical Education and Research, Rochester, MN.)

irreparable posterosuperior RCTs.

A recent anatomic cadaver study demonstrated that both isolated and simultaneous latissimus dorsi and teres major transfers were feasible and safe for the management of irreparable subscapularis tears. Therefore, in patients with subscapularis tears, the author of this chapter prefers to transfer the latissimus dorsi (with or without the teres major) to the insertion of the subscapularis tendon.

 Case Presentations

Case 1

A 44-year-old man who works in construction and participates in sports, including hockey and basketball, sustained trauma to his right shoulder while playing hockey 8 years earlier. He had substantial loss of function associated with pain at that time. He was treated with physical therapy, which resulted in marginal improvement in pain and function. He was able to return to work and sports activity approximately 6 months after the injury; however, he noticed weakness when using his shoulder. In the year before his visit to the clinic of the author of this chapter, his pain and weakness worsened and began to affect his daily activities and sleep.

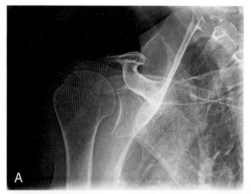
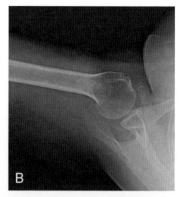
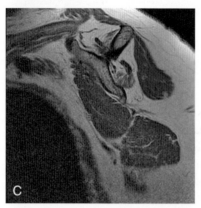
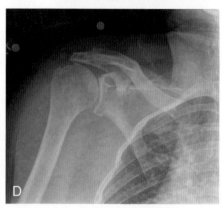

Figure 2 **A,** AP shoulder radiograph demonstrates proximal humeral head migration in a patient with a massive rotator cuff tear. **B,** Axillary radiograph demonstrates no anterior-superior subluxation. **C,** Sagittal T1-weighted MRI demonstrates a posterosuperior rotator cuff tear with advanced fatty infiltration of the supraspinatus and infraspinatus. **D,** AP shoulder radiograph obtained 13 months after lower trapezius transfer demonstrates substantial improvement in the position of the humeral head. The remaining mild proximal migration of the humeral head did not affect the outcome. (Reproduced with permission from the Mayo Foundation for Medical Education and Research, Rochester, MN.)

Physical examination reveals mild atrophy of the muscles around the right shoulder. The patient has normal function of the deltoid and periscapular muscles. He has 50° of shoulder flexion, 50° of abduction, and 30° of external rotation with a lag of 30°. Internal rotation is to L1, and the results of the belly-press and lift-off tests are negative. Shoulder radiographs demonstrate proximal migration of the humeral head with mild degenerative changes and no anterior-posterior subluxation (**Figure 2, A** and **B**). MRI demonstrates a massive irreparable RCT with advanced fatty atrophy of the supraspinatus and infraspinatus (**Figure 2, C**).

Because of the young age of the patient, he is not a good candidate for reverse shoulder arthroplasty. A lower trapezius muscle transfer is performed to reconstruct the rotator cuff. A lower trapezius muscle transfer was selected because it is biomechanically superior in restoring normal shoulder biomechanics and kinematics compared with other muscle transfers. In addition, a recent clinical outcomes study reported that lower trapezius muscle transfers for reconstruction of massive irreparable posterosuperior RCTs led to substantial improvements in pain and shoulder ROM.

At the 13-month postoperative

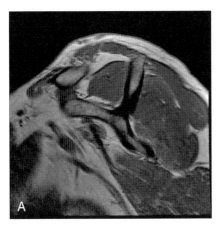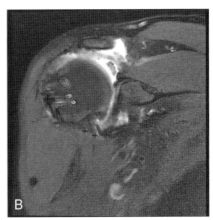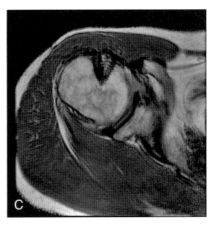

Figure 3 **A,** Sagittal T1-weighted MRI of the shoulder demonstrates advanced fatty atrophy of the subscapularis muscle in a patient with a massive anterosuperior rotator cuff tear. **B,** Coronal T1-weighted MRI demonstrates substantial deficiency of the supraspinatus tendon. **C,** Axial T1-weighted MRI demonstrates a subscapularis tendon tear with advanced fatty atrophy. (Reproduced with permission from the Mayo Foundation for Medical Education and Research, Rochester, MN.)

follow-up examination, the patient reports substantial improvement of pain and ROM. His pain is minimal or nonexistent with heavy activities. His ROM includes flexion of 150°, abduction of 130°, external rotation of 60°, and internal rotation to L2. AP shoulder radiographs demonstrate substantial improvement in the humeral head position, although minimal loss of the Gothic arch remains (**Figure 2, D**). The patient reports subjectively that his shoulder strength has improved but he continues to perceive more weakness in the surgical shoulder than in the contralateral shoulder during heavy overhead lifting activities. He was able to return to construction work and participation in hockey and basketball with minimal limitations.

Case 2

A 48-year-old, right-hand–dominant man who works as a manual laborer has a 13-month history of right shoulder pain and progressive loss of ROM. A previous RCT sustained at the age of 31 years was managed with open rotator cuff repair, and the patient recovered within 7 months after the procedure. His recent symptoms began after he fell from a height of 5 feet and tried to break the fall with his right upper extremity.

His symptoms suggested substantial painful tearing in his right shoulder. He reported no associated numbness or tingling. Original radiographs were negative. The patient was treated with several months of physical therapy, which improved his symptoms only minimally. He returned to work but generally relied on his left shoulder for lifting and used the right hand only to support the load. Progressive worsening of his pain and weakness prompted him to seek treatment. He reports substantial disability and rates his pain at an average of 7 on a scale of 1 to 10. His subjective shoulder value is 30%.

Physical examination reveals limited flexion of 100°, abduction of 90°, external rotation of 70° (compared with 50° in the left shoulder), and internal rotation to L3. The Jobe, belly-press, and lift-off tests are positive. The left shoulder is normal on examination. MRI reveals evidence of a massive irreparable anterosuperior RCT with advanced fatty atrophy of the subscapularis and substantial deficiency of the supraspinatus tendon that is associated with proximal migration of the humeral head (**Figure 3**). A transfer of the pectoralis major muscle to the greater tuberosity is performed.

At a 15-month follow-up, the patient reports substantial improvement of pain

(averaging 2 on a scale of 1 to 10), and the subjective shoulder value is 80%. An examination reveals shoulder flexion to 130°, abduction to 120°, external rotation to 50°, and internal rotation to T12. The results of the belly-press test are improved but still partly positive. The lift-off test is negative. Radiographs demonstrate the humeral head centered on the glenoid.

 ## Indications

Patients indicated for lower trapezius muscle transfer include those who are young (chronologically and/or physically) with symptomatic, massive, irreparable, posterosuperior RCT and minimal or no arthritis. A subscapularis tear is not a contraindication for surgical reconstruction.

 ## Controversies and Alternative Approaches

Surgical treatment options for symptomatic patients who are not candidates for implant arthroplasty include arthroscopic débridement with or without suprascapular nerve release, biceps

Table 1 Results of Muscle Transfer to Manage Massive Rotator Cuff Tear

Authors	Journal (Year)	Technique (No. of Patients)	Outcomes	Comments
Wirth and Rockwood	*J Bone Joint Surg Am* (1997)	Pectoralis major transfer (7) Pectoralis minor transfer (5) Pectoralis major and minor transfer (1)	10 of 13 patients obtained satisfactory outcomes according to the Neer/Foster grading system	Pectoralis muscle is effective for reconstruction of the shoulder in patients who have loss of the subscapularis
Celli et al	*J Shoulder Elbow Surg* (1998)	Teres major transfer (6)	1 patient was very satisfied, and 5 were satisfied	Good improvement of pain and shoulder flexion/abduction and external rotation on short-term follow-up
Resch et al	*J Bone Joint Surg Am* (2000)	The superior one-half or two-thirds of the pectoralis major was transferred for irreparable subscapularis tear (12)	9 patients had excellent or good results, and 3 had fair results based on functional and Constant scores	Repair technique recommended for reconstruction in elderly patients with irreparable subscapularis tears
Galatz et al	*J Shoulder Elbow Surg* (2003)	Pectoralis major transfer (14)	11 patients had a satisfactory result Pain scores improved from 6.9 to 3.2 American Shoulder and Elbow Surgeons scores improved from 27.2 to 47.7 Shoulder forward elevation improved from 24.4° to 60.8°	Transfer of the pectoralis major deep to the conjoint tendon is a viable option for and results in a low complication rate in patients with irreparable subscapularis tears
Jost et al	*J Bone Joint Surg Am* (2003)	Pectoralis major transfer for irreparable subscapularis tear (28)	13 patients were very satisfied, 10 were satisfied, 2 were disappointed, and 3 were dissatisfied	Pectoralis major transfer leads to good outcomes in patients with isolated irreparable subscapularis tears Results are less favorable and pectoralis major transfer may not be warranted if a subscapularis tear is associated with an irreparable supraspinatus tear
Aldridge et al	*J Shoulder Elbow Surg* (2004)	Combined latissimus dorsi and pectoralis major tendon transfer for massive rotator cuff deficiency (11)	5 patients improved substantially, 2 improved minimally, and 4 had no improvement	Combined transfer may improve shoulder motion in patients with massive combined anterior and posterior rotator cuff tear; however, it is difficult to conclude which patients will have a successful outcome
Elhassan et al	*J Bone Joint Surg Br* (2008)	Pectoralis major transfer for irreparable subscapularis tear (30)	Group 1: 11 patients with irreparable subscapularis tear and instability; group 2: 8 patients with failed arthroplasty; and group 3: 11 patients with massive anterosuperior rotator cuff tear Pain improved in 7 patients in groups 1 and 3 but only 1 patient in group 2 A high failure rate was reported in patients with preoperative anterior shoulder subluxation	Worse results in patients with a history of anterior instability or those with prior failed arthroplasty procedures

Table 1 Results of Muscle Transfer to Manage Massive Rotator Cuff Tear (*continued*)

Authors	Journal (Year)	Technique (No. of Patients)	Outcomes	Comments
Henseler et al	*Bone Joint J* (2013)	Teres major transfer (28)	Mean abduction improved from 79° to 105° and mean external rotation improved from 25° to 55° Significant improvement in Constant and visual analog scale scores	Good improvement of pain and shoulder flexion/abduction and external rotation on short-term follow-up
Paladini et al	*J Shoulder Elbow Surg* (2013)	Pectoralis minor tendon transfer (27)	Improved shoulder flexion, decreased external rotation, and improved simple shoulder test and Constant scores but no improvement in strength	Pectoralis minor transfer is feasible as well as safe and may improve shoulder function and pain if performed for upper subscapularis irreparable lesions, even in patients who have an irreparable supraspinatus tear Improvement is most likely related to the tenodesis effect

tenotomy with or without tenodesis, use of an allograft patch for augmentation, and partial rotator cuff repair.

 Results

The available literature is summarized in **Table 1**. As noted, latissimus dorsi transfer is the most commonly described and reported transfer. Results of teres major and lower trapezius transfers have not been well reported. The author of this chapter is not aware of any clinical studies comparing the different transfer options.

Studies on latissimus dorsi transfer have reported that patients maintain lasting pain relief and improved ROM at long-term follow-up. Fatty infiltration of the teres minor less than grade 2 has been reported to correlate with improved outcomes. Negative prognostic factors include progression of osteoarthritis, subscapularis insufficiency, female sex, and preoperative elevation less than 90°.

The outcomes of teres major transfer for the management of posterosuperior RCTs have been reported in a study of 28 patients and another study of 6 patients. Both studies reported good improvements in pain, shoulder flexion/abduction, and external rotation at short-term follow-up.

The author of this chapter recently reported on the outcomes of 33 patients who underwent lower trapezius muscle transfer for the management of massive irreparable posterosuperior RCTs. At a mean follow-up of 47 months, 32 patients had substantial improvements in pain, subjective shoulder values, Disabilities of the Arm, Shoulder and Hand scores, and shoulder ROM. Patients who had a preoperative ROM more than 60° had more substantial gains in postoperative ROM.

The outcomes of pectoralis major transfer for the management of anterosuperior cuff tears or deficiencies have not been entirely successful. In one of the first studies on this transfer, researchers reported in 1997 on 13 patients with subscapularis tears who underwent pectoralis major transfer, pectoralis minor transfer, or transfer of both tendons, with 10 patients obtaining satisfactory outcomes according to the grading system of Neer and Foster. In a study published in 2003 on 14 patients who underwent pectoralis major transfers for the treatment of massive anterior RCTs and resultant anterior instability,

11 patients had a satisfactory result, with improvement in pain, function, and shoulder forward elevation. Other studies have demonstrated worse outcomes, with only modest improvements in shoulder function and stability. A study examining the results of this transfer in 30 patients who had irreparable subscapularis tears reported worse results in patients with a history of anterior instability or those with prior failed arthroplasty procedures. One biomechanical study suggested that transfer of the pectoralis major tendon in front of rather than behind the conjoint tendon better restored the line of pull of the subscapularis. However, in an attempt to perform a similar biomechanical study, the author of this chapter was not able to justify these conclusions. Regardless whether the pectoralis major was passed deep or superficial to the conjoint tendon, the line of pull of the transfer did not replicate that of the subscapularis. In abduction-internal rotation, a pectoralis major transfer becomes a medial translator rather than an internal rotator of the humeral head. Anatomic and intraoperative studies have reported that passing a pectoralis major transfer deep to the conjoint tendon may increase the risk for traction or compression injury to the

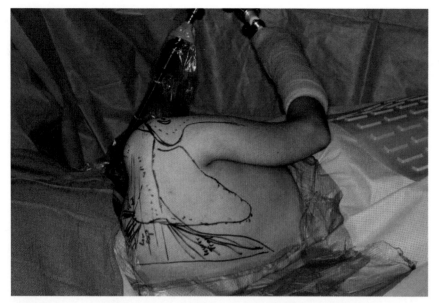

Figure 4 Intraoperative photograph of a patient placed in the lateral decubitus position with the arm attached to a dynamic arm holder to help position the shoulder throughout the procedure. Anatomic structures are marked, including the scapula, humeral head, and proximal humerus. The marked muscles include the lower trapezius, the levator scapulae, and the upper serratus anterior. (Reproduced with permission from the Mayo Foundation for Medical Education and Research, Rochester, MN.)

musculocutaneous nerve. The author of this chapter does not use a pectoralis major transfer for irreparable subscapularis tears; however, based on the data in the literature, the author performs a pectoralis major transfer superficial to the conjoint tendon to avoid injury to the musculocutaneous nerve.

Pectoralis minor transfers to the lesser tuberosity that address subscapularis insufficiency have been less widely reported than other transfers. One study reported good outcomes in five patients. In a study of this transfer in 27 patients with irreparable tears of the upper two-thirds of the subscapularis and associated irreparable supraspinatus tears, researchers reported improved shoulder flexion, decreased external rotation, and improvement in simple shoulder test and Constant scores but no improvement in strength.

Outcomes of latissimus dorsi transfer with transfer of the teres major have not been published. The experience of the author of this chapter with this

transfer in a small number of patients has been promising. Outcomes tend to be best in patients with prior shoulder arthroplasty and chronic symptomatic subscapularis insufficiency but no major proximal bone deficiency that would result in less predictable repair and healing of the latissimus (and/or teres major) to the lesser tuberosity.

 Technical Keys to Success

Latissimus Dorsi Transfer
SETUP/EXPOSURE
- The patient is placed in the lateral decubitus position on a standard surgical table (**Figure 4**).
- All bony prominences around the hip, knee, and ankle are well cushioned.
- The affected arm is prepared in its entirety and draped in sterile fashion. Draping should allow access from the midline of the spine to

the sternum, inferiorly to the iliac crest and superiorly to the base of the neck.
- The forearm is covered with a sterile stockinet that covers the hand and allows the attachment of the hand and forearm to a dynamic arm holder.

INSTRUMENTS/EQUIPMENT/ IMPLANTS REQUIRED
- A dynamic arm holder is needed.
- Tools required include an oscillating saw, osteotomes, an electric burr, a 2-mm drill bit, and a Houston suture passer.
- No. 2 nonabsorbable sutures, anchors, and EndoButtons (Smith & Nephew) are used for fixation.

PROCEDURE
- The procedure begins with exposure of the rotator cuff via a superior approach.
- An incision is made just medial to the lateral acromial border from anterior to posterior.
- The middle deltoid is identified, and the intervals between the anterior and middle deltoid and between the middle and posterior deltoid are identified and partially developed (**Figure 5, A**).
- Osteotomy of the lateral 5 mm of the acromion, which contains the origin of the middle deltoid, is done (**Figure 5, B**).
- Dissection is carried 2 to 3 cm distally in line with the deltoid fibers between the anterior-middle and middle-posterior deltoid (**Figure 5, C**). This dissection allows full exposure of the lateral aspect of the rotator cuff without the need for further distal separation of the deltoid fibers (**Figure 5, D**). This technique decreases tension on the axillary nerve during retraction for exposure and thereby decreases the risk of traction injury.
- In patients with massive irreparable

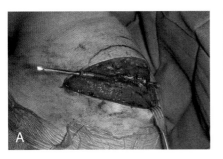
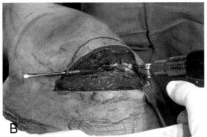
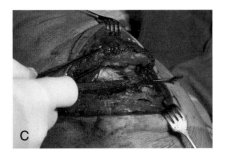
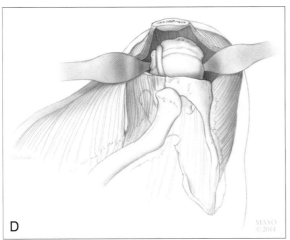
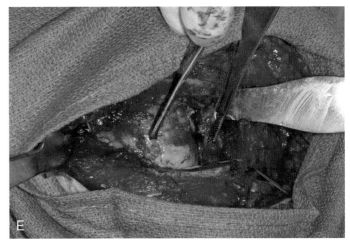

Figure 5   **A,** Intraoperative photograph shows exposure through a so-called saber incision, at the level of the lateral acromion. No elevation of skin flaps is necessary because the exposure will be through a lateral acromial osteotomy. **B,** Intraoperative photograph shows osteotomy of the lateral 5 mm of the acromion, which contains the origin of the middle deltoid. **C,** Intraoperative photograph shows reflection of the osteotomized lateral acromion laterally to expose the subacromial space and the rotator cuff insertion. **D,** Illustration depicts the surgical exposure through the lateral acromial osteotomy. **E,** Intraoperative photograph shows a bare humeral head at the site of rotator cuff insertion in a patient with a massive posterosuperior rotator cuff tear. (Reproduced with permission from the Mayo Foundation for Medical Education and Research, Rochester, MN.)

RCTs, especially those with proximal migration of the humeral head, a humeral head free of the posterosuperior rotator cuff will be visible after the middle deltoid origin has been detached and retracted (**Figure 5, E**).

- A thickened subacromial bursa will be present and is typically excised to allow a better view of the edge of the remaining rotator cuff.
- If the biceps tendon is present, tenotomy is routinely performed. Tenodesis may be performed, depending on the age of the patient. In patients who are younger than 60 years or very active, tenodesis of the biceps tendon to the proximal aspect of the biceps groove is performed.

- If the RCT extends to the subscapularis tendon, the subscapularis tendon is repaired in a standard double-row fashion.
- If the subscapularis tendon is irreparable, an additional transfer (discussed elsewhere in this chapter) may be necessary.
- The lateral edge of the torn rotator cuff tendon is trimmed to achieve a healthy tendon end.
- Nonabsorbable No. 2 sutures are placed in the supraspinatus and infraspinatus in Krackow fashion.
- Mobilization of the tendons is accomplished by performing superficial and deep dissection with the use of a blunt instrument, such as a Cobb elevator, to gain excursion laterally.

- Special care should be taken during deep dissection, especially medial to the glenoid, because the suprascapular nerve may be located within 15 mm of the glenoid surface.
- Although some studies have advocated separating the supraspinatus and infraspinatus through a lateral split to gain better excursion, the author of this chapter prefers to keep the rotator cuff in continuity to better maintain the rotator cuff cable effect.
- If the RCT appears difficult to repair or if the surgeon observes intraoperatively that the repair cannot be achieved without excessive tension on the repair site, the decision to proceed with partial or complete rotator cuff repair with or without

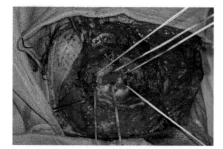

Figure 6 Intraoperative photograph shows placement of suture anchors at the level of the footprint of the supraspinatus and infraspinatus in preparation for tendon transfer. (Reproduced with permission from the Mayo Foundation for Medical Education and Research, Rochester, MN.)

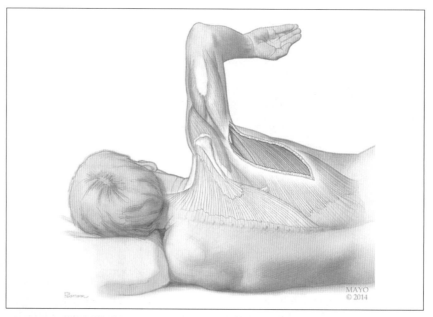

Figure 7 Illustration depicts positioning of the shoulder in abduction and internal rotation in preparation for harvest of the latissimus dorsi tendon. The incision is shown as well. (Reproduced with permission from the Mayo Foundation for Medical Education and Research, Rochester, MN.)

tendon transfer depends on the surgeon's preference.

- In the experience of the author of this chapter, most massive RCTs are associated with an advanced fatty atrophy retear if they are repaired under tension. Therefore, in these patients, or in patients with a chronic massive RCT with fatty atrophy and proximal humeral migration, the author prefers to attempt partial or full repair of the infraspinatus and augment the repair with tendon transfer. This method decreases the extent of dissection and surgical time.
- To facilitate the tendon transfer portion of the procedure, the tuberosity is repaired and the appropriate sutures and anchors are placed before the transfer is performed.
- The posterosuperior aspect of the uncovered greater tuberosity is burred to healthy bone to accept the transferred tendon.
- Three or four double No. 2 nonabsorbable sutures are placed in a transosseous fashion through the greater tuberosity in preparation for fixation of the transferred tendon (**Figure 6**).
- The latissimus dorsi tendon is harvested in the standard fashion.
- The shoulder is positioned in

abduction and internal rotation with the use of the dynamic arm holder, and a 15-cm incision is made over the palpable lateral posterior border of the latissimus dorsi muscle, extending across the axilla along one of the axillary skin folds (**Figure 7**).
- Full-thickness skin flaps are raised.
- The latissimus dorsi muscle is easily identifiable over the distal aspect of the incision. It is the most anterior muscle at that level, and toward the scapula it is accompanied by the teres major muscle, which is located just posterior to it (**Figure 8**).
- The interval between the latissimus dorsi and teres major muscles is identified. This interval can be visualized by following the latissimus dorsi muscle from distal to proximal.
- In the axillary region proximal to the level of the humeral insertion, the latissimus dorsi tendon is intimately draped over the teres major muscle.
- The latissimus dorsi tendon is

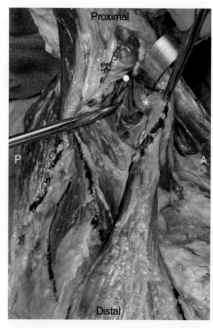

Figure 8 Photograph of anatomic dissection shows the latissimus dorsi muscle and its tendinous insertion anteriorly (*) and the teres major muscle and its tendinous insertion (circle) posterior to the latissimus tendon. A = anterior, P = posterior. (Reproduced with permission from the Mayo Foundation for Medical Education and Research, Rochester, MN.)

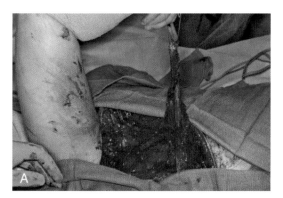 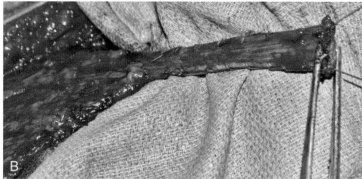

Figure 9 **A,** Intraoperative photograph shows harvesting of the latissimus dorsi tendon and dissection of the latissimus dorsi muscle more proximally to obtain full excursion. The pedicle is visualized, dissected, and protected. **B,** Intraoperative photograph demonstrates a closer view of the detached latissimus dorsi tendon and its bony insertion. (Reproduced with permission from the Mayo Foundation for Medical Education and Research, Rochester, MN.)

separated from the teres major muscle, and dissection is followed proximally and distally to fully separate the latissimus dorsi muscle and its tendon from the teres major muscle.

- In 30% of patients, the latissimus dorsi tendon is confluent with the teres major tendon at its insertion onto the humerus. In these patients, sharp dissection can be performed to separate the two tendons.

- After the latissimus dorsi and teres major tendons are fully separated, the latissimus dorsi tendon is detached from the humerus with appropriate retraction (**Figure 9, A**).

- The anterior circumflex humeral artery and the axillary nerve lie proximal to the latissimus dorsi insertion, and the radial nerve lies distal to it. These structures should be protected.

- The latissimus dorsi tendon is detached from its insertion on the humerus by performing sharp, direct laceration of the tendon with the use of a blade or by performing a 5-mm osteotomy at the latissimus dorsi tendon insertion (**Figure 9, B**). The latter technique provides slightly more length of the tendon and allows for bone-on-bone repair, which may result in better healing.

- No. 2 nonabsorbable sutures are placed in Krackow fashion in the

tendinous portion of the latissimus dorsi. These sutures help place traction on the tendon when it is mobilized to obtain better excursion and are later used to augment the repair.

- As traction is applied to the sutures and directed more proximally, the neurovascular bundle of the latissimus dorsi muscle is identified. This bundle is usually located approximately 2 cm medial or distal to the musculotendinous portion on its deep border. In order to safely identify the neurovascular bundle, dissection and elevation of the latissimus dorsi muscle is performed from proximal to distal while slight proximal traction is placed on the tendon. The undersurface of the latissimus dorsi muscle is inspected, approximately 2 to 4 cm distal to the musculotendinous junction, to identify the neurovascular bundle entering the muscle.

- After these structures are visualized, the neurovascular bundle is dissected from distal to proximal, close to the chest wall where the neurovascular bundle is located, to the level of its origin from the axillary region.

- All communicating branches with the main vascular pedicle are tied or stapled and cut to allow for unrestricted mobilization of the pedicle

without traction or impingement (**Figure 9, A**).

- With the neurovascular bundle protected, the latissimus dorsi muscle is further mobilized to separate it from the surrounding soft tissue.

- It is crucial to release the latissimus dorsi from the scapula to obtain further excursion of the muscle, which in turn allows easier transfer of the tendon to the proximal edge of the subscapularis insertion. Detachment of the latissimus dorsi from the scapula is safe because the pedicle is located more anterior and farther from the lateral scapular border.

- If mobilization of the latissimus dorsi tendon is performed appropriately, augmentation of the transferred tendon with tendon allograft or autograft is usually not necessary.

- The tendon is now ready for transfer. Because the necessary preparation at the level of the humeral insertion has already been done, the next step is to pass the tendon from the distal to the proximal wound. To do so, a subdeltoid path is created with the use of a large, curved blunt clamp passed between the deltoid and the remaining posterior rotator cuff.

- A fascial attachment is often present

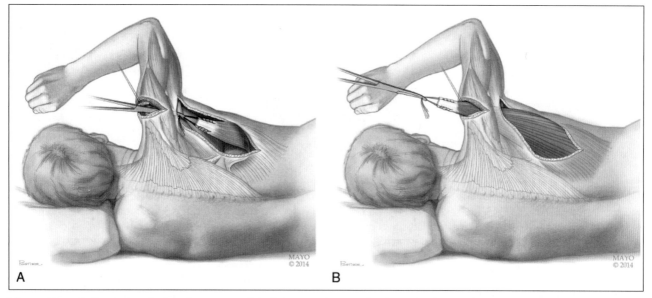

Figure 10   **A,** Illustration depicts the passage of the latissimus dorsi tendon from the distal wound to the proximal wound deep to the posterior deltoid. **B,** Illustration depicts the latissimus dorsi tendon retrieved from the proximal wound and ready to be attached. (Reproduced with permission from the Mayo Foundation for Medical Education and Research, Rochester, MN.)

between the posterior deltoid and infraspinatus distally. This attachment must be released to widen the path and facilitate the passage of the latissimus tendon.

- The clamp is passed from the proximal wound to the distal wound and is used to grasp the sutures from the latissimus dorsi and pull them through to the superior incision (**Figure 10**). The tendon and muscle belly should pass smoothly.
- The arm is placed in 45° of abduction and 30° of external rotation.
- The tendon is brought over the top of the humeral head, and the transosseous sutures previously placed over the greater tuberosity are used to repair the tendon to the proximal humerus.
- The sutures that were placed in a Krakow fashion in the latissimus dorsi tendon are used to repair the most proximal end of the tendon to the subscapularis tendon.
- If the latissimus dorsi was harvested together with its bony insertion, a shallow bony trough aimed laterally should be created just proximal to

the subscapularis insertion, and the repair should be done from bone to bone with the use of transosseous nonabsorbable sutures.
- The remaining rotator cuff is repaired to the medial aspect of the footprint of the supraspinatus if possible (**Figure 11**).
- If repair to the footprint of the supraspinatus is not possible, the author of this chapter does not routinely attempt to repair the remaining rotator cuff to the medial aspect of the attached latissimus dorsi tendon because the thick, retracted remaining rotator cuff tendon is not likely to heal to the thin medial aspect of the latissimus tendon and may tear when the patient starts motion. In addition, failure of such an attempt could affect the integrity of the latissimus dorsi tendon.

WOUND CLOSURE
- The wound is irrigated.
- The deltoid is secured to the acromion with multiple No. 2 nonabsorbable transosseous sutures.
- The deltoid split is approximated

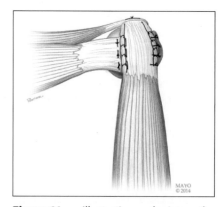

Figure 11   Illustration depicts the transfer of the latissimus dorsi muscle proximally and laterally, with the most proximal edge attached at the level of the upper border of the subscapularis. The rotator cuff is repaired medially if possible. (Reproduced with permission from the Mayo Foundation for Medical Education and Research, Rochester, MN.)

with No. 2-0 absorbable braided suture.
- The skin is closed in routine fashion over a suction drain.

Teres Major Transfer
- The transfer and attachment steps of the teres major transfer procedure

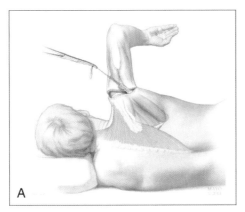
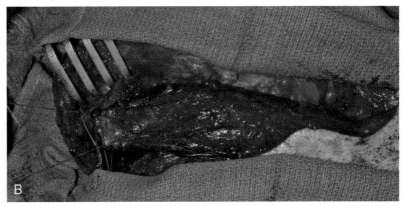

Figure 12   **A,** Illustration depicts harvesting of the teres major with the shoulder positioned in abduction and internal rotation. **B,** Intraoperative photograph demonstrates the teres major muscle and tendon harvested and ready for transfer. (Reproduced with permission from the Mayo Foundation for Medical Education and Research, Rochester, MN.)

are the same as those of the latissimus dorsi transfer procedure. The incision and dissection steps differ.

- The surgical incision for harvest of the teres major is usually a distal extension of the incision that is placed lateral to the acromion. The incision is usually extended to the level of the posterior axillary fold.

- With the shoulder placed in abduction and internal rotation, the deltoid is retracted laterally and the teres major insertion is exposed.

- The teres major muscle is the first muscle identified in the axilla through the posterior approach. The teres major tendon is either detached from its bony insertion or detached together with 5 mm of its bony insertion (**Figure 12**).

- The teres major muscle is separated proximally from the latissimus dorsi. Because of the short length of the muscle and the medial-proximal location of its pedicle, in most patients it is not necessary to identify and dissect the neurovascular pedicle (**Figure 13**).

- Double Krackow sutures are placed in the tendinous/musculotendinous portion of the teres major in preparation for transfer.

- The remaining steps of the procedure, including passage of the

muscle to the site of attachment and the repair (**Figure 14**), are the same as those of a latissimus dorsi transfer.

Lower Trapezius Tendon Transfer
SETUP/EXPOSURE

- The patient is positioned in the lateral decubitus position.

- The proximal humerus at the site of the posterosuperior rotator cuff is exposed as described in the latissimus dorsi and teres major transfer procedures.

- Instruments, equipment, and implants are similar to those listed for latissimus dorsi transfer.

PROCEDURE

- The greater tuberosity is prepared, and the transosseous sutures that will be used for tendon transfer repair are placed.

- A vertical incision is made starting 2 cm medial to the medial aspect of the scapular spine and extending approximately 5 to 7 cm distally.

- Sharp skin and subcutaneous dissection is performed to expose the lower trapezius (**Figure 15, A**).

- To facilitate dissection of the lower trapezius, the lateral border of the muscle is followed from the level

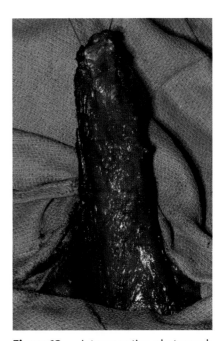

Figure 13   Intraoperative photograph of the teres major muscle. Its tendinous portion is small compared with that of the latissimus dorsi muscle. (Reproduced with permission from the Mayo Foundation for Medical Education and Research, Rochester, MN.)

medial to the medial border of the scapula to the level of the insertion of the muscle on the medial 2 to 3 cm of the scapular spine.

- The tendinous insertion of the lower trapezius is detached from the

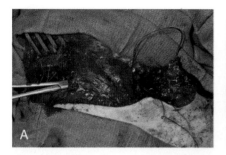
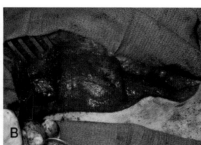

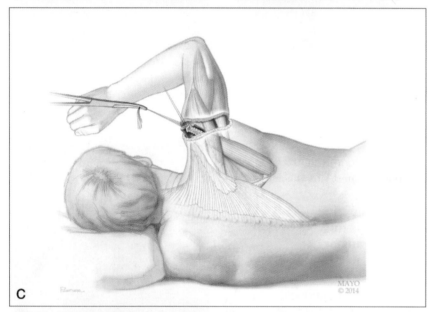

Figure 14 Intraoperative photographs demonstrate passage of the teres major deep to the posterior deltoid from the distal wound to the proximal wound (**A**) and the teres major passed to the proximal wound and ready for attachment (**B**). **C,** Illustration depicts transfer of the teres major to the proximal humerus. (Reproduced with permission from the Mayo Foundation for Medical Education and Research, Rochester, MN.)

medial spine of the scapula (**Figure 15, B**).

- The lower trapezius tendon has a triangular shape at the level of its insertion. Typically, if the horizontal top portion of the tendon is followed medially, it indicates the proximal border of the lower trapezius and the separation between the lower and middle trapezius. This interval is developed and followed medially to separate the middle trapezius from the lower trapezius. The dissection should be performed between the muscle fibers without entering the deep fascia on the trapezius to protect the neurovascular bundle, which is located in the deep fascial level.

- The spinal accessory nerve is typically located approximately two finger widths from the medial spine of the scapula (**Figure 15, C**). If necessary, a nerve stimulator can be used to identify this nerve.

- A No. 2 nonabsorbable suture is placed in a Krackow fashion into the tendinous and musculotendinous portion of the lower trapezius.

- In patients with shoulder paralysis, direct transfer of the lower trapezius tendon to the infraspinatus tendon can be performed (**Figure 16**).

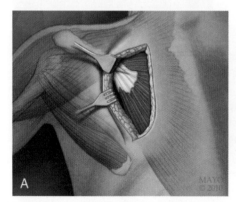
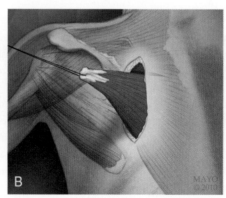
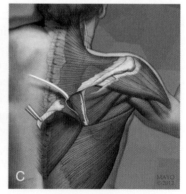

Figure 15 **A,** Illustration depicts exposure of the lower trapezius attachment through a medial incision. **B,** Illustration depicts detachment of the lower trapezius from the medial spine of the scapula and separation of the lower trapezius from the middle trapezius. **C,** Illustration depicts the location of the spinal accessory nerve, approximately two finger widths from the medial border of the scapula. (Reproduced with permission from the Mayo Foundation for Medical Education and Research, Rochester, MN.)

- In patients with massive irreparable RCTs, augmentation of the transfer with tendon graft is necessary. The author of this chapter prefers to use Achilles tendon allograft because the length of the Achilles tendon and its anatomic division into a wide, thin part and a long, thick part make it ideal for transfer. The

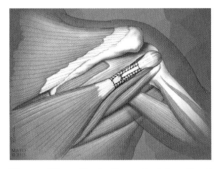

Figure 16 Illustration depicts direct transfer of the lower trapezius tendon to the infraspinatus. The line of pull of the muscle fibers of the lower trapezius is a mirror image of that of the infraspinatus muscle fibers. (Reproduced with permission from the Mayo Foundation for Medical Education and Research, Rochester, MN.)

thin portion of the Achilles tendon is wrapped around the tendinous and musculotendinous portions of the lower trapezius and secured with multiple nonabsorbable No. 2 sutures. The suture that was placed in the lower trapezius tendon also is passed through the allograft to reinforce the repair (**Figure 17, A**).

- A tunnel is created between the medial and lateral wounds deep to the posterior deltoid.
- With the shoulder positioned in 45° of abduction and 50° of external rotation, the tendon is passed from the medial wound to the lateral wound with the use of a blunt clamp and is repaired to the prepared lateral aspect of the posterosuperior greater tuberosity with multiple transosseous sutures (**Figure 17, B**).
- After the transfer is performed, the spinal accessory nerve is inspected at the level of the medial edge of the scapular spine to ensure that the medial spine of the scapula

does not impinge on the nerve.

- In patients with an irreparable musculotendinous tear of the infraspinatus, a limited posterior exposure is used. An inverted L-shaped incision is made with the horizontal portion of the incision starting at the level of the posterior origin of the posterior deltoid (approximately 3 cm medial to the medial border of the scapula) to a level posterior to the acromion. The vertical portion of the incision is extended distally toward the posterior axillary fold. After sharp dissection through skin and subcutaneous tissues, the posterior half of the posterior deltoid origin is detached together with 2 mm of its bony attachment from the spine of the scapula to enable a more complete exposure of the infraspinatus (**Figure 18, A**). In these patients, most of the tendinous portion of the infraspinatus typically remains intact and can be used for direct transfer to the lower trapezius tendon using nonabsorbable No. 2 sutures (**Figure 18, B**). If

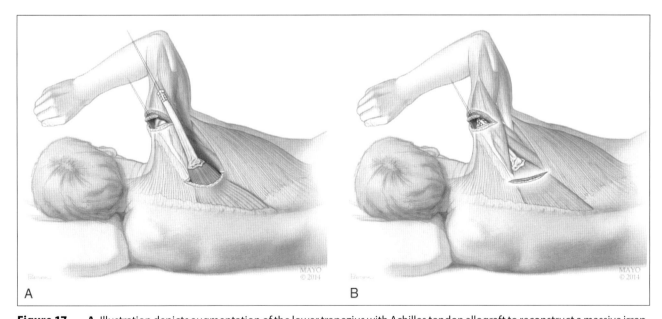

Figure 17 **A,** Illustration depicts augmentation of the lower trapezius with Achilles tendon allograft to reconstruct a massive irreparable posterosuperior rotator cuff tear. **B,** Illustration depicts transfer of the lower trapezius augmented with Achilles tendon allograft to the proximal humerus at the level of the proximal insertion of the subscapularis tendon. (Reproduced with permission from the Mayo Foundation for Medical Education and Research, Rochester, MN.)

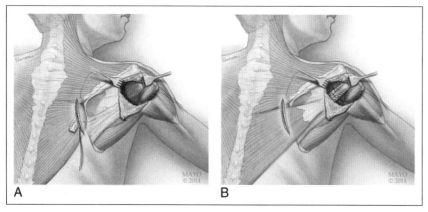

Figure 18 Illustrations depict preparation of the lower trapezius for transfer to the infraspinatus tendon (**A**) and direct transfer of the lower trapezius to the infraspinatus tendon (**B**). (Reproduced with permission from the Mayo Foundation for Medical Education and Research, Rochester, MN.)

the tendon is insufficient, augmentation with tendon allograft may be necessary. The shoulder is placed in adduction and maximal external rotation during the transfer.

WOUND CLOSURE
- The wound is irrigated.
- The deltoid is repaired with transosseous No. 2 nonabsorbable sutures, and a deep suction drain is placed.
- The wounds are closed in layered fashion.
- The patient is placed in a custom-made shoulder spica brace that is adjusted to match the shoulder position that was used during the tendon transfer.

Pectoralis Major Transfer
SETUP/EXPOSURE
- The patient is placed in the beach-chair position on a standard surgical table.
- The affected arm is prepared in its entirety and draped in sterile fashion.
- Draping should allow access from the midline of the scapula to the sternum, inferiorly to the middle of the chest wall and superiorly to the base of the neck.

- The forearm is covered with a sterile dressing that keeps the hand contained and allows for attachment of a dynamic arm holder.
- A standard deltopectoral approach is used, and the cephalic vein is taken laterally.
- Instruments, equipment, and implants are similar to those listed for latissimus dorsi transfer.

PROCEDURE
- The deltoid is freed from the humerus, and a retractor is placed beneath the deltoid to expose the proximal humerus.
- The detached and retracted subscapularis tendon can usually be identified in the subcoracoid space.
- The borders of the subscapularis are identified and dissected.
- The tendon may be torn and have an intact sleeve of tissue both anteriorly and posteriorly that remains attached to the lesser tuberosity. This sleeve and scar tissue should be incised.
- Multiple No. 2 nonabsorbable retention sutures are placed into the lateral aspect of the remaining subscapularis tendon if possible.
- The circumflex humeral artery is identified on the humerus and

ligated at the junction of the upper two-thirds and lower one-third of the subscapularis.
- The axillary nerve is identified as it passes from the posterior cord toward the anterior distal aspect of the subscapularis and posteriorly around the humeral neck. The nerve is dissected, and a vessel loop is placed around it for protection.
- The biceps tendon is examined. If pathology is observed, tenotomy is performed.
- The subscapularis is released circumferentially to allow better mobilization of the muscle and tendon.
- A direct partial or full repair of the subscapularis tendon should be attempted. If repair is not possible, a pectoralis major tendon transfer is performed.
- Numerous transfer techniques have been described, all of which begin with identification of the inferior and superior borders of the pectoralis tendon at the humeral insertion.
- One transfer technique uses the upper half of the pectoralis major tendon for transfer to the lesser tuberosity.
- The cephalad one-half to two-thirds of the pectoralis major tendon is released from the insertion on the humerus. Care must be taken to protect the biceps tendon, which runs adjacent to the pectoralis major insertion.
- The pectoralis muscle is split in line with its fibers to allow adequate mobilization of the tendon to the lesser tuberosity. To avoid placing the medial pectoral nerve at risk, the surgeon should not dissect more than 6 cm in the medial direction.
- The tendon is mobilized and sutured to bone with multiple No. 2 nonabsorbable sutures using a Mason-Allen stitch.
- If a partial pectoralis major tendon transfer will be insufficient, the

entire tendon can be transferred in a similar fashion.

- In addition, the sternal and clavicular heads can be separated with the sternal head detached, transferred deep to the clavicular head, and attached to the proximal aspect of the lesser tuberosity or to the greater tuberosity to create a better moment arm of rotation (**Figure 19, A**). Dissection in the interval between the sternal and clavicular heads should begin medially, where the interval can be easily identified.
- Alternatively, the transfer can be modified by passing the pectoralis major deep to the conjoint tendon (**Figure 19, B**). After the pectoralis major is detached from its humeral insertion, No. 2 nonabsorbable sutures are placed through the detached pectoralis major tendon for passage. The space between the conjoint tendon and the deeper pectoralis minor muscle is developed. The musculocutaneous nerve must be protected because it lies 2 to 5 cm distal to the medial border of the conjoint tendon. The nerve should remain deep to the pectoralis major during the transfer. The tendon is repaired to bone as described previously.

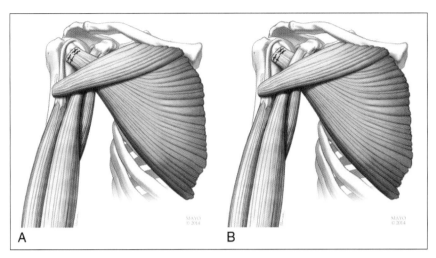

Figure 19   Illustrations depict transfer of the sternal head of the pectoralis major muscle deep to the clavicular head (**A**) or deep to the conjoint tendon (**B**) to reconstruct a subscapularis tear. (Reproduced with permission from the Mayo Foundation for Medical Education and Research, Rochester, MN.)

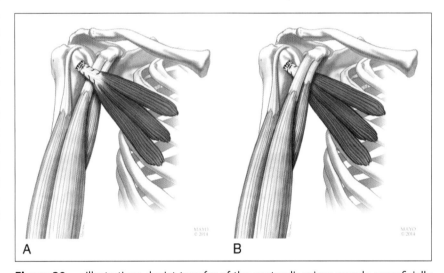

Figure 20   Illustrations depict transfer of the pectoralis minor muscle superficially (**A**) and deep (**B**) to the conjoint tendon to reconstruct a subscapularis tear. (Reproduced with permission from the Mayo Foundation for Medical Education and Research, Rochester, MN.)

WOUND CLOSURE
- The wound is irrigated.
- Deep closure is not required.
- The skin is closed in routine fashion over a deep drain.
- The patient's arm is placed in a sling.

Pectoralis Minor Transfer
- Through the deltopectoral approach, the coracoid is exposed.
- The pectoralis minor is detached from its insertion on the medial aspect of the coracoid.
- A No. 2 nonabsorbable suture is placed in a Krackow fashion in the tendinous and musculotendinous

portions of the pectoralis minor.
- Exposure and preparation of the lesser tuberosity is performed as described for the pectoralis major transfer procedure.
- The pectoralis minor is passed either superficially or deep to the conjoint tendon (**Figure 20**) and is repaired to the upper part of the lesser tuberosity.

Latissimus Dorsi and Teres Major Transfer
SETUP/EXPOSURE
- The patient is placed in the beach-chair position.
- The arm, shoulder, and upper back are prepared and draped.
- A deltopectoral approach is used, with a skin incision of approximately 5 to 7 cm.

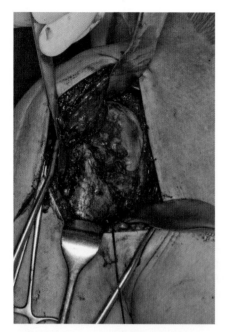

Figure 21 Intraoperative photograph shows the tendinous insertion of the latissimus dorsi through the anterior approach to the shoulder. (Reproduced with permission from the Mayo Foundation for Medical Education and Research, Rochester, MN.)

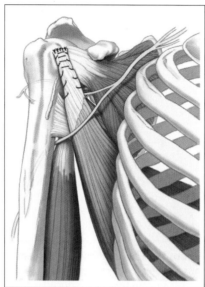

Figure 22 Illustration depicts transfer of the tendinous insertion of the latissimus dorsi to the subscapularis insertion without impingement on the axillary or radial nerves. (Reproduced with permission from the Mayo Foundation for Medical Education and Research, Rochester, MN.)

- Skin and subcutaneous dissections are performed.
- The deltopectoral interval is identified with the cephalic vein used as a landmark.
- Instruments, equipment, and implants are similar to those listed for latissimus dorsi transfer.

PROCEDURE

- The first part of the procedure is the same as that described for pectoralis major transfer. If the subscapularis is deemed irreparable, attention is directed toward harvesting the latissimus dorsi tendon.
- Through the same exposure, the proximal one-third of the pectoralis major is lacerated, with a small cuff of tendon left attached to the humerus to be used later for tendon repair.
- The latissimus dorsi tendon lies immediately deep to the pectoralis major tendon (**Figure 21**).
- Dissection of the tendinous insertion of the latissimus dorsi is performed. The tendon should be separated from the teres major before it is detached from the humerus.
- If the partial conjoint tendon is located between the latissimus dorsi and the teres major, sharp dissection with scissors or a knife is performed to separate the latissimus dorsi from the teres major.
- The tendon is either detached from the bone or detached together with 5 mm of its bony insertion.
- A nonabsorbable No. 2 suture is placed in a Krackow fashion in the tendinous portion to facilitate muscle mobilization and later tendon repair.
- The neurovascular bundle is identified proximally and protected.
- After the tendon is sufficiently mobilized, it is transferred to the proximal aspect of the lesser tuberosity (**Figure 22**). However, in patients with proximal migration of the humeral head resulting from an anterosuperior RCT, the author of this chapter prefers to transfer the tendon to the anterior aspect of the greater tuberosity.

- If transfer of the teres major is planned, the same exposure is used, and the latissimus dorsi tendon is retracted to expose the teres major. The teres major is detached with or without small bony insertion. The remaining steps of the transfer to the lesser tuberosity are the same as those of latissimus dorsi transfer, except that the site of the transfer should be the central or distal aspect of the lesser tuberosity. This recommendation is based on a cadaver model study that demonstrated potential impingement of the teres major on the axillary nerve with a more proximal transfer.
- A double transfer of the latissimus dorsi proximally on the lesser tuberosity and the teres major medially or distally on the lesser tuberosity is feasible, does not risk nerve impingement, and can be considered in patients with difficult anterior subluxation associated with irreparable anterosuperior RCTs, especially if an isolated latissimus dorsi transfer is insufficient to achieve reduction.

WOUND CLOSURE

- The pectoralis major tendon that was partly lacerated is repaired with nonabsorbable No. 2 sutures.
- The deltopectoral interval is approximated with No. 0 Vicryl sutures.
- The wound is closed in layers in a subcuticular fashion.
- The patient is placed in a shoulder immobilizer with the shoulder in internal rotation.

Table 2 Rehabilitation Protocol After Muscle Transfer to Manage Massive Rotator Cuff Tear

Postoperative Week	Range of Motion	Strengthening	Return to Play	Comments/ Emphasis
0-2	None	None	None	—
2-6	None	None	None	—
6-12	Active assisted	None	None	No passive stretching
12-24	Full active	Progressive	After 6 mo	—

 Rehabilitation

The rehabilitation protocol is summarized in **Table 2**. All patients who undergo tendon transfer to reconstruct posterosuperior RCTs follow a similar postoperative rehabilitation protocol. A custom-made shoulder abduction/external rotation brace is placed postoperatively, with the arm held in the same position as during the surgical procedure. The drain is removed after the drainage is less than 30 mL per 24 hours. Patients remain in the brace for 8 weeks postoperatively. Passive forward flexion and external rotation are allowed under the supervision of a physical therapist between 6 and 8 weeks postoperatively while patients are still in the brace; this motion consists of additional passive motion to the position in which the shoulder was placed at the time of brace application. Active-assisted ROM with hydrotherapy is initiated at 8 weeks postoperatively, and the use of biofeedback is encouraged at this time. Gentle strengthening is begun at 14 weeks postoperatively and progressed until 6 months postoperatively, at which time unrestricted activities are allowed.

After pectoralis major transfer, passive ROM may be initiated immediately. Limits should be set based on passive external rotation of the arm intraoperatively under direct visualization of the repair. The author of this chapter takes the shoulder through gentle ROM during surgery to determine the degree at which external rotation places tension on the pectoralis repair. The author considers this level of rotation as the maximum passive ROM allowed postoperatively. Passive elevation may be performed with the arm internally rotated. Active-assisted ROM is delayed until 6 weeks postoperatively. Light strengthening of the shoulder flexors, abductors, and external rotators can begin at 10 weeks postoperatively as tolerated. Internal rotation against resistance is delayed until 12 weeks postoperatively.

After combined latissimus dorsi and teres major transfer, the patient remains in a shoulder immobilizer with the shoulder in internal rotation for 6 weeks postoperatively. At 4 weeks postoperatively, passive shoulder exercises are begun, with external rotation restricted to neutral. An active-assisted exercise program is begun at 8 weeks postoperatively. Gentle strengthening is begun at 12 weeks postoperatively and progresses slowly for 2 to 3 months. The patient is allowed to return to full activity at 6 months postoperatively.

 Avoiding Pitfalls

In the experience of the author of this chapter, a number of steps can be taken to avoid pitfalls during surgery, the most important of which are patient setup and the availability of all necessary instruments/equipment. Whether placed in the beach-chair position for anterior transfers or the lateral position for posterior transfers, the patient should be well positioned, and all of the areas that may be involved in surgery should be included in the surgical field. A dynamic arm holder helps position the arm throughout surgery and maintain the shoulder in the position necessary for closure and the application of the shoulder brace. Knowledge of shoulder anatomy is crucial because it helps the surgeon achieve the desired exposure and may help avoid potential complications if visualization is not adequate. Adequate muscle mobilization for transfer, protection of the neurovascular pedicle, and knowledge on how to prepare the recipient location for transfer are essential to avoid potential complications.

 Bibliography

Aldridge JM III, Atkinson TS, Mallon WJ: Combined pectoralis major and latissimus dorsi tendon transfer for massive rotator cuff deficiency. *J Shoulder Elbow Surg* 2004;13(6):621-629.

Aoki M, Okamura K, Fukushima S, Takahashi T, Ogino T: Transfer of latissimus dorsi for irreparable rotator-cuff tears. *J Bone Joint Surg Br* 1996;78(5):761-766.

Celli A, Marongiu MC, Rovesta C, Celli L: Transplant of the teres major in the treatment of irreparable injuries of the rotator cuff (long-term analysis of results). *Chir Organi Mov* 2005;90(2):121-132.

Celli L, Rovesta C, Marongiu MC, Manzieri S: Transplantation of teres major muscle for infraspinatus muscle in irreparable rotator cuff tears. *J Shoulder Elbow Surg* 1998;7(5):485-490.

Costouros JG, Espinosa N, Schmid MR, Gerber C: Teres minor integrity predicts outcome of latissimus dorsi tendon transfer for irreparable rotator cuff tears. *J Shoulder Elbow Surg* 2007;16(6):727-734.

Elhassan B: Lower trapezius transfer for shoulder external rotation in patients with paralytic shoulder. *J Hand Surg Am* 2014;39(3):556-562.

Elhassan B, Bishop A, Shin A: Trapezius transfer to restore external rotation in a patient with a brachial plexus injury: A case report. *J Bone Joint Surg Am* 2009;91(4):939-944.

Elhassan B, Bishop A, Shin A, Spinner R: Shoulder tendon transfer options for adult patients with brachial plexus injury. *J Hand Surg Am* 2010;35(7):1211-1219.

Elhassan B, Christensen TJ, Wagner ER: Feasibility of latissimus and teres major transfer to reconstruct irreparable subscapularis tendon tear: An anatomic study. *J Shoulder Elbow Surg* 2014;23(4):492-499.

Elhassan B, Ozbaydar M, Massimini D, Diller D, Higgins L, Warner JJ: Transfer of pectoralis major for the treatment of irreparable tears of subscapularis: Does it work? *J Bone Joint Surg Br* 2008;90(8):1059-1065.

Elhassan BT, Wagner ER, Werthel JD: Outcome of lower trapezius transfer to reconstruct massive irreparable posterior-superior rotator cuff tear *J Shoulder Elbow Surg* 2016; Mar 8 [Epub ahead of print].

Galatz LM, Connor PM, Calfee RP, Hsu JC, Yamaguchi K: Pectoralis major transfer for anterior-superior subluxation in massive rotator cuff insufficiency. *J Shoulder Elbow Surg* 2003;12(1):1-5.

Gartsman GM: Massive, irreparable tears of the rotator cuff: Results of operative debridement and subacromial decompression. *J Bone Joint Surg Am* 1997;79(5):715-721.

Gavriilidis I, Kircher J, Magosch P, Lichtenberg S, Habermeyer P: Pectoralis major transfer for the treatment of irreparable anterosuperior rotator cuff tears. *Int Orthop* 2010;34(5):689-694.

Gerber C: Latissimus dorsi transfer for the treatment of irreparable tears of the rotator cuff. *Clin Orthop Relat Res* 1992;(275):152-160.

Gerber C, Maquieira G, Espinosa N: Latissimus dorsi transfer for the treatment of irreparable rotator cuff tears. *J Bone Joint Surg Am* 2006;88(1):113-120.

Gerber C, Rahm SA, Catanzaro S, Farshad M, Moor BK: Latissimus dorsi tendon transfer for treatment of irreparable posterosuperior rotator cuff tears: Long-term results at a minimum follow-up of ten years. *J Bone Joint Surg Am* 2013;95(21):1920-1926.

Gerber C, Vinh TS, Hertel R, Hess CW: Latissimus dorsi transfer for the treatment of massive tears of the rotator cuff: A preliminary report. *Clin Orthop Relat Res* 1988;(232):51-61.

Hartzler RU, Barlow JD, An K-N, Elhassan BT: Biomechanical effectiveness of different types of tendon transfers to the shoulder for external rotation. *J Shoulder Elbow Surg* 2012;21(10):1370-1376.

Henseler JF, Nagels J, van der Zwaal P, Nelissen RG: Teres major tendon transfer for patients with massive irreparable posterosuperior rotator cuff tears: Short-term clinical results. *Bone Joint J* 2013;95(4):523-529.

Iannotti JP, Hennigan S, Herzog R, et al: Latissimus dorsi tendon transfer for irreparable posterosuperior rotator cuff tears: Factors affecting outcome. *J Bone Joint Surg Am* 2006;88(2):342-348.

Jost B, Puskas GJ, Lustenberger A, Gerber C: Outcome of pectoralis major transfer for the treatment of irreparable subscapularis tears. *J Bone Joint Surg Am* 2003;85(10):1944-1951.

Kim SJ, Lee IS, Kim SH, Lee WY, Chun YM: Arthroscopic partial repair of irreparable large to massive rotator cuff tears. *Arthroscopy* 2012;28(6):761-768.

Knudsen ML, Hibbard JC, Nuckley DJ, Braman JP: Anatomic landmarks for arthroscopic suprascapular nerve decompression. *Knee Surg Sports Traumatol Arthrosc* 2014; Jul 4 [Epub ahead of print].

Konrad GG, Sudkamp NP, Kreuz PC, Jolly JT, McMahon PJ, Debski RE: Pectoralis major tendon transfers above or underneath the conjoint tendon in subscapularis-deficient shoulders: An in vitro biomechanical analysis. *J Bone Joint Surg Am* 2007;89(11):2477-2484.

Moursy M, Forstner R, Koller H, Resch H, Tauber M: Latissimus dorsi tendon transfer for irreparable rotator cuff tears: A modified technique to improve tendon transfer integrity. *J Bone Joint Surg Am* 2009;91(8):1924-1931.

Omid R, Lee B: Tendon transfers for irreparable rotator cuff tears. *J Am Acad Orthop Surg* 2013;21(8):492-501.

Paladini P, Campi F, Merolla G, Pellegrini A, Porcellini G: Pectoralis minor tendon transfer for irreparable anterosuperior cuff tears. *J Shoulder Elbow Surg* 2013;22(6):e1-e5.

Pearle AD, Kelly BT, Voos JE, Chehab EL, Warren RF: Surgical technique and anatomic study of latissimus dorsi and teres major transfers. *J Bone Joint Surg Am* 2006;88(7):1524-1531.

Resch H, Povacz P, Ritter E, Matschi W: Transfer of the pectoralis major muscle for the treatment of irreparable rupture of the subscapularis tendon. *J Bone Joint Surg Am* 2000;82(3):372-382.

Walch G, Edwards TB, Boulahia A, Nové-Josserand L, Neyton L, Szabo I: Arthroscopic tenotomy of the long head of the biceps in the treatment of rotator cuff tears: Clinical and radiographic results of 307 cases. *J Shoulder Elbow Surg* 2005;14(3):238-246.

Warner JJ, Higgins L, Parsons IM IV, Dowdy P: Diagnosis and treatment of anterosuperior rotator cuff tears. *J Shoulder Elbow Surg* 2001;10(1):37-46.

Wirth MA, Rockwood CA Jr: Operative treatment of irreparable rupture of the subscapularis. *J Bone Joint Surg Am* 1997;79(5):722-731.

Chapter 24

The Massive Rotator Cuff Tear: Patches and Augmentation Devices

Marc R. Labbé, MD

Introduction

Treatment of massive rotator cuff tears can be a challenge. Failure rates significantly exceed those for smaller tears. Chronic tears can be especially challenging because the bone and soft tissues change over time. Without mechanical stress, the tendons, which have minimal blood flow to begin with, degenerate further and become friable. The muscles lose volume and undergo fatty replacement. The greater tuberosity loses density, making anchor retention more difficult. Without a superior restraint, the deltoid pulls the humeral head into the acromion, and the inferior capsule becomes contracted and stiff. The articular cartilage begins to degrade and arthropathy develops.

Open rotator cuff augmentation was first described in 1978 using freeze-dried rotator cuff. Results of subsequent studies were mixed but mostly negative. As a result, augmentation fell out of favor. In the early 2000s, arthroscopic augmentation and bridging techniques were developed.

A growing body of clinical and laboratory data now support the use of biologic grafts in rotator cuff repair. Augmentation serves to reinforce the repair by attaching the graft to the cuff medial to the tear and the tuberosity laterally covering the repair. Grafts also have been used as interposition devices to bridge a gap for tears that are irreparable or only partially repairable. The graft is sewn to the edges of the irreparable tendons medially and the tuberosity laterally, essentially replacing a portion of the cuff.

More recently, techniques for reconstruction of the superior capsule have been developed. The concept behind superior capsule reconstruction is to rebuild a superior restraint that centers the humeral head within the glenoid, allowing the deltoid and remaining teres minor and subscapularis to create glenohumeral motion. The technique involves attaching a graft directly to the superior glenoid neck and the humeral head laterally. The remaining rotator cuff remnant is attached to the patch. With the graft helping to center the humeral head, a balanced cuff and the deltoid can flex and abduct the shoulder. As surgical techniques have evolved, so have grafting materials. Synthetic graft, xenograft, and allografts in various configurations are currently available. The specific properties, laboratory data, and clinical data vary for each type and should be considered before use.

Case Presentation

The following case example describes the first arthroscopic grafting procedure performed by the author of this chapter in 2003. Four months after undergoing repair of a massive rotator cuff tear, a 67-year-old woman was seen for reevaluation. The repair had clearly failed; the patient continued to experience dysfunction and often had pain while riding in the car on the rural roads near her home. A repeat MRI showed retracted tears of the supraspinatus and infraspinatus with moderate fatty infiltration. Hemiarthroplasty was considered, but the author of this chapter thought that it would not adequately address the problem or improve the patient's function. Reverse arthroplasty was not as popular at the time, and the patient was resistant to arthroplasty regardless. A standard surgical revision procedure could have been attempted, but it likely would have failed. The patient did not want to live with her dysfunction. She had been participating in a formal rehabilitation program and was not progressing. After lengthy discussion with the patient, arthroscopic cuff augmentation was chosen. The author of this chapter had experience with glenoid resurfacing using a graft made from porcine small intestine submucosa and converted that technique for the rotator cuff augment procedure. Four months after revision surgery, the patient had regained active

Dr. Labbé or an immediate family member has received royalties from and is a member of a speakers' bureau or has made paid presentations on behalf of Mitek Sports Medicine and serves as a paid consultant to ConMed Linvatec, Mitek Sports Medicine, and Rotation Medical.

motion without pain, and her strength was returning.

Indications

Patient selection starts with a detailed history and physical examination. The patient should be asked about total duration of symptoms, specific injuries, and treatments attempted. A history of trauma and a sudden decrease in function can indicate an acute or acute-on-chronic tear. The surgeon should ask if the patient had symptoms before the injury. Usually, traumatic tears have better quality and more mobile tendons and are more amenable to repair compared with chronic tears. If a patient has a history of previous surgical treatment, the surgeon should review intraoperative images and surgical notes. Physical examination should include visualization of the shoulder. The surgeon should evaluate the patient for muscle wasting in the scapular fossa. If the patient previously underwent surgical treatment, careful examination of the deltoid and assessment of its function is warranted. Active and passive motion are evaluated. If the examination is inhibited by patient pain, subacromial lidocaine can be administered. Strength of the individual muscles must be tested. The lift-off test can be painful; thus, the belly-press test with the patient's wrist in neutral alignment is preferred. Supraspinatus testing is done in scaption with the patient's thumb toward the ceiling. The infraspinatus is tested in 30° of abduction and neutral flexion.

Imaging is important in understanding the extent of the disease. Plain radiographs and MRIs are the mainstays for evaluating the number of tendons involved, the extent of retraction and chondral damage, and the degree of fatty infiltration. Patients with radiographic signs of arthropathy (acetabularization of the acromion, absent or minimal joint space, and osteophytes) are not good candidates for surgical treatment. Humeral head elevation should be inferred from standing images rather than from the supine MRI. For patients who have undergone previous surgical treatment, MRI arthrography can help provide more detail. CT arthrography is helpful in patients who cannot be evaluated with MRI.

Treatment and counseling must be individualized to each patient. Repair should be pursued in younger and more active patients. For older and more sedentary patients, reverse arthroplasty is a better choice. In general, repair with graft should be considered for large or massive primary tears or revision repairs in patients aged 65 years and younger with minimal chondromalacia and no radiographic signs of arthropathy.

Contraindications

Contraindications for grafting are similar to those for rotator cuff repair. Active infections are a contraindication. Medical comorbidities that can affect healing, such as organ transplant, cancer therapy, chronic oral or intravenous steroid use, and complicated diabetes, are relative contraindications. Smoking is a relative contraindication, and patients must stop smoking before undergoing surgical treatment. NSAIDs must be stopped before surgery and should not be used during the first 6 weeks of recovery. Sensitivity to the specific graft material also should be considered and discussed prior to surgery.

Controversies and Alternative Approaches

Nonsurgical treatment, including therapy and corticosteroid injections, can help reduce pain and improve function in patients with massive rotator cuff tears. Predictably, the shoulder will become arthritic and may develop pseudoparalysis. Over time, tears that initially may have been reparable will become irreparable and require arthroplasty. Even so, nonsurgical treatment is often well tolerated and appreciated by patients who are not good candidates for repair or who are not ready for joint reconstruction. Resurfacing or replacing the humeral head can address pain related to arthritis and can be useful in patients capable of forward flexion and abduction. Muscle transfers are another treatment option. Transfers typically involve substituting the pectoralis major for the subscapularis and the latissimus dorsi for the superior cuff. Muscle transfer also has been combined with arthroplasty with good short-term results. However, these techniques are challenging, substantially alter the anatomy, and provide variable results.

Superior capsular reconstruction is another arthroscopic technique that is gaining favor. Rather than attaching the graft to the medial edge of the remaining cuff, the graft is attached directly to the glenoid neck. The posterior edge of the cuff also is sewn to the graft. This technique requires a well-functioning subscapularis, teres minor, and deltoid. Biomechanical data show that subacromial contact pressures normalize with the reconstruction compared with a torn supraspinatus. Early clinical results also are promising, although data are very limited. The sole clinical study, published in 2013, reported on 24 shoulders in 23 patients. Significant improvements in motion and American Shoulder and Elbow Surgeons shoulder outcome scores were noted. Postoperative MRI showed intact grafts in 83.3% of patients, and no progression of arthrosis was noted at an average follow-up of 34 months.

Reverse total shoulder arthroplasty is another option for the treatment of massive tears. By altering the mechanics of the glenohumeral joint, the procedure can restore a substantial amount of motion and markedly improve function. The development of a variety of implants and revision options has made this technique popular. However, the procedure irrevocably alters the normal anatomy to accommodate the implants. A thorough evaluation by the physician and thoughtful discussion with the patient is needed in deciding between an arthroscopic approach and reverse arthroplasty. Reverse arthroplasty is the preferred technique in patients with pseudoparalysis and rotator cuff arthropathy.

Results

The results of arthroscopic rotator cuff augmentation have been largely positive. A randomized, prospective study published in 2012 evaluated the use of an acellular human dermal matrix in tears measuring more than 3 cm. Functional scores and MRI arthrogram were used to evaluate the patients postoperatively. Patients treated with graft had significantly improved functional scores compared with patients who were not treated with graft. Only 40% of the nonaugmented repairs were intact on postoperative MRI, whereas 85% of the augmented repairs were intact. No adverse outcomes were noted from the graft. **Table 1** summarizes several recent clinical studies.

Video 24.1 Arthroscopic Rotator Cuff Repair and Augmentation With Acellular Human Dermal Graft. Marc Labbé, MD (8 min)

Technical Keys to Success

The FDA has approved the use of soft-tissue grafts for any rotator cuff that can be repaired either completely or to within 1 cm of the greater tuberosity.

Open or arthroscopic grafting may be performed. The number of graft options has increased tremendously in the past decade. Key factors to consider in evaluating grafts include the source material, cross-linking, and clinical data. Xenografts and artificial grafts can generate rejection reactions. Cross-linking is a chemical process that binds collagen bundles together, resulting in a more durable and stiff graft; however, cross-linking may affect the ability of the host tissue to integrate. Research on graft materials is ongoing, and surgeons are advised to stay up to date as new data are published.

To apply a graft using an open technique, a standard cuff repair is performed. The graft must be prepared and cut so that it covers the repair completely. Usually, the medial edge of the graft is placed at the muscle-tendon junction. Using high–tensile strength suture, the graft is sutured medially and on the anterior and posterior edges. The surgeon should take care to avoid any sutures from the initial repair. Laterally, the graft can be sutured with any remaining stitches in the repair anchors. Alternatively, extra anchors can be inserted laterally.

Four-Corner Arthroscopic Augmentation

This arthroscopic technique offers a simple and reproducible method. As with any surgical technique, myriad variations are available to suit the style of the individual surgeon.

STEP 1: REPAIR
- The operating room is arranged in the surgeon's usual manner.
- Hemostats, free cutting needles that fit a No. 2 suture, and an 8.5-mm cannula are needed.
- The first step is to perform either an open or arthroscopic partial or complete cuff repair and perform any bony procedures necessary (**Figure 1**).

STEP 2: THE CORNERS
- The fixation framework for the graft is created in the subacromial space. Four points of fixation are used: two are placed medial to the tear, and two are placed lateral to the tear.
- The medial fixation consists of two No. 2 high-tensile strength mattress sutures; usually, these sutures are placed at the muscle-tendon junction. The sutures should be wider than the tear anteriorly and posteriorly.
- The sutures are inserted using a margin convergence technique. With the arthroscope in the lateral portal, a retrograde suture passer is placed in the cuff in a through-and-through fashion via the posterior or anterior portal.
- A small loop of suture is brought down a cannula in the opposite portal and handed off to the grasper.
- The sutures are brought out the portal opposite the side of insertion; for example, the posterior medial corner is brought out the anterior portal. By bringing the sutures out the opposite portal, they cross in the subacromial space, which facilitates visualization and later retrieval (**Figure 2**).
- The lateral corners are created either by saving sutures in the anterior and posterior cuff repair anchors or by placing more anchors lateral to the repair or over the edge of the tuberosity at the point at which transosseous sutures would come out.
- If the bone is weak, extra anchors should be used so as not to overload the repair anchors.
- To size the graft, the distance between the corners on all four sides is measured using either a probe with markings or a suture and two graspers. If a suture is used for measurement, one grasper is used to

Table 1 Results of Graft Augmentation in the Management of Massive Rotator Cuff Tear

Authors	Journal (Year)	Technique (Number)	Graft Used	Graft Material	Outcomes	Failure Rate (%)	Comments
Audenaert et al	*Knee Surg Sports Traumatol Arthrosc* (2006)	Open interposition (41 patients)	Mersilene (Ethicon) mesh	Synthetic	Improved clinical scores, pain relief, and performance of activities of daily living	7.3 (retear)	41 patients Mean follow-up, 43 mo
Iannotti et al	*J Bone Joint Surg Am* (2006)	Open augment (15 shoulders treated with graft; 15 shoulders in control group)	Porcine small intestine xenograft (Restore; DePuy)	Biologic xenograft	No clinical improvement was noted	73.3 (graft) 40 (control group)	RCT Graft option not recommended 9 of 15 shoulders healed in the control group 4 of 15 shoulders healed in the graft group Mean follow-up, 14 mo
Moore et al	*Am J Sports Med* (2006)	Open augment (28 patients)	Cuff tendon allograft	Allograft	23 patients were satisfied with their outcome 1 infection and 1 graft rejection occurred	100[a]	Clinical use, case series Mean follow-up, 31.3 mo
Scheibel et al	*Knee Surg Sports Traumatol Arthrosc* (2007)	Open augment (20 patients)	Periosteal flap	Autograft	Improved clinical scores and moderately low retear rate (20%)	20 (retear)	Clinical use, case series Risk of rotator cuff calcification, not correlated with inferior clinical outcomes Mean follow-up, 14.4 mo
Badhe et al	*J Shoulder Elbow Surg* (2008)	Open augment (10 patients)	Porcine dermal xenograft (Permacol; Covidien)	Biologic xenograft	Improved clinical scores, pain, strength, and ROM postoperatively	20 (retear)	Mean follow-up, 54 mo
Bond et al	*Arthroscopy* (2008)	Arthroscopic interposition (16 patients)	Acellular human dermal matrix (GraftJacket; Wright Medical Technology)	Allograft	15 patients were satisfied with their outcome Improved functional scores were noted	18.8	Case series Mean follow-up, 26.8 mo
Bektaşer et al	*Acta Orthop Traumatol Turc* (2010)	Open augment (46 patients)	Free total or partial coracoacromial ligament graft	Autograft	ROM clinical scores improved	0	Clinical use, case series Mean follow-up, 26 mo

RCT = randomized controlled trial, ROM = range of motion.
[a] All 15 patients evaluated on MRI demonstrated radiographic failure of the allograft rotator cuff reconstruction.

Table 1 Results of Graft Augmentation in the Management of Massive Rotator Cuff Tear (*continued*)

Authors	Journal (Year)	Technique (Number)	Graft Used	Graft Material	Outcomes	Failure Rate (%)	Comments
Nada et al	*J Bone Joint Surg Br* (2010)	Massive arthroscopic cuff repair and Dacron ligament construction (17 patients)	Polyester fiber mesh ligament	Synthetic	Improved clinical score and ROM	11.8	Clinical use, case series
Encalada-Diaz et al	*J Shoulder Elbow Surg* (2011)	Open augment (10 patients)	Reticulated polycarbonate polyurethane patch (Biomerix)	Synthetic	Decreased pain, improved clinical scores, and low retear rate	10	Clinical use Small case series Follow-up, 12 mo
Barber et al	*Arthroscopy* (2012)	Arthroscopic augment (22 patients)	Acellular human dermal matrix (GraftJacket; Wright Medical Technology)	Allograft	Multicenter RCT found decreased retear rates and improved clinical scores compared with control subjects	15 (with graft) 60 (without graft)	Clinical use Very few participants in RCT 20 control subjects Mean follow-up, 24 mo
Gupta et al	*Am J Sports Med* (2012)	Mini-open interposition (24 patients)	Acellular human dermal matrix allograft	Biologic	Decreased pain Improved functional scores	24	Case series Mean follow-up, 36 mo
Yoon et al	*Am J Sports Med* (2016)	Arthroscopic augment with bone stimulation (22 patients)	Acellular dermis (Allocover: Hans Biomed) Tenotomized biceps tendon Control group	Allograft	Reported improvement in some aspects of ROM, strength, and image-based healing	19 (augment group) 46.3 (control group)	Clinical use, case series

RCT = randomized controlled trial, ROM = range of motion.

[a] All 15 patients evaluated on MRI demonstrated radiographic failure of the allograft rotator cuff reconstruction.

hold the end of the suture at one corner. The suture is grabbed at the other corner so that it is taut. The surgeon lets go of the suture on the end and removes the stich. The length from the end of the sutures to the grasper is measured.

- The graft is prepared according to the manufacturer's specifications and cut according to the measurements.

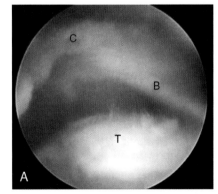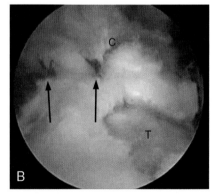

Figure 1 Arthroscopic views of a shoulder from the lateral portal demonstrate a massive recurrent rotator cuff tear before (**A**) and after (**B**) repair. Arrows indicate sutures from repair anchors. B = biceps tendon, C = rotator cuff, T = greater tuberosity.

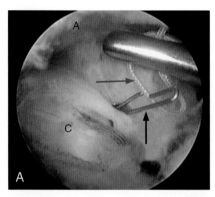 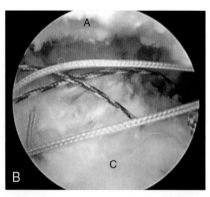

Figure 2   **A,** Arthroscopic image of a shoulder demonstrates through-and-through passage of a retrograde suture passer (black arrow) through the rotator cuff (C) and retrieval of a suture loop (red arrow), creating the posteromedial corner. The suture limbs were then retrieved through the anterior portal. **B,** Arthroscopic image of a shoulder demonstrates the anteromedial and posteromedial sutures crossing in the subacromial space for easier visualization and later retrieval. A = acromion.

STEP 3: SUTURE RETRIEVAL AND PASSAGE

- The arthroscope is moved to the posterior portal.
- The 8.5-mm cannula is placed in the lateral portal.
- One of the medial mattress suture pairs is retrieved and pulled out of the cannula.
- Using a hemostat, the suture is clamped to the drape in the same position that the suture occupies in the subacromial space. For example, the anteromedial corner sutures are clamped anteriorly and medially on the drape.
- With slight tension on the sutures just retrieved, the surgeon slides the suture retriever down the cannula away from the sutures in the cannula. The next medial pair of sutures is retrieved and clamped on the drapes. Maintaining tension on the sutures allows for retrieval and avoids crossing the sutures within the cannula. Successful outcome depends on ensuring that the sutures do not cross in the cannula.
- At this point in the procedure, the sutures are ready to be passed through the graft.
- One hemostat is placed in each corner of the graft, and one or two

assistants hold the graft over the lateral cannula in the same orientation in which it will be placed in the subacromial space.

- With a free needle, one pair of lateral sutures is passed through the graft in a mattress pattern, maintaining the same orientation as in the subacromial space. For example, the anterolateral sutures in the subacromial space are passed through the anterolateral corner of the graft.
- The limbs of the mattress suture should be approximately 1 cm apart.
- The process is repeated for the other lateral pair of sutures, taking care not to cross the sutures underneath the graft.
- Next, the medial sutures are passed. Because these sutures do not come from an anchor, each suture pair has an anterior limb and a posterior limb. One medial suture pair is prepared by gently pulling on one limb while visualizing it arthroscopically in the subacromial space to identify it as either an anterior or posterior limb.
- Using the free needle, the limb is passed through the graft in its respective corner and in the

appropriate position as either the anterior or posterior limb of the mattress stitch. The second limb is passed through the graft.

- These steps are repeated for the other medial suture pairs.
- A visual inspection is performed with the arthroscope in the subacromial space and externally to confirm that all four corners are placed through the graft and that no sutures cross as they pass through the cannula and the graft (**Figure 3**).

STEP 4: PASSING AND SECURING THE GRAFT

- An arthroscopic sliding or sliding-locking knot is tied in each of the four corners; these knots are not initially backed up. That is, no extra knots are made after the initial sliding-locking knot.
- One hemostat is placed on the post limb of each knot, and the clamps are removed from the graft (**Figure 4, A**).
- With a small grasper, the medial edge of the graft is grabbed in the middle and the graft is pushed into the cannula. The graft can be gently folded around the grasper if needed.
- After the graft is placed in the subacromial space, tension is applied to the post limbs while maintaining inward pressure with the grasper on the graft.
- The sutures are pulled in line with the cannula so that the knots slide toward the graft. A knot pusher can be used if necessary, but the hemostat should be replaced on the post limb so that the limb can be identified later. The medial sutures are tensioned first.
- Extra slack can be removed from the wrapping limbs, but the knots are left unlocked.
- At this point in the procedure, the graft should be positioned in the subacromial space and against the

cuff (**Figure 4, B**). A second cannula is placed in the anterior portal or a separate accessory lateral portal for knot tying.

- One limb of one medial mattress suture is retrieved and identified as either the post or the wrapping limb. It is important to remember that the post is being held by the hemostat. The other limb is removed, and the knot-tying procedure is completed.
- These steps are repeated on the other three corners.
- The graft should be well fixed to the cuff medially and to the tuberosity laterally. Ideally, the circumference of the graft contacts the cuff and tuberosity with no gaps (**Figure 4, C**).
- If an area needs to be further secured, a suture can be passed through the cuff and graft using the margin convergence technique. The suture passer is placed through the cuff and then the graft (or vice versa), and a suture loop is handed to the retriever. The suture limbs are retrieved and tied with an arthroscopic knot.
- The graft should be under some tension because it was cut to fit the dimensions outlined by the corner sutures.

WOUND CLOSURE
- The wounds are repaired with simple sutures, and a well-padded dressing and abduction pillow are applied.
- The dressing should be thick to absorb leakage of the arthroscopic fluid. Typically, the dressing is removed 2 to 4 days postoperatively.

Partial Repair

The technique for augmentation of a partial repair is similar to the technique for augmentation of a complete repair. The surgeon should ensure security of the graft by applying sutures as necessary to achieve structural stability and

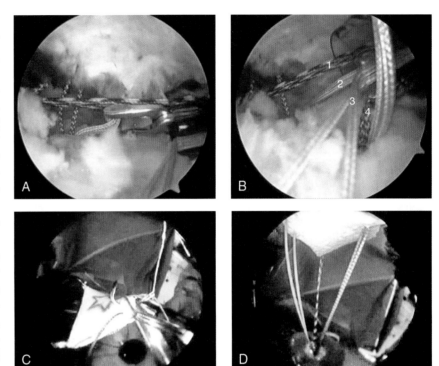

Figure 3   **A** and **B,** Arthroscopic views of a shoulder from the posterior portal during retrieval of a suture pair. **A,** Crossing of the sutures during retrieval can be avoided by tensioning the sutures already in the cannula prior to passing the suture grasper. **B,** The appearance of the sutures (numbered 1 through 4) entering the cannula after all of four pairs are retrieved; note that the sutures do not cross. Intraoperative photographs show the sutures being passed from bottom to top through the graft with a cutting needle (**C**). The sutures entering the graft in the same orientation in which they are placed in the subacromial space, without crossing (**D**).

good contact between the graft and the surrounding tissues.

Rehabilitation

Multiple studies have demonstrated that delayed therapy after rotator cuff repair offers benefits and few complications. For difficult tears, the surgeon should allow time for healing to occur before stressing the repair. Strengthening of the cuff muscle does not start until 3 months postoperatively, and gym exercises such as the bench press can be cautiously initiated at 4 months postoperatively or later. To avoid excessive cuff strain when performing bench press or overhead press motions, patients should keep a short arc of motion so that the elbow does not dip past the shoulder.

Table 2 outlines a basic protocol for rehabilitation. However, the rehabilitation protocol must be individualized to each patient. For example, in patients at risk of developing stiffness, initiation of therapy before 6 weeks postoperatively may be warranted. Patients who have difficulty healing may require a slower rehabilitation protocol to ensure the integrity of the repair construct as therapy progresses.

Avoiding Pitfalls

The surgeon attempting an arthroscopic graft should be well versed in the techniques of arthroscopic cuff repair, including suture passage, suture management, the use of margin convergence sutures, and knot tying. Maintaining

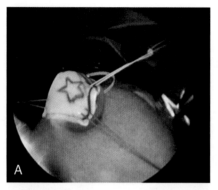 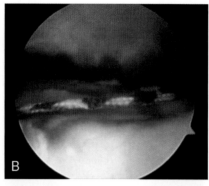 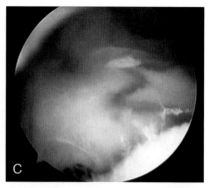

Figure 4 **A,** Intraoperative photograph of a shoulder shows the graft prepared for passage down the cannula with the sliding-locking knots tied and the post limbs held in a clamp. **B** and **C,** Arthroscopic views of a shoulder from the posterior portal. **B,** The appearance of the graft sitting against the cuff and the sutures exiting the lateral cannula after the knots have been passed and tensioned with a knot pusher. **C,** The graft is secured and has good circumferential contact with the cuff and the greater tuberosity.

Table 2 Rehabilitation Protocol After Rotator Cuff Repair With Graft Augmentation

Postoperative Week	ROM	Strengthening	Return to Play	Comments/Emphasis
0-4	Active elbow ROM, scapular retraction	None	None	Avoid active shoulder ROM, and limit weight to <2 lb
4-6	Add passive ROM	Scapular strengthening only	None	Avoid active shoulder ROM, and limit weight to <2 lb
6-12	Add active-assisted ROM, active ROM	Scapular strengthening only	None	Maintain limited weight <2-3 lb in the hand
12-16	As tolerated	Add cuff strengthening	None	Slowly increase weight in the hand during activities of daily living, but do not lift above shoulder height
≥16	As tolerated	Add gym exercises (planks, push-ups)	Sport-specific practice first, then play	Weight and resistance are increased slowly in consultation with a physical therapist

ROM = range of motion.

Reproduced with permission from Steele B, Gordon JA, Labbé M: The use of graft augmentation in the treatment of massive rotator cuff tears, in Kelly JD, ed: *Elite Techniques in Shoulder Arthroscopy.* Cham, Switzerland, Springer International Publishing, 2016, pp 255-269.

tension on the sutures while retrieving the other sutures helps avoid crossing the sutures within the cannula. It is important not to cross the sutures underneath the graft while placing the sutures through the graft with the free needle. A hemostat should be placed to mark the post limb of each knot before removing the clamps from the graft. After the graft is passed into the subacromial space, tension should be placed on the posts to help slide the graft into position. A knot pusher also can be used for this. The surgeon must start with the medial end. Placing gentle tension on the suture limbs will remove excess suture material from the subacromial space and improve visualization. The surgeon must take care not to prematurely lock the initial knots.

Bibliography

Audenaert E, Van Nuffel J, Schepens A, Verhelst M, Verdonk R: Reconstruction of massive rotator cuff lesions with a synthetic interposition graft: A prospective study of 41 patients. *Knee Surg Sports Traumatol Arthrosc* 2006;14(4):360-364.

Badhe SP, Lawrence TM, Smith FD, Lunn PG: An assessment of porcine dermal xenograft as an augmentation graft in the treatment of extensive rotator cuff tears. *J Shoulder Elbow Surg* 2008;17(1 suppl):35S-39S.

Barber FA, Aziz-Jacobo J: Biomechanical testing of commercially available soft-tissue augmentation materials. *Arthroscopy* 2009;25(11):1233-1239.

Barber FA, Burns JP, Deutsch A, Labbé MR, Litchfield RB: A prospective, randomized evaluation of acellular human dermal matrix augmentation for arthroscopic rotator cuff repair. *Arthroscopy* 2012;28(1):8-15.

Barber FA, Herbert MA, Coons DA: Tendon augmentation grafts: Biomechanical failure loads and failure patterns. *Arthroscopy* 2006;22(5):534-538.

Barber FA, Hrnack SA, Snyder SJ, Hapa O: Rotator cuff repair healing influenced by platelet-rich plasma construct augmentation. *Arthroscopy* 2011;27(8):1029-1035.

Bektaşer B, Ocgüder A, Solak S, Gönen E, Yalçın N, Kılıçarslan K: Free coracoacromial ligament graft for augmentation of massive rotator cuff tears treated with mini-open repair. *Acta Orthop Traumatol Turc* 2010;44(6):426-430.

Bond JL, Dopirak RM, Higgins J, Burns J, Snyder SJ: Arthroscopic replacement of massive, irreparable rotator cuff tears using a GraftJacket allograft: Technique and preliminary results. *Arthroscopy* 2008;24(4):403.e1-409.e8.

Chaudhury S, Holland C, Porter D, Tirlapur UK, Vollrath F, Carr AJ: Torn human rotator cuff tendons have reduced collagen thermal properties on differential scanning calorimetry. *J Orthop Res* 2011;29(12):1938-1943.

Encalada-Diaz I, Cole BJ, Macgillivray JD, et al: Rotator cuff repair augmentation using a novel polycarbonate polyurethane patch: Preliminary results at 12 months' follow-up. *J Shoulder Elbow Surg* 2011;20(5):788-794.

Flurin PH, Landreau P, Gregory T, et al; Société Française d'Artroscopie: Arthroscopic repair of full-thickness cuff tears: A multicentric retrospective study of 576 cases with anatomical assessment [French]. *Rev Chir Orthop Reparatrice Appar Mot* 2005;91(S8):31-42.

Frankle M, Siegal S, Pupello D, Saleem A, Mighell M, Vasey M: The Reverse Shoulder Prosthesis for glenohumeral arthritis associated with severe rotator cuff deficiency: A minimum two-year follow-up study of sixty patients. *J Bone Joint Surg Am* 2005;87(8):1697-1705.

Goldberg SS, Bigliani LU: Hemiarthroplasty for the rotator cuff-deficient shoulder: Surgical technique. *J Bone Joint Surg Am* 2009;91(suppl 2 pt 1):22-29.

Gupta AK, Hug K, Berkoff DJ, et al: Dermal tissue allograft for the repair of massive irreparable rotator cuff tears. *Am J Sports Med* 2012;40(1):141-147.

Iannotti JP, Codsi MJ, Kwon YW, Derwin K, Ciccone J, Brems JJ: Porcine small intestine submucosa augmentation of surgical repair of chronic two-tendon rotator cuff tears: A randomized, controlled trial. *J Bone Joint Surg Am* 2006;88(6):1238-1244.

Ito J, Morioka T: Surgical treatment for large and massive tears of the rotator cuff. *Int Orthop* 2003;27(4):228-231.

Jerosch J, Sokkar SM, Neuhaeuser C, Abdelkafy A: Humeral resurfacing arthroplasty in combination with latissimus dorsi tendon transfer in patients with rotator cuff tear arthropathy and preserved subscapularis muscle function: Preliminary report and short-term results. *Eur J Orthop Surg Traumatol* 2014;24(7):1075-1083.

Kim YS, Chung SW, Kim JY, Ok JH, Park I, Oh JH: Is early passive motion exercise necessary after arthroscopic rotator cuff repair? *Am J Sports Med* 2012;40(4):815-821.

Kluczynski MA, Nayyar S, Marzo JM, Bisson LJ: Early versus delayed passive range of motion after rotator cuff repair: A systematic review and meta-analysis. *Am J Sports Med* 2015;43(8):2057-2063.

Kokkalis ZT, Mavrogenis AF, Scarlat M, et al: Human dermal allograft for massive rotator cuff tears. *Orthopedics* 2014;37(12):e1108-e1116.

McCarron JA, Milks RA, Chen X, Iannotti JP, Derwin KA: Improved time-zero biomechanical properties using poly-L-lactic acid graft augmentation in a cadaveric rotator cuff repair model. *J Shoulder Elbow Surg* 2010;19(5):688-696.

Mihata T, Lee TQ, Watanabe C, et al: Clinical results of arthroscopic superior capsule reconstruction for irreparable rotator cuff tears. *Arthroscopy* 2013;29(3):459-470.

Mihata T, McGarry MH, Kahn T, Goldberg I, Neo M, Lee TQ: Biomechanical role of capsular continuity in superior capsule reconstruction for irreparable tears of the supraspinatus tendon. *Am J Sports Med* 2016; Mar 4[Epub ahead of print]

Mihata T, McGarry MH, Pirolo JM, Kinoshita M, Lee TQ: Superior capsule reconstruction to restore superior stability in irreparable rotator cuff tears: A biomechanical cadaveric study. *Am J Sports Med* 2012;40(10):2248-2255.

Moore DR, Cain EL, Schwartz ML, Clancy WG Jr: Allograft reconstruction for massive, irreparable rotator cuff tears. *Am J Sports Med* 2006;34(3):392-396.

Mori D, Funakoshi N, Yamashita F: Arthroscopic surgery of irreparable large or massive rotator cuff tears with low-grade fatty degeneration of the infraspinatus: Patch autograft procedure versus partial repair procedure. *Arthroscopy* 2013;29(12):1911-1921.

Nada AN, Debnath UK, Robinson DA, Jordan C: Treatment of massive rotator-cuff tears with a polyester ligament (Dacron) augmentation: Clinical outcome. *J Bone Joint Surg Br* 2010;92(10):1397-1402.

Namdari S, Voleti P, Baldwin K, Glaser D, Huffman GR: Latissimus dorsi tendon transfer for irreparable rotator cuff tears: A systematic review. *J Bone Joint Surg Am* 2012;94(10):891-898.

Omae H, Steinmann SP, Zhao C, et al: Biomechanical effect of rotator cuff augmentation with an acellular dermal matrix graft: A cadaver study. *Clin Biomech (Bristol, Avon)* 2012;27(8):789-792.

Scheibel M, Brown A, Woertler K, Imhoff AB: Preliminary results after rotator cuff reconstruction augmented with an autologous periosteal flap. *Knee Surg Sports Traumatol Arthrosc* 2007;15(3):305-314.

Sclamberg SG, Tibone JE, Itamura JM, Kasraeian S: Six-month magnetic resonance imaging follow-up of large and massive rotator cuff repairs reinforced with porcine small intestinal submucosa. *J Shoulder Elbow Surg* 2004;13(5):538-541.

Tashjian RZ: Epidemiology, natural history, and indications for treatment of rotator cuff tears. *Clin Sports Med* 2012;31(4):589-604.

Thangarajah T, Pendegrass CJ, Shahbazi S, Lambert S, Alexander S, Blunn GW: Augmentation of rotator cuff repair with soft tissue scaffolds. *Orthop J Sports Med* 2015;3(6):2325967115587495.

Wong I, Burns J, Snyder S: Arthroscopic GraftJacket repair of rotator cuff tears. *J Shoulder Elbow Surg* 2010; 19(2 suppl):104-109.

Yoon JP, Chung SW, Kim JY, et al: Outcomes of combined bone marrow stimulation and patch augmentation for massive rotator cuff tears. *Am J Sports Med* 2016;44(4):963-971.

Zingg PO, Jost B, Sukthankar A, Buhler M, Pfirrmann CW, Gerber C: Clinical and structural outcomes of nonoperative management of massive rotator cuff tears. *J Bone Joint Surg Am* 2007;89(9):1928-1934.

 Video Reference

Labbé M: Video. *Arthroscopic Rotator Cuff Repair and Augmentation With Acellular Human Dermal Graft*. Houston, TX, 2015.

Chapter 25

Tears of the Subscapularis Tendon: Recognition and Treatment

Yohei Ono, MD, PhD

Ian K.Y. Lo, MD, FRCSC

Case Presentations

Case 1: Partial-Thickness Upper Subscapularis Tendon Tear With Concomitant Supraspinatus Tendon Tear

HISTORY

A 54-year-old, right-hand–dominant man who works as a concrete finisher had pain in his right shoulder after a fall with his arm in extension and external rotation. The physical examination demonstrates active forward elevation to 140°, external rotation to 40°, and internal rotation to L5. The patient has positive impingement signs, an equivocal result on liftoff testing, an intermediate result on the Napoleon test, and pain and weakness with bear-hug testing (**Figure 1**). Sclerosis of the undersurface of the acromion is noted radiographically (**Figure 2, A**). MRI demonstrates a partial-thickness tear of the upper subscapularis tendon (**Figure 2, B**) with medial subluxation

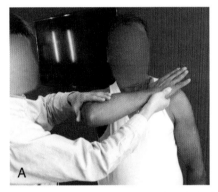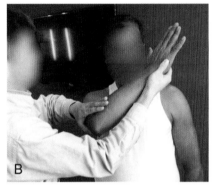

Figure 1 Clinical photographs of the bear-hug test. **A,** The patient's arm is placed in the starting position, across the body, with the hand on the opposite shoulder. The examiner then applies an external rotation force perpendicular to the forearm, pulling the hand away from the shoulder while the patient tries to hold the starting position by using an internal rotation force. **B,** This patient's inability to hold the hand against the contralateral shoulder denotes a positive bear-hug test result, which indicates a subscapularis tendon tear.

of the long head of the biceps (LHB) tendon (**Figure 2, C**) as well as a full-thickness tear of the supraspinatus tendon with retraction measuring 1.2 cm (**Figure 2, D**). After the failure of nonsurgical treatment, the patient elected to undergo surgery.

 Video 25.1 Upper Subscapularis Tear With Supraspinatus Tear. Ian K.Y. Lo, MD, FRCSC (4 min)

SURGICAL TREATMENT

Standard anterior and posterior glenohumeral portals were established, and diagnostic arthroscopy with a 30° arthroscope was performed. The LHB tendon was partially frayed and subluxated medially, secondary to an upper subscapularis tendon tear (**Figure 3, A**). A complete tear of the supraspinatus tendon was noted (**Figure 3, B**). After diagnostic arthroscopy was performed, the anterosuperolateral portal was established.

Dr. Lo or an immediate family member has received royalties from Arthrex, ArthroCare, and Smith & Nephew; is a member of a speakers' bureau or has made paid presentations on behalf of Arthrex, ArthroCare, and Smith & Nephew; serves as a paid consultant to ArthroCare and Smith & Nephew; serves as an unpaid consultant to Smith & Nephew; has stock or stock options held in Tenet Medical Engineering; has received research or institutional support from Arthrex, ArthroCare, ConMed Linvatec, and Smith & Nephew; and serves as a board member, owner, officer, or committee member of the American Shoulder and Elbow Surgeons and the Arthroscopy Association of North America. Neither Dr. Ono nor any immediate family member has received anything of value from or has stock or stock options held in a commercial company or institution related directly or indirectly to the subject of this chapter.

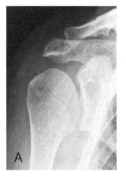
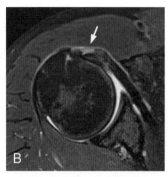
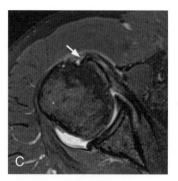
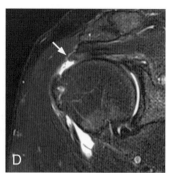

Figure 2 Preoperative imaging of a right shoulder. **A,** AP radiograph demonstrates sclerosis of the undersurface of the acromion. **B,** Axial MRI demonstrates a partial-thickness tear of the subscapularis tendon (arrow). **C,** Axial MRI demonstrates medial subluxation of the long head of the biceps tendon (arrow). **D,** Coronal oblique MRI demonstrates a retracted full-thickness tear of the supraspinatus tendon (arrow).

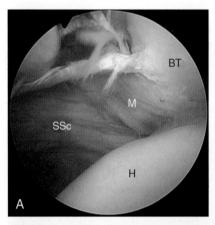
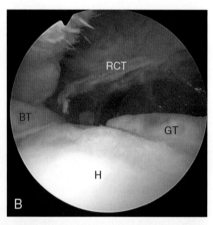

Figure 3 Arthroscopic views of the right shoulder through a posterior portal demonstrate tears of the subscapularis and supraspinatus tendons. **A,** A partial-thickness upper subscapularis tendon (SSc) tear and medially subluxated long head of the biceps tendon (BT) with some medial fraying. **B,** A full-thickness tear of the supraspinatus tendon. GT = greater tuberosity, H = humeral head, M = medial sling, RCT = posterosuperior rotator cuff tear.

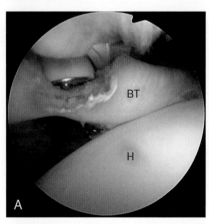
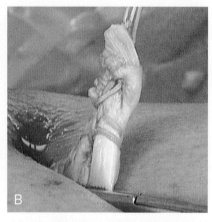

Figure 4 **A,** An arthroscopic view of the right shoulder through a posterior portal demonstrates release of the long head of the biceps tendon (BT). **B,** Intraoperative photograph demonstrates the long head of the biceps tendon with a whipstitch placed in a baseball fashion. The tendon has been brought out extracorporeally through the anterolateral portal. H = humeral head.

The LHB tendon was tagged with a racking stitch, released from its origin on the superior labrum (**Figure 4, A**), and then brought out extracorporeally through the anterolateral portal with the elbow in flexion. The tendon was markedly enlarged and flattened; therefore, approximately 2 to 3 cm of the tendon was excised to prepare for tenodesis along the bicipital groove. The tendon stump was secured with a whipstitch of No. 2 braided composite suture placed using a baseball stitch (**Figure 4, B**).

To maximize visualization of the lesser tuberosity and the subscapularis tendon, a 70° arthroscope was used from the posterior portal, and the patient's arm was positioned in forward flexion and internal rotation. This method provided a top-down view of the entire subscapularis tendon footprint and the bicipital groove. To prepare the footprint of the subscapularis tendon, the upper lesser tuberosity was débrided down to a bleeding bone surface (**Figure 5, A**). The upper portion of the transverse ligament was released to expose the bicipital groove. A 7-mm hole was drilled in the bicipital groove, and the tendon was placed in situ and fixed with a 7-mm biocomposite threaded interference screw (**Figure 5, B**).

Because this was a partial-thickness upper subscapularis tendon tear, no advanced releases were required to improve the mobility of the tendon. The comma sign, a comma-shaped arc of soft tissue located above the superolateral border of the torn subscapularis tendon, was used to identify the borders of the subscapularis tendon tear (**Figure 6, A**). A standard suture anchor was inserted on the footprint medially (**Figure 6, B**), and suture limbs were passed in a mattress fashion using a self-retrieving antegrade suture passer through the anterosuperolateral portal. The medial sutures were tied and brought out laterally in a transosseous-equivalent fashion to a lateral interference suture anchor, thus compressing the rotator cuff against the footprint (**Figure 6, C and D**).

After the subscapularis tendon was repaired, the supraspinatus tendon was similarly repaired with standard techniques in the subacromial space. In this patient, the supraspinatus tendon was repaired in a similar transosseous-equivalent fashion (**Figures 7** and **8**).

Case 2: Retracted Full-Thickness Subscapularis Tendon Tear With Concomitant Supraspinatus Tendon Tear

HISTORY

A 59-year-old, right-hand–dominant man had left shoulder pain after a fall onto his elbow. The physical examination demonstrates active forward elevation to 150°, external rotation to 80°, and internal rotation to T12. The patient has positive impingement signs and positive results on the liftoff and Napoleon tests. Biceps tension testing demonstrates a positive result on the Speed test and a negative result on the Yergason test. Ultrasonography demonstrates full-thickness tears of the subscapularis and supraspinatus tendons along with the absence of the LHB tendon in the bicipital groove. Nonsurgical treatment was unsuccessful, and the patient elected to undergo surgery.

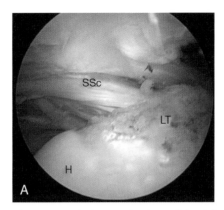
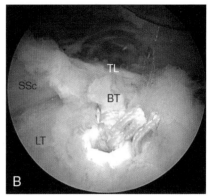

Figure 5   Arthroscopic views of the right shoulder through a posterior portal using a 70° arthroscope demonstrate bone bed preparation and biceps tenodesis. **A,** Débrided upper lesser tuberosity (LT). **B,** Tenodesis of the long head of the biceps tendon (BT). H = humeral head, SSc = subscapularis tendon, TL = transverse ligament.

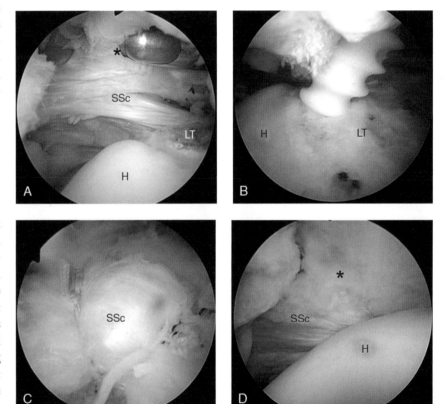

Figure 6   Arthroscopic views of the right shoulder through a posterior portal (**A**, **B**, and **D**) and a posterolateral portal (**C**) demonstrate subscapularis tendon (SSc) tear and repair. **A,** Identification of the comma sign (asterisk) helps identify the borders of the subscapularis tendon tear. **B,** An anchor is inserted medially on the débrided bone bed of the lesser tuberosity (LT). **C,** Appearance of the double-row subscapularis tendon repair from the bursal side. **D,** Appearance of the subscapularis tendon repair from the glenohumeral joint. H = humeral head.

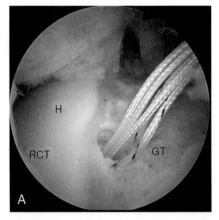
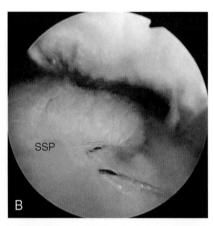

Figure 7 Arthroscopic views of the right shoulder through a posterior portal demonstrate supraspinatus tendon (SSP) repair. **A,** An anchor is inserted medially on the débrided bone bed of the greater tuberosity (GT). **B,** Appearance of the double-row supraspinatus tendon repair from the bursal space. H = humeral head, RCT = postero-superior rotator cuff tear.

Video 25.2 Complex Releases for Complete Subscapularis Tears. Ian K.Y. Lo, MD, FRCSC (3 min)

SURGICAL TREATMENT

Diagnostic arthroscopy showed the LHB tendon to be dislocated medially and posterior to the subscapularis tendon (**Figure 9, A**). The patient had a full-thickness tear of the subscapularis tendon with the tendon stump retracted and scarred to the inner deltoid fascia (**Figure 9, B**). A full-thickness tear of the supraspinatus tendon also was present (**Figure 9, C**). After diagnostic

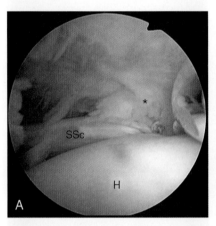
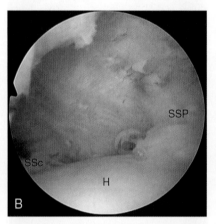
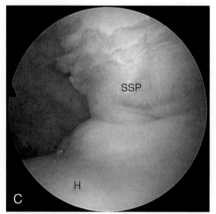

Figure 8 Sequential arthroscopic views of the right shoulder through a posterior portal demonstrate subscapularis and supraspinatus tendon repairs. **A,** Anatomically repaired subscapularis tendon (SSc) and comma sign (asterisk). **B,** Rotator interval tissue between the repaired subscapularis and supraspinatus tendons. **C,** Anatomically repaired supraspinatus tendon (SSP). H = humeral head.

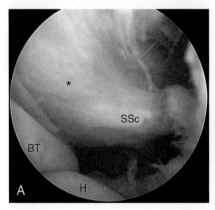
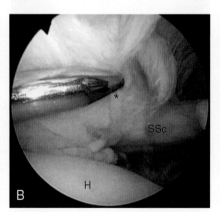
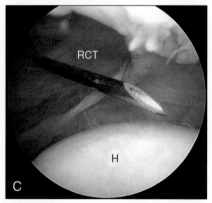

Figure 9 Arthroscopic views of the left shoulder through a posterior portal demonstrate subscapularis and supraspinatus tendon tears. The asterisk indicates the comma sign. **A,** A full-thickness subscapularis tendon (SSc) tear and a medially dislocated long head of the biceps tendon (BT). **B,** A full-thickness tear of the subscapularis tendon with the tendon stump retracted medially and scarred to the inner deltoid fascia. **C,** A full-thickness supraspinatus tendon tear. H = humeral head, RCT = posterosuperior rotator cuff tear.

arthroscopy was performed, an antero-superolateral portal was created through the supraspinatus tendon tear.

The LHB tendon was tagged and released from its origin to maximize visualization. In patients with a full-thickness tear of the subscapularis tendon, the borders of the subscapularis tendon can be difficult to identify because of scarring and adhesions to the inner deltoid fascia. To assist in identifying the subscapularis tendon, the comma sign was located. With the use of a self-retrieving antegrade suture passer introduced through the anterosuperolateral portal, a traction stitch was passed through the so-called crook of the comma (that is, the superolateral corner of the subscapularis tendon) to aid in tendon releases and reduction.

Because this patient had a complete full-thickness subscapularis tendon tear, tendon releases were required to improve mobility. A three-sided release consisting of the superior, anterior, and posterior surfaces of the subscapularis tendon was performed. The superior release was performed first by creating a window through the rotator interval. Tension was applied to the traction stitch to draw the subscapularis tendon laterally, thereby exposing the rotator interval and the superior border of the subscapularis tendon from behind the glenoid. A combination of an electrocautery device and a shaver inserted through the anterosuperolateral portal was used to perform soft-tissue resection superior to the subscapularis tendon, keeping the lateral rotator interval tissue (the comma sign) intact. As the resection progressed, the underlying coracoid was felt as a bony prominence behind the rotator interval, and the coracoid was subsequently exposed. Care was taken to stay on the posterolateral aspect of the coracoid to avoid catastrophic neurovascular injury.

After a wide rotator interval window was created, a 70° arthroscope was

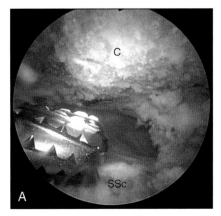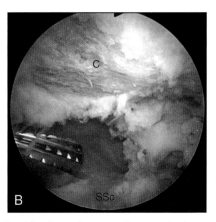

Figure 10 Arthroscopic views of the left shoulder through a posterior portal using a 70° arthroscope demonstrate coracoplasty. **A,** A burr is introduced through the antero-superolateral portal anterior to the subscapularis tendon (SSc). The subcoracoid space appears slightly narrowed. **B,** Coracoplasty is performed in line with the subscapularis tendon, creating a space of approximately 7 to 10 mm. C = coracoid.

advanced through the window, which provided a top-down view of the structures anterior to the subscapularis tendon. The coracoid was identified, and the anterior release was performed. The shaver and electrocautery instruments were introduced through the anterosuperolateral portal now directed anterior to the subscapularis tendon. Fibroadipose tissue was removed from the subcoracoid space, and the posterolateral aspect of the coracoid was skeletonized, essentially releasing the coracohumeral ligament.

The subcoracoid space was assessed by comparing the space available with a 6.0-mm oval burr (**Figure 10, A**). In this patient, a narrowed (less than 6 mm) subcoracoid space was present; therefore, coracoplasty was performed with a burr inserted through the anterosuperolateral portal. The goal of the coracoplasty was to create a 7- to 10-mm space between the posterolateral tip of the coracoid and the anterior plane of the subscapularis tendon (**Figure 10, B**). Care was taken to protect the inferior conjoint tendon and the superolateral coracoacromial ligament. Subcoracoid decompression can help increase the anterior working space, thereby improving visualization and facilitating repair.

The posterior release was performed next, and the arthroscope was withdrawn through the rotator interval window to view the posterior aspect of the subscapularis tendon. The electrocautery device and an elevator were used to release the subscapularis tendon from the middle glenohumeral ligament and the anterior capsule. After completing the three-sided release, sufficient mobility was available to repair the tendon to the bone.

After the subscapularis tendon was released, the tendon was repaired to the bone using standard rotator cuff repair techniques. For many patients, retraction of the subscapularis tendon and the use of complex releases make it impossible to perform a double-row repair because of limited tendon excursion. In this patient, a single-row repair was done, using multiple triple-loaded anchors to maximize tendon-to-bone fixation (**Figure 11**). The full-thickness tear of the supraspinatus tendon was similarly repaired, incorporating the residual comma sign.

■ Indications

The indications for arthroscopic subscapularis tendon repair are essentially

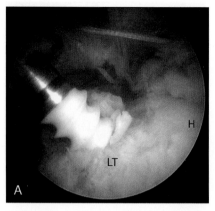
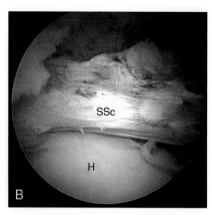

Figure 11 Arthroscopic views of the left shoulder through a posterior portal demonstrate subscapularis tendon (SSc) repair. **A,** An anchor is inserted on the center of the débrided bone bed of the lesser tuberosity (LT). **B,** A view of the subscapularis tendon repair performed using a single-row technique. C = coracoid, H = humeral head.

the same as the indications for arthroscopic rotator cuff repair. Patients experiencing substantial pain and disability despite 3 to 6 months of nonsurgical treatment are candidates for arthroscopic repair. The senior author of this chapter (I.K.Y.L.) is of the opinion that, similar to acute tears of the posterosuperior rotator cuff, acute tears of the subscapularis tendon should be treated urgently to prevent further retraction and atrophy.

Although an open technique can be used, arthroscopic subscapularis tendon repair provides improved visualization of the anterior and posterior aspects of the subscapularis tendon, thus facilitating tendon identification, releases, and repair. Furthermore, arthroscopic management allows multiple portals of entry and angles of approach when repairing massive rotator cuff tears involving the subscapularis tendon combined with posterior extension. However, because of its relative complexity, arthroscopic subscapularis tendon repair should be attempted only after the surgeon is comfortable with standard arthroscopic rotator cuff repair techniques.

The two approaches used for arthroscopic subscapularis tendon repair are the bursal approach and the articular

approach. In the bursal approach, a lateral subacromial portal is used for viewing, and the subscapularis tendon is repaired with instruments introduced through a separate anterolateral portal. This method provides improved visualization of the bursal surface of the subscapularis tendon and may be performed by using a standard 30° arthroscope. However, in the experience of the authors of this chapter, visualization and instrument spacing can be problematic.

The authors of this chapter prefer the articular approach, which maximizes instrument spacing by allowing visualization of the anterior structures from the posterior glenohumeral portal with a 30° or 70° arthroscope. The articular approach allows easy visualization, identification, and release of the subscapularis tendon and can simplify arthroscopic coracoplasty and subscapularis tendon repair. Occasionally, more complex cases (such as a lesser tuberosity avulsion) require a combined approach. In these patients, a 70° arthroscope can be used through a posterior glenohumeral portal, and a 30° arthroscope can be used through a lateral or anterolateral subacromial portal.

Controversies and Alternative Approaches

Nonsurgical management of subscapularis tendon tears is similar to that for standard posterosuperior rotator cuff tears. However, few protocols have been specifically designed to address the subscapularis tendon. In general, nonsurgical treatment may include cold and/or heat therapy, pain medications, NSAIDs, injections (for example, subacromial or glenohumeral), and/or physical therapy.

For patients with chronic tears, particularly those with substantial tendon retraction and fatty infiltration of the subscapularis tendon, arthroscopic repair may be unsuccessful. Alternative treatments, including allograft or tendon transfer (such as split pectoralis major transfer), are generally performed through an open approach.

Although arthroscopic repair of full-thickness tears of the subscapularis tendon is commonly done after nonsurgical treatment has failed, débridement with or without a biceps tenotomy or a tenodesis may be considered in carefully selected patients. In contrast to younger patients, older patients may have issues that complicate tendon repair, including larger tear sizes, concomitant disease, and delayed presentation that can lead to tendon retraction, muscle atrophy, and fatty infiltration. In addition, some older patients may be unwilling or unable to participate in the postoperative rehabilitation program. In one study, 9 of 11 such patients had good or excellent results after arthroscopic débridement of the subscapularis tendon tear and release of the LHB tendon.

Results

The results of subscapularis tendon repair are summarized in **Table 1**. These results demonstrate improvement in

Table 1 Results of Arthroscopic Subscapularis Tendon Repair

Authors	Journal (Year)	Technique	Outcomes	Failure Rate (%)	Comments
Denard et al	*Arthroscopy* (2012)	Single-row repair	Mean UCLA score improved from 16.5 to 30.1 Mean ASES score improved from 40.8 to 88.5	7.6 (poor result)	79 shoulders Mean follow-up: 104.8 mo Level IV therapeutic case series
Toussaint et al	*Orthop Traumatol Surg Res* (2012)	Single- or double-row repair	Mean Constant score improved from 48.3 to 74.1, and mean UCLA score improved from 14.6 to 30.2 in patients with a subscapularis tear Mean Constant score improved from 50.7 to 77.9, and mean UCLA score improved from 14.3 to 32.6 in patients with both subscapularis and supraspinatus tears	8 (recurrent tear) and 18.6 (muscle wasting of the upper subscapularis) at radiologic follow-up of ≥6 mo	103 patients Clinical follow-up: ≥12 mo Level III study
Lanz et al	*Arthroscopy* (2013)	Single- or double-row repair	Mean Constant score improved from 46.4 to 79.9 Mean modified UCLA score improved from 15.1 to 31.5 Mean coracohumeral distance increased from 9.7 to 10.1 mm	11 (re-rupture)	46 patients Final follow-up: 24-48 mo Level IV therapeutic case series

ASES = American Shoulder and Elbow Surgeons shoulder outcome, UCLA = University of California–Los Angeles Shoulder Rating Scale.

clinical outcome and function at short- and midterm follow-up. The reported re-rupture rate was 8% to 11%.

 Technical Keys to Success

Patient Positioning
- Although the beach-chair position can be used, the lateral decubitus position is preferred because it maximizes surgical access circumferentially around the shoulder and facilitates visualization in abduction, forward flexion, internal rotation, and posterior translation.
- The arm is placed in a limb positioner with a lateral arm attachment under longitudinal traction.

Procedure
- A posterior glenohumeral portal is established.

- Diagnostic arthroscopy is performed through the posterior portal, and the subscapularis tendon tear is identified.
- The anterosuperolateral portal is created approximately 2 cm off the anterolateral corner of the acromion, anterior to the supraspinatus tendon but posterior to the LHB tendon, and parallel to the lesser tuberosity. This is the critical working portal. It is used for releases, bone bed débridement, suture passage, and knot tying (**Figure 3**).
- A whipstitch is placed in the biceps, and a biceps tenotomy is performed in preparation for later tenodesis.
- The subscapularis tendon is identified, and releases are performed as required.
- Subcoracoid decompression and coracoplasty may be warranted, such as in a patient with a

coracohumeral distance of less than 6 mm.
- The bone bed on the lesser tuberosity is prepared.
- Biceps tenodesis is performed, if necessary.
- The subscapularis tendon is repaired to bone using standard suture anchor fixation techniques.
- Any required repairs in the subacromial area are performed, including repair of the posterosuperior rotator cuff after repair of the subscapularis tendon.
- During the procedure, the arm is manipulated into abduction, internal rotation, forward flexion, and posterior translation to draw the fibers of the subscapularis tendon away from the humeral head, thereby increasing the anterior working space and revealing the tendon insertion (**Figure 12, A**). A 70° arthroscope is used routinely

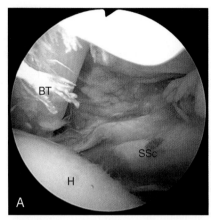
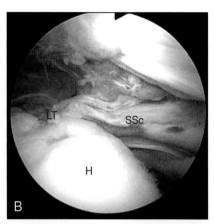

Figure 12 **A,** Arthroscopic view of a right shoulder through a posterior portal using a 30° arthroscope, with the patient's arm held in abduction, internal rotation, and posterior translation. **B,** Arthroscopic view of the same shoulder through a posterior portal using a 70° arthroscope, with the arm in the same position but after biceps tenotomy to maximize visualization. BT = biceps tendon, H = humeral head, LT = lesser tuberosity, SSc = subscapularis tendon.

in combination with arm positioning to maximize visualization (**Figure 12, B**).

- The 70° arthroscope provides a top-down view of the subscapularis tendon to improve visualization of the bone bed, the tendon insertion, and the subcoracoid space.
- The increased angle of the 70° arthroscope improves visualization of the complex releases required when the tendon is retracted medial to the glenoid.

THE COMMA SIGN

- It may be necessary to locate the comma sign to assist in identifying the margins of the subscapularis tendon. In patients with complete full-thickness tears of the subscapularis tendon or tears associated with adhesive capsulitis, the margins of the subscapularis tendon are commonly scarred to the inner deltoid fascia and the coracoid. In some patients, the margins are obliterated, and the subscapularis tendon may be assumed to be absent.
- The comma sign is a comma-shaped arc of soft tissue located above the superolateral border of the torn

subscapularis tendon (**Figure 9, A**). This tissue is composed of the medial biceps sling (that is, the medial coracohumeral ligament and the superior glenohumeral ligament) and interdigitates with the superior fibers of the subscapularis tendon at its humeral insertion. When the subscapularis tendon tears, the medial biceps sling tears along with it and remains attached to the superolateral corner of the subscapularis tendon, forming this comma-shaped soft tissue.

- Pulling on the so-called crook of the comma laterally (**Figure 9, B**) draws the subscapularis tendon laterally, thereby exposing and delineating the superior and lateral borders of the subscapularis tendon.
- Identifying the comma sign facilitates subsequent releases to expose the borders of the subscapularis tendon.

LHB TENDON

- Most patients with substantial tears of the subscapularis tendon have instability of the biceps tendon. The authors of this chapter perform

biceps tenodesis in most patients, with the exception of patients older than 70 years and patients who have lower demands, in whom a simple biceps tenotomy may suffice. Stabilization of the biceps tendon with reconstruction of the medial sling is rarely performed because of the risk of ongoing biceps instability, which may lead to failure of the subscapularis tendon repair.

- In many patients, particularly those with partial or complete full-thickness tears of the subscapularis tendon, the biceps tendon is subluxated medially, obscuring visualization of the lesser tuberosity and the residual subscapularis tendon and also lying in the way of the subsequent repair. Tagging and releasing the biceps tendon early in the procedure and retrieving the suture through the anterosuperolateral portal lateralizes the LHB tendon away from the lesser tuberosity, maximizing visualization for subsequent anterior shoulder work (releases and bone bed preparation).
- Tenodesis is performed low in the bicipital groove (suprapectoral biceps tenodesis). Tenodesis is done after subscapularis releases but before definitive tendon-to-bone fixation. Performing biceps tenodesis after tendon-to-bone fixation would be more difficult because subscapularis tendon reduction can limit visualization of the lower bicipital groove.

RELEASES AND CORACOPLASTY

- In most patients with complete subscapularis tendon tears, releases are critical for improving mobility of the retracted subscapularis tendon to allow tension-free repair to bone.
- A three-sided release, beginning superior and proceeding to anterior and posterior, provides sufficient mobility of the subscapularis

tendon, allowing tendon repair to bone (Video 25.2).

- In addition, a lateral release may be required in patients with chronic adhesive capsulitis, in whom the lateral border of the subscapularis tendon is obliterated.
- An inferior release, which can compromise the axillary nerve, is rarely required.
- To begin the releases, a traction stitch is placed through the superolateral corner of the subscapularis tendon.

Superior Release
- The superior release is performed first to create a window through the rotator interval.
- Tension on the traction stitch draws the tendon laterally and exposes the subscapularis tendon and the rotator interval to improve visualization and safety.
- The rotator interval is carefully resected superior to the subscapularis tendon, maintaining the lateral border (the comma sign).
- As resection continues, the bony prominence of the coracoid may be palpated through the rotator interval.
- The rotator interval is resected, exposing the coracoid tip.
- A 70° arthroscope can aid in visualizing the medial aspect of the superior border of the subscapularis tendon behind the glenoid, and superior adhesions are released.

Anterior Release
- After the rotator interval is resected (that is, the superior release is complete), the anterior aspect of the subscapularis tendon is visualized by advancing a 70° arthroscope through the rotator interval window.
- Instruments (such as a shaver and an electrocautery device) are introduced through the anterosuperolateral portal both posterior

and anterior to the subscapularis tendon to aid in débridement and release.

- Fibroadipose tissue is removed from the subcoracoid space, and the posterolateral aspect of the coracoid is skeletonized, essentially releasing the coracohumeral ligament. Release of the scar tissue and adhesions between the coracoid and subscapularis tendon is critical in performing a complete anterior release. It is important to stay on the posterolateral aspect of the coracoid to prevent catastrophic neurovascular injury.

Coracoplasty
- A top-down view of the subcoracoid space is obtained using a 70° arthroscope through the posterior glenohumeral portal.
- The subcoracoid space (coracohumeral interval) may be measured using an instrument of known size, such as a 6.0-mm oval burr. If the space is less than 6 mm, a coracoplasty is performed with a burr inserted through the anterosuperolateral portal to create a 7- to 10-mm space.
- The resection is performed parallel to the anterior surface of the subscapularis tendon, after which the arm is moved through a range of motion to ensure that adequate resection has been performed.
- Care is taken to protect the inferior conjoint tendon and the superolateral coracoacromial ligament during coracoplasty.

Posterior Release
- For the posterior release, the subscapularis tendon is released from the middle glenohumeral ligament and the anterior capsule.
- The arthroscope is retracted into the glenohumeral joint so that the posterior aspect of the subscapularis tendon can be viewed.

- An arthroscopic elevator and an electrocautery are used to release the posterior border of the subscapularis tendon; this technique is similar to capsular release for adhesive capsulitis.

Lateral Release
- In some patients with chronic adhesion, lateral release may be necessary when the lateral margin of the subscapularis tendon is scarred to the inner deltoid fascia, coracoid, and conjoint tendon.
- The lateral margin is defined and delineated, using the comma sign as a guide, and the soft-tissue bursal leader lateral to the tendon is débrided.
- The dissection continues inferiorly until the subscapularis tendon is released from the anterior structures and the subcoracoid space is reconstituted.

Video 25.3 The Lateral Subscapularis Release. Ian K.Y. Lo, MD, FRCSC (1 min)

REPAIR
- A burr is inserted through the anterosuperolateral portal, and the bone bed is prepared to receive the subscapularis tendon. The amount of bone bed exposed may be compared with cadaver data to estimate the percentage of tendon torn. Data from cadaver studies indicate that the average height of the bone bed is 25.8 ± 3.2 mm, and the average width is 18.1 ± 1.6 mm. Knowledge of these dimensions helps determine the amount of bone bed that must be exposed.
- Standard suture anchor techniques are used for definitive fixation of tendon to bone.
- Starting inferiorly, suture anchors are percutaneously inserted in the lesser tuberosity at the

Table 2 Rehabilitation Protocol After Arthroscopic Subscapularis Tendon Repair

Postoperative Week	Range of Motion	Strengthening	Return to Play	Comments/Emphasis
0-2	Passive external rotation to 0° Hand, wrist, and elbow motions are performed	None	None	Sling immobilization during ambulation and sleep Active motion of the elbow is restricted if biceps tenodesis was performed
2-6	Passive external rotation to 0° Hand, wrist, and elbow motions are performed	Parascapular muscle strengthening	None	Sling immobilization during ambulation and sleep Active motion of the elbow is restricted if biceps tenodesis was performed
6-12	Forward elevation progresses from active-assisted to active	Biceps, triceps, and isometric rotator cuff strengthening	None	Active elbow motion allowed in patients treated with biceps tenodesis
12-24	Terminal end range-of-motion stretching; all planes, no restrictions	Rotator cuff and deltoid strengthening	Integrate into sport- and work-specific activities	—

deadman angle with the use of needle localization.

- Sutures are passed antegrade through the anterosuperolateral portal. The use of a self-retrieving antegrade suture-passing device is critical.
- In addition, the percutaneous anchor portal may be used for suture management.
- The repair proceeds superiorly with subsequent anchor insertion, suture passage, and knot tying.
- Usually, two or three double-loaded anchors are required for a complete subscapularis tendon tear. Sufficient tendon excursion is required to achieve double-row repair. However, single-row repair may be the only option, particularly in patients with full-thickness complete tears. The use of single-row repair has generally had good clinical results.

Rehabilitation

A general rehabilitation protocol after arthroscopic subscapularis tendon repair is noted in **Table 2**. Sling immobilization during ambulation and sleep is recommended for 6 weeks postoperatively. Hand, wrist, and elbow motions are performed immediately postoperatively; however, active motion of the elbow is restricted for 6 weeks in patients who underwent biceps tenodesis. Passive external rotation also is performed immediately postoperatively, but it is limited to 0° or as assessed intraoperatively. Forward elevation is started 6 weeks postoperatively and progresses from active-assisted to active range of motion. Rotator cuff and deltoid strengthening may begin 12 weeks postoperatively.

Avoiding Pitfalls

Although arthroscopic subscapularis tendon repair can be difficult, it can be done effectively and efficiently by knowing and applying several key principles. Subscapularis tendon repair should be performed before any other procedures. Visualization is best prior to substantial swelling of the shoulder, which can obscure visualization and the working space available for subscapularis tendon repair.

Visualization of the subscapularis tendon is maximized by placing the patient's arm in abduction, forward flexion, internal rotation, and posterior translation and using a 70° arthroscope. To maximize visualization and facilitate repair, biceps pathology should be addressed by tagging and releasing the tendon early in the procedure. The comma sign can be used to identify the superior and lateral borders of the subscapularis tendon. It is important to avoid resecting the comma sign, which facilitates reduction of the subscapularis and supraspinatus tendons and can be incorporated into the repair of the supraspinatus tendon. A traction stitch can be placed in the superolateral corner of the subscapularis tendon to draw the retracted subscapularis tendon from behind the glenoid neck and into view.

It is important to perform adequate releases. Inadequate releases can lead to high tissue tension and failure of the repair. Releases of the subscapularis tendon should be started superiorly and progress anteriorly and posteriorly. A lateral release also may be necessary in patients with adhesion. If tension remains after the releases, the bone bed should be medialized. Inferior dissection should be avoided to protect the axillary nerve. Standard suture anchor repair techniques using antegrade suture passage are easiest for tendon-to-bone fixation.

Bibliography

Burkhart SS, Brady PC: Arthroscopic subscapularis repair: Surgical tips and pearls A to Z. *Arthroscopy* 2006;22(9):1014-1027.

Burkhart SS, Lo IK: Arthroscopic rotator cuff repair. *J Am Acad Orthop Surg* 2006;14(6):333-346.

Burkhart SS, Tehrany AM: Arthroscopic subscapularis tendon repair: Technique and preliminary results. *Arthroscopy* 2002;18(5):454-463.

Curtis AS, Burbank KM, Tierney JJ, Scheller AD, Curran AR: The insertional footprint of the rotator cuff: An anatomic study. *Arthroscopy* 2006;22(6):609.e1.

D'Addesi LL, Anbari A, Reish MW, Brahmabhatt S, Kelly JD: The subscapularis footprint: An anatomic study of the subscapularis tendon insertion. *Arthroscopy* 2006;22(9):937-940.

Denard PJ, Burkhart SS: Medialization of the subscapularis footprint does not affect functional outcome of arthroscopic repair. *Arthroscopy* 2012;28(11):1608-1614.

Denard PJ, Jiwani AZ, Lädermann A, Burkhart SS: Long-term outcome of a consecutive series of subscapularis tendon tears repaired arthroscopically. *Arthroscopy* 2012;28(11):1587-1591.

Edwards TB, Walch G, Nové-Josserand L, et al: Arthroscopic debridement in the treatment of patients with isolated tears of the subscapularis. *Arthroscopy* 2006;22(9):941-946.

Lanz U, Fullick R, Bongiorno V, Saintmard B, Campens C, Lafosse L: Arthroscopic repair of large subscapularis tendon tears: 2- to 4-year clinical and radiographic outcomes. *Arthroscopy* 2013;29(9):1471-1478.

Lo IK, Burkhart SS: Arthroscopic coracoplasty through the rotator interval. *Arthroscopy* 2003;19(6):667-671.

Lo IK, Burkhart SS: The comma sign: An arthroscopic guide to the torn subscapularis tendon. *Arthroscopy* 2003;19(3):334-337.

Lo IK, Burkhart SS: The interval slide in continuity: A method of mobilizing the anterosuperior rotator cuff without disrupting the tear margins. *Arthroscopy* 2004;20(4):435-441.

Lo IK, Nelson AA, Burkhart SS: Lateral releases of the subscapularis tendon. *Int J Shoulder Surg* 2013;7(4):139-142.

Lo IK, Parten PM, Burkhart SS: Combined subcoracoid and subacromial impingement in association with anterosuperior rotator cuff tears: An arthroscopic approach. *Arthroscopy* 2003;19(10):1068-1078.

Ticker JB, Burkhart SS: Why repair the subscapularis? A logical rationale. *Arthroscopy* 2011;27(8):1123-1128.

Toussaint B, Audebert S, Barth J, et al: Arthroscopic repair of subscapularis tears: Preliminary data from a prospective multicentre study. *Orthop Traumatol Surg Res* 2012;98(8 suppl):S193-S200.

Video References

25.1. Lo IK: Video. *Upper Subscapularis Tear with Supraspinatus Tear.* Calgary, Alberta, Canada, 2015.

25.2. Lo IK: Video. *Complex Release for Complete Subscapularis Tears.* Calgary, Alberta, Canada, 2015.

25.3. Lo IK: Video. *Lateral Subscapularis Release.* Calgary, Alberta, Canada, 2015.

Chapter 26

Tears of the Pectoralis Major: Repair and Augmentation

Mandeep S. Virk, MD

Akshay Jain, MD

Nikhil N. Verma, MD

 Introduction

Pectoralis major tear is an uncommon injury that has been increasingly recognized and indicated for surgical repair in the past 20 years. Pectoralis major tear most often occurs in men aged 20 to 40 years. The most common mechanism of injury is indirect trauma during a sports activity (often bench-press weight training) in which the musculotendinous unit of the pectoralis major fails under heavy load during the eccentric contraction phase of the muscle. Most pectoralis major tears are complete tears involving the sternal head and commonly occur near the tendon insertion on the humerus and at the musculotendinous junction. Partial tears are less common than complete tears. Assessment of partial tears includes determining the tear location, percentage of tendon and/or muscle involved, and patient age and activity level. Typically, examination and decision-making must be individualized to each patient. Bone avulsion and intramuscular tears are less common.

No consensus exists on the time frame for pectoralis major tears to be labeled as acute or chronic, and clinical studies have used the term acute repair for surgical procedures performed up to 4 to 6 weeks after injury. Chronic tears are characterized by substantial adhesions of the pectoralis major to the surrounding structures and retraction of the tendon into the substance of the muscle. Acute injuries are characterized by pain, swelling, and substantial ecchymosis in the arm and chest region. The classic deformity resulting from pectoralis major tear is easily missed in the acute phase because of swelling. Subacute and chronic complete tears of the pectoralis major result in loss of symmetry of the chest contour and weakness in adduction. The asymmetry of the chest can be accentuated with resisted adduction of the arm and can result in webbing or a prominent skin fold in the anterior axilla, loss of thickness of the anterior axillary fold, and medialization of the muscle belly of the pectoralis major. Occasionally, palpation reveals a tender lump in the chest, which represents the rolled-up tendon in the substance of the muscle. Associated neurovascular injuries are rare.

Understanding the relevant anatomy of the pectoralis major musculotendinous unit and the pathoanatomy of pectoralis major tears is critical for reconstruction and repair. The pectoralis major has two origins: the clavicular head and the sternocostal head. The clavicular head is a single, anatomically distinct unit, whereas the sternocostal head can be divided along fascial planes into multiple muscle segments. The two heads of the pectoralis major unite to form a common tendon that inserts on the lateral lip of the bicipital groove. Anatomic cadaver studies have demonstrated that the width of the common tendon at the level of the footprint is typically 4 to 6 cm. The clavicular head has minimal tendon tissue before its insertion into the common tendon. The sternocostal head is posterior to the clavicular head near its common insertion. The two bellies can be separated superiorly by a fat plane but are usually continuous at the inferior border.

The neurovascular supply of the pectoralis major muscle is segmented. The motor nerve supply comes from the lateral and medial pectoral nerves, which are branches of the lateral and medial cord of the brachial plexus, respectively. The lateral pectoral nerve supplies the clavicular head and upper portion of

Dr. Verma or an immediate family member has received royalties from Smith & Nephew; serves as a paid consultant to MinInvasive and Smith & Nephew; has stock or stock options held in Cy-Medica, MinInvasive, and Omeros; has received research or institutional support from Athletico, Arthrex, Arthrosurface, ConMed Linvatec, Mitek Sports Medicine, DJO, MioMed, and Smith & Nephew; and serves as a board member, owner, officer, or committee member of the Arthroscopy Association of North America. Neither of the following authors nor any immediate family member has received anything of value from or has stock or stock options held in a commercial company or institution related directly or indirectly to the subject of this chapter: Dr. Virk and Dr. Jain.

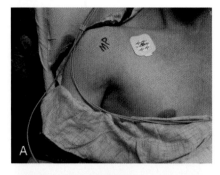

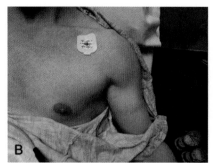

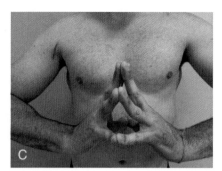

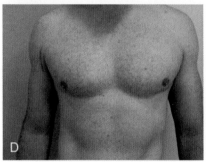

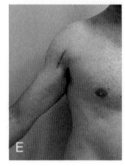

Figure 1 Preoperative photographs of the affected arm (**A**) and uninjured arm (**B**) of a patient with a complete tear of the sternocostal head of the pectoralis major. **C,** through **E,** Postoperative clinical photographs of the upper extremity of the same patient shown in panels A and B show restoration of the contour of the pectoralis major (inferior border) on the injured side.

the sternocostal head (manubrial part), and the medial pectoral nerve supplies the remainder of the sternocostal head. A cadaver model study demonstrated that the lateral pectoral nerve enters the pectoralis major muscle at a mean distance of 12.5 cm from its humeral insertion. This location is consistently medial to the pectoralis minor tendon. In contrast, the medial pectoral nerve commonly travels through the pectoralis minor tendon before entering the pectoralis major muscle at a mean distance of 11.9 cm from its lateral humeral insertion and 2 cm proximal to the inferior border of the pectoralis major. The vascular supply to the pectoralis major predominantly derives from the thoracoacromial artery (superior vascular branch and pectoral branch), with contributions from the lateral thoracic artery (inferior branch). The neurovascular pedicles enter the undersurface of the pectoralis major muscle in the middle third region. Thus, it is critical to avoid performing blind, deep medial dissection on the undersurface of the pectoralis major muscle medial to the medial margin of the coracoid because

doing so can result in inadvertent damage to the neurovascular pedicles.

Case Presentation

While bench-pressing with heavy weights, a 48-year-old, right-hand–dominant man heard a pop in his left arm, followed by severe, sharp pain. He noticed substantial ecchymosis developing over his left axilla and spreading into the region of his upper arm and biceps within 24 hours after the injury. The swelling and ecchymosis gradually resolved over 2 to 3 weeks, but the patient continued to have pain in his arm and had a noticeable cosmetic deformity. His primary care physician ordered an MRI of the left shoulder and chest, which demonstrated a left pectoralis major tear. The patient's pain had decreased by the time he presented to the institution of the authors of this chapter 4 weeks after his injury, but he expressed concern about weakness in his arm and was dissatisfied with the asymmetry in his chest.

A physical examination performed 4 weeks after injury demonstrated

minimal ecchymosis and swelling. A visible difference was observed in the contour of the left pectoralis major muscle compared with the right, and this difference was further accentuated if the patient isometrically contracted the muscle. A small, round, firm mass was felt in the retracted muscle belly, which was tender on palpation (**Figure 1**). The anterior axillary fold was thin and less robust compared with the contralateral side. The patient had pain on resisted adduction with the arm at his side and in forward flexion. He displayed full active range of motion (ROM) of his shoulder, and his rotator cuff strength was comparable with the contralateral side. No Popeye deformity was observed. Plain radiographs of the left humerus and shoulder were normal. An MRI of the shoulder and chest demonstrated avulsion of the footprint of the pectoralis major with retraction of torn tendon into the muscle (**Figure 2**). The long head of the biceps (LHB) and rotator cuff musculotendinous units were normal. Because of the patient's young age and active lifestyle and the presence of a complete tear on clinical examination and imaging, he was offered surgical repair of the torn pectoralis major. The risks, benefits, and alternatives to the surgical treatment were explained to him. The patient underwent open surgical repair of his left pectoralis major with three suture anchors. At his latest follow-up, the patient reported restoration of chest symmetry, the ability to return to weight training, and no pain.

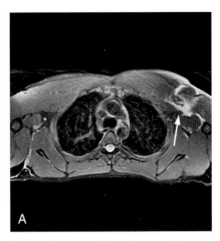
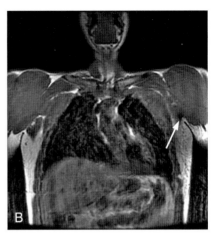

Figure 2 Axial (**A**) and coronal (**B**) proton density MRIs of an upper extremity demonstrate a retracted pectoralis major tear (arrow).

Indications

Open surgical repair of a pectoralis major tear is indicated in active individuals with complete tears (acute and chronic) and in patients in whom nonsurgical management of partial or complete tears has failed.

Controversies and Results

Nonsurgical treatment is indicated in older or sedentary individuals; patients who have partial tears or intramuscular tears; and patients who wish to avoid surgical treatment. Nonsurgical treatment is associated with deficits in peak torque and adduction strength in the affected arm and persistent cosmetic deformity. The general consensus in the orthopaedic literature is that complete pectoralis major tears should be surgically repaired in young, active individuals. Better clinical and cosmetic outcomes have been achieved after surgical repair compared with nonsurgical management (**Table 1**).

Several small case series with long-term results (greater than 5 years) have demonstrated reproducible good-to-excellent outcomes in most patients treated with surgical repair of the torn pectoralis major (**Table 2**). In most patients, results of postoperative isometric and isokinetic testing of pectoralis major repairs are comparable with those of the uninjured arm in terms of peak torque and work performed. The optimal timing of surgical management and ideal method of reattachment of the tendon are not known. Pectoralis major tear is not a common injury; therefore, high-quality studies with large patient numbers are not available. The available scientific literature, which predominantly includes small level III and IV studies, suggests that pectoralis major tears are easy to repair within 4 to 6 weeks after injury. Repair of chronic, retracted tears commonly requires the use of autograft or allograft augmentation. Pectoralis major tears occurring through the midsubstance of the tendon can be repaired primarily via a tendon-to-tendon repair with or without graft augmentation. If the quality of tendon tissue in the stump is suboptimal, then allograft or autograft tendon is required to perform a tendon-to-bone repair.

No consensus exists regarding the optimum method of fixation of the pectoralis major tendon to its footprint. Historically, the tendon was reattached to its footprint with the use of a transosseous trough and sutures tied over the bone bridge. In this technique, a cortical trough is created at the pectoralis major footprint, and two or three bicortical drill holes are made adjacent to the trough with an intervening bone bridge of sufficient size. The torn tendon is secured with heavy nonabsorbable sutures, and these sutures are shuttled through the drill holes and tied to each other over a bony bridge. Newer fixation techniques include the use of suture anchors and endosteal or cortical buttons. In a study of experimentally created complete tears of the pectoralis major in fresh-frozen cadaver specimens, the biomechanical characteristics of three methods of fixation (transosseous repair, suture anchor, and endosteal button) were compared. The biomechanical strength of three fixation techniques was inferior to the pullout strength of the native pectoralis major tendon. No significant differences were found in any of the biomechanical outcomes among the three types of fixation. There are no clinical studies that compare different fixation techniques for pectoralis major repair.

Graft augmentation is required in patients who have chronic pectoralis major tears if sufficient tendon length or tissue is not available to achieve primary repair. However, some studies suggest that the pectoralis major can be lengthened sufficiently through extensive adhesion release and mobilization of the musculotendinous unit even if the pectoralis major tear is repaired a few years after injury. In a series of 16 patients with pectoralis major tears, researchers

Table 1 Results of Surgical and Nonsurgical Management of Pectoralis Major Tears

Authors	Journal (Year)	Treatment (No. of Patients)	Outcomes	Comments
Wolfe et al	*Am J Sports Med* (1992)	Surgical (7), nonsurgical (7)	Isokinetic testing Higher deficit in the peak torque and work/repetition in the nonsurgical group Higher satisfaction rate in the surgical group	Mean follow-up, 21.5 mo (surgical group)
Schepsis et al	*Am J Sports Med* (2000)	Surgical (13), nonsurgical (4)	Subjective questionnaire and objective evaluation Lower satisfaction rate ($P = 0.004$), poor pain relief ($P = 0.013$), and dissatisfaction with cosmesis ($P = 0.013$) in the nonsurgical group Isokinetic testing performed in 8 patients (3 acute, 3 chronic, and 2 in nonsurgical group) Significant improvements in recovery of peak torque ($P = 0.0001$) and work performed (acute, $P = 0.0003$; chronic, $P = 0.0015$) in surgical group compared with the nonsurgical group	Mean follow-up, 28 mo
Hanna et al	*Br J Sports Med* (2001)	Surgical (10), nonsurgical (12)	Functional evaluation and isokinetic testing Significant recovery of peak torque ($P = 0.007$) and work performed ($P = 0.02$) in surgical group compared with nonsurgical group	Mean follow-up, 15 mo
de Castro Pochini et al	*Am J Sports Med* (2014)	Surgical (31), nonsurgical (29)	Functional evaluation and isokinetic testing Superior outcomes in the surgical group ($P = 0.05$) Mean peak torque deficit was significantly higher in the nonsurgical group ($P < 0.05$)	Mean follow-up, 48.3 mo

performed primary repairs in 7 patients at least 4 months after injury (2 of these tears were repaired more than 12 months after injury). No graft augmentation was required, and the authors of the study did not find any substantial difference in outcomes (isokinetic strength testing and failure rate between the chronic tears [>3 months] and the acute tears [<3 months]). However, in patients who underwent tear repair more than 1 year after injury, full restoration of chest symmetry was not achieved.

No clinical studies have compared the surgical repair of chronic tears with graft augmentation versus primary repair. Multiple studies report favorable outcomes with use of allograft (Achilles tendon, fascia lata) and autograft (hamstring tendon) tissues for reconstruction in chronic tears. However, these clinical studies have small patient numbers, and there are no comparative control groups.

The largest study to date on graft augmentation was published in 2014. Of 60 patients with pectoralis major tears, 19 patients underwent surgical repair using hamstring graft at least 3 months after their initial injury. At a mean follow-up of 48.2 months, 12 excellent and 5 good results were achieved. The authors of that study recommend using graft augmentation between 3 weeks and 3 months after injury in patients who have tendinopathy of the torn tendon. In a study published in 2015, four patients with pectoralis major tears underwent delayed repair (mean, 131 days after injury) consisting of fascia lata allograft reconstruction and suture anchor fixation of the graft. At a mean follow-up of 62.5 months, there were two excellent and two good results, and all repairs were intact on ultrasound imaging.

As with most tendon tears, acute repair should be performed if possible. When treating patients whose injury occurred at least 3 months prior to surgical repair, the authors of this chapter always make sure to have a graft available in case it should be needed. The decision regarding mobilization and tendon quality is made intraoperatively. Typically, an Achilles allograft is used.

Technical Keys to Success

Setup/Exposure

- General or regional anesthesia is administered.
- A preoperative intravenous antibiotic such as cefazolin, clindamycin (if the patient has penicillin allergy), or vancomycin (if the patient is allergic to both clindamycin and cefazolin) is administered.
- To prevent intraoperative deep vein thrombosis, pneumatic compression boots are used on both lower extremities during the procedure.
- The patient is placed in a modified beach-chair or supine position, and the patient's head and body

Table 2 Long-Term Outcomes of Pectoralis Major Repair

Authors	Journal (Year)	Technique (No. of Patients)	Outcomes	Comments
Pavlik et al	*Knee Surg Sports Traumatol Arthrosc* (1998)	Tendon-tendon repair (5), transosseous repair (2)	Clinical evaluation and strength testing Results were excellent in 5 patients and good in 2 6 patients returned to sports participation at their preinjury level	Mean follow-up, 6.5 yr
Aärimaa et al	*Am J Sports Med* (2004)	Transosseous repair (10), suture anchor (12), tendon-tendon repair (11)	Functional evaluation (subjective and objective) Results were excellent in 8 patients, good in 12, fair in 10, and poor in 3	Mean follow-up, 4.4 yr
He et al	*Chin Med J (Engl)* (2010)	Transosseous repair (4), tendon-muscle repair (8)	Clinical evaluation, outcome scores, and strength testing Results were excellent in 3 patients, good in 5, and fair in 1 11 patients returned to their preinjury activities	Mean follow-up, 6.7 yr
Merolla et al	*Eur J Orthop Surg Traumatol* (2015)	Primary repair (8), allograft (4)	Ultrasonography and isometric strength testing Results were excellent in 9 patients and good in 3 High satisfaction rate, acceptable cosmesis, and maintenance of strength compared with the uninjured arm All repairs were intact on ultrasonography	Mean follow-up, 5 yr

are safely secured to the surgical table.

- The arm is draped free, and a padded Mayo stand is used to support the arm during the procedure. Alternatively, an articulated arm holder may be used.

Procedure

SKIN INCISION AND SUPERFICIAL DISSECTION

- The skin incision (measuring approximately 6 to 8 cm) is made on the anterior aspect of the shoulder, medial to the most distal aspect of the standard deltopectoral approach (**Figure 3, A**). This approach allows access to the medially retracted pectoralis major muscle belly and tendon as well as to the footprint laterally. Alternatively, an anterior axillary approach may be used.
- Full-thickness flaps are elevated above the deltopectoral fascia

(medial more than lateral) using a needle-tipped Bovie.

DEEP DISSECTION

- The deltopectoral interval is identified, and the cephalic vein is retracted laterally (**Figure 3, B**). Typically, the tendon is approached inferiorly in the plane between the remaining pectoralis major and short head of the biceps.
- Inferiorly, the short head of biceps is identified, and the torn tendon is approached from below (**Figure 3, C**). The torn pectoralis major musculotendinous unit is identified and freed of adhesions to surrounding tissue.
- The use of traction sutures through the pectoralis major muscle or an atraumatic soft-tissue clamp helps hold the tendon under tension during dissection and mobilization. Care is taken to preserve the

fascia overlying the pectoralis major during dissection. Adhesions to the underlying chest wall and overlying subcutaneous tissue are released meticulously, especially in patients with chronic tears, to adequately mobilize the pectoralis major musculotendinous unit and bring it to the lateral footprint. The pectoralis major tendon is often retracted in the depth of the muscle and must be retrieved during dissection.

FOOTPRINT PREPARATION AND PECTORALIS MAJOR REPAIR

- After the pectoralis major has been adequately mobilized, the insertional footprint is prepared. The bicipital groove is exposed, and the LHB and any remaining tendon stump of the pectoralis major are identified.
- A Hohmann retractor can be used to retract the LHB in a medial

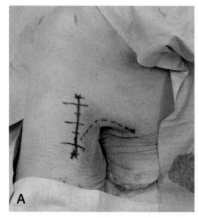
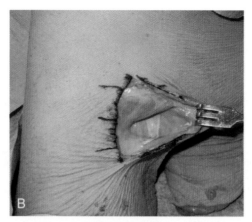
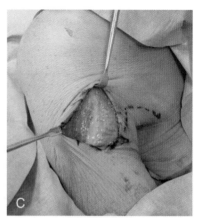

Figure 3 Photographs of the shoulder of a cadaver specimen show the skin incision used for pectoralis major repair (**A,** solid line; dotted line indicates the inferior border of the pectoralis major), the deltopectoral interval (**B**), and the inferior border of the pectoralis major (**C**).

direction so that it is not trapped in the repair.

- The lateral lip of the bicipital groove is decorticated to produce a bleeding bed.
- Depending on the extent of the tear, two to four suture anchors are used. These anchors are loaded with one or two No. 2 ultra–high-strength nonabsorbable sutures. One suture limb is passed in a running, nonlocking Krackow fashion starting from the torn end of the tendon and advanced toward the musculotendinous junction and then brought back in a nonlocking fashion through the tendon. The other suture limb is then used as a post limb to pull and reduce the tendon to the bone. After all the sutures have been passed in this fashion and with the patient's arm in neutral and mild internal rotation, the two suture limbs from each anchor are tied to each other. Alternatively, drill holes or cortical buttons can be used for fixation. Care is taken not to incarcerate the LHB in the pectoralis major repair because doing so will lead to postoperative anterior arm pain. After the repair is completed, the LHB tendon is inspected for impingement. It can be palpated inferiorly

to confirm adequate restoration of tension and normalization of the inferior axillary fold.

- According to the senior authors of this chapter (N.N.V. and M.S.V.), in most patients with chronic tears, adequate mobilization of the pectoralis major and primary repair to the footprint can be achieved. However, if the tendon cannot be brought to the native footprint despite extensive mobilization or if an extensive tear is present at the musculotendinous junction, augmentation with allograft, autograft, or synthetic graft is necessary (**Figure 4**). Use of Achilles allograft is preferred by the senior authors of this chapter. However, fascia lata, autograft (hamstring), or synthetic grafts have been used with equally good results.
- A sufficient length (5 cm) of the broad proximal part of the Achilles allograft is secured to the pectoralis major using high-tensile–strength sutures. Various configurations of sutures have been described. The authors of this chapter prefer to secure the allograft at the superior border, inferior border, and midsubstance of the pectoralis major using interrupted or short running locking sutures. In addition, the

donor tendon is weaved through the muscle.

- The narrow end of the allograft is tubularized over the native tendon for a more secure interface between the allograft and native tendon tissue. The allograft is then repaired to the pectoralis major footprint. The authors of this chapter prefer to use suture anchors, but bone tunnels or other fixation devices such as cortical button can be used.

Wound Closure

- The deep fascia is closed with interrupted absorbable braided suture.
- Absorbable monofilament suture is used for subcutaneous and subcuticular closure.

Rehabilitation

Postoperative rehabilitation is critical to the surgical management of pectoralis major tears. The timing and general guidelines for rehabilitation are outlined in **Table 3**. The shoulder is immobilized for approximately 6 weeks postoperatively. Active-assisted forward flexion of the shoulder is initiated at 4 weeks postoperatively, but no passive ROM is allowed until 6 weeks postoperatively. Shoulder external rotation, abduction,

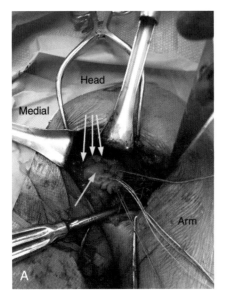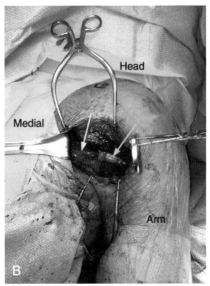

Figure 4 Intraoperative photographs of the shoulder of a patient with a chronic, retracted pectoralis major tear show the use of allograft. **A,** The allograft is draped over the native muscle and tendon remnant (blue arrow) and secured to the pectoralis major with multiple sutures (yellow arrows). **B,** The allograft (blue arrow) is fixed to the footprint with suture anchors. The yellow arrow in panel B points to the native pectoralis major.

and extension should be restricted to protect the repair. Because the repair is an extra-articular procedure, the risk of postoperative stiffness is low. Active ROM of the shoulder is introduced at 6 weeks postoperatively, with the goal of achieving near full ROM by 3 months postoperatively. Strengthening, which includes progression through submaximal isometrics, pulleys, isotonic and eccentric strengthening, is begun at 12 weeks postoperatively and continues through the remainder of the rehabilitation period. Weight lifting and bench-press activity are introduced at submaximal (light) weights between 4 and 6 months postoperatively and gradually worked up to 50% of the patient's previous single-repetition maximum. During the early strengthening phase, it is important to avoid using heavy weights with extended elbows on

Table 3 Rehabilitation Protocol After Pectoralis Major Repair

Postoperative Week	ROM	Strengthening	Return to Play	Comments/ Emphasis
0-6	At 4 wk, active-assisted ROM is begun (supine shoulder flexion with wand; start with 45° and gradually advance to 120° over the next 4 wk)	At 4 wk, start shoulder shrugs and scapular retraction (without resistance)	Active use of hand, wrist, and elbow	The shoulder is immobilized
6-12	At 6 wk, active-assisted ROM is begun (external rotation and abduction of shoulder with wand) At 6 wk, active ROM of the shoulder is begun in the pain-free range, with a goal of full active ROM at 12 wk	Submaximal isometrics	Active use of hand, wrist, and elbow	—
12-24	Passive ROM and mobilization at terminal shoulder ROM	Strengthening of shoulder (light strengthening with elastic resistance bands with gradually increasing resistance, push-up progression [wall, table, chair, and regular], and light weight training) Gradual return to full, unrestricted weight lifting or bench-press activity at 6 mo	Return to play or contact sports at 6 mo	—

ROM = range of motion.

chest-fly machines or during dumbbell-fly exercises because these activities place excessive stress on the repair. After 6 months postoperatively, gradual progression to full, unrestricted weight lifting or bench-press activity is allowed.

 ## Avoiding Pitfalls

A thorough understanding of the surgical anatomy and pathoanatomy of pectoralis major tears is critical for performing surgical repair of a torn pectoralis major tendon. In patients with chronic pectoralis major tears, it is important to release adhesions of the pectoralis major to the overlying subcutaneous tissue and underlying chest wall and thoroughly mobilize the pectoralis major musculotendinous unit. The surgeon should be mindful of the neurovascular pedicles during deep dissection and mobilization of the pectoralis major.

If a transosseous technique is used to fix a torn tendon, the surgeon should avoid making deep troughs or large drill holes because doing so increases the risk of fracture. After the pectoralis major repair, the surgeon should check for incarceration of the LHB tendon in the repair to avoid a tenodesis effect and postoperative anterior arm pain.

 ## Bibliography

Aärimaa V, Rantanen J, Heikkilä J, Helttula I, Orava S: Rupture of the pectoralis major muscle. *Am J Sports Med* 2004;32(5):1256-1262.

Bak K, Cameron EA, Henderson IJ: Rupture of the pectoralis major: A meta-analysis of 112 cases. *Knee Surg Sports Traumatol Arthrosc* 2000;8(2):113-119.

Carey P, Owens BD: Insertional footprint anatomy of the pectoralis major tendon. *Orthopedics* 2010;33(1):23.

Chomiak J, Dungl P: Reconstruction of elbow flexion in arthrogryposis multiplex congenita type I: Part I. Surgical anatomy and vascular and nerve supply of the pectoralis major muscle as a basis for muscle transfer. *J Child Orthop* 2008;2(5):357-364.

de Castro Pochini A, Andreoli CV, Belangero PS, et al: Clinical considerations for the surgical treatment of pectoralis major muscle ruptures based on 60 cases: A prospective study and literature review. *Am J Sports Med* 2014;42(1):95-102.

de Castro Pochini A, Ejnisman B, Andreoli CV, et al: Pectoralis major muscle rupture in athletes: A prospective study. *Am J Sports Med* 2010;38(1):92-98.

Dehler T, Pennings AL, ElMaraghy AW: Dermal allograft reconstruction of a chronic pectoralis major tear. *J Shoulder Elbow Surg* 2013;22(10):e18-e22.

Dodds SD, Wolfe SW: Injuries to the pectoralis major. *Sports Med* 2002;32(14):945-952.

ElMaraghy AW, Devereaux MW: A systematic review and comprehensive classification of pectoralis major tears. *J Shoulder Elbow Surg* 2012;21(3):412-422.

Fung L, Wong B, Ravichandiran K, Agur A, Rindlisbacher T, Elmaraghy A: Three-dimensional study of pectoralis major muscle and tendon architecture. *Clin Anat* 2009;22(4):500-508.

Haley CA, Zacchilli MA: Pectoralis major injuries: Evaluation and treatment. *Clin Sports Med* 2014;33(4):739-756.

Hallock GG: The total pectoralis major muscle myocutaneous free flap. *J Reconstr Microsurg* 2013;29(7):461-464.

Hanna CM, Glenny AB, Stanley SN, Caughey MA: Pectoralis major tears: Comparison of surgical and conservative treatment. *Br J Sports Med* 2001;35(3):202-206.

He ZM, Ao YF, Wang JQ, Hu YL, Yin Y: Twelve cases of the pectoralis major muscle tendon rupture with surgical treatment: An average of 6.7-year follow-up. *Chin Med J (Engl)* 2010;123(1):57-60.

Joseph TA, Defranco MJ, Weiker GG: Delayed repair of a pectoralis major tendon rupture with allograft: A case report. *J Shoulder Elbow Surg* 2003;12(1):101-104.

Kang RW, Mahony GT, Cordasco FA: Pectoralis major repair with cortical button technique. *Arthrosc Tech* 2014;3(1):e73-e77.

Klepps SJ, Goldfarb C, Flatow E, Galatz LM, Yamaguchi K: Anatomic evaluation of the subcoracoid pectoralis major transfer in human cadavers. *J Shoulder Elbow Surg* 2001;10(5):453-459.

Kretzler HH Jr, Richardson AB: Rupture of the pectoralis major muscle. *Am J Sports Med* 1989;17(4):453-458.

Lee J, Brookenthal KR, Ramsey ML, Kneeland JB, Herzog R: MR imaging assessment of the pectoralis major myotendinous unit: An MR imaging-anatomic correlative study with surgical correlation. *AJR Am J Roentgenol* 2000;174(5):1371-1375.

Manske RC, Prohaska D: Pectoralis major tendon repair post surgical rehabilitation. *N Am J Sports Phys Ther* 2007;2(1):22-33.

Merolla G, Campi F, Paladini P, Porcellini G: Surgical approach to acute pectoralis major tendon rupture. *G Chir* 2009;30(1-2):53-57.

Merolla G, Paladini P, Artiaco S, Tos P, Lollino N, Porcellini G: Surgical repair of acute and chronic pectoralis major tendon rupture: Clinical and ultrasound outcomes at a mean follow-up of 5 years. *Eur J Orthop Surg Traumatol* 2015;25(1):91-98.

Metzger PD, Bailey JR, Filler RD, Waltz RA, Provencher MT, Dewing CB: Pectoralis major muscle rupture repair: Technique using unicortical buttons. *Arthrosc Tech* 2012;1(1):e119-e125.

Naderi NM, Funk L: Chronic bilateral pectoralis major ruptures and reconstruction with allograft. *Injury Extra* 2009;40:267-269.

Pavlik A, Csépai D, Berkes I: Surgical treatment of pectoralis major rupture in athletes. *Knee Surg Sports Traumatol Arthrosc* 1998;6(2):129-133.

Petilon J, Carr DR, Sekiya JK, Unger DV: Pectoralis major muscle injuries: Evaluation and management. *J Am Acad Orthop Surg* 2005;13(1):59-68.

Porzionato A, Macchi V, Stecco C, Loukas M, Tubbs RS, De Caro R: Surgical anatomy of the pectoral nerves and the pectoral musculature. *Clin Anat* 2012;25(5):559-575.

Provencher MT, Handfield K, Boniquit NT, Reiff SN, Sekiya JK, Romeo AA: Injuries to the pectoralis major muscle: Diagnosis and management. *Am J Sports Med* 2010;38(8):1693-1705.

Schachter AK, White BJ, Namkoong S, Sherman O: Revision reconstruction of a pectoralis major tendon rupture using hamstring autograft: A case report. *Am J Sports Med* 2006;34(2):295-298.

Schepsis AA, Grafe MW, Jones HP, Lemos MJ: Rupture of the pectoralis major muscle: Outcome after repair of acute and chronic injuries. *Am J Sports Med* 2000;28(1):9-15.

Sherman SL, Lin EC, Verma NN, et al: Biomechanical analysis of the pectoralis major tendon and comparison of techniques for tendo-osseous repair. *Am J Sports Med* 2012;40(8):1887-1894.

Wolfe SW, Wickiewicz TL, Cavanaugh JT: Ruptures of the pectoralis major muscle: An anatomic and clinical analysis. *Am J Sports Med* 1992;20(5):587-593.

Zacchilli MA, Fowler JT, Owens BD: Allograft reconstruction of chronic pectoralis major tendon ruptures. *J Surg Orthop Adv* 2013;22(1):95-102.

Zafra M, Muñoz F, Carpintero P: Chronic rupture of the pectoralis major muscle: Report of two cases. *Acta Orthop Belg* 2005;71(1):107-110.

Arthroscopic Distal Clavicle Resection: Optimizing Technique

Benjamin S. Shaffer, MD

Introduction

Since it was first described in 1941, excision of the distal clavicle has been a recognized and largely effective technique in managing chronic painful conditions of the acromioclavicular (AC) joint, most commonly osteoarthritis (OA) and distal clavicle osteolysis. With the advent of arthroscopy, surgical excision via less invasive arthroscopic techniques has led to decreased postoperative morbidity and soft-tissue injury to the deltoid, capsule, and ligaments; less pain; and quicker recovery. Attention to outcomes has helped refine the ideal indications, technique, and amount of distal clavicle excision necessary.

Recent data suggest that the historic standard of resecting 1 to 2 cm of the distal clavicle may be excessive, and indicate that AC joint decompression may be achieved with removal of as little as 2.5 mm of the distal clavicle and with resection of the acromial facet without compromising capsular or soft-tissue ligamentous integrity. Consensus seems to be emerging with regard to ideal indications and contraindications, the optimal methods to achieve resection without iatrogenic soft-tissue injury, and the appropriate amount and location of bone resection to achieve predictable, excellent results.

Case Presentation

A 43-year-old left-hand–dominant man presents with a 6-month history of intermittent activity-related pain of his left shoulder. Pain in the region of the AC joint is one of the most common findings in patients with AC joint pathology. The pain is predominantly localized to the area of the AC joint (**Figure 1**), but occasionally refers to his left trapezius and neck. He has no history of prior injuries, no problems with most activities of daily living, and does not experience nocturnal awakening. He experiences pain when weight lifting, especially when performing bench presses, dips, and shoulder flies. Treatment has included avoiding the most provocative exercises, using acetaminophen and various NSAIDs, and attending a brief course of physical therapy (stretching, strengthening, and modalities), all of which proved ineffective. He has received two corticosteroid injections, each in the subacromial space, which provided partial and temporary improvement. He is frustrated with his ongoing symptoms and physical limitations, and wants to return to his previous level of activity.

Physical examination demonstrates subtle asymmetric prominence of the left AC joint compared with the opposite shoulder. The patient has no scapular

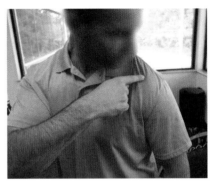

Figure 1 Clinical photograph shows a left-hand–dominant man pointing to the location at which he feels pain over the acromioclavicular joint of his left shoulder.

dysrhythmia or motion restriction in any plane. He has mildly positive results for the Neer and Hawkins impingement tests, in which pain is referred to the deltoid and posterior cuff. He has negligible pain and normal strength on testing his supraspinatus (empty can test on the plane of the scapula), infraspinatus (maintaining external rotation against resistance with the elbow at the side) and subscapularis (belly-press test). He has no tenderness along the course of the long head of the biceps tendon. Speed and O'Brien (active compression) tests results are negative. He has moderate AC joint tenderness on palpation, with discomfort reproducing his symptoms on both passive and active cross-body adduction (**Figure 2, A**). He also has pain in the AC joint if he actively internally rotates his arm behind his back (**Figure 2, B**). He has only mild discomfort on the resisted shoulder

Dr. Shaffer is deceased. At the time this chapter was written, Dr. Shaffer or an immediate family member served as a board member, owner, officer, or committee member of the American Orthopaedic Society for Sports Medicine and the Arthroscopy Association of North America.

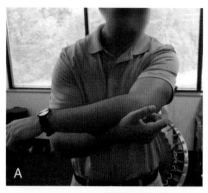 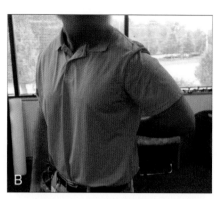

Figure 2 Clinical photographs show a cross-body adduction test (**A**) and active internal rotation (**B**) to evaluate for pain in the area of the acromioclavicular (AC) joint. Pain on either test is indicative of AC joint pathology.

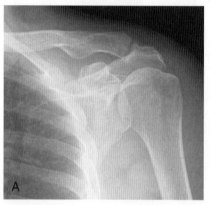 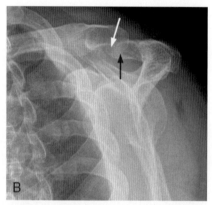

Figure 3 **A,** Zanca view radiograph of a shoulder obtained with the x-ray beam angled approximately 10° caudally and with approximately one-half the radiation required to obtain an AP view demonstrates a clear appreciation of an osteoarthritic acromioclavicular joint. **B,** Outlet view radiograph demonstrates a Bigliani type II acromion. The white arrow points to the flattened acromial profile, and the black arrow points to the AC joint.

extension test (if he tries to extend his 90° forward-flexed arm against resistance). He has no findings of instability (that is, he displays no apprehension, mechanical click or clunk, or asymmetric laxity with load-and-shift or drawer tests). He has no generalized laxity. His cervical spine examination is normal without any restriction or Spurling sign.

Radiographic evaluation, including AP, Zanca, outlet, and axillary views, demonstrates OA of the AC joint, including joint space narrowing, subchondral sclerosis, and osteophyte formation (**Figure 3, A**). A Bigliani type II/III acromion is demonstrated on the outlet view. This finding is indicative of possible subacromial impingement

(**Figure 3, B**). There is no discernable glenohumeral arthritis. After discussing the treatment alternatives for OA of the AC joint, the patient elected to undergo an additional corticosteroid injection but this time directed into the AC joint.

To facilitate targeting, the obliquity of the AC joint was discerned on a Zanca view radiograph and the joint was palpated and outlined with a marking pen. The needle entry point was determined by palpating the sulcus, which is often palpable over the anterior and superior aspect of the joint and sometimes is enhanced by translating the distal clavicle anteriorly and posteriorly. Ethylene chloride spray was used to anesthetize the skin. Using an anterior-superior

approach, a 23-gauge 1-inch needle on a 1-mL syringe was directed into the joint. A pop was felt as the needle penetrated the capsule. A combination of 5 mL of betamethasone and 0.5 mL of 1% plain lidocaine was injected; resistance increased after injection of approximately 0.5 mL of fluid, as the limit of the capacity of the joint was approached.

The patient had near-immediate appreciable pain relief after the injection, had no perceptible tenderness over the AC joint, and could perform push-ups without pain. This improvement in symptoms lasted approximately 2 weeks, after which his symptoms gradually recurred on resumption of his previous activities, including weight lifting. Arthroscopic excision of the distal clavicle is the ideal approach to manage this patient's problem. He hopes to return to his previous level of activity of recreational athletics and weight lifting. He understands and accepts the surgical risks and benefits of as well as the postoperative convalescence required after AC joint resection.

Indications

The clinical presentation, physical examination findings, radiographic findings, and injection response of the patient presented in the case study are consistent with isolated AC joint pathology. These include failure of nonsurgical management over a 6-month period, including activity modification; use of analgesics; a trial of physical therapy; and two cortisone injections that provided substantial but only temporary relief.

Surgical excision of the distal clavicle also may be beneficial for the small number of patients who may have a history of trauma and who develop posttraumatic arthritis in the AC joint. Care must be taken to identify patients with a history of trauma and those with an occult AC joint capsule injury that may be inadvertently exacerbated by distal clavicle resection.

Another common indication for distal clavicle resection is a younger patient with distal clavicle osteolysis in whom repetitive stresses lead to breakdown of cartilage tissue of the AC joint. Typically, these patients are weight-lifting athletes who present with activity-related pain over the AC joint, which is often prominent and tender. Radiographs demonstrate enlargement of the often osteopenic distal clavicle, accompanied by resorptive subchondral cysts and joint space widening.

 Contraindications

Contraindications to distal clavicle resection include posttraumatic AC joint pathology (following a type II or greater AC separation); in these patients, resection can lead to exacerbation of underlying instability and worsening of symptoms. Patients with concomitant subacromial pathology or rotator cuff tears may benefit from concomitant distal clavicle excision if the AC joint is contributing to the symptoms. The prevalence of age-related radiographic changes in the AC joint by age 50 years mandates careful clinical correlation to determine whether these changes are the cause of a patient's pain. In many patients, arthritis of the AC joint that is detected radiographically or on MRI is incidental and does not require resection.

 Controversies and Alternative Approaches

The amount of distal clavicle to excise is controversial. Historically, resection of 1 to 2 cm of bone was advocated, but outcome and biomechanical studies suggest that this standard may be excessive, violates important proximate soft-tissue structures, and risks unmasking or iatrogenically precipitating AC joint instability. Recent data suggest that although a minimum of 5 mm of distal clavicle resection is likely necessary to eliminate joint contact in most patients, even this nominal amount begins to encroach on the distal insertion of the trapezoid on the underside of the clavicle. The width of the AC joint space must be taken into consideration when determining the amount of bone to resect. This width varies from bone-on-bone in a typical osteoarthritic joint to a space as large as 5 to 6 mm in a patient who has distal clavicle osteolysis.

Removal of a portion of the acromial facet during AC joint decompression recently was proposed as a strategy to limit the amount of distal clavicle excision required. Reduced excision of the distal clavicle would minimize the risk of destabilizing the joint that would be caused by releasing or resecting important proximate soft-tissue ligament attachments. Performing a symmetric resection, in which the medial acromial facet and distal clavicle are removed, is an appealing option in patients who are undergoing concomitant subacromial decompression and in whom the acromial facet is already exposed.

An alternative to the indirect or bursal-sided technique is the direct approach, in which only the AC joint is instrumented. The direct approach offers the advantages of limiting unnecessary injury to the potentially normal subacromial space, possibly preserving some of the important surrounding capsule and ligamentous tissue, and minimizing the risk of scar tissue and stiffness. In addition, some data show that use of the direct approach results in faster recovery and return to activities compared with the indirect approach. This difference may be particularly relevant for select athletes who are eager to minimize their recovery timetable. There are disadvantages to the direct technique, however. It is more technically demanding in terms of instrumentation and technique. Because the AC joint space is often only 2 to 3 mm wide, smaller instruments are necessary to access the joint. Typically, a 2.7-mm camera (with 30° and 70° lenses) and a smaller shaver and blades (2.9 and 3.5 mm, respectively) are required.

 Results

A high percentage of good and excellent results have been achieved after arthroscopic resection of the distal clavicle (**Table 1**). Complications are infrequent, with the most commonly cited reasons for clinical failure being residual pain consequent to inadequate resection and exacerbation of underlying occult or unrecognized posttraumatic instability. Results must be carefully interpreted, however, because the literature is replete with level IV data reporting heterogeneous cohorts mixing atraumatic OA, posttraumatic AC joint pain, and distal clavicle osteolysis; variable concomitant surgical procedures (most commonly subacromial decompression); varied surgical technique with direct and indirect approaches and with varying amounts of distal clavicle and/or acromion resected; and variable and often not validated outcome measurement tools.

 Technical Keys to Success

Indirect Approach

- In most patients with AC joint pathology, surgery is performed via an indirect or bursal-sided approach to the distal clavicle. The indirect approach affords access to the less biomechanically vulnerable inferior and anterior joint capsule, preserving the more important posterior and superior soft-tissue ligaments. This access to the AC joint also facilitates treatment of concomitant

Table 1 Results of Isolated Arthroscopic Distal Clavicle Excision

Author(s)	Journal (Year)	Technique (No. of Shoulders)	Outcomes	Failure Rate (%)	Comments
Bigliani et al[a]	*Orthop Clin North Am* (1993)	Direct or indirect (42 total)	Results were compromised with retained posterior cortical ridge or posttraumatic AC instability	9	Diagnosis was mixed Avg amount resected, 5 mm
Gartsman[a]	*Am J Sports Med* (1993)	Indirect (20)	Ratings for pain, ADLs, work, and sports improved in 17 patients	15	Diagnosis: OA of the AC joint Amount resected: 10-15 mm from distal clavicle; 5 mm from medial acromion 3 patients underwent open surgery for inadequate distal clavicle bone resection Mean patient age, 51.3 yr Follow-up, ≥24 mo
Tolin and Snyder[a]	*Orthop Clin North Am* (1993)	Indirect (23)	3 poor results	13	Diagnosis: Painful AC joint Avg amount resected, 14 mm Mean patient age, 39 yr Follow-up, 25 mo
Kay et al[a]	*Clin Orthop Relat Res* (1994)	Indirect (10)	All patients had a satisfactory outcome, and all returned to their preinjury occupation	0	Diagnosis: Arthritis Amount resected: 10-15 mm 4 patients underwent concomitant arthroscopic subacromial decompression Mean patient age, 44 yr Avg follow-up, 14 mo
Auge II and Fischer[a]	*Am J Sports Med* (1998)	Direct (10)	Returned to previous training level at avg of 9.1 d	0	Diagnosis: DCO Avg amount resected: 4.5 mm Mean patient age, 30.4 yr Follow-up, 18.7 mo
Zawadsky et al[a]	*Arthroscopy* (2000)	Direct (41)	Good or excellent result in 38 shoulders (pain decreased considerably; no significant compromise in function)	7	Diagnosis: DCO Amount resected: 4-7 mm All 3 failures were posttraumatic and were subsequently managed with AC joint stabilization procedures Mean patient age, 39 yr Avg follow-up, 74.4 mo
Charron et al[b]	*Am J Sports Med* (2007)	Direct (18) or indirect (16)	Faster return to sports with direct approach compared with indirect approach (mean, 21 and 42 d, respectively)	3	Diagnosis: Osteolysis or arthrosis Amount resected: 8-10 mm Mean patient age, 28 yr 1 patient developed heterotopic ossification Follow-up, 27 mo
Freedman et al[b]	*J Shoulder Elbow Surg* (2007)	Indirect (7) or open (10)	Both procedures provided significant pain relief and return to function	0	Diagnosis: Mixed pathology (OA, PTA, DCO) Avg amount resected, 10 mm Mean patient age, 40 yr Follow-up, 6 mo and 12 mo

AC = acromioclavicular, ADLs = activities of daily living, DCO = distal clavicle osteolysis, OA = osteoarthritis, PTA = posttraumatic arthritis.

[a] Level IV study.

[b] Level II study.

[c] Level III study.

Table 1 Results of Isolated Arthroscopic Distal Clavicle Excision (*continued*)

Author(s)	Journal (Year)	Technique (No. of Shoulders)	Outcomes	Failure Rate (%)	Comments
Robertson et al[c]	*Am J Sports Med* (2011)	Indirect (32)	Less residual pain was noted after arthroscopic treatment compared with open treatment	3	Diagnosis: OA (27 patients), DCO (5 patients) Amount resected: 10 mm Mean patient age, 47 yr Follow-up, avg 50.4 mo

AC = acromioclavicular, ADLs = activities of daily living, DCO = distal clavicle osteolysis, OA = osteoarthritis, PTA = posttraumatic arthritis.

[a] Level IV study.

[b] Level II study.

[c] Level III study.

subacromial pathology, including impingement with a prominent anteroinferior acromion (Bigliani type II or III morphology), and/or rotator cuff pathology.

- The patient is brought to the operating room and undergoes induction with general anesthesia after an interscalene block has been placed under ultrasound guidance for postoperative pain control.

- The patient is placed in the beach-chair position, and the head, neck, and torso are carefully secured in neutral alignment. This position permits free access to the entire shoulder girdle. Although the author of this chapter preferred the beach-chair position because it affords an easy anatomic orientation, lateral decubitus positioning may be used.

- Examination under anesthesia is performed to exclude the unlikely possibility that the AC joint demonstrates unexpected asymmetric translation compared with the opposite shoulder (particularly in patients with a history of trauma) and to assess glenohumeral range of motion for the finding of adhesive capsulitis.

- Preoperative antibiotics are administered, and the shoulder is prepped and draped in a sterile manner.

- Three standard arthroscopic portals

are used in the indirect approach: the standard posterior scope portal, a lateral para-acromial portal (3 cm directly lateral to the anterolateral acromion), and an anterior AC joint portal (1 to 2 cm anterior to the AC joint; **Figure 4**).

- An anterior rotator interval portal, established approximately 1.5 cm inferior to and in line with the AC joint, helps in glenohumeral assessment and treatment. It also serves to provide subsequent access directly to the distal clavicle and the AC joint.

- A 4-mm 30° arthroscope is introduced into the glenohumeral joint via the posterior portal.

- A comprehensive diagnostic evaluation is performed and any glenohumeral pathology addressed.

- The arthroscope is positioned within the subacromial space and directed toward the coracoid. A pop is felt as the scope sleeve and obturator penetrate the posterior subacromial veil.

- While still viewing from the posterior portal, a 4.5-mm shaver blade and/or a bipolar device from the lateral para-acromial portal are used to débride and/or ablate just enough obscuring soft tissues to permit visualization and assessment of the undersurface of the coracoacromial ligament and the rotator cuff.

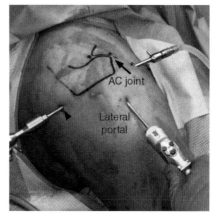

Figure 4 Photograph of a shoulder shows arthroscopic portals used in the indirect (subacromial or bursal-sided) approach to distal clavicle resection. The posterior portal (arrowhead) is used for glenohumeral arthroscopy, the lateral para-acromial portal is used to access the subacromial space, and the anterior acromioclavicular (AC) joint portal (asterisk), which initially serves as the anterior glenohumeral joint portal through the rotator interval, later allows direct access to the distal clavicle and AC joint.

- The bipolar probe is used to identify and mobilize the soft tissues inferior to and including the AC joint capsule. Pushing down on the distal clavicle helps identify the location of the joint.

- A percutaneous spinal needle introduced at the anteroposterior extent of the AC joint can facilitate orientation if necessary.

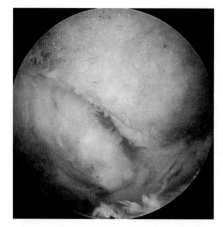

Figure 5 Arthroscopic image from the posterior portal obtained after débridement of the subacromial soft tissues from the lateral para-acromial portal to expose the undersurface of the acromioclavicular joint.

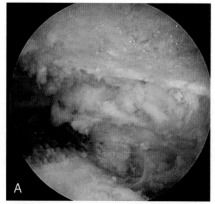
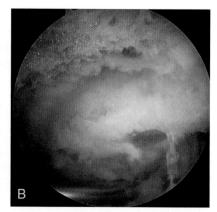

Figure 6 Arthroscopic images of a clavicle obtained from the lateral portal show the obstructing medial acromial facet before (**A**) and after (**B**) facet exposure with a bipolar device and resection with a burr to permit visualization of the exposed acromioclavicular joint and distal clavicle.

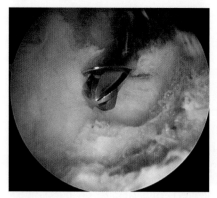

Figure 7 Arthroscopic image of a clavicle obtained from the posterior portal shows distal clavicle resection performed using a 5.5-mm burr placed through the anterior portal.

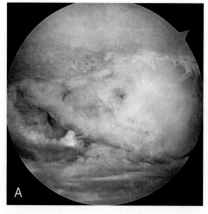
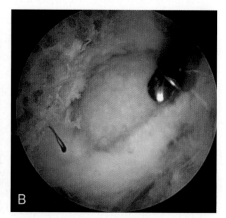

Figure 8 **A,** Arthroscopic image of a clavicle from the lateral portal with a 30° lens shows a bipolar device shelling out the anterior and inferior acromioclavicular joint margins. The distal clavicle is delivered into the field by pushing inferiorly. **B,** Arthroscopic end-on view of a distal clavicle after removal of soft tissues and the medial acromial facet, exposing the circumferential bone margins.

- Resection begins by inserting an oval 5.5-mm burr from the lateral para-acromial portal.
- The acromial facet is taken down sufficiently to visualize the anteroposterior extent of the AC joint (**Figure 5**). In a patient with concomitant subacromial decompression, this step has likely already been done.
- In the absence of subacromial pathology, only sufficient medial acromial facet is débrided to ensure direct AC joint visualization (**Figure 6**).

- Initial distal clavicle resection is performed using a 5.5-mm burr, resecting no more than 6 mm (**Figure 7**). The extent of resection achievable with this initial approach varies, but satisfactory resection nearly always requires portal and instrument repositioning for procedure completion.
- The scope is positioned over a switching stick in the lateral portal, permitting an end-on view of the distal clavicle.
- A switching stick is introduced

through the previously established anterior AC joint portal (that had provided initial access during glenohumeral arthroscopy through the rotator interval), confirming direct and perpendicular access to the AC joint and distal clavicle.
- While viewing from the lateral portal, remnant degenerative meniscus as well as inferior capsule and soft tissue are removed using the 4.5-mm shaver blade and/or bipolar device, preserving the posterior and superior capsule (**Figure 8**). Soft-tissue cautery helps

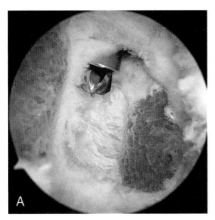 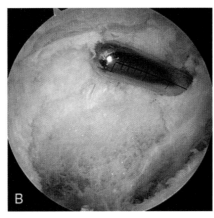

Figure 9   **A,** Arthroscopic image of a clavicle from the posterior portal shows that distal clavicle has been resected from the anterior acromioclavicular joint portal. **B,** Arthroscopic image of a clavicle from the posterior portal shows distal clavicle resection examination for evenness and adequate joint space decompression, confirming preservation of the important posterior and superior capsular tissue attachments.

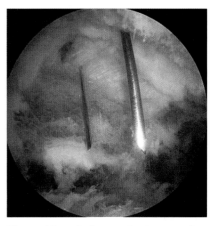

Figure 10   Arthroscopic image of a clavicle shows percutaneous placement of needles that are used to assess the degree of bone resection and joint decompression.

limit bleeding and improves visualization of the AC joint margins.

- The 5.5-mm burr is then brought in through the anterior AC joint portal and used to evenly resect the distal clavicle, working systematically in a windshield wiper motion, sweeping from inferior to superior and from anterior to posterior (**Figure 9, A**).

- A 4-mm switching stick or 5.5-mm instrument in the anterior AC joint portal is used to assess the dimensions of the joint space, and by palpation, to ensure a parallel, smooth, and even resection (**Figure 9, B**).

- A switch is made to a 70° lens in the lateral portal to allow for visualization of the superior extent of the resection, ensuring completeness of the resection and preservation of the superior capsular fibers.

- A series of percutaneously placed needles is used to assess the adequacy of the resection, with a goal of AC joint space measuring between 6 and 10 mm (**Figure 10**).

- A 30° lens is introduced over the switching stick in the anterior AC joint portal for visual confirmation of the adequacy of resection (**Figure 11, A**).

- Despite the perception of even

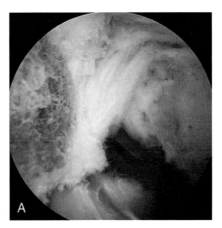 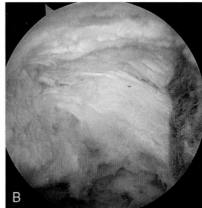

Figure 11   **A,** Arthroscopic image of a clavicle obtained with the arthroscope placed directly into the acromioclavicular joint through an anterior portal. This view allows for direct visualization of the joint for assessing adequacy of the decompression. **B,** Arthroscopic image of a clavicle shows an A-shaped residual space, a common finding after what has been perceived to be an adequate decompression.

resection, an A-shaped space is often appreciated at this point in the procedure, and fine-tuning with additional planing of the superior distal clavicle is required to ensure that the walls of the resection space are parallel (**Figure 11, B**).

- Further resection is accomplished under lateral visualization using a 70° lens, and passive cross-body arm positioning is performed to confirm the absence of bony abutment.

- Excess fluid is removed and the scope portals are closed with No. 3-0 nylon sutures.

- A sterile compressive dressing is applied, and the patient's arm is placed in a simple sling (or sling and swathe).

Direct Approach

- The direct approach begins by outlining the AC joint and marking the posterosuperior and anterosuperior portals (**Figure 12**).

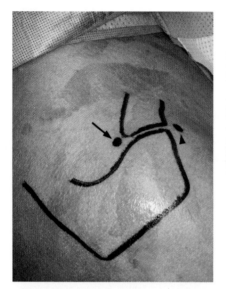

Figure 12 Photograph of a shoulder shows the posterior acromioclavicular (AC) joint portal (arrow) and the anterior AC joint portal (arrowhead), which are used for direct resection of the distal clavicle.

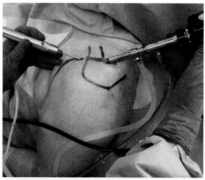

Figure 13 Intraoperative photograph of a shoulder shows a 2.7-mm arthroscope positioned in the posterosuperior portal and use of a small shaver to débride the acromioclavicular joint through the anterosuperior portal.

- From a superior approach, the joint is penetrated with an 18-gauge, 1.5-inch (or spinal) needle.
- After mixing 1 to 2 mL of 1% lidocaine with epinephrine, a small incision is made at the posterosuperior aspect of the joint, into which the 2.7-mm scope sheath with obturator is introduced.
- The sheath pops into the joint, and the obturator is exchanged for the 2.7-mm 30° arthroscope.
- Gravity-assisted fluid inflow is achieved via the scope sheath. Fluid outflow is temporarily accomplished using the needle that was used for joint injection. This setup enables preliminary visualization of the joint space, which typically exhibits degeneration.
- A second incision is made at the anterosuperior corner of the joint, and a small, motorized shaver with blades is inserted to begin joint débridement (**Figure 13**).
- Under direct visualization from the posterosuperior portal, a 2.9- or

3.5-mm abrader or a 3.5-mm barrel burr is used to progressively remove distal clavicle from anterior to posterior (**Figure 14**).
- A small arthroscopic wand with suction is often helpful in delineating the joint margins.
- After the anterior joint space has been decompressed, the scope and shaver portals are exchanged, and the posterior joint and distal clavicle are decompressed (**Figure 15**).
- After the AC joint space has been sufficiently enlarged, the 4-mm scope and conventional shaving blades or burr are exchanged, and the procedure is completed.
- As with the indirect approach, the goal is to achieve a decompressed AC joint space of between 6 and 10 mm.
- Although the author of this chapter did not routinely resect the medial acromial facet, such resection has merit. After confirming that the joint has been satisfactorily decompressed (using percutaneous spinal needles and a ruler, or an intra-articular measurement guide or reference to known instrument dimension), instrumentation is removed, and the scope portals are closed with No. 3-0 nylon sutures,

after which a sterile dressing is applied, and the patient's arm is placed in a sling.
- An intraoperative AP radiograph or fluoroscopic view obtained after distal clavicle resection may aid in recognizing residual pathology, which is common along the superior distal clavicle.
- Recently, the use of a sterile intraoperative ultrasonography probe to directly measure the space during and/or after the procedure has been discussed. The author of this chapter had no personal experience with this tool, however. Currently, a postoperative Zanca radiograph of the resection is preferred to measure the AC joint space (**Figure 16**).

Rehabilitation

A shoulder sling is applied postoperatively. The patient is permitted to remove the sling for hygiene, comfort, and rehabilitation exercises. Rehabilitation is begun the day after surgery, at which time icing and gentle pendulum exercises are initiated. The patient uses his or her unaffected arm to begin assisted forward flexion and external rotation range of motion. As comfort allows, the patient progresses to unassisted forward flexion and external rotation. Strengthening exercises are delayed until 2 to 6 weeks postoperatively to allow for capsular healing. Cross-chest stretching and internal rotation stretching are initiated as pain permits. Additional strengthening exercises are begun 6 weeks postoperatively and are progressed based on pain, swelling (which should be minimal), and activity demands.

Use of the arm as soon as it is comfortable is encouraged, with restrictions based solely on tolerance. Sling use is discontinued as soon as the patient thinks it is no longer needed, and the patient may proceed with activities of daily living and even easy exercises

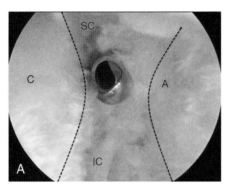 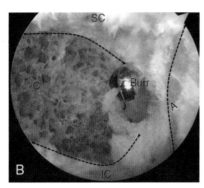

Figure 14 Arthroscopic images obtained from the posterosuperior portal show early stages in resection of the distal clavicle using a small burr. **A,** Appearance before resection. **B,** The appearance of progressive burring of the distal clavicle using a small burr. A = acromion, C = clavicle, IC = inferior capsule, SC = superior capsule.

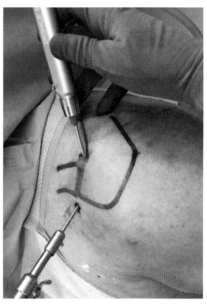

Figure 15 Intraoperative photograph of a shoulder shows the instruments exchanged. This is done after satisfactory anterior joint decompression has been achieved. The remaining joint débridement and distal clavicle resection are evaluated and completed.

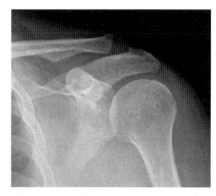

Figure 16 Postoperative Zanca radiograph of a shoulder demonstrates even resection of the distal clavicle.

depending on her or his symptoms. Typically, formal physical therapy is unnecessary unless concomitant procedures, such as subacromial decompression, rotator cuff repair, superior labrum anterior to posterior repair, or biceps tenodesis, were performed.

Avoiding Pitfalls and Complications

A thorough preoperative clinical evaluation is necessary to identify other causes of shoulder pain and any occult posttraumatic AC joint instability and to confirm the role of the AC joint. Attention to several key steps is helpful in optimizing treatment via the indirect approach. The surgeon should ensure complete visualization of the joint margin by performing adequate soft-tissue débridement on the inferior and anterior distal clavicle margins. Soft-tissue cautery and ablation of possible vascular inferior-capsular soft tissue help limit bleeding and expose the inferior joint. Sufficient medial acromial facet must be resected to ensure adequate visualization of and access to the distal clavicle. Accurate placement of the anterior AC joint portal provides a perpendicular approach for distal clavicle resection. The distal clavicle must be evenly resected

using a windshield wiper motion, viewing from the lateral or posterior portals and working from anterior to posterior. The surgeon should use a 70° arthroscope from the lateral portal and/or a 30° arthroscope from the anterior portal to confirm the evenness of the resection. The biomechanically important superior and posterior capsular ligament tissue must be preserved. When performing via the direct approach, it is important to ensure that sufficient joint space exists to accommodate small instrumentation. The joint space must be at least 3 mm wide.

Iatrogenic instability can be prevented by avoiding resection in patients with posttraumatic AC injury in whom occult instability may be discovered and exacerbated by even modest resection of the distal clavicle. The risk of persistent or increased postoperative pain can be mitigated by limiting the amount of distal clavicle excision and/or resecting some of the medial acromial facet. The most common cause of postoperative pain is inadequate resection, and the pain is usually the result of residual abutment at the posterior aspect of the joint. Residual impingement can be avoided by using a 70° arthroscope during resection to ensure that the resection is even and by carefully inspecting the excision from the anterior AC joint portal. Adequacy

of resection can be assessed in a variety of ways, including visual inspection in comparison with instruments of known dimensions (such as a 5.5-mm shaver blade), placement of spinal needles on either side of the joint resection and measurement of the space along the site of skin penetration with a ruler, or use of a sterile ultrasonography probe to directly measure the space.

Bibliography

Alluri RK, Kupperman AI, Montgomery SR, Wang JC, Hame SL: Demographic analysis of open and arthroscopic distal clavicle excision in a private insurance database. *Arthroscopy* 2014;30(9):1068-1074.

Auge WK II, Fischer RA: Arthroscopic distal clavicle resection for isolated atraumatic osteolysis in weight lifters. *Am J Sports Med* 1998;26(2):189-192.

Bigliani LU, Nicholson GP, Flatow EL: Arthroscopic resection of the distal clavicle. *Orthop Clin North Am* 1993;24(1):133-141.

Boehm TD, Barthel T, Schwemmer U, Gohlke FE: Ultrasonography for intraoperative control of the amount of bone resection in arthroscopic acromioclavicular joint resection. *Arthroscopy* 2004;20(6 suppl 2):142-145.

Charron KM, Schepsis AA, Voloshin I: Arthroscopic distal clavicle resection in athletes: A prospective comparison of the direct and indirect approach. *Am J Sports Med* 2007;35(1):53-58.

Edwards SL, Wilson NA, Flores SE, Koh JL, Zhang LQ: Arthroscopic distal clavicle resection: A biomechanical analysis of resection length and joint compliance in a cadaveric model. *Arthroscopy* 2007;23(12):1278-1284.

Freedman BA, Javernick MA, O'Brien FP, Ross AE, Doukas WC: Arthroscopic versus open distal clavicle excision: Comparative results at six months and one year from a randomized, prospective clinical trial. *J Shoulder Elbow Surg* 2007;16(4):413-418.

Gartsman GM: Arthroscopic resection of the acromioclavicular joint. *Am J Sports Med* 1993;21(1):71-77.

Gurd FB: The treatment of complete dislocation of the outer end of the clavicle: An hitherto undescribed operation. *Ann Surg* 1941;113(6):1094-1098.

Kay SP, Ellman H, Harris E: Arthroscopic distal clavicle excision: Technique and early results. *Clin Orthop Relat Res* 1994;(301):181-184.

Mall NA, Foley E, Chalmers PN, Cole BJ, Romeo AA, Bach BR Jr: Degenerative joint disease of the acromioclavicular joint: A review. *Am J Sports Med* 2013;41(11):2684-2692.

Pandhi NG, Esquivel AO, Hanna JD, Lemos DW, Staron JS, Lemos SE: The biomechanical stability of distal clavicle excision versus symmetric acromioclavicular joint resection. *Am J Sports Med* 2013;41(2):291-295.

Pensak M, Grumet RC, Slabaugh MA, Bach BR Jr: Open versus arthroscopic distal clavicle resection. *Arthroscopy* 2010;26(5):697-704.

Robertson WJ, Griffith MH, Carroll K, O'Donnell T, Gill TJ: Arthroscopic versus open distal clavicle excision: A comparative assessment at intermediate-term follow-up. *Am J Sports Med* 2011;39(11):2415-2420.

Stine IA, Vangsness CT Jr: Analysis of the capsule and ligament insertions about the acromioclavicular joint: A cadaveric study. *Arthroscopy* 2009;25(9):968-974.

Tolin BS, Snyder SJ: Our technique for the arthroscopic Mumford procedure. *Orthop Clin North Am* 1993;24(1):143-151.

Walton J, Mahajan S, Paxinos A, et al: Diagnostic values of tests for acromioclavicular joint pain. *J Bone Joint Surg Am* 2004;86(4):807-812.

Zawadsky M, Marra G, Wiater JM, et al: Osteolysis of the distal clavicle: Long-term results of arthroscopic resection. *Arthroscopy* 2000;16(6):600-605.

Chapter 28

Management of Os Acromiale

Jia-Wei Kevin Ko, MD

Joseph A. Abboud, MD

 ## Introduction

Os acromiale results from a failure of osseous union at one of the four ossification centers of the acromion. These ossification centers are the basiacromion, meta-acromion, mesoacromion, and preacromion. Os acromiale is named after the anterior-most segment at the site of nonunion. Mesoacromion is the most common type of os acromiale.

Most patients with os acromiale can be treated nonsurgically. Often, os acromiale is discovered during the workup of another shoulder problem. Although os acromiale can be detected with plain radiography, most commonly on the axillary view, it is easily missed. MRI is more sensitive than radiography and may reveal adjacent edema or cysts in addition to other shoulder pathology. MRI is preferred over CT because of the high incidence of rotator cuff tears in patients with symptomatic os acromiale.

Os acromiale may become symptomatic for reasons including gross motion at the site of the synchondrosis,

subacromial impingement resulting from flexion of the anterior segment, and the presence of a prominent subacromial bone spur. The mechanism of pain resulting from micromotion is similar to that at any other site of nonunion. A history of injury or trauma before the onset of symptoms is common. Such inciting events are thought to induce subtle instability at the synchondrosis site, leading to increased micromotion and pain. Impingement pain in these instances results from a dynamic process in which the subacromial space can lessen with arm elevation as the deltoid contraction pulls the anterior fragment downward. Because of this dynamic impingement, it may not be possible to fully visualize the impingement potential of the shoulder on static imaging of acromial morphology. Bone spurs are sometimes present at the nonunion site and act as a more centrally located impingement spur. Bone spurs may worsen over time as the synchondrosis adapts to the stresses placed on it and because of the micromotion that occurs.

 ## Case Presentation

A 32-year-old man presents with unremitting pain localized to his nondominant shoulder. He reports having felt a "pop" when performing shoulder presses at the gym approximately 1 month earlier. The pain is localized to the superolateral shoulder over a small bony prominence on the acromion. The pain has persisted despite activity modifications and the use of anti-inflammatory medications. The patient reports no previous dysfunction of or injury to the affected shoulder.

No neurovascular deficits are noted on physical examination. The patient has full passive range of motion and rotator cuff strength, with the exception of Medical Research Council grade 4+/5 strength in the supraspinatus. Exquisite point tenderness without radiation is elicited over the bony prominence on the acromion, and minimal tenderness is noted at the acromioclavicular (AC) joint. The pain is re-created with cross-body adduction testing and any overhead activity. Results of the Neer impingement test and the Jobe test are moderately positive. The remainder of the examination is unremarkable.

Radiographic evaluation of the shoulder reveals an os acromiale at the mesoacromion (**Figure 1**). The patient is referred for MRI of the affected shoulder to further characterize the os acromiale and to evaluate for additional

Dr. Abboud or an immediate family member has received royalties from Integra LifeSciences; serves as a paid consultant to Integra LifeSciences and Tornier; has stock or stock options held in MinInvasive; has received research or institutional support from DePuy Synthes, Integra LifeSciences, Tornier, and Zimmer; and serves as a board member, owner, officer, or committee member of the American Shoulder and Elbow Surgeons and the Mid-Atlantic Shoulder and Elbow Society. Neither Dr. Ko nor any immediate family member has received anything of value from or has stock or stock options held in a commercial company or institution related directly or indirectly to the subject of this chapter.

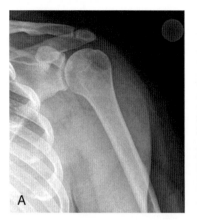
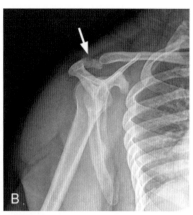
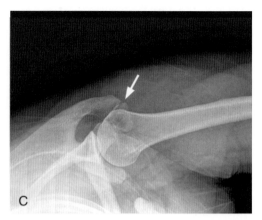

Figure 1   AP (**A**), scapular Y (**B**), and axillary (**C**) radiographs of the left shoulder of a patient with os acromiale (arrows in panels B and C) demonstrate a mesoacromion with adjacent sclerosis and periarticular cysts.

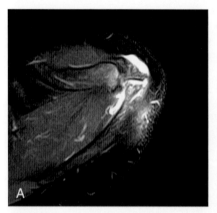
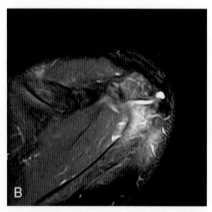

Figure 2   **A** and **B,** Consecutive T2-weighted axial MRIs of the affected left shoulder of the same patient described in Figure 1 demonstrate substantial adjacent edema, cyst formation, and peripheral osteophytes about the synchondrosis.

intra-articular pathology. A gentle progressive physical therapy protocol is initiated.

Several weeks after the initial clinical examination and after continued nonsurgical treatment, the patient had not experienced substantial improvement in symptoms. MRI revealed substantial adjacent bony and soft-tissue edema, cyst formation, and peripheral osteophytes about the os acromiale (**Figure 2**). High-grade tendinopathy of the supraspinatus tendon without a definite discrete full-thickness tear was also noted. Because nonsurgical management was unsuccessful, the patient was offered surgical treatment. The surgeon and patient discussed the

options of fixation of the os acromiale and excision of the synchondrosis. The patient elected to proceed with arthroscopic excision of the synchondrosis. He returned to full duty as a police officer 3 months postoperatively.

 Indications

The symptoms associated with an os acromiale can be difficult to distinguish from the symptoms associated with subacromial impingement. Additionally, both conditions can coexist in the same patient. Patients with a symptomatic os acromiale typically have point tenderness directly at the synchondrosis site,

much like that noted in patients with symptomatic arthritis of the AC joint. Patients with subacromial impingement may demonstrate classic Neer and Hawkins impingement signs. However, some may not demonstrate symptoms until they perform active shoulder elevation; these symptoms are caused by dynamic impingement.

All patients with an isolated symptomatic os acromiale should undergo a trial of nonsurgical management. Nonsurgical management typically entails activity modification, physical therapy using a graduated protocol similar to that used for shoulder impingement, and the use of NSAIDs. Subacromial corticosteroid injections can be helpful in particularly symptomatic patients. Additionally, injection directly into the synchondrosis can be attempted. Because the physical examination findings can be difficult to distinguish between the two sources of pathology, these injections have the potential to be both therapeutic and diagnostic. Nonsurgical measures may obviate or delay the need for surgical treatment. However, the patient described in this chapter had undergone 2 months of nonsurgical treatment without lasting relief of symptoms and continued to have point tenderness at the nonunion site. The patient was dissatisfied with his inability to return to his previous level

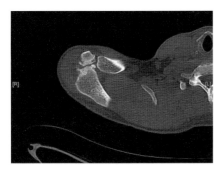

Figure 3 CT scan of a symptomatic os acromiale demonstrates peripheral osteophytes, subchondral sclerosis, and periarticular cysts; these findings are typically seen in arthritic joints.

of functioning and his work as a police officer. Therefore, the patient opted for surgery.

The authors of this chapter prefer to manage symptomatic os acromiale with subacromial decompression and arthroscopic resection of the synchondrosis. Patients who most benefit from this approach typically have point tenderness at the site of the os acromiale and/or pain that is elicited on manual stressing of the nonunion site. The rationale behind the authors' approach is that the synchondrosis is analogous in many ways to an AC joint. That is, symptoms are generated by the micromotion leading to localized inflammation. The theory that the symptoms associated with an os acromiale are analogous to those of symptomatic AC joint arthropathy is reinforced by the increased fluid signal seen on MRI in many cases of symptomatic os acromiale. Additionally, examinations of patients with symptomatic os acromiale have demonstrated hypertrophy, cysts, and sclerosis of the pseudojoint (**Figure 3**). Therefore, similar to a distal clavicle resection, excision of the synchondrosis is a resection arthroplasty of a pseudarthrosis.

The use of subacromial decompression and arthroscopic resection of the synchondrosis stems from dissatisfaction with alternative approaches. The authors of this chapter acknowledge that

few data support this approach and that resection of the synchondrosis may lead to increased flexion instability of the anterior segment with shoulder elevation. However, data to support alternative approaches are also lacking, and promising early results have been achieved with this method in appropriately selected patients.

Controversies and Alternative Approaches

As noted previously, the optimal surgical treatment of os acromiale is controversial because of the lack of quality evidence to guide treatment decisions and the limited number of os acromiale that become persistently symptomatic. The three main treatment types are excision, decompression, and fusion.

Excision

Excision of the anterior fragment has been reported by several authors. However, the results of this approach have been inconsistent because of persistent deltoid dysfunction after removal of the fragment. Variable rates of success have been reported in many small series of open excision of os acromiale. It is difficult to draw definitive conclusions from these studies because of the significant heterogeneity in the patient populations and because the largest series contains only nine patients. However, one common finding is that the larger the fragment, the greater the risk of postoperative deltoid dysfunction. In one series, the only os acromiale that was successfully managed with open excision involved a small preacromion. The authors of another study concluded that all larger fragments should be retained. Similarly, in yet another study, no satisfactory outcomes were reported after the excision of larger mesoacromions.

More recent series have reported the results of arthroscopic excision of

os acromiale. The results of these studies demonstrate better function after arthroscopy than after open approaches. In a study of younger athletes aged 18 to 25 years with symptomatic mesoacromions, all patients returned to play by 14 weeks postoperatively with minimal deltoid dysfunction. The authors of another study reported no loss of deltoid function with arthroscopic excision of mesoacromions and preacromions. The benefits of arthroscopic excision likely stem from the ability to preserve the superior deltoid periosteal attachment. These findings suggest that if excision of the fragment is attempted, it should be performed arthroscopically. In general, excision seems to be best reserved for smaller preacromions; however, in select patients, perhaps in younger athletes, mesoacromions can also be excised.

Decompression

Subacromial decompression has been used in the management of symptomatic os acromiale, particularly in the presence of impingement symptoms or rotator cuff disease. Considerable variation in outcomes has been reported with this procedure as well. The rate of satisfactory results ranges from 33% to 84%. However, in patients with exquisite point tenderness at the synchondrosis, results of subacromial decompression alone can be unsatisfactory. Several series have reported recurrent pain and worse outcomes compared with routine subacromial decompression without the presence of os acromiale. In theory, this is because nothing is done to directly manage the pain at the synchondrosis site. In the patient reported on in this chapter, pain at the synchondrosis site was the most prominent symptom. Therefore, the authors of this chapter did not think that subacromial decompression alone would adequately address the patient's condition. It can be difficult to differentiate between subacromial impingement and a symptomatic os acromiale. In this patient, the os

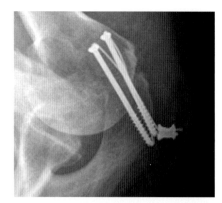

Figure 4 Axillary radiograph demonstrates a symptomatic os acromiale managed with cannulated screws and tension-band wiring. A deep hardware infection requiring débridement and hardware removal later developed.

acromiale was clearly the source of pathology. If there is any doubt, however, the authors of this chapter sometimes use a subacromial injection to discern the primary source of pain.

Fusion

Techniques for fusion of the synchondrosis were developed in response to the inconsistent results of os acromiale excision. Techniques described in the literature include the use of tension-band wiring and compression screws. Many authors have advocated the use of bone graft. Although fusion demonstrated more consistent initial results than open excision, enthusiasm for it has waned because of the high rate of hardware complications and secondary surgical procedures.

Obtaining a satisfactory outcome with fusion depends on obtaining a successful osseous union between the two fragments. Nonunion rates as high as 33% have been reported in some small series using tension-band wiring. However, more rigid fixation techniques have demonstrated union rates approaching 100%. Even if union is achieved, hardware prominence or irritation can cause persistent postoperative symptoms and irritation. Hardware complication rates

greater than 80% have been reported in many series; these rates are defined by the need for hardware removal. Overall satisfaction rates of 38% to 100% have been reported across several studies, with dissatisfaction resulting, in part, from the need for secondary procedures.

In terms of fixation techniques, the use of compression screws with or without tension-band wiring and bone graft seems to provide the best results. The authors of one series reported better union rates with the use of cannulated screws and tension-band wiring (**Figure 4**) than with the use of Kirschner wires with tension-band wiring. The authors of another study reported more nonunions with the deltoid-off approach, in which the deltoid and its superficial periosteal sleeve are detached from the anterior segment. Those authors hypothesized that disruption of these soft-tissue attachments disrupts the blood supply to the acromion. Arthroscopic fixation techniques have also been described, with union achieved in seven of eight patients studied.

Regardless of the specific method used, rigid fixation with preservation of acromial vascularity seems to offer the best chance of union. Unfortunately, union may not reduce the need for further intervention because of the high incidence of hardware-related symptoms. Given these concerns, the authors of this chapter elected to perform arthroscopic subacromial decompression and synchondrosis excision in the patient discussed previously, leaving the remnant anterior segment and all its superior periosteal attachments intact. This approach can allow for an expeditious recovery and does not prevent the use of fixation or complete excision as a salvage procedure in the event of failure.

 Results

Current literature on the surgical treatment of os acromiale is summarized

in **Tables 1**, **2**, and **3**. Although many approaches have been reported, too few high-quality studies are available to enable definitive conclusions regarding treatment. In the only study of the synchondrosis excision technique discussed in this chapter, six patients demonstrated average improvement in the Penn Shoulder Score from 50.6 preoperatively to 78.5 postoperatively and had an average reduction in the pain portion of the Penn score from 5.6 preoperatively to 1.3 postoperatively. All patients demonstrated resolution of point tenderness over the synchondrosis site, and no additional procedures were required to address the os acromiale. The treatment algorithm in **Figure 5** is based on the experience of the authors of this chapter and the results reported in the literature.

 Technical Keys to Success

Excision of the Synchondrosis

- The surgical approach for excision of the synchondrosis is similar to any other arthroscopic approach to the shoulder.
- After performing a routine diagnostic arthroscopy of the shoulder, the subacromial space is entered through the standard posterior portal.
- Adequate visualization is obtained through a bursectomy and partial release of the coracoacromial ligament to identify the leading edge of the acromion.
- Given the relatively high incidence of associated rotator cuff tears, the posterosuperior rotator cuff should be evaluated carefully and any associated tears repaired.
- The lateral portal is established under direct visualization and in line with the os acromiale to optimize eventual excision of the synchondrosis. This portal may be made

Table 1 Results of Excision of Symptomatic Os Acromiale

Authors	Journal (Year)	Type of Os Acromiale	Outcomes	Failure Rate (%)	Comments
Mudge et al	*J Bone Joint Surg Am* (1984)	N/A	Excellent results in 4 of 6 shoulders	33	Authors concluded in retrospect that larger fragments should be retained All presented with RCT
Edelson et al	*J Bone Joint Surg Br* (1993)	N/A	Satisfactory results in 4 of 5 shoulders	20	Lateral deltoid-splitting approach All presented with RCT Follow-up, 1.5–3.3 yr
Armengol et al	*J Shoulder Elbow Surg* (1994)	Mesoacromion and preacromion	No satisfactory results in the 5 shoulders studied	100	All fragments were considered to be large
Warner et al	*J Bone Joint Surg Am* (1998)	Mesoacromion and preacromion	Good outcome in 1 of 3 shoulders	66	The successful case involved preacromion excision 1 patient presented with RCT Mean follow-up, 2.8 yr
Boehm et al	*J Bone Joint Surg Br* (2003)	Mesoacromion and preacromion	Good to excellent results in all 6 shoulders Mean Constant pain score improved from 3.3 to 13.4	0	3 preacromion, 1 bipartite mesoacromion, and 2 small soft mesoacromion not amenable to fixation 1 deep infection All presented with RCT Mean follow-up, 3.2 yr
Pagnani et al	*J Shoulder Elbow Surg* (2006)	Mesoacromion	All returned to play by 14 wk	0	Arthroscopic excision in 12 young athletes (14 shoulders) Technique involved meticulous preservation of the deltoid No patient presented with RCT
Campbell et al	*Orthopedics* (2012)	Mesoacromion and preacromion	ASES score improved from 33.7 to 80.3 in 31 shoulders	0	Arthroscopic excision Deltoid periosteal sleeve preserved No loss of deltoid function 16 of 31 shoulders presented with RCT Mean follow-up, 3.4 yr

ASES = American Shoulder and Elbow Surgeons shoulder outcome, N/A = not available, RCT = rotator cuff tear.

slightly more posterior than the typical anterolateral portal.

- The os acromiale is clearly delineated using an electrocautery device (**Figure 6**).
- Next, an acromioplasty is performed. The burr is introduced from the posterior portal, and the newly established lateral portal is used for visualization.
- The authors of this chapter prefer to use a so-called cutting block technique described by Caspari, in which the burr is brought in through the posterior portal and

used to create a smooth transition between the posterior acromion and the anterior acromion.

- A substantial subacromial spur may or may not be present.
- Impingement symptoms of os acromiale may result from a dynamic process that occurs with elevation of the shoulder and flexion of the anterior acromion through the synchondrosis. Therefore, an anterior acromion with a normal appearance can be symptomatic. Thus, the authors of this chapter advocate a relatively aggressive acromioplasty

to ensure that the portion of the acromion anterior to the nonunion site is well decompressed.

- After the acromioplasty has been completed, the arthroscope is moved back to the posterior portal, and the shaver is introduced through the lateral portal.
- The excision of the synchondrosis is initiated with the shaver. After enough space has been created, the burr is introduced to complete the excision.
- The goal with this technique is to create approximately 5 to 7 mm of

Table 2 Results of Decompression of Symptomatic Os Acromiale

Authors	Journal (Year)	Type of Os Acromiale	Outcomes	Failure Rate (%)	Comments
Hutchinson and Veenstra	*Arthroscopy* (1993)	Mesoacromion and preacromion	Satisfactory results in 1 of 3 shoulders	66	Subacromial decompression Converted to excision in 1 patient after poor result All patients had recurrent pain by 1 yr postoperatively No patient presented with RCT
Armengol et al	*J Shoulder Elbow Surg* (1994)	Mesoacromion and preacromion	Good or excellent results in 19 of 22 shoulders	34	Aggressive anterior acromioplasty was done, leaving just a superior cortical shell to preserve the deltoid attachment (almost an excision)
Jerosch et al	*Unfallchirurg* (1994)	N/A	12 shoulders; results were excellent in 43%, good in 17%, and fair in 25%	15	Subacromial decompression Patients with os acromiale had slightly worse outcomes after subacromial decompression compared with patients without os acromiale No patient presented with RCT Follow-up, 1-3 yr
Wright et al	*Arthroscopy* (2000)	Mesoacromion	Mean UCLA score improved from 17 to 31 in 13 shoulders	0	Anterior acromioplasty, more bone resection than typical acromioplasty 1 patient presented with RCT Mean follow-up, 2.4 yr
Boehm et al	*J Bone Joint Surg Br* (2003)	Mesoacromion	Good to excellent results in 3 of 5 shoulders Mean Constant pain score improved from 4.6 to 12.2	0	Open anterior acromioplasty 2 deep infections All presented with RCT Mean follow-up, 3.1 yr
Abboud et al	*J Shoulder Elbow Surg* (2006)	Mesoacromion	Satisfactory results in 7 of 11 shoulders	0	Acromioplasty Workers' compensation associated with worse outcomes 36% (4 shoulders in 4 patients) presented with RCT Mean follow-up, 3.3 yr
Johnston et al	*Orthop Clin North Am* (2013)	Mesoacromion	In the 6 shoulders studied, mean Penn Shoulder Score improved from 50.6 to 78.5; pain component decreased from mean 5.6 to 1.3	0	Synchondrosis excision (current preferred technique) 67% of shoulders presented with RCT Mean follow-up, 2.1 yr

N/A = not available, RCT = rotator cuff tear, UCLA = University of California–Los Angeles Shoulder Rating Scale.

space between the anterior and posterior fragments, removing bone in equal amounts from either side of the synchondrosis.

- The integrity of the superior periosteum should be maintained to prevent postoperative deltoid dysfunction.

- Additionally, the acromial attachments of the posterior AC capsular ligaments should be preserved at the medial aspect of the resection.

- The adequacy of the resection is best evaluated from the lateral portal (**Figure 7**). The amount of resection is judged with the use of two spinal needles or by comparing the resection with the size of the burr.

- The authors of this chapter do not excise the medial portion unless the

Table 3 Results of Fusion of Symptomatic Os Acromiale[a]

Author(s)	Journal (Year)	Type of Os Acromiale	Outcomes	Failure Rate (%)	Comments
Norris et al	*Orthopaedic Transactions* (1983)	N/A	Excellent or satisfactory results in 7 of 10 shoulders	30	80% of shoulders had hardware complications
Edelson et al	*J Bone Joint Surg Br* (1993)	N/A	2 patients treated; both had a satisfactory result 100% union	0	Compression screws All hardware removed Neither patient presented with RCT Follow-up: first pt, 1.5 yr; second pt, 3 yr
Warner et al	*J Bone Joint Surg Am* (1998)	Meta-acromion and meso-acromion	Good outcome in 6 of 12 shoulders Nonunion in 4 of 12 shoulders	50	Bone graft used Use of tension band with cannulated screws resulted in better union rate (6 of 7 shoulders) and outcome (5 of 7 shoulders had a good outcome) 3 nonunions resulting from failure of the wire construct in the tension-band group 7 of 12 shoulders had RCTs
Hertel et al	*J Shoulder Elbow Surg* (1998)	Mesoacromion	8 of 15 shoulders had minimal to no pain 10 shoulders successfully united	13	Tension-band wiring construct More nonunions occurred after the deltoid-off approach Functional outcome better when union achieved 12 shoulders had RCT Mean follow-up, 3.6 yr
Ryu et al	*Orthopedics* (1999)	Mesoacromion	UCLA score improved from 19 to 35 Union achieved in all 4 shoulders	0	Compression screws No patient presented with RCT Mean follow-up, 2.8 yr
Satterlee	*J Shoulder Elbow Surg* (1999)	Mesoacromion	Excellent outcomes in all 6 shoulders 100% union	0	Herbert screws Anterior fragment tilted upward before ORIF 3 shoulders had RCT Follow-up, 3-6 yr
Boehm et al	*J Bone Joint Surg Br* (2003)	Mesoacromion	Good to excellent results in 19 of 22 shoulders 15 shoulders successfully united	0	Tension-band technique with wires 1 deep infection Hardware removal was performed in 21 of 22 shoulders All presented with RCT Follow-up, 3-3.5 yr
Peckett et al	*J Shoulder Elbow Surg* (2004)	Mesoacromion	Satisfactory results in 24 of 26 shoulders 25 shoulders united	8	Fixation with Kirschner wires or screws and tension banding with wire or suture Bone graft used Hardware removal was performed in 8 of 26 shoulders 17 shoulders (65%) presented with RCT

N/A = not available, ORIF = open reduction and internal fixation, RCT = rotator cuff tear, UCLA = University of California–Los Angeles Shoulder Rating Scale.

[a] All studies in this table used ORIF except as noted.

Table 3 Results of Fusion of Symptomatic Os Acromiale[a] (continued)

Author(s)	Journal (Year)	Type of Os Acromiale	Outcomes	Failure Rate (%)	Comments
Abboud et al	*J Shoulder Elbow Surg* (2006)	Mesoacro-mion	Satisfactory results in 3 of 8 shoulders 100% union rate	0	Tension-band technique with wires or compression screws Hardware removal was required in 7 shoulders Workers' compensation was associated with worse outcomes 4 shoulders presented with RCT Mean follow-up, 3.3 yr
Atoun et al	*J Shoulder Elbow Surg* (2012)	Mesoacro-mion	Mean Constant score improved from 49 to 81 7 of 8 shoulders united	12.5	Arthroscopic fixation Absorbable cannulated screws 5 shoulders (63%) presented with RCT Mean follow-up, 1.8 yr

N/A = not available, ORIF = open reduction and internal fixation, RCT = rotator cuff tear, UCLA = University of California–Los Angeles Shoulder Rating Scale.

[a] All studies in this table used ORIF except as noted.

AC joint is symptomatic. Mobility is not assessed intraoperatively because the surgical decision making was done based on the preoperative evaluation.

- In patients with a rotator cuff tear that is noted at the time of diagnostic arthroscopy, the tear is addressed in standard arthroscopic fashion before completion of the procedure.

Fusion of the Os Acromiale

- The authors of this chapter prefer to use a transacromial approach in which a longitudinal incision is made in line with the synchondrosis. This helps to preserve the blood supply to the anterior and posterior segment. Large, full-thickness subcutaneous flaps are developed anteriorly and posteriorly, but the deltoid attachments should be preserved as much as possible except for directly at the synchondrosis site.
- The deltoid can be split in line with its fibers laterally to allow exposure of the subacromial space and evaluation of the rotator cuff.

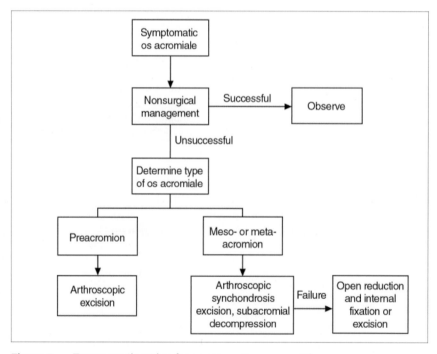

Figure 5 Treatment algorithm for symptomatic os acromiale.

- The synchondrosis must be fully resected to expose bleeding bone on both the anterior and posterior segments.
- Care should be taken to avoid introducing flexion at the synchondrosis site; preferably, the shape of the acromion should be flattened by fusing the segments in extension slightly greater than was present initially.
- The authors of this chapter prefer

to use cannulated screws with tension-band wiring.

- All patients should be counseled preoperatively that they likely will require secondary surgery in the future for hardware removal.

 Rehabilitation

The postoperative rehabilitation protocol may be influenced by procedures performed along with the synchondrosis excision, such as rotator cuff repair. The rehabilitation protocols in the absence of additional procedures are outlined in **Tables 4** and **5**.

 Avoiding Pitfalls

The surgeon should maintain as much stability of the anterior fragment as possible while performing an adequate resection of the synchondrosis. To do this, the superior periosteal attachment and the posterior AC ligaments should be

maintained. Most of the coracoacromial ligament should be preserved to provide additional stability to the anterior fragment. Preservation of this ligament is key to maintaining deltoid function and preventing secondary shoulder dysfunction, such as AC joint instability.

Adequate anterior acromioplasty should be performed to prevent dynamic impingement. With resection of the

synchondrosis, the anterior fragment becomes less stable and more prone to flexion with elevation of the arm. An adequate acromioplasty can help to prevent this effect. Although the amount of acromion that needs to be resected varies from patient to patient, the authors of this chapter advocate a slightly more aggressive acromioplasty than is typically undertaken, with the goal of

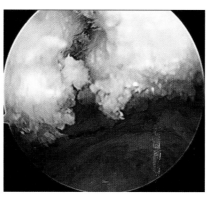

Figure 6 Intraoperative arthroscopic image demonstrates the appearance of the os acromiale from the lateral viewing portal.

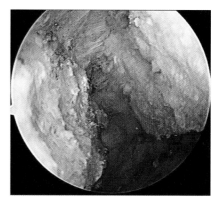

Figure 7 Intraoperative arthroscopic image demonstrates the appearance of the os acromiale from the lateral viewing portal after excision of the synchondrosis.

Table 4 Rehabilitation Protocol After Either Excision or Fusion to Manage Os Acromiale

Postoperative Week	ROM	Strengthening	Return to Play	Comments/Emphasis
0-2	Sling	None	No	Activities of daily living permitted
2-4	As tolerated	None	No	Formal therapy only if restricted ROM at postoperative visit
4-12	As tolerated	Yes	No	Progressive strengthening within limits of comfort
>12	As tolerated	Yes	Yes	No restrictions

ROM = range of motion.

Table 5 Rehabilitation Protocol After Decompression to Manage Os Acromiale

Postoperative Week	ROM	Strengthening	Return to Play	Comments/Emphasis
0-2	Sling	None	No	Sling at all times
2-6	Passive only	None	No	Sling except for ROM exercises
6-12	As tolerated	Progressive	No	Progressive ROM and strengthening as tolerated
>12	As tolerated	Functional	When pain free	Activity as tolerated

ROM = range of motion.

creating a smooth and completely flat transition with the posterior acromion.

It is important to identify associated conditions, such as rotator cuff tear. An association between rotator cuff tears and os acromiale has been established in the literature. Although a patient may have point tenderness over the os acromiale, failure to identify and manage a rotator cuff tear can have substantial implications regarding long-term function for the patient. Additionally, pain related to a cuff tear and pain related to the os acromiale may be difficult to distinguish. Therefore, thorough evaluation of the rotator cuff is imperative during any surgical intervention for os acromiale, even if MRI is inconclusive.

Having point tenderness over the synchondrosis site is a requisite for synchondrosis excision to be successful. This approach may not be as effective if the patient presents with more vague symptoms that could be attributable to a rotator cuff tear/tendinitis or impingement-type symptoms. Synchondrosis excision should be done only in patients who exhibit point tenderness over the synchondrosis site. Excision may not be effective for patients who present with vague symptoms that could be attributable to rotator cuff tear, tendinitis, or impingement.

The optimal treatment of symptomatic os acromiale remains controversial. The benefits of arthroscopic synchondrosis excision are substantiated by only a single small published study, but, anecdotally, the authors of this chapter have found the procedure to work well in their own experience. The benefits of arthroscopic excision of the synchondrosis include reliable relief of pain at the synchondrosis site, less risk of deltoid dysfunction, and limited risk of complications. Given these benefits and the potential complications of other procedures described in the literature, the authors of this chapter find arthroscopic excision to be most satisfactory. Additionally, the use of this procedure does not prevent the use of other options, such as excision and fixation, in the event that it is unsuccessful.

Bibliography

Abboud JA, Silverberg D, Pepe M, et al: Surgical treatment of os acromiale with and without associated rotator cuff tears. *J Shoulder Elbow Surg* 2006;15(3):265-270.

Armengol J, Brittis D, Pollack R: The association of unfused acromial epiphysis with tears of the rotator cuff: A review of 42 cases. *J Shoulder Elbow Surg* 1994;3:S14.

Atoun E, van Tongel A, Narvani A, Rath E, Sforza G, Levy O: Arthroscopically assisted internal fixation of the symptomatic unstable os acromiale with absorbable screws. *J Shoulder Elbow Surg* 2012;21(12):1740-1745.

Boehm TD, Matzer M, Brazda D, Gohlke FE: Os acromiale associated with tear of the rotator cuff treated operatively: Review of 33 patients. *J Bone Joint Surg Br* 2003;85(4):545-549.

Campbell PT, Nizlan NM, Skirving AP: Arthroscopic excision of os acromiale: Effects on deltoid function and strength. *Orthopedics* 2012;35(11):e1601-e1605.

Caspari RB, Thal R: A technique for arthroscopic subacromial decompression. *Arthroscopy* 1992;8(1):23-30.

Edelson JG, Zuckerman J, Hershkovitz I: Os acromiale: Anatomy and surgical implications. *J Bone Joint Surg Br* 1993;75(4):551-555.

Hertel R, Windisch W, Schuster A, Ballmer FT: Transacromial approach to obtain fusion of unstable os acromiale. *J Shoulder Elbow Surg* 1998;7(6):606-609.

Hutchinson MR, Veenstra MA: Arthroscopic decompression of shoulder impingement secondary to os acromiale. *Arthroscopy* 1993;9(1):28-32.

Jerosch J, Steinbeck J, Strauss JM, Schneider T: Arthroscopic subacromial decompression: Indications in os acromiale [German]. *Unfallchirurg* 1994;97(2):69-73.

Johnston PS, Paxton ES, Gordon V, Kraeutler MJ, Abboud JA, Williams GR: Os acromiale: A review and an introduction of a new surgical technique for management. *Orthop Clin North Am* 2013;44(4):635-644.

Mudge MK, Wood VE, Frykman GK: Rotator cuff tears associated with os acromiale. *J Bone Joint Surg Am* 1984;66(3):427-429.

Norris TR, Fischer J, Bigliani L, Neer CS II: The unfused acromial epiphysis and its relationship to impingement syndrome. *Orthopaedic Transactions* 1983;7:505-506.

Pagnani MJ, Mathis CE, Solman CG: Painful os acromiale (or unfused acromial apophysis) in athletes. *J Shoulder Elbow Surg* 2006;15(4):432-435.

Peckett WR, Gunther SB, Harper GD, Hughes JS, Sonnabend DH: Internal fixation of symptomatic os acromiale: A series of twenty-six cases. *J Shoulder Elbow Surg* 2004;13(4):381-385.

Ryu RK, Fan RS, Dunbar WH 5th: The treatment of symptomatic os acromiale. *Orthopedics* 1999;22(3):325-328.

Sammarco VJ: Os acromiale: Frequency, anatomy, and clinical implications. *J Bone Joint Surg Am* 2000;82(3):394-400.

Satterlee CC: Successful osteosynthesis of an unstable mesoacromion in 6 shoulders: A new technique. *J Shoulder Elbow Surg* 1999;8(2):125-129.

Warner JJ, Beim GM, Higgins L: The treatment of symptomatic os acromiale. *J Bone Joint Surg Am* 1998;80(9):1320-1326.

Wright RW, Heller MA, Quick DC, Buss DD: Arthroscopic decompression for impingement syndrome secondary to an unstable os acromiale. *Arthroscopy* 2000;16(6):595-599.

Chapter 29

Acromioclavicular Joint Repair and Reconstruction: Anatomic Considerations and Technical Tips

John Apostolakos, BS

Michael B. O'Sullivan, MD

Monica Shoji, BA

Jessica DiVenere, BS

Mark P. Cote, DPT, MSCTR

Augustus D. Mazzocca, MS, MD

 ## Case Presentation

A 43-year-old right-hand–dominant man presents to the physician 2 weeks after falling headfirst over the handlebars of his mountain bike and sustaining a direct blow to the anterosuperior aspect of his left shoulder. The patient describes severe shoulder pain with movement, and shoulder deformity is noted with the patient in the upright position.

Standard shoulder radiographs and a 15° bilateral cephalad radiograph of both acromioclavicular (AC) joints reveal widening of the left coracoclavicular (CC) interval measuring approximately 20 mm, compared with widening of 5 mm on the right side. There is no indication of fracture to the left AC joint (**Figure 1**). Physical examination reveals an inability to reduce the left AC joint when shrugging the shoulders (shrug test) or while contracting the trapezius

muscle. The patient has substantial pain on forward elevation greater than 90°, considerable pain posteriorly, and substantial weakness.

A Rockwood type V separation is diagnosed based on the severity of radiographic CC displacement and the inability of the patient to reduce the joint while shrugging. The physician explains that type V injuries typically are managed with early surgical treatment to address tearing of the deltotrapezial fascia and the CC and AC ligaments. Nonsurgical treatment options also are discussed, but the patient opts to undergo surgery.

 ## Indications

Type I and II AC separations typically are managed nonsurgically, type III separations are managed on a case-by-case basis, and type IV through VI injuries

are managed surgically because of the severity of soft-tissue damage and the substantial morbidity of a persistently dislocated AC joint. It is generally agreed that type III injuries should be managed nonsurgically for 8 to 12 weeks, after which the patient should be examined for residual pain and/or dysfunction. Many patients report improvement in pain and motion with nonsurgical management. The presence of residual pain is of utmost importance in the evaluation of patients with AC joint injury. In the practice of the senior author (A.D.M.), substantial residual pain is the primary indicator for surgery. Secondary factors that may be indicators for surgery include weakness and loss of motion in the extremity.

A history of a direct blow to the anterosuperior aspect of the AC joint such as in the case presented in this chapter should raise immediate suspicion of AC joint injury. Generalized anterosuperior shoulder pain or pain localized to the AC joint in combination with visual evidence of a dramatic deformity compared with the contralateral side further validates an initial diagnosis of AC joint separation. As in

Dr. Mazzocca or an immediate family member serves as a paid consultant to and has received research or institutional support from Arthrex. None of the following authors or any immediate family member has received anything of value from or has stock or stock options held in a commercial company or institution related directly or indirectly to the subject of this chapter: Mr. Apostolakos, Dr. O'Sullivan, Ms. Shoji, Ms. DiVenere, and Dr. Cote.

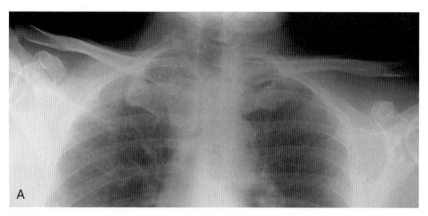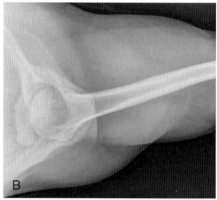

Figure 1   Preoperative radiographs obtained from a 43-year-old man 2 weeks after he fell over the handlebars of his mountain bike and onto the anterosuperior aspect of his left shoulder. **A,** Bilateral Zanca view of the acromioclavicular joints. **B,** Axillary view of the injured left shoulder, which was used to rule out a posteriorly displaced type IV dislocation.

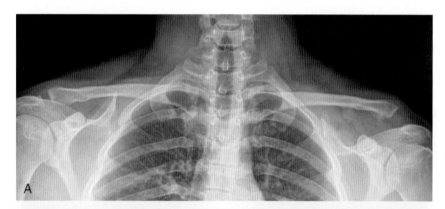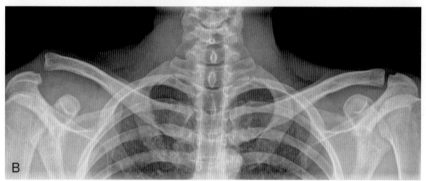

Figure 2   Bilateral Zanca radiographs obtained from two patients with acromio-clavicular joint separation. Neither radiograph is from the patient discussed in the case study in this chapter. **A,** Rockwood type III separation is evident on the left side. **B,** Rockwood type V separation is evident on the right side.

helpful during physical examination. In patients with type III injury, the AC joint may reduce during the shrug test, but in patients with type V injury, a deltotrapezial fascia tear makes reduction of the AC joint impossible.

Controversies and Alternative Approaches

Uncertainty regarding the optimal management of AC joint injury can be traced to Galen and Hippocrates, with the first "modern" treatments performed in the 1860s. Since the 1860s, various surgical and nonsurgical methods for managing the AC joint have been reported in the literature. The authors of a systematic review conducted in 2011 and published in 2013 found 120 studies describing 151 different surgical techniques for AC joint reconstruction. Rockwood was the first to note that most of these surgical techniques are simple variations and combinations of previously described procedures. In an effort to simplify decision making, Rockwood classified these procedures into four categories: AC repair, CC repair, distal clavicle excision, and dynamic muscle transfer. In addition to the lack of a single preferred surgical technique to manage AC joint injury, there is also

the case presented in this chapter, it can be difficult to differentiate between type III and type V separations. Type III separations exhibit 100% superior displacement of the clavicle above the level of the coracoid process compared with the contralateral side. In contrast, type V separations exhibit superior dislocation of the AC joint radiographically of 100% to 300% compared with the uninjured side (**Figure 2**). Although it is difficult to differentiate between type III and type V injury solely on the basis of the shrug test, this test can be uncertainty regarding surgical versus nonsurgical management, early versus delayed management, anatomic versus nonanatomic repair, and arthroscopic versus open repair.

Surgical Versus Nonsurgical Management

Although it is generally agreed that type I and II lesions should be managed nonsurgically, many differing opinions exist regarding the best nonsurgical management. Nonsurgical management involves one of two options described by Rockwood: the use of a harness or sling to promote joint immobilization, or skillful neglect. Regardless of the option used, the goal of nonsurgical management is uninterrupted continuous pressure on the superior surface of the distal clavicle to allow ligamentous healing. On the other end of the spectrum, consensus regarding surgical management of type IV through VI injuries is based on the presence of extensive soft-tissue damage and substantial joint deformity.

Type III lesions present the greatest challenge in terms of determining the best management approach. Athletes require individualized evaluation, with treatment based on the demands placed on the shoulder (type of sport, position played), timing of the injury relative to the athletic season, and level of play. In the practice of the senior author, nonathletes with type III injuries are treated with 12 weeks of nonsurgical care and then are evaluated for pain and function. In nonathletes, surgery may be warranted to manage persistent pain and/or functional limitations after the period of initial nonsurgical management.

Early Versus Delayed Management

Few published studies have compared early with delayed surgical management of AC joint injuries. Of the 120 studies included in the systematic review discussed earlier in this chapter, only 4 reported data on early versus delayed treatment. These four retrospective reports suggested a benefit to early repair of AC injuries; however, the low quality of evidence and the varied methods of reconstruction led the authors of the systematic review to conclude that data were insufficient to determine optimal timing for intervention.

In the practice of the senior author, patients undergo 4 weeks of nonsurgical management to allow acute tears to heal on their own, followed by reevaluation of clinical symptoms. Tendon grafts or other biologic material are not used in acute repair because ruptured soft-tissue structures of the acutely injured AC joint are able to heal after reduction of the clavicle to the scapula. Tendon grafts are reserved for surgical management of chronic injury.

Anatomic Versus Nonanatomic Repair

For the purposes of this chapter, anatomic techniques are those that use graft or nonabsorbable suture to reproduce the stabilizing forces of the native conoid and trapezoid ligaments, and nonanatomic techniques are those that either reproduce a single CC ligament or are done using open reduction and internal fixation, which involves the use of hardware such as screws, pins, plates, and wires. Few outcomes studies comparing anatomic and nonanatomic procedures have been published. Although analysis of three studies that compared anatomic and nonanatomic repair suggests a slight favor for anatomic repair, the limited number of studies and their low level of evidence suggest the need for further research.

Arthroscopic Versus Open Repair

Several arthroscopic and open techniques have been described. Although joint visualization is believed to be increased in open procedures, proponents of arthroscopy note that visualization of the coracoid process remains limited even during open procedures and that there is a risk of damaging neurovascular structures during passage of the graft or suture with any type of procedure. Proponents of arthroscopy also note that arthroscopic exposure of the joint requires less soft-tissue dissection, which augments the healing process by promoting natural healing.

Conversely, despite the difficulty involved in exposing the coracoid process in open procedures, the visualization created during open repairs allows the surgeon to precisely dissect out the muscular insertions of the deltoid and trapezius onto the clavicle; this dissection is more difficult via an arthroscopic approach. In addition, the open incision allows for accurate measurement and placement of the clavicular tunnels, which has been reported to play an important role in the stability of the repair. In particular, the open technique allows proper repair of the deltotrapezial fascia. Although proponents of arthroscopy argue that the lack of soft-tissue disruption with the arthroscopic approach promotes the natural healing process, in higher grade AC lesions the deltotrapezial fascia often is disrupted, and proper repair and strengthening of the fascia provides stability to the repaired AC joint that is important to healing. The authors of this chapter are not aware of any study that compares the outcomes of open and arthroscopic procedures as the primary purpose of investigation. The authors of this chapter prefer open repair because it offers enhanced visualization for the placement of clavicular tunnels and facilitates proper repair of the deltotrapezial fascia.

Results

In the case presented in this chapter, radiographs obtained 37 months postoperatively demonstrated a 12-mm reduction in bilateral CC difference, from 15 mm preoperatively to 3 mm

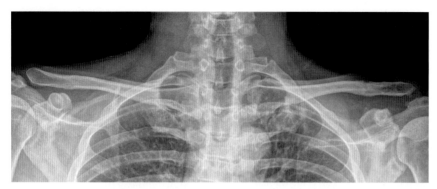

Figure 3   Bilateral Zanca radiograph obtained 37 months postoperatively demonstrates reduction in bilateral coracoacromial difference to 3 mm. The left (repaired) acromioclavicular joint displays some superior displacement of the clavicle secondary to graft loosening after reconstruction. Such displacement is concerning only if it is accompanied by clinical symptoms such as pain and/or weakness, which could indicate failure of the surgical repair. In this patient, the superior migration did not affect function or pain status.

postoperatively (**Figure 3**). Dramatic improvement also was noted clinically, with the Rowe score improving from 64 preoperatively to 100 postoperatively, the American Shoulder and Elbow Surgeons score improving from 53 preoperatively to 100 postoperatively, the Simple Shoulder Test score improving from 5 preoperatively to 12 postoperatively, and the Constant-Murley score improving from 56 preoperatively to 100 postoperatively. The postoperative Single Assessment Numeric Evaluation score was 100.

 Video 29.1 The Anatomic Coracoclavicular Reconstruction Technique (ACCR). John Apostolakos, BS; Michael B. O'Sullivan, MD; Monica Shoji, BA; Jessica DiVenere, BS; Mark P. Cote, DPT, MSCTR; Augustus D. Mazzocca, MS, MD (14 min)

 Technical Keys to Success

Based on the experience of the senior author and the results of multiple clinical and biomechanical studies on the AC joint, the authors of this chapter suggest the following anatomic principles to guide surgical management of the AC joint. First, it is important to respect the bony anatomy of the clavicle and acromion. That is, the surgeon should avoid substantial resection of the distal clavicle to prevent further instability of the joint. Second, the conoid and trapezoid ligaments should both be reconstructed to anatomically reproduce the stabilizing forces of the native CC ligaments. Finally, the reconstruction should be done in a manner that balances the need to reproduce the native three-dimensional motion pattern of the joint and the need for joint stability.

Setup/Exposure

- The operating room should be equipped with a standard operating room bed, a mini C-arm, and, if needed, the allograft preferred by the surgeon.
- After induction of anesthesia, the patient is placed in the beach-chair position and moved as far laterally on the table as can be tolerated. The ipsilateral arm should hang unimpeded at the patient's side to ensure adequate positioning and access to the surgical site.
- A bump is placed behind the ipsilateral scapula to improve surgical exposure by protracting and stabilizing the scapula.

- The patient is secured to the surgical table with a safety belt and taped as needed (**Figure 4**). The head and neck are kept relatively free to enable repositioning of the patient intraoperatively to improve exposure of the medial clavicle.
- After the patient is secured, the mini C-arm is brought in to ensure that adequate intraoperative imaging can be obtained. If imaging is suboptimal, patient positioning is reassessed.
- The patient is prepped with 2% chlorhexidine gluconate and 70% isopropyl alcohol solution and draped from the spine of the scapula posteriorly to the sternoclavicular joint medially.

Procedure
APPROACH

- The clavicle, acromion, AC joint, coracoid, and incision are marked.
- The incision is begun at the posterior aspect of the clavicle, approximately 3.5 cm medial to the AC joint, and extends inferiorly and laterally to the coracoid (**Figure 5**). If necessary to achieve adequate exposure, the incision can be extended toward the scapular spine posteriorly.
- After the skin is incised, a needle-tip Bovie electrocautery device (Bovie Medical) is used to complete the dissection and achieve strict hemostasis.
- Skin flaps are created at the level of the deltotrapezial fascia to aid in visualization.
- Self-retaining retractors can be inserted as needed to maintain exposure.
- The deltotrapezial fascia is incised in line with the clavicle along the intermuscular plane between the insertion of the trapezius on the posterior clavicle and the origin of the deltoid on the anterior clavicle.
- The fascial incision extends from

the midportion of the clavicle to the AC joint capsule laterally.

- The fascia is elevated off the clavicle in full-thickness flaps and tagged with nonabsorbable polyester suture to ensure adequate wound closure (**Figure 6**).
- After the dissection is complete, an assistant attempts provisional reduction of the AC joint by lifting the patient's arm. This reduction is confirmed on direct visualization or under fluoroscopy.
- Any soft tissue or scar tissue interposed in the AC joint is freed to allow joint reduction.
- Depending on the degree and type of AC joint separation, it may be necessary to release the distal clavicle from beneath the coracoid, beneath the acromion, or from within the deltotrapezial fascia to achieve joint reduction.

CLAVICLE TUNNELS

- It may be necessary to turn the patient's head to the contralateral side or grasp the clavicle with a towel clip to improve exposure for tunnel preparation.
- After sufficient exposure of the clavicle and provisional reduction of the AC joint are attained, the tunnels are drilled from superior to inferior.
- Care must be taken to avoid plunging when placing guidewires or drilling tunnels.
- To create the conoid ligament tunnel, a guidewire is started 40 to 45 mm medial to the distal clavicle at the posterior aspect of the clavicle and directed toward the inferior clavicle.
- To create the trapezoid ligament tunnel, a second guidewire is started 20 to 25 mm medial to the distal clavicle. The guidewire should be inserted into the anterior aspect of the clavicle directed inferiorly.
- A 5.0-mm cannulated reamer is

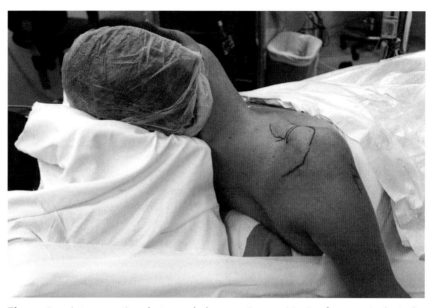

Figure 4   Intraoperative photograph shows patient positioning for acromioclavicular joint repair, with a bump placed beneath the ipsilateral shoulder to improve surgical exposure.

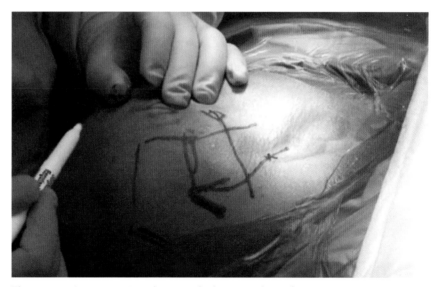

Figure 5   Intraoperative photograph shows markings for surgery to manage acromioclavicular joint injury. Markings of the borders of the acromion are shown on the left side of the photograph, and the circle at the top of the image marks the coracoid process. The vertical line that extends through the coracoid and the posterior aspect of the clavicle indicates the planned dissection site.

advanced over each guidewire until penetration of the distal cortex is achieved. Irrigation is used during drilling to prevent thermal necrosis. To prevent eccentric reaming,

the reamer is turned off, disconnected, and manually pulled out.

- A 5.5-mm tap is used in the conoid and trapezoid tunnels to create thread holes for the screw.

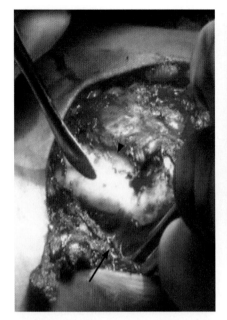

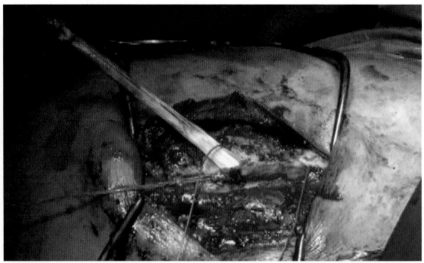

Figure 7   Intraoperative photograph shows a graft passed through both bone tunnels.

Figure 6   Intraoperative photograph shows the insertion of the trapezius muscle peeled back from the posterior clavicle (arrow). The deltoid insertion (arrowhead) has yet to be removed to achieve complete visualization of the clavicle.

GRAFT PREPARATION, PASSAGE, AND FIXATION

- The authors of this chapter prefer to use peroneus longus allograft for reconstruction.
- Looped high-strength, nonabsorbable suture is sewn through both ends of the graft; this tapers the graft edges to facilitate passage through the bone tunnel and serves as an internal brace during the healing process. This is considered to be the nonbiologic portion of the repair.
- The graft is passed using a curved suture passer, and a No. 2 high-strength, nonabsorbable suture is passed underneath the coracoid process. Although it is possible to pass the suture in either direction, the senior author prefers to pass the graft from medial to lateral under direct visualization.
- A suture passer is used to shuttle the graft from inferior to superior through the conoid tunnel. The

graft should fit snugly in the tunnel, and moderate force should be required to pass the graft.
- The graft is pulled until approximately 2 cm of graft exits the conoid tunnel superiorly.
- The remaining graft end is passed through the trapezoid tunnel in the same manner (**Figure 7**).
- To achieve anatomic reduction of the AC joint, as determined by the relationship of the distal end of the clavicle to the acromion, a clamp is used to achieve provisional anatomic fixation of the clavicle. Reduction is verified via direct visualization and radiographically using a mini C-arm.
- After adequate reduction is achieved using the clamp, both ends of the graft are cyclically tightened to remove slack from the system.
- The ends of the graft are held taught, and a 5.5- × 8-mm cannulated polyetheretherketone (PEEK) interference screw is placed in the anterior aspect of the conoid ligament tunnel.
- The graft is secured and then retensioned, after which a second 5.5- × 8-mm cannulated PEEK interference screw is placed in the

trapezoid ligament tunnel (**Figure 8**). The senior author of this chapter prefers to use screws measuring 8 mm in length.
- The No. 2 high-strength, nonabsorbable suture is passed through the cannulated PEEK screws and tied together to act as a nonbiologic splint.

AC Joint Reconstruction and Wound Closure

- After the graft is secured, the excess conoid graft tissue (short end) is sutured to the excess trapezoid graft tissue (long end) with high-strength, nonabsorbable suture (**Figure 9**).
- Primary repair of the AC joint capsule and ligaments is done with interrupted absorbable suture.
- The excess trapezoid graft is brought laterally to the AC joint. This graft is wrapped superiorly over the AC joint from medial to lateral and then posteriorly across the AC joint from lateral to medial, then sutured in place with high-strength, nonabsorbable suture to reinforce the AC joint repair.
- The deltotrapezial fascia is sutured closed with interrupted

nonabsorbable polyester suture.

- Braided absorbable suture is used for deep dermal closure, and absorbable monofilament suture is used for running subcuticular wound closure.

Rehabilitation

The rehabilitation protocol for anatomic coracoclavicular reconstruction is described in **Table 1**. The shoulder is immobilized in a platform brace for 6 to 8 weeks, and the patient is instructed to follow a home exercise program that consists of elbow, forearm, wrist, and hand exercises. At 8 weeks postoperatively, active-assisted range-of-motion exercises such as table or wall slides are initiated. Closed chain exercises such as table or wall slides have been shown to stimulate low amounts of shoulder muscle activity. At 12 weeks postoperatively, full range of motion is allowed and strength exercises are begun to target scapular stabilizers to help retract the scapula and thereby decrease the load across the AC joint. Patients may return to their sports activities and to work 24 to 28 weeks after surgery. Typically, peak strength is regained by 9 to 12 months postoperatively.

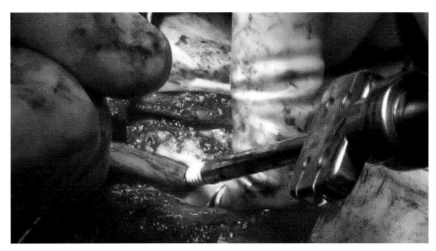

Figure 8   Intraoperative photograph shows fixation of the trapezoid ligament under tension.

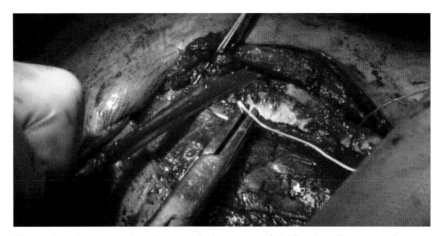

Figure 9   Intraoperative photograph shows superficial fixation of excess graft.

Avoiding Pitfalls

The surgeon must take care when raising skin flaps. In particular, the surgeon must avoid penetrating through the skin with vigorous dissection under electrocautery when raising the medial skin flap superior to the clavicle. The deltotrapezial fascia must be elevated carefully as well. The deltoid has a broad origin along the anterosuperior and inferior surfaces of the clavicle. During dissection, it is crucial to raise the deltotrapezial fascia as full-thickness flaps for wound closure by dissecting directly off the clavicle until the most inferior

margin is reached. To do this, the dissection must curve along the underside of the clavicle to prevent violation of the deltoid muscular substance.

Tunnels should measure 5 mm in diameter to prevent fracture of the clavicle. The tunnel that is too small for graft passage or screw placement should be re-reamed in 0.5-mm increments until sufficient diameter is achieved. Respectively, the conoid and trapezoid tunnels should be positioned 40 to 45 mm and 20 to 25 mm medial to the distal clavicle. Lateralization of the tunnels must be avoided because bone mineral density of the clavicle and the load-to-failure value decreases from medial to lateral. The bone tunnels must be placed

at least 2 cm apart to prevent fracture (**Figure 10**).

Graft options include peroneus longus allograft, tibialis anterior allograft, and semitendinosus allograft or autograft. The authors of this chapter prefer to use allograft in general to avoid donor site morbidity and issues related to patient positioning that are associated with graft harvest. The authors prefer peroneus longus allograft in particular because it is easily available and more appropriately sized than are the larger tibialis anterior and semitendinosus grafts.

Closure of the deltotrapezial fascia is imperative for adequate wound closure. Tagging sutures should be placed to aid

Table 1 Rehabilitation Protocol After Surgical Management of Acromioclavicular Joint Injury

Postoperative Week	ROM	Strengthening	Return to Sports/Work	Comments
0-8	Elbow, forearm, wrist, and hand motion are allowed as part of an HEP	None	None	The shoulder is immobilized in a platform brace that supports the AC joint and protects it from the pull of gravity. The patient is instructed to remove the brace only for self-care and to do the HEP.
8-12	Active-assisted, progressing to active as pain allows	Closed chain scapular exercises and kinetic chain activities	None	Rehabilitation primarily is focused on restoration of ROM and scapular control. Motions that may increase stress on the AC joint, specifically internal rotation behind the back, cross-body adduction, and end-range forward elevation, should be initiated cautiously and only as pain allows. Resistance strengthening exercises are avoided.
12-24	Full	Rowing exercises using resistance bands, progressing to isotonic scapular strength exercises (Blackburn exercises)	None	Strength exercises should target the scapular muscles to promote stabilization and retraction of the scapula, thereby decreasing the load across the AC joint. When the patient can demonstrate active forward elevation without scapular asymmetry (that is, symmetric protraction of the medial border of the scapula during shoulder flexion and upward rotation and retraction during abduction), T exercises and Y exercises are prescribed.
24	Full	No restrictions	Full-contact sports and heavy labor are allowed	Higher-load exercises, including shoulder press, bench press, pullovers, and pectoral fly exercises are begun. Full-contact sports are not allowed until week 24.

AC = acromioclavicular, HEP = home exercise program, ROM = range of motion.

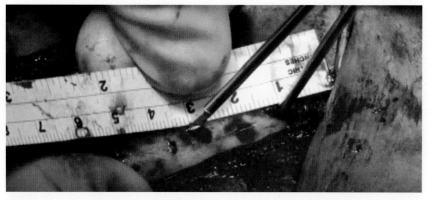

Figure 10 Intraoperative photograph shows measurement of the 20-mm distance between the bone tunnels drilled to receive the coracoclavicular ligament.

in reapproximation. Nonabsorbable polyester suture should be used for this layer. Knots should be tied as far posteriorly as possible to prevent skin irritation. During reconstruction of the AC joint capsule and ligaments, the excess trapezoid graft tissue should be used to reinforce the repair to provide increased horizontal stability. The authors of this chapter avoid performing distal clavicle resection in conjunction with anatomic CC ligament reconstruction because of the risk of increased anterior-to-posterior instability at the AC joint.

Bibliography

Beitzel K, Cote MP, Apostolakos J, et al: Current concepts in the treatment of acromioclavicular joint dislocations. *Arthroscopy* 2013;29(2):387-397.

Beitzel K, Obopilwe E, Apostolakos J, et al: Rotational and translational stability of different methods for direct acromioclavicular ligament repair in anatomic acromioclavicular joint reconstruction. *Am J Sports Med* 2014;42(9):2141-2148.

Beitzel K, Obopilwe E, Chowaniec DM, et al: Biomechanical comparison of arthroscopic repairs for acromioclavicular joint instability: Suture button systems without biological augmentation. *Am J Sports Med* 2011;39(10):2218-2225.

Beitzel K, Obopilwe E, Chowaniec DM, et al: Biomechanical properties of repairs for dislocated AC joints using suture button systems with integrated tendon augmentation. *Knee Surg Sports Traumatol Arthrosc* 2012;20(10):1931-1938.

Beitzel K, Sablan N, Chowaniec DM, et al: Sequential resection of the distal clavicle and its effects on horizontal acromioclavicular joint translation. *Am J Sports Med* 2012;40(3):681-685.

Bishop JY, Kaeding C: Treatment of the acute traumatic acromioclavicular separation. *Sports Med Arthrosc* 2006;14(4):237-245.

Carofino BC, Mazzocca AD: The anatomic coracoclavicular ligament reconstruction: Surgical technique and indications. *J Shoulder Elbow Surg* 2010;19(2 suppl):37-46.

Cote MP, Wojcik KE, Gomlinski G, Mazzocca AD: Rehabilitation of acromioclavicular joint separations: Operative and nonoperative considerations. *Clin Sports Med* 2010;29(2):213-228, vii.

Eschler A, Gradl G, Gierer P, Mittlmeier T, Beck M: Hook plate fixation for acromioclavicular joint separations restores coracoclavicular distance more accurately than PDS augmentation, however presents with a high rate of acromial osteolysis. *Arch Orthop Trauma Surg* 2012;132(1):33-39.

Fraschini G, Ciampi P, Scotti C, Ballis R, Peretti GM: Surgical treatment of chronic acromioclavicular dislocation: Comparison between two surgical procedures for anatomic reconstruction. *Injury* 2010;41(11):1103-1106.

Geaney LE, Beitzel K, Chowaniec DM, et al: Graft fixation is highest with anatomic tunnel positioning in acromioclavicular reconstruction. *Arthroscopy* 2013;29(3):434-439.

Mazzocca AD, Arciero RA, Bicos J: Evaluation and treatment of acromioclavicular joint injuries. *Am J Sports Med* 2007;35(2):316-329.

Mazzocca AD, Santangelo SA, Johnson ST, Rios CG, Dumonski ML, Arciero RA: A biomechanical evaluation of an anatomical coracoclavicular ligament reconstruction. *Am J Sports Med* 2006;34(2):236-246.

Mazzocca AD, Spang JT, Rodriguez RR, et al: Biomechanical and radiographic analysis of partial coracoclavicular ligament injuries. *Am J Sports Med* 2008;36(7):1397-1402.

Murena L, Canton G, Vulcano E, Cherubino P: Scapular dyskinesis and SICK scapula syndrome following surgical treatment of type III acute acromioclavicular dislocations. *Knee Surg Sports Traumatol Arthrosc* 2013;21(5):1146-1150.

Rios CG, Mazzocca AD: Acromioclavicular joint problems in athletes and new methods of management. *Clin Sports Med* 2008;27(4):763-788.

Rockwood C, Green D: *Fractures in Adults,* ed 2. Philadelphia, PA, Lippincott, 1984.

Salzmann GM, Walz L, Buchmann S, Glabgly P, Venjakob A, Imhoff AB: Arthroscopically assisted 2-bundle anatomical reduction of acute acromioclavicular joint separations. *Am J Sports Med* 2010;38(6):1179-1187.

Tauber M, Gordon K, Koller H, Fox M, Resch H: Semitendinosus tendon graft versus a modified Weaver-Dunn procedure for acromioclavicular joint reconstruction in chronic cases: A prospective comparative study. *Am J Sports Med* 2009;37(1):181-190.

Trainer G, Arciero RA, Mazzocca AD: Practical management of grade III acromioclavicular separations. *Clin J Sport Med* 2008;18(2):162-166.

Wise MB, Uhl TL, Mattacola CG, Nitz AJ, Kibler WB: The effect of limb support on muscle activation during shoulder exercises. *J Shoulder Elbow Surg* 2004;13(6):614-620.

 Video Reference

Apostolakos J, O'Sullivan MB, Shoji M, DiVenere J, Cote MP, Mazzocca AD: Video. *The Anatomic Coracoclavicular Reconstruction Technique (ACCR).* Farmington, CT, 2015.

Chapter 30

Sternoclavicular Joint Reconstruction for the Management of Anterior and Posterior Sternoclavicular Joint Instability

John E. Kuhn, MD, MS

 ## Case Presentation

A 15-year-old, right-hand–dominant boy has a recurrent sternoclavicular joint injury resulting from a traumatic injury 1 year previously. The initial injury occurred during a wrestling meet in which the patient's opponent jumped on him, forcing the patient to fall onto his right side. The patient immediately developed posterior pain in his right shoulder and was subsequently referred for treatment. At the time of the initial physical examination, the patient had no difficulty breathing, and the neurovascular status of his upper extremity was normal. A posterior Salter-Harris type II fracture-dislocation of the clavicle was demonstrated on advanced imaging, which included radiographs, a CT scan, and a three-dimensional CT reconstruction (**Figure 1**). The patient was treated with open reduction that included primary repair of the capsule and periosteum using nonabsorbable sutures. The patient's shoulder was immobilized postoperatively, and activity was prohibited for 5 weeks. At 3 months postoperatively, the patient reported some tenderness at the sternoclavicular joint, and a 12-week course of physical therapy was prescribed. Seven months postoperatively, the patient developed prominence, a popping sensation, and pain, and a repeated CT scan demonstrated slight posterior subluxation of the joint (**Figure 2**).

Approximately 1 year postoperatively, the patient experienced pain and a popping sensation in the sternoclavicular joint while playing basketball. On presentation to the clinic of the author of this chapter, the patient describes some numbness and tingling in the ulnar digits of the right hand. Persistent posterior subluxation of the sternoclavicular joint is noted on CT (**Figure 3**). The patient's symptoms include substantial pain with shoulder motion, resulting in absences from school and difficulty sleeping. On physical examination, the patient demonstrates mild static scapular winging, and the scapular assistance test yields positive results. Motion of the clavicular head is noted with elevation of the arm from a resting posterior position to an anterior reduced position. A scapula brace and a second 12-week course of physical therapy focused on strengthening the serratus and lower trapezius muscles is prescribed. As a result of the physical therapy, the patient's symptoms worsen, and his function is limited by pain. Based on the clinical findings, reconstruction of the sternoclavicular joint using a figure-of-8 semitendinosus autograft is identified as the best treatment option.

 ## Indications

Reconstruction of the sternoclavicular joint is indicated to manage acute, irreducible posterior dislocations and chronic posterior dislocations. A patient with chronic, anterior instability with substantial symptoms also may benefit from reconstruction of the sternoclavicular joint.

Three of the most popular procedures used to reconstruct the sternoclavicular joint are the Burrows technique (transfer of the subclavius tendon; **Figure 4**), transfer of the intra-articular disk and ligament into the resected end of the clavicle as described by Rockwood (**Figure 5**), and reconstruction of the anterior and posterior capsules using a figure-of-8 semitendinosus autograft as described later in this chapter. The figure-of-8 reconstruction has substantially better mechanical properties compared with the other reconstruction techniques; for this reason, it is the preferred technique of the author of this chapter.

Dr. Kuhn or an immediate family member serves as a board member, owner, officer, or committee member of the American Orthopaedic Society for Sports Medicine and the American Shoulder and Elbow Surgeons.

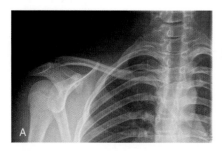 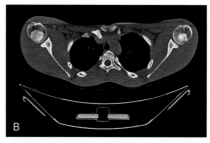 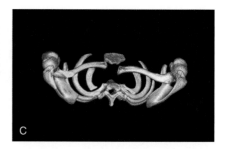

Figure 1 Initial advanced imaging of the upper extremity of a 15-year-old boy with a recurrent sternoclavicular joint injury. Initial radiograph (**A**), CT scan (**B**), and three-dimensional CT reconstruction (**C**) demonstrate a Salter-Harris type II fracture through the physis of the right medial clavicle with posterior displacement of the right clavicle shaft.

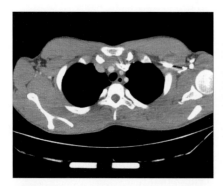

Figure 2 Axial CT scan of an upper extremity demonstrates posterior subluxation of the clavicular head 7 months after open reduction and primary repair of the capsule and periosteum with nonabsorbable sutures. Fracture healing is evident.

 ## Contraindications

Atraumatic, voluntary sternoclavicular joint instability is a contraindication to surgery. The presence of a connective tissue disorder, such as Ehlers-Danlos syndrome, is a relative contraindication to surgery.

 ## Controversies and Alternative Approaches

Various surgical techniques have been described for reconstruction of the sternoclavicular joint. Resection of the sternal head of the clavicle yields poor results in the management of anterior and posterior sternoclavicular joint instability. Techniques to reconstruct the

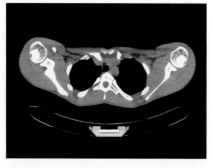

Figure 3 Axial CT scan of an upper extremity demonstrates posterior subluxation of the right clavicular head 1 year postoperatively.

ligamentous structures have included tendon grafts, fascial loops, and synthetic substitutes. Myoplasty, tenodesis of the sternal head of the sternocleidomastoid muscle, and tenodesis of the subclavius tendon also have been described. In the management of acute instability, the reduced sternoclavicular joint has been held with large-bore cannulated screws, temporary screws with an anterior plate, and external fixation. Historically, the use of temporary Kirschner wires or Steinmann pins was recommended; however, this method is currently contraindicated because the pins have been reported to break and migrate into vital structures, resulting in severe and even fatal injuries.

 ## Results

The literature describing the figure-of-8 autograft technique and its

modifications is summarized in **Table 1**. Modifications to the technique include alterations to the manner of weaving the tendon and the use of allograft and double-loaded suture anchors. Decreased pain and improved shoulder function with return to sports (including contact sports) are typically achieved with the figure-of-8 technique. The largest study included 27 patients, and the results demonstrated considerable improvement in patient-reported outcome scores. In that study, surgical complications included failure, donor site morbidity, and discomfort at the surgical site in some patients.

 ## Technical Keys to Success

The figure-of-8 hamstring autograft technique for the reconstruction of chronic sternoclavicular joint dislocation is performed in an anatomic region in which vital retrosternal vascular and other structures are at substantial risk. This procedure must be performed with the assistance of a thoracic surgeon. The thoracic surgeon is instrumental in developing the retrosternal plane and helping to pass sutures, which are then used to pass the graft. The presence of a thoracic surgeon also is vital because chronic and acute sternoclavicular joint dislocations may include vascular injury that is not apparent until the clavicle is reduced.

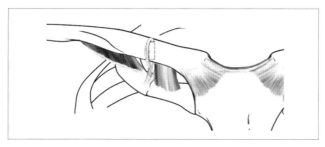

Figure 4   Illustration shows the Burrows technique for reconstruction of the sternoclavicular joint. The tendon of the subclavius muscle is dissected from the muscle belly, leaving its insertion on the first rib intact. The tendon of the subclavius muscle is passed through a drill hole in the anterior clavicle and secured to itself. (Adapted with permission from Spencer EE Jr, Kuhn JE: Biomechanical analysis of reconstructions for sternoclavicular joint instability. *J Bone Joint Surg Am* 2004;86[1]:98-105.)

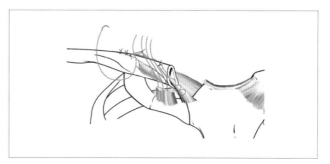

Figure 5   Illustration shows the step in the Rockwood technique for reconstruction of the sternoclavicular joint in which the medial end of the clavicle is resected, the intra-articular disk and ligaments are passed into the intramedullary space, and sutures are passed through small drill holes on the top of the clavicle and tied. (Adapted with permission from Spencer EE Jr, Kuhn JE: Biomechanical analysis of reconstructions for sternoclavicular joint instability. *J Bone Joint Surg Am* 2004;86[1]:98-105.)

Table 1   Results of Figure-of-8 Graft Techniques for the Management of Sternoclavicular Joint Instability

Authors	Journal (Year)	Technique (No. of Patients)	Outcomes	Failure Rate (%)	Comments
Standard technique					
Bae et al	*J Pediatr Orthop* (2006)	Semitendinosus figure-of-8 (8), reconstruction with sternocleidomastoid fascia (1)	Mean SST score improved to 10.9	0	Mean follow-up, 55 mo
Singer et al	*J Shoulder Elbow Surg* (2013)	Figure-of-8 hamstring autograft (6)	Mean DASH score improved 25 points No recurrence of instability	16.7	Follow-up, >22 mo All patients returned to full activity, including contact sports The 1 failure consisted of postoperative infection
Modified technique					
Guan and Wolf	*J Shoulder Elbow Surg* (2013)	Hamstring autograft placed in Roman numeral X pattern anteriorly using figure-of-8 strands as well as transverse strands placed inferiorly and superiorly (6)	No pain in 5 patients, mild pain in 1 (VAS score)	16.7	Mean follow-up, 40 mo All patients returned to preoperative activities, including sports The 1 failure occurred 4 yr postoperatively
Bak and Fogh	*J Shoulder Elbow Surg* (2014)	Suture anchor placed in the sternum: palmaris autograft (7), gracilis autograft (25)	Median WOSI score improved 31%	7.4	Median follow-up, 54 mo 5 patients were lost to follow-up 68% of patients had donor site morbidity 40% of patients had some discomfort at the surgical site
Sabatini et al	*J Shoulder Elbow Surg* (2015)	Figure-of-8 allograft with tenodesis screws (10)	Mean ASES score improved 49 points	30	Mean follow-up, 38 mo 1 postoperative hematoma, 1 postoperative superficial infection, 1 patient had pain and osteoarthritis

ASES = American Shoulder and Elbow Surgeons-shoulder outcome; DASH = Disabilities of the Arm, Shoulder and Hand; SST = Simple Shoulder Test; VAS = visual analog scale; WOSI = Western Ontario Shoulder Instability Index.

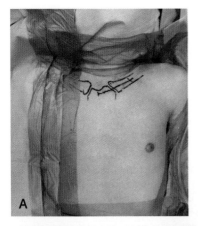

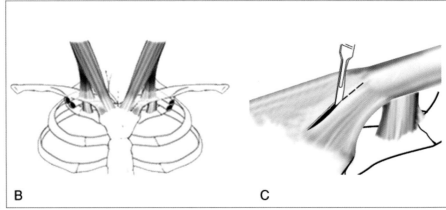

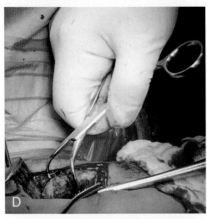

Figure 6 Images depict steps related to incision in reconstruction of the sterno-clavicular joint. **A,** Intraoperative photograph shows the outlines of the clavicle and ma-nubrium as well as the planned incision marks in preparation for incision of the anterior capsule of the joint parallel to the clavicle and dissection of the anterior capsule from the clavicle and manubrium. **B** and **C,** Illustrations show the skin incision made follow-ing Langer lines, following a necklace-shaped pattern over the sternoclavicular joint. **D,** Intraoperative photograph shows the medial shaft of the clavicle after it has been mobilized and moved anteriorly. Gentle technique is used to leave tissue for later clo-sure. (Panels B and C reproduced from Kuhn JE: Sternoclavicular joint reconstruction for chronic dislocation, in Zuckerman JD, ed: *Advanced Reconstruction: Shoulder*. Rosemont, IL, American Academy of Orthopaedic Surgeons, 2007, pp 255-262.)

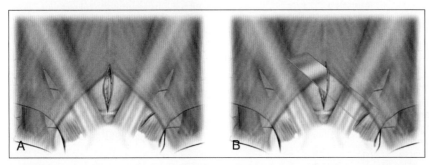

Figure 7 Illustrations show the steps for incision in the sternal notch and substernal dissection. **A,** The platysma muscle above the sternal notch is incised vertically, similar to the approach for a mediastinoscopy. Blunt dissection with a finger is performed to free the soft tissues from the back of the manubrium and sternoclavicular joint. **B,** A malleable ribbon retractor is placed behind the sternoclavicular joint. (Reproduced from Kuhn JE: Sternoclavicular joint reconstruction for chronic dislocation, in Zuckerman JD, ed: *Advanced Reconstruction: Shoulder*. Rosemont, IL, American Academy of Orthopaedic Surgeons, 2007, pp 255-262.)

Setup/Exposure

- General anesthesia is administered.
- The patient is placed in the supine position, with a small towel placed beneath the spine between the scapulae.
- The entire chest and neck are prepared and draped free. Wide exposure is recommended in case injury to substernal structures occurs.

Procedure

- An incision is made along the Langer lines, which follow a necklace-shaped curve over the sternoclavicular joint to the midline (**Figure 6, A**).
- The skin and subcutaneous tissues are undermined to identify the pla-tysma muscle, which is incised and reflected in the same direction as the skin incision. The sternoclei-domastoid muscle and the sternal notch are exposed (**Figure 6, B**).
- The capsule of the sternoclavicular joint is incised, and the medial head of the clavicle is exposed and re-duced (**Figure 6, C**).
- The retrosternal space is exposed. This step is usually performed by

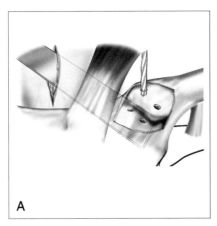 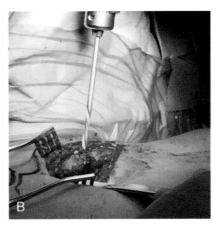 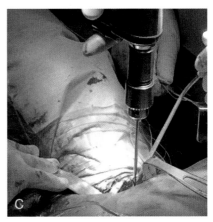

Figure 8   Illustration (**A**) and intraoperative photograph (**B**) of a sternoclavicular joint show proper placement of four parallel drill holes using a 0.25-inch drill bit. Two holes are drilled in the clavicle, and two holes are drilled in the manubrium. **C,** Intraoperative photograph of a sternoclavicular joint shows a malleable ribbon retractor placed behind the joint to protect the underlying structures during drilling. (Panel A reproduced from Kuhn JE: Sternoclavicular joint reconstruction for chronic dislocation, in Zuckerman JD, ed: *Advanced Reconstruction: Shoulder.* Rosemont, IL, American Academy of Orthopaedic Surgeons, 2007, pp 255-262.)

a thoracic surgeon. A vertical incision is made in the platysma muscle above the sternal notch (**Figure 7, A**).

- The retrosternal tissue is bluntly dissected from the back of the sternum using a finger in a sweeping motion. The back of the sternum and the back of the medial clavicle must be cleared of all underlying soft tissue. A malleable ribbon retractor may be placed behind the sternoclavicular joint to protect the underlying structures during drilling (**Figure 7, B**).

- A 0.25-inch drill is used to create two holes in the medial clavicle and two parallel holes in the manubrium behind the subchondral plate of the articular surface of the joint (**Figure 8, A** and **B**). To avoid plunging the drill into the mediastinum, the drill is advanced slowly, and the malleable ribbon retractor or a finger is placed behind the sternoclavicular joint (**Figure 8, C**). The drill also may be used to start the hole in the distal cortex. A curette can be inserted to gently complete the drill hole. The drill holes are placed as parallel as possible to prevent rotation of the clavicle as

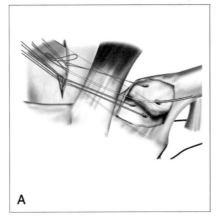 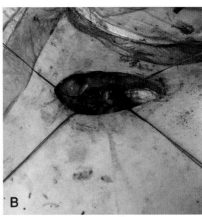

Figure 9   Illustration (**A**) and intraoperative photograph (**B**) of a sternoclavicular joint show four loops of No. 2 permanent suture passed through the drill holes and out through the incision in the sternal notch. These loops of suture will be used to pass the tendon graft later in the procedure. (Panel A reproduced from Kuhn JE: Sternoclavicular joint reconstruction for chronic dislocation, in Zuckerman JD, ed: *Advanced Reconstruction: Shoulder.* Rosemont, IL, American Academy of Orthopaedic Surgeons, 2007, pp 255-262.)

the graft is secured later in the procedure. Some patients have symptoms with anterior subluxation, and the author of this chapter has used a technique in which two unicortical holes are drilled in the manubrium and clavicle without drilling through the posterior cortex. When this approach is used, the graft is passed in a box-shaped pattern.

- A smooth wire loop or a suture passer is inserted into one of the drill holes (**Figure 9, A**). The bent end of the wire is identified behind the sternoclavicular joint and delivered through the incision above the scapular notch. A loop of No. 2 suture is passed through the hole; this suture will be used later in the procedure to pass the tendon graft. This step is repeated for the two drill holes in the manubrium

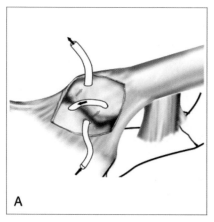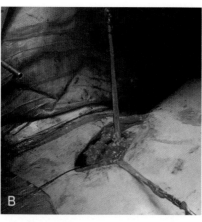

Figure 10 Illustration (**A**) and intraoperative photograph (**B**) of a sternoclavicular joint show a semitendinosus graft passed in a figure-of-8 fashion. The arrows depict the direction of graft passage. The graft is passed so that the parallel limbs of the graft are on the side of the direction of the instability (in this case, posterior). (Panel A reproduced from Kuhn JE: Sternoclavicular joint reconstruction for chronic dislocation, in Zuckerman JD, ed: *Advanced Reconstruction: Shoulder.* Rosemont, IL, American Academy of Orthopaedic Surgeons, 2007, pp 255-262.)

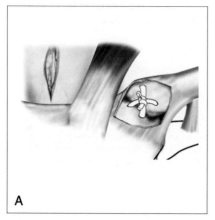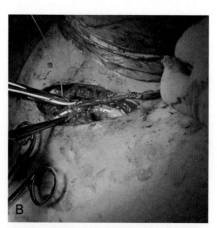

Figure 11 Illustration (**A**) and intraoperative photograph (**B**) of a sternoclavicular joint show the graft tied in a knot and secured to itself with No. 2 permanent sutures. (Panel A reproduced from Kuhn JE: Sternoclavicular joint reconstruction for chronic dislocation, in Zuckerman JD, ed: *Advanced Reconstruction: Shoulder.* Rosemont, IL, American Academy of Orthopaedic Surgeons, 2007, pp 255-262.)

and the two drill holes in the clavicle, for a total of four loops of suture (**Figure 9, B**).

- A semitendinosus graft is harvested. The author of this chapter prefers to use autograft if possible; however, an allograft can be used. The graft is passed in a figure-of-8 fashion such that the parallel fibers are on the side of the sternoclavicular joint instability because the parallel orientation of the graft strands is a

more stable construct (**Figure 10**). Occasionally, it is necessary to widen the drill holes using a curet to facilitate graft passage.

- The graft is tied and sutured to itself with the sternoclavicular joint reduced (**Figure 11**). Overtightening of the graft must be avoided because it can lead to limited joint motion and/or static scapular winging resulting from rotational positioning of the clavicle.

Wound Closure

- After the graft is secured, the capsule is repaired with permanent sutures. If the sternal head of the sternocleidomastoid muscle was detached during exposure, then the sternal head must be securely and anatomically repaired (**Figure 12**).
- The subcutaneous tissues and skin are closed.

Rehabilitation

Patients are discharged from the hospital after they are in a stable condition and comfortable, usually 1 to 2 days postoperatively. The postoperative rehabilitation protocol is outlined in **Table 2**. The shoulder is immobilized in a brace. For a patient with posterior instability, the scapula should be retracted, and the patient should be fitted with a figure-of-8 brace or a sling with a pillow that maintains the arm in external rotation (to prevent it from crossing the midline). For a patient with anterior instability, the scapula should be protracted, and use of a sling and swathe is recommended. The author of this chapter recommends that patients with both anterior and posterior instability use a sling for 8 weeks postoperatively, after which the sling may be worn for comfort only.

Passive range of motion is begun at 6 weeks postoperatively, and active range of motion is begun at 8 weeks postoperatively. Patients are expected to achieve normal motion approximately 12 weeks postoperatively. Strengthening exercises can be initiated at 12 weeks postoperatively and progressed as tolerated by the patient. Patients can return to normal work or sports activity (including contact sports) after approximately 5 months. There are no permanent restrictions from activity.

Avoiding Pitfalls

Complications are relatively rare with the figure-of-8 procedure, but they can be life-threatening because of the proximity of several vital structures in the retrosternal area. The assistance of a thoracic surgeon is critical to avoid complications during the retrosternal dissection. A sternum saw should be readily available intraoperatively in case damage to the great vessels is encountered, requiring rapid access. In addition, the use of a malleable retractor behind the sternum and clavicle prevents penetrating injuries during drilling and suture passage.

To gain normal motion after surgery and to prevent rotational misalignment of the clavicle, drill holes should

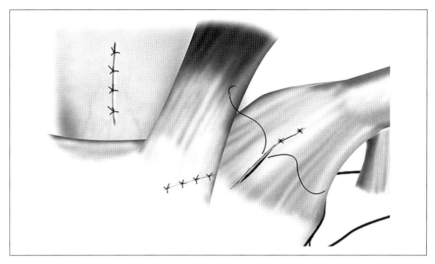

Figure 12 Illustration of a sternoclavicular joint shows closure of the anterior capsule and repair of the sternocleidomastoid muscle. The anterior capsule is closed over the construct with No. 2 permanent sutures. If the sternocleidomastoid muscle has been incised for exposure, then it must be repaired. (Reproduced from Kuhn JE: Sternoclavicular joint reconstruction for chronic dislocation, in Zuckerman JD, ed: *Advanced Reconstruction: Shoulder*. Rosemont, IL, American Academy of Orthopaedic Surgeons, 2007, pp 255-262.)

Table 2 Rehabilitation Protocol After Anterior and Posterior Sternoclavicular Joint Reconstruction

Postoperative Week	ROM	Strengthening	Return to Play	Comments/Emphasis
0-8	None for the first 5 wk. At 6 wk, passive ROM is begun; however, the patient should avoid extremes of extension and cross-body adduction	None	None	The patient's shoulder is immobilized to prevent scapular motion. For posterior instability, a figure-of-8 brace or sling with a pillow that places the arm in external rotation is used. For anterior instability, a sling and swathe that places the arm in internal rotation is used.
8-12	Active ROM is begun at 8 wk	None	None	Sling is worn for comfort only
12-16	Full shoulder motion is expected at 12 wk	Strengthening is begun at 12 wk and progressed as tolerated. Strengthening should include periscapular muscles, especially the lower trapezius muscles.	—	Immobilization is discontinued
16-20	Full	Progressed as tolerated	Sport-specific drills are begun	—
20-24	Full	Progressed as tolerated	Return to play (including contact sports)	—

ROM = range of motion.

be placed parallel to each other and perpendicular to the sternum. Use of parallel drill holes will prevent uneven tensioning of the graft, which may cause a rotational moment to the clavicle or restrict motion. Similarly, the surgeon must be careful to avoid overtensioning the graft, which may make the restoration of motion at the sternoclavicular joint difficult.

Occasionally, in patients with chronic sternoclavicular dislocations, the sternoclavicular joint is filled with scarring, and the cartilage on the medial head of the clavicle is of poor quality. In these patients, the end of the clavicle may be resected, and the space in the sternoclavicular joint may be filled with either a tendon graft or an allograft tendon tissue rolled into the shape of an anchovy.

Bibliography

Acus RW III, Bell RH, Fisher DL: Proximal clavicle excision: An analysis of results. *J Shoulder Elbow Surg* 1995;4(3):182-187.

Bae DS, Kocher MS, Waters PM, Micheli LM, Griffey M, Dichtel L: Chronic recurrent anterior sternoclavicular joint instability: Results of surgical management. *J Pediatr Orthop* 2006;26(1):71-74.

Bak K, Fogh K: Reconstruction of the chronic anterior unstable sternoclavicular joint using a tendon autograft: Medium-term to long-term follow-up results. *J Shoulder Elbow Surg* 2014;23(2):245-250.

Booth CM, Roper BA: Chronic dislocation of the sternoclavicular joint: An operative repair. *Clin Orthop Relat Res* 1979;(140):17-20.

Brinker MR, Bartz RL, Reardon PR, Reardon MJ: A method for open reduction and internal fixation of the unstable posterior sternoclavicular joint dislocation. *J Orthop Trauma* 1997;11(5):378-381.

Burrows HJ: Tenodesis of subclavius in the treatment of recurrent dislocation of the sterno-clavicular joint. *J Bone Joint Surg Br* 1951;33(2):240-243.

Cooper GJ, Stubbs D, Waller DA, Wilkinson GA, Saleh M: Posterior sternoclavicular dislocation: A novel method of external fixation. *Injury* 1992;23(8):565-566.

Eskola A, Vainionpää S, Vastamäki M, Slätis P, Rokkanen P: Operation for old sternoclavicular dislocation: Results in 12 cases. *J Bone Joint Surg Br* 1989;71(1):63-65.

Guan JJ, Wolf BR: Reconstruction for anterior sternoclavicular joint dislocation and instability. *J Shoulder Elbow Surg* 2013;22(6):775-781.

Leighton RK, Buhr AJ, Sinclair AM: Posterior sternoclavicular dislocations. *Can J Surg* 1986;29(2):104-106.

Lunseth PA, Chapman KW, Frankel VH: Surgical treatment of chronic dislocation of the sterno-clavicular joint. *J Bone Joint Surg Br* 1975;57(2):193-196.

Lyons FA, Rockwood CA Jr: Migration of pins used in operations on the shoulder. *J Bone Joint Surg Am* 1990;72(8):1262-1267.

Martínez A, Rodríguez A, González G, Herrera A, Domingo J: Atraumatic spontaneous posterior subluxation of the sternoclavicular joint. *Arch Orthop Trauma Surg* 1999;119(5-6):344-346.

Reilly P, Bruguera JA, Copeland SA: Erosion and nonunion of the first rib after sternoclavicular reconstruction with Dacron. *J Shoulder Elbow Surg* 1999;8(1):76-78.

Rockwood CA Jr, Groh GI, Wirth MA, Grassi FA: Resection arthroplasty of the sternoclavicular joint. *J Bone Joint Surg Am* 1997;79(3):387-393.

Sabatini JB, Shung JR, Clay B, Oladeji LO, Minnich DJ, Ponce BA: Outcomes of augmented allograft figure-of-eight sternoclavicular joint reconstruction. *J Shoulder Elbow Surg* 2015;24(6):902-907.

Singer G, Ferlic P, Kraus T, Eberl R: Reconstruction of the sternoclavicular joint in active patients with the figure-of-eight technique using hamstrings. *J Shoulder Elbow Surg* 2013;22(1):64-69.

Spencer EE Jr, Kuhn JE: Biomechanical analysis of reconstructions for sternoclavicular joint instability. *J Bone Joint Surg Am* 2004;86(1):98-105.

SECTION 5
The Stiff Shoulder
Jeffrey S. Abrams, MD

Chapter 31

Arthroscopic Capsular Release for the Management of Adhesive Capsulitis

Bruce S. Miller, MD, MS

 ## Introduction

Supportive observation is the mainstay in the management of adhesive capsulitis. Pain can be managed with oral analgesics and intermittent intra-articular corticosteroid injections. As the patient's pain decreases, a gentle stretching program, either a therapist-led program or a self-directed home program, may be considered.

Additional intervention should be reserved for truly recalcitrant cases. In patients requiring intervention, the two most common treatment options are manipulation under anesthesia and arthroscopic capsular release followed by manipulation. In general, patients with adhesive capsulitis should be treated with supportive therapies for 6 months before an intervention, either manipulation or surgical release, is considered. The author of this chapter prefers arthroscopic capsular release followed by manipulation over manipulation alone for several reasons. An arthroscopic approach allows the surgeon to perform selected releases dictated by the patient's physical examination and allows for release of the biceps tendon (described later in this chapter). In addition, iatrogenic

complications such as proximal humerus fractures, nerve injuries, and rotator cuff tears may be less likely to occur when releases are performed before manipulation.

 ## Case Presentation

A 49-year-old woman has a 2-year history of shoulder pain and stiffness. She describes an insidious onset of increasing pain that was followed by increasing stiffness. Although the pain has subsided over the past few months, she continues to have limited shoulder motion with resultant dysfunction. Two intra-articular corticosteroid injections have provided substantial, but transient, pain relief. She has grown increasingly frustrated with her shoulder dysfunction and desires an intervention that might accelerate her recovery. Her medical history is notable for diabetes mellitus, which has been controlled by diet, and lack of thyroid disorders.

Physical examination demonstrates marked restriction of range of motion, with both active and passive forward elevation to 95°, external rotation with the arm at the side to 10°, external rotation in the abducted position to 45°,

and internal rotation to the belt line. The patient describes substantial pain at the extremes of motion.

The patient underwent arthroscopic capsular release followed by manipulation under anesthesia, as described later. Six weeks after this intervention, the patient demonstrated marked improvement in both pain and function. At 3 months postoperatively, the patient was pain-free and demonstrated near symmetric motion and was discharged from care.

 ## Indications

The indications for intervention in the management of adhesive capsulitis should take into account the natural history of this disorder, which often includes spontaneous resolution. Thus, most patients with adhesive capsulitis should be treated nonsurgically. However, patients are often frustrated by the unpredictable nature of this resolution, as well as by the magnitude of dysfunction that can be associated with severe pain and stiffness of the shoulder. In addition, adhesive capsulitis can have a recalcitrant course in patients with diabetes. A recent systematic review suggests that patients with risk factors such as diabetes mellitus benefit from early surgical treatment.

Neither Dr. Miller nor any immediate family member has received anything of value from or has stock or stock options held in a commercial company or institution related directly or indirectly to the subject of this chapter.

Table 1 Results From Select Studies From a Systematic Review of Manipulation Versus Capsular Release in the Management of Recalcitrant Adhesive Capsulitis

Author(s)	Journal (Year)	Technique	Outcomes[a]
Chen et al	*Kaohsiung J Med Sci* (2002)	Capsular release and MUA	FE, 42° ERS, 35° IRA, 30° ASES, 46
Jerosch	*Knee Surg Sports Traumatol Arthrosc* (2001)	Capsular release and MUA	ABD, 92° ERS, 64° ERA, 81° IRA, 46° Constant score, 41
Elhassan et al	*J Shoulder Elbow Surg* (2010)	Capsular release	FE, 40° ERS, 21° Constant score, 55
Ramesh et al	*Journal of Orthopaedic Medicine* (2003)	MUA	FE, 139° ERS, 32°
Kivimäki et al	*J Shoulder Elbow Surg* (2007)	MUA	FE, 53° ABD, 83° ERS, 47°
Jacobs et al	*J Shoulder Elbow Surg* (2009)	MUA	Constant score, 42

ABD = abduction, ASES = American Shoulder and Elbow Surgeons shoulder outcome, ERA = external rotation in abduction, ERS = external rotation at the side (in adduction), FE = forward elevation, IRA = internal rotation in abduction, MUA = manipulation under anesthesia.

[a] Reported as the change from pre-procedure to final follow-up.

Adapted from Grant JA, Schroeder N, Miller BS, Carpenter JE: Comparison of manipulation and arthroscopic capsular release for adhesive capsulitis: A systematic review. *J Shoulder Elbow Surg* 2013;22(8):1135-1145.

Controversies and Alternative Approaches

The controversy in the management of adhesive capsulitis lies in the fact that this disease is often self-limiting and, in most patients, resolves with time alone. However, adhesive capsulitis in patients with poorly controlled diabetes is often recalcitrant and does not result in spontaneous resolution.

Most patients with adhesive capsulitis can be followed with supportive observation, including clear communication from the first encounter that this disorder will improve on its own with time. Patients often benefit from pain control. Options include NSAIDs, narcotics, and the judicious use of intra-articular corticosteroid injections.

Formal physical therapy is often ineffective and can be frustrating for both the therapist and the patient if initiated too early in the disease process. Therapy should be delayed until the patient's pain has subsided and only a stiff shoulder remains.

Early in the course of the disease, the pain and stiffness associated with adhesive capsulitis can be nonspecific, subtle, and often indistinguishable from other shoulder conditions. Thus, evaluations should be repeated until the diagnosis becomes more clearly defined.

In patients for whom supportive observation is not an attractive strategy, manipulation under anesthesia without surgical release has been the benchmark against which all other interventions should be measured. Little evidence is available to favor one intervention over the other.

Results

In a recent systematic review comparing the outcomes of arthroscopic capsular release versus manipulation alone for the management of adhesive capsulitis, minimal benefit was noted in range of motion and patient-reported outcomes of capsular release (**Table 1**). The authors of this systematic review reported a low level of evidence as well as limited comparative studies when investigating the results of surgical capsular release versus isolated manipulation. Thus, there was no clear evidence in support of one intervention over the other.

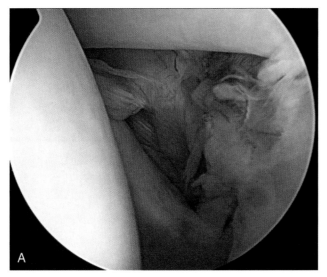
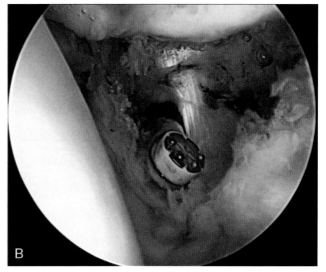

Figure 1 Arthroscopic images from the posterosuperior portal demonstrate the rotator interval capsule before release (**A**) and after release (**B**).

 Technical Keys to Success

The author of this chapter recommends the use of a postoperative indwelling scalene catheter for all patients who undergo arthroscopic capsular release. The catheter delivers local anesthesia to the brachial plexus, affording excellent pain control in the postoperative period and facilitating maintenance of the range of motion that is achieved during the procedure. The long-lasting catheter may require redosing of medication or replacement of the medication reservoir by a medical professional. Because the catheter is not placed in the intraarticular space, the risk of drug-induced chondrolysis is low. In patients who undergo manipulation without arthroscopic capsular release, a catheter is not routinely used.

Setup/Exposure

- A catheter is placed under ultrasound guidance by the anesthesia team on the day of the surgical procedure and may remain in place for as long as 7 to 12 days after the procedure.
- The author of this chapter prefers

to perform arthroscopic capsular release with the patient in the beach-chair position. This position allows for an efficient transition to the examination and manipulation under anesthesia as soon as the arthroscopic portion of the procedure has been completed.
- A standard posterior viewing portal and an anterior working portal are created. The anterior portal is created using needle localization under direct arthroscopic visualization through the rotator interval.

Procedure

- Routine diagnostic arthroscopy, in which the joint is visualized from both the anterior and posterior portals, is performed.
- The biceps tendon is inspected, palpated, and displaced into the joint with a probe to allow visualization of as much of the extra-articular portion of the tendon as possible. The biceps tendon is often diffusely injected, and the synovium associated with the tendon sheath may appear thickened and inflamed. In severe cases, adhesions may be present within the sheath, resulting

in limited excursion and a tenodesis effect that, when severe, can contribute to limited motion at the shoulder. For this reason, the author of this chapter often performs tenotomy of the long head of the biceps tendon at the time of arthroscopic capsular release if evidence of biceps tendon disease or diminished excursion of the tendon is observed.
- The surgical release begins in the rotator interval.

 Video 31.1 Arthroscopic Capsular Release: Keys to Safe and Effective Restoration of Motion. Bruce S. Miller, MD, MS (2 min)

- An ablation probe is used to resect the capsular tissue of the rotator interval, including all capsule from the anterior edge of the supraspinatus tendon to the leading edge of the subscapularis tendon. This step also involves division of the superior and middle glenohumeral ligament complexes. The rotator interval capsule is resected until the deep surface of the conjoint tendon is clearly visualized (**Figure 1**).

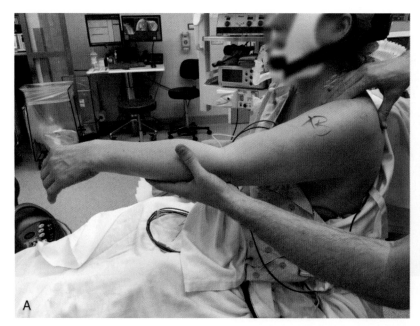
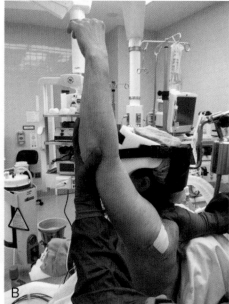

Figure 2 Photographs show forward elevation preoperatively (**A**) and after manipulation under anesthesia (**B**).

- After release of the rotator interval, releases should be continued in a timely fashion because arthroscopic fluid can extravasate through the interval into the anterior soft tissues.
- The anterior and anteroinferior capsule is released. Starting from a point in the capsule approximately 1 cm medial to the labrum, the capsule is divided either with the ablation probe or with a standard meniscal biter. Care must be taken to achieve full-thickness division of the capsule.
- To avoid inadvertent injury to the axillary nerve, the use of the radiofrequency ablation probe should be avoided when progressing from the middle capsule to the inferior capsule. The meniscal biter offers better tactile control of the release in this area.
- The release should proceed no farther than the 5-o'clock position of the anterior capsule. The most inferior aspect of the capsule will be easily ruptured during gentle manipulation after the surgical procedure.

- The posterior capsule often appears thin and may demonstrate less involvement in the adhesive capsulitis process than is observed on the anterior side. Restriction of internal rotation in the abducted shoulder on preoperative examination may suggest involvement of the posterior capsule. With the anterior portal used for visualization, the posterior capsule is easily released with the ablation probe placed through the posterosuperior portal.
- In general, the subacromial space is not entered during this surgical procedure because the disease process does not appear to affect this space.

Wound Closure
- Arthroscopy portals are closed with a simple suture pattern using nonabsorbable suture material.

Manipulation Under Anesthesia
- After the arthroscopic portals are closed, attention is immediately turned to manipulation.
- To minimize the risk of iatrogenic fracture, care must be taken to

stabilize the scapula and maintain short lever arms by securing the humerus as proximally as possible.
- Forward elevation is performed first and is often accompanied by an audible and palpable release of the remaining inferior capsule (**Figure 2**).
- The adducted arm is manipulated into external rotation (**Figure 3**).
- The abducted arm is gently manipulated through internal and external rotation (**Figure 4**).
- The range of motion gained through manipulation should be quantified and recorded to clearly communicate rehabilitation goals to the physical therapy team.

 Rehabilitation

Formal physical therapy begins on postoperative day 1, and daily visits are recommended for the first 2 weeks after capsular release to help maintain the increased range of motion achieved during the surgical procedure. The early therapy sessions should be focused on manual passive stretching, guided

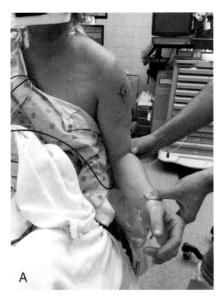 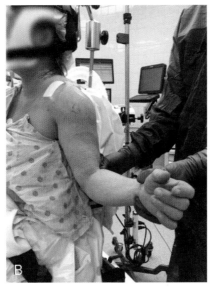

Figure 3 Photographs show external rotation in adduction preoperatively (**A**) and after manipulation under anesthesia (**B**).

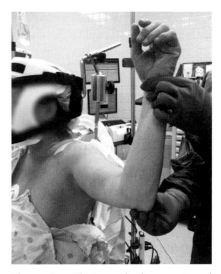

Figure 4 Photograph shows external rotation in abduction after manipulation under anesthesia.

Table 2 Rehabilitation Protocol After Arthroscopic Capsular Release for the Management of Adhesive Capsulitis

Postoperative Week	ROM	Strengthening	Return to Play/Work	Comments/Emphasis
0-2	Aggressive daily stretching sessions to maintain ROM	None	None	Daily physical therapy sessions with the goal of maintaining ROM achieved in the surgical procedure
2-6	Focus on improvement and maintenance of ROM	None	None	Therapy sessions three times per wk Maintenance stretching
6-12	Maintain ROM	Initiate as needed	As tolerated	—
12-24	Maintain ROM	Maintain strengthening	—	—

ROM = range of motion.

by the range of motion achieved in the surgical procedure. Thus, the surgeon must communicate clearly with the rehabilitation team and provide quantitative measures and goals to guide the therapy. Formal therapy sessions should be supplemented with a patient-directed home stretching program, which can be facilitated by a pulley system.

The use of an indwelling scalene catheter affords pain relief for an extended period after the procedure and facilitates rehabilitation because it improves the likelihood of maintaining the increased range of motion achieved

in the surgical procedure. Because the indwelling catheter invariably creates a motor block, it is challenging to achieve anything other than passive motion while the catheter remains in place. As soon as the catheter is discontinued, the patient can initiate active-assisted and active range of motion to supplement the passive stretching.

The author of this chapter finds that most patients benefit from formal therapy sessions three times per week for weeks 2 through 6 after the procedure, followed by one or two sessions per week or maintenance for an additional

6 weeks (**Table 2**). Although no evidence is available to support postoperative corticosteroid use, an intra-articular injection may be considered several weeks postoperatively.

 Avoiding Pitfalls

The success of arthroscopic capsular release depends on careful patient selection, clear communication of expectations, meticulous surgical technique, and appropriate postoperative rehabilitation. Although most patients respond

well to this intervention, the management of adhesive capsulitis in patients with diabetes mellitus, especially those with poorly controlled diabetes, can be challenging. The author of this chapter finds that the results of treatment are less predictable in this patient population than in patients with idiopathic adhesive capsulitis.

 ## Bibliography

Baums MH, Spahn G, Nozaki M, Steckel H, Schultz W, Klinger HM: Functional outcome and general health status in patients after arthroscopic release in adhesive capsulitis. *Knee Surg Sports Traumatol Arthrosc* 2007;15(5):638-644.

Beaufils P, Prévot N, Boyer T, et al; French Society for Arthroscopy: Arthroscopic release of the glenohumeral joint in shoulder stiffness: A review of 26 cases. *Arthroscopy* 1999;15(1):49-55.

Chen J, Chen S, Li Y, Hua Y, Li H: Is the extended release of the inferior glenohumeral ligament necessary for frozen shoulder? *Arthroscopy* 2010;26(4):529-535.

Chen SK, Chien SH, Fu YC, Huang PJ, Chou PH: Idiopathic frozen shoulder treated by arthroscopic brisement. *Kaohsiung J Med Sci* 2002;18(6):289-294.

Çinar M, Akpinar S, Derincek A, Circi E, Uysal M: Comparison of arthroscopic capsular release in diabetic and idiopathic frozen shoulder patients. *Arch Orthop Trauma Surg* 2010;130(3):401-406.

De Carli A, Vadalà A, Perugia D, et al: Shoulder adhesive capsulitis: Manipulation and arthroscopic arthrolysis or intra-articular steroid injections? *Int Orthop* 2012;36(1):101-106.

Dodenhoff RM, Levy O, Wilson A, Copeland SA: Manipulation under anesthesia for primary frozen shoulder: Effect on early recovery and return to activity. *J Shoulder Elbow Surg* 2000;9(1):23-26.

Elhassan B, Ozbaydar M, Massimini D, Higgins L, Warner JJ: Arthroscopic capsular release for refractory shoulder stiffness: A critical analysis of effectiveness in specific etiologies. *J Shoulder Elbow Surg* 2010;19(4):580-587.

Eljabu W, Klinger HM, von Knoch M: Prognostic factors and therapeutic options for treatment of frozen shoulder: A systematic review. *Arch Orthop Trauma Surg* 2015; Oct 17 [Epub ahead of print].

Flannery O, Mullett H, Colville J: Adhesive shoulder capsulitis: Does the timing of manipulation influence outcome? *Acta Orthop Belg* 2007;73(1):21-25.

Gerber C, Espinosa N, Perren TG: Arthroscopic treatment of shoulder stiffness. *Clin Orthop Relat Res* 2001;(390):119-128.

Grant JA, Schroeder N, Miller BS, Carpenter JE: Comparison of manipulation and arthroscopic capsular release for adhesive capsulitis: A systematic review. *J Shoulder Elbow Surg* 2013;22(8):1135-1145.

Hannafin JA, Chiaia TA: Adhesive capsulitis: A treatment approach. *Clin Orthop Relat Res* 2000;(372):95-109.

Hsu JE, Anakwenze OA, Warrender WJ, Abboud JA: Current review of adhesive capsulitis. *J Shoulder Elbow Surg* 2011;20(3):502-514.

Jacobs LG, Smith MG, Khan SA, Smith K, Joshi M: Manipulation or intra-articular steroids in the management of adhesive capsulitis of the shoulder? A prospective randomized trial. *J Shoulder Elbow Surg* 2009;18(3):348-353.

Jerosch J: 360 degrees arthroscopic capsular release in patients with adhesive capsulitis of the glenohumeral joint: Indication, surgical technique, results. *Knee Surg Sports Traumatol Arthrosc* 2001;9(3):178-186.

Kivimäki J, Pohjolainen T, Malmivaara A, et al: Manipulation under anesthesia with home exercises versus home exercises alone in the treatment of frozen shoulder: A randomized, controlled trial with 125 patients. *J Shoulder Elbow Surg* 2007;16(6):722-726.

Massoud SN, Pearse EO, Levy O, Copeland SA: Operative management of the frozen shoulder in patients with diabetes. *J Shoulder Elbow Surg* 2002;11(6):609-613.

Neviaser RJ, Neviaser TJ: The frozen shoulder: Diagnosis and management. *Clin Orthop Relat Res* 1987;(223):59-64.

Nicholson GP: Arthroscopic capsular release for stiff shoulders: Effect of etiology on outcomes. *Arthroscopy* 2003;19(1):40-49.

Quraishi NA, Johnston P, Bayer J, Crowe M, Chakrabarti AJ: Thawing the frozen shoulder: A randomised trial comparing manipulation under anaesthesia with hydrodilatation. *J Bone Joint Surg Br* 2007;89(9):1197-1200.

Ramesh R, Smith S, Bunker T: Long term follow up after manipulation for frozen shoulder: A resolving disease or not? *Journal of Orthopaedic Medicine* 2003;25(2):46-48.

Wang JP, Huang TF, Hung SC, Ma HL, Wu JG, Chen TH: Comparison of idiopathic, post-trauma and post-surgery frozen shoulder after manipulation under anesthesia. *Int Orthop* 2007;31(3):333-337.

Wang JP, Huang TF, Ma HL, Hung SC, Chen TH, Liu CL: Manipulation under anaesthesia for frozen shoulder in patients with and without non-insulin dependent diabetes mellitus. *Int Orthop* 2010;34(8):1227-1232.

Warner JJ, Allen A, Marks PH, Wong P: Arthroscopic release for chronic, refractory adhesive capsulitis of the shoulder. *J Bone Joint Surg Am* 1996;78(12):1808-1816.

Waszczykowski M, Fabiś J: The results of arthroscopic capsular release in the treatment of frozen shoulder: Two-year follow-up. *Ortop Traumatol Rehabil* 2010;12(3):216-224.

Yamaguchi K, Sethi N, Bauer GS: Postoperative pain control following arthroscopic release of adhesive capsulitis: A short-term retrospective review study of the use of an intra-articular pain catheter. *Arthroscopy* 2002;18(4):359-365.

 ## Video Reference

Miller BS: Video. *Arthroscopic Capsular Release: Keys to Safe and Effective Restoration of Motion*. Ann Arbor, MI, 2015.

Chapter 32

Arthroscopic Management of Glenohumeral Osteoarthritis: Nonarthroplasty Options for Joint Preservation

Maximilian Petri, MD

Joshua A. Greenspoon, BSc

Peter J. Millett, MD, MSc

 ## Introduction

Osteoarthritis (OA) of the shoulder is less prevalent than OA of the hip or knee, but it typically occurs earlier, at an average age of 60 years. The incidence of both idiopathic and posttraumatic OA is increasing. Typical symptoms include activity-related shoulder pain, night pain, and limited range of motion (ROM). Initial treatment is nonsurgical, consisting of physical therapy, activity modification, NSAIDs, and intra-articular injections with local anesthetics and corticosteroids.

In a patient with advanced glenohumeral OA in whom nonsurgical management is unsuccessful, arthroplasty can provide pain relief and a high level of satisfaction. Arthroplasty options include hemiarthroplasty, biologic osteoarticular replacement, and total shoulder arthroplasty (TSA). TSA is the most effective procedure for managing glenohumeral OA. Reverse TSA

is typically used in patients who have rotator cuff deficiency.

Several studies, however, have shown inferior clinical outcomes and low patient satisfaction after TSA in patients younger than 50 years. These outcomes may be explained by higher patient expectations before surgery and the limited longevity of current implants. Implant failure may result in the need for revision surgery. Patients who participate in high-demand activities, which accelerate implant wear, are at particular risk for revision surgery.

Increasing numbers of patients with glenohumeral OA want to avoid—or at least delay—arthroplasty, and arthroscopic management continues to evolve to meet this patient demand. The risk of perioperative complications is lower with arthroscopy than with total joint arthroplasty, which is of particular importance for patients who are elderly, have multiple morbidities, or are chronically ill. Furthermore, the activity

modifications required after arthroplasty may not be acceptable to young, active patients who are otherwise healthy or older patients who want to remain active in their later years.

Many patients with glenohumeral OA report lateral arm pain and exhibit large inferior osteophytes (so-called goat's beard osteophytes) on the inferior humeral head on imaging studies. Axillary nerve entrapment caused by these osteophytes and the resulting posterior and lateral arm pain may be a manifestation of glenohumeral OA. Atrophy of the teres minor muscle, which is innervated by the axillary nerve, has an increased prevalence in patients with large goat's beard osteophytes, which lends support to the belief that axillary nerve entrapment contributes to pain in patients with glenohumeral OA. Axillary nerve neurolysis is indicated in patients with evidence of nerve impingement on either cross-sectional imaging or direct arthroscopic visualization and those with posterior or lateral shoulder pain that corresponds to the area of innervation by the axillary nerve.

The comprehensive arthroscopic management (CAM) procedure was developed to address the pathology of humeral head osteophytes and axillary nerve entrapment and build on

Dr. Petri or an immediate family member has received nonincome support (such as equipment or services), commercially derived honoraria, or other non–research-related funding (such as paid travel) from Arthrex. Dr. Millett or an immediate family member has received royalties from Arthrex; serves as a paid consultant to Arthrex and MYOS; has stock or stock options held in Game Ready and VuMedi; and has received research or institutional support from Arthrex, Össur, Siemens, and Smith & Nephew. Neither Mr. Greenspoon nor any immediate family member has received anything of value from or has stock or stock options held in a commercial company or institution related directly or indirectly to the subject of this chapter.

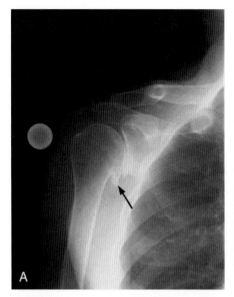 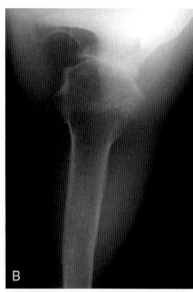

Figure 1   Preoperative AP (**A**) and axillary (**B**) radiographs of a right shoulder demonstrate extensive glenohumeral arthritis (Kellgren-Lawrence grade 4). **A,** The glenohumeral joint space measures 2.4 mm centrally and 0.5 mm inferiorly. **B,** The humeral head is concentrically located (Walch A2 glenoid). In addition, a type III acromion and a large inferior humeral osteophyte with the typical goat's beard shape (arrow in panel A) are noted.

previously described arthroscopic procedures, such as glenohumeral débridement, chondroplasty, synovectomy, capsular release, and removal of loose bodies. In many patients, microfracture to manage circumscribed cartilage lesions, subacromial decompression with or without acromioplasty, and biceps tenodesis also are needed. The CAM procedure includes these steps and adds osteoplasty of the humeral head to remove the goat's beard osteophyte and neurolysis of the axillary nerve, the combination of which decompresses the axillary nerve. Biceps tenodesis is performed in patients with pathology of the long head of the biceps. The subacromial space and the acromioclavicular joint also are addressed as indicated. Short-term and midterm results of the CAM procedure have been encouraging.

The authors of this chapter have considerable experience performing the joint-preserving CAM procedure in patients with advanced glenohumeral OA. Substantial clinical improvement and high rates of survivorship have been noted at short-term and midterm follow-up, with follow-up approaching 10 years in some patients. Patients who were converted to arthroplasty were found to have notably narrower glenohumeral joint spaces preoperatively and an increased likelihood of having Walch B and C glenoids. A glenohumeral joint space of 2 mm or more and a critical shoulder angle greater than 30° also correlate with good clinical results of the CAM procedure. Although additional studies with longer follow-up are needed to determine the longevity and durability of the CAM procedure, early clinical results at the institution of the authors of this chapter indicate that the CAM procedure can be effective at decreasing pain, improving function, and delaying the need for TSA.

 Case Presentation

A very active 58-year-old man who works as a contractor presents with bilateral shoulder pain. The right shoulder is more problematic than the left. Even after more than 10 months of nonsurgical treatment, which included physical therapy, NSAIDs, and injections, the patient continues to experience persistent stiffness, activity-related pain, night pain, and weakness with all activities.

Clinically, the patient exhibits passive forward elevation to 125°, abduction to 70°, external rotation to 15°, and internal rotation to the level of the buttocks. On active ROM, he exhibits forward flexion to 130°, abduction to 85° with positive impingement signs, and external rotation to 10°. His rotator cuff strength score is 5 of 5. Tenderness to palpation is elicited at the posterior glenohumeral joint line and on the lateral aspect of the shoulder. Tenderness is present over the long head of the biceps tendon; however, no acromioclavicular joint tenderness and no signs of instability are found. The patient has strength measuring 5 of 5 in all planes, although strength was limited by pain. Neurovascular examination findings are normal.

AP, lateral, outlet, and axillary radiographs of the right shoulder demonstrate extensive glenohumeral arthritis (Kellgren-Lawrence grade 4). In addition, a type III acromion and a large inferior humeral osteophyte with the typical goat's beard shape are noted (**Figure 1**). Advanced degenerative changes of the glenohumeral joint are confirmed on preoperative MRI; these changes consist of diffuse loss of cartilage on both the glenoid and the humeral head, cystic degenerative changes and osseous edema of the humeral head with hypertrophic bone overgrowth, and almost complete degeneration of the labrum. The rotator cuff, including the subscapularis, appears to be intact. Intra-articular visualization of the long head of the biceps tendon is not possible; the tendon appears to be scarred in the bicipital groove.

Treatment options and their respective risks and benefits were extensively discussed with the patient. The patient thought that he had exhausted all his nonsurgical treatment options and wanted to proceed with surgical management. Although his age made him a candidate for either TSA or arthroscopy, he chose the CAM procedure because of his young age, otherwise good health status, unwillingness to modify his active lifestyle, desire for functional gain and pain relief, and wish to avoid or delay arthroplasty.

End-stage OA with severe thickening of the inferior glenohumeral ligament complex, capsular contracture, and large inferior, posterior, and anterior osteophytes on the humeral head were confirmed on arthroscopy. The patient also had a degenerative labrum, synovitis, and subacromial bursitis. The rotator cuff was intact. The patient was not treated with microfracture. After anterior and posterior capsular releases were performed, the shoulder demonstrated 60° of external rotation, 110° of abduction, and 150° of forward flexion. With the arm in 90° of abduction, 90° of external rotation and 70° of internal rotation were achieved.

The patient was very satisfied with the results of the CAM procedure on his right shoulder, and he underwent the same procedure on his left shoulder several months later. At 5-year follow-up, he demonstrated improved American Shoulder and Elbow Surgeons scores on both shoulders.

Indications and Contraindications

Appropriate patient selection and well-matched patient and physician expectations are critical to success. In a Markov decision analysis published in 2014, arthroscopic management was reported to be the preferred treatment for patients younger than 47 years, whereas TSA was the preferred treatment for patients older than 66 years. Both options were deemed reasonable for patients aged 47 to 66 years. Intra-articular glenohumeral joint injection may be helpful in the diagnosis and management of glenohumeral OA. However, although pain relief after injection may seem to implicate the glenohumeral joint as the source of the pain, the predictive value of injection in patients who are candidates for the CAM procedure has not been studied. The ideal candidate for the CAM procedure has a Walch A1, A2, or B1 glenoid; a critical shoulder angle greater than 30°; a glenohumeral joint space greater than 2 mm; and a high gain of forward elevation after manipulation under anesthesia and capsular release.

Controversies and Alternative Approaches

Nonsurgical management, hemiarthroplasty, and TSA are alternatives to arthroscopy. Nonsurgical management consisting of physical therapy, activity modification, NSAIDs, and joint injections with local anesthetics and corticosteroids addresses symptoms of glenohumeral OA but does not alter the disease progression. Judicious use of corticosteroid injections can provide temporary pain relief. Physical therapy is used to improve ROM by stretching the contracted periarticular joint capsule and to improve load absorption by strengthening the surrounding musculature. Other less well-studied nonsurgical options include platelet-rich plasma injections and prolotherapy, neither of which has proved to be of notable benefit.

Although nonsurgical treatment avoids the risks associated with surgery, it is not without risk. For example, the long-term use of NSAIDs is associated with the risk of cardiovascular, gastric, and renal complications. In addition, repeated joint injections carry the risk of weakening periarticular tissues, such as the rotator cuff, and may place the patient at risk for chondral toxicity from the local anesthetics, thereby potentially accelerating the progression of glenohumeral OA.

Historically, hemiarthroplasty was the arthroplasty method of choice for the shoulder. However, TSA has been shown to provide better functional outcomes regarding pain, mobility, and activity. In addition, continuous degeneration of the glenoid after hemiarthroplasty is a serious concern. Hemiarthroplasty combined with a biologic interpositional glenoid resurfacing allograft has been suggested for younger patients. However, revision rates ranging from 17% to 77% within 2 years postoperatively led to a recommendation against these procedures in young, active patients with glenohumeral OA. Osteoarticular autografts or allografts might be considered in managing focal osteochondral defects; however, clinical results are sparse. In a study published in 2011, promising short-term results after osteochondral allograft resurfacing of the humeral head and glenoid were reported. It may be possible to perform such resurfacing using an all-arthroscopic approach. In a study published in 2014, limited improvement in outcomes and a 44% conversion rate to TSA were reported after soft-tissue interposition grafting of the glenoid in 16 patients.

TSA offers predictably good clinical results and pain relief. However, outcomes are inferior in younger patients who put increased demands on the prostheses and have high functional expectations. Implant wear is often accelerated in active patients with high physical demands, which can necessitate revision and lead to glenoid bone loss. Therefore, the authors of this chapter believe that in properly selected younger patients, the CAM procedure is a good alternative to TSA.

Table 1 Results of Arthroscopic Management of Glenohumeral Osteoarthritis

Authors	Journal (Year)	No. of Patients (Shoulders)	Technique	Outcomes	Comments
Weinstein et al	*Arthroscopy* (2000)	25	Débridement	No revisions or complications Pain improved in all patients	Mean patient age, 46 yr Worse results with humeral head osteophytes
Cameron et al	*J Shoulder Elbow Surg* (2002)	70	Débridement ± capsular releases	Revisions and complications NR Mean functional score improved from 24 to 38.7 (60-point scale) Mean patient satisfaction score improved from 0.67 to 6.28 (10-point scale) Mean FE improved from 119° to 157° Mean IR improved from L2 to T11	6 of the 61 patients available for follow-up progressed to arthroplasty Mean patient age, 50 yr Mean follow-up, 34 mo
Richards and Burkhart	*Arthroscopy* (2007)	8 (9)	Débridement ± capsular releases	Revisions and complications NR Mean FE improved from 131.9° to 153.3° Mean IR improved from 17.2° to 48.3° Mean ER improved from 42.8° to 59.4°	Mean patient age, 55 yr Mean follow-up, 13.7 mo
Kerr and McCarty	*Clin Orthop Relat Res* (2008)	19 (20)	Débridement ± tenotomy, microfracture	Revisions and complications NR Mean final scores: ASES, 75.3; Marx, 12.6; SANE, 63%; WOOS, 0.64	3 shoulders progressed to arthroplasty Mean patient age, 38 yr
de Beer et al	*Knee Surg Sports Traumatol Arthrosc* (2010)	32	Débridement, glenoid resurfacing, tenotomy	5 complications: 1 axillary paresis, 2 material failures, 1 synovitis, 1 contusion from MUA Median Constant score improved from 40 to 64.5	Median patient age, 57.5 yr

ASES = American Shoulder and Elbow Surgeons shoulder outcome, ER = external rotation, FE = forward elevation, IR = internal rotation, MUA = manipulation under anesthesia, NR = not reported, PCS = physical component summary, ROM = range of motion, SANE = Single Assessment Numeric Evaluation, SF-12 = Medical Outcomes Study 12-Item Short Form, SST = Simple Shoulder Test, TSA = total shoulder arthroplasty, UCLA = University of California–Los Angeles Shoulder Rating Scale, VAS = visual analog scale, WOOS = Western Ontario Osteoarthritis of the Shoulder Index.

[a] Survivorship analysis used TSA as the marker of failure.

Results

Results of arthroscopic management of glenohumeral OA are summarized in **Table 1**. The authors of a systematic review published in 2013 concluded that there is a lack of high-quality evidence regarding arthroscopic débridement in patients with glenohumeral OA. However, level IV evidence suggested at least short-term improvement in pain relief and patient satisfaction.

Historically, arthroscopy was typically recommended for younger patients with minimal to moderate shoulder OA but not for patients with advanced OA or large osteophytes. In a study published in 2000, patients with large inferior osteophytes had unsatisfactory outcomes after simple débridement. However, the authors of that study did not attempt to remove the osteophytes. The distance between the inferior humeral osteophyte and the axillary neurovascular bundle has been shown to be inversely correlated to the size of the inferior humeral osteophyte.

Table 1 Results of Arthroscopic Management of Glenohumeral Osteoarthritis (*continued*)

Authors	Journal (Year)	No. of Patients (Shoulders)	Technique	Outcomes of Interest	Comments
Van Thiel et al	*Arthroscopy* (2010)	71	Débridement ± capsular releases, tenotomy, microfracture, acromioplasty	Mean ASES score improved from 51.8 to 72.7 Mean SST score improved from 6.1 to 9.0 Mean VAS score improved from 4.8 to 2.7 Mean SF-12 score improved from 35.9 to 36.1 Mean final scores: Constant, 72.0; UCLA, 28.3; SANE, 71.1 Mean final ROM: FE, 137°; abduction, 129°; ER, 48°	Subjective data were reported on 55 patients (mean follow-up, 27 mo) 16 patients progressed to arthroplasty Mean patient age, 47 yr
Millett et al	*Arthroscopy* (2013)	30	Débridement ± capsular releases, humeral osteoplasty, axillary neurolysis, acromioplasty	6 of 30 shoulders progressed to TSA at a mean 1.9 yr follow-up and are excluded from these outcomes Median patient satisfaction was 9 of 10 Mean ASES score improved from 58 to 83 Mean SF-12 PCS score improved from 42.8 to 49.4 Mean FE improved from 98.2° to 152.9° Mean ER improved from 13.4° to 62.2° Mean ER at 90° of abduction improved from 27.3° to 75.4° Mean IR improved from 23.8° to 60.8°	Mean patient age, 52 yr Subjective outcome scores were available from 18 patients (mean follow-up, 2.6 yr) Survivorship rate of 92% at 1 yr and 85% at 2 yr postoperatively[a] Glenohumeral joint space <2 mm associated with an eight-fold increased risk of eventual arthroplasty

ASES = American Shoulder and Elbow Surgeons shoulder outcome, ER = external rotation, FE = forward elevation, IR = internal rotation, MUA = manipulation under anesthesia, NR = not reported, PCS = physical component summary, ROM = range of motion, SANE = Single Assessment Numeric Evaluation, SF-12 = Medical Outcomes Study 12-Item Short Form, SST = Simple Shoulder Test, TSA = total shoulder arthroplasty, UCLA = University of California–Los Angeles Shoulder Rating Scale, VAS = visual analog scale, WOOS = Western Ontario Osteoarthritis of the Shoulder Index.

[a] Survivorship analysis used TSA as the marker of failure.

That is, the larger the osteophyte, the more it encroaches on and changes the course of the axillary nerve. The size of the osteophyte also has been shown to correlate significantly with fatty degeneration of the teres minor muscle. This fatty infiltration could be considered a surrogate marker of axillary neuropathy because the teres minor muscle is innervated by branches of the axillary nerve. The larger the osteophyte, the greater the degree of fatty infiltration of the teres minor. The senior author of this chapter (P.J.M.) believes that in the patient with a large osteophyte, axillary nerve compression also may be a source of pain posteriorly and laterally as a result of sensory distribution. This may explain why removal of the osteophyte during the CAM procedure results in decreased pain postoperatively and why results after the CAM procedure are better than those after earlier series of arthroscopic treatment in which the goat's beard deformity was not addressed.

In a 2013 study on the CAM procedure, the survivorship rate (patients not converted to TSA) was 92% at 1 year postoperatively and 85% at 2 years postoperatively. Unpublished data from the institution of the senior author of this chapter (P.J.M.) indicate high rates of survivorship and suggest that critical shoulder angle and glenohumeral joint space have an effect on outcomes.

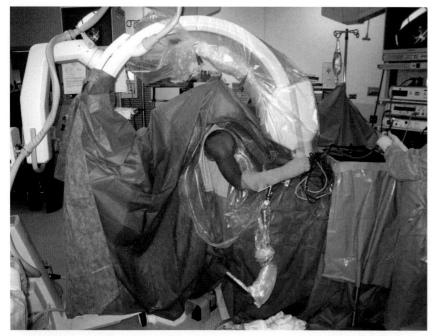

Figure 2 Intraoperative photograph shows a patient placed in the modified beach-chair position in preparation for a comprehensive arthroscopic management procedure to address glenohumeral osteoarthritis. The fluoroscopic C-arm has been draped into the surgical field using sterile technique.

 Video 32.1 Arthroscopic Management of Glenohumeral Osteoarthritis: Nonarthroplasty Options for Joint Preservation. Maximilian Petri, MD; Joshua A. Greenspoon, BSc; Peter J. Millett, MD, MSc (7 min)

Technical Keys to Success

Setup/Exposure

- The patient is placed under general anesthesia, and an interscalene nerve catheter is placed to provide analgesic agents during the initial phases of postoperative rehabilitation.
- The patient is placed in the modified beach-chair position to enable intraoperative manipulation of the arm as well as fluoroscopic and arthroscopic visualization of the goat's beard osteophyte.
- A C-arm fluoroscopy machine is draped into the surgical field using

sterile technique. Fluoroscopy is used intraoperatively for visualization and resection of the inferior humeral osteophyte (**Figure 2**).

- Bilateral examination under anesthesia is performed to evaluate any limitations in ROM. A loss of motion greater than 15° in any plane is usually consistent with capsular contracture, which is managed with arthroscopic capsular release. Loss of abduction seems to correlate with the size of the goat's beard osteophyte, and excision of the osteophyte seems to improve internal rotation, external rotation, and abduction. The right shoulder of the patient discussed in the case presentation demonstrated the following on examination under anesthesia: 20° of abduction, 50° of forward flexion, and external rotation to neutral. In addition, with the arm maximally abducted, the patient had 10° of external rotation and 10° of internal rotation.

The 2013 publication on the CAM procedure reported significant improvement in ROM on examination under anesthesia. Forward elevation improved from 98° to 152° ($P < 0.001$), external rotation improved from 13° to 62° ($P < 0.001$), external rotation at 90° of abduction improved from 27° to 75° ($P < 0.001$), and internal rotation improved from 23° to 60° ($P < 0.001$).

- Standard posterior and anterosuperior portals are established, and diagnostic arthroscopy is performed. Typically, end-stage OA with severe thickening of the inferior glenohumeral ligament complex, capsular contracture, and large inferior, posterior, and anterior osteophytes on the humeral head are confirmed. Other common findings are a degenerative labrum, synovitis, subacromial bursitis, and an intact rotator cuff.

Glenohumeral Débridement and Lysis of Adhesions

- Unstable glenohumeral articular cartilage and degenerative labral tissue are débrided to a stable border using an arthroscopic shaver to prevent mechanical irritation and the acceleration of joint degeneration. Loose bodies are removed.
- Microfracture is performed to manage focal, full-thickness chondral defects with stable borders. Microfracture is not routinely performed because it is not appropriate for managing the more common severe presentation of diffuse glenohumeral OA.
- Areas of synovial hypertrophy are resected using radiofrequency ablation.
- Scar tissue is removed from the rotator interval to restore motion at the coracohumeral interface.
- The capsule is otherwise preserved to avoid soft-tissue swelling caused

by fluid excursion and to protect the axillary nerve, which lies deep to the capsule.

Humeral Head Osteoplasty and Axillary Nerve Neurolysis

- An accessory posteroinferolateral portal is established under arthroscopic visualization to allow access to the inferior axillary recess, humeral neck, and axillary nerve (**Figure 3**).
- A spinal needle is inserted into the axillary recess near the junction of the medial and central thirds of the inferior capsule just anterior to the margin of the posterior band of the inferior glenohumeral ligament.
- A skin incision is made, taking care to incise only the skin to avoid injury to branches of the axillary nerve.
- A 2.6-mm switching stick is carefully placed in the axillary pouch using the blunt end to avoid iatrogenic injury to the axillary nerve, which passes through the inferior recess from anteromedial to posterolateral.
- Cannula dilators are placed over the switching stick to dilate the soft tissues and protect the axillary nerve.
- An 8.25-mm cannula with two deployable low-profile wings (Gemini

cannula; Arthrex) is inserted. The wings secure the cannula in the capsule and prevent the cannula from falling out during resection of the goat's beard osteophyte. Securing the cannula in place helps protect the axillary nerve. The cannula facilitates insertion and removal of the bone resection instruments, shavers, and curets used in the osteoplasty.
- The thickened capsule of the axillary pouch is preserved to protect the axillary nerve.
- The intra-articular inferior humeral osteophyte is resected using a shielded arthroscopic burr, arthroscopic shavers, and handheld curets (**Figure 4**).
- Bony resection is performed under fluoroscopic guidance. To ensure adequate bony resection, the patient's arm is internally and externally rotated to bring all areas of the osteophyte into view of the arthroscope or within the plane of the fluoroscope. Curets also can be used to remove hypertrophic bone from the anteroinferior areas that are more difficult to access with motorized instruments.
- Complete removal of hypertrophic bone is desired but is not always

possible. The surgeon should remove enough bone to decompress the axillary nerve throughout the range of shoulder motion and restore full mobility to the shoulder.
- Release of the inferior capsule is performed after humeral head osteoplasty because the intact capsular tissue can help protect the axillary nerve from iatrogenic injury.
- Arthroscopic punches and a monopolar radiofrequency probe are used in the inferior capsular release.

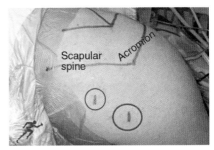

Figure 3 Intraoperative photograph shows localization of the posteroinferolateral portal (circled in red) used for humeral head osteoplasty, axillary nerve neurolysis, and inferior capsular releases. Other standard landmarks for shoulder arthroscopy are marked; the outlines of the scapular spine, acromion, and clavicle are shown, and the standard posterior portal is circled in blue.

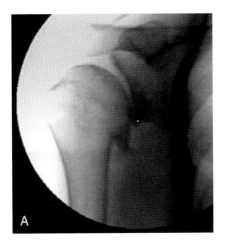
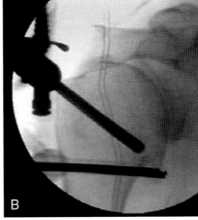
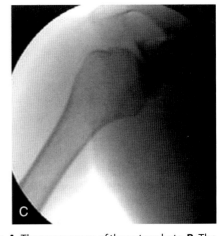

Figure 4 Fluoroscopic images demonstrate the removal of a goat's beard osteophyte. **A,** The appearance of the osteophyte. **B,** The appearance of the osteophyte during the procedure with the arthroscope placed in the posterior portal and an arthroscopic burr placed in the posteroinferolateral portal. **C,** The appearance of the humeral head after resection of the osteophyte.

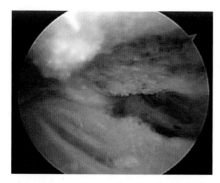

Figure 5 Arthroscopic image from the posterior portal after neurolysis of the axillary nerve demonstrates branching and arborization of the nerve.

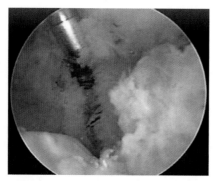

Figure 6 Arthroscopic image from the posterior portal demonstrates the appearance of the fibers of the subscapularis muscle after anterior capsular release.

- The release is started posteriorly near the insertion site of the posteroinferolateral cannula, and the capsule is released from proximal to distal. A blunt trocar can be used to help distinguish tissue planes. When radiofrequency ablation is used, care should be taken to ensure that there is excellent outflow to decrease the risk of thermal injury to the axillary nerve.
- After the axillary nerve is identified, careful dissection is performed from proximal to distal to avoid damaging branches of the nerve. Extensive branching and arborization of the axillary nerve is common (**Figure 5**).
- Dynamic examination of the shoulder throughout ROM is performed to confirm that neurolysis is complete. The axillary nerve should be clearly visible along its entire course between the subscapularis and teres minor muscles, and there should be no soft-tissue adherence or bony impingement.

Anterior and Posterior Capsular Releases

- After the nerve has been visualized and safely released, anterior and posterior capsular releases can be performed using typical techniques used in frozen shoulder procedures.

- The rotator interval, which lies medial to the biceps reflection pulley and inferior to the superior glenohumeral ligament, is released using electrocautery and a motorized shaver. The release continues until the coracoid and the coracoacromial ligament are clearly visible.
- The anterior capsule is released medially along the capsulolabral junction, posterior to the subscapularis, to allow visualization of the subscapularis muscle fibers (**Figure 6**).
- If the posterior capsule is tight, it too is released.
- The arthroscope is placed in the anterosuperior portal to achieve visualization of the posterior capsule and capsulolabral junction. The patient's arm is placed in slight internal rotation to avoid damage to the posterior rotator cuff tendinous insertions on the humerus, and the posterior capsule is released via the posterior portal from inferior to superior along the capsulolabral junction.
- Dynamic examination and manipulation are performed under arthroscopic and fluoroscopic visualization to evaluate shoulder ROM.
- Typically, after capsular release, shoulder ROM improves substantially to a mean of 48° of external

rotation, 50° of external rotation with the arm in 90° of abduction, 57° of forward elevation, and 41° of internal rotation.

Subacromial Decompression and Long Head of the Biceps Tendon Tenodesis

- The arthroscope is placed into the posterior portal to access the subacromial space. Arthroscopic subacromial decompression with complete bursectomy typically is performed. All patients undergo subacromial bursoscopy and bursectomy.
- The rotator cuff is carefully visualized from the bursal side. Adhesions in the subdeltoid plane are removed to restore the normal scapulohumeral motion interface. An impingement lesion with visible fraying or scuffing of the coracoacromial ligament, or a large anterolateral acromial spur, is managed with acromioplasty performed with an arthroscopic burr through the lateral portal.
- The biceps tendon is visualized. Pathology of the long head of the biceps tendon that compromises the ability of the tendon to glide freely in the bicipital groove is thought to be a major source of pain. Therefore, arthroscopic release and subpectoral tenodesis are often performed. Examples of biceps pathology include tendinitis, pulley lesions, degenerative superior labrum anterior to posterior tears, and hourglass deformity. The authors of this chapter prefer to perform biceps tenodesis instead of tenotomy because they think that muscle strength and cosmesis are better with tenodesis and because of the decreased occurrence of muscle cramping. Biceps tenodesis can be performed in several ways, but the senior author of this chapter (P.J.M.) prefers to perform

Table 2 Rehabilitation Protocol After Comprehensive Arthroscopic Management of Glenohumeral Osteoarthritis

Postoperative Week	Range of Motion	Strengthening	Return to Work/Play
0-6	Passive with early use of CPM, active assisted Cautious stretching is allowed as tolerated	None	Only office work is allowed
6-12	No limitations	Functional, with elastic resistance bands	Return to work depends on profession and pain
>12	No limitations	Advanced exercises (eg, specific motion sequences used in overhead sports)	Return to sports is allowed at 4-6 mo

CPM = continuous passive motion.

subpectoral tenodesis with an interference screw.

- The shoulder is copiously lavaged and drained.
- The portal sites are closed with 3-0 nylon sutures, and dry sterile dressings are applied.
- A moderate amount of swelling is common because of the capsulectomy and the duration of the procedure.

 Rehabilitation

The primary goals of postoperative rehabilitation are to maintain asymptomatic joint motion and improve overall shoulder kinematics. Rehabilitation follows a phasic approach that is individualized to each patient based on concomitant pathologies and procedures (**Table 2**). Early, aggressive stretching is important to maintain function after the CAM procedure or any other arthroscopic procedure for the management of glenohumeral OA.

 Avoiding Pitfalls

Risks and complications of the CAM procedure include iatrogenic damage to the axillary nerve, incomplete osteoplasty and neurolysis, reformation of scar tissue with arthrofibrosis, glenohumeral instability resulting from excessive capsular releases, and soft-tissue damage caused by excessive swelling after fluid excursion. These complications can usually be avoided using meticulous surgical technique.

The axillary nerve is protected by the capsule and the muscle fibers of the triceps. After these structures are released, great care must be taken to avoid damage to the axillary nerve. Working from proximal to distal during axillary neurolysis aids in visualization of distal arborizations of the nerve. Performing anterior and posterior capsular releases after osteoplasty and neurolysis prevents fluid excursion or leakage into the axillary space. Leakage impedes visualization during neurolysis. To protect the axillary nerve, the capsule is preserved until after the osteoplasty is completed. Then, the inferior capsule is released and the axillary neurolysis is performed. After neurolysis is completed, the anterior and posterior capsules are released.

Incomplete humeral osteoplasty can be avoided by using the C-arm and varying the position of the patient's arm throughout the resection. However, safe removal of the entire spur arthroscopically is not always possible. Postoperative instability is a theoretical risk because of the extended capsular releases. However, the authors of this chapter have seen postoperative instability only once, in a patient who had a traumatic dislocation after a high-speed crash while waterskiing. Persistent stiffness is the most common complication after the CAM procedure.

The natural history of glenohumeral OA is one of progression. In most patients treated at the institution of the authors of this chapter, the CAM procedure effectively alleviates pain or restores function. However, in some patients the CAM procedure is ineffective because of the severity of the disease, the patient's ability to tolerate the joint degeneration, or the postoperative progression of the glenohumeral OA. These factors should be carefully discussed with the patient preoperatively. Studies are ongoing to identify patient-related and pathoanatomic factors that will help optimize patient selection for the CAM procedure.

Bibliography

Bartelt R, Sperling JW, Schleck CD, Cofield RH: Shoulder arthroplasty in patients aged fifty-five years or younger with osteoarthritis. *J Shoulder Elbow Surg* 2011;20(1):123-130.

Bishop JY, Flatow EL: Management of glenohumeral arthritis: A role for arthroscopy? *Orthop Clin North Am* 2003;34(4):559-566.

Black EM, Roberts SM, Siegel E, Yannopoulos P, Higgins LD, Warner JJ: Reverse shoulder arthroplasty as salvage for failed prior arthroplasty in patients 65 years of age or younger. *J Shoulder Elbow Surg* 2014;23(7):1036-1042.

Boileau P, Ahrens PM, Hatzidakis AM: Entrapment of the long head of the biceps tendon: The hourglass biceps. A cause of pain and locking of the shoulder. *J Shoulder Elbow Surg* 2004;13(3):249-257.

Bryant D, Litchfield R, Sandow M, Gartsman GM, Guyatt G, Kirkley A: A comparison of pain, strength, range of motion, and functional outcomes after hemiarthroplasty and total shoulder arthroplasty in patients with osteoarthritis of the shoulder: A systematic review and meta-analysis. *J Bone Joint Surg Am* 2005;87(9):1947-1956.

Buchbinder R, Green S, Youd JM: Corticosteroid injections for shoulder pain. *Cochrane Database Syst Rev* 2003;1:CD004016.

Cameron BD, Galatz LM, Ramsey ML, Williams GR, Iannotti JP: Non-prosthetic management of grade IV osteochondral lesions of the glenohumeral joint. *J Shoulder Elbow Surg* 2002;11(1):25-32.

Cole BJ, Yanke A, Provencher MT: Nonarthroplasty alternatives for the treatment of glenohumeral arthritis. *J Shoulder Elbow Surg* 2007;16(5 suppl):S231-S240.

de Beer JF, Bhatia DN, van Rooyen KS, Du Toit DF: Arthroscopic debridement and biological resurfacing of the glenoid in glenohumeral arthritis. *Knee Surg Sports Traumatol Arthrosc* 2010;18(12):1767-1773.

Denard PJ, Raiss P, Sowa B, Walch G: Mid- to long-term follow-up of total shoulder arthroplasty using a keeled glenoid in young adults with primary glenohumeral arthritis. *J Shoulder Elbow Surg* 2013;22(7):894-900.

Dines JS, Fealy S, Strauss EJ, et al: Outcomes analysis of revision total shoulder replacement. *J Bone Joint Surg Am* 2006;88(7):1494-1500.

Edwards TB, Kadakia NR, Boulahia A, et al: A comparison of hemiarthroplasty and total shoulder arthroplasty in the treatment of primary glenohumeral osteoarthritis: Results of a multicenter study. *J Shoulder Elbow Surg* 2003;12(3):207-213.

Elhassan B, Ozbaydar M, Diller D, Higgins LD, Warner JJ: Soft-tissue resurfacing of the glenoid in the treatment of glenohumeral arthritis in active patients less than fifty years old. *J Bone Joint Surg Am* 2009;91(2):419-424.

Gobezie R, Lenarz CJ, Wanner JP, Streit JJ: All-arthroscopic biologic total shoulder resurfacing. *Arthroscopy* 2011;27(11):1588-1593.

Green A, Norris TR: Shoulder arthroplasty for advanced glenohumeral arthritis after anterior instability repair. *J Shoulder Elbow Surg* 2001;10(6):539-545.

Gross C, Dhawan A, Harwood D, Gochanour E, Romeo A: Glenohumeral joint injections: A review. *Sports Health* 2013;5(2):153-159.

Kerr BJ, McCarty EC: Outcome of arthroscopic débridement is worse for patients with glenohumeral arthritis of both sides of the joint. *Clin Orthop Relat Res* 2008;466(3):634-638.

Millett PJ, Gaskill TR: Arthroscopic management of glenohumeral arthrosis: Humeral osteoplasty, capsular release, and arthroscopic axillary nerve release as a joint-preserving approach. *Arthroscopy* 2011;27(9):1296-1303.

Millett PJ, Horan MP, Pennock AT, Rios D: Comprehensive Arthroscopic Management (CAM) procedure: Clinical results of a joint-preserving arthroscopic treatment for young, active patients with advanced shoulder osteoarthritis. *Arthroscopy* 2013;29(3):440-448.

Millett PJ, Sanders B, Gobezie R, Braun S, Warner JJ: Interference screw vs. suture anchor fixation for open subpectoral biceps tenodesis: Does it matter? *BMC Musculoskelet Disord* 2008;9:121.

Millett PJ, Schoenahl JY, Allen MJ, Motta T, Gaskill TR: An association between the inferior humeral head osteophyte and teres minor fatty infiltration: Evidence for axillary nerve entrapment in glenohumeral osteoarthritis. *J Shoulder Elbow Surg* 2013;22(2):215-221.

Muh SJ, Streit JJ, Shishani Y, Dubrow S, Nowinski RJ, Gobezie R: Biologic resurfacing of the glenoid with humeral head resurfacing for glenohumeral arthritis in the young patient. *J Shoulder Elbow Surg* 2014;23(8):e185-e190.

Nakagawa Y, Hyakuna K, Otani S, Hashitani M, Nakamura T: Epidemiologic study of glenohumeral osteoarthritis with plain radiography. *J Shoulder Elbow Surg* 1999;8(6):580-584.

Namdari S, Skelley N, Keener JD, Galatz LM, Yamaguchi K: What is the role of arthroscopic debridement for glenohumeral arthritis? A critical examination of the literature. *Arthroscopy* 2013;29(8):1392-1398.

Nicholson GP, Goldstein JL, Romeo AA, et al: Lateral meniscus allograft biologic glenoid arthroplasty in total shoulder arthroplasty for young shoulders with degenerative joint disease. *J Shoulder Elbow Surg* 2007;16(5 suppl):S261-S266.

Noël E, Hardy P, Hagena FW, et al: Efficacy and safety of Hylan G-F 20 in shoulder osteoarthritis with an intact rotator cuff: Open-label prospective multicenter study. *Joint Bone Spine* 2009;76(6):670-673.

Nové-Josserand L, Walch G, Adeleine P, Courpron P: Effect of age on the natural history of the shoulder: A clinical and radiological study in the elderly [in French]. *Rev Chir Orthop Reparatrice Appar Mot* 2005;91(6):508-514.

Radnay CS, Setter KJ, Chambers L, Levine WN, Bigliani LU, Ahmad CS: Total shoulder replacement compared with humeral head replacement for the treatment of primary glenohumeral osteoarthritis: A systematic review. *J Shoulder Elbow Surg* 2007;16(4):396-402.

Raiss P, Aldinger PR, Kasten P, Rickert M, Loew M: Total shoulder replacement in young and middle-aged patients with glenohumeral osteoarthritis. *J Bone Joint Surg Br* 2008;90(6):764-769.

Rasmussen JV: Outcome and risk of revision following shoulder replacement in patients with glenohumeral osteoarthritis. *Acta Orthop Suppl* 2014;85(355):1-23.

Richards DP, Burkhart SS: Arthroscopic debridement and capsular release for glenohumeral osteoarthritis. *Arthroscopy* 2007;23(9):1019-1022.

Snow M, Boutros I, Funk L: Posterior arthroscopic capsular release in frozen shoulder. *Arthroscopy* 2009;25(1):19-23.

Sperling JW, Cofield RH, Rowland CM: Minimum fifteen-year follow-up of Neer hemiarthroplasty and total shoulder arthroplasty in patients aged fifty years or younger. *J Shoulder Elbow Surg* 2004;13(6):604-613.

Spiegl UJ, Faucett SC, Horan MP, Warth RJ, Millett PJ: The role of arthroscopy in the management of glenohumeral osteoarthritis: A Markov decision model. *Arthroscopy* 2014;30(11):1392-1399.

van der Meijden OA, Gaskill TR, Millett PJ: Glenohumeral joint preservation: A review of management options for young, active patients with osteoarthritis. *Adv Orthop* 2012;2012:160923.

Van Thiel GS, Sheehan S, Frank RM, et al: Retrospective analysis of arthroscopic management of glenohumeral degenerative disease. *Arthroscopy* 2010;26(11):1451-1455.

Walker M, Willis MP, Brooks JP, Pupello D, Mulieri PJ, Frankle MA: The use of the reverse shoulder arthroplasty for treatment of failed total shoulder arthroplasty. *J Shoulder Elbow Surg* 2012;21(4):514-522.

Warth RJ, Briggs KK, Dornan GJ, Horan MP, Millett PJ: Patient expectations before arthroscopic shoulder surgery: Correlation with patients' reasons for seeking treatment. *J Shoulder Elbow Surg* 2013;22(12):1676-1681.

Weinstein DM, Bucchieri JS, Pollock RG, Flatow EL, Bigliani LU: Arthroscopic debridement of the shoulder for osteoarthritis. *Arthroscopy* 2000;16(5):471-476.

Zoric BB, Horn N, Braun S, Millett PJ: Factors influencing intra-articular fluid temperature profiles with radio-frequency ablation. *J Bone Joint Surg Am* 2009;91(10):2448-2454.

 ## Video Reference

Petri M, Greenspoon JA, Millett PJ: Video. *Arthroscopic Management of Glenohumeral Osteoarthritis: Nonarthroplasty Options for Joint Preservation.* Vail, CO, 2016.

Chapter 33

Glenohumeral Resurfacing

Felix H. Savoie III, MD

Michael J. O'Brien, MD

 Introduction

Glenohumeral arthritis in the young, active patient (younger than 60 years) is a challenging problem to manage. If function is not restored and pain is not decreased with nonsurgical management, then surgical options may be considered. For most patients with shoulder arthritis, total shoulder arthroplasty (TSA) is the preferred treatment to alleviate pain and improve function. However, not all patients are ideal candidates for TSA because of age, activity level, or associated pathology. In one study of shoulder arthroplasty in patients younger than 50 years, high rates of glenoid lucency after TSA and glenoid erosion after hemiarthroplasty were reported. Most importantly, patient satisfaction with the procedure was poor.

In the past 15 years, resurfacing has emerged as a potential surgical option to decrease pain and preserve bone stock in the young, active patient with arthritis. Improvements in arthroscopic techniques and instrumentation enabled the development of arthroscopic biologic resurfacing of the glenoid as a temporary, intermediate step in the surgical management of arthritis in these young patients (**Table 1**).

 Case Presentations

Case 1

A 36-year-old man who works as an offshore welder presents with substantial pain and restricted motion in his left shoulder. He reports that he underwent surgery approximately 15 years earlier to address a shoulder dislocation. The patient is not sure precisely what was repaired in the previous surgery. The surgery was successful, which enabled him to pursue a career as an offshore welder. In the several years after the initial surgery, the shoulder has become progressively more stiff and painful. Initial treatment, first by his family physician and then by an orthopaedic surgeon, consisted of medications, injections, physical therapy, and, eventually, arthroscopic débridement. Although all the treatments helped somewhat, none resulted in prolonged relief. When the patient became unable to work because of the state of his shoulder, he was referred to the authors of this chapter to consider alternative options. His stated goal was to resume work as a welder. He listed his hobbies as weight lifting, hunting, fishing, and eating. He rated his functional level as 30% of normal, and his visual analog scale scores for pain were 1 to 2 at rest, 6 at night, and 10 with attempted heavy activity.

The patient is 5 feet 6 inches tall and weighs approximately 300 lb. Physical examination reveals no substantial muscle atrophy, and all scars are well healed. Active and passive motion are 120° of flexion, 90° of abduction, 0° of external rotation, and 0° of internal rotation. Strength is Medical Research Council grade 5 of 5 on manual muscle testing in the limited range of motion the patient was able to perform. Radiographs demonstrate a relatively rounded humeral head with an inferior spur and a concentric joint that on the axillary view appears to exhibit bone-on-bone contact, and no articular cartilage damage to the glenoid is evident on arthroscopy (**Figures 1** and **2**).

Several treatment options were considered, including TSA, humeral head replacement, humeral head resurfacing,

Dr. Savoie or an immediate family member is a member of a speakers' bureau or has made paid presentations on behalf of Mitek Sports Medicine and Smith & Nephew; serves as an unpaid consultant to Biomet, Exactech, Mitek Sports Medicine, Rotation Medical, and Smith & Nephew; has received research or institutional support from Mitek Sports Medicine; and serves as a board member, owner, officer, or committee member of the American Shoulder and Elbow Surgeons and the Arthroscopy Association of North America. Dr. O'Brien or an immediate family member serves as a paid consultant to Smith & Nephew; has received research or institutional support from Mitek Sports Medicine and Smith & Nephew; has received nonincome support (such as equipment or services), commercially derived honoraria, or other non–research-related funding (such as paid travel) from DePuy Synthes, Mitek Sports Medicine, and Smith & Nephew; and serves as a board member, owner, officer, or committee member of the Arthroscopy Association of North America and the Association of American Medical Colleges.

Table 1 Approaches to Glenohumeral Resurfacing

Indication	Approaches
Primary loss of glenoid articular cartilage	Microfracture/abrasion for small defects (<1 cm)
	Local tissue coverage (for rim lesions)
	Complete glenoid coverage using autograft or allograft
	The authors of this chapter currently use thick dermal allografts
Primary humeral cartilage loss with loss of normal round contour of the humeral head	Spur excision and microfracture
	Resurfacing (subscapularis-preserving approach or subscapularis takedown)
Combined lesions with deformity on both the humeral and glenoid sides	Arthroscopic-assisted glenoid and humeral resurfacing via a combined approach that includes complete glenoid coverage using autograft or allograft as well as glenoid resurfacing
	Open total shoulder arthroplasty

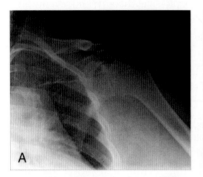
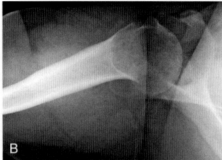

Figure 1 PA (**A**) and axillary (**B**) radiographs of a left shoulder demonstrate loss of articular cartilage but no substantial deformity. (Copyright Felix H. Savoie III, MD, New Orleans, LA.)

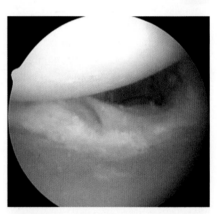

Figure 2 Arthroscopic view of a left shoulder from the posterior portal demonstrates loss of articular cartilage from the glenoid. (Copyright Felix H. Savoie III, MD, New Orleans, LA.)

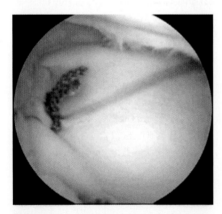

Figure 3 Arthroscopic view from the posterior portal of a dermal patch in place on the glenoid. (Copyright Felix H. Savoie III, MD, New Orleans, LA.)

and glenoid resurfacing. After discussing with the patient the options, the length of the recovery process, and the longevity of each procedure, the patient agreed to undergo biologic glenoid resurfacing.

Outpatient arthroscopic surgery was performed, with extensive microfracture and glenoid resurfacing (**Figure 3**). The patient was instructed to use an abduction sling for 4 weeks to immobilize the shoulder and to do prescribed home exercises during this time. Physical therapy, which consisted primarily of distraction stretching followed by strengthening, was initiated at 4 weeks postoperatively and continued for an additional 8 weeks. The patient then progressed to 4 weeks of work conditioning, after which he passed a strenuous physical examination and qualified to return to work as an offshore welder. He has maintained this activity level for the past 6 years with no apparent problems and has achieved active flexion of 170°, active abduction of 160°, active external rotation of 80°, and active internal rotation of 60° (**Figure 4**).

Case 2

A 28-year-old man who works in construction, serves as a volunteer firefighter, and is an avid weight lifter presents with activity-related pain and loss of motion in his right shoulder that caused him to modify his activities. He used anti-inflammatory drugs for years to manage pain. In addition, he received two corticosteroid injections, each of which provided pain relief lasting approximately 1 month but resulted in no improvement in motion. Radiographs demonstrate humeral head deformity with minimal glenoid changes (**Figure 5**).

After discussing treatment options with the patient, including change of work and hobbies, continuing injections, humeral head resurfacing via a subscapularis-sparing approach, humeral hemiarthroplasty with biologic resurfacing, and TSA, the patient elected to undergo subscapularis-sparing humeral head surface replacement arthroplasty (**Figures 6** and **7**). Home exercises were started 1 week postoperatively. In postoperative week 3, use of the sling was discontinued, and active rehabilitation was begun. The patient resumed training at the gym in postoperative week 4 and returned to work in postoperative week 6. He passed the fitness test for firefighters in postoperative week 7. By 4 years postoperatively, he had maintained the motion he gained after surgery (that is, 85% of normal motion) and had maintained a very heavy work and weight lifting program. Radiographs demonstrated a concentric glenohumeral joint with no eccentric wear.

 ## Indications

Glenoid resurfacing is indicated for a young patient with concentric glenohumeral arthritis in which most of the wear is on the glenoid side. Contraindications include Walch type B2 or C glenoid configuration or humeral head deformity. The aim of glenoid resurfacing is to resurface the glenoid with a soft-tissue patch to create a permanent, durable, biologically active surface to decrease friction and pain and improve range of motion and function. In the best scenarios, the patch may function as a hyaline-like tissue. Glenoid resurfacing preserves glenoid bone, avoids the problems related to glenoid component loosening, and leaves open the possibility of later conversion to TSA.

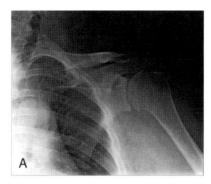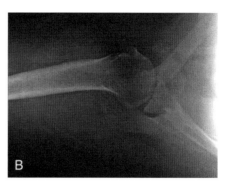

Figure 4   PA (**A**) and axillary (**B**) radiographs of a left shoulder demonstrate loss of glenoid articular cartilage; most of the deformity is on the humeral side. (Copyright Felix H. Savoie III, MD, New Orleans, LA.)

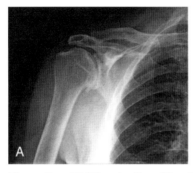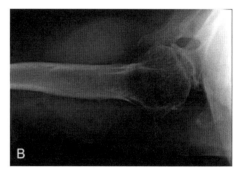

Figure 5   PA (**A**) and axillary (**B**) radiographs of a right shoulder demonstrate a square humeral head with loss of articular cartilage. (Copyright Felix H. Savoie III, MD, New Orleans, LA.)

In short, glenoid resurfacing delays the need for TSA, which is unlikely to provide satisfactory results in young, active patients.

Humeral surface replacement arthroplasty is indicated for a young, active patient with humeral deformity in which subscapularis takedown or glenoid replacement would affect the patient's activity level. Subscapularis-preserving humeral head resurfacing is reserved for active individuals with humeral deformity whose activity level requires both an alternative to polyethylene glenoid replacement and a normally functioning subscapularis.

 ## Controversies and Alternative Approaches

Biologic resurfacing of the glenoid is a controversial technique. First proposed

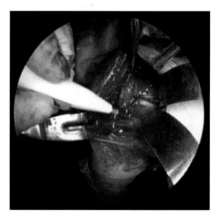

Figure 6   Intraoperative photograph of the initial incision into the subscapularis muscle demonstrates the level of the split in the muscle. Subscapularis-sparing surface replacement arthroplasty is being performed. (Copyright Felix H. Savoie III, MD, New Orleans, LA.)

in the late 1980s using fascia lata autograft and allograft, biologic resurfacing of the glenoid with or without

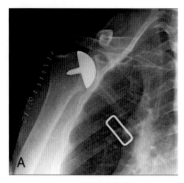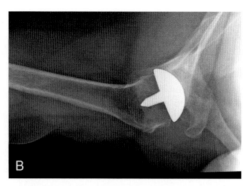

Figure 7 PA (**A**) and Bernageau (**B**) radiographs of a right shoulder after humeral head resurfacing demonstrate a balanced articulation between the humeral head and the glenoid. (Copyright Felix H. Savoie III, MD, New Orleans, LA.)

hemiarthroplasty to manage glenohumeral arthritis in young, active patients has had variable results. In the earliest published study on the technique, good to excellent results were achieved in 86% of patients; however, more recent studies in which lateral meniscus tissue was used had failure rates as high as 50%. Use of the lateral meniscus would seem to be problematic because the rim of the meniscus limits movement around the glenoid track and concentrates force into the center of the glenoid, thereby increasing the risk of glenoid deterioration.

Biologic resurfacing may also be considered in patients for whom adequate pain relief was not achieved after previous arthroscopic débridement or capsular release. Patients in this group are often laborers or persons whose work and sporting activities would not allow them to abide by the restrictions associated with placement of a polyethylene glenoid component. Although chronologic age is an important factor in determining the best treatment option, physiologic age and patient expectations are perhaps more important decision-making variables. Contraindications to glenoid resurfacing are substantial humeral head deformity or spurring, advanced glenoid bone loss, failed previous glenoid resurfacing, and active infection. Although the authors of this chapter currently prefer

to use dermal allograft patches, there is no standard material for soft-tissue interposition. Various techniques using a variety of tissues, including capsule autograft, fascia lata autograft, Achilles tendon allograft, lateral meniscal allograft, and a variety of commercially available grafts and scaffolds, have been described.

Resurfacing of the glenoid with an interposition soft-tissue graft may be performed arthroscopically or in conjunction with humeral head arthroplasty. Resurfacing has been proposed as an option to improve outcomes and avoid the potential complications associated with TSA, such as glenoid component loosening and polyethylene wear. Soft-tissue glenoid resurfacing should always be considered a temporary solution until the patient reaches an age at which TSA is appropriate.

Initial reports of humeral resurfacing were excellent, and subsequent reports indicated satisfactory results at mid- to long-term follow-up. Resurfacing without subscapularis takedown has the advantage of avoiding subscapularis insufficiency in a young, active patient population.

An approach to the young arthritic shoulder in which an open humeral hemiarthroplasty was combined with gentle concentric reaming of the glenoid to create a symmetrical glenohumeral joint was described in 2007.

The surgeon who introduced this ream-and-run approach postulated that reaming of the glenoid would produce a fibrocartilage surface, allowing high-level activity without the risk of glenoid loosening associated with TSA. In the initial study, 35 patients treated with the ream-and-run technique were compared with a similar group of patients who underwent TSA. No differences were noted between the two groups 3 years postoperatively, as measured by the Simple Shoulder Test (SST). In a study published in 2015, the use of the ream-and-run technique to manage painful, posteriorly subluxated, arthritic shoulders resulted in an increase of five tasks on the SST at 3-year follow-up. In a separate study published in 2015, specific indications, technique, and results were reported for the young, active patient with glenoid deformity. In 2012, a study of prognostic factors that predict better outcomes in patients undergoing the ream-and-run procedure indicated that older men with no previous surgery and with "reasonable" preoperative SST scores were most likely to improve after surgery. The authors of that study stressed the importance of postoperative rehabilitation compliance for optimal results. The role of the ream-and-run technique has yet to be defined.

Results

Published results of glenoid resurfacing and humeral head resurfacing are varied, with success rates as high as 81% after arthroscopic or open glenoid resurfacing to address glenohumeral osteoarthritis. Results also indicated an overall failure rate as high as 51.2% in patients treated with hemiarthroplasty or humeral head prosthetic resurfacing with either lateral meniscus allograft or human acellular dermal tissue matrix (**Table 2**). The authors of a 2014 study concluded that because of the results published in these studies, biologic resurfacing of the glenoid with humeral head resurfacing is no longer their primary treatment option for young patients with arthritis, and it should be used with caution.

Technical Keys to Success

Patient selection is the key to success. A sedentary 65-year-old patient is much better treated with TSA than with a limited joint-preserving technique. Resurfacing of the glenoid requires smoothing of the surface via a posterior portal, with microfracture to decompress any subchondral cysts. The graft should be securely anchored at four main quadrants: anterosuperior, anteroinferior, posterosuperior, and posteroinferior, with additional sutures as needed.

It has long been the policy of the authors of this chapter to separate the glenoid resurfacing and the humeral head surgery in young patients. The initial reconstructive surgery may be arthroscopic glenoid resurfacing, followed several years later by humeral resurfacing and then, eventually, TSA. In some patients, humeral resurfacing may be performed as the initial reconstructive option and followed later by either biologic resurfacing or TSA. In one study, promising results were achieved with arthroscopic treatment of the arthritic shoulder by extensive débridement, removal of humeral spurs, and an axillary nerve neurolysis. This procedure is similar to the one presented in this chapter, with the additional step of biologic resurfacing of the glenoid.

Surgical Technique

Glenoid Resurfacing
- Surgery is performed arthroscopically with the patient in the lateral decubitus position. This position offers the advantages of full access to the anterior and posterior compartments of the shoulder, access to the inferior humeral head should osteophyte resection be required, and 360° access to the glenoid rim and labrum.
- The surgical arm is placed in an arm-positioning device, and 10 lb (4.5 kg) of traction is applied to distract the glenohumeral joint.
- Standard arthroscopic portals are used: posterior, anteroinferior, and anterosuperior.
- The arthroscope is placed through the posterior portal.
- Diagnostic arthroscopy is performed, and the presence of glenohumeral arthritis is confirmed.
- The anteroinferior portal is established just above the subscapularis tendon as the primary working portal.
- An accessory anterosuperior portal is established as the viewing portal.
- It is important to maintain a wide skin bridge between the two anterior portals to create adequate working space for the passage of instruments through the anteroinferior cannula.
- The arthroscope is placed in the anterosuperior viewing portal, which allows full visualization of the glenohumeral joint in the anterior and posterior compartments.
- An 8.5-mm cannula is placed in the anteroinferior portal. Use of the larger cannula here is necessary to allow for later graft passage.
- A 5-mm cannula is placed in the posterior portal.
- Hypertrophic synovium is resected with a shaver, and all degenerative fraying of the labrum, rotator cuff, and biceps is débrided. Loose bodies are removed.
- If substantial stiffness is present, a complete capsular release outside the labrum is performed.
- A flat, concentric surface is created for placement of the graft.
- A motorized burr is introduced through the posterior portal, and the glenoid face is burred to a smooth, uniform surface. Occasionally, it may be necessary to alternate the burr between the anterior and posterior portals to ensure that the entire glenoid surface is burred smooth and flat.
- Bony ridges are removed, and limited biconcavity is planed to a flat surface.
- Residual cartilage is removed.
- Microfracture of the glenoid face is performed. The authors of this chapter prefer to use Steadman microfracture awls. The microfracture must be deep enough to allow the release of marrow contents, which facilitates healing of the biologic interposition graft to the native glenoid.
- One single-loaded, bioabsorbable suture anchor is placed anteroinferiorly, one is placed anterosuperiorly, and another is placed posterior to the labrum. The labrum is usually hypertrophic or is used for posteroinferior and posterosuperior sutures. These sutures are typically placed at the 1-, 4-, 8-, and 11-o'clock positions (either shoulder). Alternatively, in a shoulder with inadequate posterior labral tissue, suture anchors may be placed posteriorly as well.
- The anterior anchors may be placed through the anteroinferior cannula.
- The posterior anchors are usually placed percutaneously via a small posterolateral portal.
- As each anchor is placed, the sutures are retrieved without tangling and are maintained in a separate quadrant of the cannula.
- Suture management is paramount throughout the procedure to avoid crossing or twisting of the sutures.
- Using a hemostat, each suture is secured to the drapes in the corresponding position inside the

Table 2 Results of Glenoid Resurfacing and Humeral Head Arthroplasty

Authors	Journal (Year)	Technique	Outcomes	Failure Rate (%)	Comments
Krishnan et al	*J Bone Joint Surg Am* (2007)	Fascia lata autograft and allograft	85% good to excellent results	14	36 patients treated Follow-up, 2-15 yr Glenoid erosion occurred, but it stabilized by 5 yr postoperatively
Lee et al	*J Shoulder Elbow Surg* (2009)	Meniscal allograft glenoid resurfacing and shoulder hemiarthroplasty	Complication rate, 32%	32	19 shoulders treated Mean follow-up, 4.25 yr All 6 patients with complications underwent additional surgery (3 TSAs, 1 revision hemiarthroplasty, 1 synovectomy, 1 lysis of adhesions and capsular release) Study authors recommended strong consideration of TSA in all patients in whom nonsurgical treatment has been unsuccessful
Savoie et al	*Arthroscopy* (2009)	All-arthroscopic resurfacing using a biologic patch	75% satisfaction rate at last follow-up (3-6 yr) 5 patients had progressed to surface replacement arthroplasty All patients had statistically significant improvement in pain, ROM, ASES, UCLA, Rowe, Constant, and SF-12 scores	22	23 patients treated Mean patient age, 32 yr
de Beer et al	*Knee Surg Sports Traumatol Arthrosc* (2010)	Biologic resurfacing with acellular human dermal scaffold	Results were excellent in 28% of patients, satisfactory in 44%, and unsatisfactory in 28% Mean Constant score increased from 40 to 64.5 ($P < 0.0001$)	28	32 patients treated Results reported based on intermediate follow-up 5 patients had complications, including 1 reaction to graft material and 1 case of synovitis 5 patients were converted to prosthetic arthroplasty

ASES = American Shoulder and Elbow Surgeons shoulder outcome, DVT = deep vein thrombosis, N/A = not available, OA = osteoarthritis, ROM = range of motion, SF-12 = Medical Outcomes Study 12-Item Short Form, SST = Simple Shoulder Test, TSA = total shoulder arthroplasty, UCLA = University of California–Los Angeles Shoulder Rating Scale, VAS = visual analog scale.

shoulder joint. The sutures are secured under tension.
- A grasper is run along each suture individually to confirm that no tangles have occurred.
- A calibrated probe is placed across the face of the glenoid from the posterior portal. The width from anterior to posterior is measured at the widest part of the glenoid. The average height-to-width ratio of the glenoid is 3:2. The width

measurement is used to calculate the height from superior to inferior.
- At a separate table in the operating room, the graft is marked and an oval is drawn onto it to match the dimensions of the native glenoid.
- Scissors are used to cut a graft of appropriate size from the human dermal matrix. It is important to mark the subcutaneous side of the graft, which should be placed against the native glenoid bone. The

dermal side faces upward.
- With a free needle, one limb of each suture is passed through the graft corresponding with the anchor location on the glenoid. A mulberry knot, or short-tailed interference knot, can be tied and pulled to sit flush against the graft.
- The graft is rolled up and placed into the 8.5-mm anteroinferior cannula.
- The posteroinferior suture is passed

Table 2 Results of Glenoid Resurfacing and Humeral Head Arthroplasty (*continued*)

Authors	Journal (Year)	Technique	Outcomes	Failure Rate (%)	Comments
Namdari et al	*J Shoulder Elbow Surg* (2011)	Arthroscopic or open glenoid resurfacing to address glenohumeral OA	81% of patients satisfied with outcomes Mean VAS pain score improved from 7.5 to 2.5 Mean active forward elevation improved from 82° to 136° Mean active external rotation improved from 12° to 44° Improvement was noted on ASES, Constant, SST, UCLA, and Rowe scores In the 2 studies that used the Neer criteria, 27 excellent, 27 satisfactory, and 14 unsatisfactory results were reported	N/A	Systematic review of 180 patients across 7 level IV studies Mean age, 46.4 yr Mean follow-up, 46.6 mo Primary OA was the most common surgical indication (59.4%) 50.6% of patients underwent previous surgery on the affected shoulder Complication rate, 13.3% (infection, stiffness, instability, brachial neuritis, graft reaction/synovitis, DVT) No postoperative infection with arthroscopy; 6.6% postoperative infection rate with open procedures No difference in functional outcomes between arthroscopic treatment (2 studies) and open approaches (5 studies) 26% of patients required revision surgery
Muh et al	*J Shoulder Elbow Surg* (2014)	Open humeral head arthroplasty with soft-tissue interposition graft of the glenoid (human acellular dermal matrix [7 patients], Achilles tendon allograft [9 patients])	Modest improvements in pain, ROM, and ASES scores 7 patients were converted to TSA at a mean follow-up of 36 mo	44	Mean follow-up, 5 yr Because of these results, the study authors no longer use this as the primary treatment method for young, active patients with arthritis; they recommend using this technique with caution
Strauss et al	*J Shoulder Elbow Surg* (2014)	Hemiarthroplasty or humeral head prosthetic resurfacing with lateral meniscus allograft (31 patients) or human acellular dermal tissue matrix (10 patients)	Significant improvements were noted in pain, ROM, ASES, and SST scores (*P* < 0.05) High clinical failure rates were observed at intermediate time frames	Overall, 51.2 at mean 2.8-yr follow-up Lateral meniscal allograft, 45.2 at mean 3.2-yr follow-up Human acellular dermal tissue matrix, 70 at mean 2.2-yr follow-up	Mean age, 42.2 yr

ASES = American Shoulder and Elbow Surgeons shoulder outcome, DVT = deep vein thrombosis, N/A = not available, OA = osteoarthritis, ROM = range of motion, SF-12 = Medical Outcomes Study 12-Item Short Form, SST = Simple Shoulder Test, TSA = total shoulder arthroplasty, UCLA = University of California–Los Angeles Shoulder Rating Scale, VAS = visual analog scale.

Table 3 Rehabilitation Protocol After Glenoid Resurfacing

Postoperative Week	Range of Motion	Strengthening	Return to Activity	Comments/Emphasis
0-2	None	None	No activity	Work on posture
2-6	Exercises that include joint distraction	Isometric	Light activity; aquatics encouraged	—
6-12	Exercises that include joint distraction	Progressive resistance exercises	As tolerated; aquatics and yoga encouraged	—
12-24	As tolerated	As tolerated	As tolerated	—

Table 4 Rehabilitation Protocol After Humeral Head Resurfacing

Postoperative Week	Range of Motion	Strengthening	Return to Activity	Comments/Emphasis
0-2	Yes	No	No	Emphasis on home stretching exercises
2-6	Yes	Yes	As tolerated	Emphasis on range of motion and strength
6-12	Yes	Yes	Yes	No limitations; full activity allowed
12-24	Yes	Yes	Yes	No limitations

down the cannula and retrieved under the posteroinferior labrum. The posterosuperior stitch is passed the same way and retrieved under the posterosuperior labrum. These two sutures are gently tensioned to pull the graft into the joint.

- An assistant maintains appropriate tension on the posterior sutures while the anterior sutures are individually tensioned.
- With careful pulling on all four sutures, the graft is laid flat on the glenoid. A probe can be used to assist with graft positioning to ensure that the graft lies flush with the glenoid.
- The four individual sutures are tied sequentially. The authors of this chapter tie the anteroinferior suture first, followed by the anterosuperior stitch. When a short-tailed interference knot is used, the posterior sutures can be retrieved through the posterior cannula and each suture tied sequentially. Alternatively, the posterior sutures may be tied to

each other outside the posterior labrum. Compression of the humeral head on the glenoid holds the graft flush against the glenoid.

Humeral Resurfacing

- The patient is placed in the beach-chair position with a rolled sheet placed behind the scapula to keep it protracted, allowing improved visualization of the glenohumeral joint.
- A limited deltopectoral approach is used to expose the subscapularis muscle tendon unit.
- The middle or lower raphe of the subscapularis is split horizontally along the muscle plane and then is extended distally along the medial ridge of the biceps to detach and reflect the lower one-third to one-half of the muscle and tendon.
- The soft-tissue attachments to the humerus, including the capsule, are released as the arm is slowly externally rotated and abducted.
- After the posteroinferior

attachments are released, a Cobb elevator can be used to flip the subscapularis over the humeral head as it dislocates anteriorly, exposing the humeral head.
- The humeral head is reamed and resurfaced.
- The humerus is reduced, and the inferior part of the subscapularis is repaired.

 Rehabilitation

After glenoid resurfacing, rehabilitation must be delayed until after the patch has adhered to the glenoid (**Table 3**). The patient is immobilized for at least 4 weeks postoperatively while working on periscapular muscles and posture to achieve and maintain scapular retraction. Physical therapy is initiated 4 to 5 weeks postoperatively, emphasizing posture and distraction stretching (excluding manual glides and load-and-shift motion). Advanced exercises are begun approximately 8 weeks postoperatively and progress as tolerated over the next 8 weeks. Typically, sports and work conditioning is initiated 12 to 16 weeks postoperatively and is continued until function is restored, usually 5 to 6 months postoperatively.

One advantage of subscapularis-sparing replacement arthroplasty is rapid rehabilitation (**Table 4**). The patient is immobilized in a pillow sling for 1 week postoperatively, after which passive motion and scapular exercises are begun. Two weeks postoperatively, nonsubscapularis (that is, stressful) exercises are started and immobilization is discontinued. Physical therapy is started 3 weeks postoperatively, and at 4 weeks

postoperatively the patient is allowed to resume physical workouts, work-related activity, and other activities of daily living as tolerated.

 Avoiding Pitfalls

The most common pitfall with glenoid resurfacing is improper patient selection. The patient must be a young, active individual who understands that this will not be the last surgery on the affected shoulder. Other inappropriate candidates for humeral resurfacing are patients in whom the greatest amount of arthritis and deformity are on the

humeral side, as well as patients with Walch type B2 or C glenoids. Meticulous intraoperative organization is required to avoid excessive swelling that limits the ability to place and secure the graft in the joint.

The most common pitfall in humeral head resurfacing is failure to reconstitute the normal anatomy of the proximal humerus, which can be a result of oversizing the humeral head as a result of failure to remove all spurs before sizing, eccentric reaming in varus or anteversion caused by lack of full inferior release limiting exposure, and/or a failure to appreciate substantial glenoid deformity preoperatively.

 Bibliography

Bryant D, Litchfield R, Sandow M, Gartsman GM, Guyatt G, Kirkley A: A comparison of pain, strength, range of motion, and functional outcomes after hemiarthroplasty and total shoulder arthroplasty in patients with osteoarthritis of the shoulder: A systematic review and meta-analysis. *J Bone Joint Surg Am* 2005;87(9):1947-1956.

Burkhead WZ Jr, Hutton KS: Biologic resurfacing of the glenoid with hemiarthroplasty of the shoulder. *J Shoulder Elbow Surg* 1995;4(4):263-270.

Clinton J, Franta AK, Lenters TR, Mounce D, Matsen FA III: Nonprosthetic glenoid arthroplasty with humeral hemiarthroplasty and total shoulder arthroplasty yield similar self-assessed outcomes in the management of comparable patients with glenohumeral arthritis. *J Shoulder Elbow Surg* 2007;16(5):534-538.

de Beer JF, Bhatia DN, van Rooyen KS, Du Toit DF: Arthroscopic debridement and biological resurfacing of the glenoid in glenohumeral arthritis. *Knee Surg Sports Traumatol Arthrosc* 2010;18(12):1767-1773.

Edwards TB, Kadakia NR, Boulahia A, et al: A comparison of hemiarthroplasty and total shoulder arthroplasty in the treatment of primary glenohumeral osteoarthritis: Results of a multicenter study. *J Shoulder Elbow Surg* 2003;12(3):207-213.

Elhassan B, Ozbaydar M, Diller D, Higgins LD, Warner JJP: Soft-tissue resurfacing of the glenoid in the treatment of glenohumeral arthritis in active patients less than fifty years old. *J Bone Joint Surg Am* 2009;91(2):419-424.

Gartsman GM, Roddey TS, Hammerman SM: Shoulder arthroplasty with or without resurfacing of the glenoid in patients who have osteoarthritis. *J Bone Joint Surg Am* 2000;82(1):26-34.

Gilmer BB, Comstock BA, Jette JL, Warme WJ, Jackins SE, Matsen FA: The prognosis for improvement in comfort and function after the ream-and-run arthroplasty for glenohumeral arthritis: An analysis of 176 consecutive cases. *J Bone Joint Surg Am* 2012;94(14):e102.

Krishnan SG, Nowinski RJ, Harrison D, Burkhead WZ: Humeral hemiarthroplasty with biologic resurfacing of the glenoid for glenohumeral arthritis: Two to fifteen-year outcomes. *J Bone Joint Surg Am* 2007;89(4):727-734.

Lee BK, Vaishnav S, Rick Hatch GF III, Itamura JM: Biologic resurfacing of the glenoid with meniscal allograft: Long-term results with minimum 2-year follow-up. *J Shoulder Elbow Surg* 2013;22(2):253-260.

Lee KT, Bell S, Salmon J: Cementless surface replacement arthroplasty of the shoulder with biologic resurfacing of the glenoid. *J Shoulder Elbow Surg* 2009;18(6):915-919.

Matsen FA III: The ream and run: Not for every patient, every surgeon or every problem. *Int Orthop* 2015;39(2):255-261.

Matsen FA III, Warme WJ, Jackins SE: Can the ream and run procedure improve glenohumeral relationships and function for shoulders with the arthritic triad? *Clin Orthop Relat Res* 2015;473(6):2088-2096.

Millett PJ, Gaskill TR: Arthroscopic management of glenohumeral arthrosis: Humeral osteoplasty, capsular release, and arthroscopic axillary nerve release as a joint-preserving approach. *Arthroscopy* 2011;27(9):1296-1303.

Millett PJ, Horan MP, Pennock AT, Rios D: Comprehensive arthroscopic management (CAM) procedure: Clinical results of a joint-preserving arthroscopic treatment for young, active patients with advanced shoulder osteoarthritis. *Arthroscopy* 2013;29(3):440-448.

Muh SJ, Streit JJ, Shishani Y, Dubrow S, Nowinski RJ, Gobezie R: Biologic resurfacing of the glenoid with humeral head resurfacing for glenohumeral arthritis in the young patient. *J Shoulder Elbow Surg* 2014;23(8):e185-e190.

Namdari S, Alosh H, Baldwin K, Glaser D, Kelly JD: Biological glenoid resurfacing for glenohumeral osteoarthritis: A systematic review. *J Shoulder Elbow Surg* 2011;20(7):1184-1190.

Nicholson GP, Goldstein JL, Romeo AA, et al: Lateral meniscus allograft biologic glenoid arthroplasty in total shoulder arthroplasty for young shoulders with degenerative joint disease. *J Shoulder Elbow Surg* 2007;16(5 suppl):S261-S266.

Savoie FH III, Brislin KJ, Argo D: Arthroscopic glenoid resurfacing as a surgical treatment for glenohumeral arthritis in the young patient: Midterm results. *Arthroscopy* 2009;25(8):864-871.

Smith KL, Matsen FA III: Total shoulder arthroplasty versus hemiarthroplasty: Current trends. *Orthop Clin North Am* 1998;29(3):491-506.

Sperling JW, Cofield RH, Rowland CM: Minimum fifteen-year follow-up of Neer hemiarthroplasty and total shoulder arthroplasty in patients aged fifty years or younger. *J Shoulder Elbow Surg* 2004;13(6):604-613.

Sperling JW, Cofield RH, Rowland CM: Neer hemiarthroplasty and Neer total shoulder arthroplasty in patients fifty years old or less: Long-term results. *J Bone Joint Surg Am* 1998;80(4):464-473.

Strauss EJ, Verma NN, Salata MJ, et al: The high failure rate of biologic resurfacing of the glenoid in young patients with glenohumeral arthritis. *J Shoulder Elbow Surg* 2014;23(3):409-419.

Wirth MA: Humeral head arthroplasty and meniscal allograft resurfacing of the glenoid. *J Bone Joint Surg Am* 2009;91(5):1109-1119.

Wong I, Burns J, Snyder S: Arthroscopic GraftJacket repair of rotator cuff tears. *J Shoulder Elbow Surg* 2010;19(2 suppl):104-109.

▮ Introduction

Humeral head resurfacing was introduced in the late 1970s, and it has become a reliable treatment option in the armamentarium of shoulder joint reconstruction. The original procedure used a hip resurfacing implant, and first-generation implants lacked a central stem and used cement fixation. Second-generation implants evolved with the introduction of a central stem secured by a screw to the lateral humeral cortex and the incorporation of an ingrowth contact surface to improve long-term component fixation. Third-generation implants allowed for more anatomic humeral head sizing with greater sizing options along with cruciate stem designs for rotational stability. A porous hydroxyapatite or ceramic coating was also added to the undersurface to improve osseointegration and reduce the incidence of loosening.

One of the main advantages of humeral head resurfacing is the preservation of bone stock. In the revision setting, the stemless design allows for implant removal with minimal metaphyseal bone loss or risk of humeral shaft fracture. This minimal loss of bone stock preserves the option to convert to a standard stemmed humeral component if later hemiarthroplasty or total shoulder arthroplasty is required. With indications for reverse shoulder arthroplasty expanding, this also remains a viable option in future revision situations without concern for proximal bone loss. Another advantage of proximal bone preservation is the ability to perform an arthrodesis as a salvage procedure without the need for bone grafting. Humeral resurfacing may also be performed in patients with humeral shaft deformities that would otherwise preclude the insertion of a humeral stem in the intramedullary canal. It may also be performed in patients with retained hardware in the humerus (that is, intramedullary nails, screws) that would restrict the passage of a humeral stem.

Another advantage of humeral head arthroplasty is the decreased risk of periprosthetic fractures because there is no stem passing through the surgical neck as there would be in standard stemmed implants. This is of particular advantage in younger patients, who are more active and thus at increased risk for periprosthetic fracture. Compared with hip resurfacing implants, humeral resurfacing implants have less offset, and thus the rates of humeral neck fracture are lower than those of femoral neck fracture. In addition, the humeral head has a greater range of motion (ROM) and is much less constrained than the femoral head, and thus soft tissues play a predominant role in stabilization.

Normal proximal humeral anatomy (that is, version, offset, inclination) varies from individual to individual. The stemless design used in humeral resurfacing allows for anatomic placement of the component without the additional steps of matching humeral height, version, and head-shaft angle in the case of fracture or when intramedullary stemmed implants are used. After the anatomic neck is defined, accurate placement of the guide pin is achieved under direct visualization to re-create the anatomic version and inclination. Studies have shown that humeral resurfacing allows for the anatomic restoration of the humeral head offset and the supraspinatus and deltoid lever arms, which may contribute to improved function. Alterations leading to nonanatomic placement of stemmed humeral components may affect the biomechanics of the shoulder joint by changing the tension and/or lever arm of the deltoid and rotator cuff, which may lead to decreased ROM, weaker flexion, or instability.

Dr. Higgins or an immediate family member serves as a board member, owner, officer, or committee member of the American Academy of Orthopaedic Surgeons, the American Shoulder and Elbow Surgeons, and the Arthroscopy Association of North America. Neither of the following authors nor any immediate family member has received anything of value from or has stock or stock options held in a commercial company or institution related directly or indirectly to the subject of this chapter: Dr. Sood and Mr. Daniels.

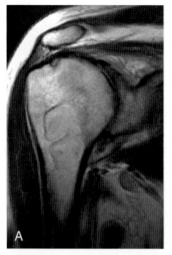
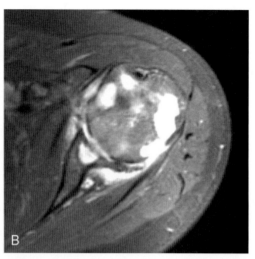

Figure 1 T1-weighted axillary (**A**) and T2-weighted coronal (**B**) MRIs demonstrate extensive osteonecrosis of the humeral head and proximal humerus. The patient presented with pain of approximately 5 months' duration. The remaining bone stock was sufficient; thus, resurfacing was not performed.

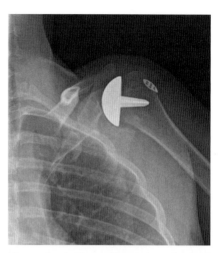

Figure 2 AP radiograph obtained 3 months after humeral head resurfacing demonstrates implant fixation.

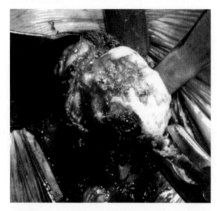

Figure 3 Intraoperative photograph demonstrates substantial osteonecrosis, which is a common indication for humeral head resurfacing.

Altered humeral head offset may also lead to impingement on the acromion or glenoid rim. It has been reported that up to 30% of unsatisfactory results from shoulder replacements are due to component malpositioning.

Case Presentation

A 30-year-old right-hand–dominant woman presents with left shoulder pain of approximately 6 months' duration that has worsened over time. On physical examination, the patient is found to have limited ROM and persistent pain, even at rest. Active forward flexion is to 30° and active external rotation to 20°. Using the Oxford scale, the patient demonstrates 4/5 rotator cuff strength in all planes of motion.

Initial radiographic imaging was obtained 1 month before the patient presented to the authors' clinic. MRIs demonstrate radiographic imaging was obtained 1 month before the patient presented to the authors' clinic. MRIs demonstrate extensive osteonecrosis of the humeral head (**Figure 1**). A partial tear of the supraspinatus with mild muscular atrophy is noted. The remaining rotator cuff muscles are intact. It was decided that the patient would benefit from a humeral head resurfacing procedure. Radiographs obtained 3 months after surgery demonstrated stable implant fixation (**Figure 2**).

Indications

The indications for humeral resurfacing have historically included the active young patient with osteoarthritis (OA) and a concentric glenoid, rheumatoid arthritis, or osteonecrosis with adequate subchondral bone support (**Figure 3**). Indications have expanded to include other forms of arthropathy, such as instability or trauma, provided there is a concentric or resurfaced glenoid. Patient age is becoming less of a consideration than it was previously, whereas the quality and amount of subchondral bone support is an increasingly relevant factor. Typically, at least 60% to 70% of the subchondral surface should be intact and stable. In the absence of adequate humeral head bone, a stemmed humeral component may be necessary to ensure early component stability (**Figure 3**).

Because resurfacing functions as a hemiarthroplasty, a concentric glenoid and stable rotator cuff kinematics must be preserved. Glenoid deficiencies such as hypoplasia, eccentric wear, and rim deficiencies must be addressed to produce a stable and congruent surface with which the resurfacing implant can articulate. Options for the glenoid include bone grafting, local tissue interposition, biologic resurfacing with soft-tissue grafts, and polyethylene components. The presence of rotator cuff tears is not an absolute contraindication provided that kinematics are stable. Anterior stability must be preserved with an intact subscapularis or transfer of the pectoralis major muscle.

Controversies and Alternative Approaches

There are multiple alternatives to resurfacing procedures. Nonsurgical management has the advantage of avoiding the risks associated with surgical intervention. Arthroscopic débridement of the chondral surface in patients with established glenohumeral OA has generally had poor results. Another option is glenohumeral joint arthrodesis. Although this method may provide substantial pain relief, the resulting limited functional ROM may make this procedure a less appealing alternative to patients. Nonetheless, in an active young patient, glenohumeral joint arthrodesis allows for the preservation of bone stock, good pain relief, and relatively good motion in those who are able to compensate through scapulothoracic motion.

Standard stemmed hemiarthroplasty is the most commonly performed procedure for humeral head replacement. However, the reduced number of steps required to perform a humeral head resurfacing compared with a standard stemmed hemiarthroplasty allows for decreased surgical time, blood loss, and pain. All these factors may contribute to an easier rehabilitation process. Resurfacing also reduces the chances for periprosthetic fracture because broaching and stem insertion are not required. Stemmed humeral implants may also cause stress risers or produce a stress-shielding effect that may lead to periprosthetic fractures or loosening—consequences typically avoided with resurfacing implants. In addition, because of the limited amount of implant material, infections are easier to address. The least favorable outcomes

and highest revision rates for resurfacing are seen in patients undergoing this procedure in the presence of rotator cuff tear arthropathy. These patients may be better treated with reverse shoulder arthroplasty.

The decision whether to resurface the glenoid is controversial. The choice is multifactorial and must take into account adequate exposure, glenoid erosion, and the condition of the glenoid articular cartilage. Progressive development of glenoid erosion and arthrosis are among the most common reasons for revision. These complications have been reported to occur in up to 12% of patients who underwent isolated humeral head resurfacing for primary OA, particularly in patients in whom an oversized humeral component was implanted. Furthermore, erosion may compromise glenoid bone stock, which could compromise future revision. In a study with 7-year follow-up, mean Constant scores increased from 33 to 93 for patients with OA who underwent total shoulder resurfacing and from 40 to 73 for patients with OA who underwent hemiresurfacing. Humeral head resurfacing in conjunction with glenoid resurfacing, that is, total shoulder resurfacing, may be performed under specific indications. However, problems with glenoid loosening may occur in up to 10% of patients. Resurfacing the glenoid also lateralizes the humeral head, which may increase tension on the rotator cuff and decrease ROM, a potential consequence that must be taken into consideration when choosing to perform this additional procedure. The higher revision rates of polyethylene glenoid components in resurfacing are likely a result of the decreased visualization achieved during resurfacing compared with that in conventional shoulder arthroplasty.

Hardware failure is one complication associated with humeral resurfacing. Because of the reduced fixation area of humeral resurfacing prostheses compared with stemmed implants, it has

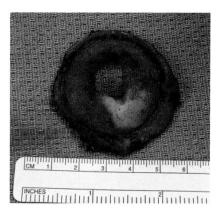

Figure 4 Clinical photograph shows fibrous ingrowth without bony ingrowth in a retrieved resurfacing implant.

been suggested that humeral resurfacing prostheses may loosen and fail over time. In revision cases, the authors of this chapter have often observed that the undersurface of the implant has minimal bone ingrowth. In some instances, the authors have observed only fibrous ingrowth to the undersurface, lacking any bone ingrowth (**Figure 4**). Other complications include humeral neck fracture and humeral head collapse, as seen in hip resurfacing. Subluxation and dislocation are rare occurrences that can result from incorrect sizing and version of the humeral component placed on the native humeral head.

In some instances, increased ROM may lead to postoperative symptoms of impingement. Consequently, a subacromial decompression is recommended at the time of surgery. However, further studies are needed to validate this additional procedure. Humeral head migration may also occur on serial postoperative imaging as a result of rotator cuff failure, glenoid erosion, or both, leading to pain and ultimately necessitating revision.

Results

Humeral resurfacing has been shown to have good clinical outcomes, with many studies reporting results comparable with those following the use of stemmed prostheses (**Table 1**). In some studies, rates of revision for humeral resurfacing have also been similar to or better than those for stemmed components. The rate of revision to total shoulder arthroplasty is reportedly as high as 12% in patients treated with stemmed humeral hemiarthroplasty. Conversion rates at midterm follow-up may be less with resurfacing; revision rates as low as 1% to 2% have been reported. Some of the greater success with shoulder resurfacing compared with hemiarthroplasty may be attributed to technique and the release of soft-tissue contractures intraoperatively. Soft-tissue releases in conjunction with correct version/sizing of the humeral head may result in better spacing of the joint and improved kinematics, leading to less glenoid wear and pain.

Early outcomes from patients with rheumatoid arthritis have also been promising, with a 94% patient satisfaction rate reported at a mean follow-up of 4 years in one study. Although complications such as glenoid erosion and proximal migration of the cup resulting from extensive rotator cuff disease may occur, patients with rheumatoid arthritis typically have good functional results comparable with those of patients with OA. However, studies have shown better Constant scores, Oxford Shoulder Scores, satisfaction levels, pain scores, and Medical Outcomes Study 12-Item Short Form scores after resurfacing in patients with OA than after resurfacing in patients with rheumatoid arthritis.

Technical Keys to Success

Preoperative imaging includes plain radiography consisting of AP, lateral, and axillary views. Advanced imaging such as CT may be obtained to better assess glenoid erosion and version. In patients with osteonecrosis, MRI is typically performed to evaluate the extent of humeral head involvement. The type of implant used is determined by the preference of the surgeon.

Setup/Exposure

- The patient is induced under general anesthesia in the operating room and is placed in the supine beach-chair position.
- The extremity is prepped and draped in the usual sterile fashion.
- Either a deltopectoral or an anterosuperior approach may be used. The authors of this chapter prefer the extended deltopectoral approach.

Procedure

- The skin incision is begun just medial to the coracoid process and is extended distally in the deltopectoral interval for approximately 8 cm.
- The cephalic vein is identified and retracted laterally with the deltoid.
- The biceps tendon is palpated in the bicipital groove, opened with electrocautery, and tagged with sutures in preparation for tenodesis at the end of the procedure.
- The bicipital groove is opened proximally through the rotator interval to the glenoid margin.
- The insertion of the subscapularis to the lesser tuberosity is identified. A wide, thin osteotome is used to perform a lesser tuberosity osteotomy to remove a 5-mm–thick wafer of bone.
- The subscapularis tendon is tagged with a suture.
- Electrocautery is used to release the remaining subscapularis and inferior capsule off of the humerus. This is performed while gently moving the extremity into adduction, extension, and external rotation to help deliver the humeral head.
- Osteophytes are removed circumferentially with osteotomes and rongeurs to define the true anatomic orientation of the humeral head at the anatomic neck interface.
- A head sizer is used to approximate the appropriately sized humeral head reamer that will be used (**Figure 5, A**).
- A pin-positioning guide is placed on the humeral head in correct alignment, and complete contact with the articular surface is confirmed. A guidewire is drilled into the center of the humeral head as close to the anatomic inclination as possible with respect to the shaft of the humeral head. The lateral cortex is penetrated with the guidewire to prevent migration of the guidewire (**Figure 5, B**).
- The pin-positioning guide is removed, and correct placement of the guidewire in the center of the humeral head is confirmed, along with confirmation of an acceptable neck/shaft angle.
- Reaming is performed using the appropriately sized humeral head reamer. Depth of the reaming is gauged by visualization through windows in the reamer and evaluation of the peripheral positioning of the reamer on the humeral neck.
- Defects in the humeral head may be filled with the bone graft shavings from the humeral head reamer. Trial heads are placed over the guidewire to confirm sizing. Any remaining osteophytes are removed with a rongeur.
- A stem punch or drill is placed over the guidewire to create a path for the stem of the final implant.
- A trial stemmed implant is impacted into place, and direct visualization is used to ensure appropriate fit and contouring of the humeral head.
- The humerus is reduced into the glenohumeral joint, and the extremity is taken through all planes

Table 1 Results of Humeral Head Resurfacing

Author(s)	Journal (Year)	No. of Shoulders	Outcomes	Complications	Comments
Thomas et al	*J Shoulder Elbow Surg* (2005)	56	Mean Constant score improved from 16 to 54	3 subsequent SADs, for impingement 1 revision for aseptic loosening 2 with nonprogressive osteolysis 1 periprosthetic humeral neck fracture managed nonsurgically 1 intraoperative glenoid fracture	52 patients Mean follow-up, 2.8 yr
Mullett et al	*J Bone Joint Surg Br* (2007)	29	Mean Constant score improved from 15 to 77 Mean FF increased from 48° to 105°	1 revision to reverse prosthesis in a patient with previous RCT arthropathy who had increasing pain and worsening function	Patient age, >80 yr Mean follow-up, 4.5 yr
Bailie et al	*J Bone Joint Surg Am* (2008)	36	Significant improvements in VAS, SANE, and ASES scores (*P* < 0.001) 35 patients returned to desired athletic activities No radiographic loosening at latest follow-up	1 traumatic subscapularis rupture 3 cases of arthrofibrosis 1 deep hematoma 1 revision to TSA for pain	Mean age, 42 yr (range, 28-54 yr) Avg follow-up, 3.2 yr
Buchner et al	*Arch Orthop Trauma Surg* (2008)	22	Mean time of surgery, estimated blood loss, and length of hospital stay significantly decreased compared with TSA group (*P* < 0.05)	Mean Constant score and ROM were better after TSA at 12-mo follow-up 2 revisions to TSA for glenoid erosion	Mean age, 61 yr Avg last follow-up, 1 yr
Pritchett	*J Shoulder Elbow Surg* (2011)	74	96% long-term survivorship 95% satisfaction No fractures, dislocations, or infections	7 revision procedures, 6 with good results 12 cemented polyethylene glenoid prostheses had radiolucencies, 3 of which produced symptoms requiring revision	61 patients (mean age, 58 yr) Technique included glenoid resurfacing Mean follow-up, 28 yr
Al-Hadithy et al	*J Shoulder Elbow Surg* (2012)	53	Mean Constant score improved from 38 to 75 Mean OSS improved from 22 to 42	1 anterosuperior escape after rotator cuff failure 12% glenoid erosion, associated with oversizing 1 revision for fracture	46 patients Mean follow-up, 4.2 yr
Alizadeh-khaiyat et al	*J Shoulder Elbow Surg* (2013)	111	85% satisfactory; 6.5% unsatisfactory Significantly higher Constant score in OA group compared with RA group Improvements in OSS, satisfaction level, pain score, and SF-12 score	1 infection 1 loosening with no clinical correlation Revision rate: 12.9% for standard shell, 54.5% for extended articular surface RCA had highest failure rate (63%), followed by RA (27.5%) and OA (10.4%)	No glenoid resurfacing performed in this study Mean follow-up, 4 yr

ASES = American Shoulder and Elbow Surgeons shoulder outcome, FF = forward flexion, OA = osteoarthritis, OSS = Oxford Shoulder Score, RA = rheumatoid arthritis, RCA = rotator cuff arthropathy, RCT = rotator cuff tear, ROM = range of motion, SAD = subacromial decompression, SANE = Single Assessment Numeric Evaluation, SF-12 = Medical Outcomes Study 12-Item Short Form, TSA = total shoulder arthroplasty, VAS = visual analog scale.

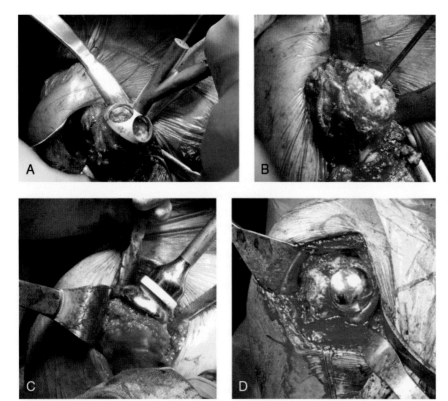

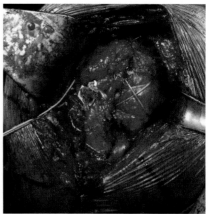

Figure 6 Intraoperative photograph shows closure of the interval; a button was positioned to reinforce the subscapularis.

Figure 5 Intraoperative photographs show key steps in the humeral head resurfacing procedure. **A,** Sizing of the humeral head reamer. **B,** Insertion of a guidewire for reaming and subsequent HemiCAP implant (Arthrosurface) sizing. **C,** Impaction of the HemiCAP implant with stem into place. **D,** Appearance of the fixed HemiCAP implant before closure.

of motion to assess soft-tissue balancing. Soft-tissue releases are performed as necessary.

- The humeral head is re-dislocated, and the trial implant is removed.
- The final implant is impacted into place (**Figure 5, C** and **D**).
- After confirmation of appropriate seating, the humeral head is reduced into the joint. Fluoroscopy may be used throughout the procedure to confirm adequate positioning of the component.
- Using a Mason-Allen stitch, four No. 2 nonabsorbable sutures are passed around the subscapularis tendon. These sutures are passed through drill holes just over the lateral edge of the intertubercular groove and tied down, anatomically repairing the tuberosity

osteotomy back to its base.
- An additional nonabsorbable suture is passed vertically in the subscapularis tendon just medial to the previously inserted sutures. These sutures are then crossed and passed lateral to the intertubercular groove through the holes that were used to pass the previously tied sutures. This suture is tied down onto the metaphyseal cortex of the humerus to create a tension-band construct over the lesser tuberosity for additional stability. If the lateral metaphyseal cortex is weak, a button may be used to prevent suture penetration through the cortex when the suture is tied down (**Figure 6**).
- The shoulder is copiously lavaged with irrigation. The authors of this chapter typically do not place a

drain for this procedure.
- The deltopectoral interval is closed using a No. 2 nonabsorbable suture. This nonabsorbable suture allows for easier identification of the deltopectoral interval in the revision setting.
- Deep soft-tissue layers are closed with a No. 0 absorbable suture followed by subcutaneous closure with a 2-0 absorbable suture and skin closure with a 3-0 absorbable suture.

Wound Closure

- A topical skin adhesive is used over the incision for final closure.
- A sterile dressing is applied. The authors of this chapter typically place a cold therapy wrap on the shoulder for comfort.
- The shoulder is placed in an immobilizer sling.

Rehabilitation

The postoperative rehabilitation protocol may involve early mobilization with specific restrictions or a period of immobilization (**Table 2**). Patients treated by the authors of this chapter begin inpatient physical therapy following a hemiarthroplasty protocol in which forward

Table 2 Rehabilitation Protocol After Humeral Head Resurfacing

Postoperative Week	Range of Motion	Strengthening	Return to Play	Comments/Emphasis
0-6	Forward flexion is limited to 125° External rotation is limited to 30°	None	None	Physical therapy is begun immediately postoperatively for passive range of motion
6-12	Full motion is allowed at 6 wk	None	None	Active-assisted and active range of motion exercises are begun
≥12	No restrictions	Strengthening exercises are begun	Sport-specific, graduated return-to-play program is begun	Graduated strengthening program

flexion is limited to 125° and external rotation is limited to 30° for 4 to 6 weeks to allow for lesser tuberosity healing. Healing of the lesser tuberosity may be confirmed on axillary radiographs at subsequent postoperative visits. The ROM restrictions are lifted after 6 weeks. Patients may begin strengthening exercises 3 months postoperatively.

Avoiding Pitfalls and Complications

Obtaining appropriate imaging is important for assessing the humeral head and the glenoid. An axillary plain radiograph may be helpful to assess the concentricity of the humeral head in the glenoid. In patients in whom glenoid bone loss is suspected, a CT scan should be obtained to determine whether an additional glenoid procedure is required. For patients with osteonecrosis, an MRI is obtained to assess the amount of stable bone available to support the resurfacing implant. Typically, at least 60% to 70% of the humeral head must be viable to achieve appropriate fixation.

All osteophytes should be removed on exposure of the proximal humerus to enable clear identification of the anatomic neck of the humerus. Reconstruction that closely approximates the natural anatomy is a substantial benefit of humeral head resurfacing. Any osteophytes that may interfere with the identification of normal anatomy must be resected to enable correct positioning of the resurfacing on the humeral head.

When inserting the initial guidewire centered on the humeral head, bicortical penetration is required to ensure that the guidewire does not change position during subsequent reaming and trialing. Of similar importance, care must also be taken to avoid bending the guidewire when reaming and trialing, which may lead to wire breakage or nonanatomic reaming.

It is also important to ensure proper reaming of the humeral head by constantly checking the depth of reaming through reamer windows and by reamer positioning on the humeral neck; overzealous reaming may lead to changes in offset and height that counteract the anatomic nature of humeral resurfacing. These changes may lead to instability or purely cancellous bone support of the implant, which may cause subsidence of the implant. However, inadequate reaming may result in insufficient subchondral bone support and early failure.

Bibliography

Al-Hadithy N, Domos P, Sewell MD, Naleem A, Papanna MC, Pandit R: Cementless surface replacement arthroplasty of the shoulder for osteoarthritis: Results of fifty Mark III Copeland prosthesis from an independent center with four-year mean follow-up. *J Shoulder Elbow Surg* 2012;21(12):1776-1781.

Alizadehkhaiyat O, Kyriakos A, Singer MS, Frostick SP: Outcome of Copeland shoulder resurfacing arthroplasty with a 4-year mean follow-up. *J Shoulder Elbow Surg* 2013;22(10):1352-1358.

Alund M, Hoe-Hansen C, Tillander B, Hedén BA, Norlin R: Outcome after cup hemiarthroplasty in the rheumatoid shoulder: A retrospective evaluation of 39 patients followed for 2-6 years. *Acta Orthop Scand* 2000;71(2):180-184.

Bailie DS, Llinas PJ, Ellenbecker TS: Cementless humeral resurfacing arthroplasty in active patients less than fifty-five years of age. *J Bone Joint Surg Am* 2008;90(1):110-117.

Buchner M, Eschbach N, Loew M: Comparison of the short-term functional results after surface replacement and total shoulder arthroplasty for osteoarthritis of the shoulder: A matched-pair analysis. *Arch Orthop Trauma Surg* 2008;128(4):347-354.

Burgess DL, McGrath MS, Bonutti PM, Marker DR, Delanois RE, Mont MA: Shoulder resurfacing. *J Bone Joint Surg Am* 2009;91(5):1228-1238.

Cameron BD, Galatz LM, Ramsey ML, Williams GR, Iannotti JP: Non-prosthetic management of grade IV osteochondral lesions of the glenohumeral joint. *J Shoulder Elbow Surg* 2002;11(1):25-32.

Constant CR, Murley AH: A clinical method of functional assessment of the shoulder. *Clin Orthop Relat Res* 1987;(214):160-164.

Copeland S: The continuing development of shoulder replacement: "Reaching the surface." *J Bone Joint Surg Am* 2006;88(4):900-905.

Fink B, Singer J, Lamla U, Rüther W: Surface replacement of the humeral head in rheumatoid arthritis. *Arch Orthop Trauma Surg* 2004;124(6):366-373.

Fuerst M, Fink B, Rüther W: The DUROM cup humeral surface replacement in patients with rheumatoid arthritis. *J Bone Joint Surg Am* 2007;89(8):1756-1762.

Harryman DT, Sidles JA, Harris SL, Lippitt SB, Matsen FA III: The effect of articular conformity and the size of the humeral head component on laxity and motion after glenohumeral arthroplasty: A study in cadavera. *J Bone Joint Surg Am* 1995;77(4):555-563.

Hill HA, Sachs MD: The grooved defect of the humeral head: A frequently unrecognized complication of dislocations of the shoulder joint. *Radiology* 1940;35(6):690-700.

Jensen KL: Humeral resurfacing arthroplasty: Rationale, indications, technique, and results. *Am J Orthop (Belle Mead NJ)* 2007;36(12 suppl 1):4-8.

Levy O, Copeland SA: Cementless surface replacement arthroplasty of the shoulder: 5- to 10-year results with the Copeland mark-2 prosthesis. *J Bone Joint Surg Br* 2001;83(2):213-221.

Levy O, Copeland SA: Cementless surface replacement arthroplasty (Copeland CSRA) for osteoarthritis of the shoulder. *J Shoulder Elbow Surg* 2004;13(3):266-271.

Levy O, Funk L, Sforza G, Copeland SA: Copeland surface replacement arthroplasty of the shoulder in rheumatoid arthritis. *J Bone Joint Surg Am* 2004;86(3):512-518.

Mullett H, Levy O, Raj D, Even T, Abraham R, Copeland SA: Copeland surface replacement of the shoulder: Results of an hydroxyapatite-coated cementless implant in patients over 80 years of age. *J Bone Joint Surg Br* 2007;89(11):1466-1469.

Pritchett JW: Long-term results and patient satisfaction after shoulder resurfacing. *J Shoulder Elbow Surg* 2011;20(5):771-777.

Raiss P, Aldinger PR, Kasten P, Rickert M, Loew M: Humeral head resurfacing for fixed anterior glenohumeral dislocation. *Int Orthop* 2009;33(2):451-456.

Rydholm U, Sjögren J: Surface replacement of the humeral head in the rheumatoid shoulder. *J Shoulder Elbow Surg* 1993;2(6):286-295.

Thomas SR, Sforza G, Levy O, Copeland SA: Geometrical analysis of Copeland surface replacement shoulder arthroplasty in relation to normal anatomy. *J Shoulder Elbow Surg* 2005;14(2):186-192.

Thomas SR, Wilson AJ, Chambler A, Harding I, Thomas M: Outcome of Copeland surface replacement shoulder arthroplasty. *J Shoulder Elbow Surg* 2005;14(5):485-491.

Williams GR Jr, Wong KL, Pepe MD, et al: The effect of articular malposition after total shoulder arthroplasty on glenohumeral translations, range of motion, and subacromial impingement. *J Shoulder Elbow Surg* 2001;10(5):399-409.

Chapter 35

Shoulder Arthroplasty: Advances and Controversies in Prosthetic Design

Adam J. Lorenzetti, MD

Brent C. Stephens, MD

Geoffrey P. Stone, MD

Mark A. Frankle, MD

 Introduction

Since the advent of shoulder arthroplasty, advances in prosthetic design have improved clinical outcomes and expanded the range of indications for the procedure. Recent advances in both anatomic total shoulder arthroplasty (TSA) and reverse shoulder arthroplasty (RSA) have led to the evolution of humeral and glenoid implants and fixation for each procedure. Humeral head resurfacing is not discussed in this chapter.

 Total Shoulder Arthroplasty

Humeral Fixation

The humeral implant has undergone continuous evolution since its introduction in 1955 by Neer for use in the management of proximal humerus fractures.

The humeral implant was first used for TSA in 1974 with the advent of glenoid resurfacing. Advances in stem design have improved implant fixation and function and decreased implant-related complications. Progression from Neer's original cemented monoblock design has led to implants that better re-create anatomy and preserve bone stock to facilitate initial implantation as well as future revision.

Studies of cemented humeral implants have shown low rates of radiolucent lines and loosening at long-term follow-up. However, noncemented press-fit stems have gained popularity. Noncemented fixation may allow for improved revision in patients with periprosthetic fracture, implant malposition, implant loosening, or infection. The authors of this chapter find that a well-fixed cemented stem can be difficult to remove for revision and may result in

increased bone loss, the requirement of a humeral window, or compromised fixation of a new implant. Press-fit fixation has been improved through proximal geometric alterations such as a metaphyseal taper, which allows impaction into metaphyseal bone, as well as the application of grit-blasted or porous-coated surface finishes to facilitate bone ingrowth or ongrowth at the metaphysis (**Figure 1**). These design improvements have yielded clinical loosening rates similar to those of cemented stems. However, higher rates of stress shielding can be seen in patients with noncemented stems, likely as a result of the increased stem diameter in the proximal humerus. Stress shielding can result from the substantial mismatch in stiffness between the metal stem and the metaphyseal bone.

In an attempt to enhance noncemented metaphyseal fixation, several manufacturers have decreased the stem length in newer designs. A new generation of humeral implants has eliminated the diaphyseal stem entirely; the use of these implants requires humeral head osteotomy, which differentiates their use from humeral head resurfacing. The term stemless is widely used in the literature to refer to humeral implants that lack a diaphyseal component. However,

Dr. Frankle or an immediate family member has received royalties from, is a member of a speakers' bureau or has made paid presentations on behalf of, and serves as a paid consultant to DJO Surgical; has received research or institutional support from BioMimetic Therapeutics and DJO Surgical; has received nonincome support (such as equipment or services), commercially derived honoraria, or other non–research-related funding (such as paid travel) from DJO Surgical; and serves as a board member, owner, officer, or committee member of the American Academy of Orthopaedic Surgeons and the American Shoulder and Elbow Surgeons. None of the following authors or any immediate family member has received anything of value from or has stock or stock options held in a commercial company or institution related directly or indirectly to the subject of this chapter: Dr. Lorenzetti, Dr. Stephens, and Dr. Stone.

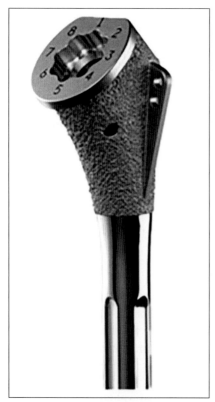

Figure 1 Photograph shows a humeral stem with a proximal plasma coating to promote bone ingrowth and a metaphyseal taper (Turon Modular Shoulder System, DJO Surgical, Vista, CA).

this term is a misnomer because these devices still contain a short, wide stem that is fixed within the metaphysis. The authors of this chapter prefer to refer to implants by the portion of bone to which they are attached; that is, resurfacing implants are designed for fixation at the epiphysis via a small peg and an undercoated humeral head cap, stemless implants achieve fixation at the metaphysis via a metaphyseal stem designed for bone ingrowth, and stemmed implants are attached at the metaphysis via geometry and ingrowth and/or at the diaphysis via interference fit or cementation.

Metaphyseal fixation systems offer several potential advantages. They avoid instrumentation of the diaphysis, which transfers the stress concentration effect of the mismatch between the prosthetic tip and the bone, from the cortical bone of the diaphysis in a stemmed implant, to the cancellous metaphyseal bone in metaphyseal fixation systems. This design also minimizes the influence of the diaphyseal stem on placement of the humeral articulation, which is a concern if the humeral articular surface is translated from the diaphysis as a result of severe malunion. These factors improve the ease of revision, eliminate the risk of periprosthetic humeral shaft fractures, and improve the ability to implant the fixation system in patients who have proximal humerus deformities, whereas previous systems required a humeral osteotomy or modification of the implant. In theory, metaphyseal fixation implants also allow a point of implant fixation that is closer to the joint center of rotation rather than farther down the metaphysis, which may reduce stress through the implant. In a finite element analysis study published in 2016, reducing stem length produced humeral stresses that more closely matched the intact stress distribution in proximal humerus cortical bone.

Metaphyseal fixation TSA was first introduced to the market in Europe in 2004 in the form of the Total Evolutive Shoulder System (TESS; Biomet). Subsequently, four other metaphyseal fixation designs were released in Europe, two of which have entered US FDA Investigational Device Exemption (IDE) clinical trials—the Eclipse (Arthrex) and the Nano (Biomet), which is the second-generation TESS. A third metaphyseal fixation system, the Simpliciti Shoulder System (Tornier), completed the FDA IDE and entered the US market in 2015 (**Figure 2**). The Eclipse achieves metaphyseal fixation via a threaded design that allows screw-in implantation, whereas the other prostheses are impacted and have coatings to encourage bone ingrowth for fixation. All available designs incorporate a modular humeral head, with the Nano enabling conversion to reverse arthroplasty, and a collar to prevent overimpaction of the prosthesis.

Published clinical data are available on all three implants discussed in the previous paragraph. The earliest study of metaphyseal fixation shoulder arthroplasty, published in 2011, followed 63 TESS implants for a minimum of 3 years. A mean 45-point improvement in the Constant score was reported, in addition to improvement of 49° in forward elevation without evidence of subsidence, loosening, osteolysis, stress shielding, or radiolucent lines around the humeral implant; however, an 11.1% revision rate and five intraoperative fractures of the lateral humeral cortex were reported. The authors of that study attributed their findings to technical errors in the initial implantation protocol, which required using the largest possible size of the corolla (one manufacturer's term for the implant wings that are impacted into the metaphysis) so that it would contact the metaphyseal cortex. Those authors subsequently advocated undersizing this component to preserve bone and avoid this complication. A prospective longitudinal study published in 2013 compared the Neer II prosthesis (Smith & Nephew), a second-generation prosthesis; the Bigliani/Flatow prosthesis (Zimmer), a third-generation prosthesis; and the TESS. No statistical difference in outcome scores was found between the groups, but higher rates of radiolucent lines were seen around the stemmed Neer II prosthesis at minimum 2-year follow-up. The largest published study on the Eclipse, which included 78 patients followed for at least 5 years, showed improvements in Constant score and range of motion and a 9% revision rate. No revisions were necessary to address the humeral component. In 149 patients treated with the Simpliciti Shoulder System, significant improvement in Constant, Simple Shoulder Test, and American Shoulder and Elbow Surgeons shoulder outcome scores was noted at minimum follow-up of 2 years. No signs of loosening, osteolysis, or subsidence were noted, and

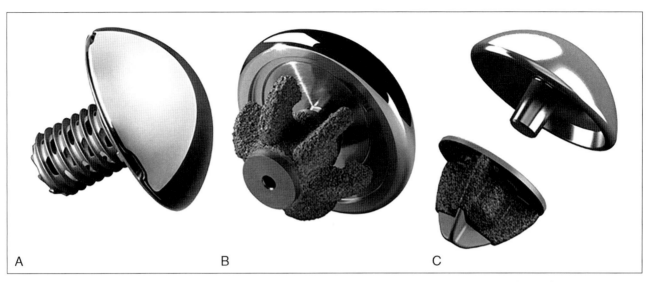

Figure 2   Photographs show the Eclipse (Arthrex; **A**), Nano (Biomet; **B**), and Simpliciti (Tornier; **C**) metaphyseal fixation total shoulder arthroplasty implants.

the three complications that occurred required revision.

Metaphyseal fixation systems require adequate bone quality for implant stability. Bone quality may be compromised by substantial bone deformity, severe osteoporosis, or inadequate surgical technique. These fixation systems should not be seen as a panacea solving the problem of humeral stem complications. Surgical experience and decision making are vital in avoiding improper placement of noncemented implants, regardless of stem length. The substantial learning curve related to surgical decision making in the use of these systems may lead to an increased complication rate for surgeons who are not familiar with such systems. Intraoperative assessment of bone quality and initial implant stability are essential because conversion to a stemmed prostheses may be necessary to achieve adequate fixation. Although metaphyseal fixation systems offer the ability to match the patient's anatomy, anatomic implantation may not be the best strategy in terms of soft-tissue balancing. Asymmetric soft-tissue contractures, such as in patients with static posterior subluxation, may require alteration of humeral anatomy to

appropriately rebalance the shoulder. Published outcomes of TSA with metaphyseal fixation are limited; however, several IDE clinical trials are ongoing.

Additional factors to consider in the choice of stem design are the degree of proximal humeral bone loss and possible stress shielding that can occur with short, thicker metaphyseal fixation stems. A biomechanical study evaluating the relationship between torsional stability and proximal humeral bone loss showed significant decreases in micromotion with an intact proximal humerus. Because many patients who undergo TSA are older and have osteoporosis, the amount of proximal humerus support must be taken into consideration. In these patients, longer stems with diaphyseal fixation may better withstand the increased stress placed on them, providing greater long-term stability than short stems with metaphyseal fixation would provide.

Another concern is whether the increased thickness of short metaphyseal fixation stems will lead to stress shielding and, ultimately, bone loss in the proximal humerus. Although no long-term studies have addressed this concern in shoulder arthroplasty, the hip

and knee arthroplasty literature contains several long-term studies investigating femoral stems with metaphyseal fixation. In a study of short femoral stems with metaphyseal fixation in patients with greater than 11-year follow-up, the authors reported little stress shielding, with no patients having greater than grade 2 stress shielding. Although these results are promising, whether they will hold true for humeral stems with metaphyseal fixation remains to be seen.

Glenoid Fixation

Since the introduction of the cemented all-polyethylene implant, glenoid loosening has become the most common cause of TSA failure. The most commonly used prostheses have been cemented, all-polyethylene implants with pegged or keeled design. Although good clinical results have been achieved with both types, significant rates of radiolucent lines and potential loosening have been found, with higher rates in keeled implants. Design improvements, including noncemented fixation, metal-backed implants, and hybrid fixation, have been introduced in an attempt to yield more stable, longer-lasting implants. Updated surgical techniques include the use of mechanical reaming, which can improve conformity of the implant and bone while preserving subchondral bone support, and improvements in cement preparation, such as the weep hole technique. In the weep hole technique, a drill hole is placed just lateral to the coracoid and medial to the glenoid rim. This hole penetrates to the central glenoid cancellous bone, after which suction is applied to help remove blood from the glenoid surface during cementing. Suction also aids in pulling cement into the cancellous bone and peg holes.

As with noncemented humeral implants, metal-backed noncemented glenoid implants offer the advantage of eliminating the cemented interface in favor of theoretically stronger bone ingrowth as well as increased immediate fixation with additional compression screws. Most designs incorporate a polyethylene liner set into a metal component and include backside compression screws, press-fit geometry, and surface treatments to encourage ingrowth. Most large, long-term studies of metal-backed implants have shown lower survival rates and higher rates of revision compared with cemented all-polyethylene implants.

As implant designs have evolved, new glenoid-related complications have occurred as a result of design characteristics intended to improve outcomes. An implant with a polyethylene insert theoretically allows a worn polyethylene component to be replaced without removal of the baseplate, but several studies have reported dissociation resulting from this increased complexity. The additional interface also has been implicated as a source of osteolysis and failure attributed to suspected backside wear resulting from motion between the baseplate and the polyethylene component, which is well documented in the knee arthroplasty literature. Screw breakage and implant loosening also have been reported in patients with delayed or incomplete bone ingrowth.

Metallosis, which can exacerbate the effect of glenoid implant failure, occurs if the metallic head component contacts the baseplate as a result of either polyethylene failure or excessive wear. Implant thickness has been a major concern because two-piece implants are thicker than one-piece all-polyethylene implants and can affect soft-tissue tensioning, raising the risk of overstuffing and putting increased stress on the glenoid implant. The increased forces and the need for thinner polyethylene inserts to reduce the size of the implant are potential causes of the increased wear, osteolysis, and failure seen with metal-backed glenoid implants.

The ease of revision also is a concern with metal-backed glenoid implants. The authors of this chapter find that the defect created by failure of a metal-backed glenoid implant can be larger compared with that created by failure of an all-polyethylene implant because of the larger size of the metal-backed implant. In contrast, failure of an all-polyethylene implant often produces a central defect that is contained. Also, in patients requiring revision surgery because of infection or rotator cuff failure, a well-fixed bone ingrowth prosthesis can be difficult to remove without substantial bone destruction. A well-fixed all-polyethylene implant can be removed with the use of an osteotome followed by removal of the remaining implant via direct visualization, without substantial damage to the surrounding bone. One potential benefit of a well-fixed metal-backed implant is the modular nature of some systems, which allows the implant to be converted to a glenosphere component and thereby eases revision to RSA in patients with instability or rotator cuff failure.

The latest generation of metal-backed glenoid implants have monoblock or hybrid designs in an attempt to eliminate backside wear, polyethylene dissociation, and overstuffing of the joint, but published data are limited. One study

reported the technique and short-term experience with the use of a cemented, non–metal-backed monoblock glenoid implant with an interference-fit plasma-coated cage peg and titanium peripheral pegs; however, the report did not include formal clinical review of cases or clinical and radiographic follow-up. In a study of a porous, tantalum-backed, press-fit monoblock glenoid implant with 2-year follow-up, researchers reported an unacceptably high complication rate, with fracture of the implant in 21% of patients. The authors of a different study found an unacceptably high failure rate (13.6% rate of implant fracture) at minimum 2-year follow-up with a noncemented, soft metal–backed monoblock glenoid implant. Modular hybrid prostheses, such as the Regenerex system (Biomet), offer the choice of a polyethylene implant with a modular, central porous metal peg to promote bone ingrowth or a standard polyethylene implant; however, clinical data have not been reported. Manufacturers have attempted to increase survival of all-polyethylene pegged implants by offering a central stem anchor peg with fins to allow the application of bone graft to the implant. Several small series have shown promising early results with either limited cement fixation around the outer pegs or noncemented fixation; however, the superiority of the use of a fully cemented pegged implant has not been demonstrated.

Articulation

One of the most difficult problems in shoulder arthroplasty is posterior glenoid wear. Historically, surgeons have corrected implant version through the use of posterior bone grafting and asymmetric reaming, but the literature has shown inconsistent results. Asymmetric reaming of the anterior glenoid can result in decreased glenoid bone stock, thereby compromising fixation, and can medialize the joint, thereby decreasing the range of motion. Posterior bone grafting has resulted in complications such as graft resorption and instability. To address these problems, step-cut or augmented glenoid implants that alter the version of the implant without affecting bone stock have been developed. Several biomechanical and computer modeling studies have suggested that augmented glenoid implants have the potential to conserve bone, correct version, and improve glenoid force relationships. However, clinical results have shown increased rates of loosening, poor long-term survival, and difficulty of correcting instability.

Techniques that focus on glenoid version alone are unable to correct the balance of forces in a shoulder with posterior subluxation and wear. Although biomechanical models predict that the restoration of anatomic version would improve the force relationships in the shoulder, these models ignore the pathology that led to the posterior subluxation and the forces that predisposed the shoulder to posterior wear. Correction of the deforming forces may be necessary. In one study of patients with glenohumeral osteoarthritis and a biconcave glenoid, researchers reported improved, consistent clinical results of RSA compared with TSA for attempts to correct the glenoid surface. The authors of this chapter have not had success with augmented implants or glenoid bone grafting in primary TSA and prefer conversion to RSA if the balance of forces cannot be corrected during glenoid preparation and the posterior subluxation persists. The intraoperative decision to perform RSA instead of anatomic TSA is based on factors including patient age, the degree of subluxation observed on preoperative imaging, intraoperative assessment of the potential to achieve glenoid bone/implant congruency while maintaining subchondral support, and the ability to center the humeral head during intraoperative trials. RSA should be considered if the surgical goals of TSA cannot be achieved.

The design of the glenoid implant also affects glenohumeral articular forces after TSA, and the articular congruity is complex. The native glenoid has a slightly larger radius of curvature than the native humeral head, but the pliable cartilage and labral complex improve conformity. This translation inherent to the glenohumeral joint is difficult to replicate in prosthetic design. A congruent glenoid implant offers a larger contact area and thereby reduces contact pressure, which theoretically should improve joint stability and reduce stress within the implant. However, this conformity reduces translation of the joint and thus exposes the implant to eccentric edge loading, which may lead to early loosening. A mismatch in curvature allows some translation while reducing eccentric loads, but may decrease joint stability and result in eccentric posterior loading. In one study that demonstrated the importance of articular congruity, researchers found significantly lower radiolucency scores if radial mismatch was greater than 5.5 mm. They recommended a mismatch of 6 to 10 mm but were unable to show a significant effect of mismatch on clinical loosening or revision rates. The ideal radial mismatch remains elusive because of the difficulty of replicating anatomy. Biomechanical studies of hybrid designs with a more conforming central region and less conforming periphery have shown promise in combining the advantages of both designs, but the results have not yet been validated in clinical studies.

Modularity

Revision of failed anatomic TSA is difficult and complicated. As indications for revision to RSA grow, the ease of revision of a well-fixed TSA has become a concern. Removal of a well-fixed stemmed prosthesis can lead to intraoperative complications, such as radial nerve palsy, bone loss, humeral fractures, and cement extravasation. Many device manufacturers currently offer modular systems that either use the same stem for both anatomic TSA and RSA or use a conversion device to allow attachment of a modular humeral cup (**Figure 3**). The ease of revision to RSA with stem retention has been touted in several small series, with findings including avoidance of neurologic and stem-removal complications. The authors of one study found significantly less blood loss and reduced surgical times during revision to RSA with humeral stem retention compared with revision to RSA with stem removal and replacement. However, they noted that removal of a well-fixed modular stem was necessary in some patients with substantial stem malposition.

Although modular prostheses offer many benefits, they have other disadvantages in addition to the inability to fully correct stem malposition. The authors of one study found mean lengthening of 2.6 cm during conversion to RSA with a modular stem in a review of 14 procedures. No neurologic complications were reported, but the risk of excessive lengthening was highlighted. Overtensioning of the deltoid may result in adduction contractures, affect joint kinematics, and increase glenoid forces, potentially increasing the risk of early glenoid loosening. Alteration of the relationship of the humerus to the surrounding structures may have unforeseen consequences (**Figure 4**). Modular systems also are associated with risk of failure at the component interfaces, which is not a concern with monoblock implants (**Figure 5**). Modularity brings a burden of choice that can potentially overcomplicate some procedures.

 # Reverse Shoulder Arthroplasty

Humeral Fixation

Although humeral loosening does not seem to be a major issue with anatomic TSA, the risk of this complication is

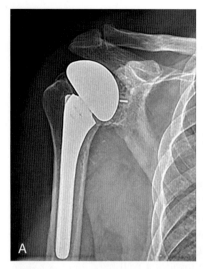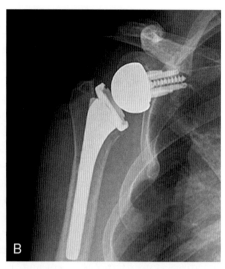

Figure 3 Preoperative (**A**) and postoperative (**B**) AP radiographs demonstrate revision of failed total shoulder arthroplasty to reverse shoulder arthroplasty with retention of the humeral implant and the use of a conversion device.

greater in RSA. In one study, patients who underwent anatomic TSA had a humeral loosening rate of 1.5% in a period of 8 years, whereas the rate was 3.6% in RSA patients. This significant difference may be attributable to the semiconstrained design of RSA prostheses, which increases the forces placed on the bone-implant interface. Historically, both TSA and RSA prostheses have been cemented to minimize humeral loosening.

As in TSA, the trend in RSA has been the use of press-fit humeral fixation. Advantages include decreased surgical time, the potential of biologic prosthetic fixation, and the avoidance of cement-related complications. Several recent studies have yielded results of noncemented humeral fixation comparable with those of cemented humeral fixation. In a study that compared noncemented, porous-coated humeral RSA stems with cemented humeral RSA stems in patients with 2- to 5-year follow-up, researchers found no significant differences in radiographic evidence of humeral loosening or functional scores. Both groups showed significant improvement over preoperative functional

scores and range of motion. The noncemented stems had the added benefit of a simplified surgical technique and no cement-related complications. In a study of the radiographic results of an noncemented trabecular metal RSA prosthesis at 1- and 2-year follow-up, researchers found minimal radiographic evidence of humeral stem loosening or subsidence, with 90% of humeral stems having no radiolucent lines at 2-year follow-up. In both studies, researchers attributed the improved results of the noncemented prostheses to the increased sophistication of the implant designs, which allowed for better bone ingrowth into the stem.

Given the decreased surgical time and the ease of implantation of noncemented prostheses, surgeons may be tempted to leave all humeral RSA implants noncemented, but this decision should be balanced with intraoperative surgical judgment. Although the authors of this chapter prefer to use press-fit fixation in most primary RSA procedures, a cemented humeral stem may be necessary in some patients, such as when the normal mechanical support provided by the proximal humerus is absent as

a result of bone loss. In addition, if the stability of the humeral implant is a concern in primary RSA, the threshold for the use of cement should be low.

Stem Length

General controversies surrounding stem length are discussed in the TSA section of this chapter. The following issues are specific to RSA.

RSA implants with short, metaphyseal fixation humeral stems have recently been introduced. No long-term data are available, but recent short-term results are encouraging. In a study of primary RSA with short, noncemented humeral stems with at least 2-year follow-up, short stems provided reliable pain relief with improved movement. At 2 years postoperatively, all humeral implants showed evidence of adequate fixation and no signs of loosening. In a different study examining the clinical and radiographic short-term outcomes of RSA with short, metaphyseal fixation humeral stems, researchers found promising results in 21 patients at minimum 2-year follow-up. Patients had significant improvements in pain, activities of daily living, and range of motion with no complications related to humeral implant fixation. In this study, four periprosthetic humeral fractures occurred in the metaphysis, three of which were managed nonsurgically and healed with good function. Although these studies reported encouraging results, they were both small, short-term studies and did not address possible complications that can arise with longer follow-up or a greater number of patients.

In a different study, researchers reported the results of 56 "stemless" metaphyseal fixation RSA implants with nearly 5-year follow-up. Results were comparable with those of stemmed implants, with improvements in each portion of the Constant-Murley score and in active forward flexion. The authors reported one intraoperative humeral metaphyseal crack, which did not

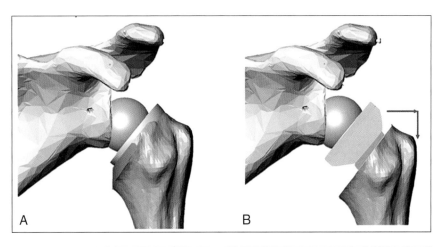

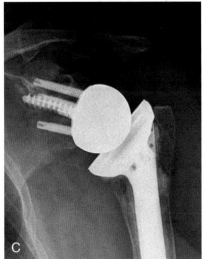

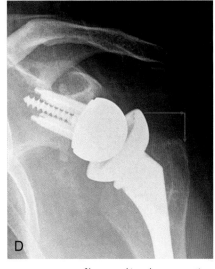

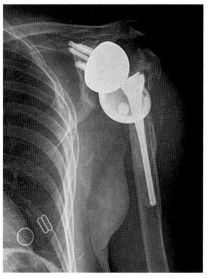

Figure 5 AP radiograph demonstrates failure of a humeral implant at a modular junction because of increased forces resulting from poor proximal bone stock.

Figure 4 Illustrations (**A** and **B**) show the consequences of humeral implant retention or conversion during revision to reverse shoulder arthroplasty. Replacement of the stem (**A**) allows for a more anatomic humeral position, whereas conversion of the stem (**B**) leads to distalization and lateralization of the humerus (indicated by red arrows). These consequences are visible in AP radiographs, which demonstrate humeral stem replacement (**C**) or humeral stem conversion, resulting in distalization and lateralization of the humerus (indicated by red arrows; **D**).

require revision, and one postoperative displacement of the stemless humeral implant, which necessitated revision to a stemmed implant. A larger study examined the same implant system in 91 RSA procedures in 87 patients and showed favorable clinical results at minimum 2-year follow-up and no radiographic evidence of loosening. The authors of the study reported three complications: recurrent instability attributed to inadequate soft-tissue tensioning, a scapular spine fracture, and a traumatic

clavicle fracture resulting from a fall. Of note, because the device used in these studies requires metaphyseal fixation through the reverse corolla (an impacted surface-coated cup), it would be classified as an inset design, discussed in the next section. Although these results of metaphyseal fixation RSA are encouraging, these two studies had a limited number of patients and short-term to intermediate-term follow-up. The authors of this chapter prefer to use a device that allows for both diaphyseal and

metaphyseal fit, providing the greatest amount of fixation.

Humeral Design

The two main humeral implant types are inset and onset. An inset design requires a surgeon to ream the metaphysis, creating a shell in which the humeral implant sits, whereas onset designs are placed on the cut surface of the humerus (**Figure 6**). This difference may affect patient outcomes and complications. Proponents of the onset design suggest that it allows for lateralization of the humerus without the need to lateralize the center of rotation. In addition, a larger glenosphere can be used because the size of the proximal humerus does not dictate the size of the glenosphere when these designs are used. A larger glenosphere and lateralized humerus theoretically provide additional stability and greater deltoid force. However, humeral lengthening increases the risk of stretch neurapraxia and makes repair of the subscapularis difficult. Although the importance of the subscapularis after RSA is heavily debated, the authors of this chapter believe that an intact subscapularis increases both stability and internal rotation strength. The authors of this chapter therefore prefer to use an inset design that allows the humeral socket to sit in the epiphyseal/metaphyseal shell. This design minimizes humeral lengthening, thereby reducing the risk of stretch neurapraxia and allowing for nearly anatomic repair of the subscapularis. The inset design also allows the center of rotation to be in line with the center of the humeral shaft, whereby the hinge is closer to the opposite edge of the implant, unlike the onset designs (**Figure 7**). An inset design can be lateralized using modular polyethylene implants in patients with soft-tissue laxity, whereas the ability to medialize an onset design to adjust soft-tissue tensioning is limited.

Glenoid Fixation

As indications for RSA continue to expand, more manufacturers are offering RSA prostheses. One characteristic that differentiates these prostheses is the type of fixation used to secure the baseplate to the glenoid. Some early RSA designs offered only peg fixation in different lengths. Unfortunately, peg fixation provides limited compression because it relies on an initial interference fix, with compression provided by additional peripheral screws. Because the loads across the bone-implant interface are multifactorial, compression is necessary to enhance initial stability and facilitate bony healing to the metal undersurface. During early recovery after shoulder arthroplasty, joint loads can reach body weight. Failure to achieve adequate fixation can result in micromotion between the baseplate and glenoid, resulting in early failure. One study comparing methods of baseplate fixation found 200 N of compressive force provided by peg fixation with peripheral screws, whereas central screw fixation provided 2000 N of compression. In situations in which bony healing is critical, such as in patients requiring

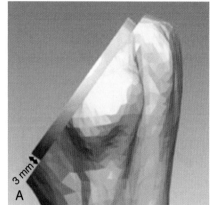
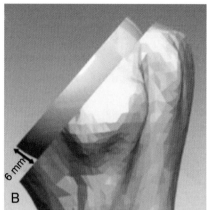

Figure 6   Illustrations show the two main humeral implant types. **A,** Inset designs require metaphyseal reaming for placement. **B,** Onset designs require no metaphyseal reaming and increase the distance from the humeral neck cut to the rim of the socket.

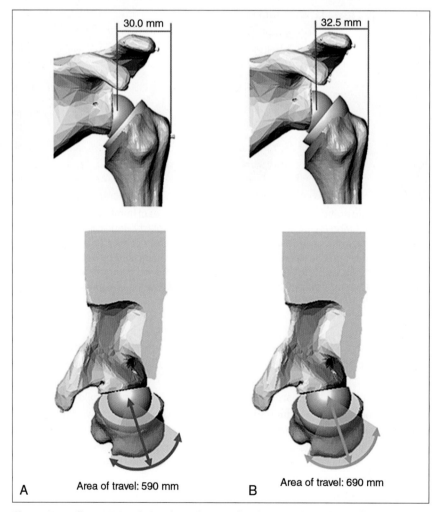

Figure 7   Illustrations show the substantially decreased rotation of the humeral greater tuberosity with an inset humeral implant design (**A**) compared with an onset humeral design (**B**).

bone graft, this increased compressive force provides a better platform for bone ingrowth.

The authors of this chapter use a system with a compressive lag screw. The compression results from variation in the thread pitch, with the screw having a 3.2-mm central core and a 6.5-mm outer thread diameter. This difference provides substantial compression of the undersurface of the baseplate to the bone. An added benefit is the intraoperative tactile feedback provided from the friction between the baseplate and bone, which helps a surgeon assess the adequacy of implant placement. This feedback can be helpful in patients with severe glenoid bone loss, in whom sufficiency of purchase is often difficult to determine. The benefits of compression and the ability to intraoperatively assess fixation strength help maximize bone ingrowth and minimize glenoid-side failures.

Articulation

The complex interplay of glenosphere design and surgical technique creates a difficult problem in attempts to maximize RSA function and longevity. Whereas the aim of TSA is to replicate anatomy, the RSA implant is nonanatomic; however, the principles of anatomy cannot be discounted. Attempts to improve glenosphere design

to maximize impingement-free range of motion, muscle tension relationships, and implant longevity and decrease the rate of notching have led many manufacturers to move from concentric to eccentric glenosphere designs. A concentric glenosphere has the center of rotation at the point of fixation, whereas an eccentric glenosphere has the center of rotation shifted laterally or inferiorly in an attempt to reduce impingement and improve range of motion.

Inferior eccentric glenospheres were developed specifically to avoid glenoid notching, which occurred at high rates with Grammont-style prostheses. In one study, researchers found a reduction in the rate of notching with an inferior eccentric design compared to a concentric design at minimum 2-year follow-up; however, the small difference in clinical outcome scores between the two groups was not statistically significant. The authors of a different study reported no difference in the incidence of notching with an inferior eccentric glenosphere but found decreased severity of notching at early follow-up. A randomized controlled trial also did not reveal a difference in notching rates or clinical outcomes with the use of an inferior eccentric glenosphere. A computer model of an inferiorly eccentric glenosphere showed a poor force distribution profile, which could result in shear forces at

the bone-implant interface and increase the risk of early failure. In addition, an inferior eccentric glenosphere positions the humerus more distally if the arm is adducted, which can adversely affect deltoid contour, stability, and soft-tissue tensioning.

Lateral eccentric glenospheres provide a more anatomic center of rotation while avoiding overdistalization of the humerus. Lateralization of the glenosphere offers many benefits, including reduced impingement during adduction and abduction and improved stability. As the humerus is shifted laterally, intact posterior cuff muscle is lengthened and tensioned to improve the external rotation force. Although some surgeons expressed initial concerns about increased shear forces with a lateralized design, studies of current prosthetic designs have shown improved fixation and low rates of mechanical failure and notching. The addition of a bone graft spacer behind the glenoid baseplate to lateralize a medial glenoid design has resulted in decreased notching; however, at 19% the rate of notching remains higher compared with that of lateralized prosthetic designs, and the procedure may be more technically demanding compared with the use of a lateralized design because it requires additional preparation of the glenoid.

 Bibliography

Ansari F, Major C, Norris TR, Gunther SB, Ries M, Pruitt L: Unscrewing instability of modular reverse shoulder prosthesis increases propensity for in vivo fracture: A report of two cases. *J Shoulder Elbow Surg* 2014;23(2):e40-e45.

Atoun E, Van Tongel A, Hous N, et al: Reverse shoulder arthroplasty with a short metaphyseal humeral stem. *Int Orthop* 2014;38(6):1213-1218.

Ballas R, Béguin L: Results of a stemless reverse shoulder prosthesis at more than 58 months mean without loosening. *J Shoulder Elbow Surg* 2013;22(9):e1-e6.

Berhouet J, Garaud P, Favard L: Evaluation of the role of glenosphere design and humeral component retroversion in avoiding scapular notching during reverse shoulder arthroplasty. *J Shoulder Elbow Surg* 2014;23(2):151-158.

Bogle A, Budge M, Richman A, Miller RJ, Wiater JM, Voloshin I: Radiographic results of fully uncemented trabecular metal reverse shoulder system at 1 and 2 years' follow-up. *J Shoulder Elbow Surg* 2013;22(4):e20-e25.

Bohsali KI, Wirth MA, Rockwood CA Jr: Complications of total shoulder arthroplasty. *J Bone Joint Surg Am* 2006;88(10):2279-2292.

Boileau P, Avidor C, Krishnan SG, Walch G, Kempf JF, Molé D: Cemented polyethylene versus uncemented metal-backed glenoid components in total shoulder arthroplasty: A prospective, double-blind, randomized study. *J Shoulder Elbow Surg* 2002;11(4):351-359.

Boileau P, Moineau G, Roussanne Y, O'Shea K: Bony increased-offset reversed shoulder arthroplasty: Minimizing scapular impingement while maximizing glenoid fixation. *Clin Orthop Relat Res* 2011;469(9):2558-2567.

Budge MD, Nolan EM, Heisey MH, Baker K, Wiater JM: Results of total shoulder arthroplasty with a mono-block porous tantalum glenoid component: A prospective minimum 2-year follow-up study. *J Shoulder Elbow Surg* 2013;22(4):535-541.

Castagna A, Delcogliano M, de Caro F, et al: Conversion of shoulder arthroplasty to reverse implants: Clinical and radiological results using a modular system. *Int Orthop* 2013;37(7):1297-1305.

Churchill RS: Stemless shoulder arthroplasty: Current status. *J Shoulder Elbow Surg* 2014;23(9):1409-1414.

Churchill RS, Chuinard C, Wiater JM, et al: Clinical and radiographic outcomes of the Simpliciti canal-sparing shoulder arthroplasty system: A prospective two-year multicenter study. *J Bone Joint Surg Am* 2016;98(7):552-560.

Cil A, Sperling JW, Cofield RH: Nonstandard glenoid components for bone deficiencies in shoulder arthroplasty. *J Shoulder Elbow Surg* 2014;23(7):e149-e157.

Cuff D, Clark R, Pupello D, Frankle M: Reverse shoulder arthroplasty for the treatment of rotator cuff deficiency: A concise follow-up, at a minimum of five years, of a previous report. *J Bone Joint Surg Am* 2012;94(21):1996-2000.

Cuff D, Levy JC, Gutiérrez S, Frankle MA: Torsional stability of modular and non-modular reverse shoulder humeral components in a proximal humeral bone loss model. *J Shoulder Elbow Surg* 2011;20(4):646-651.

Cuff D, Pupello D, Virani N, Levy J, Frankle M: Reverse shoulder arthroplasty for the treatment of rotator cuff deficiency. *J Bone Joint Surg Am* 2008;90(6):1244-1251.

De Biase CF, Ziveri G, Delcogliano M, et al: The use of an eccentric glenosphere compared with a concentric glenosphere in reverse total shoulder arthroplasty: Two-year minimum follow-up results. *Int Orthop* 2013;37(10):1949-1955.

De Wilde L, Dayerizadeh N, De Neve F, Basamania C, Van Tongel A: Fully uncemented glenoid component in total shoulder arthroplasty. *J Shoulder Elbow Surg* 2013;22(10):e1-e7.

Favard L, Katz D, Colmar M, Benkalfate T, Thomazeau H, Emily S: Total shoulder arthroplasty—arthroplasty for glenohumeral arthropathies: Results and complications after a minimum follow-up of 8 years according to the type of arthroplasty and etiology. *Orthop Traumatol Surg Res* 2012;98(4, suppl):S41-S47.

Frankle M, Virani N, Pupello D, Gutierrez S: Rationale and biomechanics of the reverse shoulder prosthesis: The American experience, in Frankle, MA, ed: *Rotator Cuff Deficiency of the Shoulder.* New York, NY, Thieme, 2008, pp 76-104.

Fucentese SF, Costouros JG, Kühnel SP, Gerber C: Total shoulder arthroplasty with an uncemented soft-metal-backed glenoid component. *J Shoulder Elbow Surg* 2010;19(4):624-631.

Giuseffi SA, Streubel P, Sperling J, Sanchez-Sotelo J: Short-stem uncemented primary reverse shoulder arthroplasty: Clinical and radiological outcomes. *Bone Joint J* 2014;96(4):526-529.

Grey SG: Use of a caged, bone ingrowth, glenoid implant in anatomic total shoulder arthroplasty technique and early results. *Bull Hosp Jt Dis (2013)* 2013;71(71, suppl 2):S41-S45.

Guery J, Favard L, Sirveaux F, Oudet D, Mole D, Walch G: Reverse total shoulder arthroplasty: Survivorship analysis of eighty replacements followed for five to ten years. *J Bone Joint Surg Am* 2006;88(8):1742-1747.

Gutiérrez S, Keller TS, Levy JC, Lee WE III, Luo ZP: Hierarchy of stability factors in reverse shoulder arthroplasty. *Clin Orthop Relat Res* 2008;466(3):670-676.

Gutiérrez S, Levy JC, Frankle MA, et al: Evaluation of abduction range of motion and avoidance of inferior scapular impingement in a reverse shoulder model. *J Shoulder Elbow Surg* 2008;17(4):608-615.

Gutiérrez S, Walker M, Willis M, Pupello DR, Frankle MA: Effects of tilt and glenosphere eccentricity on baseplate/bone interface forces in a computational model, validated by a mechanical model, of reverse shoulder arthroplasty. *J Shoulder Elbow Surg* 2011;20(5):732-739.

Habermeyer P, Lichtenberg S, Tauber M, Magosch P: Midterm results of stemless shoulder arthroplasty: A prospective study. *J Shoulder Elbow Surg* 2015;24(9):1463-1472.

Henninger HB, Barg A, Anderson AE, Bachus KN, Burks RT, Tashjian RZ: Effect of lateral offset center of rotation in reverse total shoulder arthroplasty: A biomechanical study. *J Shoulder Elbow Surg* 2012;21(9):1128-1135.

Huguet D, DeClercq G, Rio B, Teissier J, Zipoli B, TESS Group: Results of a new stemless shoulder prosthesis: Radiologic proof of maintained fixation and stability after a minimum of three years' follow-up. *J Shoulder Elbow Surg* 2010;19(6):847-852.

Iannotti JP, Lappin KE, Klotz CL, Reber EW, Swope SW: Liftoff resistance of augmented glenoid components during cyclic fatigue loading in the posterior-superior direction. *J Shoulder Elbow Surg* 2013;22(11):1530-1536.

Jost PW, Dines JS, Griffith MH, Angel M, Altchek DW, Dines DM: Total shoulder arthroplasty utilizing mini-stem humeral components: Technique and short-term results. *HSS J* 2011;7(3):213-217.

Katz D, Kany J, Valenti P, Sauzières P, Gleyze P, El Kholti K: New design of a cementless glenoid component in unconstrained shoulder arthroplasty: A prospective medium-term analysis of 143 cases. *Eur J Orthop Surg Traumatol* 2013;23(1):27-34.

Kim YH, Park JW, Kim JS, Kang JS: Long-term results and bone remodeling after THA with a short, metaphyseal-fitting anatomic cementless stem. *Clin Orthop Relat Res* 2014;472(3):943-950.

Matsen FA III, Iannotti JP, Rockwood CA Jr: Humeral fixation by press-fitting of a tapered metaphyseal stem: A prospective radiographic study. *J Bone Joint Surg Am* 2003;85(2):304-308.

Mizuno N, Denard PJ, Raiss P, Walch G: Reverse total shoulder arthroplasty for primary glenohumeral osteoarthritis in patients with a biconcave glenoid. *J Bone Joint Surg Am* 2013;95(14):1297-1304.

Papadonikolakis A, Matsen FA III: Metal-backed glenoid components have a higher rate of failure and fail by different modes in comparison with all-polyethylene components: A systematic review. *J Bone Joint Surg Am* 2014;96(12):1041-1047.

Patel RJ, Choi D, Wright T, Gao Y: Nonconforming glenoid increases posterior glenohumeral translation after a total shoulder replacement. *J Shoulder Elbow Surg* 2014;23(12):1831-1837.

Poon PC, Chou J, Young SW, Astley T: A comparison of concentric and eccentric glenospheres in reverse shoulder arthroplasty: A randomized controlled trial. *J Bone Joint Surg Am* 2014;96(16):e138.

Raiss P, Edwards TB, Deutsch A, et al: Radiographic changes around humeral components in shoulder arthroplasty. *J Bone Joint Surg Am* 2014;96(7):e54.

Razfar N, Reeves JM, Langohr DG, Willing R, Athwal GS, Johnson JA: Comparison of proximal humeral bone stresses between stemless, short stem, and standard stem length: A finite element analysis. *J Shoulder Elbow Surg* 2016; Jan 22 [Epub ahead of print].

Razmjou H, Holtby R, Christakis M, Axelrod T, Richards R: Impact of prosthetic design on clinical and radiologic outcomes of total shoulder arthroplasty: A prospective study. *J Shoulder Elbow Surg* 2013;22(2):206-214.

Sabesan V, Callanan M, Sharma V, Iannotti JP: Correction of acquired glenoid bone loss in osteoarthritis with a standard versus an augmented glenoid component. *J Shoulder Elbow Surg* 2014;23(7):964-973.

Sanchez-Sotelo J, O'Driscoll SW, Torchia ME, Cofield RH, Rowland CM: Radiographic assessment of cemented humeral components in shoulder arthroplasty. *J Shoulder Elbow Surg* 2001;10(6):526-531.

Simovitch RW, Zumstein MA, Lohri E, Helmy N, Gerber C: Predictors of scapular notching in patients managed with the Delta III reverse total shoulder replacement. *J Bone Joint Surg Am* 2007;89(3):588-600.

Sirveaux F, Favard L, Oudet D, Huquet D, Walch G, Molé D: Grammont inverted total shoulder arthroplasty in the treatment of glenohumeral osteoarthritis with massive rupture of the cuff: Results of a multicentre study of 80 shoulders. *J Bone Joint Surg Br* 2004;86(3):388-395.

Strauss EJ, Roche C, Flurin PH, Wright T, Zuckerman JD: The glenoid in shoulder arthroplasty. *J Shoulder Elbow Surg* 2009;18(5):819-833.

Teissier P, Teissier J, Kouyoumdjian P, Asencio G: The TESS reverse shoulder arthroplasty without a stem in the treatment of cuff-deficient shoulder conditions: Clinical and radiographic results. *J Shoulder Elbow Surg* 2015;24(1):45-51.

Terrier A, Büchler P, Farron A: Influence of glenohumeral conformity on glenoid stresses after total shoulder arthroplasty. *J Shoulder Elbow Surg* 2006;15(4):515-520.

Valenti P, Sauzières P, Katz D, Kalouche I, Kilinc AS: Do less medialized reverse shoulder prostheses increase motion and reduce notching? *Clin Orthop Relat Res* 2011;469(9):2550-2557.

Vavken P, Sadoghi P, von Keudell A, Rosso C, Valderrabano V, Müller AM: Rates of radiolucency and loosening after total shoulder arthroplasty with pegged or keeled glenoid components. *J Bone Joint Surg Am* 2013;95(3):215-221.

Walch G, Edwards TB, Boulahia A, Boileau P, Mole D, Adeleine P: The influence of glenohumeral prosthetic mismatch on glenoid radiolucent lines: Results of a multicenter study. *J Bone Joint Surg Am* 2002;84(12):2186-2191.

Werner BS, Boehm D, Gohlke F: Revision to reverse shoulder arthroplasty with retention of the humeral component. *Acta Orthop* 2013;84(5):473-478.

Wiater JM, Moravek JE Jr, Budge MD, Koueiter DM, Marcantonio D, Wiater BP: Clinical and radiographic results of cementless reverse total shoulder arthroplasty: A comparative study with 2 to 5 years of follow-up. *J Shoulder Elbow Surg* 2014;23(8):1208-1214.

Wieser K, Borbas P, Ek ET, Meyer DC, Gerber C: Conversion of stemmed hemi- or total to reverse total shoulder arthroplasty: Advantages of a modular stem design. *Clin Orthop Relat Res* 2015;473(2):651-660.

Williams GR, Abboud JA: Total shoulder arthroplasty: Glenoid component design. *J Shoulder Elbow Surg* 2005; 14(1, suppl):122S-128S.

Wirth MA, Loredo R, Garcia G, Rockwood CA Jr, Southworth C, Iannotti JP: Total shoulder arthroplasty with an all-polyethylene pegged bone-ingrowth glenoid component: A clinical and radiographic outcome study. *J Bone Joint Surg Am* 2012;94(3):260-267.

Young AA, Walch G: Fixation of the glenoid component in total shoulder arthroplasty: What is "modern cementing technique?" *J Shoulder Elbow Surg* 2010;19(8):1129-1136.

Zhang J, Yongpravat C, Kim HM, et al: Glenoid articular conformity affects stress distributions in total shoulder arthroplasty. *J Shoulder Elbow Surg* 2013;22(3):350-356.

Chapter 36

Uncomplicated Total Shoulder Arthroplasty: Technical Pearls for Exposure, Preparation, and Insertion

Joseph D. Zuckerman, MD

Brent Mollon, MD, FRCSC

 ## Introduction

Shoulder arthroplasty implants have evolved from early monoblock designs to modular designs that reliably re-create native anatomy and platform stems that enable conversion from anatomic to reverse shoulder prostheses. The demand for anatomic and reverse shoulder arthroplasty is rising in the United States, and increasing numbers of surgeons are being trained in the technique. Although total shoulder arthroplasty (TSA) is a rewarding procedure for both patient and surgeon, it is not without risk for complications. An understanding of individual implant design is important; however, a systematic and meticulous approach to the main procedural steps is integral to success.

 ## Case Presentation

A 72-year-old right-hand–dominant woman presents with pain in her right shoulder that has progressively worsened over several years. She rates her pain at rest as 5 to 6 on a 10-point scale. Pain is aggravated during overhead lifting, pushing, and pulling. The patient's sleep is disturbed. The right shoulder symptoms interfere with all activities of daily living, and the patient requires occasional assistance for dressing and grooming. Attempts at physical therapy proved to be too painful. The patient received an intra-articular steroid injection 2 months before assessment, which provided 1 month of relief. She denied having neck or elbow pain, upper extremity radiculopathy, or previous injury or surgery to the shoulder. She has type 2 diabetes mellitus.

The patient appears healthy on physical examination. Inspection of the affected shoulder reveals no swelling, deformity, or muscular atrophy. The anterior and posterior aspects of the glenohumeral joint are tender to palpation. Active range of motion (ROM) measures 130° of forward elevation, 25° of external rotation with the arm at the side, and internal rotation to the lumbosacral area. Results of deltoid strength, external rotation strength, and specific supraspinatus testing all measure 4+/5. Shoulder movement and muscle testing are limited by pain. No motor or sensory deficits are elicited on cervical spine and upper extremity neurologic examination.

Radiographs of the right shoulder demonstrate substantial joint-space narrowing, osteophyte formation, and subchondral sclerosis consistent with severe glenohumeral osteoarthritis. No substantial bony deformity of the humeral head or glenoid is present. Preoperative CT confirms the aforementioned findings, with glenoid retroversion of 10° (**Figure 1**).

At the time of presentation, the patient thought that she had exhausted reasonable nonsurgical modalities and that her symptoms were serious enough to warrant surgical management. Informed consent was obtained for an anatomic TSA.

 ## Indications

TSA is an established, successful, and reliable procedure for the management of glenohumeral arthritis. A successful surgical outcome is predicated on appropriate patient selection and meticulous surgical technique to produce adequate exposure for correct implant positioning. Anatomic TSA is indicated for patients with glenohumeral arthritis

Dr. Zuckerman or an immediate family member has received royalties from Exactech; serves as a paid consultant to the Musculoskeletal Transplant Foundation; serves as an unpaid consultant to J3Personica/Residency Select; has stock or stock options held in AposTherapy and Hip Innovation Technology; has received research or institutional support from SLACK, Thieme, and Wolters Kluwer Health/Lippincott Williams & Wilkins; and serves as a board member, owner, officer, or committee member of the American Orthopaedic Association. Neither Dr. Mollon nor any immediate family member has received anything of value from or has stock or stock options held in a commercial company or institution related directly or indirectly to the subject of this chapter.

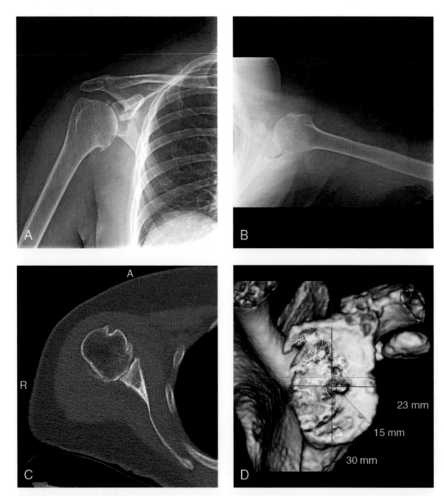

Figure 1 Images show a right shoulder with glenohumeral arthritis. **A,** Preoperative AP radiograph demonstrates joint space narrowing, osteophyte formation, and bone sclerosis corresponding to glenohumeral arthritis. **B,** Axillary radiograph demonstrates no substantial glenoid deformity. **C,** Axial CT scan obtained two slices, or 6 mm, inferior to the tip of the coracoid measures glenoid retroversion as 10°. **D,** Three-dimensional CT reconstruction used to estimate the center of the glenoid and the maximal glenoid dimensions.

osteophyte location and humeral neck morphology that can be missed when only one view is obtained. The external rotation view more accurately demonstrates humeral head height, and comparison of the preoperative radiographs is useful when assessing component positioning. The authors of this chapter routinely obtain three-dimensional CT images to definitively assess glenoid morphology and facilitate preoperative planning.

The absence of substantial bony deformities, erosion, and/or prior surgical intervention, along with clinical and radiographic evidence of rotator cuff integrity, suggest that the intraoperative course will follow the standard surgical protocol. Any bony deformities noted on radiographs may necessitate further imaging studies. Concerns regarding rotator cuff insufficiency, including muscular weakness or proximal migration of the humeral head on radiographs or CT, should prompt further evaluation with MRI. Previous surgical intervention may require the use of a modified approach to accommodate existing surgical incisions, and it raises the possibility of occult infection. C-reactive protein level, erythrocyte sedimentation rate, bone or indium scans, and joint aspiration should be obtained preoperatively when clinically indicated. One goal of the preoperative evaluation is to minimize the possibility of unexpected intraoperative findings.

Controversies and Alternative Approaches

Management of the arthritic glenohumeral joint in a young patient remains challenging. TSA consistently has been found to have superior clinical results compared with hemiarthroplasty in all age groups. Other treatment options include arthroscopic débridement, soft-tissue glenoid resurfacing combined

in whom nonsurgical management has failed and who are willing and able to comply with postoperative management. Contraindications include active infection, rotator cuff insufficiency, deltoid palsy, severe bony abnormality, and an inability to comply with postoperative instructions.

The case presentation described previously is typical of a patient with primary glenohumeral arthritis. Clinical assessment is focused on understanding the severity of the pain, the effect of arthritis on function, and the

effect of previous surgical and nonsurgical interventions. In addition, ROM and strength are quantified, a screening neurologic assessment is performed, and neck-related or other pathologies that may be responsible for referred pain to the shoulder are identified. Preoperative radiographic imaging should include a scapular AP view with the humerus in maximal internal and external rotation, a scapular Y view, and a supine axillary lateral view. The scapular AP view in both internal and external rotation provides important information about with hemiarthroplasty or humeral head resurfacing, the ream-and-run procedure, humeral head resurfacing alone, and fusion. A deficient rotator cuff can be treated with rotator cuff repair during TSA (if the tear is repairable), hemiarthroplasty, or reverse TSA (for irreparable tears).

The surgical approach and bony preparation for a standard anatomic TSA follow a predictable sequence; however, different component systems have specific associated procedures that are required for successful implantation. Although rotator cuff–sparing approaches are considered, the most common approach involves a transsubscapularis approach that uses tenotomy, subscapularis peel, or lesser tuberosity (LT) osteotomy. No technique has been shown to be superior; thus, surgeons should perform meticulous repair using the technique with which they are most comfortable.

A variety of implant designs is available. Humeral options include stemmed or stemless, eccentric heads, and variable angles of versions. Glenoid options include keel, pegged, and caged designs. Cemented and noncemented constructs are available. There are different options for glenoid component augmentation, and there are platform humeral components that allow conversion to reverse TSA. No evidence exists to show a clear superiority of one humeral design or method of proximal fixation. Although the cemented all-polyethylene glenoid component is considered superior to metal-backed components, newer glenoid designs also show promise. Surgeons should use a system with which they are familiar to improve procedural efficiency and reliability.

 Results

Table 1 lists the results and complications of the recent literature on primary TSA. These data suggest that, when performed by experienced surgeons, TSA has 5-, 10-, and 15-year survival rates of 90% to 95%, 85% to 90%, and 80% to 85%, respectively. Complication rates are acceptably low.

 Video 36.1 Uncomplicated Total Shoulder Arthroplasty. Joseph D. Zuckerman, MD; Brent Mollon, MD, FRCSC; William E. Ryan, Jr, BS (9 min)

 Technical Keys to Success

Anesthesia

- The choice of anesthesia is determined by the anesthesiologist in consultation with the patient and the surgeon. The authors of this chapter prefer regional interscalene block anesthesia combined with sedation to achieve appropriate muscular relaxation during the procedure and well-controlled analgesia postoperatively.
- If endotracheal anesthesia is indicated, it often can be combined with preoperative or postoperative interscalene block for pain control.
- Regardless of the primary choice of anesthesia, complete muscular relaxation is required if adequate exposure is to be achieved.

Instruments/Equipment/ Implants Required

- The authors of this chapter use a surgical table that allows beach-chair positioning, secure attachment of the head to the table, and free movement of the arm. An arm board or pneumatic arm positioner may be used to support the arm.
- The authors of this chapter prefer to use a padded Mayo stand, because after the initial exposure and glenoid preparation it can be removed to facilitate humeral preparation. It is important to ensure that the

Mayo stand can be positioned low enough to accommodate the surgeon's desired height for the surgical table.

- It is helpful to have a variety of self-retaining and shoulder retractors; the chapter authors' preferences are shown in **Figure 2**.
- The surgeon should confirm that all necessary implant trays and the final components are available in the operating room before skin incision.

Patient Positioning

- After anesthesia is complete, the patient is moved up the table so that the hips are positioned just superior to the point at which the bed hinges.
- The patient's head is secured in a padded holder, ensuring neutral neck alignment and confirming that the ears are not folded on themselves. The eyes are protected, and the forehead is padded.
- Pillows are placed under the legs to maintain 30° to 40° of flexion. An ipsilateral kidney rest support is placed to prevent any change in the patient's position when traction is applied during the procedure.
- The contralateral arm is placed in an arm holder in neutral position, ensuring that the shoulders remain level. The backing under the surgical shoulder is removed to allow an unobstructed extension of the shoulder with the shoulder adducted, which is critically important for adequate humeral exposure.
- Prior to preparation and draping, the arm is placed through a ROM to confirm that the aforementioned motions are possible and to document passive motion. Inability to externally rotate more than 20° suggests that subscapularis mobilization may be required in addition to capsular releases and osteophyte resection.

Table 1 Results of Primary Total Shoulder Arthroplasty With Cemented Glenoid Components

Authors	Journal (Year)	Glenoid Implant Type	Number	Survivorship	Comments
Deshmukh et al	*J Shoulder Elbow Surg* (2005)	Multiple types: all were cemented all-polyethylene	Survivorship: 320 Clinical: 72 TSAs (clinical follow-up)	1 yr, 99%; 5 yr, 98%; 10 yr, 93%; 15 yr, 88%; 20 yr, 85%	Survivorship data are based on all 320 TSAs performed Mean follow-up, 14 yr (SD ± 2.7; minimum, 10 yr)
Raiss et al	*J Bone Joint Surg Br* (2008)	Flat-backed, keeled	21 shoulders	5 yr, 100%	Mean follow-up, 7 yr (range, 5-9 yr)
Khan et al	*J Bone Joint Surg Br* (2009)	Flat-backed, keeled	39 patients	Humerus: 10 yr, 100% Glenoid: 10 yr, 92%	Mean follow-up, 10.6 yr (range, 10-12 yr)
Kasten et al	*J Bone Joint Surg Br* (2010)	Flat-backed, keeled	96 TSAs	100% (both components)	Mean follow-up, 7.4 yr (range, 5-10.6 yr)
Walch et al	*J Shoulder Elbow Surg* (2011)	Convex-backed, keeled	333 TSAs	5 yr, 99.7%; 10 yr, 98.3%	Mean follow-up, 7.5 yr (range, 5.1-12.7 yr)
Young et al	*J Bone Joint Surg Br* (2011)	Flat-backed, keeled	226 shoulders	5 yr, 99.1%; 10 yr, 94.5%; 15 yr, 79.4%	Mean follow-up, 10.2 yr (range, 5.1-18.3 yr)
Raiss et al	*J Bone Joint Surg Am* (2012)	Flat-backed, keeled	39 TSAs	100% after 13 yr (revision as end point)	Mean follow-up, 11 yr (range, 10-14 yr)
Denard et al	*J Shoulder Elbow Surg* (2013)	Flat-backed, keeled	50 patients	5 yr, 98%; 10 yr, 62.5%	Patient age, ≤55 yr Mean follow-up, 9.6 yr (range, 5-17.6 yr)
Raiss et al	*J Bone Joint Surg Am* (2014)	Flat-backed, keeled	45 shoulders in 40 patients	5 yr, 98%; 10 yr, 89%; 15 yr, 73%; 20 yr, 70%	Minimum follow-up, 15 yr

TSA = total shoulder arthroplasty.

- The table is positioned to maximize operating room working space, and the arm is prepared and draped in the usual manner (**Figure 3**).

Approach
- The deltopectoral approach is the standard approach for shoulder arthroplasty because it is familiar to all orthopaedic surgeons, and it allows adequate exposure of the glenoid and proximal humerus without damaging the deltoid, axillary nerve, or rotator cuff. Adjunctive procedures such as rotator cuff repair, bone grafting, acromioplasty, distal clavicle excision, or muscle transfers can be performed through this incision. Although some surgeons use an anterior axillary incision combined with deltopectoral dissection to reduce scar prominence, the authors of this chapter think that this incision is less desirable because it does not provide all the benefits of a deltopectoral incision.
- With the patient's arm in neutral position and resting on a padded Mayo stand, a straight line is marked, beginning just lateral to the coracoid process and extending distally toward the deltoid insertion (**Figure 4, A**). The length of the incision varies somewhat depending on the patient's body habitus, but typically, an incision measuring 12 to 14 cm is used.
- Dissection is carried down to the deep fascial layer overlying the musculature. Generous full-thickness subcutaneous flaps are developed in all directions to facilitate exposure.
- Two angled self-retaining retractors are inserted at 90° to one another, with the handles placed inferiorly and laterally.
- The deltopectoral interval is identified, most simply by identifying the fat stripe covering the cephalic vein (**Figure 4, B**). In addition, the orientation of the deltoid fibers differs from that of the pectoralis major

fibers, and this difference can be accentuated by placing the pectoralis major on stretch with shoulder external rotation.

- The anterior border of the lateral clavicle and the coracoid process mark the superior-most origin of the interval and are both useful landmarks if scarring obscures the tissue planes. After the deltopectoral interval is identified, it is developed proximally and distally. The authors of this chapter prefer to mobilize the cephalic vein laterally, because most of the cephalic branches enter the deltoid. If the vein is mobilized medially, care must be taken to coagulate these branches. The cephalic vein is protected throughout the procedure, avoiding damage from retractors or tension particularly where the vein crosses the superior aspect of the incision.

- The internervous plane between the deltoid and pectoralis major muscles is developed proximally and distally. The clavipectoral fascia is identified and incised lateral to the conjoined tendon from the pectoralis major tendon inferiorly to the coracoacromial (CA) ligament superiorly (**Figure 4, C**). The conjoined tendon is mobilized bluntly with digital dissection. A bladed self-retaining retractor such as a Kolbel retractor is inserted medially under the conjoined tendon and laterally under the deltoid. It is secured to the drape around the arm with a piercing towel clip to prevent it from rotating out of position (**Figure 4, D**).

- The anterior few millimeters of the CA ligament or the superior 1 cm of the pectoralis tendon can be released at any subsequent point for additional exposure, if necessary. Cautious release of the anterior CA ligament using electrocautery, while protecting the underlying rotator cuff with a Darrach retractor, allows better access to the rotator

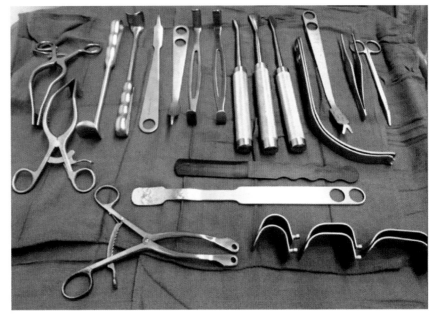

Figure 2   Photograph shows retractors and other equipment required for total shoulder arthroplasty.

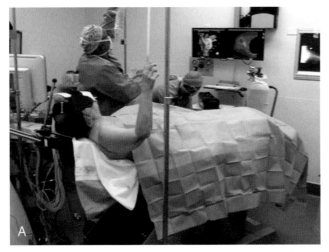
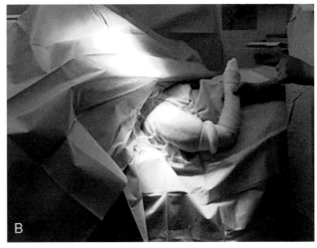

Figure 3   Preoperative photographs show patient positioning for total shoulder arthroplasty (TSA). The patient set-up for TSA is shown before (**A**) and after (**B**) draping. The table shown allows complete mobility of the shoulder, while ensuring that the patient remains stable during manipulation. The head of the table is raised 30°.

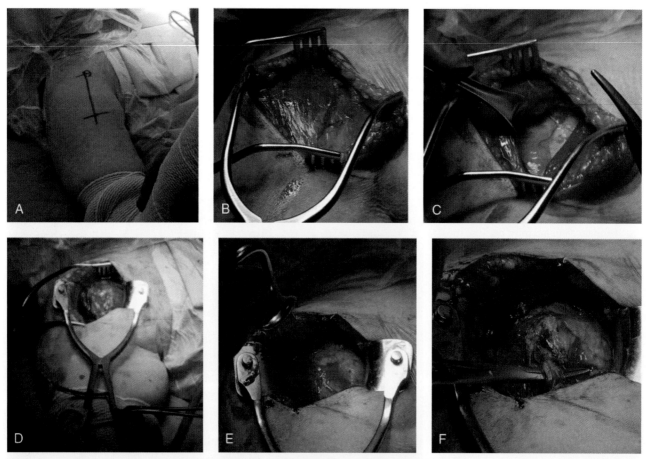

Figure 4 Intraoperative photographs show the surgical approach for uncomplicated total shoulder arthroplasty. **A,** The skin incision is marked lateral to the coracoid, extending toward the deltoid incision, with the arm in neutral position. **B,** The skin incision is made to the fascia, and the deltopectoral interval is identified by a fat stripe overlying the cephalic vein. **C,** The clavipectoral fascia lateral to the conjoined tendon is identified and incised. **D,** A self-retaining retractor is placed. **E,** A blunt elevator is placed under the coracoacromial ligament for subacromial release. **F,** The bicipital groove is opened, and a tenodesis is performed.

interval if initial visualization is inadequate. Release of the superior pectoralis major tendon allows improved mobilization of the proximal humerus, which can enhance glenoid exposure by enabling greater posterior displacement of the proximal humerus.

- Additional mobilization of the subacromial or subdeltoid spaces is performed. This step is important not only for exposure but also the restoration of postoperative ROM. The subdeltoid space is mobilized initially with finger dissection, although blunt elevators such as the Darrach elevator may be required.
- A Darrach elevator is placed under

the CA ligament and on top of the supraspinatus tendon into the supraspinatus fossa (**Figure 4, E**). This elevator then is passed into the infraspinatus fossa in a similar fashion.

- The arm is placed in external rotation and electrocautery used to release adhesions at the base of the coracoid in the area of the origin of the rotator interval. This release may result in increased humeral external rotation.
- Many surgeons perform biceps tenodesis during TSA. The authors of this chapter perform this procedure during the initial dissection.
- The bicipital groove is palpated, and

the bicipital sheath is opened with electrocautery just superior to the pectoralis major tendon.

- The biceps tendon is identified (**Figure 4, F**), and two No. 2 nonabsorbable sutures are used for tenodesis of the biceps tendon to the pectoralis major tendon.
- The biceps tendon is divided proximal to the tenodesis, and dissection proceeds to the rotator interval, where the tendon is resected.

Humeral Exposure

- After biceps tenodesis, the subscapularis tendon and the insertion site on the LT are identified. Inferior to the tendon, the anterior circumflex humeral artery and its venae comitantes, also called the three sisters, are isolated and cauterized to prevent bleeding during subscapularis release.

- Exposure of the humeral head through the subscapularis is performed using one of three techniques, which is largely determined by surgeon preference and the degree to which external rotation is limited preoperatively. The authors of this chapter prefer to perform a subscapularis tenotomy, leaving a portion of the tendon aside laterally for a tendon-to-tendon repair. Another option is subperiosteal release or peel of the subscapularis tendon off the LT and later repair using transosseous sutures.

- An LT osteotomy can be performed with suture fixation to bone and around the humeral stem at the time of component impaction.

- Irrespective of the technique chosen, these steps should be performed with the arm in external rotation, which improves visualization and reduces the potential for injury to the axillary nerve by moving it farther away from the area of dissection.

- If performing a subscapularis tenotomy, the incision is marked 1 cm medial to the insertion on the LT to allow sufficient tissue for tendon-to-tendon repair (**Figure 5, A**). As the tendon is divided, No. 2 nonabsorbable sutures are used to tag the medial tendon. Inferiorly, the tendon is less evident, and muscle fibers predominate. For more severe internal rotation contractures, the authors of this chapter perform a subperiosteal release of the subscapularis directly from the LT and tag it as described previously. An LT osteotomy also would be acceptable, because both techniques allow a more medial reattachment of the subscapularis if necessary.

This step effectively lengthens the subscapularis tendon and allows approximately 20° of increased external rotation for each 1 cm of medialization.

- Subscapularis mobilization should be completed at this time rather than after implant insertion. The goal of the 360° release is to obtain as much lateral excursion of the tendon as possible to maximize external rotation.

- A systematic release of the subscapularis tendon, beginning at the anterior glenoid margin, is performed by dividing capsular attachments to the glenoid.

- The subscapularis is freed of any adhesions at the anterosuperior glenoid, including the base of the coracoid process.

- The capsular release proceeds along the anterior glenoid margin to the inferior border of the tendon.

- The aforementioned steps for anterior soft-tissue releases are repeated until adequate excursion is obtained.

- After subscapularis tenotomy, it is important to open the rotator interval, in line with the biceps tendon, to the anterosuperior margin (**Figure 5, B**). This step defines and frees the superior aspect of the subscapularis tendon.

- The inferior capsular attachment is freed carefully from the humeral neck. To accomplish this step, the humerus is positioned in maximal external rotation and a small, flat Darrach elevator is placed on the inferior capsule within the joint (**Figure 5, C**). These maneuvers tension the anteroinferior capsule, which is released off the bone via electrocautery. Further external rotation allows a complete anterior-to-posterior capsular release to the posteroinferior aspect of the humeral neck. External rotation to 90° should be achieved.

- Osteophytes from the inferior portion of the humeral head and neck also should be removed at this time to facilitate soft-tissue releases and the later exposure of both the humerus and the glenoid.

- The use of systematic releases described previously should now enable a safe and accurate humeral neck osteotomy. Experienced surgeons perform this step in various ways. The authors of this chapter have an assistant hold the humerus parallel to the floor and in 20° to 25° of external rotation. With the humerus in this position, the osteotomy can be performed with the saw blade perpendicular to the floor to create the desired humeral retroversion.

- The osteotomy guide is placed on the proximal humerus at the level of the osteotomy, just medial to the rotator cuff insertion.

- Electrocautery is used to mark the osteotomy.

- A large Darrach retractor is placed medially between the glenoid and the humeral head to protect the axillary nerve and other medial and inferior structures.

- A small Hohmann retractor is placed superiorly to protect the rotator cuff.

- The surgeon confirms the placement of the arm as described previously and performs the osteotomy (**Figure 5, D** and **E**).

- The osteotomized humeral head is levered out and can be used for sizing and/or bone graft as needed.

- Other options for performing the humeral osteotomy include using an intramedullary guide or dislocating the humeral head and resecting it at the anatomic neck. These different approaches reflect surgeon preference and do not affect the outcome of the procedure as long as the osteotomy is performed appropriately.

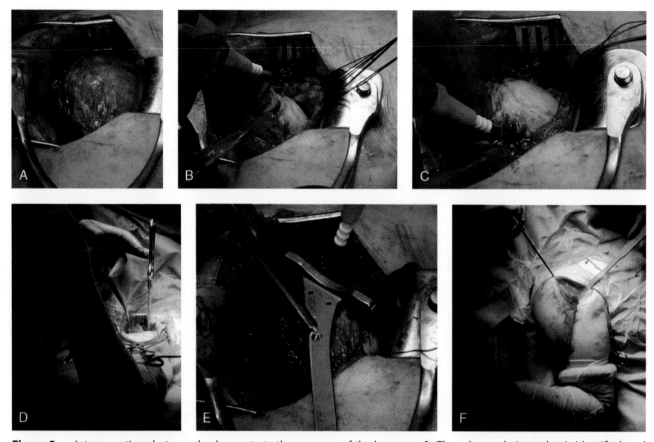

Figure 5 Intraoperative photographs demonstrate the exposure of the humerus. **A,** The subscapularis tendon is identified, and the tenotomy location is marked 1 cm medial to the lesser tuberosity insertion. The tenotomy is performed and the medial tendon is tagged. **B,** The rotator interval is divided. **C,** Inferior capsular tissue is carefully released off the inferomedial proximal humerus. **D,** The patient's arm is positioned parallel to the floor in approximately 30° of retroversion. **E,** The humeral cut is marked, and an osteotomy is performed. **F,** An assistant holds the humerus in adduction, extension, and external rotation in preparation for reaming and broaching.

- The self-retaining retractor and padded Mayo stand are removed, and the arm is placed in adduction, extension, and external rotation to deliver the proximal humerus.
- The deltoid is retracted posteriorly, and a small Hohmann retractor is placed underneath the superior rotator cuff insertion.
- A Darrach retractor is placed posteromedially to further expose the metaphysis and maintain the position of the humeral head.
- Osteophytes are removed, and the osteotomy can be modified if necessary.
- An assistant maintains the humerus in adduction, extension, and external rotation for reaming and broaching (**Figure 5, F**), but forward flexes and internally rotates the arm when these actions are not being performed to prevent traction on the brachial plexus.
- The humeral canal is entered posterior to the bicipital groove at the junction between the middle and superior thirds of the cut surface of the humeral head and as superior as possible.
- Sequential reaming and broaching are performed according to the particular implant used. The authors of this chapter prefer hand reaming because it affords more control and decreases the risk of intraoperative humeral fracture. Some systems allow the final implant to be inserted at this stage. In all instances, a metaphyseal protective plate should be used to minimize any potential for damage to metaphyseal bone of the humerus when the humerus is retracted posteriorly during glenoid preparation.

Glenoid Exposure

- The preliminary steps for exposure of the glenoid—including subdeltoid and subacromial mobilization, capsular release from the humeral neck, removal of proximal humeral osteophytes, and osteotomy of the humeral neck at the appropriate level—already have been performed in the preceding steps.
- Retractors are placed. A posterior

retractor is placed over the posterior glenoid rim. A broad, flat Darrach retractor is used for this purpose, although other retractors can be used. By placing this retractor to the midportion of the posterior glenoid neck, a limited posterior capsular release also can be achieved.

- The capsular attachment to the anterior glenoid is released, and a spiked Bankart-type retractor is placed carefully along the anterior glenoid neck directly on the bone.

- A small Hohmann retractor is placed over the superior glenoid, exposing the remainder of the biceps tendon (**Figure 6, A**).

- With these retractors in place, lighting and patient positioning can be adjusted to optimize visualization.

- The arm is placed on a padded Mayo stand in approximately 30° of abduction and neutral rotation. The table can be raised to allow the proximal humerus to be retracted posteriorly with greater ease.

- This sequence should allow circumferential excision of the remaining glenoid labrum and biceps tendon.

- A Kocher clamp is used to tension the labrum and resect it with electrocautery.

- Special care should be taken when dissecting around the inferior glenoid because of the close proximity of the axillary nerve.

- Release of the inferior capsule from the glenoid is a critically important step in glenoid preparation. This release completes a bipolar inferior capsular release of the glenoid and humerus and a 360° release of the glenoid. These releases also will have a potential effect on achieving ROM postoperatively. The authors of this chapter prefer to place the inferior capsule under tension with a flat Darrach retractor and then release the capsule from the inferior glenoid using electrocautery. A blunt elevator can be used

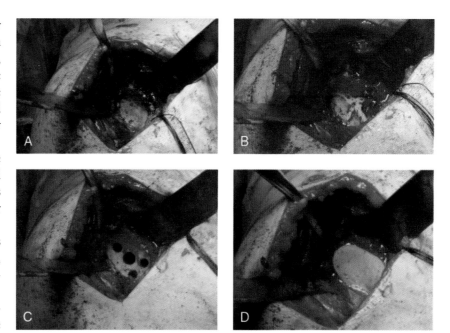

Figure 6 Intraoperative photographs demonstrate glenoid exposure. **A,** Proper retractor placement for adequate glenoid exposure is shown (anterior is on the right). **B,** After circumferential labral resection, the quadrants of the glenoid are marked. **C,** The appropriate drill holes are made. **D,** The final appearance of the impacted cemented glenoid component.

to complete the inferior capsular release, extending medially to the insertion of the long head of the triceps on the inferior glenoid neck.

- Minor retractor adjustments should enable an adequate view of the glenoid. If adequate posterior displacement of the humeral head still cannot be achieved, additional posterior capsular releases may be required.

- These additional posterior capsular releases are performed by first removing all retractors and placing a lamina spreader between the glenoid and the proximal humerus to tension the posterior capsule. The capsule then is released 1 cm lateral to the posterior glenoid margin, with care taken to avoid compromise of the posterior rotator cuff. Then, retractors can be replaced as described.

- Glenoid reaming and component insertion largely depends on which components are being used. The

specific step for each system should be well-known to the surgeon. The challenges related to glenoid component insertion include identifying the center point of the glenoid, where the best bone is available, and determining the orientation for drilling and reaming to achieve the desired version. To accomplish these goals, an understanding of glenoid anatomy, based on preoperative imaging and adequate intraoperative glenoid exposure, is essential.

- The superior-inferior and anterior-posterior quadrants of the glenoid are marked (**Figure 6, B**).

- The glenoid guide is placed, and the center of glenoid reaming is marked with a drill bit or cautery. A small-diameter drill is used to assess glenoid depth and confirm the proper angle for reaming.

- Sequential glenoid reaming is performed, with eccentric reaming used as necessary to correct small

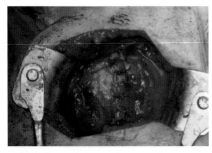

Figure 7 Intraoperative photograph of a shoulder shows the repaired subscapularis tendon, including the rotator interval closure.

degrees of glenoid retroversion. After reaming, glenoid osteophytes and any additional soft tissue that could interfere with component insertion are removed.

- Using the appropriate guides, the holes for the implant are drilled (**Figure 6, C**).

- Trial components are used to confirm the proper glenoid preparation before cementing.

- Copious irrigation of the wound is performed and the glenoid drill holes filled with thrombin-soaked absorbable gelatin powder.

- One bag of viscous antibiotic cement is mixed and used to fill a vented syringe, which is used to pressurize cement into the drill holes and impact the appropriately sized components (**Figure 6, D**).

Humeral Implant and Soft-Tissue Balancing

- If humeral reaming and broaching have not been performed, they are performed now, in the manner described previously. The final implant is inserted and seated fully.

- A noncemented press-fit stem is routinely used. Most systems have a cemented option, which can be used based on surgeon preference or if there is concern about implant fixation. In such cases, the humeral canal is irrigated and dried, and

a cement restrictor is placed 1 to 2 cm distal to the tip of the stem. A cement gun can be used to fill the humeral canal and pressurize the cement. Then, the implant is inserted fully.

- An appropriately sized humeral head trial is selected. Current modular systems have various means of adjusting for humeral offset to allow maximal coverage of the metaphysis and to reproduce the patient's humeral anatomy.

- After the appropriate trial implant is in place, the humeral head is reduced by traction, forward flexion, and internal rotation.

- Soft-tissue tension is assessed. The authors of this chapter prefer to first inspect the implant in varying degrees of internal and external rotation, with the arm in adduction to assess muscle tension and soft-tissue laxity or instability. A posteriorly and then inferiorly directed force is applied and then released. Up to 50% translation of the humeral head on the glenoid is preferred, with prompt reduction after the force is removed.

- Component height is assessed carefully to ensure that the relationship between the greater tuberosity and the superior aspect of the humeral head is anatomic. Excessive head height can cause rotator cuff problems and eventual failure, whereas inadequate positioning can result in greater tuberosity impingement on the underside of the acromion. Excessive tension indicates an inadequate humeral neck cut, improper positioning of the humeral component (varus), or an improper choice of the humeral head component.

- Instability is addressed by confirming appropriate component positioning, assessing the soft-tissue releases, and increasing the lateral offset. After balancing and height are optimized, the final implant is

secured, and the humeral head is reduced. Stability is tested again.

Wound Closure

- Copious irrigation of the joint is performed.

- The subscapularis tendon is repaired with No. 2 nonabsorbable suture, and the rotator interval is closed to reduce the tension on the repair (**Figure 7**). A subscapularis peel will require tendon-to-bone repair through drill holes. LT osteotomy also will require sutures passed through drill holes and/or around the humeral stem.

- A closed suction drain is used in all TSAs to reduce the risk of postoperative hematoma, although this step is a matter of surgeon preference.

- The deltopectoral interval is closed with a No. 0 braided absorbable suture, and the subcutaneous tissue is closed with a No. 2.0 absorbable suture.

- The skin is closed with a running subcuticular closure with No. 3.0 nonabsorbable propylene suture, and thin adhesive strips are applied.

- A full set of radiographs is obtained in the operating room to assess the position of the component. These radiographs include an AP view with the humerus in internal rotation, an AP view with the humerus in external rotation, and an axillary view.

- The upper extremity is placed in a sling for immobilization.

 Rehabilitation

Rehabilitation begins in the recovery room while regional anesthesia is still in effect (**Table 2**). Starting rehabilitation immediately postoperatively enables repeated patient reinforcement of the initial 6-week rehabilitation protocol during the 1- to 2-day hospital stay.

Table 2 Rehabilitation Protocol After Routine Total Shoulder Arthroplasty

Postoperative Week	ROM	Strengthening	Return to Work/Play	Comments/Emphasis
0-6	Passive forward flexion in the scapular plane as tolerated Passive, active-assisted external rotation with end ranges of motion determined intraoperatively based on subscapularis tension; typically, neutral to 30° is possible Active finger, wrist, and elbow motion	None	May work if able to do so in sling	Avoid shoulder extension beyond neutral with the arm in adduction, external rotation past a specified point, active internal rotation, and weight bearing
6-12	Active and active-assisted shoulder motion in all planes is begun, including internal rotation behind the back	Isometric strengthening is begun	Desk work and light duties only Cardiovascular exercise is allowed, but resisted/forceful shoulder motions are not allowed	Avoid resisted strengthening exercises
≥12	Active ROM of the shoulder is continued with more aggressive stretching exercises	Resisted strengthening exercises may begin	Graduated return to duties in the context of lifetime restrictions Gradual return to exercise in the context of lifetime restrictions	Lifetime restrictions: Avoid weight bearing >15 lb as well as strenuous, repetitive, or overhead activities

ROM = range of motion.

During the early postoperative phase, subscapularis tendon healing begins and stiffness is avoided. Later, active ROM and strengthening exercises are implemented. Rehabilitation instructions are reinforced throughout the postoperative period.

 Avoiding Pitfalls

Attention to the aforementioned surgical techniques should help avoid the most common pitfalls. The patient should be positioned so as to be held stable by the surgical table and to obtain unobstructed shoulder motion, thereby avoiding iatrogenic positioning injuries and blocked shoulder motion (especially adduction) caused by the table itself. Inadequate soft-tissue releases complicate later exposure. The surgeon should use a deltopectoral approach and carefully manage the subscapularis tendon. Soft-tissue release of the deltoid, subdeltoid, and subscapularis facilitates later steps in the procedure.

To facilitate humeral preparation, the patient's arm should be adducted and externally rotated to deliver the humeral head. Osteophyte removal is important as well, as is appropriate humeral cut and implant sizing. Problems related to humeral preparation are caused by inadequate soft-tissue release or osteophyte resection; improper cut (angle or height); improper implant version and alignment; traction neurapraxia caused by prolonged adduction and external rotation of the humerus; and fracture caused by forceful manipulation, aggressive reaming, or improper sizing.

Appropriate retractor placement, circumferential exposure of the glenoid, resection of the labrum, and careful implant insertion are important steps in glenoid preparation. During inferior releases, the surgeon must take care to avoid inadequate soft-tissue release, improper retractor placement, excessive glenoid reaming, improper component position, glenoid fracture, and axillary nerve damage.

Soft-tissue balancing involves clinical assessment with trialing and final implants and may require soft-tissue releases before final implant placement. Inadequate balancing, whether too tight or too loose, must be avoided, along with implant malposition. Meticulous subscapularis closure is required, and a drain must be placed. Complications related to closure include failed subscapularis repair, excessive repair that limits external rotation, hematoma, and infection.

Bibliography

Denard PJ, Raiss P, Sowa B, Walch G: Mid- to long-term follow-up of total shoulder arthroplasty using a keeled glenoid in young adults with primary glenohumeral arthritis. *J Shoulder Elbow Surg* 2013;22(7):894-900.

Deshmukh AV, Koris M, Zurakowski D, Thornhill TS: Total shoulder arthroplasty: Long-term survivorship, functional outcome, and quality of life. *J Shoulder Elbow Surg* 2005;14(5):471-479.

Kasten P, Pape G, Raiss P, et al: Mid-term survivorship analysis of a shoulder replacement with a keeled glenoid and a modern cementing technique. *J Bone Joint Surg Br* 2010;92(3):387-392.

Khan A, Bunker TD, Kitson JB: Clinical and radiological follow-up of the Aequalis third-generation cemented total shoulder replacement: A minimum ten-year study. *J Bone Joint Surg Br* 2009;91(12):1594-1600.

Raiss P, Aldinger PR, Kasten P, Rickert M, Loew M: Total shoulder replacement in young and middle-aged patients with glenohumeral osteoarthritis. *J Bone Joint Surg Br* 2008;90(6):764-769.

Raiss P, Edwards TB, Deutsch A, et al: Radiographic changes around humeral components in shoulder arthroplasty. *J Bone Joint Surg Am* 2014;96(7):e54.

Raiss P, Schmitt M, Bruckner T, et al: Results of cemented total shoulder replacement with a minimum follow-up of ten years. *J Bone Joint Surg Am* 2012;94(23):e1711-e10.

Walch G, Young AA, Melis B, Gazielly D, Loew M, Boileau P: Results of a convex-back cemented keeled glenoid component in primary osteoarthritis: Multicenter study with a follow-up greater than 5 years. *J Shoulder Elbow Surg* 2011;20(3):385-394.

Young A, Walch G, Boileau P, et al: A multicentre study of the long-term results of using a flat-back polyethylene glenoid component in shoulder replacement for primary osteoarthritis. *J Bone Joint Surg Br* 2011;93(2):210-216.

Video Reference

Zuckerman JD, Mollon B, Ryan WE Jr: Video. Uncomplicated Total Shoulder Arthroplasty. New York, NY, 2015.

Chapter 37

Reaming and Bone Grafting Techniques for Long-Term Glenoid Stability After Total Shoulder Arthroplasty

David M. Dines, MD

Joshua S. Dines, MD

 ## Introduction

Total shoulder arthroplasty (TSA) has proved to be an outstanding treatment for refractory osteoarthritis, resulting in good to excellent outcomes in up to 95% of patients. These results have been observed in several large series, with the revision-free survivorship of up to 20 years reported to be approximately 80%. Most of these large series reported on first- and second-generation implant designs. Given these results, the number of TSA procedures being performed continues to increase at a substantial rate.

Although the results of TSA have been impressive, the most common indications for revision remain soft-tissue failure and glenoid component wear and/or loosening. Shoulder implant failure has been associated with component malposition, soft-tissue imbalance, and insufficient bone support or morphology. In patients in whom glenoid components fails, preoperative glenoid morphology may predict outcomes.

Glenoid morphology is most commonly classified according to the Walch system. The classification is based on CT scans and includes five categories based on bone loss, version, wear, and deformity (**Figure 1**). Type A morphology denotes a centered humeral head with varied degrees of central erosion described as minor (type A1) or major (type A2). This pattern is the most common and seen in approximately 60% of patients. Type B morphology is characterized by posterior wear and/or subluxation. Type B1 has posterior narrowing without erosion, whereas type B2 has overt posterior erosion or bone loss associated with posterior subluxation. Type C morphology is a dysplastic deformity with more than 25° of glenoid retroversion.

Patients with types B2 and C have the greatest degree of deformity and bone loss and are, therefore, the most difficult to treat. Recent studies have demonstrated that in some patients, these deformities may be best treated with hemiarthroplasty or reverse shoulder arthroplasty (RSA) as the index procedure.

The surgeon needs to completely understand the glenoid deformity, including the degree of bone loss, retroversion, and humeral head subluxation, to determine and execute the appropriate surgical procedure. Ultimately, the surgical treatment of patients with deformity and bone loss depends on the severity of deformity. Options include reducing the posterior bone loss with eccentric or asymmetric anterior reaming of the high side to a more neutral version, bone grafting to address the posterior bone loss, or, more recently, the use of an augmented glenoid component. In many patients with severe deformity, RSA may be the best surgical option.

 ## Case Presentation

A 64-year-old woman, active in recreational sports, has severe refractory osteoarthritis of her right (dominant) shoulder. She has no substantial comorbidities. Trials of NSAIDs, intra-articular cortisone, lifestyle modification, and physical therapy over the previous 5 years failed. The patient has pain at night and at rest. Her active range of motion (ROM) is diminished by 50% in abduction, forward elevation, and external rotation. Her passive external rotation measures 30°. Plain radiographs, including an axillary view, demonstrate severe bone-on-bone joint space narrowing with humeral osteophytes.

Dr. David Dines or an immediate family member has received royalties and nonincome support (such as equipment or services), commercially derived honoraria, or other non–research-related funding (such as paid travel) from Zimmer Biomet and serves as a board member, owner, officer, or committee member of the American Shoulder and Elbow Surgeons. Dr. Joshua Dines or an immediate family member has received royalties from Zimmer Biomet, is a member of a speakers' bureau or has made paid presentations on behalf of Arthrex, and serves as a paid consultant to Arthrex and ConMed Linvatec.

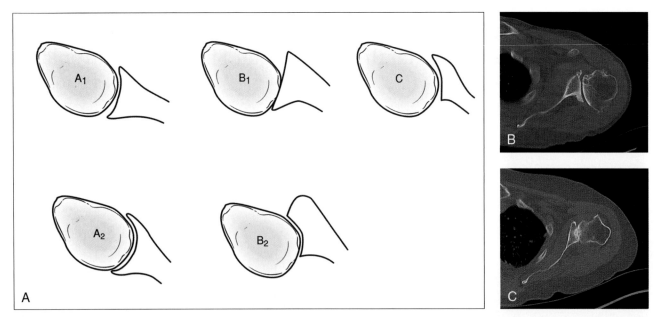

Figure 1 **A,** Illustration shows the Walch classification of posterior glenoid bone wear/deficiency. Type A1 has a well-centered humeral head. Type A2 has a well-centered head with medial glenoid erosion. Type B1 has posterior subluxation of the humeral head with minimal posterior wear. Type B2 has substantial posterior glenoid erosion. Type C has glenoid retroversion greater than 25°, irrespective of erosion and caused principally by dysplasia. CT scans demonstrate a Walch type B2 glenoid deformity (**B**) and a Walch type C glenoid deformity (**C**). (Panel A adapted with permission from Walch G, Badet R, Boulahia A, Khoury A: Morphologic study of the glenoid in primary glenohumeral osteoarthritis. *J Arthroplasty* 1999;14[6]:756-760.)

CT demonstrates substantial posterior bone loss and retroversion deformity measuring 15°. The patient underwent successful anatomic TSA with asymmetric glenoid surface reaming using a patient-specific guide system based on three-dimensional (3D) CT reconstruction with excellent clinical outcome (**Figure 2**).

 Indications

Indications for glenoid component replacement depend on several factors, including the age and activity level of the patient, soft-tissue quality, and the degree of bone deformity. In older, sedentary patients, longevity of the implant may be less important. However, in younger, active patients, such as middle-aged weight lifters, glenoid component durability is an important consideration.

Soft-tissue insufficiencies are particularly worrisome in the context of glenoid replacement. Rotator cuff insufficiencies and posterior capsular laxity play a well-documented role in implant longevity. Excessive posterior laxity, if not corrected, can result in eccentric glenoid component loading and, ultimately, loosening and/or failure. Rotator cuff insufficiencies are best treated with RSA.

The decision to perform TSA depends on many factors, such as the patient's age, activity level, morbid anatomy, and lifestyle. Contraindications may include physical or psychologic issues that may compromise healing and/or postoperative rehabilitation such as dementia. Active infection, previous nerve injury, and severe medical comorbidities should be considered contraindications. Severe bone loss and soft-tissue insufficiencies are relative contraindications and may be best treated with RSA. Another contraindication to TSA may be a Walch B2 glenoid with retroversion greater than 26° and fixed humeral head subluxation of more than 80%. A study of anatomic TSA reported a poor survival rate at 5-year follow-up in patients with Walch B2 glenoid deformity.

 Controversies and Alternative Approaches

In some patients with extreme glenoid deformity with retroversion greater than 25° to 30° and associated bone loss and soft-tissue laxity, hemiarthroplasty may be the only viable surgical option to prevent complications.

For patients with less severe posterior bone loss, the use of posteriorly augmented glenoid components, in addition to eccentric reaming and bone grafting, has generated renewed interest. These components were used in first-generation implant systems, but their use was discontinued because of a high incidence of associated posterior instability. Recently, several companies have released newer implants to treat posterior bone loss. These implants,

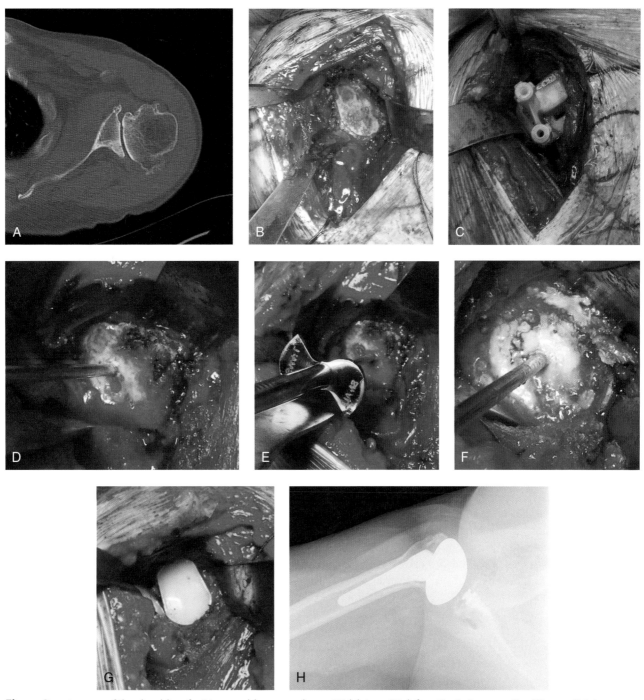

Figure 2 Images of the shoulder of a 64-year-old woman show a Walch type B2 deformity. **A,** Preoperative CT scan. **B,** Intraoperative photograph of proper glenoid exposure shows posterior glenoid bone wear and deformity. **C,** Intraoperative photograph shows a patient-specific guide used to ensure proper guidewire placement based on three-dimensional CT reconstruction. **D,** Intraoperative photograph shows a guidewire placed in proper orientation for optimum eccentric reaming. **E,** Intraoperative photograph shows a reamer inserted over the guidewire. **F,** Intraoperative photograph shows eccentric reaming to remove bone from the anterior high side to create a neutral glenoid surface. **G,** Intraoperative photograph shows the implant placed in neutral glenoid version. **H,** Axillary radiograph demonstrates the glenoid implant in a neutral position.

Table 1 Results of Autogenous Posterior Bone Grafting to Correct Posterior Glenoid Deficiency in Total Shoulder Arthroplasty

Authors	Journal (Year)	No. of Patients	Outcomes	Failure Rate (%)	Comments
Neer and Morrison	*J Bone Joint Surg Am* (1988)	19	Results were excellent in 16 patients, satisfactory in 1, and unsatisfactory in 2	0	Mean follow-up, 4.4 yr Complications included 6 radiolucent lines, 2 screw failures, and 1 loose glenoid
Steinmann and Cofield	*J Shoulder Elbow Surg* (2000)	28	Results were excellent in 13 patients, satisfactory in 10, and unsatisfactory in 5 Two-thirds of patients had normal range of motion	18	Mean follow-up, 5.1 yr Complications included 3 loose glenoids and 2 patients with instability
Hill and Norris	*J Bone Joint Surg Am* (2001)	17	According to Neer criteria, results were excellent in 3 patients, satisfactory in 6, and unsatisfactory in 8	29	Complications included 3 failed grafts, 2 rotator cuff tears, 2 patients with instability, and 1 malposition
Sabesan et al	*J Bone Joint Surg Am* (2013)	12	Results were satisfactory in 10 patients and poor in 2 patients requiring revision	16	Mean follow-up, 4.4 yr 10 grafts incorporated without resorption 2 patients had minor resorption Complications included 1 *Propionibacterium acnes* infection and 1 failure as a result of trauma

which use polyethylene or titanium posterior augmentation, are an alternative to symmetric reaming and bone grafting. However, no long-term studies of these implants are available. Even with these newer implants, many surgeons continue to advocate RSA in patients with severe deformity, such as Walch B2 deformities with more than 70° of posterior subluxation.

 Results

The results of autogenous posterior bone grafting for glenoid deficiency are summarized in **Table 1**. Reports of anatomic TSA in conjunction with eccentric reaming to correct glenoid version are limited. Two studies of asymmetric glenoid reaming reported that the humeral head was re-centered on the glenoid component in almost every patient.

In patients with more severe deformity and in younger patients, the posterior bone deformity or erosion may be treated with bone grafting. This technique showed outstanding results in 89% of 19 patients at a follow-up of 4.4 years, but long-term results were less encouraging. Recently, more encouraging midterm results were reported for clinical outcome and durability in 12 patients who underwent primary anatomic TSA with autogenous bone grafting.

 Technical Keys to Success

Preoperative Planning

Successful glenoid component replacement begins with proper preoperative workup and imaging. The clinical workup should include any history of infection, nerve injury, or comorbidities that could affect outcomes. Advanced imaging is necessary to ensure the best results, especially in patients with substantial to severe glenoid deformity

(**Figure 3**). Humeral osteophytes and glenohumeral joint space narrowing can be easily identified on plain radiographs; however, glenoid deformity, erosion, and excessive version are difficult to assess even on axillary radiographs. CT with 3D reconstruction is a better method for evaluating glenoid version, vault anatomy, and bone loss. Glenoid version also can be assessed with axial CT. The use of 3D CT not only helps define the degree of bone loss and deformity but also plays a role in technique because many patient-specific guides and instrument techniques incorporate this technology.

MRI may be helpful in patients with mild glenoid bone loss or deformity; however, it is primarily used to assess soft-tissue quality. In addition, MRI is not adaptable to patient-specific guide and instrumentation technologies.

Video 37.1 The Difficult Glenoid in Total Shoulder Arthroplasty: Reaming and Bone Grafting Techniques to Ensure Long-Term Stability. David M. Dines, MD; Joshua S. Dines, MD (8 min)

Surgical Techniques

After a careful preoperative workup and imaging, successful outcomes depend on surgical planning, instrumentation, and technique. Excellent glenoid exposure is mandatory for successful component replacement, especially in patients with difficult glenoid deformity requiring substantial asymmetric reaming and/or posterior bone graft (**Figure 4**).

Excellent glenoid exposure begins with proper anesthesia for relaxation. Surgically, it requires subscapular releases as necessary, adequate humeral head resection, and humeral osteophyte removal. Inadequate resection and retained osteophytes restrict the ability to retract the humerus posteriorly. Proper retractors, including Hohmann, "Playboy" (pitch-forked), and Fukuda posteriorly and Bankart anteriorly are necessary to adequately expose the glenoid surface (**Figure 5**).

With the selected retractors in place, careful and meticulous resection of the anterior capsule, labrum, and biceps insertion helps achieve excellent visualization. This resection should include all anterior capsular structures, the rotator interval, and the long head of biceps insertion from the 12-o'clock position down to the 6-o'clock position and beyond in the inferior glenoid, being aware of the proximity of the axillary nerve. The inferior capsule must be resected carefully to ensure sufficient exposure and postoperative motion. Inferior dissection of the capsule off the glenoid can be facilitated with the use of electrocautery, which can excise the tissue and act as a nerve stimulator if close to the nerve.

In some patients with severe deformity, a preliminary resection or reaming

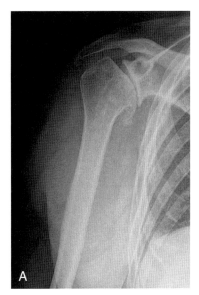
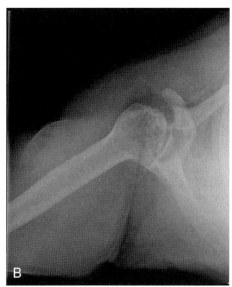

Figure 3   **A,** AP shoulder radiograph demonstrates osteoarthritis. **B,** Axillary shoulder radiograph demonstrates osteoarthritis with joint space narrowing and glenoid wear.

of the anterior or high side may be necessary before formal glenoid preparation to facilitate this exposure. Careful resection is even more important in patients with more severe glenoid deformity because posterior glenoid exposure is critical in these patients. In addition, because of the increased risk of posterior instability in patients with more severe glenoid retroversion, it is imperative to protect the posterior capsulolabral attachments to prevent postoperative instability.

ASYMMETRIC POSTERIOR GLENOID REAMING

Posterior glenoid defects are most commonly addressed with eccentric reaming. The anterior glenoid high side is reamed down to create a concentric glenoid surface for the polyethylene glenoid component.

Historically, this reaming was performed using a visual technique, which used flat reamers and, in some patients, prereaming resection with high-speed burrs or osteotomes. More detailed imaging provides a better understanding of the degree of deformity in all directions to better guide the reaming.

Several instrument systems have been developed to improve the surgeon's ability to place the glenoid component centrally in the best possible position after version correction. These computerized systems use 3D CT reconstruction to generate a patient-specific guide or provide angle measurements for version correction. Because most of these systems use a cannulated instrumentation system, the central guidewire not only establishes the best possible degree of version correction but also indicates the optimal position of the glenoid component and its fixation system (pegged or keeled; **Figure 6**).

Exposure is critical in patients with glenoid deformity. Eccentric reaming techniques, especially in patients with more substantial deformities, often require prereaming or bone tapering with a high-speed burr to provisionally lower the high side and provide an en face view. At this point, a more accurate assessment of the degree of bone loss is possible. To avoid potentially removing too much of the glenoid vault bone stock, the authors of this chapter try not to ream more than 10 mm of anterior bone or more than 15° of retroversion

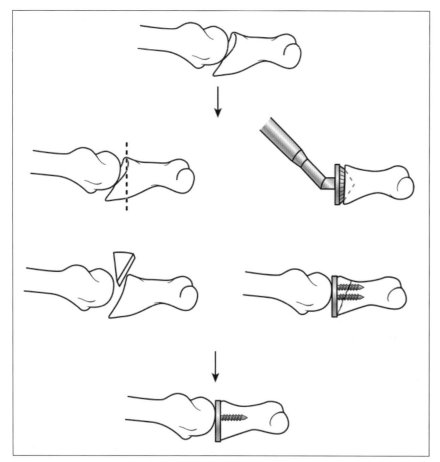

Figure 4 Illustration depicts surgical options for the treatment of posterior glenoid bone loss/wear from top to bottom. Posterior wear can be treated with eccentric bone removal or reaming to neutralize the glenoid. If bone loss is substantial, a posterior bone graft is necessary. In either situation, the result should be a well-fixed glenoid component in neutral to 7° of retroversion. (Reproduced from Dines DM: Posterior glenoid wear and bone loss: Treatment options, in Zuckerman JD, ed: *Advanced Reconstruction: Shoulder.* Rosemont, IL, American Academy of Orthopaedic Surgeons, 2007, pp 557-565.)

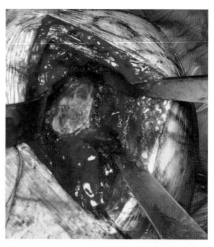

Figure 5 Intraoperative photograph of the shoulder of a patient with posterior glenoid bone wear shows excellent glenoid exposure.

deformity when using "eyeball" techniques. For patient-specific guide systems, this degree of resection is built into the instrumentation. The goal is to create a glenoid surface that is more neutral and congruent to the posterior surface of the glenoid component. In patients with substantial deformity, the area of posterior wear is usually a hard, eburnated surface; the goal is to neutralize the anterior resected surface to this surface without too much further medial resection of the glenoid vault bone stock.

Eccentric reaming techniques, although improved by the use of advanced guide systems and instrumentation, are still limited by the degree of correction possible without the risk of implant failure. As the surgeon reams asymmetrically, the glenoid vault narrows medially and bone loss increases, leaving less bone stock for implantation and fixation. Excessive reaming may require downsizing to a smaller glenoid component, resulting in concomitant soft-tissue/implant mismatch, leading to less capsular restraint and possible instability. An additional concern is that with substantial reaming, the center of rotation is medialized, resulting in abnormal tensioning in the rotator cuff

and deltoid musculature. This tensioning can result in subsequent functional loss. Another concern is that medialization of the glenoid vault can result in cortical penetration of the pegs or keel of the glenoid component. Cadaver model studies and computer simulations have indicated that the maximum extent of correction possible without the risk of perforation is 15° or less than 1 cm of bone resection.

Cadaver model studies and computer simulations have shown significant improvements in glenoid component placement with the use of patient-specific guide systems currently available with almost all commercial TSA systems. A clinical study reported the best results in patients with more than 16° of glenoid retroversion.

In addition to treating the bone deformity, the surgeon must be mindful of soft-tissue considerations. Difficult cases require thoughtful and creative soft-tissue balancing for appropriate joint mechanics. Patients with posterior bone loss typically have concomitant soft-tissue contracture anteriorly and laxity of the capsule posteriorly. These issues must be treated intraoperatively. Subscapularis tendon lengthening with a 360° release is important for

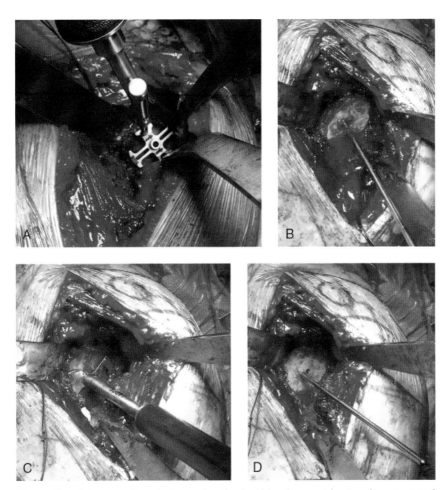

Figure 6 Intraoperative photographs of a shoulder show guidewire placement and glenoid reaming. **A,** The glenoid guidewire is positioned using a guide based on preoperative CT scans. **B,** The guidewire is in the proper position to ensure the appropriate amount of anterior reaming. **C,** A reamer is used over the guidewire. **D,** Successful asymmetric reaming of the glenoid resulted in a more neutral position.

In these patients, the natural joint line and center of rotation must be reestablished because no anterior bone is removed. The soft-tissue mechanics may undergo less alteration but still must be considered.

Although bone grafting offers a biologic solution, the risks of nonunion and graft dissolution remain substantial. Different types of graft material have been described. The authors of this chapter prefer to use the resected humeral head as a structural graft if possible. The graft is readily available and is already contoured for the glenoid deformity. A guided, cannulated system is used to place a central pin lying perpendicular to the glenoid axis in neutral position. The high side is then slightly reamed to create a flat surface for lateral attachment of the bone graft.

Next, the defect surface is prepared with light burring to create a bleeding surface. The humeral head graft is prepared and contoured to fit the defect. The graft is placed to re-create a flush surface with the anterior glenoid. The graft is fixed with 3.5-mm screws over the previously placed guidewires. The authors of this chapter prefer to use an arthroscopic cannula posteriorly to allow easier access for the instrumentation and improve access for pin and screw placement. With the graft well fixed, a cannulated system is used to create the appropriate pegs or slots for fixation of the glenoid component, which is then cemented into place in a standard fashion (**Figure 7**). After glenoid component replacement, the TSA is completed in a standard manner. Prior to final humeral component placement, trials are used, and closed reduction is carried out to test for ROM, translation, and stability. If instability persists, humeral head component offset or sizing and, in rare patients, possible posterior capsular plication may be considered.

restoration of motion and stability. In these patients, the anterior capsule is severely contracted and must be carefully released to improve motion, stability, and glenoid exposure.

Treating posterior subluxation and laxity can be difficult. Posterior capsular repair to bone and capsular plication have been described. Plication techniques include removing redundancy with the use of a "purse-string" technique or splitting the capsule and repairing it in a pants-over-vest manner. Techniques such as placing the humeral component in less retroversion or increasing the humeral head component

size also have been attempted in some patients.

BONE GRAFT

In patients with more severe deformity and in younger patients, the posterior bone deformity or erosion can be treated with bone grafting. Indications for bone grafting include glenoid wear deformities that cannot be corrected by eccentric reaming, insufficient glenoid vault bone, more than 15° of retroversion, and/or potential penetration of the vault by the component pegs or keel. Bone graft offers a biologic solution for extreme glenoid bone loss or deformity.

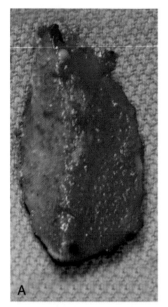
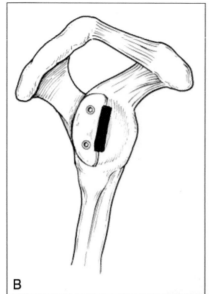
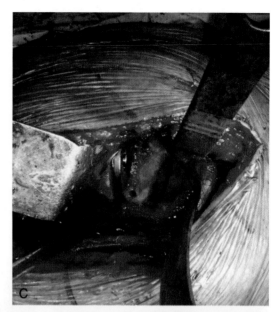
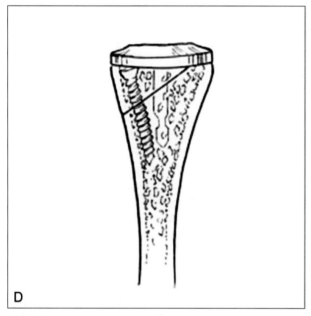
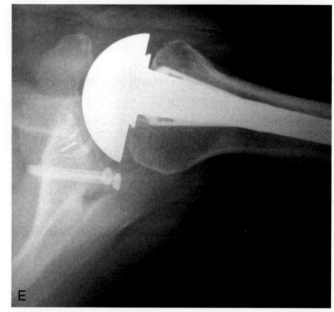

Figure 7 Images show correction of posterior glenoid deficiency with a posterior bone block. **A,** Photograph shows a bone block harvested from a humeral head segment and trimmed to fit the defect. **B,** Illustration shows a bone graft fixed to the posterior surface with cannulated screws in a provisional slot that is later finished. The screws must not interfere with the fixation device of the glenoid component. **C,** Intraoperative photograph shows a humeral head graft being contoured to fit the defect. After the surface is prepared and a preliminary slot is created, the graft is fixed with cannulated cancellous screws. **D,** Illustration shows proper screw placement. The screws must not impinge on the fixation pegs or keel of the glenoid implant. **E,** Postoperative axillary radiograph demonstrates a well-fixed, neutralized glenoid reconstruction with posterior bone graft. (Panels A, C, and E courtesy of Joseph Iannotti, MD, PhD, Cleveland, OH. Panels B and D adapted with permission from Neer CS, Morrison DS: Glenoid bone-grafting in total shoulder arthroplasty. *J Bone Joint Surg Am* 1988;70[8]:1154-1162.)

 ## Rehabilitation

After TSA, the patient is placed in a sling with or without swathe for 3 to 6 weeks, depending on the security of the soft-tissue reconstruction. Early passive ROM is begun to prevent adhesions and regain maximum ROM. These exercises include passive forward flexion, internal rotation, and external rotation limited by the security of the subscapularis tendon repair. After substantial passive

Table 2 Standard Rehabilitation Protocol After Total Shoulder Arthroplasty

Postoperative Week	ROM	Strengthening	Return to Play	Comments/Emphasis
0-2	Passive forward flexion, internal rotation, and external rotation	None	Walking	A sling with or without swathe is used
2-6	After substantial passive ROM has been achieved, progress to active-assisted and then active ROM in the first 6 to 8 wk	None	Walking/ stationary bike	Use of a sling with or without swathe is continued for 3 to 6 wk Arm may be removed from sling several times per day for active-assisted ROM and Codman exercises
6-12	—	After soft-tissue healing is sufficient and active ROM has been achieved, protected strengthening exercises are initiated and progressed through isometric and isotonic exercise programs	Non–upper extremity sports activity with limited fall risks	—
12-24	—	—	Upper extremity sports activities	—

ROM = range of motion.

ROM has been achieved, therapy is progressed to active-assisted and, ultimately, active ROM in the first 6 to 8 weeks postoperatively. Thereafter, protected strengthening exercises are initiated and progressed to isometric and then isotonic exercise programs. The standard rehabilitation protocol is summarized in **Table 2**.

In patients with substantial bone deficiency and associated substantial posterior capsular laxity who undergo eccentric reaming and posterior capsular repair or plication, the postoperative therapy regimen must be adjusted. Exercises that increase strain on the posterior structures must be limited in the early rehabilitation period. In these patients, passive ROM in the straight anterior-posterior plane should be avoided. All passive exercises should be performed in the scapular plane instead of the frontal plane.

Similarly, in patients undergoing posterior bone grafting, especially if a large graft has been used, therapy may need to be altered until evidence of graft incorporation is observed. In these patients, passive ROM should be performed in the scapular plane for the first 6 weeks postoperatively. Thereafter, active-assisted and, eventually, active ROM exercises should continue for 2 to 4 months postoperatively.

In all patients, ROM exercises should continue until full ROM and strength are attained. Strengthening exercises are begun after soft-tissue reconstruction is deemed secure enough to support this aspect of rehabilitation.

 Avoiding Pitfalls

Appropriate treatment of glenoid bone loss during TSA is technically demanding. Ensuring a successful long-term outcome begins with thoughtful preoperative planning. As noted previously, advanced imaging, especially 3D CT, is critical. Although imaging helps guide the surgeon, intraoperative findings often influence the treatment decision. Mild-to-moderate posterior bone loss can often be treated with eccentric reaming without affecting implant stability. Patients with more advanced bone loss or incongruity may require bone grafting or even posteriorly augmented glenoid components. Despite technical and technologic advances in TSA, patients with extensive bone loss may require RSA or hemiarthroplasty for optimal results.

Bibliography

Bohsali KI, Wirth MA, Rockwood CA Jr: Complications of total shoulder arthroplasty. *J Bone Joint Surg Am* 2006;88(10):2279-2292.

Cil A, Veillette CJ, Sanchez-Sotelo J, Sperling JW, Schleck CD, Cofield RH: Survivorship of the humeral component in shoulder arthroplasty. *J Shoulder Elbow Surg* 2010;19(1):143-150.

Clavert P, Millett PJ, Warner JJ: Glenoid resurfacing: What are the limits to asymmetric reaming for posterior erosion? *J Shoulder Elbow Surg* 2007;16(6):843-848.

Day JS, Lau E, Ong KL, Williams GR, Ramsey ML, Kurtz SM: Prevalence and projections of total shoulder and elbow arthroplasty in the United States to 2015. *J Shoulder Elbow Surg* 2010;19(8):1115-1120.

Denard PJ, Walch G: Current concepts in the surgical management of primary glenohumeral arthritis with a biconcave glenoid. *J Shoulder Elbow Surg* 2013;22(11):1589-1598.

Farron A, Terrier A, Büchler P: Risks of loosening of a prosthetic glenoid implanted in retroversion. *J Shoulder Elbow Surg* 2006;15(4):521-526.

Franklin JL, Barrett WP, Jackins SE, Matsen FA III: Glenoid loosening in total shoulder arthroplasty: Association with rotator cuff deficiency. *J Arthroplasty* 1988;3(1):39-46.

Friedman RJ, Hawthorne KB, Genez BM: The use of computerized tomography in the measurement of glenoid version. *J Bone Joint Surg Am* 1992;74(7):1032-1037.

Gerber C, Costouros JG, Sukthankar A, Fucentese SF: Static posterior humeral head subluxation and total shoulder arthroplasty. *J Shoulder Elbow Surg* 2009;18(4):505-510.

Habermeyer P, Magosch P, Lichtenberg S: Recentering the humeral head for glenoid deficiency in total shoulder arthroplasty. *Clin Orthop Relat Res* 2007;(457):124-132.

Hendel MD, Bryan JA, Barsoum WK, et al: Comparison of patient-specific instruments with standard surgical instruments in determining glenoid component position: A randomized prospective clinical trial. *J Bone Joint Surg Am* 2012;94(23):2167-2175.

Hill JM, Norris TR: Long-term results of total shoulder arthroplasty following bone-grafting of the glenoid. *J Bone Joint Surg Am* 2001;83(6):877-883.

Iannotti J, Baker J, Rodriguez E, et al: Three-dimensional preoperative planning software and a novel information transfer technology improve glenoid component positioning. *J Bone Joint Surg Am* 2014;96(9):e71.

Iannotti JP, Greeson C, Downing D, Sabesan V, Bryan JA: Effect of glenoid deformity on glenoid component placement in primary shoulder arthroplasty. *J Shoulder Elbow Surg* 2012;21(1):48-55.

Iannotti JP, Norris TR: Influence of preoperative factors on outcome of shoulder arthroplasty for glenohumeral osteoarthritis. *J Bone Joint Surg Am* 2003;85(2):251-258.

Mizuno N, Denard PJ, Raiss P, Walch G: Reverse total shoulder arthroplasty for primary glenohumeral osteoarthritis in patients with a biconcave glenoid. *J Bone Joint Surg Am* 2013;95(14):1297-1304.

Moskal MJ, Duckworth D, Matsen FA: Abstract: An analysis of 122 failed shoulder arthroplasties. *J Shoulder Elbow Surg* 1999;8:554.

Neer CS II, Morrison DS: Glenoid bone-grafting in total shoulder arthroplasty. *J Bone Joint Surg Am* 1988;70(8):1154-1162.

Neer CS II, Watson KC, Stanton FJ: Recent experience in total shoulder replacement. *J Bone Joint Surg Am* 1982;64(3):319-337.

Norris TR, Iannotti JP: Functional outcome after shoulder arthroplasty for primary osteoarthritis: A multicenter study. *J Shoulder Elbow Surg* 2002;11(2):130-135.

Nyffeler RW, Jost B, Pfirrmann CW, Gerber C: Measurement of glenoid version: Conventional radiographs versus computed tomography scans. *J Shoulder Elbow Surg* 2003;12(5):493-496.

Rice RS, Sperling JW, Miletti J, Schleck C, Cofield RH: Augmented glenoid component for bone deficiency in shoulder arthroplasty. *Clin Orthop Relat Res* 2008;466(3):579-583.

Rouleau DM, Kidder JF, Pons-Villanueva J, Dynamidis S, Defranco M, Walch G: Glenoid version: How to measure it? Validity of different methods in two-dimensional computed tomography scans. *J Shoulder Elbow Surg* 2010;19(8):1230-1237.

Sabesan V, Callanan M, Ho J, Iannotti JP: Clinical and radiographic outcomes of total shoulder arthroplasty with bone graft for osteoarthritis with severe glenoid bone loss. *J Bone Joint Surg Am* 2013;95(14):1290-1296.

Scalise JJ, Codsi MJ, Brems JJ, Iannotti JP: Inter-rater reliability of an arthritic glenoid morphology classification system. *J Shoulder Elbow Surg* 2008;17(4):575-577.

Shapiro TA, McGarry MH, Gupta R, Lee YS, Lee TQ: Biomechanical effects of glenoid retroversion in total shoulder arthroplasty. *J Shoulder Elbow Surg* 2007;16(3 suppl):S90-S95.

Singh JA, Sperling JW, Cofield RH: Revision surgery following total shoulder arthroplasty: Analysis of 2588 shoulders over three decades (1976 to 2008). *J Bone Joint Surg Br* 2011;93(11):1513-1517.

Steinmann SP, Cofield RH: Bone grafting for glenoid deficiency in total shoulder replacement. *J Shoulder Elbow Surg* 2000;9(5):361-367.

Walch G, Badet R, Boulahia A, Khoury A: Morphologic study of the glenoid in primary glenohumeral osteoarthritis. *J Arthroplasty* 1999;14(6):756-760.

Walch G, Moraga C, Young A, Castellanos-Rosas J: Results of anatomic nonconstrained prosthesis in primary osteoarthritis with biconcave glenoid. *J Shoulder Elbow Surg* 2012;21(11):1526-1533.

Young A, Walch G, Boileau P, et al: A multicentre study of the long-term results of using a flat-back polyethylene glenoid component in shoulder replacement for primary osteoarthritis. *J Bone Joint Surg Br* 2011;93(2):210-216.

 Video Reference

Dines DM, Dines JS: Video. *The Difficult Glenoid in Total Shoulder Arthroplasty: Reaming and Bone Grafting Techniques to Ensure Long-Term Stability.* New York, NY, 2015.

Chapter 38

Reverse Total Shoulder Arthroplasty for Rotator Cuff Tear Arthropathy

Richard J. Hawkins, MD

Jeffrey R. Backes, MD

Jared C. Bentley, MD

Michael J. Kissenberth, MD

 ## Introduction

The rotator cuff muscles provide a dynamic and balanced force couple to center the humeral head on the glenoid during all ranges of shoulder motion. This arrangement allows the deltoid and larger muscles to efficiently generate a rotary force to elevate and rotate the arm with power and direction. With a massive rotator cuff tear, the balanced axial and coronal force couples between the rotator cuff and deltoid are lost, and the deltoid loses the ability to generate effective elevation or rotational torque. Consequently, the deltoid pulls the humerus proximally, eventually resulting in anterior-superior glenohumeral instability and a pathologic articulation between the humeral head and acromion. Massive irreparable rotator cuff tear inciting the development of glenohumeral arthritis and eventual humeral head osteonecrosis was first described in 1983, and this phenomenon was termed rotator cuff tear arthropathy. In some instances, a massive irreparable rotator cuff tear can occur without glenohumeral arthritis; however, this chapter focuses on the classic description of rotator cuff tear arthropathy.

Patients with a massive rotator cuff tear and glenohumeral arthritis can have a variety of physical examination findings. Pain and functional weakness are typically the initial complaints. The supraspinatus, infraspinatus, and teres minor muscles should be tested individually using the Jobe test, external rotation resistance test, and hornblower sign test, respectively. An external rotation lag sign and a torn teres minor have been suggested as an indication for additional tendon transfers at the time of the index reverse shoulder arthroplasty. Although the authors of this chapter carefully evaluate the preoperative functional status of the posterior rotator cuff and inform patients that it can affect the functional outcome, noticeable improvement in active external rotation is consistently observed with the use of a prosthetic system with a lateralized offset design, and tendon transfers are rarely necessary to assist with postoperative external rotation.

Crepitus is often present as a result of glenohumeral and acromiohumeral arthritic changes. Anterior-superior escape of the humeral head may be evident on visual inspection and can be exacerbated with active attempts to elevate the arm. Without the inferior and compressive action of the rotator cuff, the deltoid is unopposed, and this imbalance can result in pseudoparalysis in shoulder elevation. Pseudoparalysis has been defined as the inability to actively elevate the arm in the presence of free passive range of motion, in the absence of a neurologic lesion. Although pseudoparalysis continues to be defined in the literature as the inability to elevate the arm higher than 90°, the authors of this chapter suggest that the term is more appropriately used in instances in which no active elevation is present, and attempts at shoulder elevation result only in a shoulder shrug and anterior-superior escape.

Dr. Hawkins or an immediate family member has received royalties from Össur; serves as a paid consultant to DJO; and serves as a board member, owner, officer, or committee member of the American Shoulder and Elbow Surgeons. Dr. Kissenberth or an immediate family member has received nonincome support (such as equipment or services), commercially derived honoraria, or other non–research-related funding (such as paid travel) from Arthrex, Arthrosurface, Breg, DJO, Greenville Health System, Neurotech, Pacira, and Smith & Nephew and serves as a board member, owner, officer, or committee member of the Hawkins Foundation. Neither of the following authors nor any immediate family member has received anything of value from or has stock or stock options held in a commercial company or institution related directly or indirectly to the subject of this chapter: Dr. Backes and Dr. Bentley.

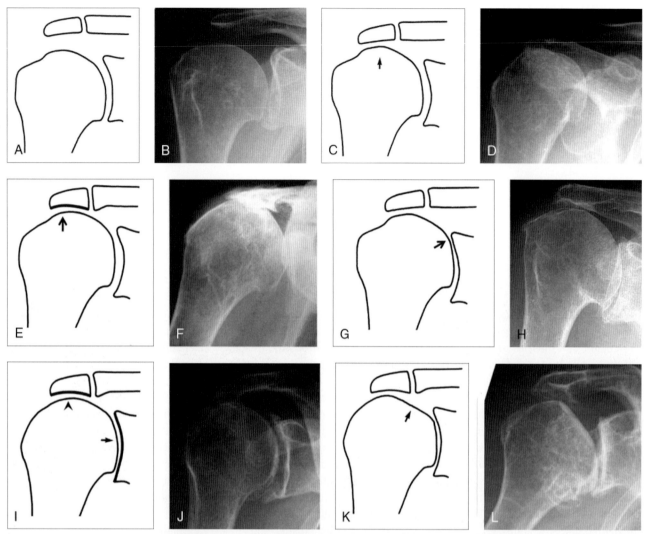

Figure 1 Illustrations (**A, C, E, G, I,** and **K**) and AP radiographs (**B, D, F, H, J,** and **L**) of a right shoulder demonstrate the Hamada classification of rotator cuff arthritis. **A** and **B,** Grade 1, acromiohumeral interval ≥6 mm. **C** and **D,** Grade 2, acromiohumeral interval (arrow) of ≤5 mm. **E** and **F,** Grade 3, acromiohumeral interval of ≤5 mm, and concave deformity (acetabularization) on the undersurface of the acromion (arrow). **G** and **H,** Grade 4A, glenohumeral arthritis without acetabularization. Note the narrowed glenohumeral joint space (arrow). **I** and **J,** Grade 4B, glenohumeral arthritis with acetabularization. Note the narrowed glenohumeral joint space (arrow, I) and acetabularization of the acromion (arrowhead, I). **K** and **L,** Grade 5, the arrow indicates collapse of the humeral head. (Reproduced with permission from Hamada K, Yamanaka K, Uchiyama Y, Mikasa T, Mikasa M: A radiographic classification of massive rotator cuff tear arthritis. *Clin Orthop Relat Res* 2011;469[9]:2452-2460.)

The Hamada radiographic classification of massive rotator cuff tears was proposed in 1990. This five-grade classification was developed to reflect the temporal evolutional radiographic changes that occur when two or more rotator cuff tendons are torn. Grade 1 is defined by the presence of an acromiohumeral interval greater than or equal to 6 mm (**Figure 1, A** and **B**). The acromiohumeral interval narrows to 5 mm or less in grade 2 (**Figure 1, C** and **D**). Acetabularization of the acromion (subacromial arthritis with a concave deformity of the undersurface of the acromion) in addition to acromiohumeral interval narrowing is classified as grade 3 (**Figure 1, E** and **F**). Glenohumeral joint narrowing is the hallmark feature of grade 4. Because massive rotator cuff tears with glenohumeral narrowing but without acromial acetabularization have been identified, Hamada grade 4 has been subdivided into grade 4A, glenohumeral arthritis without acromial acetabularization (**Figure 1, G** and **H**), and grade 4B, glenohumeral arthritis with acromial acetabularization (**Figure 1, I** and **J**). Grade 5 is characterized by humeral head collapse (**Figure 1, K** and **L**).

Four glenoid erosion patterns have been identified on the basis of radiographic appearance. In type E0, the

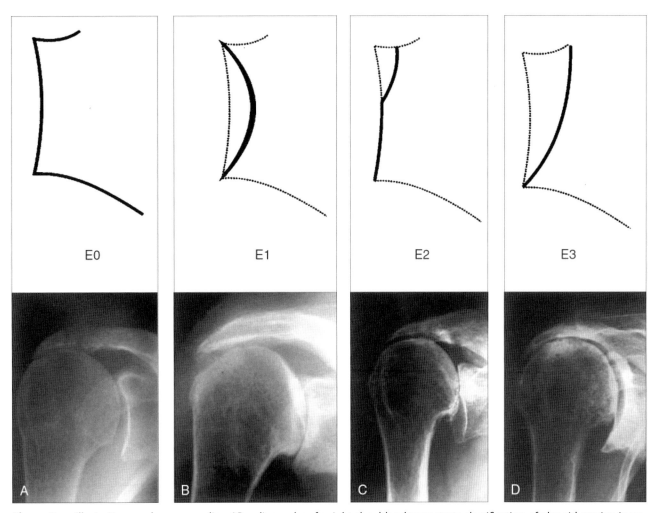

Figure 2   Illustrations and corresponding AP radiographs of a right shoulder demonstrate classification of glenoid erosion in patients with osteoarthritis and massive rupture of the rotator cuff. **A,** In type E0, the head of the humerus migrates upward without glenoid erosion. **B,** Type E1 is defined by concentric glenoid erosion. **C,** Type E2 has superior glenoid erosion. **D,** In type E3, erosion extends to the inferior part of the glenoid. (Reproduced with permission from Sireaux F, Favard L, Oudet D, Huquet D, Walch G, Molé D: Grammont inverted total shoulder arthroplasty in the treatment of glenohumeral osteoarthritis with massive rupture of the cuff: Results of a multicentre study of 80 shoulders. *J Bone Joint Surg Br* 2004;86[3]:388-395.)

humeral head migrates upward without glenoid erosion. Type E1 is defined by concentric erosion of the glenoid. Type E2 has superior glenoid erosion, and in type E3, the erosion extends to the inferior part of the glenoid (**Figure 2**).

Routine radiographs can reveal cuff tear arthropathy, decreased acromiohumeral interval, decreased glenohumeral joint space, destruction of the humeral head, and glenoid erosion. MRI and CT demonstrate the extent of rotator cuff involvement and any muscle atrophy and fatty infiltration. The degree of fatty infiltration of the teres minor has been shown to directly affect outcome scores and external rotation following reverse total shoulder arthroplasty (RTSA). In one study, fatty infiltration of the teres minor classified as Goutallier grade 3 or 4 was associated with an average net loss of 7° of external rotation, compared with a gain of 9° of external rotation with grade 0, 1, or 2 fatty infiltration of the teres minor. In a separate study, the mean active external rotation was 15° in patients with less than 50% fatty infiltration of the teres minor, compared with 0° in those with more than 50% fatty infiltration. Osseous wear of the glenoid also is better evaluated on advanced imaging modalities. Particular attention should be given to the degree of superior wear of the glenoid because it directly affects the preparation of the glenoid during the procedure.

Case Presentation

A 70-year-old woman presents with pain and diminished function that

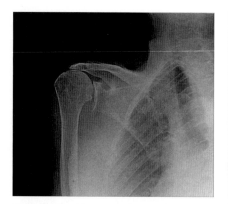

Figure 3 Plain AP radiograph of a right shoulder demonstrates a reduced acromiohumeral interval of less than 2 mm.

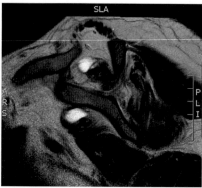

Figure 4 Sagittal T1-weighted MRI of a left shoulder demonstrates fatty degeneration of the supraspinatus and infraspinatus. Note the hypertrophied teres minor.

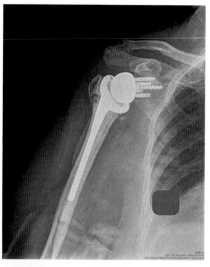

Figure 5 Postoperative AP radiograph of a right shoulder demonstrates reverse total shoulder arthroplasty using a prosthetic system with a 10-mm laterally offset glenoid center of rotation.

have progressively worsened over the past 2 years. A trial of nonsurgical management consisting of physical therapy, NSAIDs, and corticosteroid injections has failed.

Physical examination demonstrates 80° of active forward elevation and 160° of passive forward elevation. The patient has 15° of external rotation without a lag sign or hornblower sign. Active internal rotation is to T-10. The belly-press test result is negative. Plain AP radiographs demonstrate an acromiohumeral interval of less than 2 mm (**Figure 3**). In addition, early collapse of the anterior-superior humeral head is observed. Axial radiographs demonstrate degenerative changes of the glenohumeral joint. MRI demonstrates a massive 5-cm rotator cuff tear with retraction. A positive tangent sign indicates substantial supraspinatus atrophy. Goutallier grade 3 and grade 2 changes are present in the supraspinatus and infraspinatus, respectively. The teres minor is intact without any fatty changes (**Figure 4**).

RTSA is performed with a prosthetic system that has a 10-mm laterally offset glenoid center of rotation (**Figure 5**). At the 2-year follow-up examination, the patient demonstrates 130° of painless, active forward elevation. External rotation has improved to 45°, and internal rotation to T-10 remains stable.

 ## Indications

Originally designed for the management of rotator cuff tear arthropathy, the RTSA prosthesis treats the altered kinematics resulting from rotator cuff deficiency. The reverse ball-and-socket orientation shifts the center of rotation medially and the humerus distally, improving the mechanical advantage of the deltoid and decreasing the amount of force required for shoulder abduction and elevation. The capability of RTSA to restore function to the patient who has a massive irreparable rotator cuff tear with glenohumeral arthritis and pseudoparalysis has revolutionized shoulder surgery. With improved implant designs, the indications for reverse arthroplasty have expanded; nevertheless, the success of this procedure is predicated on appropriate indications and careful patient selection. Clinical evidence suggests that the results deteriorate over time even without radiographic evidence of prosthetic failure; therefore, reverse arthroplasty should be used cautiously in younger and/or high-demand patients.

Rotator cuff tear arthropathy was the original indication and remains a common indication for reverse shoulder arthroplasty. The surgical indications have expanded to include failed hemiarthroplasty or failed total shoulder arthroplasty, proximal humerus fractures, proximal humerus nonunion or malunion, severe bone loss, fixed shoulder dislocation, and irreparable rotator cuff tear without glenohumeral arthritis. Contraindications to reverse shoulder arthroplasty include active infection, axillary nerve palsy, deltoid insufficiency, insufficient bone stock, or severe neurologic deficiencies.

 ## Controversies, Alternative Approaches, and Results

Alternative treatment options for patients with irreparable rotator cuff tears associated with glenohumeral joint osteoarthritis have had varied results. Nonsurgical treatment should be attempted first and should include activity modification, oral analgesics, anti-inflammatory medications, corticosteroid injections, and fluid aspiration. Although some patients are able to tolerate the pain and maintain some shoulder function through the deltoid, some patients continue to have pain and diminished function. Arthroscopic débridement with biceps tenotomy can provide good results in patients with massive rotator cuff tears, but results are greatly inferior in patients with rotator cuff tear arthropathy. Fusion and resection have been attempted with largely disappointing results and are rarely performed except as a salvage procedure. Constrained total shoulder arthroplasty for rotator cuff tear arthropathy has resulted in complication rates up to 87% from implant loosening. Results of conventional total shoulder arthroplasty also have been poor; the authors of one study reported superior humeral head displacement, eccentric loading of the glenoid polyethylene implant (the "rocking horse" phenomenon), and a 50% rate of glenoid loosening. As a result, total shoulder arthroplasty is no longer considered an option for the management of a massive irreparable rotator cuff tear with arthritis. Although hemiarthroplasty avoids the complications of glenoid loosening and has been shown to provide pain relief and acceptable shoulder motion, it is associated with concerns of glenoid and acromion resorption, continued anterior-superior instability, and limited improvements in shoulder motion. As such, reverse shoulder arthroplasty has become the standard for surgical management of the rotator cuff–insufficient arthritic shoulder in appropriately selected patients.

Since its introduction in the late 1970s, the reverse shoulder arthroplasty prosthesis has undergone substantial design modifications. In 1987, the Grammont design medialized the center of glenohumeral rotation to the glenoid to reduce the torque on the glenoid bone-implant interface that affected early designs. The center of rotation, and subsequently the humerus, also was moved distally, maximizing the length and tension of the deltoid to increase its capability to move the shoulder and provide added stability. This design innovation was paramount in allowing the RTSA prosthesis to be FDA approved in 2003. Reverse shoulder arthroplasty is now widely used in the management of rotator cuff tear arthropathy. With major complication rates as high as 26% and limited data on long-term functional outcome and implant longevity, investigation and research into the most effective reverse arthroplasty design continues. With new-generation designs and increased experience with implantation, complication rates have decreased but remain between 10% and 30%, including infection in 2% to 4% of patients, instability (dislocation) in 2% to 8%, baseplate failure in 1% to 3%, and acromial fracture in 1% to 4%. The authors of this chapter use the Reverse Shoulder Prosthesis (DJO) because it has a lateralized center of rotation and allows excellent baseplate fixation using a 6.5-mm central locking screw and four 5.5-mm peripheral locking screws. On the basis of 10 years of experience with this prosthesis, the authors of this chapter prefer a lateralized system because of its biomechanical benefits, particularly in offering more consistent improvement of external rotation.

Much debate exists on the humeral socket version, and whether neutral or up to 40° of retroversion is most appropriate. Most systems provide a version rod and allow adjustment within that range. Preclinical investigations have demonstrated that increased retroversion allows better external shoulder rotation at the expense of internal rotation, particularly with the shoulder adducted. However, the authors of a different biomechanical study demonstrated that neutral version does not affect external rotation in the abducted position, which is used for activities such as eating, using a phone, and washing hair. The authors of this chapter prefer 30° of retroversion because it provides good glenoid baseplate coaptation at functional range of motion and allows for an appropriate arc of motion prior to impingement. Problems with inferior impingement or loss of the necessary internal rotation required to position the hand in front of or behind the body for personal hygiene have not been encountered, especially with the use of a lateralized offset glenosphere. However, if a Grammont-style prosthesis with a more medial center of rotation is used, the authors of this chapter recommend retroversion of 10° to 20°. The use of 30° retroversion with a medialized system may result in increased inferior impingement, whereas a neutral resection often misses too much articular surface because it differs too much from the native anatomy, negatively affecting the length-tension relationship of the remaining posterior cuff or teres minor.

Inferior baseplate inclination and inferior placement of the glenoid implant on the glenoid face are recommended to reduce the incidence of scapular notching, which most likely occurs from mechanical impingement of the medial aspect of the humeral implant and the lateral aspect of the scapular neck just inferior to the glenoid. Scapular notching is a particular concern with Grammont-style prostheses. Although the clinical implications of scapular notching are unclear, concerns exist regarding its effect on long-term range of motion, osteolysis, implant loosening, and pain. The authors of one study reported a 96% rate of scapular notching; in that study, 54% of the patients had grade 1 or 2 notching (grade 1a notching consists of reactive bone along the inferior scapular pillar, grade 1b notching is confined to the inferior pillar, and grade 2 notching involves an inferior screw), whereas 46% had grade 3 or 4 notching (grade 3 consists of notching beyond an inferior screw, and grade 4 consists of notching behind the baseplate; **Figure 6**). The authors of a different study using a lateralized center reverse shoulder arthroplasty prosthesis reported no

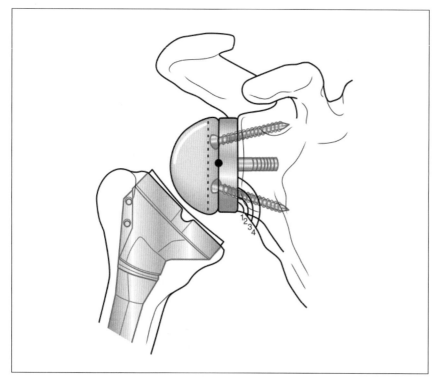

Figure 6 Illustration shows the Nerot-Sirveaux grading system for postoperative scapular notching after reverse total shoulder arthroplasty. Grade 1, defect confined to the inferior pillar of the scapular neck; grade 2, defect in contact with the inferior screw; grade 3, defect above the inferior screw; grade 4, defect extends under the baseplate.

instances of grade 3 or 4 scapular notching. Biomechanical models have demonstrated a lateralized center of rotation, a more varus neck-shaft angle (135° instead of 155°), inferior inclination of the baseplate/glenosphere, and a lowered position of the glenosphere on the glenoid, all reducing scapular notching.

Outcome studies in RTSA have demonstrated that approximately 110° to 150° of active forward flexion is achieved postoperatively. In contrast to shoulder elevation, improvement in shoulder external rotation has been varied and often minimal, especially with Grammont-style medialized implant designs (**Table 1**). The authors of this chapter prefer the DJO reverse shoulder arthroplasty system because it has different metallic glenosphere options that can lateralize the center of rotation up to 10 mm. In the experience of the authors of this chapter, this system has resulted

in more consistent improvement of external rotation (net gain of approximately 30° postoperatively) compared with initial results of a medialized system. The literature echoes those findings, with lateralized systems resulting in an average improvement in American Shoulder and Elbow Surgeons scores of 30 to 40 points, an average improvement in forward flexion of 50°, and an average improvement in external rotation of 30° (**Table 1**). The authors of one study reported improvement of external rotation from 12° preoperatively to 41° postoperatively using a reverse shoulder arthroplasty prosthesis in which the center of rotation was shifted laterally to the bony glenoid-implant interface. In a different study, researchers documented final postoperative external rotation of 51° using the DJO reverse shoulder arthroplasty prosthesis. Other researchers, in a study in which autograft bone

was used to increase the offset and lateralize the glenoid with the use of the Aequalis Bony Increased Offset Reverse Shoulder Arthroplasty prosthesis (BIO-RSA; Tornier), reported mean postoperative external rotation of 23°, a gain of 10° from the mean preoperative measurement. This finding demonstrated improvement from an earlier study of a medialized system, in which the mean final postoperative external rotation was only 14°. In contrast to implant designs in which the center of rotation is lateralized by means of the metallic glenosphere shape, in the BIO-RSA study the prosthesis was lateralized with the use of bone graft harvested from the humeral head. In this technique, the prosthesis as well as the center of rotation is shifted laterally, but the newly established center of rotation is set on the interface between the implant and the autografted extended glenoid (**Figure 7**).

Three additional studies demonstrated no improvement in external rotation postoperatively using implant designs with the center of rotation at the glenoid bone-implant interface. One of these studies demonstrated a net loss of external rotation (17° preoperatively to 12° postoperatively) with the use of the Delta III (DePuy) reverse shoulder arthroplasty prosthesis in 58 patients.

A lateralized center of rotation is theorized to reduce laxity of the external rotators and posterior deltoid, reduce prosthesis-bone impingement, and improve the cosmetic appearance of the shoulder contour. The authors of a three-dimensional CT cadaver model reported that a lateralized center of rotation in reverse shoulder arthroplasty maintained the rotational moment arms and muscle pretension length of the subscapularis and teres minor. In contrast, a similar study of a Grammont-style medialized prosthesis demonstrated decreases in the rotational moment arms of up to 36% in the subscapularis and 25% in the teres minor. These preclinical findings offer a possible explanation

Table 1 Results of Reverse Total Shoulder Arthroplasty to Manage Cuff Tear Arthropathy

Authors	Journal (Year)	Center of Rotation	Outcomes[a]	Comments
Sirveaux et al	*J Bone Joint Surg Br* (2004)	Medial	FF improved from 73° to 138° ER improved from 3° to 11° Constant score improved from 23 to 66	80 shoulders treated Status of the teres minor significantly affected the Constant score (67 if intact vs 58 if torn; *P* < 0.01) 3.8% revision rate Glenoid loosening was the most common complication, occurring in 15%
Werner et al	*J Bone Joint Surg Am* (2005)	Medial	FF improved from 42° to 100° ER decreased from 17° to 12° Constant score improved from 29 to 64	58 shoulders treated Significant negative correlation between previous operations and final Constant score (72 primary vs 58 revision; *P* < 0.01) 33% reoperation rate
Boileau et al	*J Shoulder Elbow Surg* (2006)	Medial	FF improved from 53° to 123° ER improved from 9° to 14° Constant score improved from 18 to 66	21 shoulders Results were better in patients treated for cuff tear arthropathy than in patients treated for fracture sequelae or who underwent revision arthroplasty 5% reoperation rate if the diagnosis was rotator cuff tear arthritis
Frankle et al	*J Bone Joint Surg Am* (2006)	Lateral	FF improved from 55° to 105° ER improved from 12° to 41°	68% of patients rated their outcome as good or excellent 12% revision rate
Wall et al	*J Bone Joint Surg Am* (2007)	Medial	FF improved from 76° to 142° ER improved from 5° to 7° Constant score improved from 21 to 65	74 shoulders Patients treated with primary RTSA for rotator cuff arthropathy had better functional and clinical outcomes compared with RTSA for revision arthroplasty or posttraumatic arthritis 13.3% complication rate in primary procedures
Cuff et al	*J Bone Joint Surg Am* (2008)	Lateral	FF improved from 74° to 130° ER improved from 20° to 36°	37 shoulders Substantial improvement in external rotation was achieved even though no patient underwent latissimus transfer 5.3% reoperation rate
Mulieri et al	*J Bone Joint Surg Am* (2010)	Lateral	FF improved from 53° to 134° ER improved from 27° to 51°	72 shoulders Patients with preserved motion (>90° of elevation) preoperatively had a higher complication rate compared with patients in whom preoperative elevation was <90° 90.7% survival at 52 mo
Boileau et al	*Clin Orthop Relat Res* (2011)	Lateral (BIO-RSA)	FF improved from 86° to 146° ER improved from 13° to 23° Constant score improved from 31 to 67	42 shoulders Grafting to the glenoid surface at the time of baseplate implantation resulted in excellent incorporation with minimal complications No revisions/instability or glenoid loosening at mean 28-mo follow-up)

BIO-RSA = bony increased-offset reverse shoulder arthroplasty prosthesis, ER = external rotation, FF = forward flexion, RTSA = reverse total shoulder arthroplasty.

[a] Mean values.

of the clinically improved rotation seen with the use of systems having a lateralized center of rotation. However, it is important to note both lateralized and medialized systems still create a center of rotation medial to that of the native anatomy. More anatomic nomenclature for lateralized RTSA designs would technically be less medialized (**Figure 8**).

Table 1 Results of Reverse Total Shoulder Arthroplasty to Manage Cuff Tear Arthropathy (*continued*)

Authors	Journal (Year)	Center of Rotation	Outcomes[a]	Comments
Nolan et al	*Clin Orthop Relat Res* (2011)	Medial	FF improved from 61° to 121° ER improved from 14° to 15° Constant score improved from 28 to 62	71 shoulders A two-fold increase in instability was noted in patients with preoperative subscapularis failure 23% overall complication rate No patients required reoperation
Valenti et al	*Clin Orthop Relat Res* (2011)	Lateral	FF improved from 65° to 126° ER improved from 15° to 30° Constant score improved from 24 to 59	76 shoulders ER with the elbow at the side improved 15° and abduction improved 30° at 90° without latissimus transfer 13.1% revision rate
Middleton et al	*Bone Joint J* (2014)	Lateral	FF improved from 47° to 79° ER improved from 13° to 26°	62 shoulders The implant used was a fully constrained prosthesis with a monoblock baseplate design 13.4% revision rate 20.6% reoperation rate

BIO-RSA = bony increased-offset reverse shoulder arthroplasty prosthesis, ER = external rotation, FF = forward flexion, RTSA = reverse total shoulder arthroplasty.

[a] Mean values.

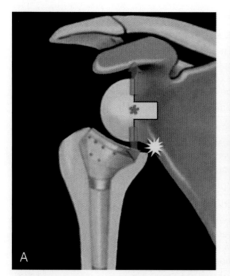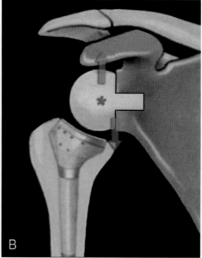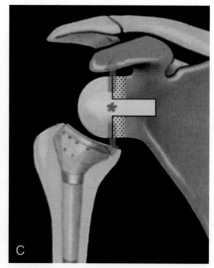

Figure 7   Diagrams of right shoulders show medialization versus lateralization in reverse shoulder arthroplasty (RSA). **A,** Medialized (Grammont) RSA (hemisphere) places the center of rotation(*) at the bone-prosthesis interface. Deltoid force applied to the center of rotation does not develop any torque because there is no lever arm; however, there is a risk of scapular notching (yellow star). **B,** Metallic lateralized RSA (two-thirds of a sphere) reduces the risk of scapular notching but creates a lever arm because a lateralized center of rotation produces shear forces detrimental to glenoid fixation. **C,** Bony increased-offset RSA (BIO-RSA) reduces the risk of scapular notching due to lateralization while maximizing glenoid fixation because the center of rotation remains at the bone-prosthesis interface and there is no lever arm. Arrows = forces on the glenoid component. (Reproduced with permission from Boileau P, Moineau G, Roussanne Y, O'Shea K: Bony increased-offset reversed shoulder arthroplasty: Minimizing scapular impingement while maximizing glenoid fixation. *Clin Orthop Relat Res* 2011;469[9]:2558-2567.)

For patients undergoing RTSA in whom severe preoperative external rotation deficits are present, concomitant latissimus dorsi and teres major transfers are often recommended. Specifically, in the presence of teres minor dysfunction as demonstrated by an external rotation lag sign, a hornblower sign, and fatty degeneration of the teres minor (Goutallier grade 2 or higher), many studies have reported that recovery of external rotation is not possible with

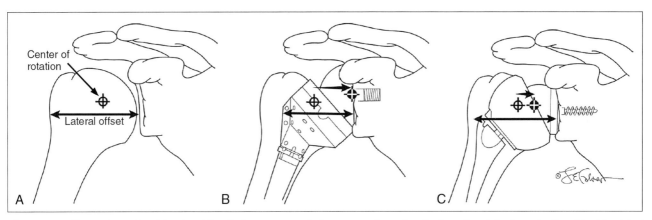

Figure 8 Illustrations of a right shoulder. **A,** Appearance of the center of rotation (bullseye) and the lateral offset (double-sided arrow). **B,** A Grammont-style implant, which causes the center of rotation and lateral offset to shift medially with respect to the anatomic shoulder. **C,** A lateralized design, which demonstrates how the device causes the center of rotation and lateral offset to shift medially with respect to the anatomic shoulder but to a smaller degree than the Grammont style. (Reproduced with permission from Frankle M, Siegal S, Pupello D, Saleem A, Mighell M, Vasey M: The reverse shoulder prosthesis for glenohumeral arthritis associated with severe rotator cuff deficiency: A minimum two-year follow-up study of sixty patients. *J Bone Joint Surg Am* 2005;87[8]:1697-1705.)

RTSA in isolation. Although external rotation motion after RTSA is inferior in the presence of advanced teres minor deficits, the authors of this chapter routinely observe external rotation gains of as much as 30° with the use of a lateralized system. A modified L'Episcopo or latissimus transfer is rarely performed in conjunction with RTSA.

Grammont-style medialized designs and more lateralized RTSA systems also shift the center of rotation distally, thereby increasing the mechanical advantage of the deltoid and reducing the force required for shoulder abduction and elevation. In addition, any inferior tilt and/or inferior position of the glenoid baseplate affects the shoulder mechanics after RTSA. In one biomechanical study, inferior placement of the glenosphere had a more substantial effect on the mechanical advantage of the deltoid than did medialization of the glenosphere. Superior placement of the glenosphere increases the glenohumeral joint reaction forces by 10% and increases the adduction deficit by 15° relative to the recommended inferior position. The authors of a biomechanical study demonstrated that tilting the glenosphere 15° inferiorly in the scapular plane created the least

amount of tensile force at the baseplate-glenoid interface and produced the most uniform compressive force. Additional benefits of an inferiorly tilted glenosphere include increased stability through improved deltoid tension and, as noted previously, reduced scapular notching. A study at the institution of the authors of this chapter examined the radiographs of more than 130 patients who underwent RTSA and demonstrated that although implantation with 15° of inferior tilt was attempted, the average actual change in inclination was 8.5°, roughly one-half of the intended change that should be produced by the instrumentation guide. Static superior migration of the humeral head can result in eccentric glenoid wear and superior erosion of the osseous glenoid in patients with massive rotator cuff tears. If this bone loss is not managed appropriately and inclination guides are blindly followed, the glenoid component may be inadvertently implanted with superior tilt, risking glenoid failure. As such, critical analysis of preoperative radiographs is required, and in patients with substantial eccentric glenoid wear, further evaluation with CT is recommended to assist in planning for baseplate implantation.

Glenoid fixation also affects the results of reverse shoulder arthroplasty. In a biomechanical study of glenoid fixation in reverse shoulder arthroplasty, the use of 5.0-mm peripheral locking screws was found to reduce micromotion at the baseplate-bone interface to less than 150 μm, allowing for osseous ingrowth. This ingrowth is particularly important when a system with a less medialized center of rotation is used because the lateral offset of the center of rotation increases the torque force at the baseplate-glenoid bone interface. One study demonstrated that lateralization of only 6 mm increased joint reaction force by 8% relative to standard medial designs. Early clinical reports reflect this increased shear force at the baseplate, with a 12% rate of early mechanical failure reported for a design with a lateralized center of rotation and 3.5-mm peripheral screws for baseplate fixation. A simple modification of that technique to incorporate 5.0-mm peripheral locking screws for the baseplate eliminated any evidence of mechanical failure at the baseplate. This finding has been further supported by a study showing that with modern fixation techniques, the shear force and micromotion at the glenoid-baseplate interface is inconsequential, even when the center of rotation is placed 10 mm lateral to the glenoid surface. The authors of this chapter use a 6.5-mm central cancellous screw with four 5.0-mm peripheral locking screws. Additionally, researchers have suggested that at least 15 mm of bone stock medial to the centering line of the glenoid is necessary to obtain adequate purchase of the central screw. Some authors have suggested orienting the drill slightly more posteriorly in patients with substantial glenoid bone loss to access the thick column of bone present at the junction of the scapular spine and the scapular body. In our experience, however, the central baseplate screw usually engages the anterior glenoid cortex.

Depending on the prosthetic system, the humeral socket-shaft angle can vary from 130° to 155°. The more valgus designs increase the deltoid tension by lengthening the acromiohumeral distance. Achieving an acromion-to-greater tuberosity distance of 38 mm has been shown to have a 90% positive predictive value of obtaining 135° of active forward elevation. Inferior placement and inferior tilt of the glenosphere also substantially lengthen the acromiohumeral distance. The system preferred by the authors of this chapter uses a 135° humeral socket-shaft angle, which more closely approximates the native shoulder anatomy. A less valgus angle also helps reduce the incidence of scapular notching.

The authors of this chapter do not routinely repair the subscapularis because, in their experience, no difference in complication rates or dislocation has been found between reverse arthroplasty patients with and without subscapularis repair. However, the authors of one published study found higher rates of implant instability with a compromised subscapularis. The use of a lateralized offset glenoid, discussed elsewhere in this chapter, often does not allow a subscapularis repair during closure; in the

experience of the authors of this chapter, the lack of subscapularis repair has had no effect on later instability. Furthermore, one theory suggests that repair of the subscapularis could actually impede the deltoid from initiating abduction. The authors of one study found that after reverse shoulder arthroplasty, the middle and inferior regions of the subscapularis function as adductors. Although this scenario may generate a compression force at the joint surface and improve implant stability, it also could limit the abduction force of the deltoid.

Video 38.1 Cuff Tear Arthropathy Reverse Shoulder Arthroplasty: Steps to Get it Right. Richard J. Hawkins, MD; Jeffrey R. Backes, MD; Jared C. Bentley, MD; Michael J. Kissenberth, MD (15 min)

Technical Keys to Success

Setup/Exposure

- The patient is positioned in the upright beach-chair position with the arm draped free and the head firmly secured.
- Two small folded towels are placed behind the scapula. The torso and the affected arm must be positioned sufficiently off the table to allow for maximal adduction and extension of the shoulder to allow the surgeon access to both the humerus and the glenoid.
- Preoperative antibiotics, typically a first-generation cephalosporin, are administered 30 minutes before incision.

Procedure

- The authors of this chapter perform reverse shoulder arthroplasty via the deltopectoral approach. The anterior superior approach can be

used; however, violation of the deltoid, inadequate glenoid exposure, and the inability to extend the approach distally are concerns.
- The topographic anatomy, particularly the coracoid process, is identified, and a standard deltopectoral incision is made. The length of the incision is typically 8 to 13 cm, depending on the size of the patient.
- The cephalic vein is located in the interval between the deltoid and the pectoralis major. A fat stripe often covers the cephalic vein and can aid in its identification.
- If the surgeon has difficulty identifying the cephalic vein or the correct plane within the deltopectoral interval, dissection should start proximally because a small triangular area devoid of muscle tissue is present between the proximal aspects of the deltoid and the pectoralis major.
- The easily palpable coracoid serves as a landmark and can further aid in correct development of the intermuscular dissection.
- The cephalic vein can be retracted medially or laterally. Although most branches of the cephalic vein are laterally based off the deltoid, the authors of this chapter prefer to take the vein medially because deltoid retraction often disrupts the vein during the procedure if the vein is retracted laterally.
- The authors of this chapter do not routinely release the pectoralis major tendon inferiorly, but the superior 1 cm of its insertion can be released to enhance visualization of the inferior aspect of the subscapularis and the anterior humeral circumflex vessels.
- The arm is moved into abduction to allow development of the subdeltoid space using a finger or a Cobb elevator, and a deltoid retractor is placed.
- With the patient's arm placed in

slight external rotation, the coracoacromial ligament is visualized and sectioned just lateral to its insertion on the coracoid.

- With the patient's arm maintained in external rotation, the shoulder is moved into neutral adduction and a space is created superior to the coracoid process using a finger, a Cobb elevator, or occasionally Mayo scissors. This technique allows a Hohmann retractor to be placed behind the base of the coracoid to provide proximal retraction.

- The conjoint tendon attaches just medial to the coracoacromial ligament on the coracoid. This tendon is retracted medially with an anterior glenoid retractor or a Richardson retractor to expose the subscapularis.

- If the subscapularis is intact, it is transected transtendinously 1.5 cm medial to the biceps. The subscapularis tendon and underlying capsule are incised as one layer.

- The medial border is tagged with two No. 2 sutures, primarily for traction. The authors of this chapter do not routinely repair the subscapularis tendon at the time of closure. When a 10-mm offset glenoid is used, subscapularis repair is often not feasible with the arm in neutral position. When a glenoid with less than 10 mm offset is used, the authors of this chapter consider subscapularis repair; however, in the authors' experience, repair has had no influence on complication or dislocation rates.

- With the arm in forward flexion and neutral rotation and after the axillary nerve is palpated, a circumferential release of the subscapularis and capsule is performed.

- The anterior humeral circumflex vessels are cauterized inferiorly.

- The humeral head is atraumatically dislocated with gentle extension and external rotation of the arm.

- A Darrach retractor is placed medial to the humeral head against the glenoid and is used as a "shoehorn" to dislocate the humeral head while the amount of external rotation and extension is progressively increased. A Hohmann retractor may be positioned superiorly to assist with this maneuver.

- The intra-articular portion of the biceps is released, and a soft-tissue biceps tenodesis is performed with No. 2 polyethylene sutures at the level of the pectoralis major tendon.

- The capsular tissue around the humeral neck is completely released, and any osteophytes present at the neck are removed. The authors of this chapter often use a combination of osteotomes and rongeurs to remove osteophytes to clearly define the head-neck juncture and, more importantly, to prevent impingement between the osteophytes and scapula.

- The humeral neck cut is made in 30° of retroversion using the forearm as a reference. The ideal humeral socket version is greatly debated. The authors of this chapter prefer 30° of retroversion because it provides good glenoid baseplate coaptation and facilitates an appropriate arc of motion. However, if a Grammont-style prosthesis with a more medial center of rotation is used, the authors of this chapter recommend retroversion of 10° to 20°. Less humeral head is resected than would be resected in a standard arthroplasty, and care should be taken to preserve as much of the existing posterior rotator cuff as possible. As noted previously, the status of the remaining posterior rotator cuff has been shown to affect outcomes in reverse shoulder arthroplasty, and in the authors' experience, an intact posterior rotator cuff (teres minor) results in superior postoperative motion.

- After the humeral neck cut is made, a handheld canal finder and sequential reamers are used to prepare the humeral canal. The authors of this chapter prefer to use powered reamers because they provide better tactile feedback for chatter and allow more control and efficiency than hand reamers.

- Humeral broaches are inserted sequentially until a tight fit is achieved. It is important to seat the broach below the level of the osteotomy.

- The humeral broach is left in place until the final glenoid implant is placed. Final preparation of the proximal humerus with metaphyseal reamers is completed only after the glenoid is implanted. This sequence is critical because it maintains adequate humeral bone stock to support retraction during glenoid preparation. If the metaphyseal reamers are used first, the weak shell of bone in the proximal humerus can fracture and be crushed during subsequent glenoid exposure.

- Obtaining adequate glenoid exposure is paramount during reverse shoulder arthroplasty and often is the most challenging part of the procedure. An appropriate proximal humerus release to allow for retraction of the humerus (with the humeral broach in place) is a critical step in obtaining glenoid exposure. Typically, an aggressive 360° subperiosteal periglenoid capsular release is performed using a Darrach retractor posteriorly and a glenoid retractor anteriorly.

- A Cobb elevator and a knife are used to remove the superior labrum, and a Hohmann retractor is placed at the superior aspect of the glenoid.

- A finger is placed inferiorly to protect the axillary nerve while electrocautery is used to remove the remaining labrum and inferior capsule.

- After satisfactory visualization is achieved, the center hole is drilled with a 2.0-mm drill. Placement of the glenoid in an inferiorly tilted position is key to this technique. The authors of this chapter often place the guide freehand before using the 6.5-mm tap in patients with advanced superior glenoid wear.

- In patients with mild to moderate superior bone loss, inferior reaming alone can correct glenoid orientation. The appropriate eccentric reaming of the inferior glenoid often creates a rim of bone inferiorly, which can easily be removed with a rongeur, and a small area of unreamed glenoid superiorly, which can later be prepared with small drill holes if necessary.

- In patients with severe superior glenoid bony wear, superior bone grafting or augmentation may be necessary to reposition the glenoid to an inferiorly directed, or at least neutral, position. Often, the superior baseplate does not sit flush with the superior glenoid. In fact, this situation may be a visual clue that the appropriate amount of inferior tilt has been established.

- In addition to inferior tilt of the baseplate, inferior positioning of the baseplate on the glenoid is important. It is therefore critical to obtain a 360° view of the glenoid before setting the initial drill position so that both the tilt and the positioning of the baseplate can be correctly determined.

- To aid in sagittal plane alignment, the surgeon can use a finger to replace the anterior glenoid retractor and serve as a guide to ensure correct trajectory in that plane.

- A 6.5-mm tap is used to enlarge the pilot drill hole, and cannulated reamers are then used sequentially. Although inferior tilt is important, the surgeon should take care not to aggressively ream through cancellous bone because maintaining bone stock in this area is paramount. The surgeon should ream as little bone as possible and should attempt to remove only the cartilage and subchondral surface. Bone grafting is considered for severely deficient glenoids as noted on preoperative imaging, particularly in patients in whom superior attritional wear limits baseplate surface contact to 50% or less, prepared at appropriate inferior tilt. Augmented baseplates can be used in shoulders in which attritional wear compromises baseplate fixation and position.

- A fixed-angle glenoid baseplate is affixed. The authors of this chapter use a 6.5-mm central cancellous screw with four 5.0-mm peripheral locking screws.

- Bicortical fixation is attempted with each peripheral screw. If good fixation is not achieved when the central 6.5-mm screw is inserted, the drill is redirected and the step is repeated. Obviously, the number of attempts must be minimized.

- If the purchase of the central screw is less than ideal, the surgeon may consider, with hesitation, relying on the four peripheral screws. In the rare procedure in which no glenoid fixation can be achieved, reverse arthroplasty should be abandoned.

- Glenosphere selection is based on the size of the patient, the quality of glenoid bone, the degree of soft-tissue contracture, and the expected degree of instability. The Reverse Shoulder Prosthesis system preferred by the authors of this chapter has the following glenosphere options: 32-mm neutral offset (center of rotation lateralized 10 mm from glenoid), 32 mm with −4-mm offset (6-mm lateralized center of rotation), 36-mm neutral offset (6-mm lateralized center of rotation), 36 mm with −4-mm offset (2-mm lateralized center of rotation), 40-mm neutral offset (4-mm lateralized center of rotation), and 40 mm with −4-mm offset (center of rotation at glenoid interface). In routine procedures, the authors of this chapter prefer to use a constrained, 32-mm neutral-offset glenosphere, which maximizes the distance between the glenoid bone and the center of rotation of the glenosphere.

- The glenosphere is placed in the baseplate using a Morse taper. A 3.5-mm retaining screw is used for added security to reduce the risk of component dissociation.

- With the final glenosphere in place, attention is returned to the humerus. The previously mentioned metaphyseal reamers are used, and a trial humeral socket is chosen on the basis of the preferred soft-tissue tension, glenohumeral range of motion, and glenohumeral joint stability. The combination of glenosphere size and humeral socket polyethylene size is determined subjectively and has a substantial effect on the stability of the prosthesis.

- After the polyethylene trial is inserted, the glenohumeral joint is reduced. This reduction should require some force to accomplish and is aided by neuromuscular paralysis from the anesthesia. Gradually flexing the arm while applying distal traction, often with a bone hook, assists in reduction.

- After the glenohumeral joint is reduced, minimal (less than 2 mm) shucking should occur between the glenosphere and the humeral socket with inferior translation.

- The arm should be moved through a range of motion to assess two aspects: First, stability must be assessed in adduction, in internal and external rotation, and in extension, the position with the highest risk of instability. Second, with the arm in forward flexion, the surgeon should assess the impaction of the greater tuberosity and the implants on the acromion. According to one theory, acromial stress fractures following reverse shoulder arthroplasty are secondary to repetitive impingement in this manner. Some researchers have suggested assessing the tautness of the deltoid and conjoint tendon to evaluate appropriate tensioning; however, the authors of this chapter have not found this method to be reliable.

- After the appropriate humeral socket size is determined, the shoulder is dislocated by using traction and extension. This dislocation should be difficult. The authors of this chapter often use a push-pull method to dislocate the prosthesis, simultaneously using a bone hook to pull the prosthesis and a Cobb elevator to push it inferiorly.

- The humeral broach is removed, and the final humeral implant is placed.

- Standard humeral implants in reverse arthroplasty have required the use of cement for adequate fixation. Newer prosthetic designs allow press-fit humeral stems, and the authors of this chapter have begun to use these designs more frequently. If bone quality is poor, however, the authors of this chapter use the largest humeral stem diameter that will allow a 2-mm circumferential cement interface around the implant. A large stem diameter is important because, if revision is required, the surgeon can remove the humeral implant, leaving the cement in place, and cement a stem with a narrower diameter into place. The authors of this chapter use antibiotic-laden cement because it has been found to reduce the risk of deep infection.

- The humeral socket-shaft angle can vary from 130° to 155°, depending on the implant system. The system preferred by the authors of this chapter uses a 135° humeral socket-shaft angle.

- For the final humeral socket, the authors of this chapter almost always use the constrained option for a particular size. Although this method decreases the theoretical range of motion, the added conformity of the deeper, semiconstrained sockets provides increased stability that outweighs a possible small decrease in the range of motion.

Wound Closure

- After final reduction of the prosthesis, the wound is irrigated with sterile saline and diluted povidone-iodine wash.

- The authors of this chapter do not routinely repair the subscapularis.

- A medium-size closed suction drain is placed on a case-by-case basis to help prevent postoperative hematoma. Drains are used routinely in patients treated for fracture or fracture sequelae (malunion) and in patients undergoing revision.

- A layered wound closure is performed.

Rehabilitation

Although the authors of this chapter use the following standard postoperative rehabilitation protocol, adjustments and modifications should be considered on an individual basis. If an implant with a medialized center of rotation is used, especially via a superior approach, the subscapularis should be repaired. This repair would affect the postoperative protocol because additional time would be needed before external rotation is allowed (**Tables 2** and **3**). After routine reverse shoulder arthroplasty procedures, the patient wears a sling for 1 to 2 weeks at all times except when performing hygiene tasks and hand, wrist, and elbow exercises. Because the authors of this chapter typically do not repair the subscapularis, activity limitations in the first 2 weeks are mainly to allow the wound to heal. Therapy is begun at 2 weeks with active elevation and external rotation. Pendulums are not allowed because they would increase the risk of dislocation. Extension posterior to the axilla also is avoided initially because extension and external rotation place the patient in a vulnerable position. Strengthening is initiated when pain is manageable and motion improves, typically at about 6 weeks. Return to activities varies: golf is allowed at 3 months, starting with chipping and putting and slowly returning to full play by approximately 4 months.

Avoiding Pitfalls

Adequate glenoid exposure begins with good exposure of the humerus. During humeral exposure, a complete inferior capsular release must be ensured while the affected arm is progressively externally rotated, adducted, and forward flexed to complete the release to the 4-o'clock position on the humeral head (right shoulder). This is followed by resection of peripheral and inferior osteophytes using an osteotome or rongeur. Additional humeral neck resection or pectoralis release are additional humeral-side techniques performed to improve glenoid exposure.

Careful and sequential glenoid exposure to achieve 360° visualization is a foundational step toward implanting a well-fixed, appropriately oriented glenosphere. The axillary nerve should be visualized and palpated during exposure of the inferior glenoid and scapular neck. Appropriate visualization of the inferior glenoid is critical to ensure appropriate implantation of the glenosphere and to reduce mechanical impingement. In addition, superior attritional wear is best appreciated if the view of the inferior glenoid is unobstructed.

Table 2 Rehabilitation Protocol After Reverse Shoulder Arthroplasty Without Subscapularis Repair

Postoperative Week	ROM	Strengthening	Return to Work/Play	Comments/ Emphasis
0-4	Passive No pendulums Supine external rotation of 0° or 20° Supine forward elevation of 90° No internal rotation	None	Return to computer use at wk 4	Advance ROM as tolerated
4-6	No pendulums Active ROM with passive stretching to prescribed limits Supine-seated external rotation; gradual increase to full Supine-seated forward elevation; progress to seated Internal rotation; gradually increase to full	None	Return to ADLs at wk 5	Standard sling discontinued at wk 5
6-12	No pendulums Achieve and maintain motion as tolerated to full ROM	Begin focused deltoid strengthening and scapular mobilization Resistance training, consisting of external and internal rotation, standing forward punch, seated rows, shoulder shrugs, biceps curls, and bear hugs	None	Resistance training introduced at wk 7
12-24	Unrestricted ROM is allowed, and ROM is advanced as tolerated, with the goal of full ROM	Weight training is begun at wk 12, keeping hands within eyesight and elbows bent Overhead activities are minimized Military press, pull-down behind head, and wide-grip bench press are not allowed	Return to golf at 3 mo, tennis at 4 mo	—

ADLs = activities of daily living, ROM = range of motion.

Baseplate version and inclination are critical in the setting of attritional bone loss. Augmentation with bone graft is necessary if appropriate baseplate position compromises baseplate contact with the prepared glenoid.

Glenoid fixation is of paramount importance. The surgeon should place a finger or Freer elevator anteriorly and palpate along the glenoid neck and coracoid base to aid in assessing native version and optimizing screw position. Bicortical fixation with excellent purchase must be achieved with central screw placement. If the central screw purchase is not ideal, the screw must be redirected. In the rare patient in whom it is not possible to achieve glenoid fixation, the RTSA should be abandoned and converted to hemiarthrodesis with consideration for glenoid grafting as plans for a staged reconstruction.

If humeral bone quality is poor, the humeral stem should be cemented. Cementing a larger diameter stem is important if revision is later required. In a revision setting, the surgeon can remove the humeral implant, leave the cement in place, and cement a stem with a narrower diameter.

Appropriate tension is achieved via careful trialing. Appropriate trials should allow minimal translation or distraction with longitudinal traction. Prosthetic impingement in extension leading to instability and bony impingement of the anterior humerus limiting forward flexion are common impediments to motion. After the appropriate humeral socket size is determined, the dislocation required to permit implantation of final components should be difficult.

Table 3 Rehabilitation Protocol After Reverse Shoulder Arthroplasty With Subscapularis Repair

Postoperative Week	ROM	Strengthening	Return to Work/Play	Comments/Emphasis
0-1	Shoulder is kept quiet in the sling, but active elbow, wrist, and hand motions are allowed Physical therapist–guided active scapular retraction/protraction exercises are begun Protraction is not allowed	None	Return to computer use at wk 4	A sling with an abduction pillow is used
1-4	Passive exercises Supine external rotation to 0° or 20° depending on tissue quality at the time of repair Supine forward elevation to 90° Neither internal rotation nor protraction is allowed	None	No change	A sling with an abduction pillow is used to wk 3, after which a standard sling is used
4-6	Active exercises No protraction until wk 6 Supine-seated external rotation; gradual increase to full Supine-seated forward elevation; progress to seated Internal rotation; gradual increase to full	None	No change	Continue use of standard sling ROM is progressed pain-free; do not push internal rotation or cross-body adduction. Avoid passive overpressure
6-12	Resisted exercises Pendulum exercises are not allowed Achieve and maintain full ROM as tolerated/unrestricted beginning at wk 8-10	Focused deltoid strengthening and scapular mobilization are begun at wk 8 Resistance training is begun, consisting of external and internal rotation, standing forward punch, seated rows, shoulder shrugs, biceps curls, and bear hugs	Return to ADLs at wk 8	Sling use is discontinued at wk 8 Resistance training is introduced at wk 10
12-24	Full ROM	Weight training is begun at wk 12, keeping the hands within eyesight and the elbows bent Overhead activities are minimized Military press, pull-down behind head, and wide-grip bench press are not allowed	Return to golf at 3 mo, tennis at 4 mo	—

ADLs = activities of daily living, ROM = range of motion.

[a] Range of motion should be progressed pain-free; do not push internal rotation or cross-body adduction. Avoid passive overpressure.

Bibliography

Ackland DC, Richardson M, Pandy MG: Axial rotation moment arms of the shoulder musculature after reverse total shoulder arthroplasty. *J Bone Joint Surg Am* 2012;94(20):1886-1895.

Arntz CT, Matsen FA III, Jackins S: Surgical management of complex irreparable rotator cuff deficiency. *J Arthroplasty* 1991;6(4):363-370.

Boileau P, Baqué F, Valerio L, Ahrens P, Chuinard C, Trojani C: Isolated arthroscopic biceps tenotomy or tenodesis improves symptoms in patients with massive irreparable rotator cuff tears. *J Bone Joint Surg Am* 2007;89(4):747-757.

Boileau P, Moineau G, Roussanne Y, O'Shea K: Bony increased-offset reversed shoulder arthroplasty: Minimizing scapular impingement while maximizing glenoid fixation. *Clin Orthop Relat Res* 2011;469(9):2558-2567.

Boileau P, Watkinson D, Hatzidakis AM, Hovorka I: The Grammont reverse shoulder prosthesis: Results in cuff tear arthritis, fracture sequelae, and revision arthroplasty. *J Shoulder Elbow Surg* 2006;15(5):527-540.

Bries AD, Pill SG, Wade Krause FR, Kissenberth MJ, Hawkins RJ: Accuracy of obtaining optimal base plate declination in reverse shoulder arthroplasty. *J Shoulder Elbow Surg* 2012;21(12):1770-1775.

Clark JC, Ritchie J, Song FS, et al: Complication rates, dislocation, pain, and postoperative range of motion after reverse shoulder arthroplasty in patients with and without repair of the subscapularis. *J Shoulder Elbow Surg* 2012;21(1):36-41.

Cuff D, Pupello D, Virani N, Levy J, Frankle M: Reverse shoulder arthroplasty for the treatment of rotator cuff deficiency. *J Bone Joint Surg Am* 2008;90(6):1244-1251.

Edwards TB, Williams MD, Labriola JE, Elkousy HA, Gartsman GM, O'Connor DP: Subscapularis insufficiency and the risk of shoulder dislocation after reverse shoulder arthroplasty. *J Shoulder Elbow Surg* 2009;18(6):892-896.

Favard L, Levigne C, Nerot C, Gerber C, De Wilde L, Mole D: Reverse prostheses in arthropathies with cuff tear: Are survivorship and function maintained over time? *Clin Orthop Relat Res* 2011;469(9):2469-2475.

Frankle M, Levy JC, Pupello D, et al: The reverse shoulder prosthesis for glenohumeral arthritis associated with severe rotator cuff deficiency: A minimum two-year follow-up study of sixty patients surgical technique. *J Bone Joint Surg Am* 2006;88(suppl 1, pt 2):178-190.

Frankle M, Siegal S, Pupello D, Saleem A, Mighell M, Vasey M: The Reverse Shoulder Prosthesis for glenohumeral arthritis associated with severe rotator cuff deficiency: A minimum two-year follow-up study of sixty patients. *J Bone Joint Surg Am* 2005;87(8):1697-1705.

Franklin JL, Barrett WP, Jackins SE, Matsen FA III: Glenoid loosening in total shoulder arthroplasty: Association with rotator cuff deficiency. *J Arthroplasty* 1988;3(1):39-46.

Gartsman GM, Edwards TB, eds: *Shoulder Arthroplasty*. Philadelphia, PA, Saunders, 2008.

Gerber C, Pennington SD, Nyffeler RW: Reverse total shoulder arthroplasty. *J Am Acad Orthop Surg* 2009;17(5):284-295.

Greiner S, Schmidt C, König C, Perka C, Herrmann S: Lateralized reverse shoulder arthroplasty maintains rotational function of the remaining rotator cuff. *Clin Orthop Relat Res* 2013;471(3):940-946.

Gulotta LV, Choi D, Marinello P, et al: Humeral component retroversion in reverse total shoulder arthroplasty: A biomechanical study. *J Shoulder Elbow Surg* 2012;21(9):1121-1127.

Gutiérrez S, Greiwe RM, Frankle MA, Siegal S, Lee WE III: Biomechanical comparison of component position and hardware failure in the reverse shoulder prosthesis. *J Shoulder Elbow Surg* 2007;16(3, suppl):S9-S12.

Hamada K, Fukuda H, Mikasa M, Kobayashi Y: Roentgenographic findings in massive rotator cuff tears: A long-term observation. *Clin Orthop Relat Res* 1990;(254):92-96.

Harman M, Frankle M, Vasey M, Banks S: Initial glenoid component fixation in "reverse" total shoulder arthroplasty: A biomechanical evaluation. *J Shoulder Elbow Surg* 2005;14(1, suppl S):162S-167S.

Herrmann S, König C, Heller M, Perka C, Greiner S: Reverse shoulder arthroplasty leads to significant biomechanical changes in the remaining rotator cuff. *J Orthop Surg Res* 2011;6:42.

Hoenecke HR Jr, Flores-Hernandez C, D'Lima DD: Reverse total shoulder arthroplasty component center of rotation affects muscle function. *J Shoulder Elbow Surg* 2014;23(8):1128-1135.

Jarrett CD, Brown BT, Schmidt CC: Reverse shoulder arthroplasty. *Orthop Clin North Am* 2013;44(3):389-408, x.

Jobin CM, Brown GD, Bahu MJ, et al: Reverse total shoulder arthroplasty for cuff tear arthropathy: The clinical effect of deltoid lengthening and center of rotation medialization. *J Shoulder Elbow Surg* 2012;21(10):1269-1277.

Kempton LB, Balasubramaniam M, Ankerson E, Wiater JM: A radiographic analysis of the effects of prosthesis design on scapular notching following reverse total shoulder arthroplasty. *J Shoulder Elbow Surg* 2011;20(4):571-576.

Middleton C, Uri O, Phillips S, et al: A reverse shoulder arthroplasty with increased offset for the treatment of cuff-deficient shoulders with glenohumeral arthritis. *Bone Joint J* 2014;96-B(7):936-942.

Mulieri P, Dunning P, Klein S, Pupello D, Frankle M: Reverse shoulder arthroplasty for the treatment of irreparable rotator cuff tear without glenohumeral arthritis. *J Bone Joint Surg Am* 2010;92(15):2544-2556.

Nam D, Kepler CK, Neviaser AS, et al: Reverse total shoulder arthroplasty: Current concepts, results, and component wear analysis. *J Bone Joint Surg Am* 2010;92(suppl 2):23-35.

Neer CS II, Craig EV, Fukuda H: Cuff-tear arthropathy. *J Bone Joint Surg Am* 1983;65(9):1232-1244.

Nolan BM, Ankerson E, Wiater JM: Reverse total shoulder arthroplasty improves function in cuff tear arthropathy. *Clin Orthop Relat Res* 2011;469(9):2476-2482.

Saltzman MD, Mercer DM, Warme WJ, Bertelsen AL, Matsen FA III: A method for documenting the change in center of rotation with reverse total shoulder arthroplasty and its application to a consecutive series of 68 shoulders having reconstruction with one of two different reverse prostheses. *J Shoulder Elbow Surg* 2010;19(7):1028-1033.

Sanchez-Sotelo J, Cofield RH, Rowland CM: Shoulder hemiarthroplasty for glenohumeral arthritis associated with severe rotator cuff deficiency. *J Bone Joint Surg Am* 2001;83(12):1814-1822.

Simovitch RW, Helmy N, Zumstein MA, Gerber C: Impact of fatty infiltration of the teres minor muscle on the outcome of reverse total shoulder arthroplasty. *J Bone Joint Surg Am* 2007;89(5):934-939.

Sirveaux F, Favard L, Oudet D, Huquet D, Walch G, Molé D: Grammont inverted total shoulder arthroplasty in the treatment of glenohumeral osteoarthritis with massive rupture of the cuff: Results of a multicentre study of 80 shoulders. *J Bone Joint Surg Br* 2004;86(3):388-395.

Stephenson DR, Oh JH, McGarry MH, Rick Hatch GF III, Lee TQ: Effect of humeral component version on impingement in reverse total shoulder arthroplasty. *J Shoulder Elbow Surg* 2011;20(4):652-658.

Valenti P, Sauzières P, Katz D, Kalouche I, Kilinc AS: Do less medialized reverse shoulder prostheses increase motion and reduce notching? *Clin Orthop Relat Res* 2011;469(9):2550-2557.

Virani NA, Cabezas A, Gutiérrez S, Santoni BG, Otto R, Frankle M: Reverse shoulder arthroplasty components and surgical techniques that restore glenohumeral motion. *J Shoulder Elbow Surg* 2013;22(2):179-187.

Walch G, Boileau P, Molé D, Favard L, Lévigne C, Sirveaux F: *Reverse Shoulder Arthroplasty: Clinical Results, Complications, Revision.* Montpellier, France, Sauramps Medical, 2006.

Wall B, Nové-Josserand L, O'Connor DP, Edwards TB, Walch G: Reverse total shoulder arthroplasty: A review of results according to etiology. *J Bone Joint Surg Am* 2007;89(7):1476-1485.

Werner CM, Steinmann PA, Gilbart M, Gerber C: Treatment of painful pseudoparesis due to irreparable rotator cuff dysfunction with the Delta III reverse-ball-and-socket total shoulder prosthesis. *J Bone Joint Surg Am* 2005;87(7):1476-1486.

Williams GR Jr, Rockwood CA Jr: Hemiarthroplasty in rotator cuff-deficient shoulders. *J Shoulder Elbow Surg* 1996;5(5):362-367.

 ## Video Reference

Hawkins RJ, Backes JR, Bentley JC, Kissenberth MJ: Video. *Cuff Tear Arthropathy Reverse Shoulder Arthroplasty: Steps to Get it Right.* Greenville, SC, 2015.

Chapter 39

Revision Shoulder Arthroplasty for the Management of Implant Wear or Loosening

Thomas R. Duquin, MD

John W. Sperling, MD, MBA

Introduction

Shoulder arthroplasty is a reliable procedure for the management of arthritic conditions of the shoulder, and good results are achieved in most patients. Improved surgical techniques and implant design have resulted in expanded indications for shoulder arthroplasty; therefore, the use of this procedure has substantially increased in the past decade and is projected to increase further in the next 10 years. The survival rate for shoulder arthroplasty is 98% at 5 years but declines to 89% at 10 years and 70% at 20 years. Results of shoulder arthroplasty have been shown to improve in the first year after the procedure and then remain stable for many years. Between 8 and 20 years postoperatively, outcome scores gradually decline and patient satisfaction decreases.

The increased prevalence of shoulder arthroplasty and the longevity of patients with shoulder arthroplasty will result in a substantial increase in the number of implant failures and revision procedures. Revision shoulder arthroplasty can be challenging because of the presence of soft-tissue contractures, bone or soft-tissue loss, infection, or well-fixed monoblock or malpositioned implants. In patients with good bone stock and soft tissues, revision arthroplasty can improve pain and function. In patients with bone or soft-tissue loss, revision to reverse shoulder arthroplasty or hemiarthroplasty should be considered.

Careful assessment of the etiology of failure is essential for successful revision. Reasons for failure of shoulder arthroplasty include implant loosening, infection, instability, rotator cuff tear, fracture, polyethylene wear, and nerve injury. Thus, evaluation of a patient with painful or failed shoulder arthroplasty must include a workup for implant loosening, implant malposition, infection, rotator cuff failure, and instability.

The most common reason for revision of shoulder arthroplasty is implant loosening and failure. Radiolucent lines around cemented glenoid implants are common, with an incidence between 20% and 95%. In some series, glenoid radiolucent lines have been identified in greater than 50% of immediate postoperative radiographs after total shoulder arthroplasty. The annualized risk of developing glenoid radiolucent lines is approximately 7% per year, whereas the risk of symptomatic glenoid loosening is approximately 1% per year. Radiolucent lines may be associated with poor surgical technique, implant malposition, polyethylene wear, instability, infection, or mechanical loosening. A static, minor radiolucent line is of little concern but should be monitored. Progressive or major radiolucent lines can indicate that an implant is at risk. Evidence of migration or subsidence indicates a loose implant. The progression from radiolucency to loosening has not been fully established, although the presence of radiolucency has been associated with the need for revision of total shoulder arthroplasty. The Deutsch modification of the Souter classification system can be used in the radiographic assessment of glenoid radiolucency (**Table 1**). Evaluation of the glenoid on AP and axillary radiographs is an essential part of routine follow-up after total shoulder arthroplasty. In patients with suspected loosening, a CT scan may be required to better visualize the interface between the prosthesis and the glenoid bone. A CT scan can also provide information regarding the extent of glenoid bone loss and the version of the glenoid and humeral implants. In patients with symptomatic, progressive radiolucent lines or a loose glenoid implant, revision may be indicated.

Humeral implant loosening is much less common than glenoid implant loosening. The reported incidence of humeral loosening at long-term follow-up is

Dr. Duquin or an immediate family member is a member of a speakers' bureau or has made paid presentations on behalf of, serves as a paid consultant to, and has received research or institutional support from Zimmer Biomet. Dr. Sperling or an immediate family member has received royalties from Zimmer Biomet and DJO and serves as a paid consultant to Tornier.

Table 1 Deutsch Classification of Glenoid Radiolucent Lines and Loosening[a]

Grade	Glenoid Lucent Lines
0	None
1	<1 mm, incomplete
2	1 mm, complete
3	1.5 mm, incomplete
4	1.5 mm, complete
5	2 mm, complete

[a] Radiographic evidence of a loose glenoid is defined as the presence of a 2-mm circumferential lucent line, progression of lucent lines, cement fragmentation, or implant migration.

Adapted with permission from Deutsch A, Abboud JA, Kelly J, et al: Clinical results of revision shoulder arthroplasty for glenoid component loosening. *J Shoulder Elbow Surg* 2007;16(6):706-716.

less than 5%, and rates of aseptic loosening are even less frequent. Patients with progressive radiolucent lines or a loose humeral implant should be considered to have infection until proved otherwise. The diagnosis of infection in patients who have undergone shoulder arthroplasty can be challenging because of the prevalence of low-virulence organisms and the unreliable nature of laboratory studies, pathology, and cultures. A high index of suspicion for infection is required in the management of failed shoulder arthroplasty because the reported incidence of unsuspected positive cultures discovered at the time of revision shoulder arthroplasty has been greater than 50% in some series. Risk factors for positive cultures at the time of revision include younger age, male sex, and the presence of humeral osteolysis or a loose humeral implant.

Although infection rates after shoulder arthroplasty are low (1% to 2%), loose implants (especially humeral implants) should be considered infected until proved otherwise. Before any revision procedure, patients should be evaluated for possible infection. A standard evaluation for infection includes blood tests (complete blood cell count, erythrocyte sedimentation rate, and C-reactive protein level) and joint aspiration sent for cell count and culture. Cultures should be held for 14 to 21 days to allow identification of low-virulence organisms such as *Propionibacterium acnes*. With standard evaluation methods, sensitivity for detecting infection is approximately 70%. In an effort to increase the rate of detection, new tests have been developed, including serum interleukin-6, α-defensin, and synovial fluid polymerase chain reaction. Even with the addition of these newer screening tests, the ability to detect infection before revision surgery remains imperfect, and the possibility of an unsuspected positive culture after revision surgery exists.

Assessment of the integrity and function of the rotator cuff is essential. A torn or dysfunctional rotator cuff may result in early loosening or wear of a glenoid implant; in these patients, revision to reverse total shoulder arthroplasty or hemiarthroplasty is required. Preoperative assessment of muscle atrophy and strength of the rotator cuff should be accompanied by either ultrasonography or CT arthrography. CT arthrography can be performed at the same time as aspiration, allowing assessment of the rotator cuff, implant position, and joint infection.

Instability after shoulder arthroplasty may be associated with early implant loosening or wear. Assessment of instability can be challenging both clinically and radiographically. The etiology of instability is typically multifactorial and can involve soft-tissue deficiency, contracture, and/or implant malposition. Radiographic evaluation of subluxation or dislocation of the humeral head is classified as mild (<25%), moderate (25% to 50%), or severe (>50%). Anterior subluxation is typically associated with rupture of the subscapularis, and superior subluxation is typically associated with rupture of the supraspinatus. In patients with posterior subluxation, implant malposition and anterior joint contractures are common.

Periprosthetic humeral fractures after shoulder arthroplasty are rare, with a reported incidence of approximately 2%. Management of these fractures depends on the fracture type and the stability of the humeral prosthesis. Fractures that involve a loose humeral stem require revision to a long-stemmed humeral component. In the absence of a loose component, treatment options often include nonsurgical management and open reduction and internal fixation.

After the etiology of the failed shoulder arthroplasty has been evaluated, a plan for the revision can be created. Preoperative planning is essential to ensure that the appropriate equipment for the revision is available. The surgical report of the initial procedure should be obtained, and the surgeon should become familiar with the characteristics of the existing implant and techniques for removal. The surgeon should have multiple options available at the time of revision, including anatomic and reverse total shoulder arthroplasty systems, as well as a plan for bone graft harvest and fixation in the event that reimplantation is not possible. An antibiotic spacer can be useful on rare occasions because infection is possible even in patients with negative aspiration and laboratory study results.

Case Presentation

A 66-year-old woman has progressive pain 10 years after undergoing total arthroplasty of the left shoulder. She had good results after the procedure until several months before presentation, when she began experiencing worsening pain and limitations in function. She reports no injury or trauma to the extremity.

Physical examination reveals limited range of motion, with active forward elevation of 40° and abduction of 30°.

Examination of the rotator cuff reveals weakness of the rotator cuff musculature. The patient has intact deltoid, biceps, and triceps function and normal neurologic examination findings in her left upper extremity.

Radiographs of the shoulder demonstrate evidence of displacement of the glenoid implant and superior subluxation of the humeral head (**Figure 1, A** and **B**). The humeral stem appears well fixed, with no visible radiolucent lines. CT arthrography reveals compromise of the rotator cuff and displacement of the glenoid implant from the glenoid (**Figure 1, C**).

The patient is evaluated for infection with aspiration and laboratory studies, and the results are negative. The glenoid implant is found to be displaced from the glenoid and trapped in scar tissue in the anterior aspect of the shoulder joint capsule. The subscapularis and supraspinatus tendons are observed to be torn and retracted. The patient undergoes removal of the humeral and glenoid implants and revision to reverse total shoulder arthroplasty (**Figures 2** and **3**).

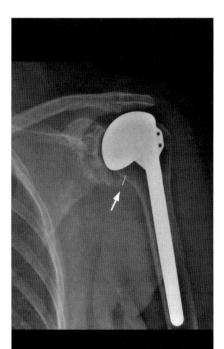
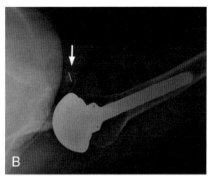
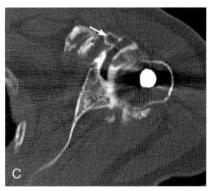

Figure 1 **A,** AP radiograph demonstrates the left shoulder of a 66-year-old woman 10 years after total shoulder arthroplasty. The arrow indicates a radiographic marker on the glenoid implant, which has displaced from the glenoid. **B,** Axillary radiograph from the same patient demonstrates the displaced glenoid implant (arrow). **C,** CT arthrogram of the shoulder. The arrow points to the glenoid implant, which has fully dislodged from the glenoid and is displaced anteriorly.

Indications

Revision shoulder arthroplasty is indicated in patients with symptomatic implant loosening or wear. Patients with

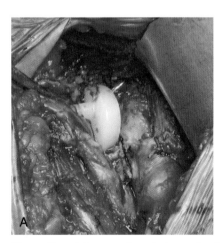
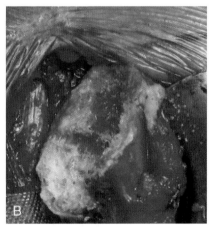
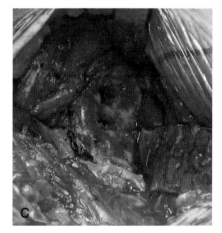

Figure 2 Intraoperative photographs show the shoulder of a patient undergoing revision to reverse total shoulder arthroplasty to address a failed previous total shoulder arthroplasty. **A,** The displaced glenoid implant is lodged in scar tissue in the anterior capsule. **B,** The humerus is depicted after removal of the humeral stem. The rotator cuff was found to be torn. **C,** The glenoid demonstrates contained mild bone loss resulting from implant loosening and displacement.

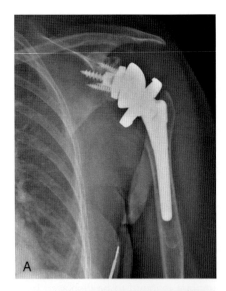

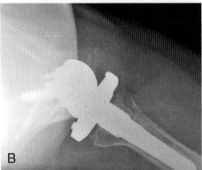

Figure 3 Radiographs from the same patient described in Figure 2 obtained 1 year after revision to reverse total shoulder arthroplasty. **A,** AP View obtained after revision. **B,** Axillary radiograph demonstrates intact implants with no evidence of loosening or failure.

failed shoulder arthroplasty associated with worn or loose implants typically report pain, loss of function, or mechanical symptoms. Many patients report a gradual decline in function and an increase in pain several years after an initially successful shoulder arthroplasty procedure. Implants that demonstrate gross loosening with displacement or subsidence on radiographs or CT scan are a clear indication for revision. In patients with symptomatic radiolucent lines in the absence of gross loosening, further workup is required to rule out other potential causes of failure, including infection, instability, and soft-tissue compromise. Radiolucent lines are frequently seen on routine follow-up radiographs in asymptomatic patients. In the absence of pain or symptoms, the patient is treated with close observation and repeat radiographs 6 months later. Development of symptoms, progressive loosening, or impending fracture warrants consideration of revision surgery.

An understanding of the etiology of the failed arthroplasty is essential in planning a successful revision procedure. Revision options in patients with a loose glenoid implant include revision of the glenoid implant in a one- or two-stage procedure, conversion to hemiarthroplasty with or without glenoid bone grafting, and revision to reverse total shoulder arthroplasty. Factors that influence the type of revision include glenoid bone loss, infection, soft-tissue quality, and patient factors, including age and activity level (**Figure 4**).

Contraindications

Absolute contraindications for revision of failed shoulder arthroplasty include associated medical conditions that prevent surgical intervention and patient inability to comply with postoperative instructions. Infection is a contraindication for primary revision and should be managed with staged débridement, followed by revision after the infection has been cleared.

Controversies and Alternative Approaches

Patients who are not candidates for revision surgery or who have asymptomatic loose implants can be treated nonsurgically. Nonsurgical management includes activity modification and pain management using NSAIDs or narcotic pain medications as needed. Physical therapy plays a limited role because exercise will likely result in the progression of implant loosening and worsening of the patient's symptoms.

Results

The available literature on revision shoulder arthroplasty is limited to retrospective reviews involving small numbers of participants (level IV evidence). Results after revision for implant loosening or wear typically reveal improvement in pain and function but are inferior to those of primary shoulder arthroplasty. Patient satisfaction after revision shoulder arthroplasty can be expected in 65% to 85% of cases. The results of revision with glenoid reimplantation have been shown to be superior to glenoid resection regarding pain relief and function. However, patients with instability or rotator cuff pathology have been shown to have poor outcomes after revision arthroplasty with glenoid reimplantation. Patients should be counseled that the results after revision may not be equal to the initial results after a successful primary shoulder arthroplasty. **Table 2** reviews the available literature on revision shoulder arthroplasty.

Technical Keys to Success

Setup/Exposure
- The patient is positioned in the beach-chair position with a bump placed medial to the scapula.
- The deltopectoral approach is used for the procedure, and the previous surgical incision can be used in most patients.

Instruments/Equipment/Implants Required
- As noted previously, the surgeon should have multiple options available at the time of revision, including anatomic and reverse total

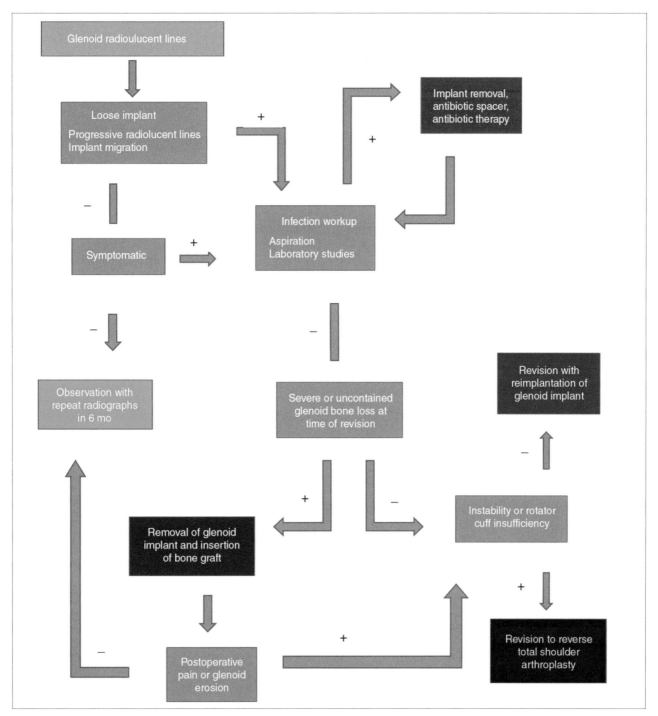

Figure 4   Decision algorithm demonstrates the evaluation and management of glenoid implant loosening. + = yes, – = no.

shoulder arthroplasty systems, as well as a plan for harvesting and fixation of bone graft to be used in the event that reimplantation is not possible.

• An antibiotic spacer can be useful

because infection is possible even in patients with negative results of aspiration and laboratory studies.

• Standard shoulder retractors are used.

• Revision tools for disassembly

of modular parts specific to the implanted prosthesis should be available.

• Stem extraction instruments include a square-tip impactor, vice grips, a slap hammer, a micropower

Table 2 Results of Revision Shoulder Arthroplasty

Authors	Journal (Year)	Technique (No. of Patients)	Outcomes[a]	Failure Rate (%)	Comments
Antuna et al	*J Shoulder Elbow Surg* (2001)	Revision of loose glenoid: reimplantation of new glenoid (30), glenoid removal and bone graft (18)	VAS pain score improved from 4.0 to 1.9 Active elevation improved from 96° to 112° Patient satisfaction was much better in 29, better in 7, same or worse in 12 Neer score was excellent in 10, satisfactory in 14, unsatisfactory in 19	25 (reoperation)	Mean follow-up, 4.9 yr Satisfactory pain relief in 86% after reimplantation and 66% after removal Better satisfaction was achieved with reimplantation 3 patients treated with removal and bone grafting underwent a second revision for implantation of the glenoid because of severe pain 2 patients treated with revision glenoid required removal because of failure 2 patients underwent reoperation to manage fracture
Dines et al	*J Bone Joint Surg Am* (2006)	Glenoid revision/ resection (22) Conversion hemiarthroplasty to TSA (16) ORIF periprosthetic fracture (4) Revision humeral stem (8) Revision humeral head (4) Rotator cuff repair (10) Treatment of instability (5) Revision of a failed tuberosity reconstruction (4) Staged reimplantation or resection arthroplasty (5)	UCLA score, 21.4 L'Insalata score, 68.73	NA	Mean follow-up, 76 mo
Neyton et al	*J Shoulder Elbow Surg* (2006)	Revision of loose glenoid with hemiarthroplasty and corticocancellous iliac crest bone graft (9)	Constant score improved from 46.3 to 49.9 Neer score was satisfactory in 5 patients and unsatisfactory in 4 Active elevation decreased from 119° to 114°	11 (reoperation)	Improved pain but limited to no improvement in function Mean medialization of the humeral head, 4.1 mm
Phipatanakul and Norris	*J Shoulder Elbow Surg* (2006)	Humeral head replacement with glenoid bone grafting (24)	Satisfactory pain relief in 92%	NA	Aseptic glenoid loosening Mean follow-up, 33.4 mo

ASES = American Shoulder and Elbow Surgeons shoulder outcome, NA = not available, ORIF = open reduction and internal fixation, TSA = total shoulder arthroplasty, UCLA = University of California–Los Angeles Shoulder Rating Scale, VAS = visual analog scale.

[a] Mean values unless otherwise noted.

Table 2 Results of Revision Shoulder Arthroplasty (*continued*)

Authors	Journal (Year)	Technique (No. of Patients)	Outcomes[a]	Failure Rate (%)	Comments
Deutsch et al	*J Shoulder Elbow Surg* (2007)	Glenoid reimplantation (15) Hemiarthroplasty (17)	Improvement in pain and ASES score in both groups Results were better after reimplantation than after hemiarthroplasty	47	Most failures were associated with soft-tissue deficiency or instability 2 patients treated with hemiarthroplasty returned for glenoid implantation because of pain
Cheung et al	*J Shoulder Elbow Surg* (2008)	Revision with implantation of glenoid component (33) Revision with removal of glenoid component and bone grafting without glenoid reimplantation (35)	Significant pain relief in 23 patients with new glenoid component and 24 patients with removal and grafting alone (*P* = 0.9203) No significant change in range of motion	9 (new component) 22 (removal)	7 reoperations after revision with implantation of glenoid component glenoid removal for loosening (2), resection arthroplasty for persistent instability (2), rotator cuff repair (2), fracture (1) 7 reoperations after removal of glenoid component and grafting: implantation of glenoid (6), resection arthroplasty for infection (1) Failure rates calculated from 5-yr survival
Elhassan et al	*Clin Orthop Relat Res* (2008)	Revision with glenoid bone grafting: anatomic TSA (3), hemiarthroplasty (5), hemiarthroplasty with biologic resurfacing (10), reverse TSA (3)	Constant scores: anatomic TSA, 69; hemiarthroplasty, 68; hemiarthroplasty with biologic resurfacing, 61; reverse TSA, 72	10 (reoperation)	Mean follow-up, 45 mo Constant scores improved in all groups, with greater improvement in patients with glenoid implantation Improved forward elevation in patients treated with reverse TSA
Scalise and Iannotti	*Clin Orthop Relat Res* (2008)	Revision to hemiarthroplasty with glenoid bone graft to manage glenoid bone loss after aseptic loosening of glenoid component (11)	Penn Shoulder Score improved from 23 to 57	18	Graft subsidence in all patients, 8 of whom had subsidence >5 mm The degree of subsidence did not correlate with outcome scores
Melis et al	*J Shoulder Elbow Surg* (2012)	Reverse TSA (37)	86% of patients were very satisfied Constant score improved from 24 to 55 Active forward elevation improved from 68° to 121°	21	Failure consisted of glenoid loosening in 9%, prosthetic anterior instability in 6%, and humeral subsidence in 6% Mean follow-up, 47 mo
Bonnevialle et al	*J Shoulder Elbow Surg* (2013)	Reimplantation of an all-polyethylene cemented glenoid implant (42)	Constant score improved from 41 to 57 Active forward elevation improved from 106° to 125°	17	Radiologic loosening in 67% Mean follow-up, 74 mo

ASES = American Shoulder and Elbow Surgeons shoulder outcome, NA = not available, ORIF = open reduction and internal fixation, TSA = total shoulder arthroplasty, UCLA = University of California–Los Angeles Shoulder Rating Scale, VAS = visual analog scale.

[a] Mean values unless otherwise noted.

Table 2 Results of Revision Shoulder Arthroplasty (*continued*)

Authors	Journal (Year)	Technique (No. of Patients)	Outcomes[a]	Failure Rate (%)	Comments
Schubkegel et al	*Am J Orthop (Belle Mead NJ)* (2014)	Revision loose glenoid with hemiarthroplasty and bone grafting glenoid defect with cancellous allograft (14 shoulders)	VAS pain score improved from 6.4 to 1.2 ASES score improved from 33 to 72 13 patients reported satisfaction Active elevation improved from 84° to 113°	7.1 (reoperation)	All patients had an intact rotator cuff at the time of revision surgery
Wagner et al	*J Bone Joint Surg Am* (2015)	Reverse TSA with glenoid bone grafting (40 shoulders)	5-yr survival, 76% ASES score, 66 Simple Shoulder Test, 6 Active abduction, 112° Satisfaction, 83%	18	Most glenoid grafting done with cancellous allograft Lateral center of rotation was found to be a poor prognostic factor Study authors recommend structural grafts for defects that result in <30% to 50% contact with host bone

ASES = American Shoulder and Elbow Surgeons shoulder outcome, NA = not available, ORIF = open reduction and internal fixation, TSA = total shoulder arthroplasty, UCLA = University of California–Los Angeles Shoulder Rating Scale, VAS = visual analog scale.

[a] Mean values unless otherwise noted.

burr with a small head or router tip, osteotomes, and cement removal tools.

- Glenoid removal instruments include a micropower saw, curets, trephines, and a micropower burr.
- Other instruments that may be needed are a pulse lavage with a canal-irrigating tip, a cerclage wire or cable system, and a plate-and-screw set.

Procedure

EXPOSURE AND IMPLANT REMOVAL

- The deltoid is mobilized from its origin on the clavicle to the insertion on the humerus. Mobilization of the deltoid in the subdeltoid and subacromial spaces is performed, with care taken to avoid injury to the axillary nerve and the rotator cuff.
- The subscapularis is carefully mobilized from the conjoint tendon, and the axillary nerve is identified at the

inferior margin of the subscapularis tendon in the subcoracoid region.

- If subscapularis insufficiency or rotator cuff tears are present, conversion of the procedure to reverse total shoulder arthroplasty (discussed later in this chapter) may be required.
- The subscapularis can be released with a standard tenotomy; alternatively, in patients with substantial internal rotation contracture, the tendon insertion can be peeled from the insertion on the lesser tuberosity.
- The inferior capsule is released from the humerus, with care taken to stay subperiosteal to avoid injury to the axillary nerve.
- After complete release of the inferior capsule, the humeral head is dislocated. In patients with modular implants, the humeral head can be dissociated from the stem.
- Culture of the synovial fluid and

three to five tissue cultures are obtained. Tissue cultures are obtained from the joint capsule as well as from the interfaces between the humeral and glenoid implants and the native bone.

- Synovial tissue is also sent for pathologic evaluation, although previous studies have shown limited sensitivity of pathology in the identification of infection. However, a recent study showed improved sensitivity (72%) and specificity (100%) of intraoperative histology for the identification of infection with *P acnes* when a revised threshold of 10 polymorphonuclear leukocytes per 5 high-power fields was used.
- Humeral stem removal may be required in patients with monoblock, loose, or malpositioned humeral implants. Removal of a loose stem can be performed with an appropriate extraction tool or a

vice grip and slap hammer. To remove a well-fixed humeral stem, the authors of this chapter prefer to use a pencil-tipped router to free the interface between the proximal aspect of the humeral stem and the bone. This can be performed from the superior aspect of the implant after removal of a modular humeral head.

- After circumferential release of the humeral implant proximally, the appropriate extraction device and slap hammer can be used to remove the implant.

- Alternatively, a square-tipped impactor may be placed at the medial neck of the humeral stem and a mallet used to drive the implant out of the humerus. This technique works particularly well in implants with a collar, but for implants without a collar, a notch can be created in the medial aspect of the implant with the use of a metal cutting burr to create a surface for the square-tipped impactor to engage.

- In patients with a prosthesis that is well fixed distally, a longitudinal split of the humerus or a humeral window may be required to remove the stem.

- After the humeral implant has been addressed, attention is turned to the glenoid. Glenoid exposure in revision arthroplasty can be difficult because of scarring of the rotator cuff, deltoid, and pectoralis major and the presence of capsular contractures.

- Mobilization of the subdeltoid and subacromial spaces and complete inferior capsule release from the humerus are essential for visualization of the glenoid.

- A humeral implant that is proud can also limit glenoid exposure, and it may be necessary to remove the implant to allow for visualization.

- The authors of this chapter typically use anterior and posterior

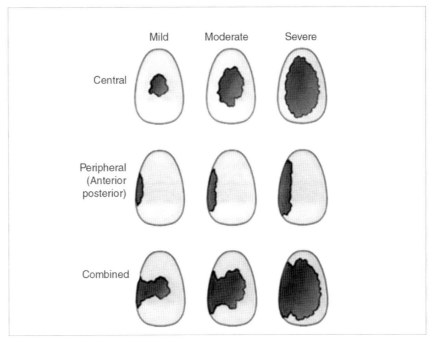

Figure 5 In the Antuna classification of glenoid bone loss, defects are classified as central, peripheral, or combined and are graded as mild, moderate, or severe. (Reproduced with permission from Antuna SA, Sperling JW, Cofield RH, Rowland CM: Glenoid revision surgery after total shoulder arthroplasty. *J Shoulder Elbow Surg* 2001;10[3]:217-224.)

Bankart glenoid retractors and a bent Hohmann retractor placed over the superior aspect of the glenoid. A variety of glenoid retractors should be available during the procedure because different retractors may be useful in certain patients.

- After adequate exposure is obtained, the glenoid implant can be examined for loosening or wear. In cases in which the implant is loose, removal of the implant is easy, and the remaining cement should be debrided, with care taken to preserve the glenoid bone stock.

- For the well-fixed glenoid that must be removed, the type of implant dictates the method of removal. Pegged implants can be cut into pieces with a small saw blade, which allows removal of each individual peg from the cement mantle with minimal damage to the surrounding bone. For a well-fixed keeled implant, the surface of the glenoid can be cut from the keel with the use of

a small saw, and the keel can then be carefully freed from the cement mantle with a pencil-tipped router to minimize bone loss during implant removal.

- After removal of the implants, the bone stock of the glenoid and humerus is evaluated. The options for revision will be influenced by the extent of glenoid bone loss (**Figure 5**) and the status of the remaining soft tissues around the shoulder.

SINGLE-STAGE REVISION WITH GLENOID IMPLANTATION

- In patients without infection who have good bone stock and an intact rotator cuff, a new glenoid component should be implanted.

- If the patient has minor or contained bone defects, the glenoid defect can be filled with cement, and a new glenoid can be implanted into the larger cement mantle. This technique can be performed with a keeled implant after the removal of a pegged implant that has become loose but has not resulted in substantial bone loss.

- In patients with larger but contained glenoid defects, the defect can be filled with the use of an impaction grafting technique and cementation of a new glenoid implant. Success with this technique requires the creation of a stable conforming surface for the new glenoid implant with meticulous preparation and cementation of the new implant. If a stable surface to support the new glenoid implant cannot be obtained, alternative procedures should be considered.

REVISION WITH GLENOID BONE GRAFTING WITH OR WITHOUT STAGED GLENOID IMPLANTATION

- In patients with severe glenoid bone loss such that the glenoid cannot support a new implant, the glenoid should be bone grafted with a structural tricortical iliac crest or allograft bone graft.
- The bone graft should be aligned so that the cortical aspect of the graft articulates with the humeral implant.
- The graft can be contoured to match the defect and allow for press-fit fixation of the glenoid implant into the glenoid defect, and additional cancellous graft can be impacted around any remaining defect.
- If the graft is stable after impaction, no additional fixation is required. If the graft is not stable after impaction, additional fixation can be achieved with the use of recessed or headless screws, bioabsorbable screws, or screws placed from anterior to posterior. Careful placement of fixation is required because articulation with the humeral implant can result in metal debris.
- Progressive wear after glenoid bone grafting has been well documented and can result in medialization of

the humeral implant. In patients with glenoid bone wear or pain after glenoid bone grafting, a two-stage revision can be performed. In the second stage, the glenoid is implanted with the use of standard techniques provided that the bone graft has incorporated and adequate bone is available for support of the glenoid implant (**Figure 6**). A CT scan should be performed before the second stage to ensure incorporation of the bone graft and adequate bone stock to allow for glenoid implantation.

HUMERAL IMPLANT REVISION

- In rare cases of humeral loosening without infection or glenoid loosening, primary revision of the humeral stem can be performed.
- A thorough workup for infection is essential because the rates of aseptic humeral loosening are extremely low and humeral implant loosening has been shown to be associated with unsuspected infection with a low-virulence organism.
- Revision options depend on the status of the humeral bone stock and the presence of cement. In patients with a well-fixed and stable cement mantle, a smaller humeral stem can be implanted using a cement-in-cement technique. This procedure is performed with the use of an implant that is at least 2 mm smaller in diameter and shorter in length, allowing the creation of a new stable cement mantle that will bond to the existing cement mantle.

REVISION TO REVERSE TOTAL SHOULDER ARTHROPLASTY

- In patients with rotator cuff insufficiency or an irreparable subscapularis tendon, or in elderly patients with life expectancy of less than 10 years, reverse total shoulder arthroplasty should be considered.
- In patients who require conversion

to reverse total shoulder arthroplasty, the authors of this chapter prefer to perform a one-stage revision with bone grafting of the glenoid defect and implantation of a reverse baseplate.

- Bone grafting of the glenoid is facilitated with a reverse baseplate that allows for compression of the graft with stable fixation and a bone ingrowth interface.
- In many patients, bone graft can be obtained from the proximal humerus because the humeral stem will require removal and a humeral osteotomy will be done 5 to 10 mm distal to the original osteotomy for conversion to reverse arthroplasty.
- If the stem is well fixed and convertible, it can be kept in place. In this scenario, bone graft can be obtained from the distal clavicle or iliac crest, or allograft bone can be used.
- One technique described for iliac crest bone grafting involves implanting the baseplate on the iliac crest, harvesting the surrounding bone, and then performing fixation of the baseplate and bone graft to the deficient glenoid. This technique can be useful in patients with massive glenoid bone deficiency.
- Because of the risk of donor site morbidity, the authors of this chapter take bone graft from the iliac crest only in cases in which no alternatives are available. The authors' preference is to use allograft iliac crest or femoral head grafts as an alternative to iliac crest autograft. Depending on the reverse baseplate design, the bone graft can be fixed using the peripheral screws of the baseplate or screws placed outside the baseplate (**Figure 7**).

Wound Closure

- After implantation of the new components is complete, a radiograph is obtained to confirm appropriate

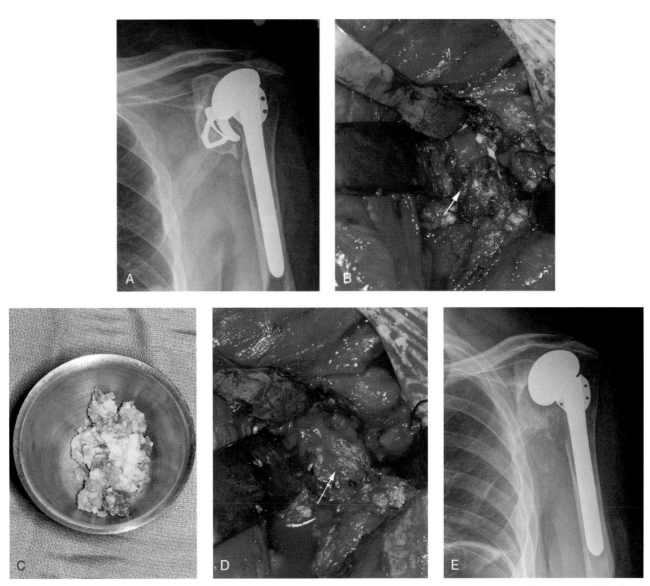

Figure 6 Images of a revision of a failed total shoulder arthroplasty obtained from a patient with glenoid loosening and displacement. **A,** Preoperative AP radiograph demonstrates glenoid and humeral bone loss secondary to osteolysis. **B,** Intraoperative photograph of the glenoid after removal of a pegged polyethylene component. The arrow points to the resulting contained cavitary bone defect from the cemented pegs of the glenoid. **C,** Intraoperative photograph shows the femoral head allograft used for bone grafting of the glenoid defect. **D,** Intraoperative photograph after bone grafting of the glenoid defect. The arrow points to the impacted femoral head allograft bone. **E,** AP radiograph demonstrates the shoulder after removal of the glenoid implant and bone grafting of the defect.

position and the absence of fractures.

- The joint is irrigated, and hemostasis is obtained.
- The subscapularis tendon is repaired using heavy nonabsorbable sutures passed through the lesser tuberosity, if possible.

- The rotator interval is closed, and the subscapularis tendon repair is augmented with heavy absorbable sutures.
- After repair of the subscapularis tendon, it should be possible to externally rotate the shoulder to at least 30°.

- A drain is left in the subdeltoid space, and the deltopectoral interval is closed with heavy absorbable sutures.
- Skin closure is performed with interrupted absorbable deep dermal sutures followed by a running subcuticular absorbable suture and a topical skin adhesive.

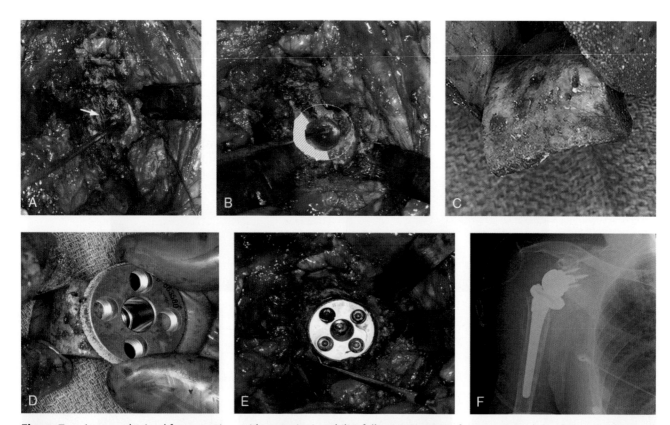

Figure 7 Images obtained from a patient with posterior instability following revision of anatomic total shoulder arthroplasty to reverse total shoulder arthroplasty and use of structural iliac crest allograft to repair the glenoid bone defect. **A,** Intraoperative photograph shows the severe posterior peripheral glenoid defect (arrow) after removal of the original glenoid component. **B,** The glenoid after reaming in preparation for placement of a glenoid baseplate (footprint outlined). Approximately 35% of the baseplate footprint is unsupported by native bone (shaded area). **C,** Appearance of the allograft iliac crest after burring to match the baseplate geometry and the size of the bone defect. **D,** The baseplate is applied to the bone graft. **E,** The glenosphere baseplate after implantation. The bone graft was fixed using a screw placed through the posterior peripheral hole of the baseplate. **F,** Postoperative radiograph demonstrates completed reverse total shoulder arthroplasty.

 ## Rehabilitation

The shoulder is placed in an immobilizer for 6 weeks after revision total shoulder arthroplasty. Physical therapy is begun in the first week and consists initially of elbow, wrist, and hand range of motion exercises and pendulum exercises of the shoulder. Gradual progression of passive and active-assisted range of motion is allowed during the 6-week immobilization period. After 6 weeks, active range of motion is initiated, and the patient is allowed to use the arm for light activities. Strengthening and gradual, progressive return to normal activity are begun after 12 weeks, depending on patient tolerance. Recovery after revision total shoulder arthroplasty is typically slower than recovery after primary total shoulder arthroplasty, and rehabilitation must proceed with care to protect the subscapularis repair.

 ## Avoiding Pitfalls

Revision shoulder arthroplasty is a difficult and technically demanding procedure. Assessment of loosening or wear of the humeral and glenoid implants is essential in the evaluation of a patient with failed shoulder arthroplasty. When revision is planned for the management of implant loosening or wear, the etiology of the failure, including infection, instability, rotator cuff dysfunction, implant malposition, or mechanical wear, should be identified. Failure to address the associated factors at the time of revision will result in early failure of the revision procedure. Preoperative planning and preparation can limit intraoperative complications. Common factors that can lead to pitfalls and complications include infection, soft-tissue deficiency, and bone deficiency.

The results of aspiration and laboratory studies are helpful when positive, but infection cannot be completely ruled out by a negative result because of the poor sensitivity of these tests. Rates of unsuspected positive cultures after revision shoulder arthroplasty have been reported to be greater than 50% in some series. If suspicious fluid, purulence, or a loose humeral implant is observed at the time of revision, the surgeon should perform irrigation and débridement, remove the implant, and place an antibiotic spacer.

Meticulous handling of soft tissues is essential for the success of anatomic arthroplasty. High rates of failure of revision shoulder arthroplasty have been reported in patients with instability or rotator cuff insufficiency. If soft-tissue deficiency is identified, a glenoid implant should not be placed, and the procedure should be converted to hemiarthroplasty or reverse total shoulder arthroplasty.

Bone deficiency is common in patients with loose glenoid or humeral implants. Reconstruction of the glenoid to create a stable foundation for the glenoid implant is essential. If a stable foundation cannot be obtained, structural bone grafting should be performed without glenoid implantation. Humeral bone defects are less common, but the surgeon should be prepared to manage humeral bone loss at the time of revision surgery. Techniques that can be used in patients with substantial humeral bone loss include revision with an allograft prosthesis composite or an endoprosthesis.

 ## Bibliography

Antuna SA, Sperling JW, Cofield RH, Rowland CM: Glenoid revision surgery after total shoulder arthroplasty. *J Shoulder Elbow Surg* 2001;10(3):217-224.

Bonnevialle N, Melis B, Neyton L, et al: Aseptic glenoid loosening or failure in total shoulder arthroplasty: Revision with glenoid reimplantation. *J Shoulder Elbow Surg* 2013;22(6):745-751.

Cheung EV, Sperling JW, Cofield RH: Revision shoulder arthroplasty for glenoid component loosening. *J Shoulder Elbow Surg* 2008;17(3):371-375.

Cil A, Veillette CJ, Sanchez-Sotelo J, Sperling JW, Schleck CD, Cofield RH: Survivorship of the humeral component in shoulder arthroplasty. *J Shoulder Elbow Surg* 2010;19(1):143-150.

Day JS, Lau E, Ong KL, Williams GR, Ramsey ML, Kurtz SM: Prevalence and projections of total shoulder and elbow arthroplasty in the United States to 2015. *J Shoulder Elbow Surg* 2010;19(8):1115-1120.

Deutsch A, Abboud JA, Kelly J, et al: Clinical results of revision shoulder arthroplasty for glenoid component loosening. *J Shoulder Elbow Surg* 2007;16(6):706-716.

Dines JS, Fealy S, Strauss EJ, et al: Outcomes analysis of revision total shoulder replacement. *J Bone Joint Surg Am* 2006;88(7):1494-1500.

Duquin TR, Sperling JW: Revision shoulder arthroplasty: How to manage the humerus? *Operative Techniques in Orthopedics* 2011;21(1):44-51.

Elhassan B, Ozbaydar M, Higgins LD, Warner JJ: Glenoid reconstruction in revision shoulder arthroplasty. *Clin Orthop Relat Res* 2008;466(3):599-607.

Franta AK, Lenters TR, Mounce D, Neradilek B, Matsen FA III: The complex characteristics of 282 unsatisfactory shoulder arthroplasties. *J Shoulder Elbow Surg* 2007;16(5):555-562.

Grosso MJ, Frangiamore SJ, Ricchetti ET, Bauer TW, Iannotti JP: Sensitivity of frozen section histology for identifying Propionibacterium acnes infections in revision shoulder arthroplasty. *J Bone Joint Surg Am* 2014;96(6):442-447.

Melis B, Bonnevialle N, Neyton L, et al: Glenoid loosening and failure in anatomical total shoulder arthroplasty: Is revision with a reverse shoulder arthroplasty a reliable option? *J Shoulder Elbow Surg* 2012;21(3):342-349.

Neyton L, Walch G, Nové-Josserand L, Edwards TB: Glenoid corticocancellous bone grafting after glenoid component removal in the treatment of glenoid loosening. *J Shoulder Elbow Surg* 2006;15(2):173-179.

Norris TR, Kelly JD, Humphrey CS: Management of glenoid bone defects in revision shoulder arthroplasty: A new application of the reverse total shoulder prosthesis. *Techniques in Shoulder & Elbow Surgery* 2007;8:37-46.

Papadonikolakis A, Neradilek MB, Matsen FA III: Failure of the glenoid component in anatomic total shoulder arthroplasty: A systematic review of the English-language literature between 2006 and 2012. *J Bone Joint Surg Am* 2013;95(24):2205-2212.

Phipatanakul WP, Norris TR: Treatment of glenoid loosening and bone loss due to osteolysis with glenoid bone grafting. *J Shoulder Elbow Surg* 2006;15(1):84-87.

Pottinger P, Butler-Wu S, Neradilek MB, et al: Prognostic factors for bacterial cultures positive for Propionibacterium acnes and other organisms in a large series of revision shoulder arthroplasties performed for stiffness, pain, or loosening. *J Bone Joint Surg Am* 2012;94(22):2075-2083.

Raiss P, Bruckner T, Rickert M, Walch G: Longitudinal observational study of total shoulder replacements with cement: Fifteen to twenty-year follow-up. *J Bone Joint Surg Am* 2014;96(3):198-205.

Rodosky MW, Weinstein DM, Pollock RG, Flatow EL, Bigliani LU, Neer CS II: Abstract: On the rarity of glenoid component failure. *J Shoulder Elbow Surg* 1995;4(suppl 1):S13-S14.

Scalise JJ, Iannotti JP: Bone grafting severe glenoid defects in revision shoulder arthroplasty. *Clin Orthop Relat Res* 2008;466(1):139-145.

Schubkegel TA, Kwon YW, Zuckerman JD: Analysis of intermediate outcomes of glenoid bone grafting in revision shoulder arthroplasty. *Am J Orthop (Belle Mead NJ)* 2014;43(5):216-219.

Singh JA, Sperling JW, Cofield RH: Risk factors for revision surgery after humeral head replacement: 1,431 shoulders over 3 decades. *J Shoulder Elbow Surg* 2012;21(8):1039-1044.

Vavken P, Sadoghi P, von Keudell A, Rosso C, Valderrabano V, Müller AM: Rates of radiolucency and loosening after total shoulder arthroplasty with pegged or keeled glenoid components. *J Bone Joint Surg Am* 2013;95(3):215-221.

Wagner E, Houdek MT, Griffith T, et al: Glenoid bone-grafting in revision to a reverse total shoulder arthroplasty. *J Bone Joint Surg Am* 2015;97(20):1653-1660.

Chapter 40
One- and Two-Stage Revision of Infected Total Shoulder Arthroplasty

Lynn A. Crosby, MD

 Introduction

Infection is one of the most common complications following shoulder arthroplasty. The incidence is less than 2% in primary anatomic total shoulder arthroplasty patients and slightly more than 2% in primary reverse total shoulder arthroplasty patients. The infection rate increases to 2.8% in anatomic total shoulder arthroplasty patients and 4.7% in reverse total shoulder arthroplasty patients when the patient has had a previous orthopaedic procedure performed on the same shoulder.

Patients with infection commonly report pain. The physical signs of infection are difficult to differentiate from those of other causes of pain in arthroplasty patients, such as implant wear, aseptic loosening, and rotator cuff pathology. Laboratory data such as the erythrocyte sedimentation rate (ESR), C-reactive protein (CRP) level, white blood cell count, and interleukin-6 (IL-6) value provide helpful information when they are abnormal but frequently are normal. The diagnosis is more straightforward in the presence of swelling, erythema, or draining sinuses. Radiographic studies are helpful when obvious signs of loosening or osteolysis are present. Any implant with radiographic loosening should be considered infected until proven otherwise. Technetium Tc-99m bone scans and indium In-111–labeled leukocyte scintigraphy are not routinely used because the sensitivity and specificity of these tests make interpretation difficult. Aspiration of the joint perioperatively and intraoperatively is recommended. Arthroscopic evaluation and tissue biopsy may be beneficial when the distinction between septic and aseptic loosening remains unclear. Multiple intraoperative biopsies are recommended, including tissue samples obtained at the bone-implant interfaces. Any specimen that has five or more leukocytes per high-power field should typically be considered infected. In these patients, the surgeon should consider placing an antibiotic spacer and delaying the revision procedure.

 Case Presentation

A 65-year-old man undergoes anatomic total shoulder arthroplasty for the management of degenerative arthritis. His recovery is uneventful, and he returns to normal activity. Six months after the procedure, he starts having mild discomfort accompanied by swelling and erythema around the surgical site (**Figure 1**). Aspiration biopsy is performed in the clinic, but no fluid is obtained. Laboratory studies disclose the following values: ESR, 35 mm/h; CRP, 11 mg/L; and IL-6, 10 pg/mL. The wound is opened surgically, revealing purulent material (**Figure 2**). Cultures are obtained, and biopsy reveals 30 leukocytes per high-power field. The implants are removed, and cultures are obtained from the humerus and glenoid at the bone-implant interfaces (**Figure 3**). Extensive irrigation and débridement is performed, and a commercially available antibiotic spacer is placed (**Figure 4**). The wound is closed over a drain. The patient is started on intravenous vancomycin at the recommendation of an infectious disease specialist.

The cultures are positive on day 14 for *Propionibacterium acnes* sensitive to vancomycin. The IL-6 value is measured weekly and returns to normal 4 weeks after implant removal. The patient undergoes revision to a reverse ball-and-socket total shoulder arthroplasty 6 weeks after placement of the antibiotic spacer. At the time of the revision surgery, biopsies reveal less than five leukocytes per high-power field in five specimens. The patient remains on an oral antibiotic for 4 weeks after the revision surgery. Postoperative

Dr. Crosby or an immediate family member has received royalties from, is a member of a speakers' bureau or has made paid presentations on behalf of, serves as a paid consultant to, and has received research or institutional support from Exactech and serves as a board member, owner, officer, or committee member of the Accreditation Council for Graduate Medical Education and the American Academy of Orthopaedic Surgeons.

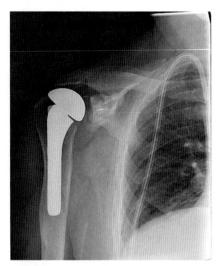

Figure 1 AP radiograph demonstrates anatomic total shoulder arthroplasty 6 months postoperatively. Swelling and erythema were noted on physical examination, and the patient reported pain.

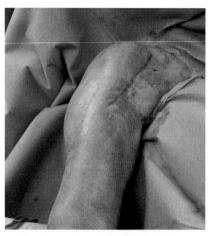

Figure 2 Intraoperative photograph shows the patient's shoulder draped free; obvious erythema and swelling are seen. (Reproduced from Crosby LA: Infected total shoulder arthroplasty: Two-stage revision, in Zuckerman JD, ed: *Advanced Reconstruction: Shoulder*. Rosemont, IL, American Academy of Orthopaedic Surgeons, 2007, pp 605-611.)

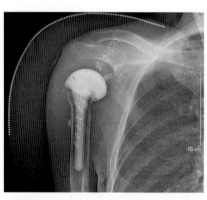

Figure 4 AP radiograph demonstrates placement of the antibiotic spacer.

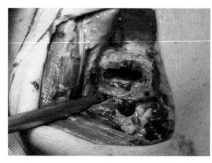

Figure 3 Intraoperative photograph shows the appearance of the surgical site after removal of the infected total shoulder arthroplasty implants. (Reproduced from Crosby LA: Infected total shoulder arthroplasty: Two-stage revision, in Zuckerman JD, ed: *Advanced Reconstruction: Shoulder*. Rosemont, IL, American Academy of Orthopaedic Surgeons, 2007, pp 605-611.)

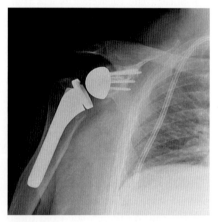

Figure 5 AP radiograph obtained after revision to reverse total shoulder arthroplasty.

rehabilitation is uneventful, and the patient remains infection free at 2-year follow-up (**Figure 5**).

 Indications

In patients with chronic infection, the goal of surgical treatment is to eradicate the infection and preserve as much function as possible. To accomplish this goal, the implants and all foreign material such as sutures and cement must be removed. In patients with long-standing infections and in patients with acute infections involving a gram-negative organism, placement of an antibiotic spacer after thorough débridement has been shown to have the best long-term results in eradicating the infection. The antibiotic spacer provides local antibiotic elution into surrounding tissue and helps support the soft-tissue envelope for later revision. A prefabricated antibiotic spacer provides a constant antibiotic elution, a smoother articular surface to prevent further bone destruction, and determined length and stem width. Consultation with an infectious disease specialist is

strongly recommended. After the causative organism has been identified and appropriate antibiotic treatment started, laboratory values can be monitored to determine when revision procedures can be safely performed. The IL-6 value, a marker of acute inflammation, has been shown to be a reliable indicator for use in the planning of revision surgery, whereas the ESR and CRP level tend to remain elevated for an extended period after an infection. Early removal of the antibiotic spacer results in a better

functional result. If the spacer is left in place for more than 100 days, the patient's pain level and functional result will be essentially the same as if the spacer were retained permanently. By monitoring the IL-6 value, the surgeon can determine when the inflammation has subsided. The IL-6 value drives the CRP level and ESR; the latter two values are much slower to return to normal. Early safe revision can provide results similar to those of the original arthroplasty; however, delaying revision may not be better than retaining the spacer because retaining the spacer may result in long-term problems similar to those seen after hemiarthroplasty, such as medial glenoid erosion and dislocation.

 ## Contraindications

Poor general medical condition of the patient is an absolute contraindication to surgical management of infected shoulder arthroplasty. Consultation with an infectious disease specialist is important in this difficult scenario. Aspiration and identification of the organism, followed by the use of suppressive antibiotics, although not ideal, may be the only treatment available for patients unable to undergo a procedure requiring general or regional anesthesia.

If the patient's medical condition improves such that he or she can tolerate anesthesia, the prosthesis can be removed and an articulating antibiotic spacer placed. Removal of the articulating spacer followed by revision total shoulder arthroplasty can then be done on an elective basis. Some patients, usually those who have low physical demands or poor general health, may prefer to avoid further surgical treatment and maintain the articulating antibiotic spacer permanently.

 ## Controversies and Alternative Approaches

Data regarding outcomes of débridement and retention of the prosthesis are limited. In patients with acute infection (3 to 6 weeks), an attempt to salvage the arthroplasty with thorough irrigation and débridement (with polyethylene exchange in reverse total shoulder arthroplasty patients) can be made. The technique can be successful, especially if the infecting organism is identified. Although no long-term outcome data are available, the author of this chapter considers this salvage technique to be a reasonable first-line approach. Removal of the polyethylene liner, when possible, allows exposure of more surface area for irrigation and débridement. After the débridement, a new polyethylene liner is placed. In anatomic total shoulder arthroplasty patients, the glenoid implant is often stabilized with cement and would be difficult to remove. In these patients, the polyethylene implant is usually left in place and not exchanged during the procedure.

A few reports of successful single-stage revision of infected total shoulder arthroplasty are available. These reports, however, are small case series; most of the literature suggests a high rate of recurrence of infection with this technique. Aspiration techniques and/or arthroscopic retrieval of cultures and biopsy specimens may be beneficial in identifying the organism before single-stage revision. If the organism cannot be identified before surgical intervention or if the organism is gram-negative, a two-stage procedure is recommended. *P acnes* is a common pathogen causing periprosthetic infections of the shoulder joint. It has unusual indolent growth characteristics that differ from those of other causative organisms such as staphylococcal or streptococcal species. *P acnes* generates little inflammation, grows slowly in the deep tissues, and avoids detection in standard wound cultures. The surgeon should request that cultures be placed on chocolate agar medium in an anaerobic environment and held for a minimum of 14 days. Removal of the implants, extensive débridement of all nonviable tissue, and placement of antibiotic-impregnated cement with revision of the implants is recommended. Knowledge of the infecting organism will dictate the antibiotic to be used in the cement. The wound should be closed over a drain and the appropriate antibiotic regimen prescribed at the recommendation of the infectious disease specialist. The antibiotic regimen should typically be continued until the IL-6 value has returned to normal and a decrease in CRP level and ESR is noted.

 ## Results

The goals of these revision procedures are to eradicate the infection and maintain as much pain-free function as possible. The recent increase in use of reverse total shoulder arthroplasty has led to improved function after revision surgery because a more aggressive initial surgical débridement that includes nonviable rotator cuff tissue can be performed in these patients. Most recurrent infections have been attributed to inadequate postoperative antibiotic treatment resulting from the inability to identify the organism. In nine studies involving 108 infected shoulders, the overall success rate was 91% with the use of a two-stage approach (**Table 1**).

 ## Technical Keys to Success in Two-Stage Revision

Stage 1
SETUP/EXPOSURE
- The patient is positioned in the modified beach-chair position (elevation of approximately 30°) with the entire involved upper extremity draped free.
- If the organism has not been identified preoperatively, the use of antibiotics should be delayed until tissue for culture, sensitivity testing, and histologic analysis has been obtained.
- An extended deltopectoral skin incision is made, incorporating the previous skin incision if possible. Care must be taken to excise all sinus tracts if present.
- The deltoid may be scarred from the previous procedure and must be protected. Palpation of the coracoid

Table 1 Infection Rates After Two-Stage Revision for the Management of Infected Shoulder Arthroplasty

Authors	Journal (Year)	Technique (No. of Patients)	Infection Rate (%)
Seitz and Damacen	*J Arthroplasty* (2002)	Anatomic TSA (8)	0
Mileti et al	*J Shoulder Elbow Surg* (2004)	Anatomic TSA (4)	0
Cuff et al	*J Bone Joint Surg Br* (2008)	Reverse TSA (12)	0
Strickland et al	*J Bone Joint Surg Br* (2008)	Anatomic TSA (19)	37
Coffey et al	*J Shoulder Elbow Surg* (2010)	Reverse TSA (10), anatomic TSA (2)	0
Jawa et al	*J Bone Joint Surg Am* (2011)	Reverse TSA (10), anatomic TSA (5)	13
Sabesan et al	*Clin Orthop Relat Res* (2011)	Reverse TSA (17)	6
Weber et al	*Int Orthop* (2011)	Reverse TSA (3), anatomic TSA (1)	0
Romanò et al	*Int Orthop* (2012)	Reverse TSA (13), anatomic TSA (4)	0

TSA = total shoulder arthroplasty.

process may aid in finding the deltopectoral interval.

- Adhesions in the subacromial space and subdeltoid bursae are released to help protect and mobilize the deltoid.
- The axillary nerve will be difficult to identify as a result of scarring. Care must be taken to localize and protect this nerve during the dissection.
- The subscapularis is released and tagged.
- All remaining suture material is removed.
- The capsular tissue is removed, and sections are sent for immediate pathologic evaluation to determine the number of leukocytes per high-power field. Specimens must be obtained for culture and sensitivity testing throughout the procedure.
- Releases are performed along the humeral neck to enable adequate external rotation of the humerus to dislocate the implant.

INSTRUMENTS/EQUIPMENT/IMPLANTS REQUIRED

- Removal of the prosthesis, cement (if present), and all nonviable tissue is essential to ensure adequate débridement. If the implant

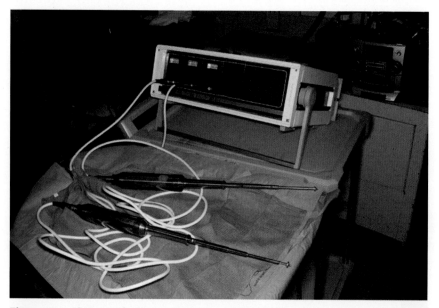

Figure 6 Photograph shows ultrasonic equipment for use in removal of humeral canal cement.

manufacturer is known, the surgeon can preorder specific instruments for removal.
- Ultrasonic cement removal equipment, handheld burrs, curets, and flexible osteotomes are helpful in extracting the implant and any retained cement (**Figures 6** and **7**). If the implant cannot be removed with this equipment, an extended humeral osteotomy or window will be necessary for extraction of the implant.

- An antibiotic spacer may be created by mixing antibiotics and cement on the back table and using a mold; however, commercially available antibiotic spacers have been shown to provide a more concentrated elution of antibiotics over an extended period (**Figure 8**).
- If the surgeon uses a mold to create the spacer, metal reinforcement should be used because the cement may break down if the spacer is left in place for an extended period.

PROCEDURE

- After adequate exposure has been obtained, the prosthetic humeral head is removed to allow visualization of the glenoid implant.
- Removal of the glenoid implant is usually not difficult and can be accomplished with a rongeur and/or osteotomes.
- All remnants of cement are removed from the vault of the glenoid. A handheld burr may be used for this removal.
- Tissue samples obtained at the glenoid bone-implant interface should be sent for culture and evaluation of the number of leukocytes per high-power field. Tissue from this location typically has the highest yield of positive cultures and needs to be obtained if at all possible.
- The humeral stem is removed with the manufacturer's recommended removal equipment if available; if such equipment is not available, standard revision instrumentation is used. If the humeral stem is well fixed, then the use of a needle-tipped burr around the implant can aid in the extraction.
- Osteotomy may be necessary in patients with well-fixed cemented implants. A straight longitudinal cut is made approximately 3 to 4 cm proximal to the tip of the distal cement plug. The cement mantle is loosened with a thin osteotome through the osteotomy site. This maneuver usually weakens the prosthesis-cement interface and/or the bone-cement interface.
- The prosthesis is removed using a bone tamp or the manufacturer's recommended instrumentation.
- Culture and biopsy specimens are obtained from the bone-implant interface.
- All cement, if present, is removed with the ultrasonic device.

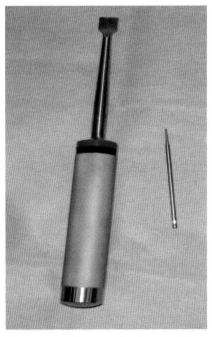

Figure 7 Photograph shows a bone tamp and a needle-tipped burr for use in implant removal.

Adequate irrigation must be used during this procedure to avoid overheating the bone. To avoid radial nerve injury, care must be taken not to penetrate the humerus during cement removal.

- The osteotomy is protected with heavy polydioxanone suture or cerclage wires.
- The wound is copiously irrigated with pulsatile lavage using antibiotic solution.
- A small amount of antibiotic-impregnated cement is used to form a collar for the spacer to sit on, and the spacer is placed. This cement also provides rotational stability.

WOUND CLOSURE

- A deep drain is placed in the glenohumeral joint space, and the deltopectoral interval is closed.
- If the rotator cuff tissue can be repaired, the repair is performed with the use of heavy monofilament suture.

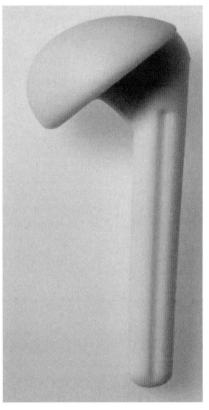

Figure 8 Photograph shows a commercially available articulating antibiotic spacer (Tecres [Verona, Italy]; distributed by Exactech).

- The deltopectoral interval is closed with monofilament suture.
- The skin is closed with a monofilament suture or skin staples.
- The shoulder is immobilized in a sling or immobilizer for comfort and wound support.

Stage 2

After the organism has been identified and the appropriate antibiotic regimen started, the patient's IL-6 value can be measured weekly to determine the timing of the second stage of the procedure. The second stage is typically performed approximately 4 to 8 weeks after the first stage.

SETUP/EXPOSURE

- Patient positioning is the same as in stage 1.

Table 2 Rehabilitation Protocol After One- or Two-Stage Revision Shoulder Arthroplasty

Postoperative Week	ROM	Strengthening	Return to Play	Comments/Emphasis
0-2	Passive ROM with the shoulder in forward flexion and external rotation Active hand, wrist, and elbow motion allowed	NA	NA	Drain removed when <20 mL of fluid is obtained in an 8-hr period Home antibiotic treatment with peripherally inserted central catheter line Patient uses sling for comfort during the day and pillow splint at night
2-6	Advance to passive/assist with pulleys and cane-assisted ROM	NA	At 4 wk, arm may be used for activities of daily living Lifting, pushing, or pulling activities should be avoided	Sling discontinued at 4 wk
6-12	Resistance exercises are begun	Resistance bands	NA	ROM and strengthening exercises are discontinued if they are painful
12-24	Normal activities of daily living	Continue resistance	As tolerated	Activity level is dictated by the presence or absence of pain

NA = not applicable, ROM = range of motion.

- The same skin incision is used as in the first stage of the procedure.
- All remnants of monofilament suture material and scar tissue are removed.

INSTRUMENTS/EQUIPMENT/IMPLANTS REQUIRED

- In most patients, reconstruction of the rotator cuff tissue is not possible, and the use of a reverse total shoulder arthroplasty prosthesis will be required.

PROCEDURE

- The antibiotic spacer is removed.
- Extensive irrigation and débridement is performed.
- The canals are dried using sponge packing and long suction tips.
- Bone grafting of the glenoid vault is performed if necessary.
- The humeral implant is placed. The use of an organism-specific antibiotic cement is recommended.

WOUND CLOSURE

- A drain is placed.
- The wound is closed in standard fashion.
- The shoulder is placed in a sling or immobilizer for 3 to 4 weeks for comfort.

 Rehabilitation

After the first stage of the procedure, the drain is kept in place until less than 20 mL of fluid is obtained in an 8-hour period. A peripherally inserted central catheter line usually is placed on postoperative day 2 for home intravenous antibiotic treatment. Physical therapy begins on day 2 with passive range of motion with the shoulder in forward flexion and external rotation. Active hand, wrist, and elbow motion are allowed with no restrictions. The patient wears a sling for comfort during the day and a pillow splint at night. At 4 weeks the sling may be discontinued during the day and the arm used for activities of daily living; however, lifting, pushing, or pulling activities should be avoided. The rehabilitation protocol is summarized in **Table 2**.

Avoiding Pitfalls

Careful handling of the deltoid during débridement and removal of the infected prosthesis is critical. If the deltoid or axillary nerve is injured, arthrodesis will be required. Removal of all cement and nonviable tissue is essential to eradicate the infection after the stage 1 débridement and to prevent recurrence of infection after the stage 2 reconstruction. Obtaining the appropriate cultures at the bone-implant interfaces and requesting placement of the specimens on chocolate agar in an anaerobic environment for a minimum of 3 weeks will help identify *P acnes* as a causative organism.

Bibliography

Coffey MJ, Ely EE, Crosby LA: Treatment of glenohumeral sepsis with a commercially produced antibiotic-impregnated cement spacer. *J Shoulder Elbow Surg* 2010;19(6):868-873.

Crosby LA, ed: *Total Shoulder Arthroplasty.* Rosemont, IL, American Academy of Orthopaedic Surgeons, 2000, pp 39-46.

Cuff DJ, Virani NA, Levy J, et al: The treatment of deep shoulder infection and glenohumeral instability with debridement, reverse shoulder arthroplasty and postoperative antibiotics. *J Bone Joint Surg Br* 2008;90(3):336-342.

Florschütz AV, Lane PD, Crosby LA: Infection after primary anatomic versus primary reverse total shoulder arthroplasty. *J Shoulder Elbow Surg* 2015;24(8):1296-1301.

Gorman MT, Crosby LA: Treatment of deep infection after total shoulder arthroplasty with an antibiotic spacer. *Techniques in Shoulder and Elbow Surgery* 2006;7(2):82-85.

Hackett DJ Jr, Crosby LA: Evaluation and treatment of the infected shoulder arthroplasty. *Bull Hosp Jt Dis (2013)* 2013;71(suppl 2):88-93.

Jawa A, Shi L, O'Brien T, et al: Prosthesis of antibiotic-loaded acrylic cement (PROSTALAC) use for the treatment of infection after shoulder arthroplasty. *J Bone Joint Surg Am* 2011;93(21):2001-2009.

Mileti J, Sperling JW, Cofield RH: Reimplantation of a shoulder arthroplasty after a previous infected arthroplasty. *J Shoulder Elbow Surg* 2004;13(5):528-531.

Romanò CL, Borens O, Monti L, Meani E, Stuyck J: What treatment for periprosthetic shoulder infection? Results from a multicentre retrospective series. *Int Orthop* 2012;36(5):1011-1017.

Sabesan VJ, Ho JC, Kovacevic D, Iannotti JP: Two-stage reimplantation for treating prosthetic shoulder infections. *Clin Orthop Relat Res* 2011;469(9):2538-2543.

Seitz WH Jr, Damacen H: Staged exchange arthroplasty for shoulder sepsis. *J Arthroplasty* 2002;17(4 suppl 1):36-40.

Singh JA, Sperling JW, Schleck C, Harmsen WS, Cofield RH: Periprosthetic infections after total shoulder arthroplasty: A 33-year perspective. *J Shoulder Elbow Surg* 2012;21(11):1534-1541.

Sperling JW, Kozak TK, Hanssen AD, Cofield RH: Infection after shoulder arthroplasty. *Clin Orthop Relat Res* 2001;(382):206-216.

Strickland JP, Sperling JW, Cofield RH: The results of two-stage re-implantation for infected shoulder replacement. *J Bone Joint Surg Br* 2008;90(4):460-465.

Weber P, Utzschneider S, Sadoghi P, Andress HJ, Jansson V, Müller PE: Management of the infected shoulder prosthesis: A retrospective analysis and review of the literature. *Int Orthop* 2011;35(3):365-373.

Chapter 41

Revision of Total Shoulder Arthroplasty to Reverse Total Shoulder Arthroplasty

Ryan M. Carr, MD

Yousef Shishani, MD

Janice Flocken, BA, MS

Reuben Gobezie, MD

 ## Case Presentation

A 62-year-old woman who underwent repair of her right rotator cuff was treated with total shoulder arthroplasty (TSA) on that same shoulder 15 months later. Both procedures were performed at an outside facility. After the TSA procedure, she experienced pain localized to her right shoulder. She describes this pain as achy in nature and aggravated with activities of daily living. She cannot dress herself and has nocturnal pain that prevents her from sleeping. The pain at night is constant; however, during the day the pain occurs with activities such as lifting, pulling, and pushing. The patient also has weakness in the shoulder. Physical therapy does not provide substantial relief.

Physical examination elicits passive forward elevation of 110°, active forward elevation of 110°, external rotation of 20°, and internal rotation to L5. Results of the Hawkins, O'Brien, and empty can tests are positive, whereas those of the Speed and belly-press tests are negative. Muscle strength is graded as 4 on forward elevation, 5 on internal rotation, and 4 on abduction.

Radiographs demonstrate a high-riding humeral head (**Figure 1**). These findings are consistent with a rotator cuff tear that has resulted in pain and loss of function. Because prior rotator cuff repair failed, any subsequent attempts likely will be unsuccessful. The rotator cuff tear is considered massive because of the superior migration of the humeral head. The patient undergoes revision to reverse total shoulder arthroplasty (RTSA; **Figure 2**).

 ## Indications

In patients with massive rotator cuff tear and failed TSA, such as in the case presented in this chapter, the options are to revise the prosthesis to a customized hemiarthroplasty or to convert to an RTSA. Multiple studies have evaluated the efficacy of these procedures, and although complication rates are higher after revision procedures than after primary arthroplasty, patient outcomes and satisfaction are better after RTSA.

 ## Controversies, Alternative Approaches, and Results

In patients with substantial medical comorbidities or deficient bone stock, salvage procedures, such as specialized hemiarthroplasty, arthrodesis, or resection arthroplasty, may be considered. However, these procedures do not reliably alleviate pain or restore function. If possible, revision arthroplasty should be performed. In patients with well-fixed humeral implants that are not easily removed using a circumferential release, osteotomies may help loosen the stem.

One study describes an alternative to vertical humeral osteotomy in which well-fixed humeral implants are removed with the use of an anterior or medial cortical window. At the conclusion of the procedure, the cortical piece

Dr. Gobezie or an immediate family member has received royalties from Arthrex; is a member of a speakers' bureau or has made paid presentations on behalf of Arthrex; serves as a paid consultant to Arthrex and Tornier; and serves as a board member, owner, officer, or committee member of the American Academy of Orthopaedic Surgeons, the American Shoulder and Elbow Surgeons, the Arthroscopy Association of North America, and the Orthopaedic Research and Education Foundation. None of the following authors nor any immediate family member has received anything of value from or has stock or stock options held in a commercial company or institution related directly or indirectly to the subject of this chapter: Dr. Carr, Dr. Shishani, and Ms. Flocken.

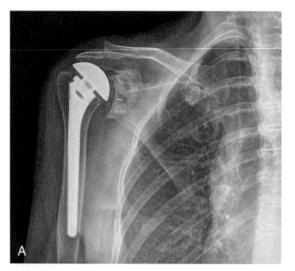
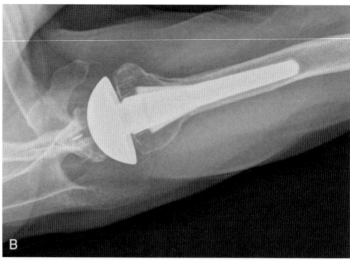

Figure 1 AP (**A**) and axillary (**B**) radiographs of a right shoulder demonstrate superior migration of the humeral head implant and no evidence of mechanical loosening.

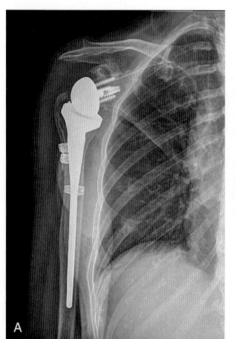
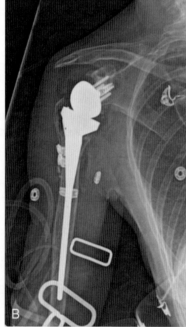

Figure 2 Postoperative AP (**A**) and axillary (**B**) radiographs of a right shoulder demonstrate revision from total shoulder arthroplasty to reverse shoulder arthroplasty.

In patients with glenoid bone loss or defects, bone grafting or augmentation has been described. In TSA, the results have been less than satisfactory, with reports of persistent instability and subluxation or glenoid loosening. The use of bone grafting in RTSA has demonstrated more successful outcomes, however. One study demonstrated no radiographic failure or graft resorption and noted improvements in all postoperative outcome measures.

Studies of the conversion of failed TSA to RTSA are summarized in **Table 1**.

 Video 41.1 Revision Total Shoulder Arthroplasty to Reverse Total Shoulder Arthroplasty. Reuben Gobezie, MD; Yousef Shishani, MD (9 min)

 Technical Keys to Success

Setup/Exposure

- The patient is placed in the beach-chair position with the medial border of the scapula overhanging the edge of the surgical table. This position allows for extension

is fixed using a heavy No. 5 suture, a cable or wire, or screws. In a series of 20 patients, 4 patients sustained intraoperative fractures (three humeral shaft fractures and one greater tuberosity fracture), and 17 patients demonstrated radiographic union. With limited radiographic follow-up, the remaining three patients demonstrated either incomplete healing or absence of healing. In comparison, a study of vertical humeral osteotomy reported no perioperative or postoperative fractures or instances of instability. All stems were cemented in place, and no cement extravasation was observed in the diaphyseal region.

Table 1 Results of Conversion of Failed Total Shoulder Arthroplasty to Reverse Total Shoulder Arthroplasty

Authors	Journal (Year)	Technique	Outcomes[a]	Complications	Comments
Van Thiel et al	*J Shoulder Elbow Surg* (2011)	Vertical humeral osteotomy	VAS score, 1.3 ASES score, 64.7 SST score, 6.3	None	No intraoperative diaphyseal or metaphyseal fractures, radiographic lucencies at the implant-cement interface, extruded cement in the diaphyseal region, or periprosthetic fractures
Johnston et al	*J Shoulder Elbow Surg* (2012)	Longitudinal split osteotomy	VAS score improved from 7.8 to 2.3 ASES score improved from 19.6 to 58.9 SST score improved from 1.4 to 4.6 FF improved from 60.6° to 89.4° External rotation improved from 24.4° to 40°	1 infection	No intraoperative fractures or postoperative nerve palsies No radiographic evidence of humeral loosening or periprosthetic fractures at latest follow-up Study authors concluded that longitudinal split osteotomy is safe and effective in the removal of well-fixed humeral implants
Patel et al	*J Shoulder Elbow Surg* (2012)	Humerus: retention of humeral stem, circumferential loosening of proximal cement/bone interface with thin osteotomies, or anterior corticotomy Glenoid: bone grafting (tibial plateau graft or cancellous bone chips)	SST score improved from 1.5 to 7.6 VAS score improved from 7.0 to 2.6 UCLA score improved from 7.4 to 23.5 ASES score improved from 24 to 66.2 FF improved from 44° to 108°	1 Vancouver type B fracture resulting from a fall at 5 mo 1 patient had persistent instability with anterosuperior dislocation 1 infection	Study authors concluded that patients can expect improved functional outcomes and decreased pain

ASES = American Shoulder and Elbow Surgeons shoulder outcome, FF = forward flexion, RTSA = reverse total shoulder arthroplasty, SST = Simple Shoulder Test, SSV = Subjective Shoulder Value, UCLA = University of California Los Angeles–Shoulder Rating Scale, VAS = visual analog scale.
[a] All outcomes are mean values unless otherwise noted.

and adduction of the arm during dislocation.

- The arm is secured with a mechanical arm holder (**Figure 3, A**).
- Multiple approaches have been described for shoulder arthroplasty; however, the authors of this chapter prefer the deltopectoral approach (**Figure 3, B**).
- The previous skin incision should be used or incorporated if possible to decrease the risk of skin necrosis.

Procedure
- The interval between the deltoid and the pectoralis major is developed using sharp dissection. Care is taken not to jeopardize the cephalic vein; however, inadvertent damage rarely results in adverse outcomes. Blunt dissection often is made difficult by the abundance of scar tissue and lack of tissue planes.
- After the interval is developed, the patient's arm is moved into 90° of abduction.

- A blunt rake is used to retract the deltoid muscle superiorly. Adhesions often are present in the subdeltoid space, and this interval should be developed posterior to the greater tuberosity (**Figure 4, A**). Care is taken not to disturb the axillary nerve, which runs on the undersurface of the deltoid muscle. Failure to develop the subdeltoid space both posteriorly and superiorly will make it difficult to obtain adequate exposure of the humeral

Table 1 Results of Conversion of Failed Total Shoulder Arthroplasty to Reverse Total Shoulder Arthroplasty (*continued*)

Authors	Journal (Year)	Technique	Outcomes[a]	Complications	Comments
Walker et al	*J Shoulder Elbow Surg* (2012)	Humerus: circumferential loosening or linear corticotomy Glenoid: easy removal of loose glenoid components or removal of well-fixed glenoid components with osteotomes or small oscillating saw	VAS score improved from 5 to 1.5 ASES score improved from 38.5 to 67.5 SST score improved from 1 to 5 FF improved from 50° to 130° External rotation improved from 12.5° to 49.5°	Complications occurred in 5 patients (22.7%): 1 scapular spine fracture resulting from a fall; 1 dislocation at 5 wk, postoperatively managed with closed reduction; 1 patient had persistent glenoid-sided loosening; 1 patient had implant loosening secondary to residual infection; and 1 patient had grade 4 scapular notching associated with glenoid loosening	Effective at reducing pain and improving function Complication rate is higher than in primary RTSA
Black et al	*J Shoulder Elbow Surg* (2014)	RTSA	SSV improved from 24% to 60% VAS score improved from 7.3 to 1.4 ASES score, 69.7 SST score, 58.8 FF, 115°	Major complications occurred in 6 patients (18.8%): 1 patient had instability, 1 patient had nerve injury, 2 patients had baseplate failure, 1 patient had hematoma, 1 patient underwent removal of painful screw in suprascapular notch Minor complications occurred in 3 patients (9.4%): 2 patients had acromial fractures, 1 patient had posterior rotator cuff deterioration requiring tendon transfer	78.1% of patients stated that they would undergo the procedure again Study authors concluded that revision RTSA is effective at improving function and reducing pain

ASES = American Shoulder and Elbow Surgeons shoulder outcome, FF = forward flexion, RTSA = reverse total shoulder arthroplasty, SST = Simple Shoulder Test, SSV = Subjective Shoulder Value, UCLA = University of California Los Angeles–Shoulder Rating Scale, VAS = visual analog scale.
[a] All outcomes are mean values unless otherwise noted.

head, which is paramount to humeral resection and revision.

- After the subdeltoid space is developed, a Browne retractor is inserted underneath the deltoid, and the arm is placed in approximately 30° of forward flexion and slight internal rotation (**Figure 4, B**).
- The conjoined tendon is identified and dissected along the lateral muscular border.

- After the interval between the conjoined tendon and the humerus is developed, a blunt Hohmann retractor is placed along the surgical neck (**Figure 4, C**).
- The subscapularis tendon is taken down with either a tenotomy or a peel technique and then tagged for later repair (**Figure 4, D**). The authors of this chapter prefer the peel technique to release the

subscapularis because the repair can be moved medially if there is substantial internal rotation contracture. However, if the subscapularis tendon is very attenuated or the internal rotation contracture is so severe that the subscapularis repair would be performed under tension, then the authors of this chapter prefer to release the subscapularis without repair.

- Care is taken not to dissect along the inferior portion of the humeral neck because of the proximity of the axillary nerve. Instead, the blunt Hohmann retractor is removed and a sharp Hohmann retractor is placed between the humeral neck and the subscapularis tendon. Retraction places the tissue under tension and can aid in tissue release.
- The humerus is moved into extension and adduction, resulting in anterior dislocation of the humeral head.
- The humeral head is extracted, and the stem is assessed for loosening (**Figure 4, E**). If the humeral or glenoid implant is sufficiently loose that suspicion for infection is high, then the authors of this chapter manage the shoulder as if there is primary infection. The published evidence suggests that intraoperative analysis of soft-tissue biopsies is not reliable for identifying infection. *Propionibacterium acnes*, the most common organism present in periprosthetic shoulder infections, is difficult to identify with intraoperative testing. If real-time polymerase chain reaction testing for *P acnes* or biomarker testing such as erythrocyte sedimentation rate, C-reactive protein level, white blood cell count, procalcitonin, tissue necrosis factor–α, and interleukin level is available at a surgeon's institution, then the authors of this chapter advocate routine use of such tests in the preoperative workup for all patients undergoing revision arthroplasty.
- If the stem is not loose, a revision humeral neck cut is performed to reveal the superior aspect of the stem (**Figure 4, F** and **G**).
- An osteotome or burr is used around the periphery of the stem to help loosen the stem. Stem disimpaction must be done carefully; the use of

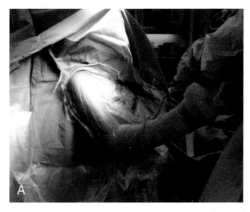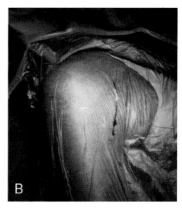

Figure 3 Intraoperative photographs show placement of the affected arm in an arm holder in slight forward flexion and external rotation (**A**) and marking of the deltopectoral approach (**B**).

too much force can fracture the humerus. A controlled osteotomy, as demonstrated in the video that accompanies this chapter, should be performed to remove the stem if it cannot be extracted using reasonable force. If the stem cannot be removed with minimal disruption to the proximal humerus bone stock, an osteotomy should be done. This technique is especially important in managing well-fixed press-fit stems, proximal porous-coated stems, and press-fit stems that are cemented in the humerus. The osteotomy should be made lateral to the bicipital groove and between the insertions of the pectoralis major and the deltoid (**Figure 4, H**). The osteotomy should not extend below the tip of the prosthesis. The authors of this chapter never use cortical windows in the extraction of humeral stems.

- An envelope is developed, and the stem is freed (**Figure 4, I**). The decision to perform an osteotomy should not be made before the entire trunnion of the humerus has been exposed anteriorly, laterally, medially, and posteriorly. Exposing the proximal aspect of the implant breaks the bond between the stem and the humerus. In patients with cemented stems, the cement

is removed. After the surgeon has cleared the trunnion and has failed to disimpact the prosthesis using reasonable force, humeral osteotomy is indicated.

- Humeral osteotomy begins with identifying the bicipital groove. Using a saw, the humerus is split between the insertion of the pectoralis major tendon and the deltoid. The length of the osteotomy along the groove is decided based on radiographic visualization and the design of prosthesis being extracted. Often, the osteotomy extends only to the point at which the coating of that particular stem ends. After the osteotomy is performed, sharp 0.25-inch osteotomes, both curved and straight, are used around the prosthesis to disrupt the ingrowth of bone onto or into the stem.
- To avoid unnecessary fractures, universal extractors may be used after the tuberosities are freed.
- If a cement mantle is present, some of it may be removed. However, in the absence of infection, removing the entire mantle is unnecessary. Instead, a new stem may be cemented into the old mantle and secured with cerclage cables. After the osteotomy has been performed and the stem has been removed, provisional fixation of the

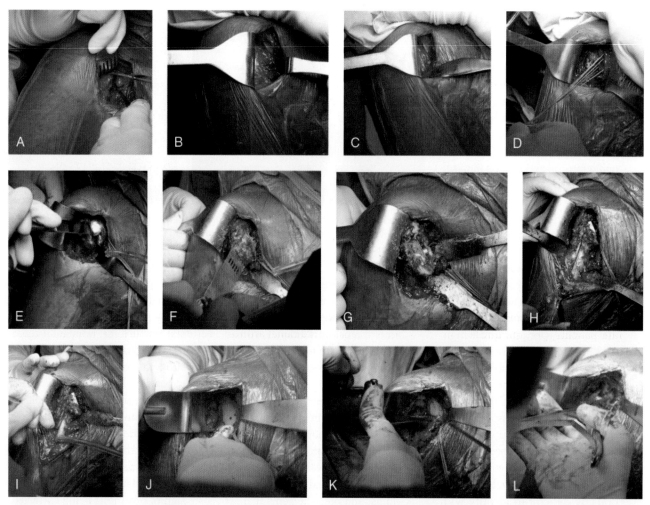

Figure 4   Intraoperative photographs of a right shoulder show exposure and removal of a primary arthroplasty prosthesis. **A,** Adhesions are released from the subdeltoid space with the use of sharp dissection and a Cobb elevator. **B,** A Browne retractor is placed in the subdeltoid space for retraction, after which the interval between the conjoined tendon and the subscapularis is developed. **C,** A blunt Hohmann retractor is placed along the surgical neck. **D,** The subscapularis tendon is taken down and tagged for later repair. **E,** The humeral head is removed. **F,** An oscillating saw is used to expose the proximal aspect of the stem. **G,** Stem extraction is attempted. **H,** An osteotomy is performed, and the original incision is extended distally to aid in stem extraction. **I,** The stem is freed with the use of an osteotome. **J,** A Fukuda retractor and an anterior glenoid retractor are used to expose the glenoid. **K,** Using an oscillating saw, the glenoid is scored in a cross fashion to facilitate removal. **L,** The polyethylene is removed with the use of a rongeur.

humerus along with use of polyethylene cables that enable the surgeon to provisionally tighten the cables, loosen them, and then definitively tension them at the end of the procedure is recommended. Cabling aids fixation of the long stem past the site of the osteotomy. At least two cables are recommended for osteotomies that extend below the meta-diaphysis of the humerus. If the osteotomy is extensive and reaches past the

spiral groove, then dissecting the radial nerve at the level of the osteotomy or distally between the brachialis and the brachioradialis, and following its course to the level at which the cables are passed should be accomplished.

- To expose the glenoid, the patient's arm is placed in an abducted and externally rotated position. The humerus rests along the posterior margin of the glenoid.
- If the posterior capsule is taut, the

use of a Fukuda retractor may facilitate exposure.

- An anterior glenoid retractor is placed beneath the lip of the anterior glenoid to help keep the capsule and subscapularis tendon out of the surgical field (**Figure 4, J**).
- If a vertical humeral osteotomy is not performed, a rongeur may be necessary during preparation for drilling and reaming to remove a small lip in the humeral neck to allow direct access to the glenoid.

If this lip is not removed, the position of the humerus may cause the surgeon to work anteriorly, leading to poor socket position.

- If there is an existing glenoid component that requires removal, it can be scored with an oscillating saw and removed with a rongeur (**Figure 4, K** and **L**). The surgeon must then assess the remaining glenoid for suitability for a revision implant. In patients in whom sufficient glenoid stock exists to enable implantation of a glenosphere, the surgeon may proceed to revision to RTSA. If glenoid stock is insufficient, the surgeon may use bone graft for later staged revision, proceed to a revision hemiarthroplasty, or, in rare patients, perform a resection arthroplasty.

- After the glenoid has been managed, the humerus is reamed and broached as necessary. The stem is inserted, and the version is assessed with the use of the alignment rod (**Figure 5, A**). In revision surgeries, the stem is placed in at least 30° of retroversion to balance the common occurrence of relative glenoid anteversion to capture the central screw or fix the baseplate between the "tables" of the scapular body.

- Cerclage cables are passed around the corticotomy and secured in place (**Figure 5, B, C, and D**). Prophylactic antibiotic cement is recommended in all revision surgeries.

- Stability can be assessed during the trial stage. The most important maneuver for assessing stability in reverse arthroplasty is checking adduction in hyperextension with external rotation to evaluate for decoaptation. Typically, instability is caused by lack of deltoid tension or version mismatch between the glenoid component and the humeral stem. Lack of deltoid tension is managed by increasing the size of the polyethylene insert. Version

mismatch is more difficult to manage. In some patients, stability can be achieved by increasing tension with or without a constrained liner. If stability cannot be achieved with these steps, however, the stem or glenoid component must be revised. Version mismatch should not be managed by increasing tension and using larger spacers because doing so results in problems with soft-tissue balancing, often resulting in a stiff shoulder (**Figure 5, E**).

Wound Closure

- Wound closure is typically accomplished in layers.
- Repair of the subscapularis is controversial in the setting of RTSA, but is critical if traditional arthroplasty is accomplished.
- Subcutaneous tissues and skin are closed and dressed in a sterile manner.
- While the patient is in the operating room, the affected shoulder is fitted with a cryotherapy device and a sling.

 Rehabilitation

The rehabilitation protocol is summarized in **Table 2**. Immediately postoperatively and continuing for 2 weeks postoperatively, the arm is protected in a sling. During that period, the sling is removed for elbow, wrist, and hand range of motion (ROM) exercises. After 2 weeks, sling use is discontinued and return to sedentary work is allowed with the arm protected at the side. Passive ROM exercises are initiated, with forward flexion to 160°, internal rotation to L5, gentle stretching, and pendulum/Codman exercises. Three weeks postoperatively, active ROM exercises are started, with forward flexion to 150° and internal rotation to L5. Physical therapy is discontinued after full and fluid active ROM is achieved. Light-duty work

is allowed 6 weeks postoperatively, and strengthening is achieved in the course of light work activities and activities of daily living. Twenty-six weeks postoperatively, restrictions on work are lifted, and the patient is allowed to return to sports participation.

 Avoiding Pitfalls

Complication rates are higher after revision shoulder arthroplasty than after primary shoulder arthroplasty. Complications include instability or dislocation, infection, humeral shaft fracture during implant removal, glenoid fracture or loosening, musculocutaneous or radial nerve palsy, symptomatic hardware, and acromial fracture. Knowledge of these potential complications can help minimize them.

Proximal bone loss can occur as the result of infection or during revision surgery and implant removal. In the proximal humerus, substantial bone loss can result in implant loosening and instability because of a lack of soft-tissue tension or soft-tissue attachment. If necessary, augmentation of the proximal humerus with an allograft composite may be beneficial. The composite provides multiple advantages. It helps increase stability by decreasing stress on the implant. It also increases bone stock, which is helpful should a subsequent procedure become necessary. It restores height and offset, which helps appropriately tension the deltoid muscle. Finally, it contains a subscapularis tendon that may be used for soft-tissue repair, thereby increasing stability and internal rotation strength.

Glenoid bone loss can result in glenoid baseplate loosening. In patients who have severe glenoid bone loss, delayed reimplantation may be preferred. In this scenario, the glenoid is grafted with the use of autologous bone graft. The humeral stem is not placed until the graft incorporates, after which

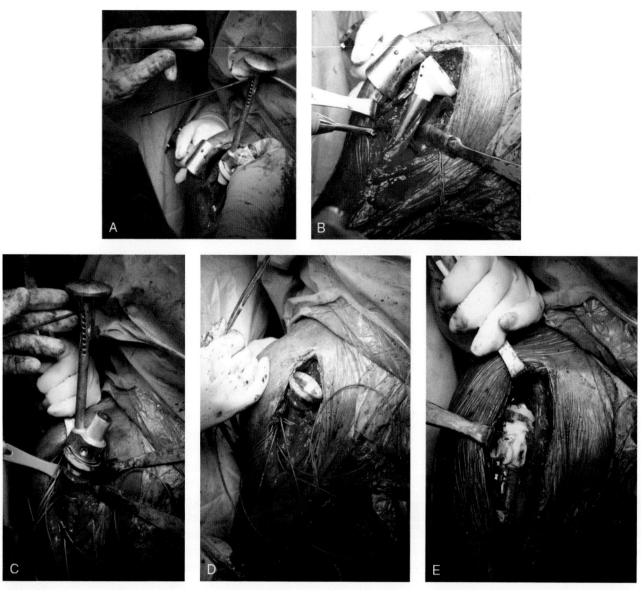

Figure 5   Intraoperative photographs of a right shoulder show placement of a reverse shoulder arthroplasty prosthesis. **A,** An alignment rod is used to assess the version of the stem. **B,** The osteotomy is secured with the use of cerclage cables. **C,** Stem version is reassessed. **D,** A trial implant is placed. **E,** The stem is reduced. Any gaps between the osteotomy and the stem can be augmented with cement.

time revision to RTSA is performed. In patients in whom glenoid bone loss is less severe, glenoid grafting may be performed at the time of the revision surgery. Most cavitary defects can be treated with a single-stage procedure. However, patients who have severe segmental defects may require a two-stage approach. Whether to perform one- or two-stage reconstruction is dictated by the type of prosthesis (baseplate) being

implanted and surgeon experience with complex glenoid reconstruction.

Instability or dislocation is a substantial problem in revision surgery. Instability or dislocation can result from humeral retroversion, glenoid anteversion, or inadequate restoration of humeral height. In addition, superior placement of the glenoid baseplate can lead to glenoid notching and loosening. Remaining cognizant of implant

position and soft-tissue tension is paramount in avoiding this problem. The optimal version of the glenoid and humerus for reverse arthroplasty is somewhat controversial. For primary reverse arthroplasty, the authors of this chapter prefer to place the glenoid in neutral version, with a slight inferior tilt and approximately 30° of retroversion on the humerus. The deltoid tension in reverse arthroplasty should not be

Table 2 Rehabilitation Protocol After Revision From Total Shoulder Arthroplasty to Revision Total Shoulder Arthroplasty

Postoperative Week	ROM	Strengthening	Return to Work/Play	Comments/Emphasis
0-2	Elbow, wrist, and hand motion out of sling	None	None	The arm is protected in a sling
2-3	Passive ROM Forward flexion to 150° Internal rotation to L5 Gentle stretching Pendulum/Codman exercises	None	Sedentary work, arm protected at the side	Sling use is discontinued
3-6	Active ROM Forward flexion to 150° Internal rotation to L5	None	Sedentary work, arm protected at the side	Forward flexion in the scapular plane After full and fluid active ROM is achieved, physical therapy is discontinued
6-26	Resume normal daily activities	None	Light-duty work	Strengthening occurs through activities of daily living and light work activities
26	Resume normal daily activities May start lifting	None	No restrictions on work May return to sports	—

ROM = range of motion.

too tight; rather, it should enable supple movement of the shoulder in most planes.

Exposure is important in every surgical procedure. If the appropriate releases are not performed, overzealous retraction or improper placement of retractors can lead to postoperative palsy of the radial or musculocutaneous nerve.

The past decade has seen substantial advances in screening tools for indolent infections in patients undergoing revision arthroplasty. The traditional screening with white blood cell count and differential, C-reactive protein level, and erythrocyte sedimentation rate is not reliable in identifying preoperative infection. As a result, biomarkers with much greater sensitivity and specificity for indolent infections by organisms such as *P acnes* are being used. In the opinion of the authors of this chapter, the use of biomarker analysis for identifying infection is critical for enhancing detection of indolent infection in revision arthroplasty.

 ## Bibliography

Black EM, Roberts SM, Siegel E, Yannopoulos P, Higgins LD, Warner JJ: Reverse shoulder arthroplasty as salvage for failed prior arthroplasty in patients 65 years of age or younger. *J Shoulder Elbow Surg* 2014;23(7):1036-1042.

Chacon A, Virani N, Shannon R, Levy JC, Pupello D, Frankle M: Revision arthroplasty with use of a reverse shoulder prosthesis-allograft composite. *J Bone Joint Surg Am* 2009;91(1):119-127.

Dimmen S, Madsen JE: Long-term outcome of shoulder arthrodesis performed with plate fixation: 18 patients examined after 3-15 years. *Acta Orthop* 2007;78(6):827-833.

Gerber C, Pennington SD, Nyffeler RW: Reverse total shoulder arthroplasty. *J Am Acad Orthop Surg* 2009;17(5):284-295.

Hill JM, Norris TR: Long-term results of total shoulder arthroplasty following bone-grafting of the glenoid. *J Bone Joint Surg Am* 2001;83(6):877-883.

Johnston PS, Creighton RA, Romeo AA: Humeral component revision arthroplasty: Outcomes of a split osteotomy technique. *J Shoulder Elbow Surg* 2012;21(4):502-506.

Klein SM, Dunning P, Mulieri P, Pupello D, Downes K, Frankle MA: Effects of acquired glenoid bone defects on surgical technique and clinical outcomes in reverse shoulder arthroplasty. *J Bone Joint Surg Am* 2010;92(5):1144-1154.

Levy J, Frankle M, Mighell M, Pupello D: The use of the reverse shoulder prosthesis for the treatment of failed hemi-arthroplasty for proximal humeral fracture. *J Bone Joint Surg Am* 2007;89(2):292-300.

Muh SJ, Streit JJ, Lenarz CJ, et al: Resection arthroplasty for failed shoulder arthroplasty. *J Shoulder Elbow Surg* 2013;22(2):247-252.

Patel DN, Young B, Onyekwelu I, Zuckerman JD, Kwon YW: Reverse total shoulder arthroplasty for failed shoulder arthroplasty. *J Shoulder Elbow Surg* 2012;21(11):1478-1483.

Rice RS, Sperling JW, Miletti J, Schleck C, Cofield RH: Augmented glenoid component for bone deficiency in shoulder arthroplasty. *Clin Orthop Relat Res* 2008;466(3):579-583.

Sperling JW, Cofield RH: Humeral windows in revision shoulder arthroplasty. *J Shoulder Elbow Surg* 2005;14(3):258-263.

Topolski MS, Chin PY, Sperling JW, Cofield RH: Revision shoulder arthroplasty with positive intraoperative cultures: The value of preoperative studies and intraoperative histology. *J Shoulder Elbow Surg* 2006;15(4):402-406.

Van Thiel GS, Halloran JP, Twigg S, Romeo AA, Nicholson GP: The vertical humeral osteotomy for stem removal in revision shoulder arthroplasty: Results and technique. *J Shoulder Elbow Surg* 2011;20(8):1248-1254.

Walker M, Willis MP, Brooks JP, Pupello D, Mulieri PJ, Frankle MA: The use of the reverse shoulder arthroplasty for treatment of failed total shoulder arthroplasty. *J Shoulder Elbow Surg* 2012;21(4):514-522.

Wall B, Nové-Josserand L, O'Connor DP, Edwards TB, Walch G: Reverse total shoulder arthroplasty: A review of results according to etiology. *J Bone Joint Surg Am* 2007;89(7):1476-1485.

 ## Video Reference

Gobezie R, Shishani Y: Video. *Revision Total Shoulder Arthroplasty to Reverse Total Shoulder Arthroplasty.* Cleveland, OH, 2015.

Chapter 42

Management of Prosthetic Instability After Shoulder Arthroplasty

Brian Grawe, MD

Frank A. Cordasco, MD, MS

 ## Introduction

Instability after arthroplasty of the glenohumeral joint is a common complication that has been reported in up to 29% of patients. The etiology of the instability is often multifactorial, and instability can occur subsequent to humeral head replacement, anatomic total shoulder arthroplasty, and reverse shoulder arthroplasty. Instability can occur in the coronal or sagittal plane and can range in time of onset and severity from early acute subluxation to chronic fixed dislocation. The direction and timing of the episode of instability often plays a critical role in discerning the underlying origin of the dislocation and guiding the surgeon to the appropriate treatment pathway.

When evaluating a patient with an unstable shoulder prosthesis, the surgeon must consider all possible reasons for dislocation, which may include implant malposition, soft-tissue imbalance, rotator cuff deficiency, bone loss, function of the nerves about the shoulder, and septic failure. A comprehensive understanding of the potential causes of instability can help the surgeon avoid potential pitfalls at the time of the index arthroplasty and can aid in the effective management of postoperative instability. Treatment must address all the contributing factors that led to the instability, and the type of correction must be individualized to each patient. The authors of this chapter present a treatment algorithm for the unstable shoulder arthroplasty, with a focus on evaluation and management. The case presentation describes a previously reported complex clinical scenario, highlighting key features that must be addressed in the evaluation of a patient with an unstable prosthesis of the glenohumeral joint.

 ## Case Presentation

A 78-year-old woman with multiple medical comorbidities presents with an exposed prosthesis (**Figure 1**). She underwent cemented humeral head replacement at another institution 4 years previously for the management of a failed closed reduction and percutaneous pinning of a two-part proximal humerus fracture, for which she underwent revision osteosynthesis subsequent to the failed percutaneous pinning (tension-band wiring). The index hemiarthroplasty with a cemented stemmed humeral head implant was uneventful. Secure fixation of the greater and lesser tuberosities was achieved with the use of nonabsorbable sutures through the prosthesis and humeral shaft. The coracoacromial ligament was not resected at the time of the hemiarthroplasty. The patient's recovery after the hemiarthroplasty was complicated by range of motion (ROM) difficulties and shoulder weakness. The patient had concomitant deltoid atrophy that prompted electrodiagnostic testing 7 months postoperatively. These studies revealed brachial plexopathy of the superior trunk. One year after the hemiarthroplasty, the patient had persistent ROM difficulties, pain, and gradual prominence of the prosthesis as well as marked atrophy of the anterior deltoid. Physical examination demonstrated prosthetic instability, with anterosuperior dislocation of the hemiarthroplasty on active arm elevation. The prosthesis remained prominent and could be grossly visualized in a subcutaneous manner on dislocation. Radiographs revealed subluxation of the humeral head with migration in the anterosuperior direction and nonunion of the greater and lesser tuberosities; the prosthesis was otherwise well fixed.

Dr. Cordasco or an immediate family member has received royalties from Arthrex and ConMed Linvatec; serves as a paid consultant to or is an employee of Arthrex; and serves as a board member, owner, officer, or committee member of the American Academy of Orthopaedic Surgeons, the American Shoulder and Elbow Surgeons, and the American Orthopaedic Society for Sports Medicine. Neither Dr. Grawe nor any immediate family member has received anything of value from or has stock or stock options held in a commercial company or institution related directly or indirectly to the subject of this chapter.

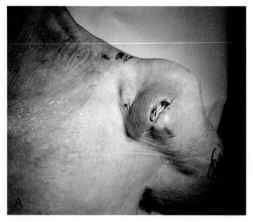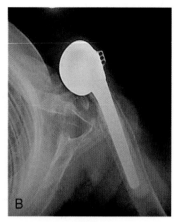

Figure 1   Clinical photograph (**A**) and AP radiograph (**B**) demonstrate severe antero-superior escape and subsequent fixed instability after hemiarthroplasty.

Surgical correction was considered at this time, and the option of reconstruction of the coracoacromial arch with revision fixation of the tuberosities, supplemented with pectoralis major transfer, was discussed with the patient. Fearing further complications, the patient elected nonsurgical treatment.

Two years later, the patient presented to the senior author of this chapter (F.A.C.) with an exposed prosthesis without antecedent trauma or drainage. She underwent hardware removal, resection arthroplasty, and irrigation and débridement, and the remnants of the rotator cuff were sutured directly to the humeral shaft. The patient was treated with a 6-week course of intravenous antibiotics because final cultures demonstrated growth of *Enterococcus faecalis* in the broth in one of four specimens. At 1-year follow-up, the patient had limited pain at rest and exhibited elevation to 70°.

The key findings of this complex case are the risks associated with the multiply-operated shoulder (infection and instability), the soft-tissue imbalance resulting from improper function of the rotator cuff, and the issues related to nerve injury and its effect on management options. This case demonstrates a calamitous example of anterosuperior instability. Although the patient initially opted for nonsurgical treatment, soft-tissue reconstruction was offered. This historical case represents an extreme outlier; currently, the patient would be treated with a reverse shoulder prosthesis.

 Indications

Anterior Instability

Anterior instability is most often the result of subscapularis tendon failure, anterior glenoid insufficiency, or incorrect anterior version of the humeral or glenoid implant. The etiologies of anterior instability often occur concomitantly and compound each other.

SOFT-TISSUE INSUFFICIENCY

Soft-tissue structures about the anterior aspect of the shoulder can become attenuated, torn, and eventually insufficient, leading to anterior instability. This type of instability can occur in patients with subscapularis ruptures, subscapularis insufficiency, and/or lesser tuberosity nonunion. These pathologies can occur on a spectrum, and treatment algorithms display substantial overlap.

Rupture of the subscapularis is a frequent cause of anterior shoulder instability after glenohumeral arthroplasty. Subscapularis rupture may occur for several reasons, including biologic failure of the repair (either failed tendon healing or nonunion of a lesser tuberosity osteotomy), poor tendon quality coupled with an inadequate repair, tendon dehiscence secondary to the use of an oversized humeral implant, excessive anterior placement of the humeral implant, glenoid implant anteversion in patients with eccentric anterior glenoid wear, and insufficient posterior capsular release resulting in soft-tissue imbalance.

The temporal sequence of the deficiency of the anterior structures must be thoroughly evaluated before surgical correction. Patients with a ruptured subscapularis that is identified in the early postoperative period may benefit from early soft-tissue repair alone. Failure is confirmed on clinical examination and evaluation of an axillary radiograph. Anterior reconstruction can involve transfer of a complete or partial (sternal head) pectoralis major tendon to allow dynamic control of the glenohumeral joint and static constraint control with the use of an allograft tendon. The goal and rationale of the muscle transfer is twofold: first, to restore active muscle power with the use of locally available healthy vascularized tissue, and second, to create a dynamic restraint for the prosthesis, thus preventing excessive anterior translation during ROM. For failures that are recognized within 3 to 6 weeks, primary repair is attempted. If the repair can be achieved with minimal to no tension, then neither allograft nor pectoralis tendon is used. Overall, the authors of this chapter recommend converting to a reverse shoulder arthroplasty if primary repair cannot be achieved. Tendon transfer and allograft reconstruction are options but are not the first line of treatment. Currently, the authors of this chapter do not recommend the use of any commercially available patches.

Soft-tissue reconstruction of the deficient coracoacromial arch can be accomplished with the aid of an allograft. Achilles tendon allograft with the attached bone plug offers the advantage of secure bony fixation of the graft onto the glenoid. Furthermore, the graft itself is typically long and broad, allowing for reconstruction of the anterior and superior capsule. This technique can be accomplished via a standard deltopectoral approach and exposure of the anterior neck of the glenoid. The bone plug of the Achilles tendon allograft is secured with a 3.5-mm screw and washer, after which the tendon is secured to the lesser tuberosity with the aid of small suture anchors. Ultimately, the tendon can be wrapped back around and oversewn to the bone plug. The superior portion of the tendon can also be secured to the supraspinatus in an attempt to re-create the static restraint of the coracoacromial arch. The combination of local tissue transfer and allograft reconstruction offers the benefit of biologic protection of the graft during its incorporation into the surrounding tissue. The authors of this chapter prefer to manage chronic anterosuperior instability with conversion to reverse shoulder arthroplasty because the results of soft-tissue reconstruction have been disappointing.

BONY INSUFFICIENCY

Anterior glenoid insufficiency is most commonly encountered in patients with rheumatoid arthritis or arthritis associated with recurrent dislocations of the shoulder. Conversely, if the bone loss is not addressed at the time of the index arthroplasty, the glenoid implant is at risk for being placed with an unacceptable amount of anterior version. Preoperative recognition of the phenomenon is paramount. Axillary radiographs and advanced osseous imaging (CT) are recommended. Management of bone loss depends on the amount of remaining viable bone stock. Eccentric posterior reaming is most commonly performed to treat asymmetric anterior wear. Advanced options include structural bone grafting or the use of a custom-designed

glenoid implant. Glenoid malpositioning resulting from excessive anteversion in the presence of native anterior glenoid insufficiency must be addressed with one of the previously mentioned strategies to eliminate anterior instability.

IMPLANT MALPOSITION

Excessive anteversion of either the humeral or glenoid implant can result in anterior instability after glenohumeral arthroplasty. Humeral anteversion alone is rarely the sole cause of anterior instability; however, it must be assessed at the time of revision surgery. With the advent of new humeral designs allowing for eccentric placement of the humeral head, anterior translation of the humeral head has become less common. Malposition of the glenoid often occurs in the presence of an unrecognized eccentric wear pattern. The surgeon must be mindful of the resulting combined version of both prosthetic components. The authors of this chapter recommend obtaining advanced three-dimensional imaging of the prosthetic components when malpositioning is suspected. The surgeon should also perform imaging studies of the contralateral side when necessary. The native humeral retroversion can range from 0° to 55°, whereas the natural retroversion of the glenoid is between 0° and 5°.

INFECTION

An infectious etiology must be considered in patients with prosthetic instability. Obtaining an accurate diagnosis can be challenging because indolent infections are often present. Appropriate evaluation includes laboratory studies (complete blood count, erythrocyte sedimentation rate, and C-reactive protein level) and the judicious use of fluid aspiration. If fluid aspiration is undertaken in either the office setting or the operative suite, consideration should be given to sending a portion of the sample for an α-defensin level test. Synovial fluid levels of α-defensin have recently been

demonstrated to have excellent sensitivity and specificity for diagnosis of prosthetic joint infection in the shoulder, hip, and knee. Its global and pervasive use should be balanced with cost, availability, and lack of longitudinal data; however, early results seem promising. Intraoperative tissue cultures have been shown to be effective and sensitive. Cultures must be held for 10 to 14 days to rule out indolent infection (*Propionibacterium acnes*).

NEUROLOGIC INJURY

Axillary nerve injury, as in the case presented previously herein, is devastating and frequently affects treatment options. The reverse shoulder arthroplasty design inherently allows for a semiconstrained joint that can compensate for any soft-tissue deficiencies leading to an unstable anatomic shoulder arthroplasty prosthesis. However, the success of the reverse shoulder arthroplasty hinges on the presence of a functioning deltoid without frank axillary nerve injury.

Posterior Instability

Posterior sagittal plane instability is most common in patients with an excessively loose posterior capsule (**Figure 2**). The posterior structures are often attenuated in patients with severe glenohumeral osteoarthrosis, and substantial wear of the posterior glenoid may be present, leading to translation of the humeral head. The morphologic characteristics of the glenoid and their relation to glenohumeral arthroplasty have received much attention in the recent literature. The Walch classification system is widely used, and the static position of the humeral head at the time of arthroplasty may affect the outcome. Other common causes include posterior rotator cuff deficiency and improper retroversion of the humeral or glenoid implant. Any of these etiologies can be further compounded by the internal rotation contracture with anterior capsular tightness that is often seen in

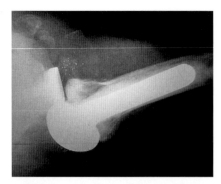

Figure 2 Axillary radiograph demonstrates posterior instability after total shoulder arthroplasty.

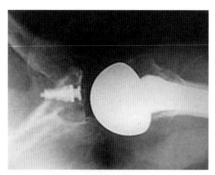

Figure 3 Axillary radiograph demonstrates posterior subluxation with resulting instability secondary to excessive retroversion of the glenoid implant.

patients with degenerative conditions of the shoulder.

Management of posterior instability is analogous to that of anterior instability. Soft-tissue balance is critical, and anterior capsular lengthening is necessary when inadequate soft-tissue balance contributes to excessive posterior subluxation. An appropriate release (anterior capsule from anterior glenoid with complete mobilization of the subscapularis) should be performed in a judicious manner, and in patients with limited external rotation, the subscapularis can be lengthened via recession off of the lesser tuberosity (medialized repair with suture anchors or bone tunnels) or Z-lengthening incorporating the capsule. Similarly, a patulous posterior capsule should be addressed with plication. The authors of this chapter prefer to use suture anchors in the glenoid after humeral head resection to achieve a true posterior capsulorrhaphy. Suture anchor fixation offers the advantage of osseous fixation; alternatively, the plication can be done with soft-tissue repair in a purse-string configuration. Anchor placement can be achieved before glenoid preparation with retraction of the osteotomized humeral head posteriorly. AP translation of 50%, measured on the basis of the width of the glenoid, is a reliable surrogate marker of physiologic intraoperative stability. After the joint is reduced and in neutral rotation,

the authors of this chapter also ensure that the center of the humeral head is pointed toward the center of the glenoid. Posterior bone wear should be addressed with eccentric reaming of the high side (anterior), which can reliably correct retroversion deficits of 10° to 15°. Larger bony voids must be filled with structural graft (allograft or autograft). The authors of this chapter prefer to use the resected humeral head or neck combined with interfragmentary compression screws or a custom glenoid implant. Grafting allows for excellent version correction without pathologic medialization of the joint. Bone voids in the glenoid can also be filled with augmented glenoid components. Many options exist when augmenting the glenoid with metal and are often produced specifically for the patient after obtaining a three-dimensional rendering of the entire scapula. Alternatively, conversion to reverse shoulder arthroplasty can be considered in patients with substantial bony architecture deficits, and some authors have advocated primary reverse shoulder arthroplasty in patients with glenoid morphology that could increase the risk of posterior instability.

Excessive retroversion of either the humeral or glenoid implant should be ruled out with imaging studies (**Figure 3**). Humeral heads with pathologic retroversion (greater than 40°) should be corrected with component revision.

Superior and Inferior Instability

Superior instability is included in the previous discussion of anterior instability, including the case presentation. Anterosuperior escape results from a deficient anterior rotator cuff with an absent coracoacromial arch. Reconstruction should occur in a stepwise manner, as previously outlined, or conversion to reverse total shoulder arthroplasty should be considered.

Inferior instability is often the direct result of prosthetic malpositioning or neurologic compromise, which must be ruled out. Specifically, inferior instability can occur after arthroplasty to manage a proximal humerus fracture when the humeral length is not adequately restored. Attention to soft-tissue tensioning and appropriate humeral head height (3 to 5 mm above the greater tuberosity) will help avoid this complication. In the management of inferior instability after shoulder arthroplasty, imaging of the contralateral extremity can help the surgeon identify the humeral length and bony architectural landmarks. Revision should include proper placement of the humeral implant with cement fixation or allograft when necessary. For patients in whom the greater tuberosity is no longer available as a reliable bony landmark because of fracture, revision surgery, or tumor, the authors of this chapter have found the superior insertion of the pectoralis major to be a valuable guide for determining appropriate prosthesis height.

Instability After Reverse Shoulder Arthroplasty

Reverse shoulder arthroplasty has become a viable option in the management of myriad shoulder pathologies, including failed shoulder arthroplasty. The understanding of the biomechanics and kinematics of the reverse design has greatly improved in the past decade; however, dislocation with subsequent instability remains a difficult clinical scenario for even the most experienced shoulder surgeon (**Figure 4**). Similar to instability after anatomic total shoulder arthroplasty, instability after reverse shoulder arthroplasty can be classified as early or late, and all associated contributing factors must be addressed to ensure successful management. Ruling out an infectious etiology is paramount because infection can be a contributing factor in up to 44% of early-onset instability cases. Appropriate tensioning of the deltoid myofascial sleeve is crucial to avoid postoperative instability and can be assessed with intraoperative monitoring of the tension placed on the conjoined tendon after implant reduction or via radiographic measurement of arm length. The authors of one study demonstrated that arm length templating based on the contralateral upper extremity can prove useful because shorter lengths of the humerus and arm were correlated with a higher incidence of postoperative instability. Repair of the subscapularis remains controversial. Some studies have shown that an intact tendon leads to lower rates of instability; however, anecdotally, many surgeons do not repair the tendon because they do not believe that it aids in stability. However, the authors of this chapter routinely repair the subscapularis after reverse shoulder arthroplasty, when possible. Other authors recommend a superior (transdeltoid) approach to avoid violation of the subscapularis; the authors of this chapter prefer not to use this approach because of the risk of erroneous tilt of the glenoid implant or superior placement.

If global decoaptation (that is, the absence of coaptation of the glenoid and humeral components) is the source of the instability, tension must be increased through surgical means. Strategies include increasing the diameter of the glenosphere, increasing the thickness of the polyethylene cup, placing a humeral neck extension beneath the humeral cup, and using a more constrained polyethylene cup. However, these strategies

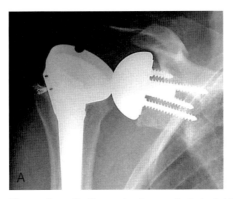
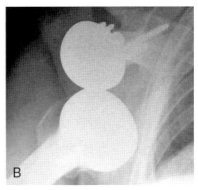

Figure 4   Radiographs demonstrate instability after reverse shoulder arthroplasty in two different patients. **A,** AP radiograph demonstrates superior placement and superior tilt of the glenoid baseplate, which may have contributed to the instability. **B,** Axillary radiograph demonstrates excessive anteversion of the glenosphere, which can result in anterior instability of the prosthesis.

must be used with caution because overtensioning of the deltoid can result in fractures of the acromion or neurapraxia of the brachial plexus. Fractures of the acromial base have also been reported to contribute to instability after reverse shoulder arthroplasty. Postoperative fracture of the acromion or scapula after reverse shoulder arthroplasty remains a challenge because such fractures can adversely affect outcomes and lead to a higher rate of revision.

Controversies

The authors of this chapter do not believe that there are any controversies regarding the management of prosthetic instability after shoulder arthroplasty.

Results

The literature includes few large case series investigating outcomes of surgical management of instability after shoulder arthroplasty (**Table 1**). The largest published series examined the options for the management of instability after shoulder arthroplasty. Soft-tissue dysfunction was the leading cause of instability, responsible for 21 of 32 cases of instability. Eleven of the 32 shoulders

had prosthetic malpositioning combined with either abnormal capsular tension or rotator cuff deficiency. Results demonstrated that revision surgery restored stability in only nine shoulders. Anterior instability was associated with a significantly higher failure rate, and 23 shoulders had unsatisfactory overall results based on the Neer rating system. No patients in this study underwent conversion to reverse shoulder arthroplasty for instability after shoulder arthroplasty.

The authors of a different series from the same institution examined reverse total shoulder arthroplasty for the management of instability following hemiarthroplasty or total shoulder arthroplasty. In a cohort of 33 shoulders, 94% were stable at average final follow-up of 42 months. The two recurrent dislocations occurred early, at 2.5 weeks and 3 months postoperatively. Importantly, 70% of patients had excellent or satisfactory results according to the Neer rating system.

One smaller series reported outcomes of revision for instability after shoulder arthroplasty. In this series, 10 patients had instability resulting from soft-tissue imbalance. Most patients had anterior instability, and in three patients, two procedures were required to restore stability. These three patients underwent

Table 1 Results After Revision of Unstable Shoulder Arthroplasty

Authors	Journal (Year)	Technique (No. of Shoulders)	Outcomes	Failure Rate (%)	Comments
Moeckel et al	*J Bone Joint Surg Am* (1993)	Subscapularis mobilization and repair (7 [anterior instability]), glenoid bone grafting and posterior capsular plication (3 [posterior instability])	3 of the 7 patients with anterior instability developed recurrent instability and were treated with allograft reconstruction of the anterior soft-tissue envelope All 3 patients with posterior instability remained stable 2 yr postoperatively	30	Allograft reconstruction of the anterior soft tissues should be reserved for patients in whom primary repair of the subscapularis cannot be achieved
Sanchez-Sotelo et al	*J Bone Joint Surg Am* (2003)	Various (32)	5 patients underwent resection arthroplasty 15 patients were stable 14 patients remained unstable	70	Most shoulders developed instability secondary to soft-tissue imbalance No patients underwent revision to a reverse shoulder arthroplasty
Abdel et al	*Bone Joint J* (2013)	Revision to reverse shoulder arthroplasty (33)	31 shoulders remained stable	6	Significant improvement in pain scores and active elevation (*P* = 0.001 for both measures)

successful allograft reconstruction of the coracoacromial arch. Nine patients maintained stability at follow-up.

Technical Keys to Success

Surgical management of prosthetic instability must be individualized to each patient. In any procedure, meticulous preoperative evaluation, including a full review of all potential causes of instability, is necessary. Liberal use of advanced imaging is important to ensure appropriate preoperative evaluation of local anatomy and implant positioning. The surgeon should also review the index surgical procedure to ensure that no errors were made during implantation or soft-tissue repair. Maintaining a high level of suspicion for infection, especially in patients with instability of a reverse shoulder arthroplasty prosthesis, is essential. The surgeon must ensure that

all etiologies of the instability, including soft-tissue imbalance, implant malposition, bony deformity, infection, and/or neurologic injury, are corrected at the time of the revision procedure.

Rehabilitation

Postoperative physical therapy and rehabilitation depend on the patient's pathoanatomy and the procedures performed to restore stability of the shoulder. Important considerations involve soft-tissue repair, tendon transfers, and the use of allograft. The authors of this chapter prefer to place the patient's arm in an abduction orthosis for 4 to 6 weeks after rotator cuff repair or pectoralis major tendon transfer. If allograft is used for reconstruction of the coracoacromial arch, it must be protected during biologic incorporation with sling immobilization and the judicious use of ROM exercises in physical therapy.

Some authors advocate immobilizing the patient's arm in neutral rotation with a gunslinger brace after posterior capsular plication; however, the authors of this chapter allow early pendulum exercises with elbow, wrist, and hand ROM directly after the surgical procedure. Motion posterior to the coronal plane is strictly avoided for at least 4 to 6 weeks postoperatively.

Avoiding Pitfalls

Inadequate recognition of a factor contributing to the instability can lead to continued instability. In particular, failure to correctly identify a septic etiology of shoulder instability after arthroplasty can result in continued instability. Careless handling of the soft tissue intraoperatively can result in an improper compensatory imbalance, resulting in further instability in a different direction.

Bibliography

Abdel MP, Hattrup SJ, Sperling JW, Cofield RH, Kreofsky CR, Sanchez-Sotelo J: Revision of an unstable hemiarthroplasty or anatomical total shoulder replacement using a reverse design prosthesis. *Bone Joint J* 2013;95-B(5):668-672.

Boileau P, Watkinson D, Hatzidakis AM, Hovorka I: The Grammont reverse shoulder prosthesis: Results in cuff tear arthritis, fracture sequelae, and revision arthroplasty. *J Shoulder Elbow Surg* 2006;15(5):527-540.

Chehab EL, Pearle AD, Cordasco FA: Exposed shoulder hemiarthroplasty as a result of anterosuperior escape: A case report. *J Shoulder Elbow Surg* 2006;15(6):e27-e30.

Clark JC, Ritchie J, Song FS, et al: Complication rates, dislocation, pain, and postoperative range of motion after reverse shoulder arthroplasty in patients with and without repair of the subscapularis. *J Shoulder Elbow Surg* 2012;21(1):36-41.

Clavert P, Millett PJ, Warner JJ: Glenoid resurfacing: What are the limits to asymmetric reaming for posterior erosion? *J Shoulder Elbow Surg* 2007;16(6):843-848.

Cofield RH, Edgerton BC: Total shoulder arthroplasty: Complications and revision surgery. *Instr Course Lect* 1990;39:449-462.

Dilisio MF, Miller LR, Warner JJ, Higgins LD: Arthroscopic tissue culture for the evaluation of periprosthetic shoulder infection. *J Bone Joint Surg Am* 2014;96(23):1952-1958.

Edwards TB, Williams MD, Labriola JE, Elkousy HA, Gartsman GM, O'Connor DP: Subscapularis insufficiency and the risk of shoulder dislocation after reverse shoulder arthroplasty. *J Shoulder Elbow Surg* 2009;18(6):892-896.

Frangiamore SJ, Gajewski ND, Saleh A, Farias-Kovac M, Barsoum WK, Higuera CA: α-Defensin accuracy to diagnose periprosthetic joint infection: Best available test? *J Arthroplasty* 2016;31(2):456-460.

Frangiamore SJ, Saleh A, Grosso MJ, et al: α-Defensin as a predictor of periprosthetic shoulder infection. *J Shoulder Elbow Surg* 2015;24(7):1021-1027.

Gallo RA, Gamradt SC, Mattern CJ, et al; Sports Medicine and Shoulder Service at the Hospital for Special Surgery, New York, NY: Instability after reverse total shoulder replacement. *J Shoulder Elbow Surg* 2011;20(4):584-590.

Hennigan SP, Iannotti JP: Instability after prosthetic arthroplasty of the shoulder. *Orthop Clin North Am* 2001;32(4):649-659, ix.

Hill JM, Norris TR: Long-term results of total shoulder arthroplasty following bone-grafting of the glenoid. *J Bone Joint Surg Am* 2001;83(6):877-883.

Hsu JE, Ricchetti ET, Huffman GR, Iannotti JP, Glaser DL: Addressing glenoid bone deficiency and asymmetric posterior erosion in shoulder arthroplasty. *J Shoulder Elbow Surg* 2013;22(9):1298-1308.

Iannotti JP, Norris TR: Influence of preoperative factors on outcome of shoulder arthroplasty for glenohumeral osteoarthritis. *J Bone Joint Surg Am* 2003;85(2):251-258.

Lädermann A, Williams MD, Melis B, Hoffmeyer P, Walch G: Objective evaluation of lengthening in reverse shoulder arthroplasty. *J Shoulder Elbow Surg* 2009;18(4):588-595.

Laver L, Garrigues GE: Avoiding superior tilt in reverse shoulder arthroplasty: A review of the literature and technical recommendations. *J Shoulder Elbow Surg* 2014;23(10):1582-1590.

Levy JC, Anderson C, Samson A: Classification of postoperative acromial fractures following reverse shoulder arthroplasty. *J Bone Joint Surg Am* 2013;95(15):e104.

Levy JC, Blum S: Postoperative acromion base fracture resulting in subsequent instability of reverse shoulder replacement. *J Shoulder Elbow Surg* 2012;21(4):e14-e18.

Moeckel BH, Altchek DW, Warren RF, Wickiewicz TL, Dines DM: Instability of the shoulder after arthroplasty. *J Bone Joint Surg Am* 1993;75(4):492-497.

Norris TR, Lipson SR: Management of the unstable prosthetic shoulder arthroplasty. *Instr Course Lect* 1998;47:141-148.

Resch H, Povacz P, Ritter E, Matschi W: Transfer of the pectoralis major muscle for the treatment of irreparable rupture of the subscapularis tendon. *J Bone Joint Surg Am* 2000;82(3):372-382.

Sanchez-Sotelo J, Sperling JW, Rowland CM, Cofield RH: Instability after shoulder arthroplasty: Results of surgical treatment. *J Bone Joint Surg Am* 2003;85(4):622-631.

Walch G, Badet R, Boulahia A, Khoury A: Morphologic study of the glenoid in primary glenohumeral osteoarthritis. *J Arthroplasty* 1999;14(6):756-760.

Warren RF, Coleman SH, Dines JS: Instability after arthroplasty: The shoulder. *J Arthroplasty* 2002;17(4 suppl 1):28-31.

Wirth MA, Rockwood CA Jr: Complications of total shoulder-replacement arthroplasty. *J Bone Joint Surg Am* 1996;78(4):603-616.

Wirth MA, Rockwood CA: Glenohumeral instability following shoulder arthroplasty. *Orthopaedic Transactions* 1995;19:459.

Chapter 43

Resection or Arthrodesis for the Management of Failed Shoulder Arthroplasty

Michael H. Amini, MD

Eric T. Ricchetti, MD

Joseph P. Iannotti, MD, PhD

 ## Introduction

Shoulder arthroplasty has become increasingly popular since the mid 1990s and offers good long-term survival with the use of modern techniques and implants. With the increased number of primary shoulder arthroplasty procedures performed, complications and revision surgery will become more common. Reasons for failure include infection, osteolysis, rotator cuff tears, stiffness, instability, aseptic loosening, implant malpositioning, and nerve injury. Revision arthroplasty, particularly reverse shoulder arthroplasty (RSA), can address these causes of failure. However, the risk of repeated failure with revision arthroplasty may be unacceptably high in patients with permanent axillary nerve or brachial plexus palsy, detachment of the deltoid muscle, intractable infection after multiple failed surgical procedures, massive bone loss, or persistent prosthetic instability. In these situations, resection arthroplasty or glenohumeral arthrodesis can be performed to salvage upper extremity function and improve pain, which is often debilitating. Although resection arthroplasty of the glenohumeral joint can provide substantial pain relief, the resulting function is limited to lightweight activities at or below waist level. Glenohumeral arthrodesis similarly improves pain and allows for modest elevation of the arm through function of the scapulothoracic articulation.

 ## Case Presentation

A 36-year-old, right-hand–dominant woman has chronic shoulder pain and poor function after multiple surgical procedures. Approximately 10 years previously, she sustained a proximal humerus fracture that was initially managed nonsurgically and resulted in malunion with dislocation of the glenohumeral joint. An open surgical procedure to correct the malunion failed.

After unsuccessful conversion to hemiarthroplasty, the patient underwent revision to RSA but had persistent pain and poor function.

The patient was first seen in the authors' clinic several years after undergoing RSA, with radiographs revealing mechanical failure of the glenoid baseplate and complete loss of the tuberosities (**Figure 1, A**). Results of an infection workup, including aspiration with a 2-week hold for *Propionibacterium acnes*, erythrocyte sedimentation rate, and C-reactive protein level, were negative. To restore humeral and glenoid bone stock and to improve pain and function, hemiarthroplasty was performed with a humeral allograft-prosthesis composite and glenoid bone grafting with a proximal femoral allograft (**Figure 1, B**). The patient developed an intractable infection postoperatively, underwent multiple débridements with eventual removal of the prosthesis and allografts, and ultimately underwent conversion to a resection arthroplasty (**Figure 1, C**).

Two years after the conversion to resection arthroplasty, she returns with debilitating pain and limited use of the arm. She has substantial bone loss of the glenoid and proximal humeral metadiaphysis, including both tuberosities and part of the deltoid insertion. This bone loss results in substantial pistoning at the shoulder with any attempted use of

Dr. Ricchetti or an immediate family member has received research or institutional support from DePuy Synthes and Tornier. Dr. Iannotti or an immediate family member has received royalties from DePuy Synthes, Integra LifeSciences, Tornier, and Zimmer; is a member of a speakers' bureau or has made paid presentations on behalf of DePuy Synthes and Zimmer; serves as a paid consultant to DePuy Synthes and Tornier; and has received nonincome support (such as equipment or services), commercially derived honoraria, or other non–research-related funding (such as paid travel) from Wolters Kluwer Health. Neither Dr. Amini nor any immediate family member has received anything of value from or has stock or stock options held in a commercial company or institution related directly or indirectly to the subject of this chapter.

the upper extremity and causes poor elbow function as a result of the loss of a stable fulcrum at the shoulder, despite maintained elbow motion and an intact neurovascular examination. Results of the infection workup are negative.

Due to the current pain and disability, multiple previous failed arthroplasties, history of recurrent infection, and substantial bone loss, the patient elects to undergo glenohumeral arthrodesis. Because of the absence of proximal bone, a vascularized fibular autograft is used (**Figure 1, D**).

 ## Indications

In most instances of failed arthroplasty, revision arthroplasty is the surgical treatment of choice and the most likely to maximize pain relief and function. Glenohumeral arthrodesis or resection arthroplasty should be reserved for patients in whom revision arthroplasty would lead to unacceptably poor outcomes or the risk of failure would be unacceptably high. If the goals of the procedure include restoration of shoulder function and creation of a stable base for distal function, arthrodesis is preferred to resection. Arthrodesis typically allows shoulder-level elevation and is more durable for high-demand patients, such as laborers, although the ability to perform labor at or above shoulder level after arthrodesis is rare. Older, low-demand patients who are not good candidates for a major surgical procedure, patients who have limited healing potential, and patients who are unable to tolerate prolonged immobilization to allow healing after arthrodesis may be better treated with resection arthroplasty.

Nerve Injury

Neuromuscular factors may provide compelling reasons to perform glenohumeral arthrodesis or resection arthroplasty. Patients with brachial plexus

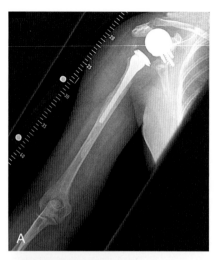
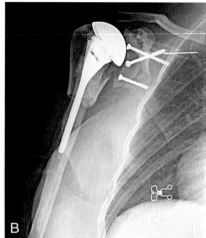
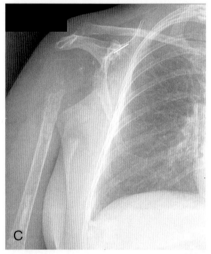
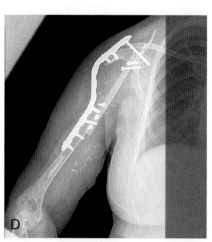

Figure 1 **A,** AP radiograph demonstrates reverse shoulder arthroplasty with mechanical failure of the glenoid baseplate and extensive bone loss of the greater and lesser tuberosities. **B,** AP radiograph demonstrates revision to hemiarthroplasty with a humeral allograft-prosthesis composite and bulk proximal femoral allograft on the glenoid to restore bone stock. **C,** AP radiograph of the shoulder of the same patient whose radiographs are shown in panels **A** and **B** after several débridements for infection and eventual removal of the implant and both the humeral and glenoid bone grafts. **D,** AP radiograph demonstrates a vascularized fibular autograft, lag screw fixation of the graft to the glenoid and humerus, and plate application from the scapular spine to the native humeral shaft.

and/or axillary nerve paralysis are unable to elevate the shoulder or create a stable platform for distal function, particularly with the arm away from the body. Most patients with failed arthroplasty and deltoid denervation also have abnormalities or major tissue loss of the rotator cuff. Although RSA is the treatment of choice in patients with substantial rotator cuff deficiency who require

revision arthroplasty, revision to RSA in patients with brachial plexus and/or axillary nerve paralysis is unlikely to produce satisfactory function and may even lead to prosthetic instability.

Before performing glenohumeral arthrodesis or resection arthroplasty, the surgeon must investigate the cause of nerve palsy to identify the potential for recovery. Electromyography and nerve conduction velocity studies are often used to evaluate the severity of the lesion. Glenohumeral arthrodesis or resection arthroplasty should be delayed until the underlying diagnosis is clear, adequate time to allow for nerve recovery has passed, and axillary nerve repair or nerve transfer has been considered or previously performed and has failed to reinnervate the deltoid.

Deltoid Failure

Dehiscence of the deltoid from previous open surgical treatment results in a functional scenario similar to axillary nerve palsy, although potentially to a lesser degree if only part of the muscle is involved. Part of the deltoid attachment is commonly taken down in open surgical rotator cuff repair, and although repair of the detached deltoid is routine, dehiscence can occur, leaving the deltoid weak or functionally impaired.

Attrition of the deltoid over the long term in patients who have undergone RSA may result in a similar situation and may become more common given the increased use of RSA. Stress fractures of the acromion or scapular spine that occur after RSA and result in nonunion may cause severe weakness of the deltoid. In patients with major rotator cuff deficiency, shoulder function is poor, and fusion may be considered.

Revision of a failed RSA in patients with atrophy, attrition, or dehiscence of the anterior and/or middle heads of the deltoid must be done cautiously, and the surgeon should consider the merits of arthrodesis or resection in this scenario. In some patients with deltoid detachment and major rotator cuff deficiency, RSA and repair of the deltoid origin or rotation deltoplasty should be considered before fusion or resection arthroplasty.

Intractable Infection

Recalcitrant prosthetic joint infection is a source of continued pain and disability for patients and remains difficult to manage. A one- or two-stage replantation strategy, including thorough débridement and targeted intravenous antibiotics, can effectively treat most patients. However, the patient and surgeon must weigh the necessity of repeated surgical procedures and multiple courses of intravenous antibiotics against the alternatives of arthrodesis and resection.

Massive Bone Loss

Substantial bone loss of the proximal humerus and/or glenoid is a common and challenging scenario in patients requiring revision surgery. Bone loss may be the result of osteolysis, infection, dissolution of unhealed tuberosities after reconstruction for fracture, or removal of ingrown or cemented implants, and bone loss may preclude placement of a new, stable implant. Humeral bone loss also may compromise the attachments of the remaining rotator cuff and can extend to involve the deltoid tuberosity. Although revision to RSA may be possible in patients with proximal humeral bone loss involving the greater and lesser tuberosities, loss of the deltoid tuberosity will compromise the functional outcome. In these patients, glenohumeral arthrodesis or resection arthroplasty may be the best option.

Persistent Prosthetic Instability

Persistent instability of an anatomic shoulder arthroplasty, depending on the etiology, is most often managed with revision to RSA. Instability after RSA typically can be addressed with implant revision to increase soft-tissue tension or correct implant malposition. However, instability may persist in these patients and can lead to substantial disability. After all other options have been exhausted, glenohumeral arthrodesis or resection arthroplasty may be effective in managing the instability.

Contraindications

Because glenohumeral arthrodesis and resection arthroplasty should be reserved for carefully selected patients, the primary contraindication to either of these procedures is the presence of a reasonable alternative treatment. Beyond this contraindication, dysfunction of the scapulothoracic joint is the most important contraindication to glenohumeral arthrodesis. Substantial scapular winging, scapulothoracic bursitis, and dysfunction of the serratus anterior, levator scapulae, and rhomboid muscles are relative contraindications to arthrodesis because function of the shoulder girdle, and thus positioning of the hand in space, occurs through scapulothoracic motion after glenohumeral fusion. Previous scapulothoracic fusion is therefore an absolute contraindication because glenohumeral arthrodesis would severely limit upper extremity function in these patients. In addition, the presence of neurologic conditions that may involve the periscapular muscles and are either progressive, such as facioscapulohumeral muscular dystrophy, or systemic, such as amyotrophic lateral sclerosis, preclude arthrodesis. Bilateral glenohumeral fusion may result in substantial functional impairment and should be considered a relative contraindication in the management of failed arthroplasty. Finally, patients with intractable infection may be best treated with resection arthroplasty because an attempt at arthrodesis in this situation will likely lead to infection and failure of the fusion.

Controversies and Alternative Approaches

One of the most controversial points in shoulder arthrodesis is the position of the glenohumeral joint for fusion. Early reports suggested 45° to 50° of abduction, 15° to 25° of forward flexion from the scapular plane, and 25° to 30° of internal rotation. Fusion with insufficient internal rotation will limit the patient's ability to reach the midline to perform self-care and activities of daily living (ADLs). Fusion in an excessively abducted position causes substantial medial winging and inferior tilting of the scapula when the patient brings the arm fully to the side, which can lead to pain and fatigue because of the abnormal stresses in the periscapular musculature. Recommendations for the amount of abduction have decreased, with the most recent recommendation being 10° to 20°. Most surgeons agree that the ideal position should allow the patient to reach the midline and subsequently the mouth with elbow flexion, comfortably adduct the arm fully to the side of the body at rest, elevate the arm approximately to shoulder level, reach the contralateral shoulder, rotate the arm to reach front and back pockets, and potentially reach the perianal area. Moreover, the ideal position for fusion varies depending on body habitus. Patients with large body habitus can undergo fusion with larger degrees of abduction or forward elevation without scapular winging. For most patients with a body mass index less than 30, the authors of this chapter recommend 10° to 20° of abduction, 10° to 20° of forward elevation, and 35° to 45° of internal rotation. In larger patients, particularly those with excess adipose tissue on the side of the body, a position with slightly more abduction is better tolerated because of the soft-tissue support for the arm and is necessary to allow the arm to clear the lateral chest wall.

Fusion techniques must be modified in patients with failed arthroplasty because of the severe bone loss on the humeral and glenoid sides that is often present. Current recommendations favor internal fixation with planned fusion of the acromiohumeral and glenohumeral articulations, known as the AO technique. This technique is commonly used in primary arthrodesis and can be modified for use in the management of failed arthroplasty with mild to moderate bone loss. Structural bone graft is often necessary in patients with failed arthroplasty because, at a minimum, the humeral head would have been removed at the time of the original arthroplasty. Sometimes, vascularized free fibular autograft may be necessary to bridge large gaps, particularly if proximal humeral bone loss exceeds 5 cm. In these patients, glenohumeral fusion is the only option because the available bone is inadequate to achieve both extra- and intra-articular fusion according to the AO technique.

Distal function of the extremity must be carefully evaluated before glenohumeral arthrodesis. The remaining joints need to function well to allow upper extremity motion and maximize hand use after the fusion. In patients with brachial plexus injury, particularly injury of the upper plexus, elbow flexion may be impaired or absent. Patients with a fused shoulder and a flail elbow will have extremely limited upper extremity function. In these patients, elbow flexorplasty can be performed concomitant with the shoulder arthrodesis. This procedure involves transfer of the pectoralis major to the biceps. The pectoralis is released off the proximal humerus, and a long graft, either autogenous fascia lata or allograft, is sewn to the pectoralis tendon proximally and to the distal biceps distally. It is important to tension the transfer after stabilizing the arthrodesis.

Results

Pain

Almost all patients experience pain relief with resection arthroplasty, although they may experience some pain postoperatively with attempted use of the arm. In the literature examining resection performed for the management of failed arthroplasty, a 2006 study reported no more than mild pain in 6 of 7 patients; a 2007 study reported the same in 13 of 18 patients, with the average visual analog scale score decreasing from 8.8 to 4.5; and a 2013 study reported that 22 of 22 patients improved, with the average visual analog scale score improving from 6 to 3.

After arthrodesis, most patients experience substantial improvement from their preoperative level of pain, although some remaining pain is common and should be expected. Because neurologic injury in patients with failed shoulder arthroplasty is an indication for arthrodesis, it is important to note that neurogenic pain is unlikely to improve even with a successful fusion. The authors of one study reported that only 4 of 16 patients were pain free after fusion. However, in the only study of arthrodesis exclusively for the management of failed arthroplasty, the senior author of this chapter (J.P.I.) and a colleague reported that pain improved in all patients, with average pain subscores of the Penn Shoulder Score improving from 8 to 26 on a 30-point scale. In studies that primarily included patients with other preoperative diagnoses, the authors of one study reported that 90% of patients with persistent infections had a marked reduction in pain, and the authors of another study reported that 75% of patients had no or mild pain.

Function

Despite good pain relief, resection leaves the shoulder girdle unstable. Positioning the hand in space becomes difficult because the humerus does not have a stable fulcrum and pistons with attempted movement. Functional outcome becomes unpredictable. Studies have reported forward elevation ranging from 28° to 70°, with one study noting an increase from 39° to 70° and another study noting a decrease from 60° to 45°. External rotation is similarly limited, with rates ranging from 8° to 31°. Patient-reported outcomes demonstrate functional limitations, with American Shoulder and Elbow Surgeons scores of 36 to 38.8 and a Constant score of 27. However, the authors of a study of seven patients noted that all patients could reach their mouth, contralateral axilla, back pocket, and perineum.

Arthrodesis provides a stable base for distal use of the upper extremity. The resulting motion remains limited but often is substantially improved from the preoperative level. In a study published by the senior author of this chapter (J.P.I.) and a colleague, patients undergoing arthrodesis after failed arthroplasty had improvement in overall Penn Shoulder Scores from 17 to 58, with mean subscores for function improving from 8 to 26 on a 60-point scale. Studies of patients with a variety of diagnoses report different rates of the ability to perform certain activities, but this variation is likely attributed to the positions used in fusion. In a study of 33 arthrodesis procedures performed mostly for the management of brachial plexus injury, 21 patients could reach shoulder level, 29 could reach waist level, 25 could wash their face, and 13 could perform self-hygiene, but none could perform overhead work. In a different study of shoulder fusions, none of 17 patients who underwent arthrodesis for osteoarthritis could perform overhead work, 4 could not return to manual labor, and 5 returned to manual labor at a lower level than they previously achieved. Another study reported that 70% of patients with fusion performed for various diagnoses could dress, eat, and perform self-hygiene, 21% could perform light shoulder-level work, and 82% found the fusion functionally beneficial. A study published in 2005 reported mean Constant scores of 57 after arthrodesis.

Complications Associated With Arthrodesis

The literature on resection arthroplasty for the management of failed shoulder arthroplasty demonstrates that complications are largely related to poor functional outcomes or fracture of the humerus during implant removal. Given the small body of literature on arthrodesis after failed arthroplasty, the surgeon must extrapolate results from studies of arthrodesis in patients with other diagnoses. The risk of nonunion, however, is substantially higher in patients with previous failed arthroplasties than in patients with other diagnoses.

NONUNION

Most studies of modern surgical techniques demonstrate union rates of approximately 90% or more after primary arthroplasty. However, because of the existing soft-tissue and microvascular disruption, as well as substantial bone loss, fusion after failed arthroplasty is more difficult. In the series published by the senior author of this chapter (J.P.I.) and a colleague, only three of seven patients had union after the first procedure, an additional two of two patients achieved healing after a bone grafting procedure, one patient had an asymptomatic nonunion, and one patient with a symptomatic nonunion was treated with resection arthroplasty. Since the date of that publication, an additional four patients healed, with one surgical procedure performed.

INFECTION

Reported infection rates vary. Studies of reconstruction and fusion after resection for the management of malignancy report infection rates of 10% to 33%. In other studies, infection rates of approximately 10% or less have been reported. In the series published by the senior author of this chapter (J.P.I.) and a colleague, of seven patients, one superficial infection developed; since the date of that publication, one deep infection developed in an additional four patients. The infection rate in patients undergoing arthrodesis after failed arthroplasty is likely higher than the rate in patients undergoing primary arthroplasty.

MALPOSITION

Opinions vary on the best position of the humerus for arthrodesis, and although each position has its own merits, the surgeon should be aware of the signs and symptoms of malposition in a given patient and the treatment of it. Increasing angles of abduction and forward flexion, particularly in combination, are associated with increasing levels of pain because of the higher strain on the periscapular muscles and the substantial winging that occurs with attempted adduction of the arm to the side. In addition, excessive abduction and forward flexion may improve the ability to perform activities above waist level but impair the ability to perform activities below waist level. Too much or too little internal rotation may cause functional limitations in ADLs. If the position makes the arthrodesis unacceptable to the patient, even after a trial period to adjust, an osteotomy can be performed distal to the fusion site, or the position can be adjusted in patients undergoing revision surgery for delayed union or nonunion. In a study of nine patients undergoing osteotomy of the humeral shaft distal to the fusion site, all patients experienced improvements in function and pain. Osteotomies distal to a fusion site have a high risk of failure or nonunion because of the proximal location of the fusion, and fixation should be protected in a spica cast or other form of rigid immobilization for 12 to 16 weeks or until radiographic and clinical healing has occurred.

IMPLANT PROMINENCE

The robust implants necessary to stabilize the large lever arm of the upper extremity are often prominent beneath the soft tissues. This scenario occurs frequently over the scapular spine and sometimes occurs in more distal sites because the soft tissues are not as robust after multiple surgical procedures. In two of the largest series, researchers reported implant removal in 20% to 24%

of patients. Although most of these patients underwent arthrodesis for other reasons, these results likely can be generalized to patients with failed arthroplasty. If the implant is prominent and the patient wishes to undergo removal, the removal should be delayed ideally until 1 year after the fusion, and if union remains questionable, a CT scan should be obtained before implant removal.

PERIPROSTHETIC FRACTURE

The upper extremity is a large lever arm, and the stiffness of the plate creates a large stress riser in the humeral diaphysis. This scenario can lead to periprosthetic fractures of the humerus around the end of the plate. Such fractures have been reported to occur in 2% to 11% of patients. Typically, a fracture of the native humerus can withstand a fairly substantial amount of malunion before causing functional limitations. However, in patients with a fused shoulder, motion and function are already so limited that any substantial change as a result of fracture can lead to decompensated upper extremity function. In addition, in patients with a fused shoulder, the entire moment arm of the upper extremity is transmitted to the fracture site, and this force may exceed the strain threshold of the union. Periprosthetic fractures with no or minimal displacement may be managed nonsurgically, but patients with displaced fractures should undergo fixation to preserve upper extremity function.

Technical Keys to Success

Before performing glenohumeral arthrodesis, the surgeon should consider the available treatment options and ensure that no reasonable alternative exists. The causes of implant failure should be carefully evaluated, and other sources of pain should be ruled out. In addition, the amount of bone loss

should be assessed preoperatively. In some patients, it may be necessary to measure long-film radiographs of both humeri with a graduated ruler to determine the loss of length of the humerus. Three-dimensional CT can be useful to define bone loss on the humeral and glenoid sides. Together, these images help the surgeon anticipate the need for bone graft. It is important to prepare for unanticipated additional bone loss during implant removal, particularly if the implant is well fixed. Often, the patient's iliac crest is insufficient to provide the amount of bone graft needed, and bulk femoral head allograft should be available. When proximal humeral bone loss exceeds 5 cm, the surgeon should plan for a vascularized fibular graft. The presence of a second surgical team, including a microvascular surgeon, allows for a more efficient surgical procedure in which the vascularized fibular autograft is harvested while the shoulder site is prepared to receive the graft.

Setup/Exposure

- The patient is placed under general anesthesia as well as an interscalene nerve block with an indwelling catheter.
- The patient is placed in the modified beach-chair position with the medial border of the scapula free.
- Before draping, the surgeon must verify the ability to maximally adduct and extend the patient's shoulder to facilitate removal of the humeral implant.
- When the surgical plan involves a vascularized fibular autograft, both lower extremities are prepared, and a second surgical team is prepared to work simultaneously.
- A curvilinear incision is made starting on the spine of the scapula proximally and posteriorly and continuing around to the anterior acromion before extending distally. The existing scar is incorporated if possible.

- The deltopectoral interval is identified and entered. The distal limb of the incision should allow for extension of the deltopectoral interval to the anterolateral interval along the lateral edge of the biceps brachii for exposure of the humeral shaft.
- The anterior and middle deltoid is detached from the acromion. Often, extensive scar tissue must be dissected to identify proper tissue planes.
- Any remaining subscapularis is released off the humerus, and the humeral head is dislocated and exposed with extension, adduction, and external rotation.
- Great care must be taken during removal of implants to avoid iatrogenic bone loss or propagation of a fracture and further compromise of already limited bone stock.

Instruments/Equipment/Implants Required

- Standard and flexible osteotomes are required.
- Cement-removing instruments may be necessary.
- Cerclage cables are used.
- A large-fragment plate set is needed.

Procedure

FIXATION AND BONE GRAFTING

- In patients with intact tuberosities, the remaining humeral bone should be placed against the native glenoid to obtain primary healing of native bone.
- Regardless of the methods of fixation and fusion, the surgeon must pay particular attention to the position of fixation. The authors of this chapter attempt to obtain 10° to 20° of abduction, 10° to 20° of forward elevation, and 35° to 45° of internal rotation. For larger patients, the arm is placed in slightly more abduction.
- Unintentional translation of the scapula while positioning the arm

for provisional fixation should be avoided because it may result in incorrect assessment of the final position of the arm.

- Provisional fixation of the remaining humerus to the glenoid is achieved with a 3-mm Steinmann pin placed lateral to medial through the proximal humerus into the glenoid.
- A second pin is placed superior to inferior from the acromion into the humerus.
- The ability to reach the mouth and contralateral shoulder with elevation and elbow flexion, to reach the front and back pockets and the groin, and to easily adduct the arm to the torso should be gently trialed. The Steinmann pins can be withdrawn to allow adjustment of the position and then replaced.
- After the optimal position is achieved, the medial side of the proximal humerus may require contouring to be parallel to the glenoid surface.
- Any intact surface of bone, including a malpositioned tuberosity, is kept intact and used for additional bone contact or a point of fixation.
- If further preparation of the glenoid face is necessary to maximize contact, it is performed at this time.
- The pins between the humerus and glenoid are removed and replaced with one or two 6.5-mm partially threaded screws to compress the humerus to the glenoid. Because of medialization of the proximal humerus, primary fixation between the acromion and the humerus is rarely possible.

USE OF BULK ALLOGRAFT IN PATIENTS WITH INTACT TUBEROSITIES
- Given the preoperative bone loss and intraoperative bony resection, compression of the humerus to the glenoid results in substantial medialization of the proximal humerus under the acromion. Bulk femoral head allograft is used to fill this void.
- The allograft is shaped to fit the lateral side of the humerus, the undersurface of the acromion, and the undersurface of the plate that will be used. The graft should project slightly lateral to the lateral edge of the acromion.
- One or two 6.5-mm partially threaded cancellous compression screws are placed through the graft into the humerus and glenoid to secure the graft.
- A 4.5-mm compression plate of an appropriate length is chosen to allow placement of at least three bicortical screws through the scapular spine and the intact humeral shaft.
- The plate is bent and contoured to the scapular spine, to the acromion, and distally to the proximal humerus.
- An attempt should be made to place additional screws through the plate to simultaneously transfix the allograft, the humerus, and the glenoid.
- Care must be taken to maximize screw fixation into the scapular spine. The longest screw should be placed through the plate proximally from the scapular spine to the glenoid neck near the base of the coracoid.
- Additional fixation through the plate enters the acromion, passes through the graft between the acromion and the proximal humerus, and extends into the proximal humeral shaft.
- Depending on the amount of proximal humeral and glenoid bone loss, the location of the screws and the allograft are modified to optimize bone contact and fixation.

USE OF VASCULARIZED FIBULAR AUTOGRAFT IN PATIENTS WITH LOSS OF THE TUBEROSITIES
- If bone loss exceeds 5 cm and the tuberosities are no longer present, a vascularized fibular autograft at least 6 cm longer than the anticipated humeral defect is harvested after implant removal and débridement.
- The defect should be measured before the autograft is harvested; however, most surgeons harvest the maximum length available, leaving the proximal and distal fibula to preserve knee and ankle function, and trim the graft after the shoulder site is prepared.
- After the microvascular team prepares the fibula with its vascular pedicle, the least possible amount of muscle is stripped from the fibula to allow fixation of the proximal and distal end of the fibula to the remaining humeral canal and glenoid (**Figure 2, A**).
- Several options are available for humeral fixation. The choice of fixation depends on the amount of humeral bone remaining and the shape and size of the fibula. With a large humeral canal, the distal 2 to 4 cm of the fibula can be placed in the humeral canal; this method provides the best inherent stability before screw fixation. Alternatively, side-to-side fixation can be performed with a step-cut technique or with bayonet apposition of the two bones.
- Two or three 4.5-mm screws are used to fix the graft to the humerus (**Figure 2, B**).
- Positioning of the arm of patients in whom a fibular autograft is used requires more estimation of proper arm position than is necessary in the previously described technique for the treatment of a patient with intact tuberosities.
- The arm length is determined with the use of traction on the arm, and

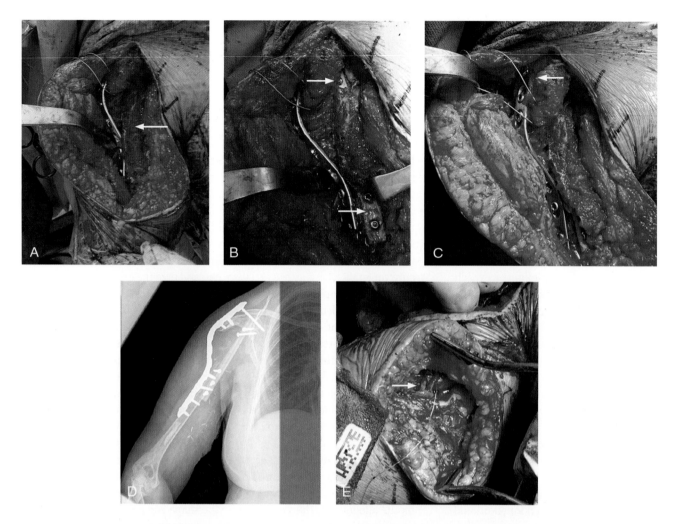

Figure 2 **A,** Intraoperative photograph of a shoulder shows the final construct with the plate applied and the fibular autograft in place, covered by muscle (arrow). **B,** Intraoperative photograph shows the proximal and distal aspects of the fibular autograft (arrows) secured with independent lag screws. **C,** Intraoperative photograph shows the proximal end of the plate applied over the superior surface of the scapular spine (arrow). **D,** AP radiograph demonstrates the final construct. **E,** Intraoperative photograph demonstrates the incision on the medial arm made for anastomosis to the brachial artery (arrow).

the fibula is cut so that at least 1 to 2 cm of additional length is available with the arm in the correct position.

- A slot is fashioned in the glenoid with the use of a burr, and the proximal part of the graft is placed into the slot.

- The graft can be held in this location with compressive pressure. If the fibula is large enough to accommodate it, a 3-mm Steinmann pin can be placed to stabilize the joint temporarily.

- The position of the arm is assessed as described previously.

- After a satisfactory position is achieved, the fibular and glenoid surfaces are assessed to determine the need for further preparation to maximize contact.

- At least one or preferably two 4.5-mm screws are placed through the graft into the glenoid (**Figure 2, B**).

- As in the previously described technique without fibular autograft, a piece of femoral head allograft is cut and placed lateral to the proximal

end of the fibula such that it fills the space between the eventual plate and the fibula.

- Alternatively, a proximal humeral allograft may be placed between the fibular autograft and the plate.

- Placing an allograft between the fibular autograft and the plate allows for additional points of fixation between the native bone and the plate, improving the overall stability of the construct. In the experience of the senior author of this chapter (J.P.I.), proximal loss of fixation occurred in some patients in whom no additional allograft was used, requiring a second procedure for grafting and fixation.

- A plate of appropriate length is chosen to allow placement of at least three bicortical screws through the scapular spine and native humeral shaft (**Figure 2, C** and **D**). This plate must be longer than that used in the previously described technique. Additional fixation should be placed through the plate, grafts, and glenoid if possible.
- After the fibula and arm are secure, the fibula is revascularized by the microvascular team (**Figure 2, E**).
- Autogenous iliac crest aspirate is mixed with allograft matrix, and the mixture is placed at the proximal and distal sites of the fibular graft.
- Some microvascular surgeons prefer to achieve vascular reperfusion of the graft before final fixation of the graft as described previously. This method is better for the graft but requires careful and gentle handling of the bone to protect the anastomosis during graft preparation and fixation.
- If graft fixation is done first, it should be completed in less than 45 minutes. Ideally, the fixation process should be started as soon as the graft is removed from the leg, with the last step of harvest being cutting the vascular supply. A well-coordinated and experienced team can accomplish this.

Wound Closure
- A deep drain is placed.
- The deltoid is repaired to the acromion with the use of bone tunnels to maximize soft-tissue coverage of the grafts and implants.
- The soft tissues are closed in layers.
- The patient is placed in an abduction brace.
- An indwelling Doppler probe is placed at the vascular anastomosis to monitor the vascularity of the graft.
- Intraoperative and postoperative anticoagulation is started based on the preference of the microvascular surgeon.
- Meticulous hemostasis of the surgical site must be achieved to avoid wound healing complications and hematoma.

 Rehabilitation

Some surgeons place the arm in an abduction brace for only 6 weeks after primary arthrodesis, and sometimes only a sling is used in reliable patients with excellent bone stock. However, in patients who undergo arthrodesis for the management of failed arthroplasty, additional immobilization is necessary because of substantial bone loss and delayed healing. After arthrodesis, the patient is placed in a shoulder abduction orthosis or spica cast for 12 to 16 weeks or until radiographic and clinical evidence of fusion is observed. Immediately postoperatively, the patient is encouraged to perform elbow, wrist, and hand motion to minimize stiffness in the remaining extremity. After union has occurred, the patient is instructed on a scapulothoracic range-of-motion exercise program and strengthening of the periscapular musculature. Despite substantial prominence, implants are left in place whenever possible. If implant removal is necessary, it should be delayed until union is achieved. The rehabilitation protocol is summarized in **Table 1**.

 Avoiding Pitfalls

Proper patient selection and exhaustion of other options are keys to success with either arthrodesis or resection. If other reasonable reconstruction options exist, even if the outcome may not be optimal, they should be weighed against the limitations in function and surgical risks associated with arthrodesis and resection. If no other reasonable option exists, the patient should be informed that arthrodesis will not restore elevation above shoulder level and that resection will not allow rotation at waist level. To help the patient reach a good preoperative understanding of the consequences of the procedure, it may be helpful for prospective patients to speak with other patients who have undergone the procedure, with both ideal and less than ideal results.

Intraoperatively, the surgeon must use caution to avoid additional bone loss during implant removal. Fracture of the humerus may substantially compromise the already limited bone stock and may complicate stabilization of the fusion. A careful longitudinal osteotomy affords control during implant removal and helps limit unintentional fractures.

Malposition of the arm without sufficient internal rotation will impair the patient's ability to perform self-care activities and ADLs, and malposition in excessive abduction will lead to fatigue and pain of the periscapular musculature. After provisionally stabilizing the glenohumeral joint with Steinmann pins, the surgeon should carefully evaluate the position of the arm intraoperatively. If malposition substantially limits the patient's arm motion, osteotomy of the humerus distal to the fusion may be done. However, this osteotomy is often not an option in patients with a free fibular graft.

The surgeon must maintain a high index of suspicion for delayed union or nonunion. Although union rates of 80% to 90% have been reported for primary glenohumeral arthrodesis, fusion rates after failed arthroplasty are substantially lower because of the limited bone stock and impaired biologic environment. Prolonged immobilization with an abduction sling, brace, or spica

Table 1 Rehabilitation Protocol After Arthrodesis to Manage Failed Shoulder Arthroplasty

Postoperative Week	ROM	Strengthening	Return to Play	Comments/Emphasis
0-2	Elbow, wrist, and hand motion	—	None	Shoulder abduction orthosis or spica cast for 12-16 wk or until radiographic and clinical evidence of fusion is observed
2-6	Elbow, wrist, and hand motion	—	None	—
6-12	Elbow, wrist, and hand motion	—	None	—
12-24	Scapulothoracic ROM exercise program after evidence of union is observed	Strengthening of periscapular musculature after evidence of union is observed	None	—

ROM = range of motion.

cast is required for 3 to 4 months postoperatively. The choice of immobilization method depends on the patient's ability to comply with restrictions, the quality of the remaining bone, and the fixation achieved. The surgeon should take a conservative approach to immobilization. Healing may be difficult to assess radiographically because of the relatively minimal callus formation. If progression of fusion remains unknown at 12 to 16 weeks postoperatively, a CT scan should be obtained. If delayed union is observed, preemptive bone grafting should be performed to avoid implant failure, which would likely require revision fixation. With recognition of delayed union and appropriate intervention, union can be achieved in most patients.

Bibliography

Braman JP, Sprague M, Bishop J, Lo IK, Lee EW, Flatow EL: The outcome of resection shoulder arthroplasty for recalcitrant shoulder infections. *J Shoulder Elbow Surg* 2006;15(5):549-553.

Codd TP, Yamaguchi K, Pollock RG, Flatow EL, Bigliani LU: Infected shoulder arthroplasties: Treatment with staged reimplantation vs resection arthroplasty. *J Shoulder Elbow Surg* 1996;5(2):S5.

Cofield RH, Briggs BT: Glenohumeral arthrodesis: Operative and long-term functional results. *J Bone Joint Surg Am* 1979;61(5):668-677.

Fuchs B, O'Connor MI, Padgett DJ, Kaufman KR, Sim FH: Arthrodesis of the shoulder after tumor resection. *Clin Orthop Relat Res* 2005;(436):202-207.

Groh GI, Williams GR, Jarman RN, Rockwood CA Jr: Treatment of complications of shoulder arthrodesis. *J Bone Joint Surg Am* 1997;79(6):881-887.

Hawkins RJ, Neer CS II: A functional analysis of shoulder fusions. *Clin Orthop Relat Res* 1987;(223):65-76.

Muh SJ, Streit JJ, Lenarz CJ, et al: Resection arthroplasty for failed shoulder arthroplasty. *J Shoulder Elbow Surg* 2013;22(2):247-252.

Richards RR: Glenohumeral arthrodesis, in Iannotti JP, Miniaci A, Williams GR, Zuckerman JD, eds: *Disorders of the Shoulder.* Philadelphia, PA, Lippincott Williams & Wilkins, 2013, vol 1, pp 523-551.

Richards RR, Waddell JP, Hudson AR: Shoulder arthrodesis for the treatment of brachial plexus palsy. *Clin Orthop Relat Res* 1985;(198):250-258.

Rispoli DM, Sperling JW, Athwal GS, Schleck CD, Cofield RH: Pain relief and functional results after resection arthroplasty of the shoulder. *J Bone Joint Surg Br* 2007;89(9):1184-1187.

Rose PS, Shin AY, Bishop AT, Moran SL, Sim FH: Vascularized free fibula transfer for oncologic reconstruction of the humerus. *Clin Orthop Relat Res* 2005;(438):80-84.

Rühmann O, Schmolke S, Bohnsack M, Flamme C, Wirth CJ: Shoulder arthrodesis: Indications, technique, results, and complications. *J Shoulder Elbow Surg* 2005;14(1):38-50.

Scalise JJ, Iannotti JP: Glenohumeral arthrodesis after failed prosthetic shoulder arthroplasty. *J Bone Joint Surg Am* 2008;90(1):70-77.

Scalise JJ, Iannotti JP: Glenohumeral arthrodesis after failed prosthetic shoulder arthroplasty: Surgical technique. *J Bone Joint Surg Am* 2009;91(suppl 2 pt 1):30-37.

Wick M, Müller EJ, Ambacher T, Hebler U, Muhr G, Kutscha-Lissberg F: Arthrodesis of the shoulder after septic arthritis: Long-term results. *J Bone Joint Surg Br* 2003;85(5):666-670.

Open Reduction and Internal Fixation of Three- and Four-Part Proximal Humerus Fractures: Plating Techniques

Sanjit R. Konda, MD

Kenneth A. Egol, MD

Introduction

Three- and four-part proximal humerus fractures have the potential to be severely debilitating injuries. Greater tuberosity displacement can result in substantial pain in overhead activities because of impingement in the subacromial space. Humeral head malalignment can result in rotational deficits of the arm and increase the risk for nonunion, which, in younger and middle-aged patients, can preclude participation in many work-related activities. In geriatric patients, malalignment can affect the ability to perform activities of daily living. Surgical management of three- and four-part proximal humerus fractures can restore normal anatomy and minimize functional deficits.

Case Presentation

A 65-year-old, right-hand–dominant woman presents with acute right shoulder pain after a ground-level fall. She currently works as a school teacher and enjoys routine recreational activities, including tennis and golf. A standard three-view shoulder trauma series of plain radiographs (AP, scapular Y, and axillary views) was obtained (**Figure 1**). Radiographs demonstrated a three-part fracture of the proximal humerus with posterosuperior displacement of the greater tuberosity and a surgical neck fracture with 100% anteromedial displacement of the humeral shaft relative to the humeral head. The humeral head remained reduced. A typical ecchymotic pattern along the course of the arm and forearm is shown in **Figure 2**. The patient was recommended for open reduction and internal fixation and underwent internal fixation via a deltopectoral approach with a proximal humerus locking plate and supplemental suture fixation of the greater tuberosity fragment. Calcium phosphate bone cement was injected into the metaphyseal region to provide axial support to the head fragment and prevent settling. Intraoperative imaging demonstrates restoration of the neck-shaft angle and reduction of the greater tuberosity fragment (**Figure 3**). The patient had an uneventful postoperative course and was discharged home on postoperative day 2. Routine follow-up at 2 weeks, 6 weeks, and 3 months postoperatively show progressive healing with complete radiographic union and clinical healing at 3 months postoperatively. At 3 months postoperatively, the shoulder range of motion (ROM) was forward elevation, 120°; internal rotation to T8; and external rotation, 45°. At final follow-up at 6 months postoperatively, shoulder ROM improved substantially to forward elevation, 160°; internal rotation, T6; and external rotation, 70°. Final radiographs show a healed proximal humerus fracture (**Figure 4**).

Indications

Most displaced three- and four-part proximal humerus fractures and fracture-dislocations require surgical treatment. Specific criteria that warrant strong consideration for surgical fixation include fractures with superiorly displaced greater tuberosity fragments (greater than 5 mm), varus angulation of the humeral head, more than 100% translation of the humeral head on the humeral shaft, fracture-dislocations of

Dr. Egol or an immediate family member has received royalties from and serves as a paid consultant to Exactech; has received research or institutional support from OMEGA, the Orthopaedic Research and Education Foundation, and Synthes; and has received nonincome support (such as equipment or services), commercially derived honoraria, or other non–research-related funding (such as paid travel) from SLACK and Wolters Kluwer Health–Lippincott Williams & Wilkins. Neither Dr. Konda nor any immediate family member has received anything of value from or has stock or stock options held in a commercial company or institution related directly or indirectly to the subject of this chapter.

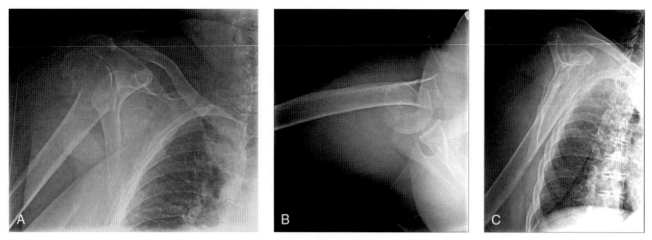

Figure 1   Plain radiographs of a right shoulder demonstrate a displaced three-part proximal humerus fracture. **A,** AP view demonstrates superior displacement of the greater tuberosity fragment into the subacromial space and medial displacement of the humeral shaft. Axillary (**B**) and scapular Y (**C**) radiographs demonstrate 100% anterior displacement of the humeral shaft relative to the humeral head. The axillary view confirms that the humeral head remains reduced.

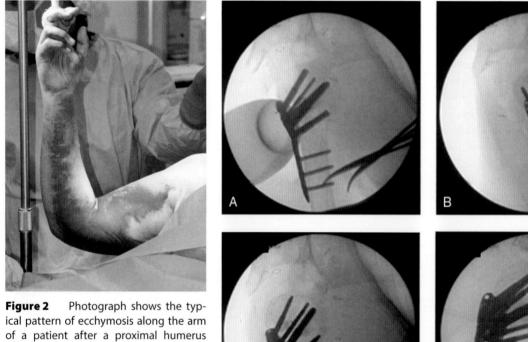

Figure 2   Photograph shows the typical pattern of ecchymosis along the arm of a patient after a proximal humerus fracture. This pattern may be more pronounced in patients being treated with chronic anticoagulation therapy.

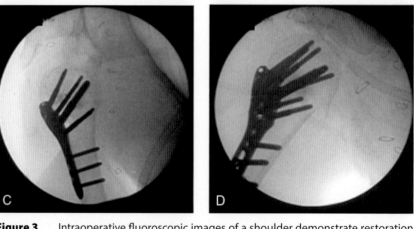

Figure 3   Intraoperative fluoroscopic images of a shoulder demonstrate restoration of the proximal humerus neck-shaft angle and reduction of the greater tuberosity fragment. AP views demonstrate external rotation (**A**) and internal rotation (**B**) of the proximal humerus. **C,** Calcium phosphate has been introduced into the head-neck junction to prevent settling of the humeral head, preventing postoperative intra-articular screw penetration. **D,** Axillary view demonstrates no intra-articular screw penetration.

the humeral head, and humeral head rotation (typically retroversion). Superior displacement of the greater tuberosity fragment will result in impingement against the acromion with overhead activities, resulting in poor functional outcome. Varus angulation of the humeral

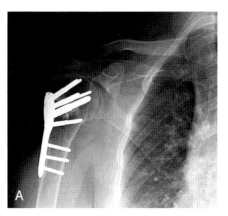 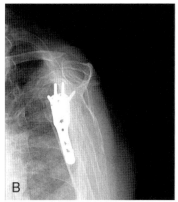 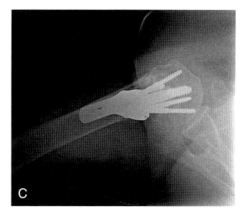

Figure 4   AP (**A**), scapular Y (**B**), and axillary (**C**) radiographs of a right shoulder obtained 6 months postoperatively demonstrate a healed three-part proximal humerus fracture. No interval settling of the humeral head or osteonecrosis has occurred, and all locking screws in the humeral head remain in their original subchondral location.

head predisposes the fracture to additional collapse and increased risk for osteonecrosis. Furthermore, one-third of fractures that heal in varus malunion will result in long-term functional deficits. Conversely, three- or four-part valgus-impacted fractures have better prognoses than other types of displaced three- and four-part proximal humerus fractures because the medial capsular blood supply remains intact. Fractures with more than 100% translation have a greater risk for nonunion or healing in malunion, causing substantial functional deficit. Three- or four-part fracture-dislocations of the proximal humerus often require open reduction of the humeral head segment to achieve reduction. In these fractures, internal fixation should be performed to achieve stability and promote healing, because the humeral head vascular supply is further compromised as the surrounding soft tissue is stripped to achieve reduction. Finally, substantial humeral head rotation (typically retroversion) will result in decreased internal rotation.

The authors of this chapter prefer to use the deltopectoral approach for exposure of the fracture. The deltopectoral approach is the so-called workhorse of shoulder surgery and allows access to all portions of a fractured proximal humerus. If fracture fixation cannot be achieved, arthroplasty can easily be performed as a "bailout" via this same approach. Precontoured proximal humeral locking plates can be placed easily onto the anterolateral aspect of the humerus for internal fixation of three- and four-part proximal humerus fractures. These implants have shown a substantial improvement in the past 15 years compared with nonlocked implants. Biomechanically, as an axial or bending force is applied, the bolts and plate act as a single construct with no angular change occurring at the bolt-plate interface. Furthermore, the construct's strength of fixation equals the total capability of all bolts to resist shear at the bolt-bone interface instead of the thread purchase of a single screw. This is a potential advantage when working with osteopenic bone.

In osteopenic bone or high-energy fractures with impaction of the metaphyseal cancellous bone, it has been shown that calcium phosphate bone substitute used to fill this void can provide resistance to compression forces at the fracture site, thereby preventing settling of the humeral head in the postoperative period. Settling of the humeral head when using a locking plate can result in screw penetration into the glenohumeral joint.

Controversies and Alternative Approaches

An alternative to the deltopectoral approach is the deltoid-splitting approach, which is used to expose the lateral aspect of the proximal humerus. The skin incision can be either a vertical incision off the lateral aspect of the acromion or an elliptical incision that flaps down to expose the deltoid. In either case, the muscle is split longitudinally beginning at the raphe at the one-third/two-thirds junction of the deltoid muscle off the lateral aspect of the acromion. It is critical to identify and protect the axillary nerve as it passes across the deltoid distally (**Figure 5**). The nerve creates two soft-tissue windows that provide access to the displaced tuberosities and head segments (above the nerve) and the humeral shaft (below the nerve). The advantage of this approach is improved access to posteriorly displaced greater tuberosity fragments. The disadvantage is potential damage to the axillary nerve.

A fibular strut allograft that is placed into the humeral shaft with the displaced head and tuberosity fragments secured to the fibular strut is an alternative to calcium phosphate bone substitute to fill the metaphyseal void in osteopenic bone or high-energy fractures. In a small

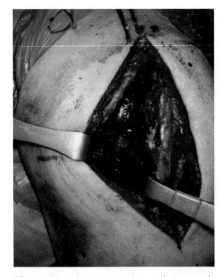

Figure 5 Intraoperative photograph of the deltoid-splitting approach, which shows the interval between the anterior one-third and posterior two-thirds of the deltoid and the underlying axillary nerve crossing from posterior to anterior approximately 5 cm distal to the lateral edge of the acromion process. The plate has been placed underneath the nerve.

cohort of patients, this technique was shown to support the humeral head, preventing collapse and intra-articular screw penetration. This strategy also has the capability to re-create the medial calcar and to buttress fractures with insufficient medial support.

Recently, studies have described the use of intramedullary nails to fix three- and four-part proximal humerus fractures using indirect reduction techniques through minimally invasive incisions. These implants may be best suited to avoid long incisions if fixing combined proximal humerus and humeral shaft fractures. However, one disadvantage of this approach is the traumatization of the rotator cuff tendon insertion necessary to place this implant, which can be avoided using traditional plate-and-screw fixation. In addition, because reduction is performed via indirect means, anatomic restoration of tuberosity fractures is

difficult to achieve and can result in residual shoulder dysfunction.

Results

Because locking plates and screws are a relatively new technology, few outcome studies reporting long-term outcomes exist; most studies have reported short-term to midterm outcomes. The literature on open reduction and internal fixation of three- and four-part humerus fractures reports that the rate of osteonecrosis following these fractures is much lower than historically reported and that the incidence of symptomatic osteonecrosis affecting function is even lower. Open reduction and internal fixation with locking plates for the treatment of three- and four-part proximal humerus fractures provides good clinical and functional results using objective outcome measures (Disabilities of the Arm, Shoulder and Hand and Constant scores) with acceptably low rates of complications compared with fixation using nonlocking plates (**Table 1**).

Technical Keys to Success

- Surgical intervention is ideally performed within the first 1 to 2 weeks after injury, before the fracture fragments have begun to heal and while the risk of heterotopic ossification remains low.
- General anesthesia, general/scalene block combination, or scalene block alone is administered for postoperative pain control. Data from the center of the authors of this chapter demonstrate improved early functional outcomes with regional anesthesia.
- The initial patient positioning and approach are of paramount importance to ensure a technically efficient surgery and optimal outcome.

The authors of this chapter place the patient in the beach-chair position with a captain's chair cutout on the surgical side. The image intensifier is placed above the patient's head to facilitate biplanar fluoroscopy (**Figure 6**). The endotracheal tube should be positioned opposite the surgical side to minimize the risk of extubation during the procedure.

- The patient's entire forequarter is prepped and draped into the sterile field.
- The deltopectoral incision is made just lateral to the coracoid process and carried distally 10 to 15 cm toward the deltoid tuberosity (**Figure 7**). Skin flaps are developed and the cephalic vein is identified at the deltopectoral interval (**Figure 8**). The vein can be moved either medially or laterally. The authors of this chapter prefer to carefully dissect the lateral branches and move the vein medially so the deltoid can be retracted laterally. The vessel is less likely to sustain damage if it is not under retractor tension throughout the procedure.
- Deep to the interval, the clavipectoral fascia, if not already torn by the injury, is incised just lateral to the conjoint tendon.
- The long head of the biceps is identified because it functions as the "lighthouse" of the proximal humerus and may be the only landmark in its anatomic position.
- The lesser tuberosity and/or subscapularis tendon are identified medially and the greater tuberosity and/or supraspinatus and infraspinatus tendons are identified superiorly and posterolaterally.
- The coracoacromial ligament can be released to gain superior exposure.
- A Brown deltoid retractor is used to expose the fracture site.
- The humeral shaft can be internally or externally rotated to provide access to the greater or lesser

Table 1 Short- and Midterm Results of Locking Plate Fixation of Three- and Four-Part Proximal Humerus Fractures

Authors	Journal (Year)	Technique (No. of Fractures)	Outcomes	Comments
Fankhauser et al	*Clin Orthop Relat Res* (2005)	ORIF with deltopectoral approach and AO locking plates (29)	Constant score, 74.6 2 patients with osteonecrosis 2 revision surgeries 1 patient had an axillary nerve injury 3 patients had postoperative subacromial impingement 3 patients had loss of fixation	Mean patient age, 64.2 yr Mean follow-up, 12 mo
Plecko and Kraus	*Oper Orthop Traumatol* (2005)	ORIF with deltopectoral approach and AO locking plates (36)	Mean Constant score, 63 (81% when corrected for age) Mean DASH, 18 3 patients with osteonecrosis (no revision surgery) 2 infections necessitating hardware removal	Mean patient age, 57.5 yr Mean follow-up, 31 mo
Papadopoulos et al	*Injury* (2009)	ORIF with deltopectoral approach and AO locking plates (29)	Mean Constant score, 86 3 patients with osteonecrosis (2 underwent plate removal) 1 patient had a malunion (>10° varus)	Mean patient age, 62.3 yr Mean follow-up, 17.9 mo
Südkamp et al	*J Bone Joint Surg Am* (2009)	ORIF with deltopectoral approach and deltoid splitting approach and AO locking plates (187)	Mean Constant score, 70.6 (85.1% of the score of the contralateral side) Mean DASH, 15.2 29 patients underwent an unplanned second surgery ≤12 mo after fracture fixation	Mean patient age, 62.9 yr Mean follow-up, 12 mo
Gaheer and Hawkins	*Orthopedics* (2010)	ORIF with deltopectoral approach and AO locking plates (55)	Overall Constant score, 72.1 1 patient had plate failure 1 patient had intra-articular screw penetration 1 subacromial impingement	Mean patient age, 68.7 yr Mean follow-up, 40 mo
Ong et al	*Am J Orthop (Belle Mead NJ)* (2012)	ORIF with deltopectoral approach and AO locking plates (51)	Mean DASH, 23.2 Mean forward elevation, 135.4° Mean external rotation, 41.7° 7 patients had screw penetration 2 patients had osteonecrosis 1 patient had hardware failure 3 patients had acute postoperative infections	Mean patient age, 62 yr Mean follow-up, 12 mo

DASH = Disabilities of the Arm, Shoulder and Hand score; ORIF = open reduction and internal fixation.

tuberosities, respectively. The greater and/or lesser tuberosity fracture fragments are identified and tagged with nonabsorbable, braided suture placed at the tuberosity/rotator cuff tendon interface and mobilized (**Figure 9**). This allows for manipulation of the fragments to achieve anatomic reduction, and

the sutures will be secured to the plate to augment tuberosity repair. Care is taken to avoid stripping the fracture fragments of their soft-tissue attachments.

- All loose hematomas are carefully curetted from the fracture bed, and the fracture site is well irrigated.
- Under fluoroscopy, the humeral

head segment is reduced to the shaft. In the setting of valgus-impacted fractures, this can be accomplished by elevating the segment using a broad osteotome (**Figure 10**).

- Care should be taken not to disrupt the medial soft-tissue hinge. For patients in whom the head is

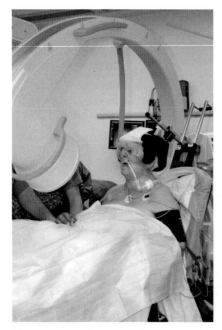

Figure 6 Photograph shows a patient placed in the beach-chair position with captain's chair cutout on the surgical side and the upper body reclined to 60°.

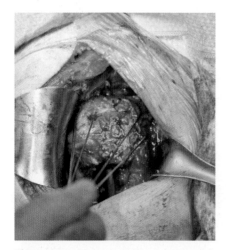

Figure 9 Intraoperative photograph of a shoulder shows braided, nonabsorbable suture placed through the greater tuberosity/rotator cuff junction to allow for manipulation of the tuberosity fragment, which will later be repaired to the proximal humerus locking plate. A Brown deltoid retractor is placed laterally to aid in fracture exposure. Note that the humerus is maximally internally rotated to bring the greater tuberosity into the middle of the surgical field.

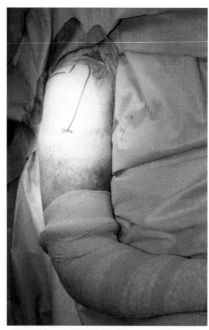

Figure 7 Photograph of a shoulder shows a planned deltopectoral skin incision. Landmarks are drawn to indicate the acromion process laterally and coracoid process medially. The skin incision starts proximal and just lateral to the coracoid process and runs distally and laterally toward the deltoid insertion on the deltoid tuberosity of the humeral shaft.

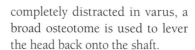

completely distracted in varus, a broad osteotome is used to lever the head back onto the shaft.

- With the head reduced, at least two Kirschner wires (K-wires) are placed provisionally to maintain the reduction while the rest of the fracture is treated. An alternate strategy for reduction is to fix a precontoured plate to the head fragment and then reduce the shaft to the plate. In either case, the tuberosities are reduced and also provisionally fixed using K-wires.
- Plate-and-screw fixation is achieved using an appropriate length precontoured locking plate placed lateral to the bicipital groove (and bicipital tendon). Care must be taken to avoid placing the plate too far proximal so that the angle-stable screw holes are positioned to

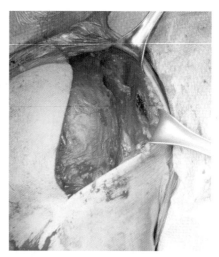

Figure 8 Intraoperative photograph of a shoulder shows development of the medial skin flap to identify the cephalic vein, which runs along the deltopectoral muscle interval.

achieve maximal bony contact. In addition, plate positioning that is too proximal will cause impingement against the acromion with arm elevation. Most plating systems have some radiographic marker for optimal plate height before screw placement.

- After reduction and plate application, the authors of this chapter prefer to begin with placement of a nonlocking screw into the slotted shaft position. This allows for proximal or distal plate positioning and allows the shaft to be pulled to the plate (**Figure 11**). This is the only nonlocking screw used in the construct preferred by the authors of this chapter.
- Four to six locking screws are drilled, measured, and placed through the targeting jig into the humeral head. Freehand placement of locking screws should be avoided to ensure proper plate/screw locking.
- Cross-threading or "cold welding" of the screw threads can make future implant removal difficult.
- All screw lengths should be checked

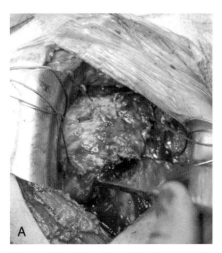 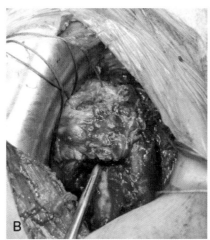

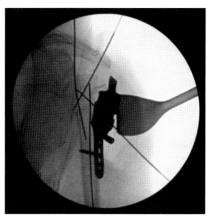

Figure 11 Intraoperative fluoroscopic image of a shoulder demonstrates provisional Kirschner wire fixation of the humeral head and tuberosity fragments to maintain reduction. The precontoured proximal humerus locking plate is then positioned lateral to the bicipital groove and secured to the shaft with one cortical screw placed in the oblong hole first to compress the plate to bone and to allow for proximal and distal translation of the plate.

Figure 10 Intraoperative photographs of a shoulder demonstrate surgical neck fracture reduction. **A,** The humeral head is reduced using a broad flat osteotome inserted into the fracture site. Levering upward reduces the valgus collapse of the humeral head. Care should be taken to keep the medial soft-tissue hinge intact to preserve the blood supply to the medial aspect of the humeral head. **B,** The humeral shaft is medialized by the pull of the pectoralis major. A bone hook that is placed in the humeral shaft can be used to lateralize the shaft into the correct position under the humeral head. Care should be taken in osteopenic bone because this maneuver can fracture the thin metaphyseal bone of the humeral shaft.

under biplanar fluoroscopy to avoid inadvertent humeral head penetration.

- Calcium phosphate bone cement can be introduced into the metaphysis either via a cortical window or a central hole in the plate through which the locking screw has been drilled but not yet placed (**Figure 12**).
- If placed through the plate, the final locking screw can be placed through the cement before it hardens.
- Range of motion should be measured intraoperatively after fixation is complete to ensure that there are no blocks to motion.
- The wound is closed in layers over a suction drain to prevent hematoma formation.

Rehabilitation

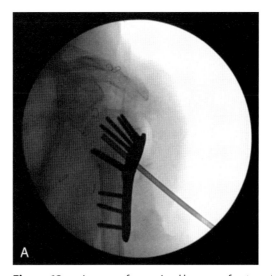 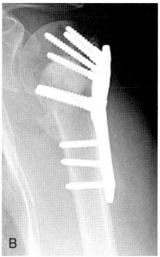

Figure 12 Images of a proximal humerus fracture. **A,** Intraoperative fluoroscopic image demonstrates injection of calcium phosphate bone cement (typically, 3 to 5 cm³ is sufficient) through a locking screw hole predrilled into a metaphyseal bone void. The cement is injected after the construct has been finalized and all screws have been checked, using biplanar fluoroscopy, to ensure that no intra-articular penetration has occurred. An additional screw can be placed into the locking screw hole through which the cement is injected before the cement hardens. **B,** AP radiograph obtained 9 months postoperatively demonstrates a healed fracture with no evidence of humeral head collapse and no intra-articular screw penetration.

The rehabilitation protocol after fixation of three- and four-part proximal humerus fractures is designed to progress from early ROM to prevent stiffness to strengthening and retraining for work and athletics (**Table 2**). Pendulum

Table 2 Rehabilitation Protocol After Fixation of Three- or Four-Part Proximal Humerus Fractures

Postoperative Week	ROM	Strengthening	Return to Play/Work	Comments/Emphasis
0-2	Pendulum exercises, active forward elevation and external rotation/internal rotation (depending on involvement of greater tuberosity or lesser tuberosity, respectively); active and passive ROM of elbow and wrist	None	N/A	Early ROM to prevent stiffness
2-6	Active and gentle passive forward elevation and external rotation/internal rotation (depending on involvement of greater tuberosity or lesser tuberosity, respectively), wall-crawling exercise; active and passive ROM of elbow and wrist	Gentle isometric strengthening of rotator cuff, scapular stabilizers	N/A	Improve ROM
6-12	Active and passive forward elevation and external rotation/internal rotation (depending on involvement of greater tuberosity or lesser tuberosity, respectively), wall-crawling exercise; active and passive ROM of elbow and wrist	Dynamic strengthening of rotator cuff, deltoid, scapular stabilizers	N/A	Focus on ROM and strengthening
12-24	Active and passive forward elevation and external rotation/internal rotation (depending on involvement of greater tuberosity or lesser tuberosity, respectively), wall-crawling exercise; active and passive ROM of elbow and wrist	Dynamic strengthening of rotator cuff, deltoid, scapular stabilizers	Gradual return to contact sports or return to work without restrictions	Focus on strengthening and athletic or work activity retraining

N/A = not applicable, ROM = range of motion.

exercises, active forward elevation, and active and passive ROM of the elbow and wrist are initiated in the first 2 weeks postoperatively. Exercises for internal and external rotation depend on the involvement of the greater and lesser tuberosities. At 2 to 6 weeks postoperatively, improving shoulder ROM is prioritized. Wall crawling exercises are initiated, along with active forward elevation and external/internal rotation (depending on the involvement of the tuberosities). From 6 to 12 weeks postoperatively, ROM and strengthening are emphasized. Passive shoulder motion is initiated, along with dynamic strengthening of the rotator cuff, deltoid, and scapular stabilizing muscles. From 3 to 6 months postoperatively, all therapy protocols are continued, emphasizing strengthening and return to athletic or work-related activity.

 Avoiding Pitfalls

Positioning and Draping

Beach-chair positioning with the captain's chair cutout on the surgical side allows full ROM of the arm intraoperatively, including arm extension. The entire forequarter is prepped and draped. The coracoid process and acromion process should be palpable in the field. For obese patients, in whom it may be difficult to palpate the coracoid process, fluoroscopy can be used to localize the coracoid process so the incision is placed in the correct interval. Some surgeons prefer to place the patient in the supine position on a radiolucent table with the image intensifier on the contralateral side. Although this is technically possible, it makes obtaining an axillary radiograph, which is needed for intraoperative assessment of the screw position,

difficult, and, therefore, the authors of this chapter do not recommend it

Intraoperative Fluoroscopy

Biplanar fluoroscopy is essential to avoid intra-articular screw placement. Positioning the C-arm at the head of the patient facilitates intraoperative AP and axillary views of the proximal humerus. Imaging should be used to ensure accurate placement of all locking screws into the humeral head and to ensure that no screws enter the intra-articular space.

Approach

Every attempt should be made to preserve the cephalic vein throughout the procedure. Although it is easier to mobilize the cephalic vein laterally, moving it medially will result in a greater likelihood of postoperative patency. This entails careful ligation of tributary branches to the deltoid. After mobilization of the vein medially, it does not have to be retracted for the remainder of the procedure, thereby preventing inadvertent laceration or thrombosis from constant pressure. Incising the coracoacromial ligament near its insertion on the lateral aspect of the coracoid process allows for superior visualization, which is helpful in the setting of greater tuberosity fragments displaced superiorly and posteriorly. In patients with metaphyseal comminution or a long metaphyseal spike extending into the proximal humeral diaphysis, the deltopectoral incision can be extended distally into the anterolateral approach for the humerus. The anterior deltoid insertion can be elevated to allow plate placement along the lateral humeral shaft without causing substantial deficit. If the biceps tendon is partially or completely torn, a soft-tissue tenodesis of the long head of the biceps tendon to the pectoralis major insertion should be considered using heavy braided, nonabsorbable suture.

Mobilization and Reduction of Tuberosity Fragments

Sequential placement of heavy sutures into the tuberosity/rotator cuff interface from anterior to posterior facilitates increased control of the tuberosity fragments. Internal rotation of the humerus will move the posterosuperiorly displaced greater tuberosity anteriorly into the surgical field. The rotator cuff should be inspected closely for evidence of a tear, for which primary repair should be performed. Intraoperative fluoroscopy should be used to ensure that the greater tuberosity is not riding high and is adequately reduced. To secure the tuberosity reductions, provisional K-wires should be placed out of the plane of the planned position of the proximal humerus locking plate. Displaced lesser tuberosity fragments may require independent anterior-to-posterior screw fixation in addition to suture fixation to the plate.

Plate Fixation

Prior to securing the plate to the bone, the tuberosity sutures are placed through the K-wire holes in the periphery of the plate (some plates allow easy passage of sutures through the plate even after the plate is secured to the bone). These tuberosity sutures will be tied after all plate screws have been placed. The plate can be provisionally fixed to the shaft with K-wires. The authors of this chapter recommend placing one of the provisional K-wires through the calcar screw portion of the plate (an inferomedial screw directed into the humeral head). The position of this K-wire will mimic the placement of the calcar screws and should be as inferior as possible along the inferomedial aspect of the proximal humerus. This position is biomechanically superior for the prevention of varus collapse in varus-displaced fractures. The first cortical screw should be placed through the oblong screw hole in the plate shaft to allow for minor adjustments in plate height. To achieve some compression of the superior aspect of the plate against the humeral head, a large, pointed bone reduction clamp can be used to directly reduce the humeral head to the proximal aspect of the plate. This maneuver will place the head into additional valgus and also can be used to eliminate any residual varus in the neck-shaft angle before locking screws are placed.

Calcium Phosphate Bone Cement Injection

If calcium phosphate bone cement is used, the authors of this chapter prefer to inject the cement through a predrilled hole in the center of the plate. Care should be taken to ensure that the cement is not injected into the intraarticular space. A locking screw can be placed through this hole after the cement is injected but before it has cured.

 Bibliography

Cornell CN: Internal fracture fixation in patients with osteoporosis. *J Am Acad Orthop Surg* 2003;11(2):109-119.

DeFranco MJ, Brems JJ, Williams GR Jr, Iannotti JP: Evaluation and management of valgus impacted four-part proximal humerus fractures. *Clin Orthop Relat Res* 2006;(442):109-114.

Egol KA, Forman J, Ong C, Rosenberg A, Karia R, Zuckerman JD: Regional anesthesia improves outcome in patients undergoing proximal humerus fracture repair. *Bull Hosp Jt Dis (2013)* 2014;72(3):231-236.

Egol KA, Sugi MT, Ong CC, Montero N, Davidovitch R, Zuckerman JD: Fracture site augmentation with calcium phosphate cement reduces screw penetration after open reduction-internal fixation of proximal humeral fractures. *J Shoulder Elbow Surg* 2012;21(6):741-748.

Esser RD: Open reduction and internal fixation of three- and four-part fractures of the proximal humerus. *Clin Orthop Relat Res* 1994;(299):244-251.

Fankhauser F, Boldin C, Schippinger G, Haunschmid C, Szyszkowitz R: A new locking plate for unstable fractures of the proximal humerus. *Clin Orthop Relat Res* 2005;(430):176-181.

Gaheer RS, Hawkins A: Fixation of 3- and 4-part proximal humerus fractures using the PHILOS plate: Mid-term results. *Orthopedics* 2010;33(9):671.

Gardner MJ, Boraiah S, Helfet DL, Lorich DG: Indirect medial reduction and strut support of proximal humerus fractures using an endosteal implant. *J Orthop Trauma* 2008;22(3):195-200.

Gerber C, Werner CM, Vienne P: Internal fixation of complex fractures of the proximal humerus. *J Bone Joint Surg Br* 2004;86(6):848-855.

Griza S, Zimmer CG, Reguly A, et al: A case study of subsequential intramedullary nails failure. *Eng Fail Anal* 2009;16(3):728-732.

Hessmann MH, Nijs S, Mittlmeier T, et al: Internal fixation of fractures of the proximal humerus with the MultiLoc nail. *Oper Orthop Traumatol* 2012;24(4-5):418-431.

Hodgson SA, Mawson SJ, Saxton JM, Stanley D: Rehabilitation of two-part fractures of the neck of the humerus (two-year follow-up). *J Shoulder Elbow Surg* 2007;16(2):143-145.

Kazakos K, Lyras DN, Galanis V, et al: Internal fixation of proximal humerus fractures using the Polarus intramedullary nail. *Arch Orthop Trauma Surg* 2007;127(7):503-508.

Kitson J, Booth G, Day R: A biomechanical comparison of locking plate and locking nail implants used for fractures of the proximal humerus. *J Shoulder Elbow Surg* 2007;16(3):362-366.

Moda SK, Chadha NS, Sangwan SS, Khurana DK, Dahiya AS, Siwach RC: Open reduction and fixation of proximal humeral fractures and fracture-dislocations. *J Bone Joint Surg Br* 1990;72(6):1050-1052.

Ong CC, Kwon YW, Walsh M, Davidovitch R, Zuckerman JD, Egol KA: Outcomes of open reduction and internal fixation of proximal humerus fractures managed with locking plates. *Am J Orthop (Belle Mead NJ)* 2012;41(9):407-412.

Papadopoulos P, Karataglis D, Stavridis SI, Petsatodis G, Christodoulou A: Mid-term results of internal fixation of proximal humeral fractures with the Philos plate. *Injury* 2009;40(12):1292-1296.

Platzer P, Thalhammer G, Oberleitner G, et al: Displaced fractures of the greater tuberosity: A comparison of operative and nonoperative treatment. *J Trauma* 2008;65(4):843-848.

Plecko M, Kraus A: Internal fixation of proximal humerus fractures using the locking proximal humerus plate [German]. *Oper Orthop Traumatol* 2005;17(1):25-50.

Südkamp N, Bayer J, Hepp P, et al: Open reduction and internal fixation of proximal humeral fractures with use of the locking proximal humerus plate: Results of a prospective, multicenter, observational study. *J Bone Joint Surg Am* 2009;91(6):1320-1328.

Szyszkowitz R, Seggl W, Schleifer P, Cundy PJ: Proximal humeral fractures: Management techniques and expected results. *Clin Orthop Relat Res* 1993;(292):13-25.

Tosounidis T, Hadjileontis C, Georgiadis M, Kafanas A, Kontakis G: The tendon of the long head of the biceps in complex proximal humerus fractures: A histological perspective. *Injury* 2010;41(3):273-278.

Wanner GA, Wanner-Schmid E, Romero J, et al: Internal fixation of displaced proximal humeral fractures with two one-third tubular plates. *J Trauma* 2003;54(3):536-544.

Chapter 45

Intramedullary Fixation of Proximal Humerus Fractures

Brian H. Mullis, MD

Jeffrey O. Anglen, MD

 ## Case Presentation

A 72-year-old woman who lives alone is brought to the emergency department for right arm, shoulder, and left hip pain after falling in her home. No history of syncope or dizziness is present. Physical examination reveals tenderness in the right shoulder, upper arm, and elbow; pain on motion of the right shoulder and elbow; a shortened, externally rotated left leg; and pain on motion of the hip. Neurovascular examination reveals normal pulses, perfusion, and motor and sensory function. Radiographs of the hip reveal an intertrochanteric fracture. Radiographs of the upper extremity reveal a displaced short oblique diaphyseal humerus fracture with a minimally displaced ipsilateral proximal humerus fracture of the surgical neck (**Figure 1, A** and **B**). After careful discussion with the patient and her family, the decision is made to manage the humeral fracture with locked intramedullary nailing. Factors considered in the decision include the need for upper extremity function for mobility given the hip fracture, the segmental nature of the fracture, and the presence of substantial osteoporosis.

Both the hip procedure and the shoulder procedure are performed in a single surgery on a fracture table. After the intertrochanteric hip fracture is reduced and fixed with the use of a sliding compression hip screw, the fracture table is rotated, and the right shoulder is positioned and prepared for surgery. An angular stable interlocking nail is used as described in the subsequent procedure section to fix the humeral fracture (**Figure 1, C** and **D**). The patient was out of bed on postoperative day 1, using the right upper extremity to assist with transfer. The patient progressed to weight bearing with a walker as tolerated.

 ## Indications

Codman described the four parts commonly involved in proximal humerus fractures, and Neer further classified these fractures to include the presence or absence of displacement and the degree of angulation, both of which are important in the prognosis and management of these fractures. Most proximal humerus fractures are nondisplaced and can be managed nonsurgically. Many forms of internal fixation have been used to manage displaced proximal humerus fractures, but no single technique has been shown to be superior or without complications. A role still exists for the closed management of displaced proximal humerus fractures in the elderly. Clinical variability and poor interobserver and intraobserver reliability in fracture classification have led to difficulty in clearly defining the indications for surgical treatment.

The factors involved in decision making for surgical management of proximal humerus fractures include the fracture pattern, the bone quality, the status of the rotator cuff, and the age and activity level of the patient. The goal of surgery is restoration of near anatomic alignment with secure fixation to allow for early range of motion (ROM). In general, displaced proximal humerus fractures in active patients are managed surgically. Many surgeons prefer open reduction with plate fixation for the treatment of patients who have displaced three- and four-part proximal humerus fractures; however, newer-generation nails allow for angular stability and suture fixation of displaced lesser or greater tuberosity fractures. Primary hemiarthroplasty, open reduction and internal fixation, and closed management of displaced three- or four-part proximal humerus fractures in elderly, low-demand patients continue to be a subject of debate.

A variety of fixation devices are available for use in the proximal humerus. Reduction and fixation with the use of an intramedullary nail may

Dr. Mullis is a member of a speakers' bureau or has made paid presentations on behalf of Daiichi Sankyo and Smith & Nephew; serves as a paid consultant to Biomet; and serves as a board member, owner, officer, or committee member of the Orthopaedic Trauma Association. Dr. Anglen or an immediate family member serves as a paid consultant to DJO and Eli Lilly.

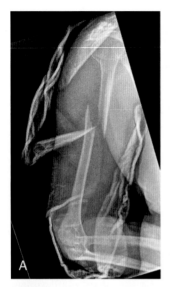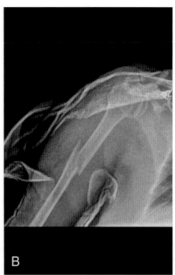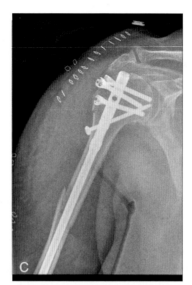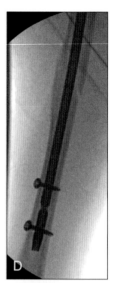

Figure 1   Images of the shoulder of a patient with a displaced short oblique diaphyseal humerus fracture with a minimally displaced ipsilateral proximal humerus fracture of the surgical neck. **A** and **B,** Preoperative radiographs demonstrate a segmental fracture of the humerus with a mid-diaphyseal displaced component and a nondisplaced two-part surgical neck fracture. Postoperative AP radiograph (**C**) and fluoroscopic image (**D**) show fixation of the humeral fracture with an interlocking nail.

be achieved in patients who have fractures with an intact humeral head. Most commonly, intramedullary nails are used for the treatment of patients who have displaced two-part surgical neck fractures; however, they also can be used for the treatment of patients who have displaced three-part proximal humerus fractures involving the greater tuberosity and displaced four-part proximal humerus fractures with minimal or no displacement of the lesser tuberosity. Intramedullary implants are particularly useful for the treatment of patients who have segmental humerus fractures in which a diaphyseal component is present in combination with a proximal fracture pattern. Intramedullary nails also can be used for the treatment of patients who have pathologic fractures or impending pathologic fractures, offering the advantage of minimal soft-tissue dissection for insertion and the ability to stabilize any potential skip lesions that occur more distal in the shaft. In a multiply injured patient, intramedullary nail fixation of a proximal humerus fracture may be a minimally invasive technique that enables early mobilization with weight bearing.

Contraindications

Contraindications to the surgical management of proximal humerus fractures include coexisting neurologic impairment sufficient to severely compromise upper extremity function (such as the hemiparetic extremity) as well as medical comorbidities that pose an extreme surgical risk, confer limited life expectancy, and involve active infection. Contraindications to intramedullary nail fixation of proximal humerus fractures are based on a surgeon's assessment of the fracture pattern, comminution, and bone quality. Other forms of management should be used for substantially displaced four-part proximal humerus fractures in elderly patients, fracture-dislocations, head-splitting fractures, anatomic neck fractures, and select three-part proximal humerus fractures in patients who have severe osteopenia because intramedullary nail fixation is unlikely to provide or maintain secure fixation.

Alternative Approaches

Most proximal humerus fractures are minimally displaced and can be managed nonsurgically with a sling and early mobilization. Surgical treatment options should be considered in patients who have displaced proximal humerus fractures, which constitute 15% to 20% of all proximal humerus fractures. Alternative surgical treatment options include open reduction and internal fixation procedures with plates and screws, tension-band wiring with heavy nonabsorbable sutures or wires, percutaneous procedures with pins or screws, unlocked intramedullary nailing with or without tension-band wiring, and prosthetic replacement.

Results

The ultimate goal of surgical management of displaced proximal humerus fractures is to achieve a comfortable and functional shoulder. Therefore, the results of intramedullary nailing of displaced proximal humerus fractures can be evaluated by the degree of pain relief, the ROM achieved, and the incidence of complications or failures requiring an additional surgical procedure.

Most patients report substantial pain relief and have improved shoulder scores after intramedullary nailing of displaced proximal humerus fractures. Outcome studies have demonstrated that a patient's fracture pattern and age correlate with pain relief and clinical outcomes. A study of 23 patients who had displaced three- or four-part proximal humerus fractures revealed that 6 of 10 patients who had three-part proximal humerus fractures reported little or no pain and no patients who had three-part proximal humerus fractures reported severe pain after intramedullary nailing. In the same study, of 10 patients who had four-part proximal humerus fractures, 2 reported little or no pain, 6 reported substantial pain, and 2 reported severe pain after intramedullary nailing. The patients with three-part proximal humerus fractures had mean Neer and Constant-Murley Shoulder Outcome scores of 83.6 and 88.4, respectively, and the patients with four-part proximal humerus fractures had mean Neer and Constant-Murley Shoulder Outcome scores of 62.5 and 67, respectively. Other studies have reported excellent or satisfactory results according to Neer and Constant-Murley Shoulder Outcome scores in 80% to 86% of patients after intramedullary nailing.

Similar to pain relief, the restoration of motion varies with the complexity of a patient's fracture pattern. In general, patients who undergo intramedullary nailing for the management of four-part proximal humerus fractures achieve less ROM compared with those who undergo intramedullary nailing for the management of three-part fractures. Good functional ROM can be achieved after locked intramedullary nailing in select displaced proximal humerus fractures.

A study reported that the mean postoperative ROM at 1-year follow-up of patients who underwent locked intramedullary nailing for the management of three-part proximal humerus fractures was 170° of forward flexion, 155° of abduction, 90° of internal rotation, and 60° of external rotation. The same study reported that the mean postoperative ROM at 1-year follow-up of patients who underwent locked intramedullary nailing for the management of four-part proximal humerus fractures was 100° of forward flexion, 120° of abduction, and 50° of both internal and external rotation. A study of 21 patients who underwent intramedullary nailing for the management of two-part proximal humerus fractures reported a mean ROM of 152° of forward flexion, 153° of abduction, 65° of internal rotation, and 48° of external rotation at a mean follow-up of 19 months.

Several different complications, including hardware failure, hardware loosening, prominent hardware, nonunion, stiffness, osteonecrosis, varus collapse, and superficial infection, have been reported in patients who undergo intramedullary nailing for the management of proximal humerus fractures. Complications that require an additional procedure are predominantly limited to loose or failed hardware and osteonecrosis. In a study of 11 patients who were treated with intramedullary nailing for two- or three-part proximal humerus fractures, 45% (5 patients, all of whom had three-part proximal humerus fractures) required additional procedures within 6 months postoperatively. Three patients required revision to cemented hemiarthroplasty as a result of failed fixation, one patient required revision intramedullary nailing, and one patient required removal of a loose proximal locking screw. Historically, a high rate of shoulder pain has been associated with humeral nails. There has been a recent trend to move the starting point more medial, using a straight nail to

potentially reduce the risk of shoulder pain, which is believed to be related to the reaming of the insertion of the rotator cuff into the greater tuberosity.

Video 45.1 Proximal Humerus Intramedullary Nail Technique. Brian H. Mullis, MD; Jeffrey O. Anglen, MD (15 min)

Technical Keys to Success

Setup/Exposure

- Preoperative planning begins with an evaluation of standard shoulder trauma radiographs, including an AP Grashey view of the glenohumeral joint, a scapular lateral view, and an axial view. Gentle traction radiographs may help delineate fracture anatomy in patients who have substantial displacement.
- Radiograph quality may vary; therefore, CT should be considered for patients who have displaced fractures that may require surgery, particularly if the humeral head is not well visualized.
- Patients, especially elderly osteoporotic patients, should be counseled that hemiarthroplasty may be required if adequate fixation cannot be achieved, and trays should be available if intraoperative conversion is necessary.
- A beach chair or a flat-top radiolucent table can be used.
- The patient is positioned with the shoulder just at the edge of the surgical table so that AP, scapular Y, and axillary lateral radiographs can be obtained (**Figure 2, A**).
- A small bump is placed at the medial border of the scapula.
- The arm can be placed on a padded Mayo stand during the procedure.
- A reverse Trendelenburg position of 30° is ideal.
- The head is secured in a headrest or

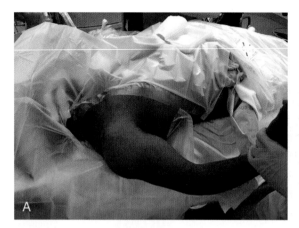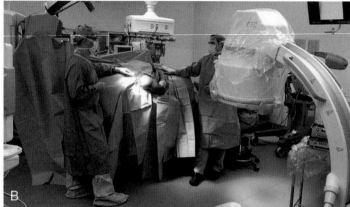

Figure 2   Photographs show patient positioning and operating room setup for intramedullary nailing of a displaced two-part surgical neck fracture. **A,** The patient is positioned with a bump under the medial scapular border. The patient's head is secured to the table, and the shoulder is positioned just at the edge of the radiolucent table so that AP, scapular Y, and axillary lateral radiographs can be obtained. **B,** The senior surgeon is positioned next to the patient's head, and an assistant is positioned at the patient's waist to help with traction. The C-arm is placed perpendicular to the patient so that all three fluoroscopic images can be obtained.

to the surgical table preoperatively, with periodic intraoperative checks to ensure that it remains secure.

- Typically, the C-arm is positioned perpendicular to the patient so that AP and axillary lateral fluoroscopic images can be obtained (**Figure 2, B**).

- A closed reduction attempt should provide confirmation of acceptable biplanar fracture visualization, assessment of fracture stability, and confirmation that no obstructions from the surgical table are present. Any necessary adjustments should be made before preparation and draping of the patient.

Instruments/Equipment/ Implants Required

- Important required technical aspects to consider are adequate patient positioning, fluoroscopic visualization of the fracture to allow for biplanar views of the shoulder and arm, fracture reduction, and implant insertion.

- In addition to the required implants, the appropriate equipment should be available.

- Fluoroscopy is integral to the procedure.

- Terminally threaded 2.5-mm Kirschner wires (K-wires) are helpful in gaining control of the proximal segments and for provisional fixation.

- An antegrade intramedullary nail device with multiple proximal locking options is necessary for closed reduction and intramedullary nailing.

- Humeral hemiarthroplasty and internal fixation devices should be available in the event that intraoperative difficulties arise during intramedullary nailing.

Procedure

- Intramedullary nailing can be accomplished via a deltoid-splitting approach.

- A longitudinal skin incision may be made in line with the greater tuberosity along the upper deltoid. Alternatively, an anterolateral saber-cut incision that follows the anterolateral aspect of the acromion may be used (**Figure 3**).

- The deltoid muscle is split in line with its fibers between the anterior and middle portions no more than 5 cm from the acromion to avoid injury to the axillary nerve. The

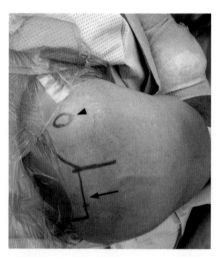

Figure 3   Preoperative photograph of a shoulder shows marking of the acromion (arrow) and coracoid (arrowhead) as well as a 4-cm incision at the anterolateral border of the acromion.

adducted arm permits access to the lateral portion of the rotator cuff.

- If an open reduction is necessary, a limited deltopectoral approach is used.

FRACTURE REDUCTION

- The expected entry point may be confirmed with the image intensifier and a K-wire before the supraspinatus tendon is incised in line with its fibers.

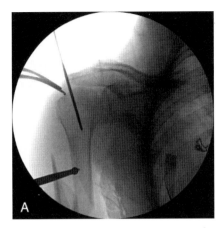
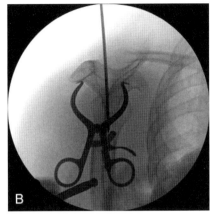
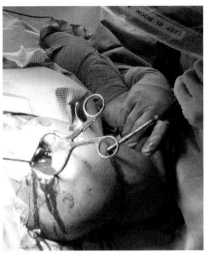

Figure 4   AP (**A**) and scapular Y (**B**) fluoroscopic images of a shoulder demonstrate guidewire placement at the lateral border of the articular cartilage. Note that a ball-spiked pusher was placed percutaneously to achieve an adducted position, which aids in the insertion of the guidewire. The scapular Y view confirms appropriate AP positioning.

Figure 5   Intraoperative photograph of a shoulder shows a ball-spiked pusher being used to hold the proximal fragment in an adducted position as the guidewire is placed. The rotator cuff was split longitudinally, and a soft-tissue protector was placed before the entry reamer was used. Alternatively, an awl can be used to open the canal.

- As with any intramedullary rod insertion, the entry point is the most important factor in avoiding malreduction. The implant insertion point is located at the lateral edge of the articular cartilage, approximately 1 cm posterior to the bicipital groove, and is confirmed on AP and scapular Y views (**Figure 4, A** and **B**).
- The entry point can be created using an entry reamer over a guidewire or using an awl.
- The guidewire position should be verified under image intensification to ensure that the guidewire has not exited through the fracture site.
- The rotator cuff should be protected during reaming or when creating the entry site with an awl to prevent damage.
- If necessary, K-wires or a ball-spiked pusher can be used to adduct the proximal humerus, aid in fracture reduction and realignment, and improve access for nail entry (**Figure 5**). If K-wires are used, it is important to ensure that they are placed anteriorly and posteriorly enough to avoid interfering with the nail insertion.

IMPLANT INSERTION

- Under fluoroscopic guidance, the implant with the attached targeting guide is inserted and aligned over the guidewire as fracture reduction is maintained with manipulation or percutaneous techniques.
- The nail is inserted with the use of manual pressure to a point at which the proximal aspect is below the cortex to avoid impingement with the subacromial structures. Care should be taken to avoid countersinking the nail more than 5 to 10 mm below the subchondral surface because doing so will place the proximal screws in a suboptimal position.
- The targeting guide and nail should be aligned to allow for optimal positioning of the screws into the tuberosities and humeral head.
- Screw length and placement are confirmed with fluoroscopy.
- In some patients, additional fixation of the tuberosities may be necessary.
- Via a limited deltopectoral approach, a suture tension-band technique may be used to augment tuberosity reduction and stability.
- Heavy nonabsorbable sutures are passed through the bone-tendon junction of the greater or lesser tuberosity. In some patients, nails also may be secured through suture holes in the interlocking screws. If no suture holes are available in the screw, the suture can be tied around the ends of interlocking screws.
- Alternatively, a unicortical small fragment screw or a hole that is drilled in the lateral cortex may serve as a post for the sutures.
- Depending on the type of implant, washers may be used in conjunction with the screws for fixation of fragmented tuberosities.
- To provide vertical and rotational stability, distal locking screws are placed in the targeting guide.
- The holes are drilled and measured, and the screws are seated under fluoroscopic guidance.
- Proximal and distal locking screws should be placed through small skin incisions in the deltoid, which is dissected bluntly with a

Table 1 Rehabilitation Protocol After Intramedullary Nailing of Displaced Proximal Humerus Fractures

Postoperative Week	ROM	Strengthening	Return to Play	Comments/Emphasis
0-4	Physician-supervised passive ROM Passive ER and FF with a 3-ft stick are done 2 to 3 times per day	None	No	A shoulder sling is used intermittently for patient comfort The hand may be used for light ADLs, such as grooming or feeding, lifting nothing heavier than a glass of water
4-6	Active and active-assisted ROM, with the goal of passive FF of 140° and ER of 30° Deltoid isometrics may be started	Grip strengthening and light resistance elbow exercises with the arm at the side	No	Advancement to these ROM exercises only after clinical and radiographic evidence of healing
6-8	Active and gentle passive ROM is continued	Strengthening is started and progressed as ROM improves Continue strengthening grip, elbow; may strengthen shoulder against gravity	Depends on sport, position, ROM, and strength Noncontact conditioning is allowed, but no throwing or contact sports at this time	—
8-12	No restrictions Continue stretching exercises until full ROM is achieved	Resistance exercises of the deltoid, rotator cuff, and scapular stabilizers are begun	Depends on sport, position, ROM, and strength Contact play can be initiated after there is radiographic evidence of healing, near full ROM, and 80% strength relative to the contralateral side	Initiation of strengthening depends on achievement of a comfortable functional ROM Radiographic evidence of healing should be expected at this time; if no healing is present, consider metabolic causes such as low vitamin D, malnutrition, and infection

ADLs = activities of daily living, ER = external rotation, FF = forward flexion, ROM = range of motion.

hemostat to provide a passage for the cannula, trocar, and screw. This step minimizes the risk of injury to the axillary nerve and its branches.

- When using long humeral nails, which may be necessary for segmental or comminuted fractures, the surgeon should consider a mini-open approach for the distal interlocking screws (making a small incision and exposing the bone) to avoid injuring the lateral antebrachial cutaneous nerve with AP distal interlocks or the radial nerve with lateral distal interlocks

because these structures are at risk in those areas.

- The humerus is taken through a ROM under fluoroscopy to assess the adequacy and stability of the reduction, ensuring that the proximal and distal segments move as a unit.
- Appropriate screw length without joint penetration is confirmed.

Wound Closure

- The defect in the supraspinatus tendon of the rotator cuff is reapproximated using heavy nonabsorbable sutures. In general, two

figure-of-8 sutures are used for the side-to-side repair.

- The deltoid fascia is reapproximated, and the skin is closed in a standard fashion.

 Rehabilitation

A rehabilitation protocol is noted in **Table 1**. Mobilization of the limb is begun in the early postoperative period. A shoulder sling is used intermittently for patient comfort. If no tuberosity fracture is present, the patient may be immediately advanced to weight bearing as tolerated. Patients who have a head injury or neuropathy should not be allowed to bear weight. Tuberosity involvement also precludes weight bearing.

Patients begin postoperative rehabilitation with a physical therapy program consisting of physician-supervised passive ROM exercises. Using a 3-foot stick and an overhead pulley, passive external rotation and forward flexion are initiated two to three times per day as tolerated. These exercises are preceded by gentle pendulum exercises. In patients who underwent lesser tuberosity fixation, external rotation is limited to neutral.

Follow-up visits should occur 2 weeks, 6 weeks, 3 months, 6 months, and 12 months postoperatively. Radiographs are obtained at each follow-up visit to assess union and implant complications. The patient is monitored for early postoperative stiffness and clinical signs of healing. If arthrofibrosis develops, it can be managed with physical therapy and the prudent use of steroid injections; however, manipulation under anesthesia is used rarely in the shoulder.

After clinical and radiographic evidence of healing is seen between 4 and 6 weeks postoperatively, the patient is advanced to active and active-assisted ROM exercises, with the goal of achieving passive forward flexion of 140° and external rotation of 30°. Deltoid isometrics also may be begun at this time. Resistance strengthening exercises of the deltoid, rotator cuff, and scapular stabilizers are delayed until 10 to 12 weeks postoperatively provided that the patient has achieved a comfortable functional ROM.

Avoiding Pitfalls

The complications of intramedullary nailing of proximal humerus fractures are similar to those of open reduction and internal fixation and arthroplasty. Most published complications are related to fixation problems. The most common complication is a malreduction with a varus deformity, which can lead to early failure. Such complications tend to occur in patients who undergo intramedullary nailing for the management of more complex proximal humerus fractures and in elderly patients who have osteopenic bone. A study that had a high revision surgery rate (45%) recommended against the use of an intramedullary nail device in patients who had displaced three- and four-part proximal humerus fractures because the authors believed that the failures were the result of insufficient purchase of the proximal locking screws in the fracture fragments. Therefore, patient selection for intramedullary nailing of proximal humerus fractures is paramount to avoid complications.

Prominent or loose proximal screws are the result of fixation within osteopenic bone or within tuberosity comminution. Several studies report the need for revision surgery to remove loose or prominent proximal screws. In patients who have osteopenic or comminuted bone, additional fixation with a suture tension band helps prevent fixation loosening. As previously discussed, a washer may be used in conjunction with the screws for fixation of fragmented tuberosities. Failure to properly seat the proximal locking screws or countersink the nail below the subchondral surface may lead to impingement within the subacromial structures.

A very low incidence of posttraumatic complications, such as osteonecrosis, nonunion, and malunion, is reported in the literature. Maintaining a closed reduction and intramedullary nailing technique minimizes disruption to the blood supply of the humeral head and soft-tissue stripping. Last, a properly positioned insertion site and the supplemental use of percutaneous K-wires optimize fracture reduction.

Bibliography

Adedapo AO, Ikpeme JO: The results of internal fixation of three- and four-part proximal humeral fractures with the Polarus nail. *Injury* 2001;32(2):115-121.

Agel J, Jones CB, Sanzone AG, Camuso M, Henley MB: Treatment of proximal humeral fractures with Polarus nail fixation. *J Shoulder Elbow Surg* 2004;13(2):191-195.

Bernard J, Charalambides C, Aderinto J, Mok D: Early failure of intramedullary nailing for proximal humeral fractures. *Injury* 2000;31(10):789-792.

Court-Brown CM, Garg A, McQueen MM: The translated two-part fracture of the proximal humerus: Epidemiology and outcome in the older patient. *J Bone Joint Surg Br* 2001;83(6):799-804.

Hauschild O, Konrad G, Audige L, et al: Operative versus non-operative treatment for two-part surgical neck fractures of the proximal humerus. *Arch Orthop Trauma Surg* 2013;133(10):1385-1393.

Hessmann MH, Hansen WS, Krummenauer F, Pol TF, Rommens P: Locked plate fixation and intramedullary nailing for proximal humerus fractures: A biomechanical evaluation. *J Trauma* 2005;58(6):1194-1201.

Iannotti JP, Ramsey ML, Williams GR Jr, Warner JJ: Nonprosthetic management of proximal humeral fractures. *Instr Course Lect* 2004;53:403-416.

Koval KJ, Blair B, Takei R, Kummer FJ, Zuckerman JD: Surgical neck fractures of the proximal humerus: A laboratory evaluation of ten fixation techniques. *J Trauma* 1996;40(5):778-783.

Lin J, Hou SM, Hang YS: Locked nailing for displaced surgical neck fractures of the humerus. *J Trauma* 1998;45(6):1051-1057.

Lopiz Y, Garcia-Coiradas J, Garcia-Fernandez C, Marco F: Proximal humerus nailing: A randomized clinical trial between curvilinear and straight nails. *J Shoulder Elbow Surg* 2014;23(3):369-376.

Maier D, Jaeger M, Izadpanah K, Strohm PC, Suedkamp NP: Proximal humeral fracture treatment in adults. *J Bone Joint Surg Am* 2014;96(3):251-261.

Neer CS II: Displaced proximal humeral fractures: I. Classification and evaluation. *J Bone Joint Surg Am* 1970;52(6):1077-1089.

Neer CS II: Displaced proximal humeral fractures: II. Treatment of three-part and four-part displacement. *J Bone Joint Surg Am* 1970;52(6):1090-1103.

Parsons M, O'Brien RJ, Hughes JS: Locked intramedullary nailing for displaced and unstable proximal humerus fractures. *Tech Shoulder Elbow Surg* 2005;6(2):75-86.

Phipatanakul WP, Norris TR: Indications for prosthetic replacement in proximal humeral fractures. *Instr Course Lect* 2005;54:357-362.

Rajasekhar C, Ray PS, Bhamra MS: Fixation of proximal humeral fractures with the Polarus nail. *J Shoulder Elbow Surg* 2001;10(1):7-10.

Ruch DS, Glisson RR, Marr AW, Russell GB, Nunley JA: Fixation of three-part proximal humeral fractures: A biomechanical evaluation. *J Orthop Trauma* 2000;14(1):36-40.

Wheeler DL, Colville MR: Biomechanical comparison of intramedullary and percutaneous pin fixation for proximal humeral fracture fixation. *J Orthop Trauma* 1997;11(5):363-367.

 ## Video Reference

Mullis BH, Anglen JO: Video. Proximal Humerus Intramedullary Nail Technique. Indianapolis, IN, 2015.

Chapter 46

Hemiarthroplasty to Manage Proximal Humerus Fractures

Kamal I. Bohsali, MD, FACS

Michael A. Wirth, MD

Introduction

Approximately 10% of proximal humerus fractures are three- or four-part injuries. The Neer classification system categorizes these fractures based on anatomic location (humeral shaft, lesser tuberosity, greater tuberosity, and articular surface), displacement of more than 1 cm, and angulation of at least 45° (**Figure 1**).

The intact humeral head receives its blood supply from the anterolateral branch of the anterior humeral circumflex artery and the posterior humeral circumflex vessel. The anterolateral artery contributes branches to the lesser tuberosity, traverses the bicipital groove, and then runs parallel to the lateral aspect of the long head of the biceps tendon. The vessel then enters the humeral head at the junction of the intertubercular groove and the greater tuberosity, where it courses in a posteromedial direction and gives rise to multiple branches that supply the subchondral bone of the humeral head. The posterior humeral circumflex artery travels posterior to the humeral head from the third segment of the axillary artery with the axillary

nerve through the quadrangular space. In patients with four-part fractures, the anterolateral ascending branch is disrupted; this disruption, combined with a denuded articular portion, may render the fracture segment avascular.

According to a 2004 study, the most important predictors of humeral head ischemia are the length of the dorsomedial metaphyseal extension, the integrity of the medial hinge, and the basic fracture pattern. The trifecta of a short medial calcar (<8 mm), medial hinge disruption, and an anatomic neck pattern demonstrated a 97% positive predictive value in assessing humeral head ischemia. More recent studies, however, have indicated that certain three- and four-part injuries may have intact blood supply through the rotator cuff attachments and the posterior humeral circumflex artery. A quantitative MRI analysis published in 2010 suggested that the posterior humeral circumflex artery provides a greater portion of the blood supply compared with the anterolateral branch of the anterior humeral circumflex artery through multiple perforating branches in proximity to the posterior humeral head (64% and

36%, respectively). In addition, valgus impacted four-part proximal humerus fractures represent a specific subtype of the proximal humerus fracture that has a much lower prevalence of osteonecrosis as a result of an intact medial hinge and capsular blood supply. These injuries may be amenable to surgical treatments, such as percutaneous pinning and formal open reduction and internal fixation.

Case Presentation

A 70-year-old, right-hand–dominant woman sustained a four-part right proximal humerus fracture as the result of a ground-level fall (**Figure 2**, **A** through **D**). The patient underwent medical optimization before surgical intervention. Hemiarthroplasty reconstruction with a modular platform-based prosthesis was performed with tuberosity reconstruction (**Figure 2**, **E** and **F**).

Indications

The primary indications for hemiarthroplasty reconstruction include four-part fractures; three-part fractures; and fracture-dislocations in older patients with osteoporosis, chronic anterior or posterior dislocation of the humeral head with involvement of more than 40% of the articular surface, and

Dr. Bohsali or an immediate family member is a member of a speakers' bureau or has made paid presentations on behalf of DePuy and serves as a board member, owner, officer, or committee member of the American Academy of Orthopaedic Surgeons. Dr. Wirth or an immediate family member has received royalties from DePuy; is a member of a speakers' bureau or has made paid presentations on behalf of and serves as a paid consultant to DePuy and Tornier; has stock or stock options held in Tornier; and serves as a board member, owner, officer, or committee member of the American Shoulder and Elbow Surgeons.

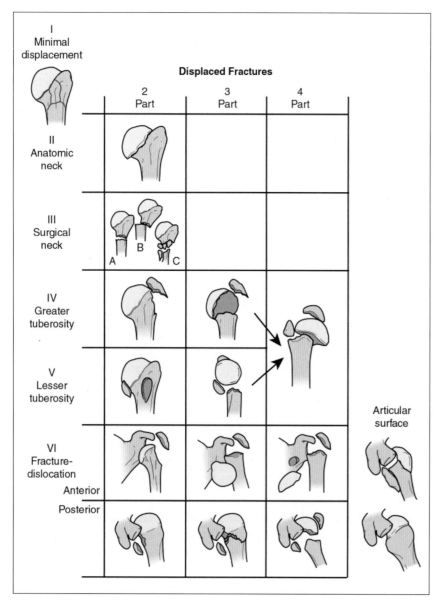

Figure 1   Illustration shows the Neer classification system, which is based on displacement and/or angulation of the four proximal humerus fracture segments: the humeral shaft, the lesser tuberosity, the greater tuberosity, and the articular surface. Displaced fractures may be two-, three-, or four-part with or without associated dislocation of the humeral head. A fracture fragment is considered displaced when separation is greater than 1 cm or angulation is greater than 45°. Articular surface injuries are typically associated with fractures of the tuberosity and the surgical neck. (Reproduced from Jones CB: Proximal humeral fractures, in Boyer MI, ed: *AAOS Comprehensive Orthopaedic Review*, ed 2. Rosemont, IL, American Academy of Orthopaedic Surgeons, 2014, pp 293-302.)

head-splitting articular segment fractures. Less commonly, some younger patients may have fracture patterns that cannot be feasibly reduced with internal fixation, thus necessitating arthroplasty. Relative contraindications to surgical treatment include medical comorbidities that preclude surgical treatment and an inability or unwillingness of the patient to follow the postoperative rehabilitation regimen, such as in patients with a closed head injury. Absolute contraindications to surgical treatment include active infection or sepsis and axillary nerve injury.

 ## Controversies and Alternative Approaches

Treatment options involve benign neglect, open reduction and internal fixation, closed reduction with percutaneous pin fixation, and reverse total shoulder arthroplasty. Nonsurgical treatment is generally reserved for patients who are medically infirm and unable to comply with postoperative restrictions and rehabilitation after hemiarthroplasty. Valgus impacted four-part proximal humerus fractures may be treated with closed reduction and pin fixation, although the forces of the rotator cuff, the pectoralis major, and the deltoid may preclude anatomic reduction. Some surgeons have recommended treating three- and four-part fractures with initial open reduction and internal fixation and reserving arthroplasty as a salvage option; however, the results of delayed arthroplasty reconstruction of three- and four-part fractures have proved inferior to the results of acute intervention, particularly in patients with malunion requiring tuberosity osteotomy. Reverse total shoulder arthroplasty has gained renewed interest as a primary option for the treatment of three- and four-part proximal humerus fractures. Several studies have demonstrated improved functional outcomes and similar short-term and midterm complication rates of reverse shoulder arthroplasty compared with hemiarthroplasty. Reverse total shoulder arthroplasty may be appropriate in patients with four-part proximal humerus fractures in which tuberosity reconstruction is not feasible because of comminution or osteoporosis. Newer implant systems allow for the conversion of hemiarthroplasty to reverse shoulder arthroplasty with stem

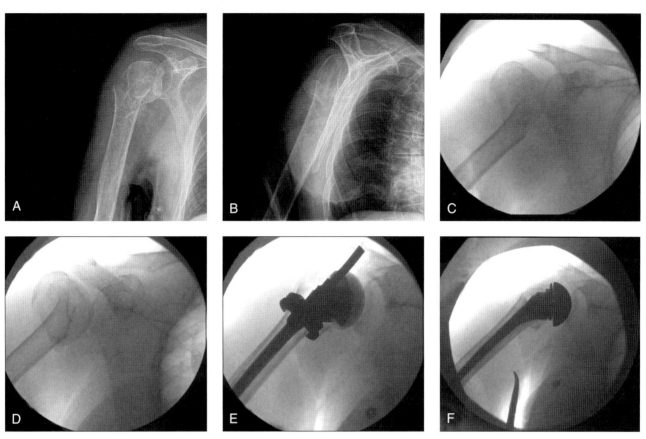

Figure 2   Preoperative AP (**A**) and scapular Y (**B**) radiographs and intraoperative fluoroscopic images (**C** and **D**) of a shoulder demonstrate a four-part proximal humerus fracture. Intraoperative AP fluoroscopic images of a shoulder demonstrate the position of a trial stem (**E**) and anatomic restoration of humeral head height and tuberosity position with the final implant in place (**F**).

retention, the use of modular implants, and adherence to the Grammont principles of reverse shoulder arthroplasty reconstruction, but data and follow-up are limited.

In the physiologically active individual, hemiarthroplasty remains a viable technique in the management of three- and four-part proximal humerus fractures with reconstructible tuberosities. The discussion of hemiarthroplasty versus reverse shoulder arthroplasty is a controversial topic because limited evidence exists to support one modality over the other. Most shoulder and elbow subspecialists would argue that reverse shoulder arthroplasty is an appropriate treatment option for patients aged 65 years or older with tuberosity comminution that precludes stable, anatomic reduction. The added benefit of hemiarthroplasty is a lack of dependence of tuberosity healing for improved shoulder function.

 Results

Clinical studies of hemiarthroplasty in patients with proximal humerus fractures are often difficult to compare because of the heterogeneity of fracture patterns, rehabilitation protocols, surgical techniques, implant designs, and functional outcome measurements. Given these limitations, results show that hemiarthroplasty provides pain relief with varying levels of shoulder function (**Table 1**).

Patient-specific and surgeon-controlled variables affect outcomes after hemiarthroplasty. Poorer outcomes have been seen in patients with advanced age (>75 years), female sex, and fracture comminution because of underlying osteoporosis and noncompliance with postoperative rehabilitation protocols. Additional patient-specific factors, such as rotator cuff deficiency, tobacco use, moderate to high levels of alcohol consumption, and neurologic injury, negatively affect functional outcomes. The timing of surgical intervention depends on patient-specific and surgeon-controlled factors because some individuals require medical optimization before definitive surgical treatment. Some surgeons have advocated intervention within 48 hours, whereas others have suggested delayed surgery to mitigate additional trauma to the acutely inflamed soft-tissue envelope. Other studies have suggested that a delay in

Table 1 Results of Hemiarthroplasty to Manage Three- and Four-Part Proximal Humerus Fractures

Authors	Journal (Year)	No. of Patients	Outcomes[a]	Comments
Prakash et al	*J Shoulder Elbow Surg* (2002)	22	20 patients were satisfied with their outcomes	Complications: 3 tuberosity malunions or nonunions, 1 loose prosthesis 1 patient required revision 7 yr postoperatively Mean age, 69 yr Mean follow-up, 33 mo (range, 6-93 mo)
Mighell et al	*J Shoulder Elbow Surg* (2003)	71	ASES score, 66 SST score, 71 Results were excellent in 35 shoulders, good in 19, satisfactory in 12, and unsatisfactory in 6	Complications: 3 tuberosity nonunions, 18 heterotopic bone formations, 6 glenoid arthroses, 1 infection, 1 aseptic humeral stem loosening, 1 ankylosis, 1 CRPS 4 patients required revision surgery Mean age, 66 yr Mean follow-up, 36 mo (range, 12-89 mo)
Antuña et al	*J Shoulder Elbow Surg* (2008)	57	Neer rating was excellent in 6 patients, satisfactory in 21, and unsatisfactory in 30	Complications: 1 posterior dislocation, 1 tuberosity malunion, 1 implant loosening 2 patients required revision surgery Mean age, 66 yr Mean follow-up, 123.6 mo (range, 60-264 mo)
Fialka et al	*J Shoulder Elbow Surg* (2008)	18 (group 1: wire cables through a medial and a lateral hole in the stem) 17 (group 2: transosseous braided sutures)	Age- and sex-adjusted Constant scores: group 1, 70.4; group 2, 46.2	Complications: 10 tuberosity resorptions, 18 heterotopic bone formations, 2 infections Mean age, 74 yr Minimum follow-up, 12 mo
Greiner et al	*J Shoulder Elbow Surg* (2008)	30	Age- and sex-adjusted Constant score, 70.7 DASH score, 39.8	Complications: NR Mean age, 74.8 yr Mean follow-up, 27.7 mo (range, 15-40 mo)
Bastian and Hertel	*J Shoulder Elbow Surg* (2009)	49	Constant score, 70 (range, 39-84) Subjective shoulder value, 90 (range, 40-100)	Complications: 6 cases of arthrofibrosis, 1 hematoma, 3 tuberosity displacements 10 patients required revision surgery Mean age, 66 yr Mean follow-up, 60 mo (range, 39.6-87.6 mo)
Kryzak et al	*Clin Orthop Relat Res* (2010)	8	Neer rating was excellent in 2 patients, satisfactory in 2, and unsatisfactory in 3	Complications: 4 tuberosity nonunions or malunions Mean age, 72 yr Mean follow-up, 118.8 mo (24-192 mo)
Boileau et al	*J Shoulder Elbow Surg* (2011)	30	Avg Constant score, 68	Complications: NR Mean age, 66 yr Mean follow-up, 45 mo (range, 24-48 mo)
Krishnan et al	*Clin Orthop Relat Res* (2011)	58 (group 1: conventional prosthesis) 112 (group 2: fracture-specific humeral prosthesis)	ASES, 66 (group 1, 72; group 2, 55) VAS: group 1, 2.1; group 2, 1.9	Complications: 3 infections, 2 periprosthetic fractures, 10 tuberosity nonunions 16 patients required revision surgery Mean age, 73 yr (group 1); 72 yr (group 2) Mean follow-up, 32 mo (range, 24-96 mo)

ASES = American Shoulder and Elbow Surgeons shoulder outcome; CRPS = complex regional pain syndrome; DASH = Disabilities of the Arm, Shoulder and Hand; EQ-5D = EuroQol Five Dimension; NR = not reported; Penn = Penn Shoulder Score; SST = Simple Shoulder Test; VAS = visual analog scale.
[a] Mean value unless otherwise noted.

Table 1 Results of Hemiarthroplasty to Manage Three- and Four-Part Proximal Humerus Fractures (*continued*)

Authors	Journal (Year)	No. of Patients	Outcomes[a]	Comments
Olerud et al	*J Shoulder Elbow Surg* (2011)	27	Constant score, 48.3 DASH score, 30.2 EQ-5D, 0.81	Complications: 8 tuberosity resorptions or displacements Mean age, 76.7 yr Mean follow-up, 24 mo
Boons et al	*Clin Orthop Relat Res* (2012)	25	Constant score, 64 SST score, 25 (range, 8-100) VAS, 23 (range, 1-65)	Complications: 1 implant dissociation, 6 tuberosity nonunions or malunions 1 patient required revision surgery Mean age, 76.4 yr Mean follow-up, 12 mo
Cai et al	*Orthopedics* (2012)	12	Constant score, 72.9 DASH score, 9.2 EQ-5D, 0.81 VAS, 13	Complications: 1 prosthetic loosening, 1 dislocation, 1 infection 3 patients required revision surgery Mean age, 71.1 yr Mean follow-up, 24 mo
Garrigues et al	*Orthopedics* (2012)	12	ASES score, 47.4 Penn, 52.5 Single Assessment Numeric Evaluation, 38.5 EQ-5D, 64.2	Complications: 2 cases of tuberosity nonunion or resorption, 2 cases of brachial plexopathy 3 patients required revision surgery Mean age, 69.3 yr Mean follow-up, 43.2 mo (range, 15.6-96 mo)
Boyle et al	*J Shoulder Elbow Surg* (2013)	313	Oxford Shoulder Score, 32.3	Complications: NR Mean age, 71.9 yr Mean follow-up, 60 mo
Fucentese et al	*J Shoulder Elbow Surg* (2014)	25	Absolute Constant score, 59 (range, 26-81) Age- and sex-adjusted Constant score, 75 (range, 31-100) 23 patients had a satisfactory result	Complications: 2 tuberosity displacements 4 failures were reported, with 2 patients requiring revision surgery Mean age, 63.3 yr Mean follow-up, 25 mo (range, 24-29 mo)

ASES = American Shoulder and Elbow Surgeons shoulder outcome; CRPS = complex regional pain syndrome; DASH = Disabilities of the Arm, Shoulder and Hand; EQ-5D = EuroQol Five Dimension; NR = not reported; Penn = Penn Shoulder Score; SST = Simple Shoulder Test; VAS = visual analog scale.
[a] Mean value unless otherwise noted.

intervention of more than 2 weeks results in reduced range of motion and functional outcomes postoperatively.

Tuberosity reduction and anatomic prosthetic height and version remain the most important factors under a surgeon's primary control. Tuberosity union partially depends on the initial anatomic reduction; the rate of healing also depends on patient characteristics, such as age, nutritional status, and medical comorbidities (such as renal disease).

In one study, the position of the greater tuberosity 5 mm above or 10 mm below the apex of the prosthetic humeral head was associated with suboptimal results. In addition, humeral lengthening greater than 10 mm and retroversion greater than 40° both correlated with reduced functional outcomes. Another study demonstrated superior range of motion (forward flexion, external rotation, and internal rotation) when the greater tuberosity was placed 10 to 16 mm below

the apex of the prosthetic humeral head. Clinical scores were lower in patients who had rotator cuff pathology, especially fatty infiltration.

Video 46.1 Fracture Platform Prosthesis. Michael A. Wirth, MD; Kamal I. Bohsali, MD, FACS (13 min)

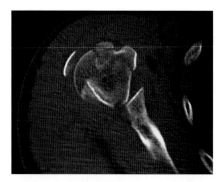

Figure 3 Axial CT scan demonstrates a comminuted right proximal humerus fracture in which the articular segment has rotated 180° counterclockwise to the glenoid articular surface.

 Technical Keys to Success

A thorough history and a complete physical examination are necessary, even in patients with an isolated injury of the proximal humerus. The history should include the mechanism of injury and the patient's occupation, hand dominance, premorbid functional status, history of malignancy, and ability to comply with postoperative restrictions and rehabilitation. A thorough examination should involve questions about loss of consciousness, paresthesias in the affected upper extremity, and pain in the ipsilateral elbow or wrist. The patient's shoulder should be evaluated for vascular status, swelling, ecchymosis, soft-tissue injuries, and deformity. In patients with acute injury, sensory deficits involving the lateral aspect of the shoulder may indicate an axillary nerve injury. Posterior fracture-dislocations result in anterior flattening of the shoulder and posterior prominence, whereas anterior fracture-dislocations demonstrate posterior flattening and anterior prominence.

Appropriate imaging includes AP and axillary radiographs of the affected shoulder. Patients may not tolerate the axillary lateral view because of pain. An alternative view, such as the Velpeau

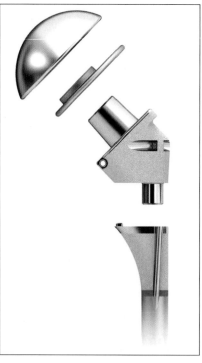

Figure 4 Graphic depiction of a modular platform-based system that allows for hemiarthroplasty reconstruction of proximal humerus fractures with stem retention and has the ability to convert to a reverse shoulder prosthesis. (Courtesy of DePuy Synthes, Warsaw, IN.)

trauma axillary view, can be used to evaluate and classify the glenohumeral articulation. CT may be used to evaluate tuberosity displacement and humeral head involvement (**Figure 3**). Radiographs of the contralateral unaffected shoulder are not mandatory, but they will guide the surgeon regarding humeral head size during reconstruction.

Hemiarthroplasty implant designs for proximal humerus fractures have evolved with regard to proximal body shape, modularity, and initial fixation. Some surgeons have demonstrated improved tuberosity healing and functional outcomes with fracture-specific implants. Generally, these implants contain a recessed proximal body with fins and multiple suture holes for tuberosity reduction and fixation. Other implants demonstrate a central cutout to facilitate bone grafting and tuberosity

union. Recently, platform-based systems with or without suture collars assist in anatomic reconstruction and can be converted to a semiconstrained device if the index procedure fails as a result of tuberosity displacement, resorption, or nonunion. When these systems are used, the reconstruction begins with secure fixation of a diaphyseal component, which allows for modular reconstruction of the proximal humerus, restoration of humeral head height and version, and tuberosity reduction (**Figure 4**).

Regardless of implant design, the key principles of hemiarthroplasty in the treatment of proximal humerus fractures are restoration of anatomic humeral head height and version and secure fixation of the shaft and tuberosities to the prosthesis and to each other.

Patient Positioning and Initial Exposure

- Perioperatively, the patient is administered appropriate intravenous antibiotics. At the surgeon's discretion, general anesthesia may be augmented with an interscalene block to provide intraoperative muscle relaxation and postoperative pain control.
- The patient is positioned on the surgical table in a modified beach-chair or semi-Fowler position (**Figure 5**). Commercially available beach-chair attachments may be used to achieve stable positioning of the patient with easy access to the affected shoulder.
- The cervical spine should be maintained in neutral alignment, and all bony prominences should be padded.
- Intraoperative C-arm fluoroscopy is strongly recommended. The C-arm may be positioned on the contralateral side at the head of the table to allow for intraoperative assessment of implant positioning and tuberosity reduction. An initial C-arm image is recommended to confirm

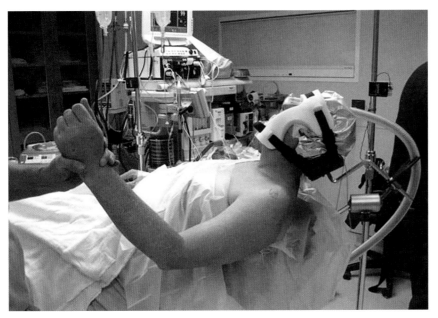

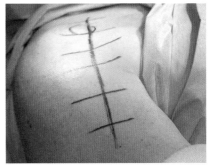

Figure 6 Preoperative photograph of a shoulder shows the location of the incision for the deltopectoral approach, which begins overlying the palpable coracoid process and extends to the topographic position of the deltoid insertion.

Figure 5 Preoperative photograph shows a patient placed in the semi-Fowler position using a commercially available beach-chair attachment.

the ability to visualize the fracture site before preparing for the surgical procedure.

- The affected extremity may be secured with a commercially available limb positioner. If sufficient support staff members are available, the authors of this chapter prefer to have the arm draped free with a padded Mayo stand.
- The affected upper extremity is prepped from the lateral aspect of the neck to the level of the wrist and draped. Unless the injury site is associated with an open wound, the authors of this chapter recommend using a commercially available preparation that contains a combination of chlorhexidine and isopropyl alcohol because this preparation has been shown to reduce staphylococcal colonization in the shoulder region compared with preparations such as povidone-iodine or iodine povacrylex with isopropyl alcohol.
- A deltopectoral approach is used, with the incision beginning superior and medial to the coracoid process and extending toward the

anterior aspect of the deltoid insertion (**Figure 6**).

- The cephalic vein is identified, preserved, and retracted laterally with the deltoid musculature.
- The pectoralis major insertion is noted and preserved to facilitate restoration of humeral head height. Several studies have estimated the humeral head apex to be 5.6 cm (± 0.5 cm) from the superior margin of the pectoralis major insertion. If necessary for exposure, the proximal 1 cm of the pectoralis major insertion may be released.
- Self-retaining soft-tissue retractors, such as Hawkins-Bell (DePuy) or Kolbel (Innomed) retractors, may be placed deep to the deltoid and the pectoralis major insertion.
- Fracture hematoma and fragments will usually be encountered after release of the clavipectoral fascia.
- The axillary and musculocutaneous nerves should be visually identified and palpated to assess integrity. The axillary nerve is located on the anteroinferior aspect of the subscapularis muscle, whereas the

musculocutaneous nerve is located approximately 3 to 6 cm from the origin of the conjoint tendon.

- Intermittent relaxation of arm position during the surgical procedure is recommended to reduce the risk of iatrogenic injury to the brachial plexus and the peripheral nerves (such as the axillary nerve).

Tuberosity Identification and Mobilization

- The surgeon should identify the long head of the biceps tendon as it extends in the bicipital groove toward the rotator interval. If the tendon is traumatically ruptured, the surgeon should attempt to locate it proximal or distal to the site of injury. This tendon is a critical landmark in the restoration of the positional relationship between the greater and lesser tuberosities (**Figure 7**).
- The rotator cuff interval and the coracohumeral ligament are incised to allow the tuberosities to be mobilized.
- If the bicipital groove is spared, then it may be necessary to use an osteotome or a sagittal saw to create a plane for tuberosity mobilization. The coracoacromial ligament

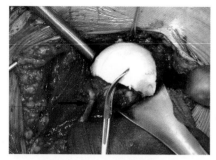

Figure 7 Intraoperative photograph of a shoulder shows a rupture of the long head of the biceps tendon (arrow) with medial dislocation.

should be retained to reduce the risk of proximal humeral head migration.

- Large-caliber, nonabsorbable sutures are placed through the rotator cuff tendon insertions adjacent to their attachment on the respective tuberosities (**Figure 8**). Multiple sutures should be threaded through the subscapularis tendon, and additional sutures should be placed through the supraspinatus in a horizontal mattress pattern. If a stem with a suture collar is used, definitive sutures may be placed with a Mayo needle after the humeral stem is implanted.

- With the tuberosities retracted, the humeral head and shaft fragments are removed. In patients with four-part fractures, the humeral head articular surface will have no soft-tissue attachments and can be removed for templating (**Figure 9**).

- All bone fragments, including the cancellous portion of the humeral head, are collected and morcellized for later grafting of the tuberosity and humeral shaft interfaces.

- The greater and lesser tuberosities may need to be reduced in volume to allow for appropriate reduction. To facilitate tuberosity healing, aggressive debulking of the tuberosities should be avoided.

- A Sonnabend retractor (DePuy Synthes), placed posteriorly, and two

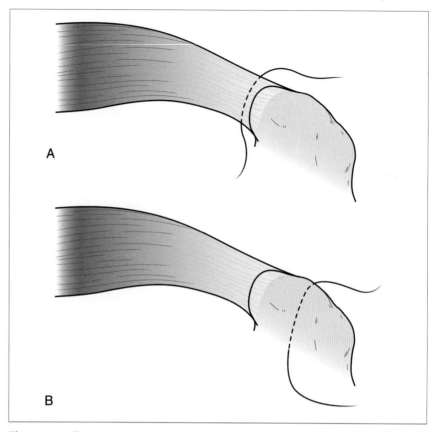

Figure 8 Illustrations show placement of large-caliber, nonabsorbable cerclage suture at the rotator cuff tendon-tuberosity attachment site (bone-tendon junction; **A**) and through the bone itself (incorrect; **B**). Suture placement through the bone-tendon junction, as shown in panel A, provides superior fixation, achieving traction and mobilization of the tuberosity.

Hohmann retractors, one placed superiorly and one placed inferiorly, may be used to achieve adequate visualization of the glenoid.

- The glenoid surface is examined for concomitant injury, and unstable fractures are addressed with internal fixation.

- Glenoid resurfacing may be required in patients with substantial glenoid wear but is contraindicated in patients with a structurally or functionally deficient rotator cuff.

Humeral Shaft Preparation

- After the tuberosities have been tagged and retracted, the surgeon delivers the humeral shaft anteriorly and superiorly.

- Fracture hematoma and detached

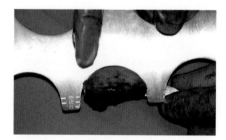

Figure 9 Clinical photograph shows a removed humeral head articular surface for size assessment and later bone grafting.

fragments of bone are extracted from the intramedullary canal of the humerus.

- Axial reamers in 1-mm increments are used on hand power to dilate the humeral shaft for trial stem implantation with or without

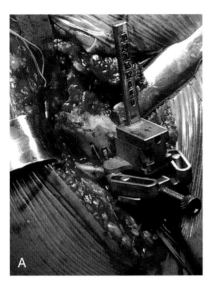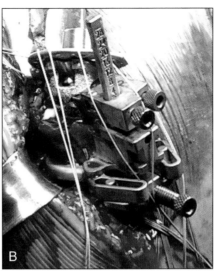

Figure 10   **A** and **B,** Intraoperative photographs of a shoulder show a commercially available clamp used for humeral stem height and version reproduction. Note the suture collar and sutures in **B**, which are used for tuberosity reduction and fixation.

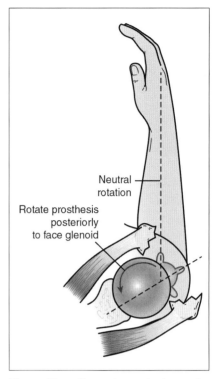

Figure 11   Illustration depicts the anatomic markers and axes used to position a humeral stem with a patient's arm in neutral rotation. The lateral fin of the prosthesis is placed approximately 8 mm posterior to the bicipital groove. The epicondylar axis also may be used to establish retroversion.

cement. Patients with osteoporotic bone require cement fixation of the humeral component to achieve implant stability for postoperative rehabilitation. Third- and fourth-generation fracture-specific stems with ongrowth and ingrowth surfaces may allow the surgeon to achieve press-fit fixation within the humeral diaphysis without using cement.

- If an implant system without a suture collar is used, the trial humeral implant should be placed with the lateral fin slightly posterior to the bicipital groove to approximate native version, and the medial aspect of the trial head should be placed at least at the height of the medial calcar. Caution should be employed when using the bicipital groove as a reference for tuberosity version because the groove internally rotates distally.
- In patients with four-part fractures and comminution involving the surgical neck region, the surgeon should take care not to inadvertently place the implant into excessive retroversion. The stem is maintained in position with a fracture clamp that sets implant height and retroversion during a trial reduction (**Figure 10**). As an alternative, a surgical sponge may be used to temporarily anchor the stem at the estimated height and version.

Humeral Stem Retroversion Determination

- Determining the correct retroversion of the humeral stem is critical in restoring the glenohumeral joint. Most surgeons suggest using 20° to 30° as a guide, although previous anthropometric studies suggest that native retroversion may vary from 10° to 50°.
- The angle can be estimated by means of the following: positioning of the lateral fin of the prosthesis 8 mm posterior to the bicipital groove; external rotation of the humerus to approximately 30°, such that the humeral head faces medially toward the glenoid; or a vertical line from the epicondylar axis that splits the prosthetic axis (**Figure 11**).

Humeral Height Restoration

- Reestablishment of prosthetic height is paramount to restore muscle tension and shoulder kinematics. The most common error is to place the stem at a reduced height, resulting in poor deltoid tension and insufficient room for the tuberosities. Visual cues, including muscle tension of the rotator cuff and deltoid and intraoperative C-arm images, will assist the surgeon in restoring prosthetic height.
- Prior to a trial reduction, two to four drill holes are placed in the proximal humerus medial and lateral to the bicipital groove, with No. 5 or equivalent nonabsorbable sutures used for fixation of the tuberosity to the shaft.

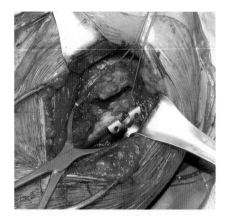

Figure 12 Intraoperative photograph of a shoulder shows the use of a commercially available tuberosity clamp situated medial and deep to the deltoid. The device is useful in performing provisional reduction and fluoroscopic assessment.

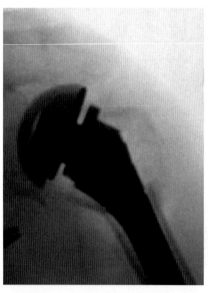

Figure 13 C-arm fluoroscopic image of a shoulder demonstrates appropriate reduction of the greater tuberosity within 1 cm of the apex of the trial humeral head.

- If the suture collar technique is used, drill holes are made through the anterolateral and posterolateral aspects of the proximal humerus, approximately 2 cm below the fracture line.
- A trial reduction is done with the mobilized tuberosities reduced below the head of the modular prosthesis or the suture collar.
- A large reduction tenaculum or proprietary clamp may be used to hold the tuberosities for fluoroscopic examination and assessment of glenohumeral stability (**Figure 12**).
- Proper head size, stem height, and version are assessed. The surgeon should be able to inferiorly displace the humeral head not more than 25% of the glenoid height. Humeral head posterior translation should not exceed 50% of the glenoid AP axis. The prosthetic head should face the glenoid surface with approximately 30° of retroversion.
- Several intraoperative adjustments may be made to improve soft-tissue tension before final implantation of the prosthesis. If the soft tissues appear tight, a smaller humeral head may be used with or without humeral stem recession. If the soft tissues appear loose, a larger (in size and/or thickness) humeral head is used. After the surgeon is satisfied with the trial construct, additional C-arm images are obtained before final stem implantation (**Figure 13**).

Final Prosthesis Implantation

- The final humeral stem should be cemented in patients with osteoporotic bone and/or poor diaphyseal fixation. Either antibiotic-impregnated cement or standard cement is used at the surgeon's discretion. Although no consensus exists on which to use, antibiotic-impregnated cement may be the best option in patients who have medical comorbidities, such as diabetes, renal disease, coexisting inflammatory arthropathy, a history of prior shoulder surgeries, and/or infections. Recent implant designs allow for press-fit placement of the humeral component with later conversion to a reverse shoulder prosthesis if necessary.
- The humeral canal is copiously lavaged with sterile saline with or without antibiotics.
- A cement restrictor is placed to prevent cement extravasation distally.
- The humeral canal is filled retrograde with a cement gun.
- The humeral component is seated into the predetermined position. Implant systems that contain a positioning device are helpful during this step.
- Excess cement is removed with curets and a Freer elevator.
- After the humeral stem has been fixed with cement or press-fit fixation, a second reduction is performed with the trial head. Soft-tissue balancing is reassessed, and repeat C-arm fluoroscopic images are obtained.
- The final head may be impacted after the cement has cured.
- If a suture collar is used, suture passage may be easier without the final humeral head in position. A No. 5 nonabsorbable so-called around-the-world suture enters the greater tuberosity at the supraspinatus tendon insertion and then passes medial or through the humeral stem and subscapularis insertion (**Figure 14**). Improved fixation with this suture has been demonstrated compared with tuberosity-to-tuberosity or tuberosity-to-fin fixation.
- Vacancies between the tuberosities, stem, and humeral shaft are filled with harvested cancellous bone from the removed humeral head (**Figure 15**).
- The order of suture tying and configuration may vary depending on surgeon preference and implant-specific instructions. In general, vertical sutures are tied first, beginning with tuberosity-to-shaft approximation, followed by horizontal sutures (tuberosity-to-tuberosity). The cerclage suture is tied next, after which the

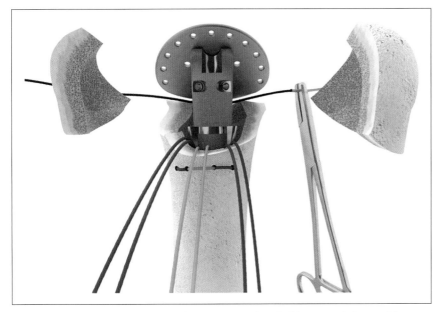

Figure 14 Graphic depiction of a No. 5 nonabsorbable around-the-world suture placed through the junctions of the rotator cuff with the lesser and greater tuberosities and medial to or through the humeral stem. (Courtesy of DePuy Synthes, Warsaw, IN.)

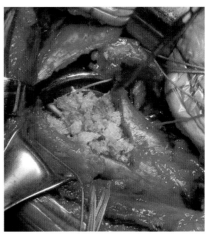

Figure 15 Intraoperative photograph of a shoulder shows autogenous bone graft harvested from the humeral head and placed between the tuberosities and the shaft before final reduction

rotator interval is approximated with No. 2 nonabsorbable sutures with the arm in approximately 30° of external rotation.

Wound Closure

- Tenodesis of the biceps tendon adjacent to the pectoralis major insertion is performed. A medium closed suction drain is placed deep to the deltoid and brought through the lateral shoulder.
- If the patient did not receive a regional block, a pain pump may be placed in a similar fashion to the drain to augment postoperative analgesia and reduce the use of narcotic medication.
- Usually, the deltopectoral interval is not closed.
- The subcutaneous tissues are reapproximated with 2-0 absorbable sutures.
- Subcuticular closure is performed with 3-0 absorbable monofilament sutures.
- Biplanar radiographs are obtained before patient extubation.

- The patient's affected extremity is placed in a padded sling or shoulder immobilizer with 30° to 45° of abduction for comfort.

Rehabilitation

The postoperative rehabilitation program is summarized in **Table 2**. Motion limitations are prescribed according to intraoperative stability and radiographic evidence of tuberosity healing. Active-assisted and active range-of-motion exercises may be initiated with tuberosity healing. Patients should be informed that functional improvement may take up to 1 year postoperatively.

Avoiding Pitfalls

Complications after hemiarthroplasty reconstruction of proximal humerus fractures include implant malposition, nonunion or malunion of tuberosities, instability, neurologic injury, wound

healing problems, heterotopic bone formation, implant loosening, regional pain syndrome, periprosthetic fracture, and glenoid arthritis. In patients undergoing treatment for an acute injury, the most common complications are related to tuberosity healing and shoulder stiffness, whereas the most common complications after delayed surgical treatment are instability, heterotopic bone formation, rotator cuff tears, and tuberosity malunion or nonunion. Infection, instability, and tuberosity healing have a direct negative effect on pain level and shoulder function.

Overall, the incidence of infection is low but is increased in patients who have renal failure or diabetes and those who have previously undergone surgical treatment for the injury (such as internal fixation). Infection risk may be reduced via timely administration of intravenous antibiotics, appropriate surgical preparation and draping, reduced duration of surgical exposure, and the gentle handling of soft tissues. Postoperative infections may require surgical débridement, long-term intravenous antibiotics specific to the causative organism, or two-stage reconstruction with revision total shoulder arthroplasty. In patients

Table 2 Rehabilitation Protocol After Hemiarthroplasty to Manage Three- or Four-Part Proximal Humerus Fractures

Postoperative Week	Range of Motion	Strengthening	Return to Play	Comments/Emphasis
0-2	Passive	None	Unable to return	At 0-10 d postoperatively, range of motion is set by the surgeon on the basis of intraoperative stability and patient-specific factors (bone quality, mentation); pendulum and passive forward flexion pulley exercises are permitted; a sling is used for immobilization; and elbow, wrist, and digital exercises are allowed. At 10-14 d postoperatively, assess surgical wound, reinforce home exercise program, and use sling for immobilization.
2-6	Passive	None	Unable to return	Evaluate tuberosity healing on radiographs Continue sling immobilization Wean off narcotic-based pain medications
6-12	Passive, active-assisted, and active	None	Focus on ability to perform activities of daily living, such as hygiene care	Evaluate tuberosity healing on radiographs Discontinue sling immobilization The physician directs the outpatient physical therapy program
12-52	Passive, active-assisted, and active	Allowed	Remove restrictions to allow return to work or play	Strengthening with graduated rubber bands; maximal improvement may take 1 yr postoperatively

with recalcitrant infection, resection arthroplasty may be necessary.

Instability in the acute setting primarily depends on initial implant positioning (humeral head height and stem version), rotator cuff deficiency, and tuberosity-related problems. The surgeon should be familiar with the specific implant system and its limitations. The implant should be placed in appropriate retroversion (approximately 20° to 30°). The height of the trial stem should be checked by using a fracture jig or a sponge for initial fixation and C-arm fluoroscopy before cement fixation is performed. If a press-fit technique is used, care must be taken to replicate the stem height and version by using intraoperative cues, such as the pectoralis major insertion and the epicondylar axis of the distal humerus. Rotator cuff deficiency

can affect initial tuberosity reduction and fixation. Displacement of the lesser tuberosity may result in anterior instability, whereas migration of the greater tuberosity can lead to anterosuperior escape and clinical pseudoparalysis.

Anatomic tuberosity union is paramount because early displacement and malunion directly correlate with poor functional outcomes. Patient-specific factors, such as fracture comminution and soft-tissue (rotator cuff) quality, may make secure reattachment of the tuberosities difficult to achieve. To reduce the risk of tuberosity migration, the authors of this chapter recommend using multiple large-caliber nonabsorbable sutures that allow for tuberosity-to-tuberosity, tuberosity-to-shaft, and stem-to-tuberosity approximation. Healing may be improved by using

cancellous autograft from the resected humeral head. Malunion is a function of initial inadequate reduction or suboptimal fixation. Malunions of the greater tuberosity with posterior or superior displacement commonly result in pain, reduced active elevation, and limited abduction. Treatment of malunion ranges from benign neglect in the medically fragile patient to revision surgery requiring tuberosity osteotomy, implant revision, or conversion to reverse shoulder arthroplasty. Although less common, excessive reduction of the greater and lesser tuberosities can lead to reduced internal and external rotation, respectively. Intraoperative and early postoperative radiographic imaging are critical because tuberosity complications often are observed during the first 6 weeks postoperatively.

Bibliography

Angst F, Schwyzer HK, Aeschlimann A, Simmen BR, Goldhahn J: Measures of adult shoulder function: Disabilities of the Arm, Shoulder, and Hand Questionnaire (DASH) and its short version (QuickDASH), Shoulder Pain and Disability Index (SPADI), American Shoulder and Elbow Surgeons (ASES) Society standardized shoulder assessment form, Constant (Murley) Score (CS), Simple Shoulder Test (SST), Oxford Shoulder Score (OSS), Shoulder Disability Questionnaire (SDQ), and Western Ontario Shoulder Instability Index (WOSI). *Arthritis Care Res (Hoboken)* 2011;63(suppl 11):S174-S188.

Antuña SA, Sperling JW, Cofield RH: Shoulder hemiarthroplasty for acute fractures of the proximal humerus: A minimum five-year follow-up. *J Shoulder Elbow Surg* 2008;17(2):202-209.

Balg F, Boulianne M, Boileau P: Bicipital groove orientation: Considerations for the retroversion of a prosthesis in fractures of the proximal humerus. *J Shoulder Elbow Surg* 2006;15(2):195-198.

Bastian JD, Hertel R: Osteosynthesis and hemiarthroplasty of fractures of the proximal humerus: Outcomes in a consecutive case series. *J Shoulder Elbow Surg* 2009;18(2):216-219.

Bohsali KI, Wirth MA: Fractures of the proximal humerus, in Rockwood CA Jr, Matsen FA III, eds: *The Shoulder,* ed 4. Philadelphia, PA, Saunders Elsevier, 2009, vol 1, pp 295-332.

Boileau P, Krishnan SG, Tinsi L, Walch G, Coste JS, Molé D: Tuberosity malposition and migration: Reasons for poor outcomes after hemiarthroplasty for displaced fractures of the proximal humerus. *J Shoulder Elbow Surg* 2002;11(5):401-412.

Boileau P, Pennington SD, Alami G: Proximal humeral fractures in younger patients: Fixation techniques and arthroplasty. *J Shoulder Elbow Surg* 2011;20(2 suppl):S47-S60.

Boileau P, Winter M, Cikes A, et al: Can surgeons predict what makes a good hemiarthroplasty for fracture? *J Shoulder Elbow Surg* 2013;22(11):1495-1506.

Boons HW, Groosen JH, van Grinsven S, van Sustante JL, van Loon CJ: Hemiarthroplasty for humeral four-part fractures for patients 65 and older: A randomized controlled trial. *Clin Orthop Relat Res* 2012;470(12):3483-3491.

Boyle MJ, Youn SM, Frampton CM, Ball CM: Functional outcomes of reverse shoulder arthroplasty compared with hemiarthroplasty for acute proximal humeral fractures. *J Shoulder Elbow Surg* 2013;22(1):32-37.

Cadet ER, Ahmad CS: Hemiarthroplasty for three- and four-part proximal humerus fractures. *J Am Acad Orthop Surg* 2012;20(1):17-27.

Cai M, Tao K, Yang C, Li S: Internal fixation versus shoulder hemiarthroplasty for displaced 4-part proximal humeral fractures in elderly patients. *Orthopedics* 2012;35(9):e1340-e1346.

Chalmers PN, Slikker W III, Mall NA, et al: Reverse total shoulder arthroplasty for acute proximal humeral fracture: Comparison to open reduction-internal fixation and hemiarthroplasty. *J Shoulder Elbow Surg* 2014;23(2):197-204.

Constant CR, Murley AH: A clinical method of functional assessment of the shoulder. *Clin Orthop Relat Res* 1987;(214):160-164.

Crosby LA, Finnan RP, Anderson CG, Gozdanovic J, Miller MW: Tetracycline labeling as a measure of humeral head viability after 3- or 4-part proximal humerus fracture. *J Shoulder Elbow Surg* 2009;18(6):851-858.

Cuff DJ, Pupello DR: Comparison of hemiarthroplasty and reverse shoulder arthroplasty for the treatment of proximal humeral fractures in elderly patients. *J Bone Joint Surg Am* 2013;95(22):2050-2055.

Fialka C, Stampfl P, Arbes S, Reuter P, Oberleitner G, Vécsei V: Primary hemiarthroplasty in four-part fractures of the proximal humerus: Randomized trial of two different implant systems. *J Shoulder Elbow Surg* 2008;17(2):210-215.

Fucentese SF, Sutter R, Wolfensperger F, Jost B, Gerber C: Large metaphyseal volume hemiprostheses for complex fractures of the proximal humerus. *J Shoulder Elbow Surg* 2014;23(3):427-433.

Garrigues GE, Johnston PS, Pepe MD, Tucker BS, Ramsey ML, Austin LS: Hemiarthroplasty versus reverse total shoulder arthroplasty for acute proximal humerus fractures in elderly patients. *Orthopedics* 2012;35(5):e703-e708.

Gerber C, Schneeberger AG, Vinh TS: The arterial vascularization of the humeral head: An anatomical study. *J Bone Joint Surg Am* 1990;72(10):1486-1494.

Greiner SH, Diederichs G, Kröning I, Scheibel M, Perka C: Tuberosity position correlates with fatty infiltration of the rotator cuff after hemiarthroplasty for proximal humeral fractures. *J Shoulder Elbow Surg* 2009;18(3):431-436.

Greiner SH, Kääb MJ, Kröning I, Scheibel M, Perka C: Reconstruction of humeral length and centering of the prosthetic head in hemiarthroplasty for proximal humeral fractures. *J Shoulder Elbow Surg* 2008;17(5):709-714.

Grönhagen CM, Abbaszadegan H, Révay SA, Adolphson PY: Medium-term results after primary hemiarthroplasty for comminute proximal humerus fractures: A study of 46 patients followed up for an average of 4.4 years. *J Shoulder Elbow Surg* 2007;16(6):766-773.

Hertel R, Hempfing A, Stiehler M, Leunig M: Predictors of humeral head ischemia after intracapsular fracture of the proximal humerus. *J Shoulder Elbow Surg* 2004;13(4):427-433.

Hettrich CM, Boraiah S, Dyke JP, Neviaser A, Helfet DL, Lorich DG: Quantitative assessment of the vascularity of the proximal part of the humerus. *J Bone Joint Surg Am* 2010;92(4):943-948.

Huffman GR, Itamura JM, McGarry MH, et al: Neer Award 2006: Biomechanical assessment of inferior tuberosity placement during hemiarthroplasty for four-part proximal humeral fractures. *J Shoulder Elbow Surg* 2008;17(2):189-196.

Kontakis G, Koutras C, Tosounidis T, Giannoudis P: Early management of proximal humeral fractures with hemiarthroplasty: A systematic review. *J Bone Joint Surg Br* 2008;90(11):1407-1413.

Krishnan SG, Bennion PW, Reineck JR, Burkhead WZ: Hemiarthroplasty for proximal humeral fracture: Restoration of the Gothic arch. *Orthop Clin North Am* 2008;39(4):441-450, vi.

Krishnan SG, Reineck JR, Bennion PD, Feher L, Burkhead WZ Jr: Shoulder arthroplasty for fracture: Does a fracture-specific stem make a difference? *Clin Orthop Relat Res* 2011;469(12):3317-3323.

Kryzak TJ, Sperling JW, Schleck CD, Cofield RH: Hemiarthroplasty for proximal humerus fractures in patients with Parkinson's disease. *Clin Orthop Relat Res* 2010;468(7):1817-1821.

Laing PG: The arterial supply of the adult humerus. *J Bone Joint Surg Am* 1956;38(5):1105-1116.

Lanting B, MacDermid J, Drosdowech D, Faber KJ: Proximal humeral fractures: A systematic review of treatment modalities. *J Shoulder Elbow Surg* 2008;17(1):42-54.

Loebenberg MI, Jones DA, Zuckerman JD: The effect of greater tuberosity placement on active range of motion after hemiarthroplasty for acute fractures of the proximal humerus. *Bull Hosp Jt Dis* 2005;62(3-4):90-93.

Mighell MA, Kolm GP, Collinge CA, Frankle MA: Outcomes of hemiarthroplasty for fractures of the proximal humerus. *J Shoulder Elbow Surg* 2003;12(6):569-577.

Murachovsky J, Ikemoto RY, Nascimento LG, Fujiki EN, Milani C, Warner JJ: Pectoralis major tendon reference (PMT): A new method for accurate restoration of humeral length with hemiarthroplasty for fracture. *J Shoulder Elbow Surg* 2006;15(6):675-678.

Namdari S, Horneff JG, Baldwin K: Comparison of hemiarthroplasty and reverse arthroplasty for treatment of proximal humeral fractures: A systematic review. *J Bone Joint Surg Am* 2013;95(18):1701-1708.

Nho SJ, Brophy RH, Barker JU, Cornell CN, MacGillivray JD: Innovations in the management of displaced proximal humerus fractures. *J Am Acad Orthop Surg* 2007;15(1):12-26.

Olerud P, Ahrengart L, Ponzer S, Saving J, Tidermark J: Hemiarthroplasty versus nonoperative treatment of displaced 4-part proximal humeral fractures in elderly patients: A randomized controlled trial. *J Shoulder Elbow Surg* 2011;20(7):1025-1033.

Prakash U, McGurty DW, Dent JA: Hemiarthroplasty for severe fractures of the proximal humerus. *J Shoulder Elbow Surg* 2002;11(5):428-430.

Richards RR, An KN, Bigliani LU, et al: A standardized method for the assessment of shoulder function. *J Shoulder Elbow Surg* 1994;3(6):347-352.

Robinson CM, Page RS, Hill RM, Sanders DL, Court-Brown CM, Wakefield AE: Primary hemiarthroplasty for treatment of proximal humeral fractures. *J Bone Joint Surg Am* 2003;85(7):1215-1223.

Saltzman MD, Nuber GW, Gryzlo SM, Marecek GS, Koh JL: Efficacy of surgical preparation solutions in shoulder surgery. *J Bone Joint Surg Am* 2009;91(8):1949-1953.

Solberg BD, Moon CN, Franco DP, Paiement GD: Surgical treatment of three and four-part proximal humeral fractures. *J Bone Joint Surg Am* 2009;91(7):1689-1697.

Torrens C, Corrales M, Melendo E, Solano A, Rodríguez-Baeza A, Cáceres E: The pectoralis major tendon as a reference for restoring humeral length and retroversion with hemiarthroplasty for fracture. *J Shoulder Elbow Surg* 2008;17(6):947-950.

Voos JE, Dines JS, Dines DM: Arthroplasty for fractures of the proximal part of the humerus. *J Bone Joint Surg Am* 2010;92(6):1560-1567.

Video Reference

Wirth MA, Bohsali KI: Video. *Fracture Platform Prosthesis.* San Antonio, TX, 2015.

Chapter 47

Reverse Shoulder Arthroplasty for Proximal Humerus Fractures: Indications, Limits, and Technique

Michael M. Hussey, MD

Brent Stephens, MD

Mark A. Frankle, MD

 Introduction

Since proximal humerus fractures were first described in the 1930s, substantial debate and controversy have occurred regarding their most effective management. Much of this controversy stems from the fact that multiple fracture patterns exist, and no single procedure or treatment modality is ideal for all fracture patterns. A substantial postsurgical complication and revision surgery rate has led the push for more effective treatments and defined the surgical procedures that are most effective in managing specific fracture patterns.

Proximal humerus fractures remain the second most common fracture of the upper extremity and the third most common fracture in patients older than 65 years. Proximal humerus fractures most commonly result from a ground-level fall onto the upper extremity in an elderly person with osteopenia.

Because substantial displacement occurs in less than 15% of such injuries, nonsurgical management is the mainstay of treatment for most proximal humerus fractures and is associated with a low nonunion rate. Most patients can resume normal activities after fracture healing has been achieved because the shoulder has a tremendous arc of motion to compensate for mild losses.

In patients in whom substantial displacement occurs, fractures often follow the characteristic patterns described by Codman and Neer. The Neer classification commonly is used to describe these injuries and is based on displacement and/or angulation of the fracture components. This classification has improved understanding of the prognostic implications of treatment and has improved therapeutic interventions. Displaced three- and four-part fractures are often associated with poor patient outcomes if left untreated, resulting in chronic

pain, loss of motion, and impairment during activities of daily living. Factors associated with humeral head ischemia and osteonecrosis include posteromedial metaphyseal head extension of less than 8 mm, loss of the medial hinge, four-fragment fractures, and angular displacement of the head greater than 45°.

Proximal humerus fractures that have substantial comminution and displacement commonly are managed surgically. In younger patients and in those with good bone quality, every effort should be made to obtain anatomic reduction and fixation of the fracture. Prosthetic replacement is considered in three-part and four-part fractures, particularly in elderly patients who have osteoporotic bone and in those with substantial articular head involvement. Hemiarthroplasty has been used most commonly but has produced mixed results because it relies heavily on correct tuberosity positioning and healing. More recently, reverse shoulder arthroplasty (RSA) has been used to manage these complex injuries, with short- and mid-term follow-up demonstrating promising results. Currently, if an elderly patient presents to the authors of this chapter with a substantially comminuted and displaced proximal humerus fracture, the preferred method of treatment is to reconstruct the injury with RSA.

Dr. Frankle or an immediate family member has received royalties from, is a member of a speakers' bureau or has made paid presentations on behalf of, serves as a paid consultant to, and has received nonincome support (such as equipment or services), commercially derived honoraria, or other non–research-related funding (such as paid travel) from DJO Surgical; has received research or institutional support from BioMimetic Therapeutics and DJO Surgical; and serves as a board member, owner, officer, or committee member of the American Academy of Orthopaedic Surgeons and the American Shoulder and Elbow Surgeons. Neither of the following authors nor any immediate family member has received anything of value from or has stock or stock options held in a commercial company or institution related directly or indirectly to the subject of this chapter: Dr. Hussey and Dr. Stephens.

Case Presentation

A 72-year-old woman presents to the clinic of the authors of this chapter 2 weeks after falling down some steps at her house. Initially, she was taken to the emergency department, where she was placed in a sling and, after being cleared for any life-threatening injuries, referred to the clinic. The patient reports severe shoulder and wrist pain on presentation. She is a relatively active, independent woman who lives alone. Her medical history is negative for any major medical comorbidities, but she is a chronic smoker. Radiographs obtained at the clinic demonstrate a four-part fracture-dislocation of the proximal humerus (**Figure 1**).

The patient's physical examination findings demonstrate that the affected extremity is neurovascularly intact, and the deltoid muscle can be activated on command. After a discussion with the patient and her family, the decision is made to perform RSA. Given the degree of fracture displacement and comminution, the authors of this chapter believe that RSA will provide the fastest return to function and independence with the fewest immediate limitations.

Intraoperative findings confirm a substantially displaced and comminuted proximal humerus fracture. The rotator cuff is found to have preserved attachments to the displaced greater and lesser tuberosities. The standard technique used by the authors of this chapter to perform RSA for acute fracture is used. A 32-mm minus 4-size glenosphere and a standard size monoblock humeral component are placed. After trialing demonstrates a completely impingement-free arc of motion, the final implants are selected, and the humeral stem is cemented into place. The tuberosities are repaired to the prosthesis and the shaft with cerclage sutures. Intraoperative fluoroscopic imaging demonstrates restoration of the scapulohumeral arch and adequate reduction

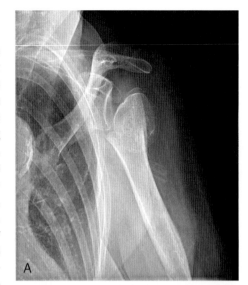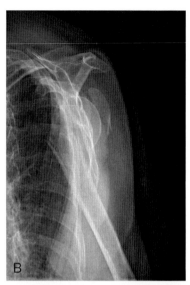

Figure 1 Preoperative shoulder radiographs demonstrate a four-part fracture-dislocation of the proximal humerus. **A,** AP view demonstrates a fracture-dislocation. **B,** Scapular lateral view demonstrates substantial displacement of the humeral head from the shaft. (Copyright the Foundation for Orthopaedic Research and Education, Tampa, FL.)

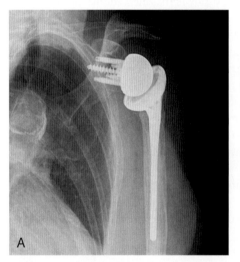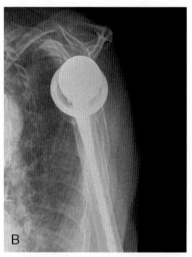

Figure 2 Postoperative shoulder radiographs obtained after reverse shoulder arthroplasty. **A,** AP view demonstrates restoration of the scapulohumeral arch and reduction of the greater tuberosity about the humeral prosthesis. **B,** Scapular Y view demonstrates the glenosphere centered on the cemented humeral component. (Copyright the Foundation for Orthopaedic Research and Education, Tampa, FL.)

of the tuberosities about the implant (**Figure 2**).

The shoulder is placed in an immobilizer postoperatively, and the patient eventually is discharged to a rehabilitation facility. Instructions are given to initiate Codman exercises and elbow, wrist, and hand exercises. The patient returns 10 days postoperatively for suture removal. At 6-week follow-up, use of the immobilizer is discontinued, and the patient is instructed in a home-based therapy regimen to include passive and active-assisted range-of-motion (ROM) exercises. Strengthening begins at 12-week follow-up, with weight bearing and lifting as tolerated.

Indications

More recently, RSA has been used for the primary management of complex proximal humerus fractures. RSA currently is indicated for elderly patients who have an acute three- or four-part proximal humerus fracture with substantial comminution and displacement or a head-split fracture with articular cartilage disruption. RSA can be an invaluable option in elderly osteoporotic patients with a comminuted fracture if tuberosity reconstruction and healing using open reduction and internal fixation are believed to be difficult and unpredictable. Good outcomes depend more on the design of the RSA prosthesis and less on tuberosity quality and healing, allowing more confidence in reconstruction if tuberosity involvement is present. The biomechanical advantage of RSA is that it allows the deltoid a greater role in arm elevation and abduction.

Another indication for RSA in the setting of a proximal humerus fracture is after failed prior nonsurgical or surgical management. Failed nonsurgical management that resulted in a painful nonunion or malunion has been successfully managed with RSA. Also, patients in whom open reduction and internal fixation or hemiarthroplasty has failed secondary to articular cartilage disruption and/or tuberosity healing complications can undergo RSA as a salvage procedure. However, the outcomes after failed prior treatment are inferior compared with those of primary RSA and have a higher complication rate.

Controversies and Alternative Approaches

After a short course of immobilization, patients are encouraged to perform daily gentle ROM exercises of the shoulder. After fracture consolidation is evident on follow-up radiographs, typically between 4 and 6 weeks postoperatively, increased passive and active ROM exercises are added to the therapy regimen. By 3 to 4 months postoperatively, strengthening is begun, and normal daily activities usually are resumed. Some ROM can be expected but is typically well tolerated because of the large arc of motion of the shoulder.

Proximal humerus fractures that have substantial comminution and displacement typically are managed surgically. In the young population and in those with good bone quality, every effort should be taken to obtain anatomic reduction and fixation of the fracture to restore the native anatomy. Frequently used methods include open reduction and internal fixation, closed reduction and percutaneous pinning, and intramedullary nail fixation.

Prosthetic replacement is considered in three- and four-part fractures, particularly in elderly patients with osteoporotic bone. Traditionally, hemiarthroplasty has been most commonly performed but has mixed results. Hemiarthroplasty typically provides adequate pain relief; however, postoperative ROM and functional outcomes have proved unpredictable because hemiarthroplasty relies greatly on correct tuberosity positioning and healing.

Results

Despite the lack of long-term published studies, RSA is a promising tool for the management of these complex injuries. RSA has been used to manage failed hemiarthroplasty performed to treat fractures. RSA can provide a reliable salvage procedure for failed hemiarthroplasty by improving ROM, functional outcomes, and patient satisfaction at short-term follow-up. RSA also appears to reliably restore motion and function in patients with acute proximal humerus fractures. Restored forward elevation and abduction can be expected irrespective of tuberosity healing; however, every attempt should be made to anatomically repair the tuberosities about the prosthesis because shoulder rotation depends more on tuberosity consolidation. The outcomes of RSA were compared in patients who underwent anatomic repair of the tuberosities and patients who had not undergone repair. A consolidated anatomic repair resulted in substantially better rotation and functional outcome scores compared with those that were not repaired.

The authors of this chapter recently evaluated their results of RSA for acute three- and four-part proximal humerus fractures (unpublished data) and have experienced promising anecdotal outcomes. In 18 patients with a mean follow-up of 27 months, the mean active forward elevation, abduction, external rotation, and internal rotation were 139.0°, 112.0°, 37.5°, and L1, respectively, at final follow-up. The mean American Shoulder and Elbow Surgeons Subjective Shoulder Scale score was 70, and the mean visual analog scale pain score was 1.7.

Recent studies comparing RSA with hemiarthroplasty for the management of these injuries appear to show superior short-term to midterm results for those managed with RSA. However, long-term prospective studies are necessary to fully assess the outcomes and potential complications of RSA for proximal humerus fractures. Patient age and the potential complications unique to RSA also should be factored into the decision surrounding treatment.

Video 47.1 Reverse Shoulder Arthroplasty for Acute Proximal Humerus Fractures. Michael M. Hussey, MD; Brent Stephens, MD; Mark A. Frankle, MD (4 min)

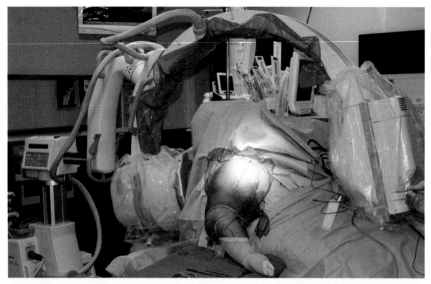

Figure 3 Preoperative photograph shows the patient positioning and setup for reverse shoulder arthroplasty. The patient is placed in the beach-chair position with the arm resting on a well-padded Mayo stand. A C-arm fluoroscopy unit with sterile covering is brought in from the head of the bed and positioned appropriately. (Copyright the Foundation for Orthopaedic Research and Education, Tampa, FL.)

 ## Technical Keys to Success

Preoperative Planning

- The assessment of deltoid function is paramount in the decision to perform RSA because the technique relies on deltoid motor function. In patients with fractures, discomfort often limits radiographic analysis.
- Typically, true scapular AP, scapular Y, and axillary radiographs are obtained to evaluate details of the fracture and determine whether a dislocation is present. A Velpeau view may be necessary if obtaining an axillary view is not possible.
- CT provides a better understanding of the fracture and enables a more detailed preoperative plan.

Patient Positioning

- The patient is placed in the beach-chair position with all bony prominences padded appropriately.
- Before starting, it is imperative that the affected extremity is draped free, with complete arm extension and adduction, to allow uninterrupted access. This helps facilitate glenoid exposure and access to the humeral canal. An assistant should be positioned behind the shoulder to aid in retraction.
- The surgical arm is allowed to rest on a well-padded Mayo stand throughout the procedure.
- A C-arm fluoroscopy unit is positioned at the head of the bed for intraoperative imaging (**Figure 3**), which allows the fluoroscope to be moved toward the contralateral shoulder when images are not being obtained for uninterrupted access to the surgical field. It should be confirmed that adequate imaging can be obtained before starting.

Procedure

- The standard deltopectoral approach is used, starting approximately 5 cm medial to the acromioclavicular joint and following the anterior edge of the deltoid muscle toward its insertion on the humerus.
- If preserved, the cephalic vein is identified and moved medially with the pectoralis major muscle, cauterizing lateral tributaries from the deltoid.
- The subdeltoid, subacromial, and subcoracoid spaces are developed and freed of all adhesions.
- Retractors are placed in the subdeltoid space, facilitating exposure of the fracture. Any overlying bursa or hematoma is removed with a rongeur to improve visualization.
- The long head of the biceps tendon is identified and tenodesed to the upper border of the pectoralis major tendon with nonabsorbable sutures. The biceps tendon is divided above the tenodesis, and the rotator interval is opened by following the tendon into the joint. After exposure, the tendon stump is amputated at its origin on the supraglenoid tubercle.
- In patients with four-part fractures, the greater and lesser tuberosities are identified and mobilized, and a tagging suture is placed at the tendon-bone interface to aid in mobilization.
- The humeral head fragment is removed through the rotator interval.
- The metaphyseal bone from the head is saved to use for bone grafting later in the procedure.
- Articular cartilage fragments that remain attached to the tuberosities are removed with a rongeur.
- Three No. 5 braided nonabsorbable sutures are placed around the tendon-bone interface of the greater tuberosity, spaced evenly apart.
- In a similar manner, two 2-mm nonabsorbable tape sutures are placed at the tendon-bone interface around the greater tuberosity in an alternating sequence between the three No. 5 sutures. All sutures are snapped together (**Figure 4, A**).
- The deltoid retractor is removed, and the Mayo stand is elevated to

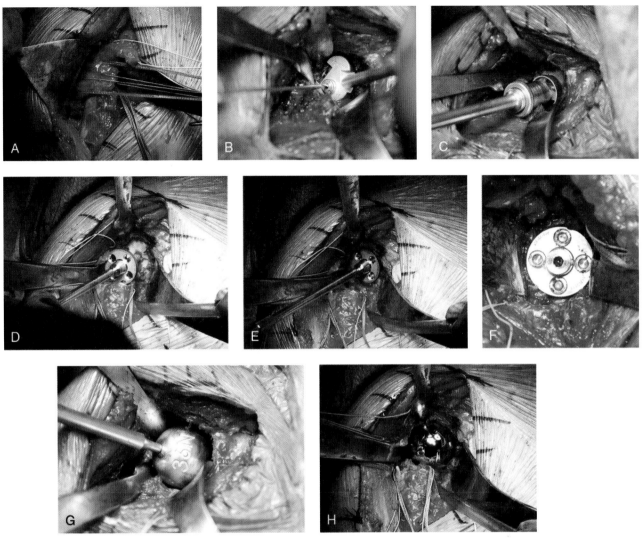

Figure 4   Intraoperative photographs show the reverse shoulder arthroplasty technique used by the authors of this chapter. **A,** Three No. 5 braided sutures with two interspersed 2-mm nonabsorbable tape sutures are positioned about the tendon-bone interface of the greater tuberosity. **B,** The guide is centered on the glenoid with 10° of inferior tilt. **C,** Sequential glenoid reaming is performed until bleeding subchondral bone is evident. **D,** A baseplate is inserted into the glenoid. Note that entry is at the same angle as the initial guide pin placement. **E,** The baseplate should be seated until it is flush with the glenoid and further advancement of the central screw is impossible. **F,** Peripheral locking screws are placed in the baseplate before glenosphere placement. **G,** Glenosphere trial placement. **H,** Final glenosphere placement. (Copyright the Foundation for Orthopaedic Research and Education, Tampa, FL.)

move the arm into abduction, re-laxing the deltoid and allowing the humerus to retract posteriorly.

- Large, sharp Hohmann retractors are placed superior and posterior to the glenoid, and a Cobra retractor is placed anteriorly.

- A 360° periglenoid release of the capsule and labrum is performed using electrocautery, with special care taken to protect the axillary

nerve during inferior capsulolabral resection.

- After excellent exposure is achieved, a 2.5-mm drill bit is used to create a center hole perpendicular to the glenoid face with 10° of inferior tilt (**Figure 4, B**). A 6.5-mm tap is inserted in the center hole.

- Sequential cannulated glenoid reamers are placed over the tap, and the glenoid is reamed until bleeding

subchondral bone is evident (**Figure 4, C**).

- After the tap is removed, a fixed-angle baseplate with an integrated central screw is inserted in line with the central hole. The baseplate should sit flush with the bone.

- Secure fixation is achieved after attempted further advancement of the screw causes the entire scapula to rotate (**Figure 4, D** and **E**).

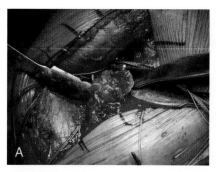
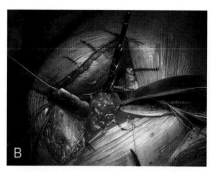

Figure 5 **A,** Intraoperative photograph of a shoulder shows humeral exposure. **B,** Intraoperative photograph of a shoulder shows a reamer placed in the center of the canal, which is reamed sequentially by hand.

- Typically, four peripheral locking screws are placed into the baseplate for additional fixation (**Figure 4, F**).
- An appropriate size glenosphere trial is selected based on the size and quality of the glenoid, the soft-tissue contracture, and the anticipated degree of instability (**Figure 4, G and H**).
- After the glenosphere is placed, attention is refocused on the humerus. The arm is moved back into adduction/extension, and the humerus is delivered from the wound (**Figure 5, A**).
- A Hohmann retractor is placed medially about the calcar, exposing the humerus.
- The humeral canal is reamed sequentially by hand in line with the humeral canal (**Figure 5, B**). Reaming is continued until cortical chatter is obtained.
- Typically, the prosthesis is undersized by one size to make room for an appropriately thick cement mantle.
- The appropriate size trial is placed down the canal. Alternatively, the actual humeral implant can be used to perform the trial reduction with the trial socket insert before cementing.
- The height of the implant can be approximated using two methods. Commonly, the fracture exits medially at the level of the surgical neck, leaving the calcar intact. The humeral socket can be allowed to sit against the calcar, providing a close estimate of normal height. The other method that can be used if substantial comminution and shaft extension are present involves obtaining bilateral full-length humeral radiographs with a radiographic ruler to approximate the humeral length on the injured side. The uninjured humerus is measured from the lateral epicondyle of the distal humerus to the top of the greater tuberosity. Next, the length from the proximal shaft fracture to the lateral epicondyle is subtracted from the uninvolved humeral measurement. The difference is the expected length that should be restored to the proximal shaft, providing a reasonable estimate of humeral height reconstruction.
- Humeral version is obtained using an alignment guide rod, placing the implant into 30° of retroversion relative to the forearm.
- The humeral socket liner trial is selected from a variety of offset sizes and constraints.
- The retractors are removed, and a trial reduction is performed, allowing soft-tissue tension to determine the prosthesis height relative to the shaft.
- The tuberosities are brought around the trial implant, approximating their normal configuration. Ideally, the trial will verify that the tuberosities can be reduced and repaired anatomically.
- The prosthesis is shucked laterally to assess the tension at the glenohumeral interface. If excessive looseness is encountered, the humeral socket liner trial can be exchanged for a thicker size, or the glenosphere can be upsized. Care should be taken when increasing component size because doing so could prevent anatomic tuberosity reconstruction. ROM also may be sacrificed in favor of stability; therefore, forward elevation should be measured whenever trial components are changed to ensure that no substantial loss of motion has occurred.
- Fluoroscopy is used to ensure that the scapulohumeral arch is restored and that the sphere and socket are well-aligned.
- After the height is deemed appropriate, the humeral stem is marked at the proximal aspect of the fractured shaft to provide a height and rotational reference during final stem implantation. The trial components are removed.
- The humeral canal is irrigated and prepared for cementing. A cement restrictor is inserted 1.5 cm below the estimated tip of the implant.
- Three drill holes are placed horizontally 1 cm below the fractured proximal humeral diaphysis, and three No. 5 braided nonabsorbable sutures are passed through the drill holes (**Figure 6**). These sutures will be used to fix the tuberosities to the shaft after the stem is implanted.
- The deep ends of the five greater tuberosity sutures are placed through the medial hole of the final humeral implant, snapped, and set aside while the cement is prepared (**Figure 7, A**).

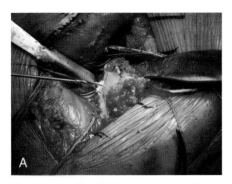
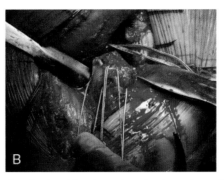
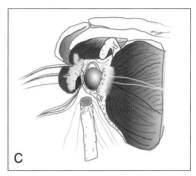

Figure 6 **A** and **B,** Intraoperative photographs of a shoulder show three horizontal nonabsorbable sutures being passed through drill holes in the humeral shaft. **C,** Illustration of a shoulder shows three sutures passed through the humeral shaft before placement of the humeral stem. (Panels A and B copyright the Foundation for Orthopaedic Research and Education, Tampa, FL.)

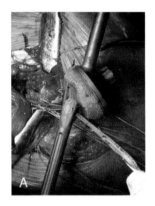
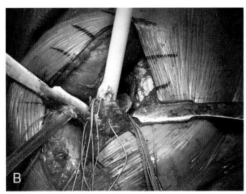
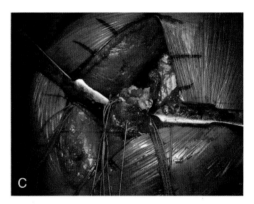

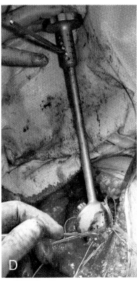
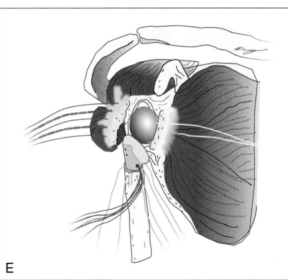

Figure 7 Images of a right shoulder. **A,** Intraoperative photograph shows the five greater tuberosity sutures shuttled through the medial islet of the stem. **B,** Intraoperative photograph shows cement introduced into the humeral canal under pressurization. **C,** Intraoperative photograph shows bone graft from the humeral head placed on top of the cement mantle using the Black-and-Tan technique. **D,** Intraoperative photograph shows a version guide, which is set at 30° of retroversion to ensure correct alignment of the humeral stem. **E,** Illustration shows the humeral stem in place with the sutures placed through the medial islet. (Panels A, B, C, and D copyright the Foundation for Orthopaedic Research and Education, Tampa, FL.)

- Antibiotic-loaded cement is pressurized down the canal with a cement gun until cement is extruding from the proximal portion of the canal (**Figure 7, B**).
- The Black-and-Tan technique for proximal bone grafting, in which the upper 1 cm of the canal is packed with cancellous bone above the cement mantle to aid in tuberosity healing, is performed (**Figure 7, C**).
- With the medial sutures already passed, the humeral stem is introduced into the cemented canal to the appropriate depth determined by the trial. The version guide attached to the stem is used to ensure that the implant is in 30° of retroversion relative to the forearm (**Figure 7, D and E**).
- After the cement has cured appropriately, the prosthesis is reduced again with the trial socket liner. Stability and motion are verified again before the final insertion of the actual humeral socket liner.
- The three No. 5 braided nonabsorbable suture limbs of the greater tuberosity that were passed through the medial hole of the prosthesis are passed individually around the bone-tendon junction of the lesser tuberosity with a free needle (**Figure 8, A**). The deep limbs of the three No. 5 shaft sutures are passed through the rotator cuff superior to the tuberosities and left untied.
- More bone graft obtained from the humeral head is packed around the humeral implant proximally. The bone graft provides an optimal environment to promote tuberosity healing after the tuberosities are reduced.
- The two 2-mm nonabsorbable tape sutures about the greater tuberosity that were not shuttled around the lesser tuberosity are tied, to reduce the greater tuberosity to the prosthesis (**Figure 8, B and C**).

- After the greater tuberosity has been reduced, the three No. 5 sutures placed about the lesser tuberosity are tied sequentially. These sutures reduce the lesser tuberosity and cerclage both tuberosities about the porous coated humeral socket, providing strong fixation (**Figure 8, D and E**).
- The last three remaining shaft sutures that were passed through the upper subscapularis and supraspinatus tendons are tied, completing closure about the prosthesis (**Figure 8, F and G**).
- Final intraoperative motion is evaluated, followed by fluoroscopic imaging to assess component positioning and tuberosity reduction.
- The wound is closed in layers, and the arm is placed in an immobilizer. Regional anesthesia of the surgical extremity frequently is used to assist in postoperative pain management.

Rehabilitation

The patient wears a shoulder immobilizer during the first 6 postoperative weeks, removing it only for hygiene purposes and to perform gentle pendulum exercises. Elbow, wrist, and hand exercises are encouraged daily. After the incision has healed completely, the patient is allowed to perform exercises in a pool. After 6 weeks postoperatively, the immobilizer is discontinued, and active-assisted ROM exercises are begun. Patients are instructed in the clinic on a home therapy regimen, which includes supine active-assisted forward elevation with a stick. Formal physical therapy is not ordered routinely; however, most of these patients are placed in a long-term rehabilitation facility postoperatively for physical therapy. At 3 months postoperatively, active ROM is allowed as tolerated. Light strengthening is begun and progressively increased over several weeks. Typically, maximal improvement in function is expected approximately 1 year postoperatively.

Avoiding Pitfalls

A common pitfall when first performing RSA for acute fracture is failure to adequately judge the tightness or laxity of the reconstructed shoulder. Surgeons new to RSA for acute fracture often place the implant in excessive tightness, resulting in restricted postoperative ROM. The passive ROM obtained intraoperatively corresponds well with the final maximum ROM at long-term follow-up. If motion is limited secondary to overstuffing the joint, downsizing of the humeral liner or glenosphere should be considered. Reducing the tuberosities fully about the trial humeral socket will provide a good estimate of postoperative joint laxity.

Several other considerations and actions can aid in optimizing results. Before beginning the procedure, it is of paramount importance to assess whether the shoulder has full ROM because uninterrupted access to the glenoid and humeral canal are absolutely necessary. Preoperatively, the fluoroscopic imaging unit is positioned so that an unobstructed image of the shoulder and humeral shaft can be obtained intraoperatively.

Every attempt should be made to repair the tuberosities about the humeral socket regardless of the selected component size. Using an RSA system with proximal porous coating will aid in osseous integration of the tuberosities to the prosthesis. The cancellous bone from the humeral head can be saved and used as autograft about the implant and tuberosities, providing a more favorable environment for healing.

All sutures must be placed before implantation and cementing of the humeral component. It is important to pass the deep ends of the greater tuberosity sutures through the medial eyelet of the

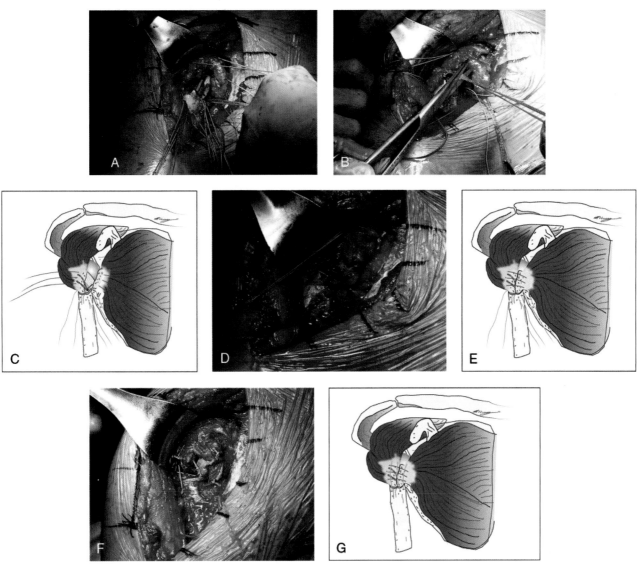

Figure 8   Images of a right shoulder. **A,** Intraoperative photograph shows three No. 5 nonabsorbable sutures placed around the bone-tendon junction of the lesser tuberosity. **B,** Intraoperative photograph shows the 2-mm nonabsorbable tape sutures tied down after all sutures have been passed into the lesser tuberosity to bring the greater tuberosity into proper alignment. **C,** Illustration shows the position of the greater tuberosity after the 2-mm nonabsorbable tape sutures have been tied in place. **D,** Intraoperative photograph shows that the three No. 5 nonabsorbable sutures passed around the lesser tuberosity have been tied, closing the tuberosities about the prosthesis. **E,** Illustration shows the position of the tuberosities after tying them down about the prosthesis. **F,** Intraoperative photograph shows that the remaining three No. 5 sutures placed from the humeral shaft into the rotator cuff are tied to create a circumferential crosshatch construct that compresses the bone graft fragments to the underlying bone and prosthesis. **G,** Illustration shows the position of all sutures after placement. The implant is secure, and the tuberosities and rotator cuff are in place. (Panels A, B, D, and F copyright the Foundation for Orthopaedic Research and Education, Tampa, FL.)

humeral implant before cementing the stem. Using large needles helps facilitate suture placement around the tuberosities. Most implant systems provide an alignment guide attached to the humeral stem to help determine version. The forearm is a convenient guide to assist in correct placement. Preoperative full-length humeral radiographs of the uninvolved side can be used as a template to restore implant height in patients who have substantial comminution and shaft involvement. Intraoperative fluoroscopy can be invaluable in reconstructing the tuberosities and achieving appropriate implant height.

Bibliography

Baron JA, Barrett JA, Karagas MR: The epidemiology of peripheral fractures. *Bone* 1996;18(3 suppl):209S-213S.

Boileau P, Krishnan SG, Tinsi L, Walch G, Coste JS, Molé D: Tuberosity malposition and migration: Reasons for poor outcomes after hemiarthroplasty for displaced fractures of the proximal humerus. *J Shoulder Elbow Surg* 2002;11(5):401-412.

Boyle MJ, Youn SM, Frampton CM, Ball CM: Functional outcomes of reverse shoulder arthroplasty compared with hemiarthroplasty for acute proximal humeral fractures. *J Shoulder Elbow Surg* 2013;22(1):32-37.

Cheung E, Willis M, Walker M, Clark R, Frankle MA: Complications in reverse total shoulder arthroplasty. *J Am Acad Orthop Surg* 2011;19(7):439-449.

Cuff DJ, Pupello DR: Comparison of hemiarthroplasty and reverse shoulder arthroplasty for the treatment of proximal humeral fractures in elderly patients. *J Bone Joint Surg Am* 2013;95(22):2050-2055.

Gallinet D, Adam A, Gasse N, Rochet S, Obert L: Improvement in shoulder rotation in complex shoulder fractures treated by reverse shoulder arthroplasty. *J Shoulder Elbow Surg* 2013;22(1):38-44.

Garrigues GE, Johnston PS, Pepe MD, Tucker BS, Ramsey ML, Austin LS: Hemiarthroplasty versus reverse total shoulder arthroplasty for acute proximal humerus fractures in elderly patients. *Orthopedics* 2012;35(5):e703-e708.

Hertel R, Hempfing A, Stiehler M, Leunig M: Predictors of humeral head ischemia after intracapsular fracture of the proximal humerus. *J Shoulder Elbow Surg* 2004;13(4):427-433.

Kralinger F, Schwaiger R, Wambacher M, et al: Outcome after primary hemiarthroplasty for fracture of the head of the humerus: A retrospective multicentre study of 167 patients. *J Bone Joint Surg Br* 2004;86(2):217-219.

Lenarz C, Shishani Y, McCrum C, Nowinski RJ, Edwards TB, Gobezie R: Is reverse shoulder arthroplasty appropriate for the treatment of fractures in the older patient? Early observations. *Clin Orthop Relat Res* 2011;469(12):3324-3331.

Levy J: Avoiding cement bone necrosis effect on tuberosity healing: The "black-and-tan" technique. *Tech Shoulder Elbow Surg* 2013;14(3):81-84.

Levy J, Frankle M, Mighell M, Pupello D: The use of the reverse shoulder prosthesis for the treatment of failed hemiarthroplasty for proximal humeral fracture. *J Bone Joint Surg Am* 2007;89(2):292-300.

Neer CS II: Displaced proximal humeral fractures: I. Classification and evaluation. *J Bone Joint Surg Am* 1970;52(6):1077-1089.

Noyes MP, Kleinhenz B, Markert RJ, Crosby LA: Functional and radiographic long-term outcomes of hemiarthroplasty for proximal humeral fractures. *J Shoulder Elbow Surg* 2011;20(3):372-377.

Schwartz DG, Cottrell BJ, Teusink MJ, et al: Factors that predict postoperative motion in patients treated with reverse shoulder arthroplasty. *J Shoulder Elbow Surg* 2014;23(9):1289-1295.

Willis M, Min W, Brooks JP, et al: Proximal humeral malunion treated with reverse shoulder arthroplasty. *J Shoulder Elbow Surg* 2012;21(4):507-513.

 ## Video Reference

Hussey MM, Stephens B, Frankle MA: Video. *Reverse Shoulder Arthroplasty for Acute Proximal Humerus Fractures.* Temple Terrace, FL, 2015.

Introduction

Nonunion after proximal humerus fracture is uncommon; it is most often seen at the level of the surgical neck. Nonunion also can result from failed internal fixation of a fracture. Surgical treatment to achieve union can be challenging because proximal humerus fracture nonunions are most commonly found in older patients with underlying osteoporosis or systemic or metabolic disorders. These comorbidities affect the potential for healing postoperatively. The nonunion site itself is complex because the humeral head is often osteoporotic and the nonunion is often associated with bone loss resulting from the cavitation effect of motion at the proximal end of the diaphyseal segment. Functional disabilities may be profound because of pain and instability at the site of nonunion, which may lead to overall limb dysfunction.

Several factors contribute to nonunion of surgical neck fractures. These fractures are subjected to the deforming forces of the surrounding musculotendinous units, with the pectoralis muscle pulling the proximal diaphyseal unit anteromedially while the rotator cuff muscles rotate and abduct the humeral head. Other reasons for failure to unite include the distraction force placed across the metaphyseal fracture site caused by the weight of the arm, soft-tissue interposition of the biceps tendon or deltoid muscle, and aggressive rehabilitation begun before the fracture has consolidated. Failure to heal also has been observed after surgical treatment of proximal humerus fractures using anatomically shaped implants featuring angular stable fixation.

Case Presentation

A 73-year-old woman has a painful nonunion of her left, nondominant proximal humerus. The original two-part surgical neck fracture of the humerus occurred 9 months before presentation after a fall from standing height. Initial treatment consisted of immobilization of the arm in a sling for 2 weeks, followed by a rehabilitation program. The patient continued to experience pain at the fracture site, limited glenohumeral motion, and limited use of her upper extremity. Serial radiographs obtained 9 months after the fracture reveal a well-defined mobile nonunion at the site of the original fracture.

Physical examination demonstrates limited forward flexion and shoulder rotation and poor ability to incorporate the left arm in activities of daily living, including personal hygiene. Review of the patient's medical history reveals systemic osteoporosis, hypertension, and thyroid dysfunction. She is married and leads an active lifestyle that includes traveling and sailing.

Radiographs obtained 9 months after the original fracture demonstrate a marked varus position of the humeral head and clearly defined margins of the nonunion. The sclerotic bony reaction is thought to be consistent with synovial pseudarthrosis. Cavitation (that is, bone resorption) in the humeral head also is suspected (**Figure 1**). The patient elected to undergo internal fixation with a 90° humeral blade plate. She demonstrated nearly completely glenohumeral motion 1 year postoperatively (**Figure 2**).

Indications

Prior to surgical treatment, the patient must be carefully evaluated regarding functional needs, medical comorbidities, and the specific characteristics of the nonunion. Despite advances in arthroplasty, including the reverse shoulder option, preservation of the humeral head in the dominant limb of an active person offers the potential for

Dr. Jupiter or an immediate family member is a member of a speakers' bureau or has made paid presentations on behalf of Synthes; serves as a paid consultant to Aptis and OHK Medical Devices; serves as an unpaid consultant to DePuy Synthes and TriMed; has stock or stock options held in OHK Medical Devices; has received research or institutional support from the AO Foundation; and serves as a board member, owner, officer, or committee member of the American Association for Hand Surgery, the American Shoulder and Elbow Surgeons, and the American Society for Surgery of the Hand.

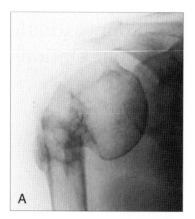 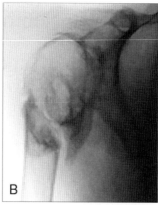 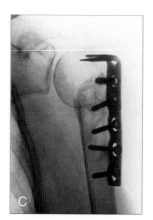 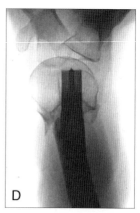

Figure 1   AP (**A**) and axillary (**B**) radiographs demonstrate a well-defined nonunion with varus deformity of the left humeral head in an active 73-year-old woman. AP (**C**) and axillary (**D**) radiographs demonstrate successful internal fixation with a 90° humeral blade plate.

good function without the associated risks of an implant. Although the patient described in this chapter was 73 years of age and had underlying osteoporosis at presentation, she was active and her life was substantially affected by her disability.

In addition to radiographic evaluation, including standard views of the glenohumeral joint, a CT scan can help identify the location of the tuberosities, the extent of bone loss in the humeral head, and the extent of sclerosis involving the proximal end of the diaphyseal segment. Although the four-part Neer classification is typically used, the Checchia classification further divides nonunion of the surgical neck into type I, in which the nonunion is located at the tuberosities, and type II, in which the nonunion is located at the lower surgical neck.

Controversies and Alternative Approaches

Because nonunion of the proximal humerus most commonly occurs at the level of the surgical neck, the alternative techniques listed herein are intended for treatment at this level. Several surgical options can provide stable internal fixation of a surgical neck nonunion in conjunction with ancillary bone grafting.

Initially, the author of this chapter used a 4.5-mm T-plate combined with an autogenous iliac crest graft and the placement of large sutures in the rotator cuff; the sutures then were tied through screw holes in the plate to provide a tension-band effect. Although some success with this method has been reported, the lack of angular stable screw fixation in the plate proves problematic in some patients with extremely osteoporotic bone. In 1990, the author of this chapter developed the 90° angled proximal humeral blade plate, which is available in 4.5- and 3.5-mm sizes with angular stable screw fixation.

A fixed-angle locked plate with intercalary strut allograft was initially described in 2006. One advantage of fibular strut allograft is that it provides increased biologic and mechanical support of the proximal humerus, which often has poor bone quality. This support is especially advantageous in patients with osteoporotic bone or loss of medial calcar bony support. The fibular strut provides better support compared with cancellous autograft or allograft. Use of the fibular strut technique also avoids the donor site morbidity that can result from iliac crest harvest, especially in older patients. Fibular allograft has a theoretical risk of disease transmission, which can be minimized with appropriate graft screening and packaging

protocols. Use of free vascularized fibular strut autograft avoids the problems associated with fibular allograft and can be used in patients who require substantial biologic support to augment mechanical stability. However, the use of free vascularized fibular strut autograft is technically demanding, requires longer surgical time, and should be performed only by experienced surgeons. Furthermore, the technique carries the risk of donor site morbidity to the lower extremity, which may not be ideal in older patients who often have medical comorbidities.

Intramedullary nailing is another option for surgical fixation of proximal humerus nonunions. However, results have been fair at best. Common problems have included violation of the rotator cuff at the insertion site and subacromial impingement, requiring a second surgery for hardware removal after union is achieved. Postoperatively, patients in whom the nonunion healed typically had good shoulder function. Recent studies have revisited intramedullary nailing, with one study of interlocked intramedullary nailing demonstrating union in all 13 patients, who were satisfied with their improved function and range of motion. However, two patients required surgical removal of proximal interlocking screws because of screw backout. Consideration of arthroplasty

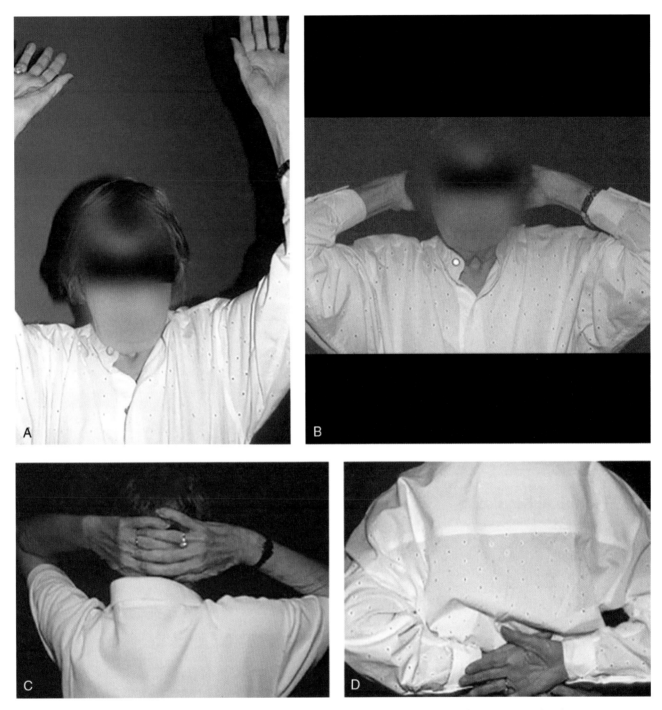

Figure 2   Clinical photographs show nearly full glenohumeral motion 1 year after internal fixation. **A,** Overhead position. **B,** External rotation, anterior view. **C,** External rotation to back of head. **D,** Internal rotation to the level of T12.

should be based on the overall patient condition and activity level, the extent of bone loss in the humeral head, and/or surgeon experience.

 Results

Studies on the use of blade plating and bone grafting for fixation of proximal humerus fracture nonunions are summarized in **Table 1**. Previous studies on this technique have demonstrated a high degree of success with limited complications and failures.

Table 1 Results of Fixation of Proximal Humerus Fracture Nonunion

Authors	Journal (Year)	Technique	Outcomes	Failure Rate	Comments
Healy et al	*J Orthop Trauma* (1990)	Nonreamed intramedullary nail or T-plate and bone graft	Better range of motion (110° forward flexion and 33° external rotation) and improved pain after T-plate fixation and bone grafting	18% (2 of 11)	Results at final follow-up were best after T-plate and bone graft with a tension-band construct to secure the rotator cuff
Jupiter and Mullaji	*Injury* (1994)	Blade plate and bone graft	Low failure rate with overall good to fair functional outcomes Results were good in 5 patients, fair in 3, and poor in 1	11%	9 patients treated Mean follow-up, 6.5 mo
Ring et al	*J Shoulder Elbow Surg* (2001)	Blade plate and autologous cancellous bone graft	Avg DASH score improved from 77 to 21 for healed fractures	8%	Better results in patients with low two-part nonunions 25 patients treated
Galatz et al	*J Orthop Trauma* (2004)	Blade plate and bone graft	Improved range of motion, pain, and function	9% (1 of 11)	10 of 11 nonunions healed within 6 mo
Badman et al	*Techniques in Shoulder and Elbow Surgery* (2006)	Blade or locked plate with fibular strut allograft	Clinical and radiographic union	0%	Heavy, nonabsorbable sutures used to fix subscapularis and supraspinatus tendons to the plate in 8 patients at final follow-up
Allende and Allende	*Int Orthop* (2009)	Locked 90° blade plate and bone graft	Avg DASH score improved from 83 to 25 Avg Constant score improved from 27.3 to 72.7	0%	100% union without complications achieved at avg 5.6-mo follow-up in all 7 patients treated

DASH = Disabilities of the Arm, Shoulder and Hand.

 ## Technical Keys to Success

- The surgical procedure is performed with the patient under general anesthesia. An additional interscalene block may be used for improved postoperative pain control, if desired.
- Patient positioning to obtain accurate intraoperative fluoroscopic imaging is important. A surgical table designed for shoulder procedures is recommended. If a standard surgical table is used, the patient is positioned with the head elevated 30° to 45° and the fluoroscopy unit positioned at the head of the bed parallel to the patient.
- Standard prepping and draping is done. The iliac crest also is sterilely prepped and included in the surgical field (**Figure 3**).
- The nonunion is approached through a standard deltopectoral interval to gain access to the clavipectoral fascia and biceps tendon.
- In some patients, the biceps tendon is interposed in the nonunion. If the tendon is deficient, tenodesis can be performed in the area of the intertubercular groove.
- The axillary and musculocutaneous nerves are located and preserved; this step is especially important if the patient has undergone a failed previous internal fixation. In these patients, the surgeon should identify both nerves and ensure strategic placement of retractors to avoid direct compression of the nerves.
- Sutures are placed into the subscapularis and supraspinatus tendons to facilitate later reattachment.

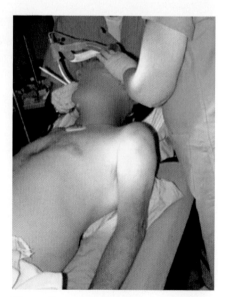

Figure 3 Intraoperative photograph shows a patient positioned on a standard surgical table with the arm and iliac crest prepped free in preparation for open reduction and internal fixation to manage nonunion of the proximal humerus.

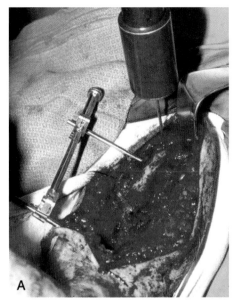
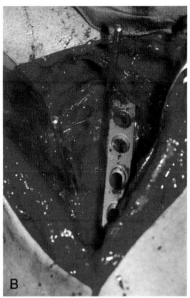

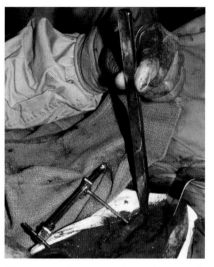

Figure 5 Intraoperative photograph shows use of a seating chisel for placement of the blade plate. The starting area on which the chisel rests was prepared by drilling several holes to allow the chisel to seat easily.

Figure 4 Intraoperative photographs show the use of a small external fixation device to stabilize nonunion of the proximal humerus after realignment of the humeral head and impaction of the diaphyseal segment. **A,** With the small external fixation device in place, a drill is used to create the seating hole for the blade plate. **B,** The humeral blade plate is positioned to sit alongside the anterolateral aspect of the humeral shaft. (Reproduced from Shin RD, Jupiter JB: Open reduction and internal fixation of surgical neck nonunion, in Zuckerman JD, ed: *Advanced Reconstruction: Shoulder.* Rosemont, IL, American Academy of Orthopaedic Surgeons, 2007, pp 307-315.)

- Proper preparation of the nonunion site is critical because the bony ends are often sclerotic, with an interposed avascular synovial membrane. Both sides of the nonunion are thoroughly débrided to bleeding surfaces.
- If use of an intramedullary fibular allograft strut is planned, the medullary canal of the humerus is sufficiently reamed to easily accept the allograft strut.
- Débridement of the humeral head segment may be particularly difficult because bony erosion may extend into the humeral head such that the synovial membrane is within the head itself. Internal fixation should not be performed in the setting of extensive cavitation in the humeral head or nonunion at a very proximal level.
- If the humeral head is rotated or in varus, as it was in the patient described in this chapter,

glenohumeral arthrolysis may be required to mobilize the head segment.
- A threaded, tipped guidewire can be used as a joystick to help maneuver the humeral head into a more anatomic position.
- A small external fixation device helps to hold the realignment in place (**Figure 4**).
- When a blade plate or a more stable anatomically shaped humeral plate with angular stable screw fixation is used, autogenous iliac crest graft is sufficient to fill any cavities in the humeral head and around the junction of the diaphyseal segment and humeral head (**Figure 5**).
- To achieve a stable nonunion construct, the proximal diaphyseal segment is impacted into the realigned humeral head whenever possible. A blade plate has been shown to be the most effective implant type to achieve a stable nonunion

construct. A 3.5- or 4.5-mm plate can be bent at 90° with the end machined down to create a narrow blade, or a commercially available 90° humeral blade plate system can be used.
- The optimal seating of the blade can be determined with the use of a guidewire under fluoroscopic guidance. The rotator interval also can be incised to visually ensure that the blade has not penetrated the articular surface.
- When securing the plate to the diaphyseal segment, the surgeon should avoid applying compression with an outrigger compression device because doing so may sink the blade distally in the humeral head, resulting in loss of the fixation point.
- If possible, the surgeon should place a screw directed obliquely from the most proximal hole aimed distally into either the diaphysis or the humeral head for added stability (**Figure 6**).
- The suture markers that were placed into the subscapularis and supraspinatus tendons earlier in the

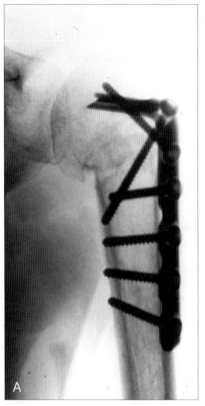 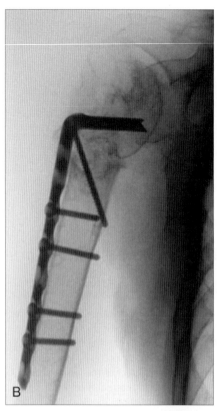

Figure 6 AP radiographs demonstrate the use of obliquely directed screws in the proximal blade plate holes to add stability to the fixation. **A,** Two oblique proximal screws were placed to add stability to the blade plate fixation. Note the very proximal placement of the blade as a result of the small humeral head. **B,** More distal placement of the blade and use of a single oblique screw.

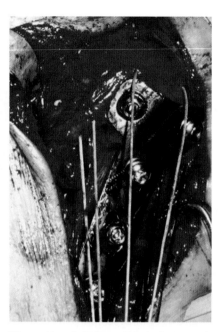

Figure 7 Intraoperative photograph shows sutures placed in the supraspinatus and subscapularis tendons in preparation for securing them to the implant to provide tension. (Reproduced from Shin RD, Jupiter JB: Open reduction and internal fixation of surgical neck nonunion, in Zuckerman JD, ed: *Advanced Reconstruction: Shoulder.* Rosemont, IL, American Academy of Orthopaedic Surgeons, 2007, pp 307-315.)

procedure are tied to the implant through screw holes to provide tension (**Figure 7**).

 Rehabilitation

The purpose of surgical treatment of proximal humerus nonunion is to create a pain-free, stable joint that will allow the patient to engage in activities of daily living. Consequently, postoperative rehabilitation should be done with the goal of restoring upper extremity function as soon as possible. Intraoperative assessment of construct stability dictates postoperative rehabilitation and motion. In the immediate postoperative period, the patient's arm is placed in a sling for comfort. Gentle passive pendulum exercises can begin immediately. Sutures are

removed 10 to 14 days postoperatively. Thereafter, gradually increasing active shoulder and elbow motion is allowed as tolerated (**Table 2**).

 Avoiding Pitfalls

Preoperatively, CT provides the best information regarding the extent of cavitation in the humeral head segment. At the time the patient is prepped for surgery, the endotracheal tube should be taped to the side of the mouth opposite the involved limb to avoid obstruction of imaging. During the procedure, glenohumeral arthrolysis should be considered if realignment of the humeral head is difficult. Passage of large sutures through the subscapularis and supraspinatus tendons aids in attaining

proper orientation of the nonunion. Later in the procedure, these sutures can be attached to the implant to provide tension. A Kirschner wire can be used as a guidewire under imaging to ensure correct placement of the blade. The surgeon should avoid placing the blade too proximally; however, in the setting of extensive bone resorption in the head, proximal placement is necessary. Whenever possible, the diaphyseal segment should be impacted into the humeral head to provide stability. When the plate is applied to the diaphyseal segment, the use of an external compression jig should be avoided because it may loosen the seating of the blade in the humeral head. Finally, if an intramedullary fibular strut technique is used, the medullary canal must be enlarged to accommodate the bone graft.

Table 2 Rehabilitation Protocol After Surgical Management of Proximal Humerus Fracture Nonunion

Postoperative Week	ROM	Strengthening	Return to Play	Comments/Emphasis
0-2	Gentle pendulum exercises	None	None	Sutures are removed 10-14 d postoperatively
2-6	Gentle passive ROM No rotation exercises	None	None	—
6-12	Internal rotation and external rotation passive ROM exercises are begun, progressing to active and active-assisted ROM as tolerated	Gentle strengthening exercises are begun	Gradual, low-impact activities	—
12-24	No restrictions	Strengthening exercises are continued	Allowed without restrictions	—

ROM = range of motion.

 Bibliography

Allende C, Allende BT: The use of a new locking 90 degree blade plate in the treatment of atrophic proximal humerus nonunions. *Int Orthop* 2009;33(6):1649-1654.

Badman B, Mighell M, Drake G: Proximal humeral nonunions: Surgical technique with fibular strut allograft and fixed-angle locked plating. *Techniques in Shoulder and Elbow Surgery* 2006;7(2):95-101.

Cadet ER, Yin B, Schulz B, Ahmad CS, Rosenwasser MP: Proximal humerus and humeral shaft nonunions. *J Am Acad Orthop Surg* 2013;21(9):538-547.

Checchia SL, Doneux P, Miyazaki AN, Spir IA, Bringel R, Ramos CH: Classification of non-unions of the proximal humerus. *Int Orthop* 2000;24(4):217-220.

Duralde XA, Flatow EL, Pollock RG, Nicholson GP, Self EB, Bigliani LU: Operative treatment of nonunions of the surgical neck of the humerus. *J Shoulder Elbow Surg* 1996;5(3):169-180.

Egol KA, Ong CC, Walsh M, Jazrawi LM, Tejwani NC, Zuckerman JD: Early complications in proximal humerus fractures (OTA Types 11) treated with locked plates. *J Orthop Trauma* 2008;22(3):159-164.

Galatz LM, Williams GR Jr, Fenlin JM Jr, Ramsey ML, Iannotti JP: Outcome of open reduction and internal fixation of surgical neck nonunions of the humerus. *J Orthop Trauma* 2004;18(2):63-67.

Healy WL, Jupiter JB, Kristiansen TK, White RR: Nonunion of the proximal humerus: A review of 25 cases. *J Orthop Trauma* 1990;4(4):424-431.

Jupiter JB, Mullaji AB: Blade plate fixation of proximal humeral non-unions. *Injury* 1994;25(5):301-303.

Ring D, McKee MD, Perey BH, Jupiter JB: The use of a blade plate and autogenous cancellous bone graft in the treatment of ununited fractures of the proximal humerus. *J Shoulder Elbow Surg* 2001;10(6):501-507.

Sonnabend DH: Blade plate fixation of humeral neck fractures and nonunions in osteoporotic bone. *J Shoulder Elbow Surg* 1993;2(suppl):49.

Walch G, Badet R, Nové-Josserand L, Levigne C: Nonunions of the surgical neck of the humerus: Surgical treatment with an intramedullary bone peg, internal fixation, and cancellous bone grafting. *J Shoulder Elbow Surg* 1996;5(3):161-168.

Yamane S, Suenaga N, Oizumi N, Minami A: Interlocking intramedullary nailing for nonunion of the proximal humerus with the Straight Nail System. *J Shoulder Elbow Surg* 2008;17(5):755-759.

Chapter 49

Technical Considerations for Nonunion and Malunion in Humeral Hemiarthroplasty

Wayne Z. Burkhead, Jr, MD

Ian G. Wilkofsky, MD

Kelly Fitzpatrick, DO

Introduction

Proximal humerus fractures account for approximately 5% of total fractures annually in the United States. Approximately 80% of proximal humerus fractures can be treated nonsurgically. Surgical intervention can be challenging because of soft-tissue disruption of the rotator cuff tendon, associated capsular disruption of the tuberosity segments, a short or comminuted metaphyseal segment, osteopenia, or a perilous blood supply that can lead to collapse of the humeral head segment.

Overwhelming evidence exists for early fixation of a displaced proximal humerus fracture. Because of a patient's age or medical comorbidities, surgical treatment is not always attempted, possibly resulting in nonunion or malunion of the tuberosities and/or the junction between the tuberosities and the humeral head. Even with surgical intervention incorporating modern locking-plate technology, fixation can fail. In addition, complex or comminuted fractures can result in suboptimal placement of the tuberosities of the humeral head (**Figure 1**). To fully treat the spectrum of proximal humerus fractures, the surgeon must be comfortable performing different types of humeral head replacement surgeries. Due to the expanding indications of the reverse prosthesis, the use of humeral head replacement surgery is decreasing.

It is imperative to manage the patient's expectations and set realistic goals when attempting a humeral head replacement for nonunion or malunion of the proximal humerus. The perceived success or failure of this surgical procedure for both the surgeon and the patient often depends on established preoperative goals. As demonstrated in the radiographs that comprise **Figure 1**, it is important to monitor patients postoperatively. Even a properly aligned, well-executed open reduction and internal fixation (ORIF) can result in a poor outcome despite optimal conditions.

Case Presentation

A 50-year-old, left-hand–dominant man who works as a mechanic reports pain, decreased range of motion (ROM), and weakness in his left arm. He had been involved in a motor vehicle accident approximately 4 years earlier. At that time, he had sustained multiple injuries, including a severely displaced fracture of the proximal humerus and an axillary nerve palsy. After clinical stability was achieved, the patient underwent ORIF with a locking plate. Several years later, in an effort to diminish pain and improve ROM, the plate was removed. The patient returned to work and wanted to remain active as long as possible, but at the time of his initial presentation, disabling pain prevented him from working.

Initial examination revealed that the patient has 80° of forward elevation, 165° of passive elevation, active external rotation of 15° with passive external rotation to 30°, a positive external rotation lag sign, internal rotation to L5, and a positive hornblower sign.

Dr. Burkhead or an immediate family member has received royalties from Tornier; is a member of a speakers' bureau or has made paid presentations on behalf of Arthrex, Arthrosurface, Lima Corporate, and Tornier; serves as a paid consultant to or is an employee of Arthrex, Arthrosurface, Lima Corporate, Stryker, Bio2 Technologies, and I-Flow; and serves as a board member, owner, officer, or committee member of the International Board of Shoulder & Elbow Surgery. Neither of the following authors nor any immediate family member has received anything of value from or has stock or stock options held in a commercial company or institution related directly or indirectly to the subject of this chapter: Dr. Wilkofsky and Dr. Fitzpatrick.

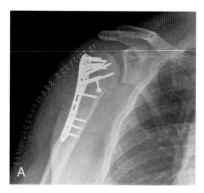
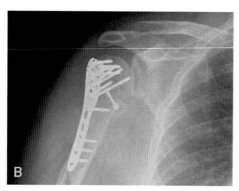
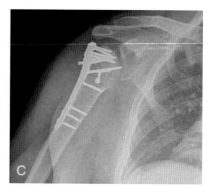

Figure 1   **A,** AP radiograph demonstrates open reduction and internal fixation of a four-part proximal humerus fracture with near-anatomic alignment. **B,** AP radiograph obtained 2 months postoperatively demonstrates slight evidence of humeral head collapse and tuberosity malunion or nonunion. **C,** AP radiograph obtained 1 year postoperatively demonstrates varus collapse of the head with altered tuberosity-to-head height.

Belly-press test results were negative. Strength testing revealed deltoid firing at 4/5 abduction strength. Supraspinatus and infraspinatus testing revealed 4/5 strength and 5/5 subscapularis strength.

Preoperative imaging demonstrates severe heterotopic ossification surrounding the glenoid and greater tuberosity (**Figure 2**). The greater tuberosity was malunited proximally and articulated with the acromion. The neck-shaft angle appeared to be in varus, measuring approximately 110°. The patient had apparent osteonecrosis of the humeral head that demonstrated moderate collapse and moderate glenohumeral joint space narrowing. A screw was present in the metaphysis of the humerus, along with ossification over the suprascapular notch. Preoperative electromyogram and nerve conduction velocity results demonstrated a chronic, although incomplete, axillary and suprascapular nerve palsy. This patient did not have complete axillary nerve palsy and wished to maintain his passive motion. Therefore, an arthrodesis was viewed as a last resort, to be performed only if there was no chance of maintaining motion and restoring function. Fusion had the potential to result in limitations at work because of the lack of passive motion.

The patient wanted to maintain his previous level of activity and did not want to be subject to lifting restrictions. Multiple surgical options were discussed. Initially, the senior author of this chapter (W.Z.B.) recommended the patient undergo a glenohumeral joint fusion, which would have resulted in a level of function comparable to that of the patient's preinjury status and eliminated joint pain. The patient would not accept the loss of passive motion inherent with this procedure, however, because it would have precluded his return to work. He expressed a desire to try anything short of a fusion to decrease the amount of pain he was experiencing and result in the same or improved motion. The patient had chronic incomplete axillary nerve palsy, but his deltoid muscle was functional and he retained the ability to raise his arm.

An arthroplasty is not an unreasonable procedure to undertake in the patient with a functioning deltoid for the goal of restoring motion and obtaining adequate pain relief. The patient ultimately underwent a humeral head resurfacing procedure and rotator cuff repair after greater tuberosity takedown to manage the malunion; suprascapular nerve release was performed as well (**Figure 3**). The implant used in this patient (HemiCAP [Arthrosurface])

relies on an interference metaphyseal fit for implant fixation. Another advantage of this particular implant is that the subscapularis repair can be performed with suture anchors. In traditional arthroplasty, bone tunnel placement typically occurs before stem placement to obtain secure fixation of this powerful rotator cuff muscle.

The patient had a suprascapular notch encased in bone, which likely led to suprascapular neuropathy. Suprascapular nerve release was performed to optimize rotator cuff function. A superior approach was used; the trapezius was split, and blunt dissection was performed inferiorly to the transverse scapular ligament. Care was taken to preserve the suprascapular artery, located superior to the ligament. In the setting of ligamentous ossification, an osteotome can be used to carefully remove the bony bridge superiorly, thus releasing the nerve.

The nonunited greater tuberosity segment was osteotomized and further mobilized; however, anatomic placement was impossible because of the inherent contracture present. Thus, a portion of the fragment was excised, and the supraspinatus tendon was mobilized. A rotator cuff repair using suture anchor fixation was performed medially at the sulcus.

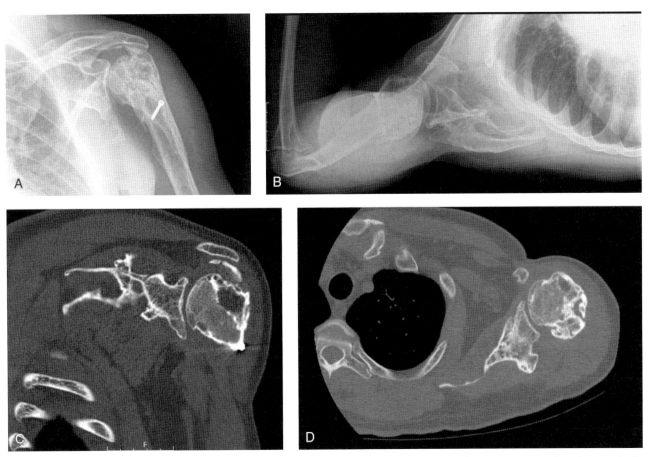

Figure 2   Images from a different patient than the one discussed in Figure 1. These images demonstrate sequelae of a chronically malunited proximal humerus fracture. AP (**A**) and axillary Y (**B**) radiographs of a left shoulder demonstrate poor bone quality and tuberosity malunion. Coronal (**C**) and axial (**D**) CT scans demonstrate heterotopic ossification of the glenoid and altered version of the humeral head.

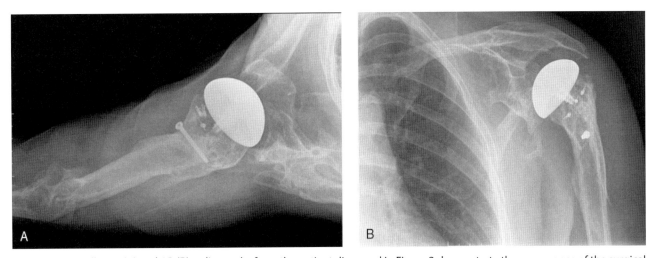

Figure 3   Axillary Y (**A**) and AP (**B**) radiographs from the patient discussed in Figure 2 demonstrate the appearance of the surgical shoulder after hemiarthroplasty.

Indications

The indications for humeral hemiarthroplasty after fracture malunion or nonunion are limited. Patients who have tuberosity malunion or nonunion may be good candidates for a hemiarthroplasty, such as in the previously discussed case. In addition, patients in whom posttraumatic arthritis has developed secondary to the initial injury, head collapse, or screw penetration into the joint may benefit from a hemiarthroplasty.

The goal of the hemiarthroplasty is to restore the mechanics of the rotator cuff by performing a tuberosity osteotomy to reposition it to a more anatomic position or by attaining adequate coverage of the humeral head. Tuberosity malposition leads to cuff dysfunction due to medialization or superior migration, which results in decreased tension of the tendon and possible superior migration of the humeral head.

Restoration of glenohumeral articulation congruency is the other advantage of humeral head resurfacing. Humeral head collapse or posttraumatic arthritis is likely to result in a painful arc of motion. Decreased pain and increased ease of mechanical rotation resulting from decreased resistance of the center of rotation are desired outcomes of a resurfaced articulation. The resurfacing may be extended to the subacromial space with use of a larger humeral head that allows articulation with the acromion (cuff tear arthropathy head), which may provide a biomechanically advantageous center of rotation.

Controversies and Alternative Approaches

A glenohumeral joint arthrodesis is an appropriate treatment of a patient who has an axillary nerve palsy with substantial pain. Patients can still maintain a certain degree of functional motion and perform activities associated with heavy labor. An arthrodesis severely limits the ability to maintain passive motion, and surgical options after arthrodesis are extremely limited should the patient be dissatisfied with the results.

Alternatively, an anatomic or reverse total shoulder arthroplasty could be attempted. In an anatomic arthroplasty, the goals are limited to pain relief and maintenance of passive ROM. The success of the glenoid component relies on the dynamic stability of the shoulder, which is primarily provided by the rotator cuff. In a patient with poor rotator cuff integrity resulting from a malpositioned tuberosity and baseline nerve damage, placement of a traditional glenoid component would not be ideal because eccentric forces likely would result in rapid component loosening. An alternative to a traditional polyethylene component is biologic resurfacing with an allograft dermal matrix. Although use of biologic resurfacing has been controversial, the senior author of this chapter (W.Z.B.) thinks it has been successful in patients with appropriate indications.

Reverse total shoulder arthroplasty is a good alternative for patients with cuff dysfunction secondary to tuberosity malunion or nonunion, and the procedure has become popular over the past decade. The primary indications for reverse total shoulder arthroplasty are cuff tear arthropathy, severe rotator cuff deficiency, primary glenohumeral arthritis with severe glenoid bone loss, and proximal humerus fractures. In patients who are active and physiologically young (younger than 60 years), however, the decision to place a reverse prosthesis becomes somewhat controversial because these patients are likely to require revision. A reverse total shoulder arthroplasty is the treatment of choice in the older, more sedentary patient. It is the preference of the senior author of this chapter (W.Z.B.) to reserve this procedure as the last resort for the young, active patient who works as a manual laborer and does not want restrictions on lifting.

Successful treatment with a hemiarthroplasty for a malunited or nonunited fracture relies on the correct placement of the tuberosities and final, overall function of the rotator cuff. This was the treatment of choice by the surgeon and the patient in the case described in this chapter, despite the presence of a questionable insertion of the rotator cuff and an equivocal function of the suprascapular nerve. Hemiarthroplasty maintains anatomic relationships throughout the glenohumeral joint. This includes the insertion of the rotator cuff and the articulation of the humeral head on the glenoid. This particular approach also preserves bone stock for future procedures if necessary. For these reasons, hemiarthroplasty was the method of treatment chosen for the patient described in this chapter (**Figure 3**).

Results

Several studies have evaluated the effectiveness of a total shoulder arthroplasty compared to a hemiarthroplasty in patients with malunited or nonunited proximal humerus fracture (**Table 1**). Both surgical approaches reliably reduce pain, but sequelae of proximal humerus fractures are difficult to manage and complications can occur. Patients treated with greater tuberosity osteotomy consistently have worse results on standardized outcome measures.

In a study of 48 patients treated for painful malunion of the proximal humerus, most patients were satisfied after treatment. However, a higher proportion of patients with severe malunions had an unsatisfactory result. This was the first study to show that greater tuberosity osteotomies resulted in significantly worse outcomes for both groups regardless whether hemiarthroplasty or total

Table 1 Results of Surgical Management of Malunited Proximal Humerus Fractures

Authors	Journal (Year)	Technique (No. of Malunions Treated)	Outcomes	Comments
Norris et al	*J Shoulder Elbow Surg* (1995)	TSA (13) HA (4)	15 complications, 5 revisions 30% of patients with previous surgery had a preexisting nerve injury Mean active FE, 92° Mean active ER, 27° Mean IR to L1	Mean age, 54 yr (range 21-80 yr) Mean follow-up, 4.1 yr (range, 2-11 yr) 23% displacement rate for patients who underwent greater tuberosity osteotomy
Beredjiklian et al	*J Bone Joint Surg Am* (1998)	Arthroplasty (22) Other procedures (17)	5 revisions Patients treated within 1 yr after injury had increased likelihood of a satisfactory result	Mean age, 53 yr (range, 27-77 yr) Mean follow-up, 3.7 yr (1-4.4 yr) 50% of patients who had an unsatisfactory result underwent a hemiarthroplasty with subsequent development of painful glenoid arthritis
Boileau et al	*J Shoulder Elbow Surg* (2001)	HA (31) TSA (17)	18 complications, 4 revisions Greater tuberosity osteotomy resulted in significantly worse function ($P < 0.005$)	Mean age, 59 yr (range 30-87 yr) Mean follow-up, 1.6 yr (range, 1-4 yr)
Antuña et al	*J Shoulder Elbow Surg* (2002)	HA (25) TSA (25)	2 revisions: 1 for fracture and 1 for persistent instability Mean active FE, 88° Mean ER, 38° 11 patients had a tuberosity nonunion or resorption	Mean age, 65 yr (range, 36-80 yr) Mean follow-up, 6 yr (range, 2-15 yr)
Mansat et al	*J Shoulder Elbow Surg* (2004)	TSA (8) HA (20)	1 complication, 1 revision Mean active FE, 107° Mean ER, 20° Mean IR to L3 85% of patients reported little pain 3 patients had greater tuberosity osteotomies, all of whom did poorly	Mean age, 61 yr (range, 36-79 yr) Mean follow-up, 3.9 yr (range, 2-13.2 yr)
Panagopoulos et al	*Adv Orthop* (2013)	HA (33)	Greater tuberosity displacement, large rotator cuff tear, and severe malunion most negatively affected outcome 60% of patients able to do activities up to shoulder level	Mean age, 61 yr (range, 36-79 yr) Mean follow-up, 9 yr (range, 2-21 yr)

ER = external rotation, FE = forward elevation, HA = hemiarthroplasty, IR = internal rotation, TSA = total shoulder arthroplasty.

shoulder arthroplasty was performed. In a study of 50 patients treated to correct a malunion of the proximal humerus, patients who underwent greater tuberosity osteotomies had significantly worse motion than their counterparts who did not undergo such an osteotomy.

 Technical Keys to Success

- For optimal success of the surgical procedure, all sources of pain, including osteonecrosis with subsequent glenohumeral incongruity and mechanical subacromial impingement of the malunited tuberosities, must be identified preoperatively.

- Proper imaging such as CT with or without arthrogram may be necessary to properly evaluate anatomic landmarks and rotator cuff tendon pathology.

- The patient is placed in the beach-chair position.
- A traditional deltopectoral approach is used, with a focus on exposing the proximal humerus as much as possible. When necessary, the incision can be taken more laterally, and extensive deltoid takedown can be conducted as described by Cofield to further optimize the visualization of this portion of the shoulder. Henry described taking down a fleck of bone with the deltoid to further visualization.
- In some patients with malunited tuberosities, it also may be necessary to perform a coracoacromial ligament takedown to assist in visualization.
- In patients with a history of lesser tuberosity fractures, this tuberosity fragment may be malunited and it may be necessary to perform an osteotomy to mobilize this fragment. An alternative is to simply excise this portion of bone and repair the remaining subscapularis either to its native insertion, just medial to the bicipital groove, or perform an even more medialized repair.
- A capsular release is performed with electrocautery started anteriorly.
- The release is extended inferiorly and posteriorly while the arm is brought into forward flexion and external rotation until it reaches beyond the 6-o'clock position. If further release is necessary, it is safe to continue beyond this 6-o'clock position while maintaining the knife or cautery on bone. This takedown and subscapularis tenotomy will lead to dislocation of the humerus and optimal visualization of the capsule.
- After the humerus is fully dislocated, attention is focused on the greater tuberosity. If an osteotomy or takedown is required, this is an optimal time to consider this technique.

- In the setting of tuberosity malposition, the surgeon may elect to use the stem of the prosthesis as an anchoring point to reinforce fixation.
- The humeral head replacement is performed using the prosthesis of choice. The surgeon should attempt to restore the Gothic arch of the proximal humerus to restore the anatomy of the humeral head.
- After the implant is in place, adequate humeral head coverage with the rotator cuff must be obtained. This may require fixation of the tuberosities to the stem or repair of the rotator cuff, which is done via suture anchors, transosseous tunnels, or circumferential stem fixation techniques.
- In patients who require takedown of the coracoacromial ligament, the ligament is repaired through two drill holes in the acromion and tied over a bony block. The senior author of this chapter (W.Z.B.) thinks that repair is necessary in these patients because rotator cuff dysfunction may lead to anterior-superior escape of the humeral head.
- The senior author of this chapter (W.Z.B.) prefers to close the deltopectoral interval with an absorbable suture. Skin closure is done using the surgeon's preferred method.

Rehabilitation

Hemiarthroplasty is essentially equivalent to repair of a massive, retracted rotator cuff tear. Thus, immobilization of the surgical arm in a sling with an abduction pillow for the first 6 weeks postoperatively is recommended, followed by gradual progression of passive ROM exercises beginning at 6 weeks postoperatively. At 8 to 10 weeks postoperatively, active-assisted ROM is begun, followed by full active motion. The patient begins gentle isometric exercises after functional ROM has been achieved.

At 12 to 16 weeks postoperatively, resistance exercises are begun, and return to activities typically is achieved 4 to 6 months postoperatively, with an expectation that continued progress will be demonstrated at 18 to 24 months postoperatively (**Table 2**).

Avoiding Pitfalls

When considering a hemiarthroplasty to manage fracture malunion or nonunion, environmental and physiologic patient factors must be accounted for, including the patient's age, medical comorbidities, overall functional requirements for work, preoperative expectations, and prior level of function. The surgeon and patient need to understand the risks involved before proceeding with definitive management. A 40-year-old, otherwise healthy construction worker who has a surgical neck nonunion may be best treated with a revision ORIF. The same injury in a 45-year-old patient who has diabetes, smokes, and is disabled may be better managed with nonsurgical treatment or arthroplasty because of the patient's lesser physiologic capability for bone healing.

Proper imaging studies are needed to aid in decision making. Orthogonal radiographs must be obtained to assess for position of key anatomic landmarks. Proper evaluation of tuberosity position, neck-shaft angle, a concentric glenohumeral joint, and degree of arthrosis is an important preoperative factor that plays a key role in surgical decision making. Another important variable to take into consideration is glenohumeral version. This condition is difficult to assess with plain radiographs, and CT may help in preoperative assessment. With recent innovative imaging techniques, three-dimensional reconstructions can be obtained to more accurately evaluate overall bony anatomy. An arthrogram also may be considered in conjunction with CT to further evaluate the rotator

Table 2 Rehabilitation Protocol After Humeral Hemiarthroplasty

Postoperative Week	ROM	Strengthening	Return to Activities	Comments/Emphasis
0-2	None	None	None	Sling immobilization with an abduction pillow
2-6	None	None	None	Sling immobilization with an abduction pillow
6-12	Passive ROM is begun at 6 wk and gradually progressed Active-assisted ROM is begun at 8-10 wk, followed by full active motion	When functional ROM is attained, gentle isometric exercises are begun	None	Focus on restoration of ROM prior to strengthening
≥12	No limitations	Resistance exercises are begun at 12-16 wk	As tolerated at 16-24 wk	Continued progress expected at 72-96 wk

ROM = range of motion.

cuff insertion. MRI also would be helpful, but it may not be necessary.

The neck-shaft angle should be taken into consideration when deciding which implant to use. The patient in the case described in this chapter had a mild to moderate varus deformity of the proximal humerus that was taken into consideration both preoperatively and intraoperatively. Correction of the neck-shaft angle can be made in instances of hemiarthroplasty, whether with a stemmed component or a resurfacing implant. In this case, varus deformity was corrected by adjusting the trajectory of the fixation component in a more valgus position. In stemmed components, this correction can be made by adjusting the cut of the humeral head as well as providing some support along the medial calcar in the form of a wedged bone graft to maintain valgus alignment with a thin or short-stemmed implant.

Normal retroversion varies among individuals. Overall, version can be assessed preoperatively with CT by using the epicondylar axis at the distal humerus and at the time of surgery by observing the direction of the humeral head in relation to this and other bony landmarks. One such relationship is the direction of the humeral head with respect

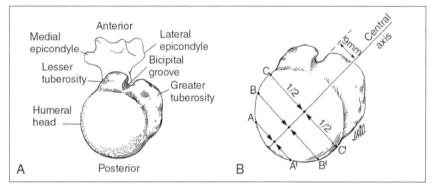

Figure 4 **A** and **B,** Illustrations depict estimation of the version of the humeral prosthesis, on the basis of cadaver studies, by placing the fin of the prosthesis approximately 9 mm posterior to the bicipital groove. **B,** To determine a central axis of the humeral head, three random points are chosen along the anterior side (A, B, C). A straight line is drawn to the posterior side at all three points (A', B', C'). The center point is measured between point A and A', B and B', and C and C'. This central line represents a central axis of the humeral head and allows a measurement to be made from the bicipital groove. (Reproduced with permission from Tillett E, Smith M, Fulcher M, Shanklin J: Anatomic determination of humeral head retroversion: The relationship of the central axis of the humeral head to the bicipital groove. *J Shoulder Elbow Surg* 1993;2[5]:255-256.)

to the bicipital groove, provided surgical neck malunion is not present. If a surgical neck malunion exists, preoperative planning should accommodate for the type of implant used and the technique for implantation should be adjusted. Traditionally, version also is measured in relation to the axis of the forearm, and many implant systems have cutting guides based on this relationship. The senior author of this chapter (W.Z.B.)

prefers to use the bicipital groove as a reference for overall version if the proximal anatomy is not disturbed. When a stemmed component is used, the fin or central portion of the broach can be placed approximately 1 cm lateral to the bicipital groove to achieve proper version. A similar technique can be used when using a resurfacing component by drawing the axis of version from this bicipital groove reference point (**Figure 4**).

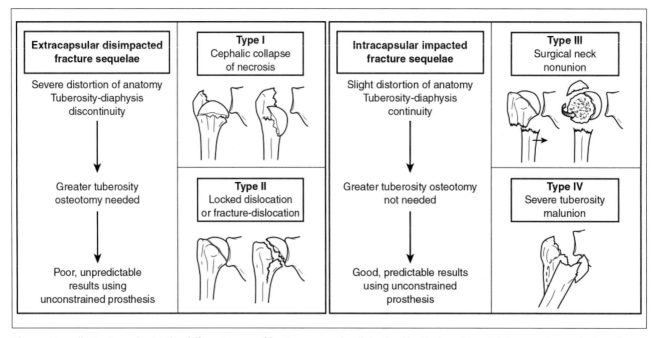

Figure 5 Illustrations depict the different types of fractures sequelae described by Boileau. Type 1, Intracapsular cephalic collapse. Type 2, Intracapsular fracture/dislocation. Type 3, Extracapsular surgical neck malunion. Type 4, Extracapsular tuberosity malunion.

It is critical to assess the location and severity of a malunion or nonunion. Boileau described a method to assess sequelae of a proximal humerus fracture, specifically focusing on the location of the fracture and outcomes associated with malunions of the tuberosities. Four groups of malunions or nonunions were stratified into two separate categories (**Figure 5**). The first category was an intracapsular or impacted fracture of the proximal humerus that was further categorized into cephalic collapse (type 1) or a fracture/dislocation of the head (type 2). The second category involved extracapsular injuries, which required an osteotomy of the greater tuberosity to restore anatomic relationships. This category was further divided into a surgical neck nonunion (type 3) or a severe tuberosity malunion (type 4). Type 4 fracture sequelae appeared to have a poorer prognosis in terms of restoration of function and ROM. This likely contributed to poor restoration of rotator cuff function. These patients are likely to experience a poorer clinical result;

therefore, a reverse prosthesis should be considered.

Being fully aware of these results from this retrospective series of patients, it is the opinion of the senior author of this chapter (W.Z.B.) that this procedure should be reserved as a last resort in healthy, active patients. The surgeon should take into consideration that patients with greater tuberosity malunions may be predisposed to a limited outcome in terms of overall function and restoration of motion.

In terms of exposure, an extended deltopectoral approach is essential when it comes to exposing the proximal humerus. The deltoid has a large insertion onto the deltoid tuberosity and takes up nearly one-third of the humeral diaphysis. A controlled takedown of the deltoid insertion with repair either proximally or distally may be necessary to obtain access to and restore the anatomic relationships of the proximal humerus. Even in the absence of previous surgery, subdeltoid scarring may be intense. The surgeon must be careful

to maintain direct contact on the bone during deltoid takedown to avoid injury to the main branch of the axillary nerve and its arborized ends. Careful takedown and repair is preferable to an uncontrolled midsubstance-deltoid laceration arising from aggressive retraction.

The coracoacromial ligament also may restrict visualization. Takedown of this important structure may be necessary to facilitate adequate exposure. Care must be taken to repair the coracoacromial ligament when closing to prevent anterior-superior escape of the humeral head in the event of future rotator cuff deficiency. The senior author of this chapter (W.Z.B.) prefers to tag the insertion of the coracoacromial ligament to the acromion with a No. 2 nonabsorbable suture after taking off the acromion and repairing the ligament over an anterior acromial bone tunnel upon closure. Visualization is critical to success. Although there is a paucity of literature supporting this technique, there is a risk of a failed repair of the coracoacromial ligament. The senior author of this chapter (W.Z.B.) thinks that the benefit of coracoacromial ligament takedown far outweighs the risk when managing a complicated case such as the one previously described.

It is critical to obtain secure fixation of the subscapularis tendon to its native insertion or just medial to this spot on the metaphysis of the proximal humerus. As noted previously, the bicipital groove can be a key landmark when assessing proper placement of the tendon. If the lesser tuberosity is in a good position without a substantial malunion, this tendon can be managed based on the surgeon's preference, much as in an anatomic arthroplasty. An osteotomy, tenotomy, or peel may be used when obtaining access to the humeral head. In the setting of malunion, an osteotomy in combination with an excision (much as in the case presented in this chapter) may be necessary to restore proper position of the insertion of the tendon. Suture anchors and/or bone tunnels should be used to obtain proper fixation to the metaphysis.

One final point when considering a hemiarthroplasty in patients with a malunion or nonunion is anticipation of a future procedure. It is critical that the surgeon be aware of the possibility of further treatment in these complex cases. In this particular case, a bone preservation technique was used with a humeral head resurfacing implant system. The preservation of the metaphyseal bone does not preclude a revision hemiarthroplasty system, allows adequate bone stock for a possible future arthrodesis, and makes the use of a reverse arthroplasty system less difficult relative to a long metaphyseal stem.

If a traditional hemiarthroplasty stem is the treatment of choice in patients with malunited or nonunited proximal humerus fracture, the surgeon should strongly consider using a convertible stem component. This allows for easy conversion of the stem from a hemiarthroplasty to a reverse component without removal of the initial stem. This is a relatively new concept, and the surgeon should be aware of the capabilities of stem conversion because this is implant dependent.

Bibliography

Antuña SA, Sperling JW, Sánchez-Sotelo J, Cofield RH: Shoulder arthroplasty for proximal humeral malunions: Long-term results. *J Shoulder Elbow Surg* 2002;11(2):122-129.

Beredjiklian PK, Iannotti JP: Treatment of proximal humerus fracture malunion with prosthetic arthroplasty. *Instr Course Lect* 1998;47:135-140.

Beredjiklian PK, Iannotti JP, Norris TR, Williams GR: Operative treatment of malunion of a fracture of the proximal aspect of the humerus. *J Bone Joint Surg Am* 1998;80(10):1484-1497.

Boileau P, Krishnan SG, Tinsi L, Walch G, Coste JS, Molé D: Tuberosity malposition and migration: Reasons for poor outcomes after hemiarthroplasty for displaced fractures of the proximal humerus. *J Shoulder Elbow Surg* 2002;11(5):401-412.

Boileau P, Trojani C, Walch G, Krishnan SG, Romeo A, Sinnerton R: Shoulder arthroplasty for the treatment of the sequelae of fractures of the proximal humerus. *J Shoulder Elbow Surg* 2001;10(4):299-308.

Bosch U, Skutek M, Fremerey RW, Tscherne H: Outcome after primary and secondary hemiarthroplasty in elderly patients with fractures of the proximal humerus. *J Shoulder Elbow Surg* 1998;7(5):479-484.

Dines DM, Warren RF, Altchek DW, Moeckel B: Posttraumatic changes of the proximal humerus: Malunion, nonunion, and osteonecrosis. Treatment with modular hemiarthroplasty or total shoulder arthroplasty. *J Shoulder Elbow Surg* 1993;2(1):11-21.

Frich LH, Søjbjerg JO, Sneppen O: Shoulder arthroplasty in complex acute and chronic proximal humeral fractures. *Orthopedics* 1991;14(9):949-954.

Henry AK: The proximal part of the humerus and the shoulder joint, in *Extensile Exposure,* ed 3. New York, NY, Churchill Livingstone, 1995, pp 29-34.

Hill J, McCann P: Prosthetic replacement for proximal humerus malunion, in Zuckerman JD, ed: *Advanced Reconstruction Shoulder.* Rosemont, IL, AAOS, 2007, pp 335-343.

Krishnan SG, Bennion PW, Reineck JR, Burkhead WZ: Hemiarthroplasty for proximal humeral fracture: Restoration of the Gothic arch. *Orthop Clin North Am* 2008;39(4):441-450, vi.

Mansat P, Guity MR, Bellumore Y, Mansat M: Shoulder arthroplasty for late sequelae of proximal humeral fractures. *J Shoulder Elbow Surg* 2004;13(3):305-312.

Norris TR, Green A, McGuigan FX: Late prosthetic shoulder arthroplasty for displaced proximal humerus fractures. *J Shoulder Elbow Surg* 1995;4(4):271-280.

Panagopoulos A, Tsoumpos P, Evangelou K, Georgiou C, Triantafillopoulos I: Late prosthetic shoulder hemiarthroplasty after failed management of complex proximal humeral fractures. *Adv Orthop* 2013;2013:403580.

Phipatanakul WP, Norris TR: Indications for prosthetic replacement in proximal humeral fractures. *Instr Course Lect* 2005;54:357-362.

Ritzman TF, Iannotti JP: Malunions of the proximal humerus, in Warner JJP, Iannotti JP, Flatow EL, eds: *Complex and Revision Problems in Shoulder Surgery.* Philadelphia, PA, Lippincott Williams & Wilkins, 2005, pp 347-364.

Siegel JA, Dines DM: Techniques in managing proximal humeral malunions. *J Shoulder Elbow Surg* 2003;12(1):69-78.

Sirveaux F, Mole D, Boileau P: The reversed prosthesis, in Warner JJP, Iannotti JP, Flatow EL, eds: *Complex and Revision Problems in Shoulder Surgery.* Philadelphia, PA, Lippincott Williams & Wilkins, 2005, pp 497-513.

Tanner MW, Cofield RH: Prosthetic arthroplasty for fractures and fracture-dislocations of the proximal humerus. *Clin Orthop Relat Res* 1983;(179):116-128.

Tillett E, Smith M, Fulcher M, Shanklin J: Anatomic determination of humeral head retroversion: The relationship of the central axis of the humeral head to the bicipital groove. *J Shoulder Elbow Surg* 1993;2(5):255-256.

Wiesel BB, Williams GR: The reverse prosthesis for failed anatomic shoulder arthroplasty, in Cofield RH, Sperling JW, eds: *Revision and Complex Shoulder Arthroplasty.* Philadelphia, PA, Lippincott Williams & Wilkins, 2010, pp 237-249.

Chapter 50

Management of Periprosthetic Fractures of the Humerus

Philipp N. Streubel, MD

Scott P. Steinmann, MD

 ## Introduction

Management of humeral shaft fractures about a shoulder arthroplasty stem is challenging. Fractures can occur intraoperatively or postoperatively. In most patients, surgical management is indicated, consisting of open reduction and internal fixation (ORIF) with or without implant revision. Surgical management is technically demanding and requires ample exposure to avoid nerve damage. Carefully planned fixation is required to ensure stability and maximize fracture healing.

 ## Case Presentation

A 62-year-old, right-hand–dominant woman reports left arm pain after a ground-level fall. Three years ago, she underwent a cemented shoulder hemiarthroplasty for a left proximal humerus fracture. Her recovery was satisfactory, and she had no pain or notable dysfunction before her recent fall. On physical examination, no neurovascular deficit is observed. Deformity and pain are noted over the proximal one-third of the arm. Radiographs demonstrate a displaced spiral fracture extending from the tip of the humeral stem proximally over 40% of the length of the proximal segment (Wright and Cofield type A). Minor lucencies are noted at the bone-cement interface proximally, but the implant is considered stable (**Figure 1, A**). Because the patient has a stable implant and no prior symptoms suggestive of rotator cuff dysfunction or glenoid pain, ORIF is selected for surgical management.

The patient received an interscalene block and was placed under general anesthesia. The fracture was exposed using an anterior brachialis-splitting approach. Humeral stem stability was confirmed intraoperatively. The fracture was reduced and stabilized with a 3.5-mm lag screw, taking care to achieve satisfactory screw purchase into the proximal cement mantle. A 10-hole, narrow, 4.5-mm locking plate was placed onto the anterior aspect of the humerus in neutralization mode. Distal fixation was obtained with five nonlocking screws, and four unicortical locking screws were placed proximally (**Figure 1, B** and **C**). Follow-up radiographs demonstrated loss of reduction at 4 weeks postoperatively with early callus formation (**Figure 1, D**). Clinically, the patient had minimal symptoms, active forward elevation to 70°, and no gross instability; therefore, the decision was made not to revise the reduction. Satisfactory healing of the fracture was observed radiographically at 9 weeks postoperatively. At 5 years postoperatively, the patient had no notable complaints, and the implant appeared radiographically stable (**Figure 1, E**).

 ## Indications

Surgical management of humeral shaft fractures about a shoulder arthroplasty stem is indicated in patients with displaced unstable fractures, patients with fractures about a loose humeral stem, and patients who are unable to tolerate nonsurgical treatment. Conversely, nonsurgical treatment is indicated in patients with stable, nondisplaced fractures and in patients in whom the risks of surgical treatment outweigh the benefits. Nonsurgical treatment is typically considered in patients with less than 20° of flexion/extension or rotation and less than 30° of angulation in the coronal plane. Surgical management options include ORIF and revision arthroplasty.

In most patients with postoperative periprosthetic fractures occurring about a stable implant, ORIF is the treatment of choice. Requirements for successful implant retention are a stable implant, lack of substantial rotator

Dr. Streubel or an immediate family member serves as a paid consultant to Acumed. Dr. Steinmann or an immediate family member has received royalties from Arthrex, Biomet, and CoorsTek Medical; serves as a paid consultant to Acumed, Arthrex, Articulinx, Biomet, and Elsevier; and serves as a board member, owner, officer, or committee member of the American Shoulder and Elbow Surgeons and the American Society for Surgery of the Hand.

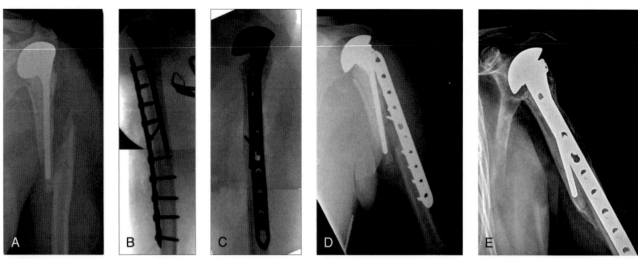

Figure 1   **A,** AP radiograph demonstrates a Wright and Cofield type A fracture about a stable shoulder hemiarthroplasty. Intraoperative axillary (**B**) and AP (**C**) fluoroscopic images demonstrate anatomic reduction and fixation with a lag screw and locking plate construct. **D,** AP radiograph demonstrates loss of reduction at 4 weeks postoperatively. Because the patient's clinical recovery was adequate, the decision was made not to revise the reduction. Satisfactory radiographic healing was observed 9 weeks postoperatively. **E,** AP radiograph demonstrates stability of the fixation 5 years postoperatively.

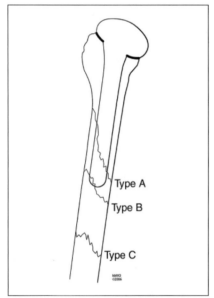

Figure 2   Illustration depicts the Wright and Cofield classification of humeral fractures after shoulder arthroplasty. Type A fractures occur at the tip of the humeral stem and extend proximally more than one-third of the length of the stem. Type B fractures are centered at the tip of the stem and extend less proximally than type A fractures. Type C fractures occur at the humeral shaft distal to the tip of the prosthesis. (Reproduced with permission from the Mayo Foundation for Medical Education and Research, Rochester, MN.)

cuff dysfunction, and absence of glenoid pain or instability. Therefore, a detailed history of shoulder symptoms and overall function before the fracture is required. Physical examination should include a detailed neurovascular examination. Assessment of rotator cuff function and glenoid pain may not be reliable in patients with periprosthetic fracture. This information may be obtained from clinical notes during routine follow-up visits and should be requested if the examination was done elsewhere. Surgical notes and information on the type of implant also should be obtained.

Radiographs consisting of two orthogonal views of the humerus and true AP, lateral scapular Y, and Velpeau axillary views of the shoulder should be obtained. An axillary view is critical to assess the glenoid surface and, if present, the glenoid implant. The position required to obtain a conventional axillary view after an acute fracture may not be well tolerated by the patient. Therefore, a Velpeau axillary view is recommended. Radiographic assessment can be used to determine the fracture location, fracture geometry, and bone quality. The Wright and Cofield system can be used

to classify postoperative periprosthetic fractures. Type A fractures occur at the tip of the humeral stem and extend proximally more than one-third of the length of the stem. Type B fractures are centered at the tip of the stem with less proximal extension. Type C fractures occur at the humeral shaft distal to the tip of the prosthesis (**Figure 2**).

Osteopenia is commonly classified according to the ratio of the combined width of the middiaphyseal cortices to the diameter of the diaphysis. Normal bone is defined as having a cortical thickness greater than 50% of the diameter of the humeral shaft. Mild osteopenia is defined as a percentage from 25% to 50%. Severe osteopenia is defined as a percentage less than 25%. Although osteopenia has been mainly studied as a risk factor for the occurrence of periprosthetic fractures, assessment of bone quality will aid in surgical planning.

Implant stability is assessed radiographically. Humeral stem loosening has been defined as the presence of a radiolucent line that is at least 2 mm wide extending along three or more of the humeral zones described by Sperling or as the presence of a change in

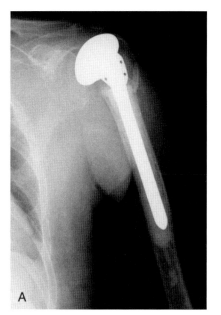 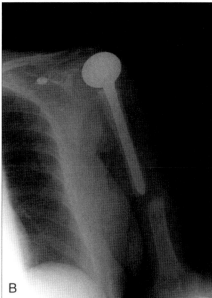 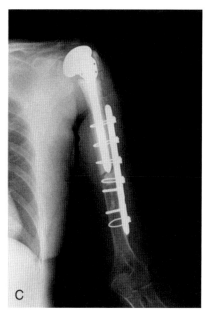

Figure 3   **A,** Preinjury AP radiograph demonstrates a cemented shoulder hemiarthroplasty. **B,** AP radiograph obtained 2 months after injury demonstrates unsuccessful nonsurgical management of a transverse humeral shaft fracture centered at the tip of the stem (Wright and Cofield type B). **C,** AP radiograph demonstrates healed fracture with a stable humeral implant 2 years after open reduction and internal fixation with plates, screws, cerclage cables, and autologous iliac crest bone graft. Note that the plate and the distal and proximal segments overlap for at least three cortical widths. Nonlocking screws and cables were used for fixation distally, whereas only cables were used proximally. (Reproduced with permission from Kumar S, Sperling JW, Haidukewych GH, Cofield RH: Periprosthetic humeral fractures after shoulder arthroplasty. *J Bone Joint Surg Am* 2004;86[4]:680-689.)

implant position as noted on subsequent radiographs. Similarly, a glenoid implant is considered to be at risk of loosening when a complete lucent line of at least 1.5 mm in width is present or when migration or tilt of the implant is observed on subsequent radiographs.

Periprosthetic fractures in the setting of an infected prosthesis pose a special treatment challenge. In patients with a stable implant, implant retention may be attempted with careful débridement and irrigation along with fracture stabilization and placement of antibiotic-impregnated cement beads. This is followed by 6 weeks of culture-specific intravenous antibiotics; frequently, the use of lifelong oral suppression antibiotics is required. However, if implant retention fails or implant loosening is noted, infected periprosthetic fractures are best managed with implant extraction, placement of an antibiotic cement spacer, and culture-specific intravenous antibiotics. After the infection

has been cleared, final treatment consists of the steps used to manage periprosthetic fracture with a loose implant.

Most patients with periprosthetic fractures are elderly and have limited functional requirements. Therefore, poor preinjury shoulder function resulting from rotator cuff pathology is rarely an indication to proceed with revision reverse shoulder arthroplasty in a patient with a stable implant. This consideration should be kept in mind during preoperative patient counseling, especially if the patient has a history of pseudoparalysis and anterosuperior escape of the humeral head.

Controversies and Alternative Approaches

Postoperative Fractures

For patients with postoperative fractures, several fixation options are

available. Locked plate fixation is considered the benchmark for the treatment of fractures in osteopenic bone. Furthermore, because of their angular stability, locking screws can provide substantial fixation, even when used unicortically. This feature is especially relevant for fixation on the proximal segment in the presence of an intramedullary implant. As in the case presented in this chapter, even the use of multiple unicortical locking screws can be insufficient to maintain fracture reduction. Alternatives to achieve stronger fixation in the presence of an intramedullary implant include the use of nonlocking and variable-angle locking screws in an attempt to bypass the humeral stem and achieve bicortical fixation. The addition of a second orthogonal plate can aid in providing further stability. Finally, cerclage wiring or cables have been used with satisfactory results with both metal plates and strut allograft (**Figures 3** and **4**). Although cerclage fixation can be obtained with

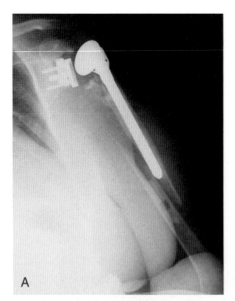
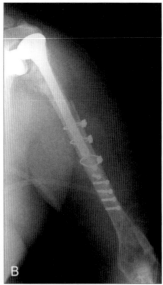
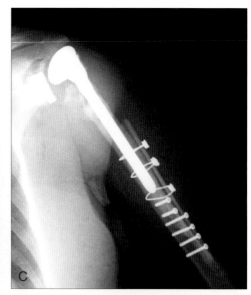

Figure 4 **A,** AP radiograph demonstrates a long, oblique Wright and Cofield type A fracture centered at the tip of the stem and extending proximally. Although the fracture extended through the distal cement mantle, the implant was stable. **B,** AP radiograph obtained after open reduction and internal fixation using lag screws, strut allograft, and cerclage cables. **C,** AP radiograph obtained 4 months postoperatively demonstrates fracture healing. (Reproduced with permission from Kumar S, Sperling JW, Haidukewych GH, Cofield RH: Periprosthetic humeral fractures after shoulder arthroplasty. *J Bone Joint Surg Am* 2004;86[4]:680-689.)

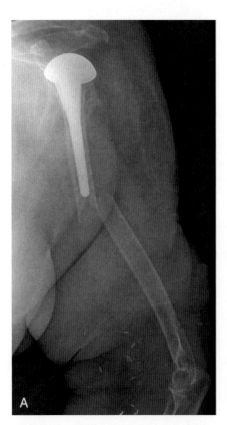
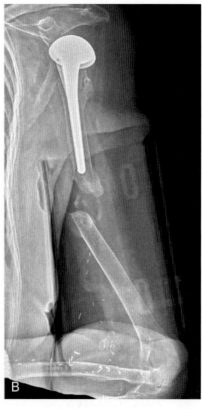

Figure 5 **A,** AP radiograph obtained in the acute period after injury demonstrates a transverse fracture at the tip of the stem (Wright and Cofield type B). Because the patient had multiple comorbidities, nonsurgical treatment was chosen. **B,** AP radiograph obtained 18 months after injury demonstrates an established nonunion.

conventional plate designs, so-called hybrid plates that allow locked screw fixation as well as cerclage fixation have been developed. In theory, using hybrid plates reduces the risk of cerclage breakage. The results of biomechanical studies suggest that periprosthetic fractures requiring surgical fixation are best stabilized with a combination of locked screws and cerclage cables proximally and locked screws distally. Locked plating alone has been shown to have a higher rate of catastrophic failure compared with cerclage fixation. In a study of femoral fracture fixation in cadaveric bone, the use of a combination of unicortical screws and cerclage cables to achieve proximal fixation resulted in a significantly higher load to failure compared with either cerclage fixation or locked screw fixation alone.

Healing rates are worse after nonsurgical management of postoperative periprosthetic humerus shaft fractures than after nonsurgical management of other humeral shaft fractures. Nonunion rates of up to 100% have been reported for periprosthetic fractures (**Figure 5**).

However, satisfactory outcomes have been reported in some series, especially for fractures distal to the tip of the humeral stem (**Figure 6**). Nonsurgical treatment should therefore be considered primarily in patients with stable, nondisplaced fractures. However, in the practice of the authors of this chapter, these fractures are managed surgically unless comorbid conditions or patient preference dictate otherwise. With the introduction of newer stemless implants, other fracture patterns may appear. Humeral surgical neck fractures adjacent to a humeral resurfacing implant may be adequately managed with immobilization and early functional rehabilitation (**Figure 7**).

Revision arthroplasty is indicated in patients with a loose humeral implant or in patients in whom prior shoulder dysfunction requires that the glenohumeral joint be addressed. This dysfunction can consist of severe rotator cuff dysfunction, glenoid erosion, glenoid implant loosening, or instability. Revision arthroplasty requires substantially more invasive surgical dissection compared with that required for ORIF.

The anterior approach is frequently required to gain access to the fracture site. In addition, a deltopectoral approach is required for access to the glenohumeral joint. It may be necessary to release the distal deltoid insertion in patients with

substantial contracture to achieve satisfactory joint exposure. Occasionally, patients with substantial subdeltoid adhesions may require an anteromedial approach to the shoulder with detachment of the anterior deltoid from the

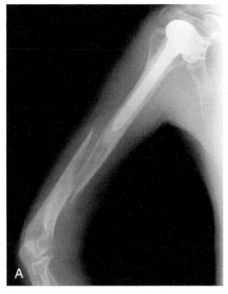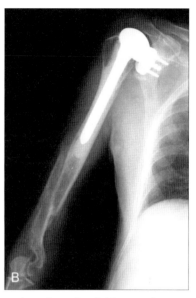

Figure 6 **A,** AP radiograph demonstrates a spiral Wright and Cofield type C fracture located distal to the tip of a stable implant. **B,** AP radiograph obtained 8 months after injury demonstrates fracture healing achieved with nonsurgical management. (Reproduced with permission from Kumar S, Sperling JW, Haidukewych GH, Cofield RH: Periprosthetic humeral fractures after shoulder arthroplasty. *J Bone Joint Surg Am* 2004;86[4]:680-689.)

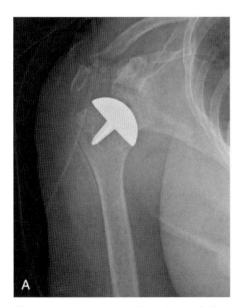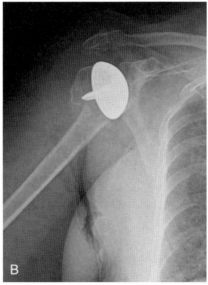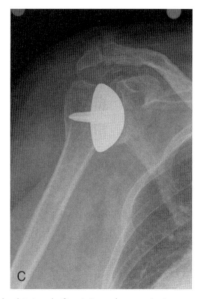

Figure 7 **A,** Preinjury AP radiograph demonstrates humeral resurfacing. **B,** AP radiograph obtained after injury demonstrates an impacted fracture of the surgical neck of the humerus. **C,** AP radiograph obtained 3 months after injury demonstrates satisfactory fracture healing with nonsurgical management (immobilization and early functional rehabilitation).

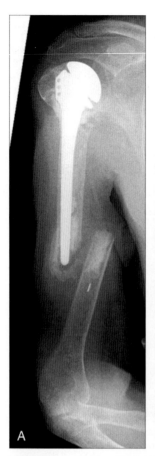
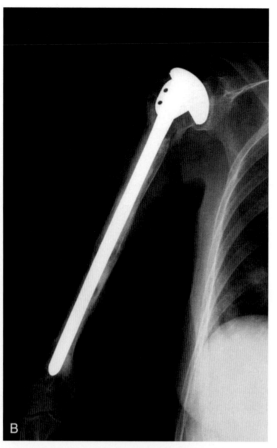

Figure 8 **A,** AP radiograph demonstrates unsuccessful nonsurgical management of a Wright and Cofield type B fracture located at the tip of a humeral stem. Radiographic concerns of implant loosening were confirmed intraoperatively. **B,** AP radiograph demonstrates revision to a long-stemmed humeral implant with cementation into both the proximal and distal humeral segments. Healing was achieved. (Reproduced with permission from Owens CJ, Sperling JW, Cofield RH: Utility and complications of long-stem humeral components in revision shoulder arthroplasty. *J Shoulder Elbow Surg* 2013;22[7]:e7-e12.)

or nonunion, a long cemented implant can be used. An intact medullary canal both distally and proximally is required to achieve satisfactory cement fixation (**Figure 8**). Care should be taken not to allow cement to extrude into the fracture site because doing so can prevent healing or cause nerve injury. Alternatively, a noncemented implant can be used. Although press-fit fixation is routinely satisfactory, distal rotational stability may be insufficient and frequently requires additional plate fixation. Rarely, periprosthetic fractures occur in patients with segmental bone loss. In these patients, standard arthroplasty implants cannot be used because of inadequate bone stock. The use of structural allograft-prosthetic composites can be helpful in these patients (**Figure 9**). Other alternatives include partial and complete humeral arthroplasty.

Intraoperative Fractures

Intraoperative fractures occur twice as frequently as postoperative fractures, as evidenced in part by data collected at the institution of the authors of this chapter over a 20-year period. The Campbell system can be used to classify intraoperative fractures into one of four regions: the tuberosities are region 1, the proximal humeral metaphysis is region 2, the proximal shaft is region 3, and the shaft distal to the humeral stem is region 4 (**Figure 10**).

Region 1 fractures almost always occur at the greater tuberosity. If any displacement is noted, the fracture is reduced and stabilized with transosseous repair using heavy nonabsorbable sutures (**Figure 11**). Stable, nondisplaced fractures can be managed with a standard implant, but it may be necessary to delay postoperative rehabilitation. Region 2 fractures may require cerclage to maintain hoop stresses during implantation of a press-fit stem. In patients with severe osteopenia, however, cerclage wiring may not provide sufficient fixation to achieve satisfactory press-fit of

acromion in an attempt to preserve the rotator cuff. Great care must be taken during extraction of the humeral implant because fracture propagation can occur.

Several revision options are available. In most patients, a long-stemmed humeral implant is indicated. Reaming of the shaft should be limited because forceful reaming may create new fractures or extend existing fracture lines. Broaching should be done carefully to avoid fracturing the proximal segment. In patients with long spiral fractures, cerclage wiring alone may provide sufficient fracture stability. Shorter fractures

or transverse fractures require stabilization with plates and/or strut allograft with screws and cerclage wires. In some patients, press fitting into the proximal humerus is not possible because of disruption of the proximal metaphyseal ring. In this setting, a long stem is cemented into the distal shaft segment. After excess cement has been removed and polymerization has concluded, the proximal humeral segment is reduced around the stem and fixed using cerclage wires or cables with or without plate and/or strut allograft augmentation. When revision arthroplasty is used in the setting of a transverse fracture

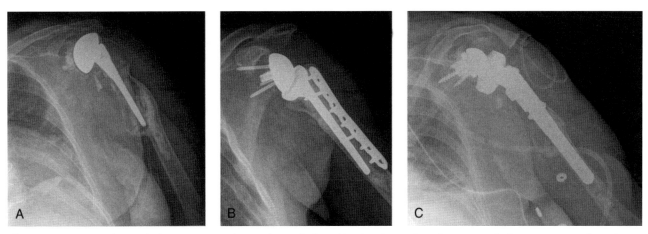

Figure 9 **A,** AP radiograph demonstrates advanced osteolysis and implant loosening after nonsurgical management of a periprosthetic fracture in a patient with a history of hemiarthroplasty for proximal humerus fracture, revision total shoulder arthroplasty, and subsequent revision to hemiarthroplasty because of glenoid bone loss. This case represents the most complex periprosthetic fracture scenario: poor bone stock at the humerus and glenoid, a loose implant, and an insufficient rotator cuff. Revision arthroplasty requires the use of either an allograft-prosthetic composite (**B**) or a tumor prosthesis (**C**), demonstrated in AP radiographs. Although reverse arthroplasty with an allograft-prosthetic composite has been approved by the FDA, reverse arthroplasty with a tumor prosthesis is considered off label. Panels A and C are of the same patient.

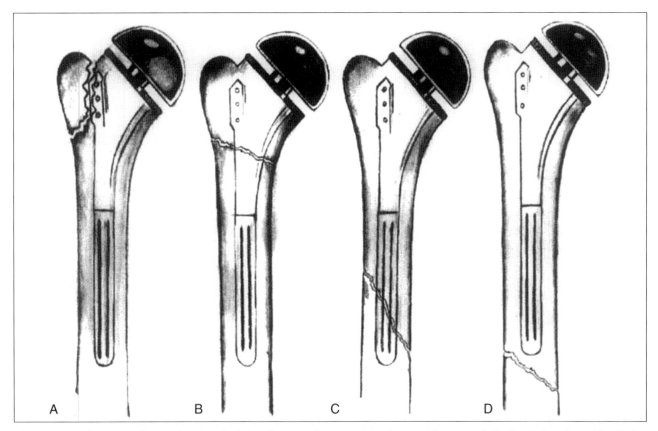

Figure 10 Illustration depicts the Campbell classification of periprosthetic humeral fractures. **A,** Region 1, the tuberosities. **B,** Region 2, the proximal humeral metaphysis. **C,** Region 3, the proximal shaft. **D,** Region 4, the shaft distal to the humeral stem. (Reproduced with permission from Campbell JT, Moore RS, Iannotti JP, Norris TR, Williams GR: Periprosthetic humeral fractures: Mechanisms of fracture and treatment options. *J Shoulder Elbow Surg* 1998;7[4]:406-413.)

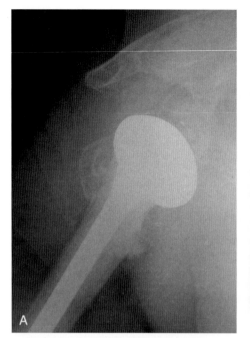
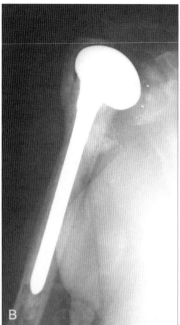

Figure 11   **A,** AP radiograph demonstrates an intraoperative greater tuberosity fracture that was managed with suture fixation and that displaced postoperatively. **B,** AP radiograph obtained 7 years postoperatively demonstrates healing of the fracture in an acceptable position and radiographic stability. (Reproduced with permission from Athwal GS, Sperling JW, Rispoli DM, Cofield RH: Periprosthetic humeral fractures during shoulder arthroplasty. *J Bone Joint Surg Am* 2009;91[3]:594-603.)

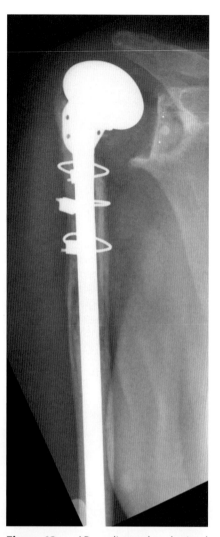

Figure 12   AP radiograph obtained 2 years postoperatively demonstrates successful management of an intraoperative periprosthetic greater tuberosity and humeral shaft fracture. The greater tuberosity was stabilized using suture fixation. The shaft was stabilized with the use of cerclage cables around a long-stemmed humeral implant. (Reproduced with permission from Athwal GS, Sperling JW, Rispoli DM, Cofield RH: Periprosthetic humeralfracturesduringshoulderarthroplasty. *J Bone Joint Surg Am* 2009;91[3]:594-603.)

a noncemented implant, and reduction and temporary stabilization followed by implantation of a cemented stem may be preferable. In general, an implant of standard length is appropriate in these patients. Fractures in regions 3 and 4 are managed in a manner similar to that of postoperative fractures. In most patients, revision to a long-stemmed implant with augmentation consisting of a plate and/or strut allograft in addition to the use of screws and cerclage is recommended (**Figure 12**). However, if the fracture is diagnosed after stem cementation, stabilization without stem revision may be performed to avoid the potential complications of cement removal.

the low frequency of these fractures. In general, the use of ORIF to manage postoperative fractures with stable implants results in failure rates ranging from zero to 17%, whereas nonsurgical management results in failure in as many as 86% of patients. The rate of infection after surgical management of periprosthetic humerus fractures is 5%. Such failures are often addressed with resection arthroplasty. Published results on the management of periprosthetic humerus fractures occurring after or during shoulder arthroplasty are summarized in **Tables 1** and **2**, respectively.

Results

The literature is composed of retrospective case series with a relatively small number of patients, underscoring

Technical Keys to Success

Setup/Exposure

- In most patients with periprosthetic fractures treated with ORIF, the

anterior approach to the humerus is used.

- Occasionally, in patients with very distal fractures, extensile anterolateral or posterior approaches may be indicated.

Table 1 Results of Management of Postoperative Periprosthetic Humerus Fractures

Authors	Journal (Year)	Technique (No. of Patients)	Outcomes	Failure Rate (%)	Comments
Boyd et al	*J Bone Joint Surg Am* (1992)	Nonsurgical (7)	1 fracture healed 2 patients had radial nerve palsy 4 patients had nonunion 5 patients required surgical treatment (2 ORIF, 3 long-stemmed revision)	86	Mean patient age, 66 yr (range, 45-78 yr) Follow-up ranged from 1.5 to 192 mo Time from arthroplasty to fracture ranged from 1.5 to 87 mo
Wright and Cofield	*J Bone Joint Surg Am* (1995)	Nonsurgical (8), ORIF (1)	In the nonsurgical group, 4 healed, 1 unacceptable alignment was managed with ORIF, and 3 non-unions were managed with ORIF (1) or revision surgery (2) The 1 surgically treated patient healed	Surgical, 0 Nonsurgical, 50	Mean patient age, 70 yr (range, 45-85 yr) Mean follow-up, 47 mo (range, 4-196 mo) Mean time from arthroplasty to fracture, 39 mo (range, 8-101 mo) All humeral stems were stable 6 fractures along stem 3 fractures distal to stem tip
Campbell et al	*J Shoulder Elbow Surg* (1998)	Nonsurgical (5)	All healed 1 patient had frozen shoulder 1 patient had skin slough	0	Mean patient age, 60 yr (range, 40-80 yr)[a] Mean follow-up, 27 mo (range, 12-72 mo)[a] Mean time from arthroplasty to fracture, 25 mo (range, 2–55 mo) All humeral stems were stable 1 fracture along stem 4 fractures distal to stem tip
Worland et al	*J Shoulder Elbow Surg* (1999)	ORIF and cerclage (1), revision with long cemented stem (4), nonsurgical (1)	All healed	0	Mean patient age, 78 yr (range, 67-94 yr) Mean follow-up, 23 mo (range, 5-62 mo) Mean time from arthroplasty to fracture, 43 mo (range, 13-85 mo) 2 humeral stems were loose 5 fractures along stem 2 fractures distal to stem tip

NA = not available, ORIF = open reduction and internal fixation.

[a] Values are for the entire study population (intraoperative and postoperative fractures).

- If revision of the implants is indicated, a glenohumeral approach is required and, in most instances, is combined with an anterior approach to the humerus (**Figure 13**).

Instruments/Equipment/Implants Required

- Surgical management of periprosthetic fractures of the humerus is technically demanding and requires a large array of tools and implants.

- Implants for both fracture fixation and revision arthroplasty, including locking plates, cerclage wires or cables, long humeral stems, and glenoid implants, should be available.

- If the fracture is around a cemented

Table 1 Results of Management of Postoperative Periprosthetic Humerus Fractures (*continued*)

Authors	Journal (Year)	Technique (No. of Patients)	Outcomes	Failure Rate (%)	Comments
Kumar et al	*J Bone Joint Surg Am* (2004)	Nonsurgical (11), ORIF (2), revision with long cemented stem (2), tumor prosthesis (1)	In the nonsurgical group, 6 healed; the 5 failures were managed with ORIF and bone graft (3) or long-stem revision (2) In the surgical group, all healed Overall, results were excellent in 3 patients, satisfactory in 4, and unsatisfactory in 9	Nonsurgical, 45 Surgical, 0	Mean patient age, 63 yr (range, 37-76 yr) Mean follow-up, 67 mo (range, 4-191 mo) Mean time from arthroplasty to fracture, 49 mo (range, 1-146 mo) 3 humeral stems were loose 12 fractures along stem 1 fracture was in the proximal metaphysis 3 fractures distal to stem tip
Groh et al	*J Shoulder Elbow Surg* (2008)	Nonsurgical (4), ORIF (3)	All healed	0	Mean patient age, 58 yr (range, 40-70 yr)[a] Mean follow-up, 25 mo (range, 6-49 mo)[a] All humeral stems were stable 6 fractures along stem 1 fracture distal to stem tip
Wutzler et al	*Arch Orthop Trauma Surg* (2009)	ORIF (6)	5 healed 1 patient had early failure and underwent eventual revision arthroplasty	17	Mean patient age, 76 yr (range, 51-83 yr) Mean follow-up, 16 mo (range, 7-39 mo) Mean time from arthroplasty to fracture, 38 mo (range, 3-180 mo) All humeral stems were stable 2 fractures along stem 3 fractures distal to stem tip 1 combined fracture was seen
Greiner et al	*Acta Chir Orthop Traumatol Cech* (2011)	ORIF (1), reverse arthroplasty with long cemented stem (3), long cemented stem cuff tear arthropathy head hemi-arthroplasty with strut graft (1)	No complications	0	Mean patient age, 69 yr (range, 51-82 yr) Mean follow-up, NA 1 humeral stem was stable 4 humeral stems were loose 4 fractures along stem 1 fracture distal to stem tip 4 acute fractures 1 nonunion after prior surgical fixation

NA = not available, ORIF = open reduction and internal fixation.

[a] Values are for the entire study population (intraoperative and postoperative fractures).

Table 1 Results of Management of Postoperative Periprosthetic Humerus Fractures (*continued*)

Authors	Journal (Year)	Technique (No. of Patients)	Outcomes	Failure Rate (%)	Comments
Martinez et al	*J Orthop Surg (Hong Kong)* (2011)	ORIF (6)	All healed	0	Mean patient age, 73 yr (range, 69-79 yr) Mean follow-up, 14 mo (range, 12-16 mo) Mean time from arthroplasty to fracture, 17 mo (range, 11-21 mo) All humeral stems were stable All fractures distal to stem tip
Sewell et al	*J Bone Joint Surg Br* (2012)	Revision arthroplasty: long stem (12), endoprosthetic replacement (8), clamshell (2)	2 patients required revision for instability 1 patient required surgical reduction for implant dissociation 1 patient required ORIF for nonunion 1 patient required screw removal 1 patient had aseptic loosening with subsequent infection requiring resection arthroplasty	10	Mean patient age, 75 yr (range, 61-90 yr) Mean follow-up, 42 mo (range, 12-91 mo) Mean time from arthroplasty to fracture, 10 mo (range, 2-56 mo) All patients had bone loss and/or an unstable implant 17 fractures along stem 5 fractures distal to stem tip
Andersen et al	*J Bone Joint Surg Am* (2013)	17 ORIF, 19 revision arthroplasty (14 long stem, 5 short stem with ORIF)	In the ORIF group, 2 patients had early failure requiring revision fixation, 1 patient had radial nerve palsy; all healed In the revision arthroplasty group, 1 patient had nonunion after multiple repeat ORIF procedures, 1 patient had implant dissociation, and 1 patient had infection requiring resection arthroplasty	ORIF, 12 Revision, 16	Minimum follow-up was 6 mo for ORIF and 2 yr for revision arthroplasty 17 humeral stems were stable 19 humeral stems were loose Allograft was used in 8 patients undergoing ORIF and in 17 patients undergoing revision arthroplasty (6 with allograft-prosthesis composite)
Mineo et al	*Injury* (2013)	ORIF (7)	All healed	0	Mean patient age, 72 yr (range, 68-75 yr) Mean follow-up, 5 mo (range, 4-6 mo) Mean time from arthroplasty to fracture, 15 mo (range, 8-21 mo) All humeral stems were stable All fractures distal to stem tip

NA = not available, ORIF = open reduction and internal fixation.

[a] Values are for the entire study population (intraoperative and postoperative fractures).

Table 2 Results of Management of Intraoperative Periprosthetic Humerus Fractures

Authors	Journal (Year)	Technique (No. of Patients)	Outcomes	Failure Rate (%)	Comments
Campbell et al	*J Shoulder Elbow Surg* (1998)	Standard length stem arthroplasty with or without internal fixation (8), long-stem arthroplasty with cerclage (8)	4 patients had transient nerve injuries (1 axillary, 3 radial) 1 patient had loss of reduction 1 patient had delayed union 1 patient had hardware failure with nonunion	13	Mean patient age, 60 yr (range, 40-80 yr)[a] Mean follow-up, 27 mo (range, 12-72 mo)[a]
Groh et al	*J Shoulder Elbow Surg* (2008)	Nonsurgical (1), cerclage (2), long-stem revision with or without cerclage (5)	All healed	0	Mean patient age, 58 yr (range, 40-70 yr)[a] Mean follow-up, 25 mo (range, 6-49 mo)[a]
Athwal et al	*J Bone Joint Surg Am* (2009)	Greater tuberosity fractures: suture fixation (11), nonsurgical management (8) Humeral shaft fractures: long-stem revision (9), nonsurgical management (5), ORIF (2) Metaphyseal fractures: bone graft (3), cerclage (2), pin and cemented stem (1) Greater tuberosity fractures extending into shaft: long-stem revision and suture fixation or cerclage (2), bone graft and suture fixation (1) Greater and lesser tuberosity fracture: cerclage (1)	6 patients had transient nerve injuries (3 brachial plexus, 2 radial nerve, 1 ulnar nerve) 2 patients had greater tuberosity displacement 2 patients required revision (1 for instability, 1 for glenoid wear)	9	Mean follow-up, 91 mo (range, 25-192 mo)[a]

ORIF = open reduction and internal fixation.

[a] Values are for entire study population (intraoperative and postoperative fractures).

stem, tools for cement removal should be available.

- A high-speed burr and osteotomes may be useful for the creation of bone windows to remove implants.
- Bone grafting materials should be available for use as structural struts and for cancellous augmentation.
- A C-arm should be readily available for intraoperative visualization of fractures. The C-arm also helps in the advancement of cement extraction tools into the distal humeral shaft and confirmation of adequate fracture reduction and implant placement.

Procedure

- A detailed description of the surgical approaches to the glenohumeral joint and humeral shaft is beyond the scope of this chapter. Thus, the main steps common to most approaches are described here, with steps applicable to specific approaches mentioned as required.
- The radial and axillary nerves must be identified during exposure to avoid inadvertent nerve damage during placement of a cerclage wire.
- When the anterior approach is used, the radial nerve is identified between the brachialis and brachioradialis muscles. This nerve can

be traced proximally to the level at which it pierces the lateral intermuscular septum.

- When the posterior approach is used, the radial nerve is best located by first identifying the lateral brachial cutaneous nerve. The brachial cutaneous nerve can be traced proximally to identify the radial nerve as it travels from the spiral groove into the lateral intermuscular septum.
- The axillary nerve is mainly at risk in the vicinity of the proximal humeral calcar. Palpation of the axillary nerve on the underside of the deltoid laterally and on the

inferior aspect of the subscapularis medially can help in locating this nerve. After the nerve enters the quadrilateral space, it is typically safe provided that wires or cables are placed directly on bone and distal to the anatomic neck of the humerus. In general, cerclage wires at the shaft should be placed from lateral to medial to protect the radial nerve. Passage of wires around the proximal humeral metaphysis should proceed from medial to lateral to protect the axillary nerve (**Figure 14**).

- When creating a bone window for implant extraction, a high-speed pencil-tip burr may be used to create a single anterior split along the proximal humeral shaft to allow gentle prying of the proximal metaphysis using two wide osteotomes. The goal of this approach is to achieve loosening of the bone-cement or bone-implant interface. Alternatively, a window may be created into the anterior cortex of the humerus. A rectangular segment 15 to 20 mm wide is delineated with the aforementioned burr. The length of the humeral stem dictates the length of the window (**Figure 14**).

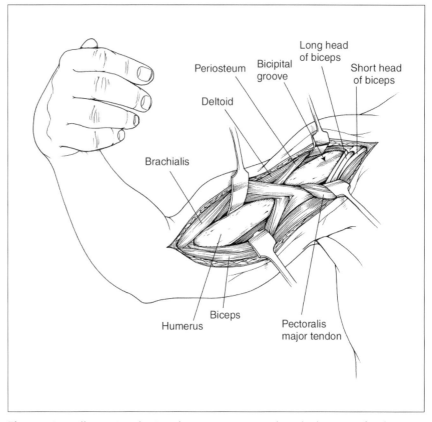

Figure 13 Illustration depicts the anterior approach to the humerus for the management of periprosthetic fracture. Proximally, the humerus is exposed through the deltopectoral interval. Distally, the biceps is retracted medially. The brachialis is split longitudinally. This technique preserves the radial innervation of the lateral segment and the musculocutaneous innervation of the medial segment of this muscle. The radial nerve is identified between the brachialis and brachioradialis muscles. (Reproduced from Steinmann SP, Cheung EV: Treatment of periprosthetic humerus fractures associated with shoulder arthroplasty. *J Am Acad Orthop Surg* 2008;16[4]:199-207.)

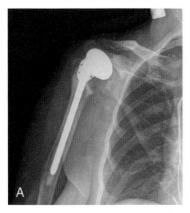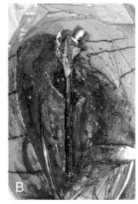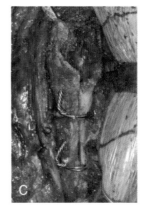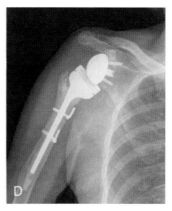

Figure 14 **A,** Preoperative AP radiograph from a patient with prior shoulder arthroplasty and severe rotator cuff dysfunction. **B,** Intraoperative photograph shows creation of an anterior bony window in a controlled manner to allow for extraction of a well-cemented implant. **C,** Intraoperative photograph demonstrates the use of a looped cerclage wire (Luque wire) to stabilize the corticotomy. Note that the wires are placed well distal to the humeral calcar. **D,** AP radiograph obtained 3 years postoperatively demonstrates adequate healing.

Table 3 Rehabilitation Protocol After Management of Periprosthetic Fracture of the Humerus

Postoperative Week	Range of Motion	Strengthening	Return to Play	Comments/Emphasis
0-6	Passive	None	Not applicable	90° forward elevation, rotation to neutral
6-12	Active assisted	None	Not applicable	Pulley and wand, unrestricted motion
12-24	Unrestricted	If required	Not applicable	—

- Because many patients with periprosthetic fractures have severe osteopenia, fracture stability should be maximized with carefully planned fixation. Locking plate constructs along with screws and cerclage wires are recommended.
- However, in patients with severe osteopenia, cerclage wires may cut through bone, leading to loss of fixation. In these patients, bone augmentation with cortical allograft struts can provide reliable stability while providing bone stock for healing.
- If structural allograft is unavailable, an additional small one-third tubular plate can be employed medially to support the cortex and prevent the cerclage wires from cutting through bone.
- To improve the healing potential of periprosthetic fractures, augmentation with morcellized cancellous autograft or allograft may be considered in any patient undergoing fracture fixation.
- For both extramedullary and intramedullary implants, the implant should be of sufficient length to allow fixation over a distance measuring three times the width of the fracture at its most distal point. If the fracture extends too distally to obtain diaphyseal fixation of at least three cortical widths in length, dual plate fixation into the lateral and medial column of the distal humerus should be performed for stabilization.

Wound Closure

- After thorough irrigation of the wound and careful confirmation of hemostasis, a drain is routinely placed deep to the muscular plane.
- The deltopectoral interval is loosely closed with interrupted absorbable sutures.
- Skin closure is achieved with subcuticular absorbable sutures and a running intradermal absorbable monofilament suture.
- The wound is covered with a layer of nonadherent dressing followed by gauze and a waterproof adhesive film.
- The surgical extremity is immobilized in a sling.
- Immediate postoperative AP and lateral radiographs of the humerus are obtained.
- The drain is removed after less than 50 mL of draining is observed over a 12-hour period.
- For pain control, patients routinely undergo preoperative interscalene block, which is followed by scheduled intravenous narcotic analgesics that are transitioned to oral medication on the first postoperative day.

 ## Rehabilitation

Rehabilitation is summarized in **Table 3**. In general, the rehabilitation protocol for fracture fixation is similar to that of revision arthroplasty. If satisfactory fracture stability has been achieved, passive range of motion of the shoulder

may be started on postoperative day 1. Range of motion is allowed to 90° of forward elevation and neutral rotation to avoid excess torque on the humeral shaft. Active-assisted range of motion is started at 6 weeks postoperatively, and strengthening is begun at 3 months postoperatively. However, because of the poor bone stock frequently found in patients with periprosthetic fractures, range-of-motion exercises are commonly delayed until the 6th postoperative week until early fracture healing has occurred.

Avoiding Pitfalls

Prevention is the best treatment for periprosthetic fractures. Risk factors for such fractures include osteopenia, rheumatoid arthritis, female sex, revision surgery, use of a press-fit humeral implant, posttraumatic arthritis, proximal humeral deformity, soft-tissue contractures, canal overreaming, placement of an oversized broach, and aggressive manipulation. Although the patient-related risk factors typically cannot be modified, multiple factors related to surgical technique should be taken into account.

Preoperative planning requires a detailed understanding of preinjury shoulder function, implant stability, and fracture geometry. Patient comorbidities and expectations play a key role in therapeutic decision making.

Fractures can be avoided with adequate capsular and soft-tissue releases to reduce the need for forceful manipulation of the extremity during shoulder arthroplasty. Furthermore, limited reaming and broaching should be performed, especially in high-risk patients. The authors of this chapter generally prefer to use hand reamers as sounds and rotate the instrument gently back and forth rather than performing forceful rotation aimed at obtaining cortical chatter.

Successful management of periprosthetic fractures requires ample exposure to allow for accurate fracture reduction, fixation, and, if necessary, implant revision. If cerclage fixation will be performed, the radial nerve should be clearly identified, and the location of the axillary nerve must be known.

Bibliography

Andersen JR, Williams CD, Cain R, Mighell M, Frankle M: Surgically treated humeral shaft fractures following shoulder arthroplasty. *J Bone Joint Surg Am* 2013;95(1):9-18.

Athwal GS, Sperling JW, Rispoli DM, Cofield RH: Periprosthetic humeral fractures during shoulder arthroplasty. *J Bone Joint Surg Am* 2009;91(3):594-603.

Boyd AD Jr, Thornhill TS, Barnes CL: Fractures adjacent to humeral prostheses. *J Bone Joint Surg Am* 1992;74(10):1498-1504.

Cameron B, Iannotti JP: Periprosthetic fractures of the humerus and scapula: Management and prevention. *Orthop Clin North Am* 1999;30(2):305-318.

Campbell JT, Moore RS, Iannotti JP, Norris TR, Williams GR: Periprosthetic humeral fractures: Mechanisms of fracture and treatment options. *J Shoulder Elbow Surg* 1998;7(4):406-413.

Chin PY, Sperling JW, Cofield RH, Schleck C: Complications of total shoulder arthroplasty: Are they fewer or different? *J Shoulder Elbow Surg* 2006;15(1):19-22.

Demos HA, Briones MS, White PH, Hogan KA, Barfield WR: A biomechanical comparison of periprosthetic femoral fracture fixation in normal and osteoporotic cadaveric bone. *J Arthroplasty* 2012;27(5):783-788.

Fulkerson E, Koval K, Preston CF, Iesaka K, Kummer FJ, Egol KA: Fixation of periprosthetic femoral shaft fractures associated with cemented femoral stems: A biomechanical comparison of locked plating and conventional cable plates. *J Orthop Trauma* 2006;20(2):89-93.

Gerwin M, Hotchkiss RN, Weiland AJ: Alternative operative exposures of the posterior aspect of the humeral diaphysis with reference to the radial nerve. *J Bone Joint Surg Am* 1996;78(11):1690-1695.

Gill DR, Cofield RH, Rowland C: The anteromedial approach for shoulder arthroplasty: The importance of the anterior deltoid. *J Shoulder Elbow Surg* 2004;13(5):532-537.

Greiner S, Stein V, Scheibel M: Periprosthetic humeral fractures after shoulder and elbow arthroplasty. *Acta Chir Orthop Traumatol Cech* 2011;78(6):490-500.

Groh GI, Heckman MM, Wirth MA, Curtis RJ, Rockwood CA Jr: Treatment of fractures adjacent to humeral prostheses. *J Shoulder Elbow Surg* 2008;17(1):85-89.

Kumar S, Sperling JW, Haidukewych GH, Cofield RH: Periprosthetic humeral fractures after shoulder arthroplasty. *J Bone Joint Surg Am* 2004;86(4):680-689.

Martinez AA, Calvo A, Cuenca J, Herrera A: Internal fixation and strut allograft augmentation for periprosthetic humeral fractures. *J Orthop Surg (Hong Kong)* 2011;19(2):191-193.

Mineo GV, Accetta R, Franceschini M, Pedrotti Dell'Acqua G, Calori GM, Meersseman A: Management of shoulder periprosthetic fractures: Our institutional experience and review of the literature. *Injury* 2013;44(suppl 1):S82-S85.

Sewell MD, Kang SN, Al-Hadithy N, et al: Management of peri-prosthetic fracture of the humerus with severe bone loss and loosening of the humeral component after total shoulder replacement. *J Bone Joint Surg Br* 2012;94(10):1382-1389.

Sperling JW, Cofield RH, O'Driscoll SW, Torchia ME, Rowland CM: Radiographic assessment of ingrowth total shoulder arthroplasty. *J Shoulder Elbow Surg* 2000;9(6):507-513.

Worland RL, Kim DY, Arredondo J: Periprosthetic humeral fractures: Management and classification. *J Shoulder Elbow Surg* 1999;8(6):590-594.

Wright TW, Cofield RH: Humeral fractures after shoulder arthroplasty. *J Bone Joint Surg Am* 1995;77(9):1340-1346.

Wutzler S, Laurer HL, Huhnstock S, Geiger EV, Buehren V, Marzi I: Periprosthetic humeral fractures after shoulder arthroplasty: Operative management and functional outcome. *Arch Orthop Trauma Surg* 2009;129(2):237-243.

Chapter 51

Midshaft Clavicular Fractures: Open Reduction and Internal Fixation

Matthew Furey, MD, MSc, FRCSC

Michael McKee, MD, FRCSC

 Introduction

Until recently, midshaft clavicular fractures were almost always managed non-surgically. This treatment was largely the result of a presumed high rate of union based on early published studies; large cohort studies published in the 1960s demonstrated nonunion rates of less than 1% with nonsurgical management and 3% to 5% with surgical management. Nonunion is defined variably in the literature as a lack of radiographic healing at the fracture site 6 months or 1 year postoperatively. Literature published since the mid 1990s has indicated that few patients with fractures of the clavicular midshaft require surgical treatment.

Review of literature published since the late 1990s, which includes patient-based outcomes that were previously unreported or unmeasured, has led to the recognition of increased residual dysfunction after nonsurgical management of midshaft clavicular fractures. Initially, the authors of a 1997 study reported unsatisfactory results in 31% of patients with displaced midshaft

clavicular fractures that were managed nonsurgically. This finding was highly correlated with fracture shortening of greater than or equal to 2 cm. A review of patients with malunion after nonsurgical treatment of displaced midshaft clavicular fractures demonstrated that, along with increased Disabilities of the Arm, Shoulder and Hand scores, statistically significant deficits in shoulder girdle strength and endurance were present. In another study, displacement of more than one bone width, comminution, and advanced age were shown to be predictors of persistent symptoms and sequelae including nonunion and malunion. A systematic review of more than 1,145 fractures managed nonsurgically found an overall nonunion rate of 6%; displaced fractures had a nonunion rate of 15%. In comparison, plating was associated with nonunion rates of 2.5% across all fractures and 2.2% for displaced fractures. High-quality randomized controlled trials (RCTs) published since 2007 have demonstrated improved functional outcomes and lower rates of malunion and nonunion with primary fixation compared with

nonsurgical management of displaced midshaft clavicular fractures.

 Case Presentation

A 24-year-old right-hand–dominant man who works as a laborer presents 1 week after a cycling accident. He is otherwise healthy with no significant medical history. The patient sustained a direct impact to the left shoulder as a result of the fall. The patient was initially seen in the emergency department and the diagnosis was an isolated left clavicular fracture. The arm was placed in a sling and the patient referred to the authors' practice for definitive management of the injury.

Clinically, the patient's arm is neurovascularly intact. The skin is bruised but intact over the fracture site. Motion is painful. The patient demonstrates obvious asymmetry of the shoulders, with the affected left shoulder positioned anteroinferomedial compared with the unaffected right shoulder (**Figure 1**).

Radiographs demonstrate substantial shortening of the clavicle measuring at 2.5 cm along with greater than 100% superior displacement of the proximal clavicle (**Figure 2, A**). No substantial comminution or angulation is present. The patient was treated surgically with a precontoured plate, with three screws placed proximally and three screws

Dr. McKee or an immediate family member has received royalties from Stryker; serves as a paid consultant to Acumed, Synthes, and Zimmer; has received research or institutional support from Wright Medical Technology and Zimmer; and serves as a board member, owner, officer, or committee member of the American Shoulder and Elbow Surgeons, the Canadian Orthopaedic Association, and the Orthopaedic Trauma Association. Neither Dr. Furey nor any immediate family member has received anything of value from or has stock or stock options held in a commercial company or institution related directly or indirectly to the subject of this chapter.

placed distally to the fracture site (**Figure 2, B**). The patient had an uneventful postoperative course and returned to modified work duties within 2 weeks after fixation. Work modifications included avoidance of pushing, pulling, or lifting greater than 5 lb with his left arm. The patient was able to resume full work duties 3 months postoperatively.

Indications

The current literature supports surgical fixation of displaced midshaft clavicular fractures, with displacement defined as greater than or equal to 2 cm of shortening, displacement in a caudal/cephalad plane of equal to or greater than one bone width, and/or substantial comminution. Other variables dictating acute surgical fixation include open fractures and fractures with underlying neurovascular injury. Relative indications include polytrauma and floating shoulder injuries. Scapular winging is an emerging indication for acute clavicular fixation.

Contraindications

Contraindications to surgical fixation of clavicular fractures include active infection, medical unfitness, the presence of substance abuse disorders, the risk for recurrent falls, and patient inability or unwillingness to comply with postoperative instructions. These risk factors are believed to be associated with increased risk of infection, refracture, and hardware compromise. Relative contraindications include minimally displaced or nondisplaced fractures.

Controversies and Alternative Approaches

Intramedullary Nailing Versus Plating

A resurgence in intramedullary fixation has occurred since 2003. The latest iteration of this technique, titanium elastic nailing, was first described for the clavicle in 2003. In an RCT, intramedullary nailing was found to be superior to nonsurgical management of displaced fractures. Results after intramedullary nailing of displaced fractures were similar to results after plating. In a recent prospective cohort study comparing flexible intramedullary nail fixation with plating, long-term outcomes were found to be similar, with lower rates of complications, including infection and revision surgery, in patients treated with intramedullary nailing. RCTs directly comparing plating with intramedullary nailing are needed.

Anterior Versus Superior Plating

Ideal positioning of the clavicular plate is controversial, with some authors promoting the use of anterior plating because of their belief that it is less likely than superior plating to cause neurovascular injury. However, no in vivo data are available to support this idea. In fact, in a cadaver study, no significant difference in distance from screws to neurovascular structures was found between anterior plating and superior plating.

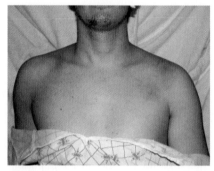

Figure 1 Preoperative clinical photograph demonstrates shoulder asymmetry in a patient with a displaced left midshaft clavicular fracture. The shoulder is displaced anteriorly, medially, and inferiorly compared with the unaffected, contralateral side.

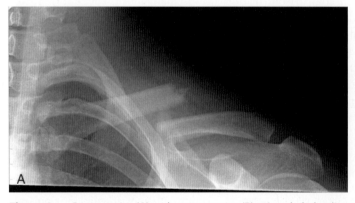
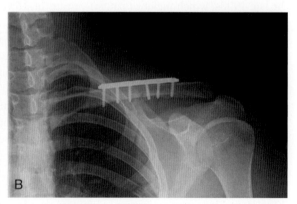

Figure 2 Preoperative (**A**) and postoperative (**B**) 15° cephalad radiographs of the left clavicle. **A,** Substantial shortening measuring approximately 2.5 cm and greater than 100% inferior displacement of the distal fragment are evident. **B,** Anatomic reduction was achieved with a precontoured compression plate applied to the midshaft clavicle with three screws placed proximal and three screws placed distal to the fracture site. Length was restored, and rotational deformity of the clavicle was corrected.

Table 1 Results of Randomized Controlled Trials Comparing Nonsurgical Management With Surgical Plating of Midshaft Clavicular Fractures

Authors	Journal (Year)	Outcomes[a]	Failure Rate[b]	Comments
Canadian Orthopaedic Trauma Society	J Bone Joint Surg Am (2007)	Plating, 5.2 Nonsurgical treatment, 13	3% after plating 14% after nonsurgical treatment	62 patients treated with precontoured plates and 49 patients treated nonsurgically
Virtanen et al	J Bone Joint Surg Am (2012)	Plating, 4.3 Nonsurgical treatment, 7.1	None after plating 24% after nonsurgical treatment	26 patients treated with reconstruction plates and 25 patients treated nonsurgically
Robinson et al	J Bone Joint Surg Am (2013)	Plating, 3.4 Nonsurgical treatment, 6.1	1% after plating 17% after nonsurgical treatment	92 patients treated with plating and 86 patients treated nonsurgically. Patients treated surgically were significantly more satisfied with the cosmetic appearance ($P < 0.0001$)

[a] Average Disabilities of the Arm, Shoulder and Hand score at 1-year follow-up.

[b] Failure is defined as nonunion.

Additionally, superior plating was found to be biomechanically superior to anterior plating in both load to failure and bending failure stiffness. Reconstruction plates were found to be biomechanically inferior to precontoured plates.

Another potential described benefit of anterior plating is decreased hardware irritation with lower hardware removal rates. Most studies have reported no association between secondary surgery and plate position.

Results

The move toward surgical fixation for displaced midshaft clavicular fractures was initiated by reports of poor patient-rated results, objectively measured clinical weakness of the shoulder, and substantially higher rates of symptomatic nonunion and malunion than were reported in previously published studies of nonsurgical treatment for displaced midshaft clavicular fractures.

The results of several RCTs comparing surgical and nonsurgical management of midshaft clavicular fractures are reported in **Table 1**. The data from these studies have been assimilated in several systematic reviews and meta-analyses.

Surgical treatment produces a relative reduction of risk for nonunion of 93% (number needed to treat, 4.6). In addition, statistically significant improvements in strength, increased range of motion (ROM), decreased chronic pain, improved cosmesis, and improved overall satisfaction with outcome have been shown in surgically treated patients.

Technical Keys to Success

Patient Positioning/Setup

- Before the skin is incised, a World Health Organization surgical time-out is performed to confirm correct patient and surgical side, with appropriate imaging prominently displayed in the operating room.
- Preoperative antibiotics are administered no more than 30 minutes before the incision is made.
- General anesthesia is administered, and the patient is placed in the beach-chair position. The involved arm may be either draped free or tucked into the side. The authors of this chapter prefer to have the arm tucked into the side.
- The patient's head is supported on a

gel head positioner or headrest with head rotation and slight tilt toward the nonsurgical side to allow unobstructed instrumentation of the clavicle. The head is then taped into position with tape placed across the forehead.

- Commercially available head restraints may be used but usually are not necessary.
- The surgical site is prepared and draped in a standard fashion (**Figure 3, A**).

Exposure

- The incision is centered anterosuperiorly over the fracture site and extended medially and laterally along the course of the clavicle. Skin and subcutaneous tissue are raised as a contiguous layer. The myofascial layer is raised as a separate flap after sharp dissection down to the clavicle is performed (**Figure 3, B**). As the surgeon gains experience with the technique, he or she may be able to dramatically reduce the length of the incision by exploiting the highly mobile skin and subcutaneous tissue of the region. The authors of this chapter use the same incision in all patients unless skin changes

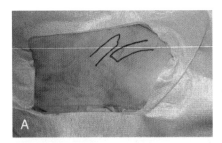
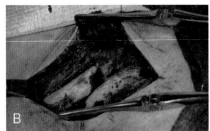
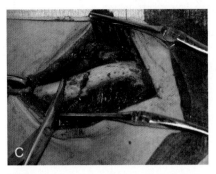
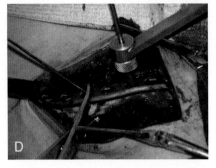
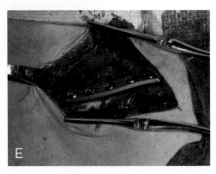

Figure 3   Intraoperative clinical photographs show open reduction and internal fixation of a midshaft clavicular fracture. **A,** Draping of the surgical site extends from the sternoclavicular region to the acromioclavicular region. The locations of the proximal and distal fragments are drawn on the skin for demonstration purposes. **B,** Exposure of the fracture was achieved after a subcutaneous layer was raised and sharp dissection was performed through the myofascial layer to bone. Fracture ends have been cleared of hematoma, taking care to minimize disruption of soft-tissue attachments including the pectoralis major. **C,** The fracture was anatomically reduced with the use of a small-fragment reduction clamp. **D,** Application of a precontoured compression plate specifically designed for the clavicle. A Kirschner wire through the plate is used to hold the fracture reduction as the plate is applied. **E,** The final position of the hardware before surgical site closure. (Reproduced with permission from Altamimi SA, McKee MD; Canadian Orthopaedic Trauma Society: Nonoperative treatment compared with plate fixation of displaced midshaft clavicular fractures: Surgical technique. *J Bone Joint Surg Am* 2008;90[suppl 2 pt 1]:1-8.)

or open wounds dictate otherwise.

- An effort is made to preserve cutaneous nerve branches of the supraclavicular nerve; however, exposure is prioritized. Some denervation is inevitable because of the quantity and variability of branching of the supraclavicular nerve. Typically, two to three nerve branches cross the surgical site.

- A recent study of chest wall numbness after surgical fixation of displaced clavicular fractures found that up to one-half of patients continue to have numbness at 1 year postoperatively; however, no correlation was found between numbness and patient-rated outcome. The authors of this chapter typically warn patients preoperatively of the potential for distal peri-incisional numbness.

Reduction and Fixation

- The medial and lateral fragments are exposed, taking care to preserve soft-tissue attachments of comminuted fragments and the anterior pectoralis major insertion.

- Interposed soft tissue is removed, after which the fracture is thoroughly irrigated and then reduced and held with a reduction clamp (**Figure 3, C**).

- In the event of comminution, intervening fragments are reduced and fixed with minifragment lag screw fixation if fragment size permits. This method allows increased accuracy in reading length and rotation and improved application of compression through the plate. If the fragments are too small for screw fixation, the authors of this chapter emphasize maintenance

of soft-tissue attachments. The fragments can be fixed to the plate with suture; many precontoured plates have holes for this purpose. Alternatively, suture can be passed around the plate or through unused screw holes.

- Depending on the orientation of the fracture, a lag screw is placed perpendicular to the fracture axis—anteriorly if the major plane of the fracture is coronal or through the plate from superior to inferior if the fracture is predominately in an axial plane.

- A precontoured 3.5-mm compression plate is centered over the fracture site to allow the placement of at least three screws medially and laterally, excluding the lag screw if placed through the plate (**Figure 3, D** and **E**).

Table 2 Rehabilitation Protocol After Surgical Management of Midshaft Clavicular Fracture

Postoperative Week	ROM	Strengthening	Return to Play	Comments/Emphasis
0-2	Passive	No	No	Sling in place Full elbow and wrist ROM exercises
2-6	Progressive active, active-assisted to full ROM	No	No	Discontinue sling Progressive return to full ROM
6-12	Full	Strengthening is begun	No	Progressive strengthening
12-24	Full	Full	Yes	Return to sport/activity, including contact sports

ROM = range of motion.

- The plate is placed over the superior surface of the clavicle. Superior plating has shown increased biomechanical stability compared with anterior plating, and superior plating is technically simpler. In addition, rates of hardware complication and required subsequent removal are the same with both superior and anterior plating. The authors of this chapter have not found anterior plating to be required or advantageous.
- The plate is applied in a compression mode. If substantial comminution is present and not amenable to compression, a bridge plating technique is used to ensure restoration of length and rotation. The typical fracture deformity involves anterior rotation or protraction of the distal fragment that must be recognized and reduced.
- In most patients who undergo acute clavicular fracture fixation, bone grafting is unnecessary. In revision fixation as well as nonunion fixation, local bone graft is usually sufficient to make distant autogenous bone grafting unnecessary. In instances of hypotrophic nonunion or bone loss, autogenous iliac crest graft may be harvested intraoperatively, if necessary, after the proximal and distal fragments have been prepared.
- Drilling from superior to inferior must be done with caution to prevent inadvertent neurovascular injury or pneumothorax. A blunt retractor may be used on the undersurface of the clavicle if necessary; however, use of a blunt retractor requires increased soft-tissue dissection, which generally should be avoided. As the surgeon's experience increases, this protection will not be necessary. If inadvertent plunging of the drill bit occurs, a postoperative chest radiograph should be obtained to evaluate for pneumothorax.

Wound Closure

- The wound is copiously irrigated and closed in layers.
- The myofascial layer is closed with 1-0 absorbable suture.
- The skin and subcutaneous tissue are closed in a separate layer with nonabsorbable suture, typically 3-0 nylon or polypropylene.
- The incision is instilled with local anesthetic.
- After the wound is dressed, the arm is placed in a removable sling.
- Because reduction and hardware application are performed under direct visualization, intraoperative imaging is generally not used. However, intraoperative fluoroscopy may be used to check reduction or screw length.
- A single AP radiograph of the clavicle is obtained in the recovery room, and another antibiotic dose is given.

Rehabilitation

Patients are instructed to use a sling for 10 to 14 days postoperatively, after which the sling is discontinued and progressive active and passive ROM is initiated. Strengthening exercises and weight bearing through the limb are begun at 6 weeks postoperatively (**Table 2**).

Return to full activity, including sports, is permitted with return of strength and motion, along with radiographic signs of union, typically at 3 months. Despite this recommendation, a large proportion of patients return to sport earlier than suggested. No published study has defined the earliest time for safe return to sport. In a study of 39 semiprofessional athletes, an average full return to sport of 45 days was reported, along with a refracture rate of 5%. Patients are made aware of this elevated risk of refracture to allow them to make an informed decision regarding return to activity.

Return to work depends largely on the patient's employment. Sedentary desk work may be resumed as early as 1 week postoperatively, whereas heavy labor employment will require a time course similar to that for return to sport.

Fracture union is defined as pain-free full ROM, no pain or motion with manual stressing of the fracture site, and radiographic bridging of the fracture site. Radiographic fracture union can be expected in most patients by 12 weeks postoperatively.

Avoiding Pitfalls

Technique Tips

Patient selection is of paramount importance in providing the greatest benefit with the lowest risk of complication. Patient factors and fracture characteristics are important considerations in the decision to proceed with surgical fixation. Because patient selection is largely based on radiographic fracture appearance, appropriate radiographs and accurate assessment of those radiographs are critical.

Radiographs should be obtained with the patient in an upright position because this position has been shown to increase displacement by an average of 89% compared with the supine position. This difference has marked implications for clinical decision making. In addition, current guidelines are based on RCTs in which radiographs were obtained with patients in the upright position.

Radiographic shortening is difficult to reliably assess, with poor interrater reliability. Shortening is particularly difficult to measure in the presence of substantial comminution. The precision of this measurement can be improved by radiographically measuring the length of the contralateral clavicle from the acromioclavicular joint to the sternoclavicular joint and comparing this measurement with that on the injured side. A recent biologic anthropology study found that 70% of people have length-symmetric clavicles, whereas 7% have a side-to-side difference greater than 1 cm. This finding indicates the need to correlate multiple measures, including clinical measurement, with a tape measure. Obvious asymmetry of the shoulder, demonstrated in **Figure 1**, usually correlates to 1.5 to 2 cm of shortening.

Shortening is used as a surrogate measure of three-dimensional deformity. It is important to quantify factors such as inferior displacement and protraction of the distal fragment as well as comminution. These factors demonstrate better interrater agreement and should be considered in the decision to proceed with fixation.

After the decision to operate has been made on the basis of clinical and radiographic findings, the surgical technique should be deliberate and consistent, resulting in the structural restoration of length and rotation, sufficient stability to allow early ROM, and avoidance of complications. The deliberate avoidance of complications begins with exposure of the fracture. Stripping of soft tissues should be limited to that required for adequate visualization and fracture reduction to minimize disruption of blood supply.

Failure to anatomically contour the applied plate can result in malreduction as well as hardware prominence and irritation. Precontoured plating systems decrease intraoperative contouring time and have been shown to improve biomechanical stability compared with reconstruction plates. The authors of this chapter prefer to use precontoured plates designed for the clavicle (**Figure 3, E**).

Fixation should use a minimum of three screws in both the proximal and distal fragments, and it should provide compression to maximize construct stability and minimize delayed union and nonunion. Locking screw fixation improves construct stiffness but is used only in patients with poor bone quality or substantial comminution requiring a bridging technique; however, these conditions typically are seen only in revision surgery. Patient selection for primary fixation would dictate that good bone quality be present. Routine use of locking screws has been associated with catastrophic implant failure. Meticulous wound closure is required to avoid wound complications and should consist of a myofascial layer and a cutaneous/subcutaneous layer to provide robust coverage.

Complications
NONUNION

Although nonunion is considerably less common after surgical treatment than after nonsurgical treatment, nonunion occurs in as many as 3% of patients treated surgically. Treatment of nonunion is relatively straightforward and consists of revision surgical fixation and bone grafting; however, infection must first be ruled out both clinically and via laboratory studies. Preoperative screening blood work is required, and the authors of this chapter approach each nonunion that proceeds to revision surgical fixation as if it may be infected. Intraoperative antibiotics are delayed until cultures have been sent, extensive irrigation is performed, and, depending on the surgeon's intraoperative judgment, powdered antibiotic is applied to the surgical site. In these patients, the incidence of infection or positive wound cultures with low-grade organisms such as *Propionibacterium acnes* is high. Patient factors also must be taken into account; smoking has been shown to be a strong risk factor in nonsurgically managed clavicular fractures and may be a factor in surgically managed fractures. Remediable risk factors must be appropriately dealt with before revision surgery.

INFECTION

Surgical site infections have been reported in up to 4.8% of surgically treated patients. The treatment algorithm includes empiric antibiotic coverage and local wound care. After fracture union occurs, irrigation and débridement with hardware removal is performed to allow complete eradication of infection. The authors of this chapter have found that *P acnes* is one of the more common organisms to cause surgical site infection. Recent studies have shown that *P acnes* can often survive standard preoperative surgical preparation including chlorhexidine as used at our institution. Cultures of this organism typically require 7 to 13 days to return a positive result. Thus, cultures should be held for longer than the typical culture period of 5 days or fewer. Typically, management of *P acnes* involves thorough débridement and appropriate antibiotic coverage (vancomycin/clindamycin). Currently, there is no role for altering preoperative prophylactic antibiotics in the fixation of acute midshaft clavicular fractures.

HARDWARE-RELATED PROBLEMS

Hardware failure occurs in as many as 1.6% of patients and warrants revision surgical fixation. In most cases, hardware failure is related to patient activity and/or reinjury. Along with revision surgical fixation, the patient should be counseled on the appropriate postoperative activity level. Hardware irritation and subsequent removal is, by far, the most common reason for revision

surgery, accounting for more than 85% of revision surgeries after surgical fixation of midshaft clavicular fractures and occurring in approximately 17% of all surgically treated patients. The authors of this chapter generally delay hardware removal until 1 year postoperatively; however, the procedure may be completed after radiographic union is observed. Hardware removal is relatively straightforward and can be accomplished as outpatient day surgery. The surgeon must take care to maintain a two-layer closure identical to that described after hardware placement, with minimal muscle stripping. Patients are advised to avoid activities that place them at risk for falling onto the shoulder for 4 to 6 weeks and to avoid contact sports for 3 months postoperatively to minimize risk of refracture.

INTRAOPERATIVE VASCULAR INJURY

Iatrogenic intraoperative vascular injury during clavicular osteosynthesis is rare, as evidenced by its absence from the reported complications in RCTs on surgical treatment of midshaft clavicular fractures. The authors of this chapter are not aware of any case reports detailing an acute limb- or life-threatening vascular injury during primary clavicular fixation. Nonetheless, multiple publications provide cadaver-based anatomic measurement of the distance of the neurovascular bundle from instrumentation or drill paths.

If substantial bleeding occurs and an underlying major vascular injury is suspected, the anesthesiologist or anesthetist should be made aware of an

imminent need for transfusion so that blood products may be mobilized. Pressure should be applied to the wound for 3 to 5 minutes. If precipitous bleeding continues, immediate intraoperative vascular surgery consultation should be obtained. Proximal and distal vascular control, achieved via the clavicular fracture site and by mobilizing the fracture fragments, will be required to prevent ongoing blood loss. If further exposure is required, a clavicular osteotomy resecting the middle third of the clavicle may be done. After dissection through the underlying subclavius muscle, the subclavian vein and artery as well as the brachial plexus are carefully identified to allow application of atraumatic vascular clips to the proximal and distal segments of the injured vessel. After vascular control has been achieved, the surgeon should assess the treatment options, including repair, ligation, and/or bypass. It is important to prevent air embolism in this setting by keeping the bleeding vessels occluded, providing aggressive fluid resuscitation, and placing the patient in the supine position.

Patients should be monitored postoperatively for signs of vascular congestion or ischemia in the surgical limb. Case reports have described delayed development of subclavian arterial aneurysms and arteriovenous fistula after clavicular surgery. However, little literature is available to guide decision making in acute vascular injury, and general principles should be followed. Decisions regarding patient discharge and initiation of ROM should be made in consultation with a vascular surgeon.

Bibliography

Altamimi SA, McKee MD; Canadian Orthopaedic Trauma Society: Nonoperative treatment compared with plate fixation of displaced midshaft clavicular fractures: Surgical technique. *J Bone Joint Surg Am* 2008;90(suppl 2 pt 1):1-8.

Althausen PL, Shannon S, Lu M, O'Mara TJ, Bray TJ: Clinical and financial comparison of operative and nonoperative treatment of displaced clavicle fractures. *J Shoulder Elbow Surg* 2013;22(5):608-611.

Ashman BD, Slobogean GP, Stone TB, et al: Reoperation following open reduction and plate fixation of displaced mid-shaft clavicle fractures. *Injury* 2014;45(10):1549-1553.

Backus JD, Merriman DJ, McAndrew CM, Gardner MJ, Ricci WM: Upright versus supine radiographs of clavicle fractures: Does positioning matter? *J Orthop Trauma* 2014;28(11):636-641.

Baker JF, Mullett H: Clavicle non-union: Autologous bone graft is not a necessary augment to internal fixation. *Acta Orthop Belg* 2010;76(6):725-729.

Brouwer KM, Wright TC, Ring DC: Failure of superior locking clavicle plate by axial pull-out of the lateral screws: A report of four cases. *J Shoulder Elbow Surg* 2009;18(1):e22-e25.

Canadian Orthopaedic Trauma Society: Nonoperative treatment compared with plate fixation of displaced midshaft clavicular fractures: A multicenter, randomized clinical trial. *J Bone Joint Surg Am* 2007;89(1):1-10.

Celestre P, Roberston C, Mahar A, Oka R, Meunier M, Schwartz A: Biomechanical evaluation of clavicle fracture plating techniques: Does a locking plate provide improved stability? *J Orthop Trauma* 2008;22(4):241-247.

Christensen TJ, Horwitz DS, Kubiak EN: Natural history of anterior chest wall numbness after plating of clavicle fractures: Educating patients. *J Orthop Trauma* 2014;28(11):642-647.

Collinge C, Devinney S, Herscovici D, DiPasquale T, Sanders R: Anterior-inferior plate fixation of middle-third fractures and nonunions of the clavicle. *J Orthop Trauma* 2006;20(10):680-686.

Cunningham BP, McLaren A, Richardson M, McLemore R: Clavicular length: The assumption of symmetry. *Orthopedics* 2013;36(3):e343-e347.

Ding M, Hu J, Ni J, Lv H, Song D, Shu C: Iatrogenic subclavian arteriovenous fistula: Rare complication of plate osteosynthesis of clavicle fracture. *Orthopedics* 2012;35(2):e287-e289.

Hill JM, McGuire MH, Crosby LA: Closed treatment of displaced middle-third fractures of the clavicle gives poor results. *J Bone Joint Surg Br* 1997;79(4):537-539.

Huh J, Posner MA, Bear RR, Banerjee R, Owens BD, Hsu JR; Skeletal Trauma Research Consortium (STReC): Performance of military tasks after clavicle plating. *Mil Med* 2011;176(8):950-955.

Hulsmans MH, van Heijl M, Houwert RM, Timmers TK, van Olden G, Verleisdonk EJ: Anteroinferior versus superior plating of clavicular fractures. *J Shoulder Elbow Surg* 2016;25(3):448-454.

Hussey MM, Chen Y, Fajardo RA, Dutta AK: Analysis of neurovascular safety between superior and anterior plating techniques of clavicle fractures. *J Orthop Trauma* 2013;27(11):627-632.

Iannotti MR, Crosby LA, Stafford P, Grayson G, Goulet R: Effects of plate location and selection on the stability of midshaft clavicle osteotomies: A biomechanical study. *J Shoulder Elbow Surg* 2002;11(5):457-462.

Jones GL, Bishop JY, Lewis B, Pedroza AD; MOON Shoulder Group: Intraobserver and interobserver agreement in the classification and treatment of midshaft clavicle fractures. *Am J Sports Med* 2014;42(5):1176-1181.

Jubel A, Andermahr J, Schiffer G, Tsironis K, Rehm KE: Elastic stable intramedullary nailing of midclavicular fractures with a titanium nail. *Clin Orthop Relat Res* 2003;(408):279-285.

Lee MJ, Pottinger PS, Butler-Wu S, Bumgarner RE, Russ SM, Matsen FA III: Propionibacterium persists in the skin despite standard surgical preparation. *J Bone Joint Surg Am* 2014;96(17):1447-1450.

Longo UG, Banerjee S, Barber J, et al: Conservative management versus open reduction and internal fixation for mid-shaft clavicle fractures in adults: The Clavicle Trial. Study protocol for a multicentre randomized controlled trial. *Trials* 2011;12:57.

McKee MD, Pedersen EM, Jones C, et al: Deficits following nonoperative treatment of displaced midshaft clavicular fractures. *J Bone Joint Surg Am* 2006;88(1):35-40.

McKee RC, Whelan DB, Schemitsch EH, McKee MD: Operative versus nonoperative care of displaced midshaft clavicular fractures: A meta-analysis of randomized clinical trials. *J Bone Joint Surg Am* 2012;94(8):675-684.

Murray IR, Foster CJ, Eros A, Robinson CM: Risk factors for nonunion after nonoperative treatment of displaced midshaft fractures of the clavicle. *J Bone Joint Surg Am* 2013;95(13):1153-1158.

Narsaria N, Singh AK, Arun GR, Seth RR: Surgical fixation of displaced midshaft clavicle fractures: Elastic intramedullary nailing versus precontoured plating. *J Orthop Traumatol* 2014;15(3):165-171.

Nathe T, Tseng S, Yoo B: The anatomy of the supraclavicular nerve during surgical approach to the clavicular shaft. *Clin Orthop Relat Res* 2011;469(3):890-894.

Neer CS II: Nonunion of the clavicle. *J Am Med Assoc* 1960;172:1006-1011.

Nordqvist A, Petersson CJ, Redlund-Johnell I: Mid-clavicle fractures in adults: End result study after conservative treatment. *J Orthop Trauma* 1998;12(8):572-576.

Nowak J, Holgersson M, Larsson S: Sequelae from clavicular fractures are common: A prospective study of 222 patients. *Acta Orthop* 2005;76(4):496-502.

Ristevski B, Hall JA, Pearce D, Potter J, Farrugia M, McKee MD: The radiographic quantification of scapular malalignment after malunion of displaced clavicular shaft fractures. *J Shoulder Elbow Surg* 2013;22(2):240-246.

Robinson CM, Goudie EB, Murray IR, et al: Open reduction and plate fixation versus nonoperative treatment for displaced midshaft clavicular fractures: A multicenter, randomized, controlled trial. *J Bone Joint Surg Am* 2013;95(17):1576-1584.

Rowe CR: An atlas of anatomy and treatment of midclavicular fractures. *Clin Orthop Relat Res* 1968;(58):29-42.

Smekal V, Irenberger A, Struve P, Wambacher M, Krappinger D, Kralinger FS: Elastic stable intramedullary nailing versus nonoperative treatment of displaced midshaft clavicular fractures: A randomized, controlled, clinical trial. *J Orthop Trauma* 2009;23(2):106-112.

Verborgt O, Pittoors K, Van Glabbeek F, Declercq G, Nuyts R, Somville J: Plate fixation of middle-third fractures of the clavicle in the semi-professional athlete. *Acta Orthop Belg* 2005;71(1):17-21.

Virtanen KJ, Remes V, Pajarinen J, Savolainen V, Björkenheim JM, Paavola M: Sling compared with plate osteosynthesis for treatment of displaced midshaft clavicular fractures: A randomized clinical trial. *J Bone Joint Surg Am* 2012;94(17):1546-1553.

Yadav V, Khare GN, Singh S, et al: A prospective study comparing conservative with operative treatment in patients with a 'floating shoulder' including assessment of the prognostic value of the glenopolar angle. *Bone Joint J* 2013;95(6):815-819.

Zlowodzki M, Zelle BA, Cole PA, Jeray K, McKee MD; Evidence-Based Orthopaedic Trauma Working Group: Treatment of acute midshaft clavicle fractures: Systematic review of 2144 fractures. On behalf of the Evidence-Based Orthopaedic Trauma Working Group. *J Orthop Trauma* 2005;19(7):504-507.

Chapter 52

Intramedullary Fixation of Middle Third Clavicle Fracture

Carl J. Basamania, MD

 ## Introduction

Although most clavicle fractures can be managed nonsurgically, a marked trend toward surgical management of displaced and shortened clavicle fractures has occurred in the past two decades. Studies of surgical management of clavicle fractures with either intramedullary fixation or plate-and-screw fixation have found significant reduction in the risk of nonunion and quicker return to full function compared with nonsurgical management. Although plate-and-screw fixation is used more commonly than intramedullary fixation, almost all studies comparing those techniques have found markedly lower complication rates with intramedullary fixation. Furthermore, intramedullary fixation can be performed as an outpatient procedure with smaller, more cosmetically pleasing incisions than those required for plate-and-screw fixation. Painful, prominent hardware is the primary complication of both intramedullary fixation and plate-and-screw fixation; however, hardware removal after intramedullary fixation is less complicated than removal of plate-and-screw constructs. The advent of better-designed, lower profile intramedullary fixation devices as well

as device-specific and clavicle-specific implantation instruments is expected to further reduce the complication rate of intramedullary fixation.

 ## Case Presentation

A 49-year-old man who is an avid bike racer crashed while traveling an estimated 35 to 40 miles per hour in a race. He was wearing a helmet, and he sustained a closed head injury with transient loss of consciousness; multiple abrasions; a comminuted, displaced, and shortened midshaft fracture of the left clavicle; and multiple segmental left-sided rib fractures with a flail chest, pneumothorax, and pulmonary contusion (**Figure 1**).

The patient was admitted to the intensive care unit for treatment of the closed head injury, flail chest, and pneumothorax. A chest tube was placed, and a CT scan of the head showed no evidence of intracranial bleeding or other abnormalities. The chest tube was discontinued after 24 hours. No evidence of posttraumatic amnesia was noted, and the patient was discharged 4 days after injury. Initial management of the clavicle fracture consisted of sling immobilization.

The patient was seen in the clinic 2 weeks after the initial injury. He reported substantial pain at the clavicle fracture site and reported difficulty breathing, describing the sensation as "my shoulder is pushing down on my chest." He also noted a tingling sensation in his left ring and small fingers. On physical examination, obvious deformity of the left shoulder girdle was noted, with the shoulder drooping downward and rotated anteriorly relative to the chest and uninvolved shoulder. An abrasion on the back of the patient's left shoulder demonstrated healing with no evidence of infection.

The patient underwent an outpatient surgical procedure for treatment of a substantially displaced midshaft clavicle fracture with compromise of the subclavicular space and suspected compression of the brachial plexus. Because of the comminution at the fracture site, a hybrid intramedullary fixation device was used, which would allow for greater length of fixation and use static fixation to prevent shortening and provide better rotational control. Surgical management with this type of device can be performed through a relatively small incision, which can help reduce the risk of infection, especially in patients with a large abrasion near the surgical site. Intramedullary fixation also allows callus healing, which occurs faster than direct healing and can be seen more easily on follow-up

Dr. Basamania or an immediate family member has received royalties from DePuy; is a member of a speakers' bureau or has made paid presentations on behalf of DePuy and Sonoma Orthopedics; serves as a paid consultant to Zimmer Biomet, DePuy, Invuity, and Sonoma Orthopedics; and has stock or stock options held in Invuity.

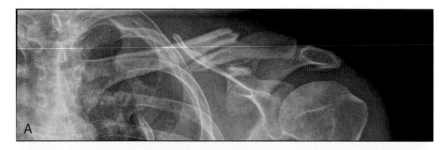

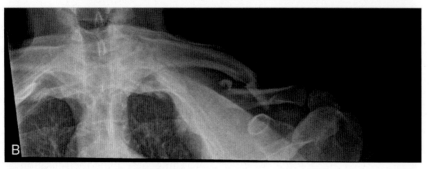

Figure 1   Initial AP (**A**) and 45° cephalic tilt AP (**B**) radiographs demonstrate a comminuted, displaced, and shortened midshaft fracture of the left clavicle.

radiographs, thereby enabling active patients to return to high-risk sports and activities as soon as possible. Furthermore, bike racing is associated with a high risk of another injury; therefore, in treating the patient described in this case study, routine deep implant removal was planned to avoid multiple stress risers in the clavicle. The presence of stress risers could increase the risk of refracture.

The patient was instructed to avoid contact sports or activities for 6 weeks that could place the clavicle at high risk; however, he resumed biking at 2 weeks postoperatively and resumed bike racing at 3 weeks postoperatively. He reported that his breathing was much improved almost immediately after the procedure. Although he had no complaints of hardware prominence or irritation, he underwent routine deep implant removal 14 weeks postoperatively to alleviate concerns of refracture in the event of another bike crash. The patient had no further problems (**Figure 2**).

 Indications

Although many low-energy, minimally displaced clavicle fractures can be managed nonsurgically, many orthopaedic surgeons assume that all clavicle fractures should be managed nonsurgically. This misconception is likely based on studies conducted in the 1960s in which lower healing rates were reported after surgical treatment. However, an author of one of these studies suggested that most instances of clavicle nonunion were caused by inadequate surgical management; the same author suggested that surgical treatment was preferred in some situations and should be accomplished with minimal damage to soft tissues, such as through the use of intramedullary fixation.

Current studies suggest that greater than 100% displacement and more than 15 mm of shortening are indications for surgical management of midshaft clavicle fractures. Additionally, the damage to the chest wall is further compromised by the loss of the normal suspensory

function of the clavicle and subsequent drooping of the shoulder onto the chest. Although these fractures could be managed nonsurgically, the risk of nonunion is 15% to 25%. In addition, because it is nearly impossible to obtain and maintain reduction of a displaced clavicle fracture without surgical treatment, the likelihood of malunion developing is 75% to 85%. In other words, two outcomes are possible after nonsurgical management of a displaced clavicle fracture: the fracture might not heal or it might heal in a malunited position. Furthermore, at least 28 weeks may be required to achieve healing with nonsurgical management, including approximately 6 weeks of sling immobilization. This treatment time could have a substantial impact on work activities and athletic training.

 Controversies and Alternative Approaches

Most clavicle fractures are managed with sling immobilization or surgery. The two primary surgical options are plate-and-screw fixation and intramedullary fixation.

Plate-and-Screw Fixation

Plate-and-screw fixation provides strong, stable fixation; offers a quick return to function; and can be performed using common internal fixation techniques. The primary disadvantages of plate-and-screw fixation are the large, cosmetically displeasing incision; soft-tissue stripping; stress shielding; the risk of infection; the potential for neurovascular injury; and the risk of refracture after plate removal. Hardware prominence resulting from the subcutaneous position of the clavicle is also a common problem. Although most plates are not intended for removal, in a recent meta-analysis of plate-and-screw fixation studies, most studies reported high

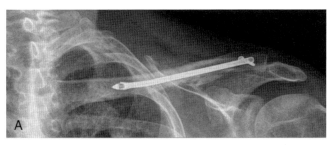

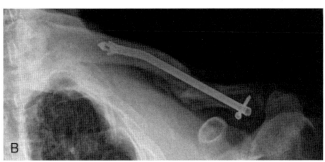

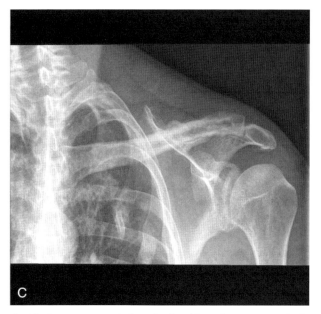

Figure 2 AP (**A**) and 45° cephalic tilt AP (**B**) radiographs from the patient in the case presentation obtained 6 weeks postoperatively demonstrate callus about the fracture site. **C,** AP radiograph from the same patient obtained 5 months after the index procedure and 6 weeks after hardware removal demonstrates anatomic alignment of the clavicle with good fracture healing.

complication rates of 9% to 64% related to prominence, irritation, or failure of the plate. Removal of the device requires a second large incision and results in the creation of multiple stress risers in the clavicle resulting from the presence of the screw holes. Furthermore, plate fixation can disrupt the blood supply to the clavicle, which is entirely periosteal. Plate fixation also relies on direct bone healing, which requires stable compression fixation. However, compression fixation can cause osteoporosis. In addition, bone healing with plate fixation can be monitored only indirectly, on the basis of the absence of adverse clinical and radiologic symptoms, rather than directly, on the basis of obvious callus. Determining when a patient can safely return to sport can be problematic when using this indirect method of monitoring.

Intramedullary Fixation

The primary advantage of intramedullary fixation is that it provides stability sufficient to allow early return to function while enabling callus healing and minimal stress shielding of the bone. Callus healing typically occurs more quickly than direct bone healing and can be easily seen on follow-up radiographs, whereas direct bone healing must be inferred rather than observed. Thus, callus healing can be an important factor in deciding when to allow the patient to return to work and resume athletic activities. With intramedullary fixation, minimal soft-tissue stripping is required, the periosteal blood supply is preserved, and the technique can be performed through small, cosmetic incisions. Because of the minimal soft-tissue stripping and small exposure, the procedure can be performed in an outpatient setting and, theoretically, is associated with a lower risk of infection than plate-and-screw fixation. Furthermore, intramedullary fixation devices can be removed easily in an outpatient setting, typically with the use of only local anesthesia and intravenous sedation. Intramedullary fixation also is associated with a lower risk of refracture than plate-and-screw fixation because the patient has few stress risers and less likelihood of relative osteoporosis of the bone after hardware removal. The lesser rigidity of intramedullary fixation can be considered an advantage rather than a limitation. Compared with plate-and-screw fixation, intramedullary fixation for the management of acute fractures is associated with minimal risk of neurovascular injury. To accommodate the medial curve of the clavicle, the drill is passed out of the anteromedial cortex in intramedullary fixation, completely away from the neurovascular structures, which can be more easily damaged during medial drilling for plate-and-screw fixation.

The primary problems with intramedullary fixation are lack of rotational control, lack of length control, hardware migration, and hardware prominence. Placement of intramedullary devices can be difficult in patients with small or almost absent medullary canals. Controversy exists as to whether the intramedullary device should be inserted in a medial to lateral direction from a medial entry point or in a retrograde fashion from a lateral entry point. It is

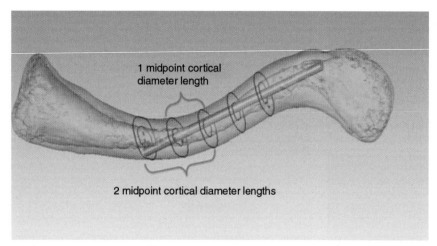

1 midpoint cortical diameter length

2 midpoint cortical diameter lengths

Figure 3 Illustration depicts the area of the clavicle that can be managed using a rigid intramedullary fixation device. (Reproduced with permission from Bachoura A, Deane AS, Kamineni S: Clavicle anatomy and the applicability of intramedullary midshaft fracture fixation. *J Shoulder Elbow Surg* 2012;21[10]:1384-1390.)

preferable to have the strongest and longest fixation in the shortest fragment. Therefore, in more lateral fractures, retrograde placement of a pin from a lateral entry point would be biomechanically preferable because this technique would allow maximum length of fixation in the shorter lateral fragment. In addition, strong cortical fixation of the intramedullary device can be achieved with the use of a lateral entry point. The strength of fixation is directly related to the length of fixation; however, the length of engagement is limited by both the curvature of the clavicle and the thickness of the fixation device. It is preferable to bypass the fracture site by at least two cortical diameters; thus, for most fractures at the junction of the middle and lateral thirds of the clavicle, a rigid device is inserted in a retrograde fashion (**Figure 3**). Fractures that are more medial may be better managed with an antegrade insertion.

TYPES OF INTRAMEDULLARY FIXATION

Intramedullary fixation devices can be classified as rigid, flexible, or hybrid and as smooth or threaded. Examples of rigid fixation devices are Herbert screws, cancellous screws, Knowles pins, Hagie pins, and Rockwood pins. Flexible fixation devices include Kirschner wires, Rush pins, and elastic nails, including the titanium elastic nail and the Nancy nail. Recently, the concept of a hybrid device has emerged, which may offer greater length of fixation, with less risk of hardware migration and soft-tissue irritation. The only hybrid fixation device currently available is flexible at the medial end to follow the normal curvature of the clavicle, but it becomes rigid after activation in the desired position. The device is rotationally stable because it has distally activated grippers on the medial side and an interlocking screw at the lateral end. The rigid medial curve also contributes to rotational stability. In theory, this stability allows for greater length of fixation compared with rigid devices combined with static locking capabilities. As a result, the device can be used for comminuted and long oblique fractures, which are difficult to manage with other types of intramedullary fixation. Because the device is designed to sit flush with the lateral cortex, the problems of hardware prominence may be reduced. The authors of a level I study published in 2015 found that a hybrid device demonstrated significantly less hardware irritation than clavicular plating (zero and 14.3%, respectively). The

hybrid device is designed to be inserted in a retrograde fashion for most fractures at the junction of the middle and lateral thirds, but it can also be inserted in an antegrade fashion such that the rigid portion of the device is in the medial fragment while the flexible portion is in the lateral fragment (**Figure 4**). The flexible end of the device must be positioned at least 50 mm into the canal to prevent excessive bending force of the rigid and flexible portions of the device on the junction.

PROBLEMS WITH FLEXIBLE INTRAMEDULLARY FIXATION

The primary problems with flexible intramedullary fixation are lack of length or rotational control and hardware migration. Passage of the nail through the canal without reaming can also be a serious problem because the narrowest portions of the canal have an average diameter of 6.7 ± 2.6 mm at the midpoint of the clavicle. Furthermore, the medullary canal is irregularly shaped, making passage of a cylindric rod difficult.

No clavicle-specific instrumentation is available to ream or open the medullary canal for flexible intramedullary fixation. Elastic intramedullary nails of 2 to 4 mm diameter are available; however, the medullary canal of the clavicle just lateral to the conoid tubercle cannot be reached with straight, rigid reamers or drills. Therefore, the application of these devices is limited in comminuted and long oblique fractures, which are common in high-energy injuries.

PROBLEMS WITH RIGID INTRAMEDULLARY FIXATION

The primary problem with rigid intramedullary fixation is the difficulty of inserting a straight, rigid device into a curved bone. The poor length and rotational control that is common with most intramedullary devices is also problematic. Some devices, such as the Rockwood pin, have different pitch threads on each end of the pin, allowing

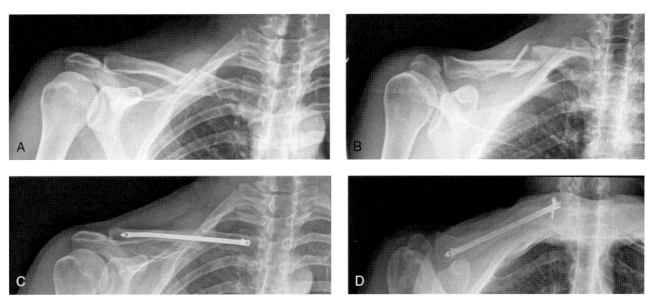

Figure 4   Preoperative AP (**A**) and 45° cephalic tilt AP (**B**) radiographs demonstrate a comminuted fracture at the medial aspect of the middle third of the clavicle. Postoperative AP (**C**) and 45° cephalic tilt AP (**D**) radiographs demonstrate antegrade intramedullary fixation with a hybrid device.

for compression at the fracture site. The Rockwood pin also has two different-size lateral nuts to prevent migration of the device, provide further compression of the fragment, and allow for relatively easy extraction after healing is achieved; however, the prominence of these nuts can cause hardware-related complications postoperatively. Another problem with rigid devices such as Herbert screws and cancellous screws is the limited number of options in length and diameter. Furthermore, because a distance of at least two cortical diameters past the fracture site should be bridged with the fixation device, the use of rigid fixation can be limited in patients with a long oblique fracture or marked comminution. Because the medullary canal is small or almost nonexistent in some patients, the relatively large diameter of rigid fixation devices can limit their use. Removal of completely intramedullary devices such as the Herbert screw is advised in patients who are at high risk of another injury, such as competitive bikers and equestrians, because the presence of the device could cause substantial problems if another fracture

occurs. However, removal of these devices is difficult because of their intramedullary position.

 Results

Although earlier studies recommended nonsurgical management of clavicle fractures, a landmark article published in 1997 suggested that patients who undergo nonsurgical treatment have poor results and that the rate of nonunion was considerably higher than previously thought. A Canadian multicenter study published in 2007 showed a significant decrease in nonunion in patients treated with plate fixation compared with sling immobilization; however, the patients treated with plate fixation had a complication rate of 31%, with 18% of patients reporting hardware irritation or pain. In a 2010 study of clavicle fractures in professional football players, almost 50% of patients with a completely displaced middle third clavicle fracture were treated successfully with acute surgical fixation and healed at an average of 8.8 weeks without sequelae. One-half

of these players were able to return to play during the same season. More than one-half of the players initially treated nonsurgically for a completely displaced middle third clavicle fracture refractured their clavicle within 1 year after the initial injury and missed an average of 1.5 seasons because of the clavicle injury. In a different study, it was shown that the overall cost of nonsurgical management was more than $5,000 higher than the cost of surgical management because of increased loss of time from work (35.2 days versus 8.4 days), increased use of pain medication, and the need for physical therapy resulting from prolonged immobilization. In addition to the higher costs, the surgically treated patients had less chronic pain (6.1% versus 25.3%), less cosmetic deformity (18.2% versus 32.5%), less weakness (10.6% versus 33.7%), less loss of motion (15.2% versus 31.3%), and fewer nonunions (zero versus 4.8%) than patients treated nonsurgically.

Table 1 shows a comparison of the different types of intramedullary fixation. In a 2015 study using hybrid fixation, no radiographic evidence of

Table 1 Results of Studies Comparing Intramedullary Fixation Techniques

Authors	Journal (Year)	Technique (No. of Patients)	Outcomes	Failure Rate (%)	Comments
Jubel et al	*Br J Sports Med* (2003)	TEN (84)	Mean Constant score in athletes, 98.3 Overall mean Constant score, 96.2	1	No complications 12 patients were high-performing athletes Athletes resumed training at a mean (± SD) of 5.9 ± 1 d postoperatively (range, 4-8 d) Participation in competition was resumed after a mean (± SD) of 16.8 ± 5 d postoperatively (range, 10-26 d) Level IV study
Jubel et al	*Clin Orthop Relat Res* (2003)	TEN (58)	Median Constant and Murley score, 98 (range, 87-100)	2	16% complication rate 1 patient had 1.5 cm shortening postoperatively 48% of patients were treated with closed reduction Most fractures were noncommi-nuted Level IV study
Kettler et al	*Acta Orthop* (2007)	TEN (87)	80 healed in an anatomic position	5	9% complication rate 3 patients healed with >30° angulation 4 patients had >100% dislocation 2 patients had shortening of >1 cm Level IV study
Frigg et al	*Am J Sports Med* (2009)	TEN (34)	Adding an end cap to the TEN did not decrease migration or complications	11	Compared standard TEN to TEN with an end cap to prevent migration 70% complication rate; 49% major complication rate Level I study
Smekal et al	*J Orthop Trauma* (2009)	TEN (30), shoulder sling (30)	Faster return to daily activities and better functional outcome in the surgical group. Constant scores were significantly higher after 6 mo and 2 yr after intramedullary stabilization	Surgical group: 0 Nonsurgical group: 10	30% complication rate in the surgical group In 2 patients treated surgically, implant failure occurred after additional trauma Level I study
Millett et al	*J Shoulder Elbow Surg* (2011)	Rockwood pin (58)	Mean ASES score improved from 42 to 89 (*P* < 0.05) Avg daily pain score decreased from 3 to 1 Mean satisfaction with surgical outcomes, 8 (10-point scale)	8.6 (all non-unions)	8.6% major complication rate 17.2% minor complication rate 5 nonunions requiring repeat surgical treatment Level IV study
Richardson et al	*Int J Shoulder Surg* (2013)	Herbert bone screw (114)	Avg time to union, 8.8 wk	2.6	15.8% complication rate 9.6% reoperation rate Level III study

ASES = American Shoulder and Elbow Surgeons shoulder outcome; DASH = Disabilities of the Arm, Shoulder and Hand; ROM = range of motion; TEN = titanium elastic nail.

Table 1 Results of Studies Comparing Intramedullary Fixation Techniques (*continued*)

Authors	Journal (Year)	Technique (No. of Patients)	Outcomes	Failure Rate (%)	Comments
King et al	*J Shoulder Elbow Surg* (2015)	Hybrid fixation (47)	No differences in ROM (*P* = 0.96), Constant score (*P* = 0.38), and DASH score (*P* = 0.33) were found among patients in the three follow-up periods	0	6% complication rate 1 infection and 2 hardware failures Both patients with hardware failure healed 34% of the fractures were comminuted Follow-up at 3-6, 6-9, and 9-12 mo Level IV study

ASES = American Shoulder and Elbow Surgeons shoulder outcome; DASH = Disabilities of the Arm, Shoulder and Hand; ROM = range of motion; TEN = titanium elastic nail.

hardware migration was found in simple or comminuted fractures. Visual and tactile examinations did not reveal any protrusion of the hybrid fixation device into the soft tissue or skin of the lateral shoulder. In a 2015 study using hybrid fixation and minimally invasive percutaneous plate osteosynthesis, there was no skin irritation in patients treated with hybrid fixation, but the incidence of skin irritation was 14.3% in patients treated with plate fixation. In a year 2000 publication comparing the use of different pins, the length of fixation of a rigid intramedullary device was found to be limited.

Multiple studies comparing plate-and-screw fixation with intramedullary fixation have typically shown equal efficacy of both techniques; however, most studies have shown lower rates of complications, especially major complications, with intramedullary fixation (**Table 2**). Similar results have been noted in meta-analyses of plate and intramedullary fixation. The authors of a study comparing plate fixation with intramedullary fixation in elderly patients found that intramedullary fixation resulted in significantly shorter surgical time (*P* < 0.001), smaller wound size (*P* < 0.001), shorter hospital stays (*P* = 0.03), less narcotic use (*P* = 0.02),

lower complication rates (*P* = 0.04), and less symptomatic hardware (*P* = 0.015).

 Technical Keys to Success

Although the technique described in this chapter is for the hybrid type of intramedullary fixation, the principles can be applied to all types of intramedullary fixation.

Setup/Exposure

- The author of this chapter performs intramedullary fixation with the patient under general anesthesia in an outpatient setting.
- General anesthesia is preferred because interscalene or regional anesthesia can cause incomplete coverage of the clavicular region and can make neurovascular examinations difficult in the recovery room.
- The general anesthesia can be supplemented with local anesthesia. The author of this chapter typically uses local infiltration of 0.5% bupivacaine with epinephrine at either the start or the end of the procedure.
- Typically, a preoperative dose of

antibiotics is administered, with an additional dose given in the recovery room.

- The patient can be placed in the supine position or the modified beach-chair position on a radiolucent surgical table. The modified beach-chair position offers easier access to the posterior aspect of the shoulder.
- Access to the clavicle and shoulder is facilitated with the use of a radiolucent shoulder-positioning device.
- The use of an image intensification device or C-arm greatly facilitates pin placement. The C-arm base is moved in from the head of the surgical table with the C-arm gantry rotated slightly away from the treated shoulder and oriented in a cephalic tilt.
- The C-arm is draped with standard split sheets, ensuring that the entire length of the clavicle can be seen and palpated after the draping.
- The arm should be draped free to allow movement, which will facilitate drilling of the lateral fragment and reduction of the fracture.
- The patient's torso should be positioned at approximately 45° relative to the floor. The C-arm gantry should be situated such that the

Table 2 Results of Plate Fixation Versus Intramedullary Fixation to Manage Clavicle Fracture

Author(s)	Journal (Year)	Techniques (No. of Patients)	Outcomes	Failure Rate	Comments
Lee et al	*Int Orthop* (2008)	IM fixation with a Knowles pin (56), DCP and reconstruction plate (32)	Significantly shorter surgical times as well as reduced scarring and decreased use of pain medication with IM fixation	No nonunion, 1% plate failure	IM fixation: No complications, painful hardware in 7.1% Plate fixation: 9.4% complication rate, painful hardware in 37.5% Level I study
Thyagarajan et al	*Int J Shoulder Surg* (2009)	IM fixation with a Rockwood pin (17), low-contact DCP (17), nonsurgical treatment (17)	100% union by 8-12 wk with IM fixation All IM procedures were outpatient Hospital stays of 2-3 d after plate fixation	IM group: No nonunion Plate group: 6% nonunion Nonsurgical group: 23.5% nonunion or malunion	IM fixation: superficial wound complications in 12% and mild pain in 12%, but all patients were satisfied with their results Plate fixation: implant failure in 12%, plate irritation in 35%, scar-related pain in 24%, and pain with activity in 35% Level III study
Ferran et al	*J Shoulder Elbow Surg* (2010)	IM fixation with a Rockwood pin (17), low-contact DCP (15)	Mean Constant score of 92.1 with IM fixation and 88.7 with plate fixation	0	IM fixation: 24% complication rate, 100% planned hardware removal Plate fixation: 80% complication rate, 53% hardware removal because of irritation and infection Level I study
Liu et al	*J Trauma* (2010)	TEN (51), straight and contoured superior plates (59)	Significantly reduced surgical time, hospital stay, incision size, and blood loss with IM fixation	Nonunion: 9.8% with IM, 10.2% with plating Malunion: 7.8% with IM, 3.4% with plating	IM fixation: 39% complication rate, 5.9% wound complication rate Plate fixation: 53% complication rate, 10.2% wound complication rate Level III study
Assobhi	*J Orthop Traumatol* (2011)	TEN (19), 3.5-mm reconstruction plate (19)	Significantly reduced hospital stay, surgical time, scar length, and blood loss with IM fixation	Nonunion: 5.3% after plating, 0 after IM fixation	IM fixation: No major complications, minor complications in 21.1%, and no refracture after hardware removal Plate fixation: Major complications in 15.8%, minor complications in 36.8%, and refracture after hardware removal in 5.3% Level I study
Böhme et al	*Z Orthop Unfall* (2011)	TEN (20); DCP, reconstruction plate, or low-contact DCP (53); nonsurgical treatment (47)	4% infection rate with plate fixation	No nonunions in surgically treated groups Results of nonsurgical management not reported	15% complication rate with IM fixation 22% complication rate with plate fixation Better pain relief, function, and cosmetic result with surgical treatment than with nonsurgical treatment Level II study

DASH = Disabilities of the Arm, Shoulder and Hand; DCP = dynamic compression plate; IM = intramedullary; MIPPO = minimally invasive percutaneous plate osteosynthesis; TEN = titanium elastic nail.

Table 2 Results of Plate Fixation Versus Intramedullary Fixation to Manage Clavicle Fracture (*continued*)

Author(s)	Journal (Year)	Techniques (No. of Patients)	Outcomes	Failure Rate	Comments
Kleweno et al	*J Shoulder Elbow Surg* (2011)	IM fixation with a Rockwood pin (18), reconstruction plate (6), locking plate (6), precontoured plate (2)	Avg time to union: 8 mo after IM fixation, 17 mo after plate fixation	0 in IM group, 7% in plate group	IM group: 28% complication rate, no delayed union or refracture Plate group: 36% complication rate, 7% delayed union rate, and 14% refracture rate Level III study
Chen et al	*J Shoulder Elbow Surg* (2012)	TEN (57), reconstruction plates (84)	Significantly reduced time to union, surgical time, and blood loss with IM fixation	2% with IM fixation, 4% with plate fixation	IM fixation: 2% infection rate, 5% hardware failure rate Plate fixation: 4% infection rate, 7% hardware failure rate 43% of patients treated with plate fixation rated their results as unsatisfactory, compared with 14% of patients treated with IM fixation Level III study
Wijdicks et al	*Int Orthop* (2012)	TEN (47), reconstruction and locking plates (43)	7% refracture rate with plate fixation, no refracture with IM fixation	Implant failure: 14% after plate fixation, 2.1% after IM fixation	IM fixation: 4% major complication rate, 2% major revision rate Plate fixation: 26% major complication rate, 12% major revision rate Level III study
Wenninger et al	*J Surg Orthop Adv* (2013)	IM fixation with a Hagie pin (33), 3.5-mm reconstruction and precontoured plates (29)	100% union rate in both the IM and plate groups All patients in both groups returned to full military duty	No nonunions	Complication rate: 31% with plate fixation, 9% with IM fixation Most symptoms were caused by the pressure of body armor and rucksack wear during training in this active-duty military population Level III study
Saha et al	*Indian J Orthop* (2014)	TEN (34), anterosuperior locking plate (37)	Significantly reduced time to union, surgical time, and blood loss with IM fixation	0 with IM fixation, 3% with plate fixation	IM fixation: No major complications, 38% minor complication rate Plate fixation: 14% major complication rate, 16% minor complication rate, and 11% infection rate; 16% of patients rated their scar as "ugly" Level I study
Zehir et al	*Arch Orthop Trauma Surg* (2015)	Hybrid fixation (24) MIPPO plate fixation (21)	Significantly shorter time to bony union with hybrid fixation Mean time of surgery and mean time of fluoroscopy were significantly shorter with hybrid fixation than with the MIPPO plate ($P < 0.001$ and $P = 0.03$, respectively) Significantly shorter time of hospital stay after hybrid fixation ($P < 0.001$)	Implant failure: 4.2% hybrid 4.8% MIPPO	Mean quick DASH scores were not significantly different between two groups Implant failure occurred in 1 patient from each group Cosmetic dissatisfaction was more common in the MIPPO group Level I study

DASH = Disabilities of the Arm, Shoulder and Hand; DCP = dynamic compression plate; IM = intramedullary; MIPPO = minimally invasive percutaneous plate osteosynthesis; TEN = titanium elastic nail.

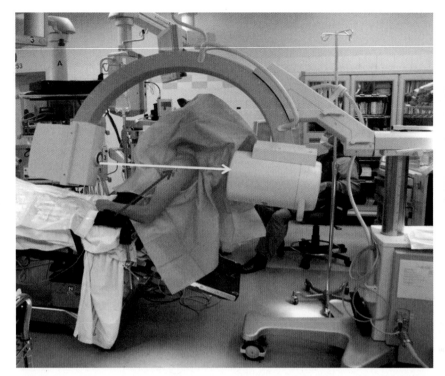

Figure 5 Photograph shows positioning of a C-arm with the beam parallel to the floor. The patient's torso is at a 45° angle relative to the floor. The yellow arrow indicates the direction of the C-arm beam, and the red arrow indicates the angle of the patient's torso.

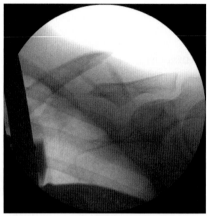

Figure 6 Fluoroscopic image from a C-arm demonstrates the equivalent of a 45° cephalic tilt radiographic view.

radiographic beam is parallel to the floor (**Figure 5**). This position gives the equivalent of a 45° cephalic tilt view of the medial clavicle, which allows the best view of the anterior curve of the clavicle (**Figure 6**).

- The positioning and orientation of the C-arm described in the previous point also allows a cephalic tilt view of the lateral fragment. This view is helpful because the placement of the pin in the lateral fragment is crucial to obtaining anatomic reduction of the fracture. If necessary, an AP-equivalent view can be obtained by extending the arm, and an axillary-equivalent view can be obtained by forward flexing the arm (**Figure 7**).
- Because of the presence of metallic or radiopaque devices on the surgical table, it may be necessary to orient the beam of the C-arm from posterolateral to anteromedial.

With this orientation, marked underestimation of the length of the fracture or overlap of the fragments can occur because the clavicle is obliquely oriented relative to the C-arm beam. If necessary, the patient's shoulder can be brought forward to better estimate the length of the fracture.

- The surgeon should ensure that the entire length of the clavicle can be viewed in one position.
- After appropriate positioning of the C-arm is achieved, a foot pedal can be used to activate the C-arm during the procedure, thereby eliminating the need for the presence of a radiology technician during the entire procedure.
- If a C-arm is not used, the surgeon must be careful when passing the drill and pin, particularly into the medial fragment, because of the close proximity of the subclavian

vessels to the junction of the medial and middle third of the clavicle.
- Alternately, radiographs can be obtained intraoperatively to verify pin position.

Instruments/Equipment/Implants Required

- Intramedullary fixation requires a few specific instruments, and most intramedullary fixation devices, including the titanium flexible nail, have device-specific instrument sets.
- A Crego elevator is needed during passage of the cerclage suture.
- Mini Hohmann retractors are used.
- Large towel clamps and small bone fracture reduction clamps are used.

Procedure

- A 2.5- to 3.0-cm incision is made in the Langer lines over the palpable distal end of the medial fragment. This technique is used because the clavicle skin is more easily moved medially than laterally.
- To minimize cosmetically displeasing scarring, the incision can be placed in the skin crease that exists in most patients.
- If the fracture has a long oblique pattern, the incision is made slightly more medially and longer

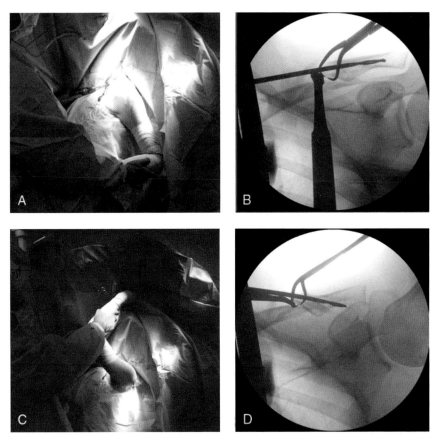

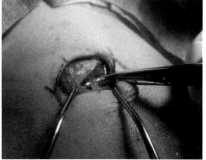

Figure 8 Intraoperative photograph shows the middle branch of the supraclavicular nerve in the clavicular fracture site.

Figure 7 Extending the patient's arm (**A**) as shown in this intraoperative photograph provides the equivalent of an AP view of the clavicle on the fluoroscopic image (**B**). Forward flexing the arm (**C**) as shown in this intraoperative photograph provides an axillary-equivalent view of the clavicle on the fluoroscopic image (**D**).

to allow elevation of the medial end of the distal fragment.

- Because the region around the mid clavicle has little subcutaneous fat, the surgeon should take care to prevent injury to the underlying platysma muscle, which inserts on the skin near the clavicle. Damage to the platysma muscle can lead to dysfunction of facial expression. Scissors are used to free the platysma muscle from the overlying skin. After the platysma muscle has been identified, its fibers are divided longitudinally.
- The surgeon must take care to prevent injury to the middle branch of the supraclavicular nerve, which is usually found directly beneath the platysma muscle near the

midportion of the clavicle. In some patients, the nerve may be found in the fracture site (**Figure 8**). Injury to the supraclavicular nerve can cause dysesthesia in the anterior shoulder, deltoid, and anterior chest wall. The nerve should be identified and retracted to prevent injury.

- In patients with acute fractures, the periosteum over the fracture site is disrupted and usually requires no further division.
- In most patients, soft tissue and/ or muscle (typically, the subclavius muscle) may be interposed in the fracture. In patients with long oblique fractures, the medial end of the lateral fragment may be embedded in the clavicular head of the pectoralis muscle. These soft tissues

should be carefully removed with an elevator or curet.

- If the medial end of the lateral fragment is embedded in muscle, the fragment can be grasped with a small reduction clamp. With lateral distraction, the medial end can be freed from the muscle with a small Key periosteal elevator.
- Small butterfly fragments should be left attached to their soft-tissue envelope. These fragments, which are usually found anteriorly and inferiorly, can be managed with cerclage fixation after the primary fixation.

PREPARATION OF THE MEDIAL FRAGMENT

- The lateral end of the medial fragment is elevated into the incision (**Figure 9**).
- Under fluoroscopic guidance, the medullary canal is identified with a 2-mm drill bit (**Figure 10**). Palpation of the medial aspect of the clavicle can aid in identifying this canal.
- After the medullary canal is identified, it can be further opened with a 3.5-mm drill bit or a straight 3-mm awl.
- Care must be taken to avoid penetrating the anterior medial cortex of the clavicle. At the point at which resistance is met, the straight drill or awl is removed.

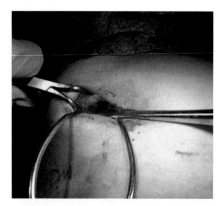

Figure 9 Intraoperative photograph shows the lateral end of the medial fragment grasped with a towel clip and elevated into the incision. A 0.5-inch (12.7-mm) Key elevator is placed under the fragment to help elevate it and prevent divergence of the drill deep to the fragment.

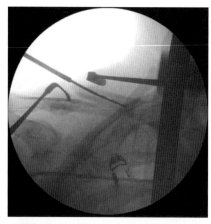

Figure 10 Fluoroscopic image of a clavicle demonstrates the 2-mm drill bit in proper orientation in the medullary canal of the medial fragment.

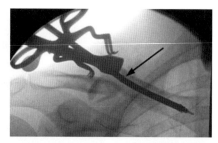

Figure 11 Fluoroscopic image of a clavicle demonstrates a 4.5-mm flexible reamer passed over a guidewire. Note the band (arrow) on the reamer, indicating a depth of 50 mm past the fracture site.

- A flexible guide pin is then passed into the medullary canal under fluoroscopic guidance until it is at least 50 mm past the fracture site. When using the hybrid fixation device, the tip of the flexible end must be placed at least 50 mm past the end of the fracture because lesser fixation may place excessive force on the junction between the rigid and flexible portions of the device and could cause early failure. Alternately, if 50 mm cannot be obtained, then the hybrid fixation device can be reversed, with the flexible portion placed in the other fragment, or the surgeon can consider using either a rigid or completely flexible device such as a titanium elastic nail or plate-and-screw fixation (**Figure 4**).
- If the bone within the canal is too dense to allow passage of the guide pin, a curved 3-mm awl can be used to further open the canal. Care must be taken to advance the awl using a short back-and-forth motion. Excessive motion can lead to eccentric reaming of the canal. The awl should be passed at least 50 mm past the fracture site. The

awl is then removed and replaced with the guide pin.
- The medial canal is reamed with a flexible 4.5-mm reamer (**Figure 11**). Care must be taken not to pass the reamer too quickly or to force the reamer into the canal because the flutes of the reamer can fill with bone, causing substantial friction that can lead to thermal necrosis of the bone.
- If resistance is encountered, the reamer should be removed and bone should be cleared from the flutes before the reaming is continued.
- After the reamer is at least 50 mm past the fracture site, reaming can be continued until resistance is encountered; however, the surgeon should be aware that when rigid fixation devices are used in older patients with large-diameter canals, a broader medial canal may compromise fixation rather than improve it.
- If the guide pin penetrates the anteromedial cortex, the tendency is for the guide pin to continue to go out the same perforation. In this situation, a small, curved Frazier suction device can be used to manipulate the guide pin past

the perforation. After the canal is reamed with the cannulated reamer, the final fixation device will follow the canal because the perforation is too small to allow passage through it.

PREPARATION OF THE LATERAL FRAGMENT

- Preparation of the lateral canal can be difficult and is critical to the technique.
- The ideal exit point in the posterolateral clavicle is halfway between the conoid tubercle and the distal clavicle and typically lies at the equator of the clavicle.
- Some patients may have an exaggerated downward lateral curve of the clavicle. In these patients, the exit point will be more superior.
- The exit point should never be below the equator of the lateral clavicle because a lower exit point would cause the distal fragment to be flexed upward relative to the medial fragment. This can cause excessive rotation of the distal fragment relative to the medial fragment or problems passing the final fixation device past the spine of the scapula.
- Although achieving the correct exit point may seem daunting, it can easily be accomplished with proper drilling under fluoroscopic guidance.

- In most patients with a lateral impact-type fracture, the lateral fragment is usually located posterior and inferior to the distal end of the medial fragment. In patients with seat belt fractures, however, the medial end of the lateral fragment may be located anterior to the medial fragment.
- After the fragment is identified, it is grasped with a towel clamp and carefully elevated into the incision. A 0.5-inch (12.7-mm) Key elevator placed under the tip of the fragment can be used to help elevate the fragment.
- As with the medial fragment, a 2-mm drill bit is used under fluoroscopic guidance to establish the orientation of the lateral canal. A 2-mm drill bit is used because the orientation can be changed without compromise of the canal.
- The drill bit should be oriented toward the midpoint of the posterior cortex of the lateral fragment. (If the lateral fragment were a hockey stick, the drill would be aimed at the midpoint of the blade.) This orientation can be facilitated by forward flexing the arm to allow an axillary view of the distal fragment.
- The surgeon can use his or her index finger as an aiming device by placing the tip of the index finger at the V formed by the junction of the lateral clavicle and the spine of the scapula, with the distal interphalangeal joint of the finger positioned at the acromioclavicular joint.
- After the correct orientation is established, the patient's arm is extended to allow an AP view of the distal fragment. On this view, the drill bit should be aiming at the equator of the clavicle (**Figures 6** and **7**).
- The canal can then be further opened with a 3-mm drill bit. After the position of the drill bit is verified, it is passed through the posterolateral cortex.

- A small incision is made over the palpable tip of the drill.
- The 3-mm drill bit is then removed and replaced with a rigid Steinmann pin, which is brought out through the posterior skin incision.
- The lateral canal is opened farther with a 4.5-mm cannulated drill bit passed in a retrograde fashion over the rigid guide pin.
- After the 4.5-mm drill bit reaches the fracture site, the rigid guide pin is removed.

FRACTURE REDUCTION

- The 4.5-mm drill bit is used to help achieve fracture reduction. With downward pressure on the medial fragment and upward force on the elbow to counteract the deformity caused by gravity, the tip of the drill bit can be placed into the canal of the medial fragment and advanced a short distance. This technique aids in temporarily holding the reduction.
- After the reduction is verified under fluoroscopy, a flexible guidewire is passed through the 4.5-mm drill bit and advanced until it is seated in the most medial aspect of the medial fragment.
- The 4.5-mm drill bit is then removed, and the entire length of the medullary canal is reamed with a 4.5-mm flexible reamer passed over the guidewire.
- In patients with a long oblique fracture, the fracture can be loosely held in a reduced position with a small bone reduction clamp to prevent shortening of the fracture.
- After the flexible reamer has been fully passed, the reduction is checked under fluoroscopy to ensure anatomic reduction. In general, if the reamer is in an intramedullary position in both the lateral fragment and the medial fragment, the fragments should be anatomically aligned.

- It is important to check the diameters of the fragments after the reduction is achieved. When viewed from any direction, the observed diameters of each fragment should appear to be the same. Different diameters are markers of rotational deformity, which must be corrected.
- After the reduction has been verified, a depth measurement is taken using the reamer.
- The reamer is removed, and a guide sleeve is passed over the guide pin.
- The guide pin is removed, and the incisions are copiously irrigated with antibiotic-laden fluid.

FINAL FIXATION

- An appropriately sized intramedullary pin is attached to the outrigger, and the tip of the final fixation device is slid along the guide sleeve until it lies in the lateral fragment.
- The sleeve is removed, and the fixation device is advanced until the tip can be seen at the medial end of the lateral fragment. It is important to advance the pin with direct pressure and not twist the device back and forth, because a twisting motion may damage the junction between the flexible and rigid portions of the pin.
- The same reduction maneuver that was used in the reaming step is performed, and the pin is advanced until it is fully seated.
- The hole in the device where the locking screw will be placed should be visualized fluoroscopically. This hole should lie just past the superior cortex to ensure adequate fixation of the locking screw.
- After the position is verified with fluoroscopy and the length is checked to ensure that the lateral end of the device is not prominent, the medial end of the pin is made rigid by inserting a torque-limiting screwdriver or actuator into the

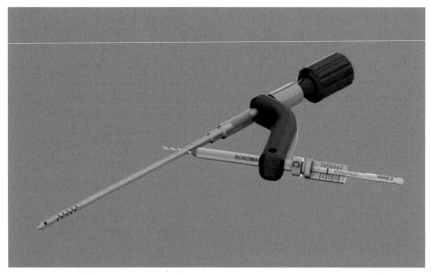

Figure 12 Photograph shows an intramedullary fixation device with outrigger and drill guide. (Courtesy of Sonoma Orthopaedics.)

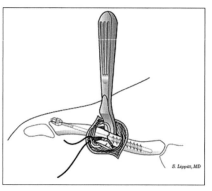

Figure 13 Illustration depicts a Crego elevator inserted under the clavicle to protect the underlying structures during passage of the cerclage suture. (Reproduced with permission from Basamania CJ, Rockwood CA Jr: Fractures of the clavicle, in Rockwood CA Jr, Matsen FA, Wirth MA, Lippitt SB, eds: *The Shoulder,* ed 3. Philadelphia, PA, Saunders, 2004, pp 381-451.)

lateral end of the pin and outrigger and turning it until the torque limit is reached and the medial grippers or talons are deployed (**Figure 12**). With this technique, the flexible portion of the device is converted to a rigid implant.

- The interlocking screw is placed by passing the guide through the outrigger until it contacts the posterolateral cortex.

- A 2-mm drill bit is passed through the drill guide, the distal clavicle, and pin until it passes through the anterior cortex.

- Because the drill bit can easily be deflected, its position in the pin should be checked by passing the actuator into the pin. The drill bit passing through the pin should prevent the actuator from fully seating. If the actuator fully seats within the device, then the drill bit did not go through the nail and thus, the drill bit must be repositioned or re-drilled in a different orientation.

- Depth is measured, and a screw of appropriate length is passed through the guide until it is fully seated. The actuator should be used to verify the passage of the screw through the pin.

MANAGEMENT OF BUTTERFLY FRAGMENTS

- After the pin is fully seated and locked into place, cerclage fixation can be used to restore the butterfly fragments to their proper place.

- A Crego elevator is passed from posterior to anterior under the clavicle and fragments.

- A No. 1 or No. 2 absorbable suture with a size 1 tapered needle is passed through the soft tissue attached to the butterfly fragments and then under the clavicle. Upward pressure should be kept on the needle to prevent it from going too deep and damaging underlying structures. Use of this particular size needle is important because it matches the curvature of the Crego elevator and makes passage of the needle easier.

- The needle is passed until it makes contact with the elevator. Because the curvature of the elevator and the size 1 needle are essentially the same, the needle should be deflected posteriorly and superiorly until it can be seen and grasped with a needle driver. This step is repeated to finish the cerclage fixation (**Figure 13**).

- The suture is tied, and the wound is irrigated again with antibiotic-laden solution.

Wound Closure

- The periosteum is closed over the fracture with multiple figure-of-8 sutures using size 0 absorbable suture.

- The platysma is repaired with size 2-0 absorbable suture, taking care not to damage the supraclavicular nerve.

- The skin is closed with size 3-0 absorbable inverted sutures and a running subcuticular nonabsorbable 3-0 suture.

- The posterior incision is closed with the same types of subcutaneous and subcuticular sutures.

- The wounds are infiltrated with a long-acting anesthetic and covered with a routine dressing.

- The patient's arm is placed in a sling for comfort.

- The patient's neurovascular status is checked and documented after the patient is alert in the recovery room.
- An additional dose of intravenous or intramuscular antibiotic is administered in the recovery room.

Alternate Approach: Medial

The same intramedullary fixation technique can be used in patients with more medial fractures or by surgeons who prefer a medial approach. It can also be used in patients in whom it is not possible to obtain at least 50 mm of fixation into the medial fragment. The only difference with this technique is that the fixation device is brought out through the medial cortex and then placed in an antegrade fashion into the lateral fragment without penetration of the lateral posterolateral cortex. The same positioning of the patient and the fluoroscopy unit can be used. However, with the medial approach, the procedure also can be performed with the patient in a supine position and the fluoroscopy unit on the patient's injured side because bringing the pin out through the posterior aspect of the shoulder is unnecessary. If the surgeon is using the hybrid device and cannot achieve at least 50 mm of fixation at the flexible end, the procedure must be performed with a medial approach to avoid locating the junction of the flexible and rigid parts of the device too close to the fracture site, where cantilever bending can cause metal fatigue and device failure.

Although both approaches can be successful in most patients, the author of this chapter has found that patients typically prefer to have only one anterior incision, rather than two as necessitated with the medial approach (**Figure 4**).

Rehabilitation

The patient is placed in a sling for comfort and is instructed to remove the sling and resume simple activities of daily living as soon as preferred postoperatively. The only restrictions are that the patient must avoid lifting more than 10 lb (4.5 kg) with the hand on the operated side, repeated use of the hand higher than shoulder level to prevent excessive torque on the fixation, and high-risk activities such as contact sports, biking, snowboarding, and horseback riding for 6 weeks. The patient is instructed to ice the surgical site for 20 minutes every 1 to 2 hours as necessary for pain control. The patient is seen in the clinic 7 to 10 days postoperatively, at which time AP and 45° cephalic tilt radiographs are obtained. The restrictions on upper extremity activity are continued until the patient is examined 6 weeks postoperatively; however, if the incisions are well healed at the first postoperative check, the patient is allowed to resume stationary bike training and running as tolerated and is cautioned to avoid falling on the surgical side. Repeat radiographs are obtained at 6 weeks postoperatively. If bridging callus is seen and the fracture site is not tender, the patient is allowed to advance upper extremity activities as tolerated. If no callus is seen, weight and motion restrictions are continued. The patient is seen again at 12 weeks postoperatively, and repeat radiographs are obtained. If the fracture appears to be completely healed, which is the case in most fractures by this time, unrestricted activity is allowed, and implant removal is scheduled if the patient desires it. The rehabilitation protocol is summarized in **Table 3**.

Implant Removal

Implant removal is usually performed in an ambulatory surgical center with intravenous sedation and local anesthesia.

The patient is placed in the beach-chair position, and a fluoroscopy unit is placed over the surgical shoulder as in the original procedure. After induction of intravenous sedation and routine prepping of the shoulder, the area around the posterior incision is infiltrated with a short-acting anesthetic with lidocaine. The incision is reopened and taken sharply down to the level of the lateral device. Under fluoroscopic guidance, the interlocking screw is localized and removed. The torque-limiting screwdriver or actuator is placed in an extraction adaptor, and the tip of the actuator is inserted into the distal end of the implant under fluoroscopic guidance. The extractor is slid down the actuator and tightened into the lateral end of the implant. The actuator is then used to deactivate the flexible portion of the implant and release tension on the grippers. A slap hammer is attached to the extraction adaptor, and the device is removed. The skin is infiltrated with long-acting anesthetic and closed using the same method as in the primary procedure.

Resumption of all activities of daily living is allowed immediately after implant removal; however, contact sports are not allowed for 4 weeks. The wound is checked in the clinic at 7 to 10 days postoperatively and again at 4 to 6 weeks postoperatively, at which time repeat radiographs are obtained. In the absence of complications, the patient is allowed to return to unrestricted activity as tolerated.

Avoiding Pitfalls

The patient should be placed in the beach-chair position to ensure that adequate fluoroscopic images of the clavicle can be obtained. Before starting the procedure, it is important to ensure that the medial and most lateral aspects of the clavicle can be visualized fluoroscopically. The shoulder

Table 3 Rehabilitation Protocol After Intramedullary Fixation of Middle Third Clavicle Fracture

Postoperative Week	Range of Motion	Strengthening	Return to Play	Comments/Emphasis
0-2	No repeated use of the hand higher than shoulder level No lifting of >10 lb	No physical therapy	Running and use of a stationary bike is allowed No contact sports	A sling is worn for comfort
2-6	Activities and lifting advanced as tolerated	Physical therapy only if necessary	No contact sports	Repeated use of the hand higher than shoulder level is not allowed
6-12	Unrestricted activity in the presence of clinical fracture healing	Physical therapy only if necessary	Contact sports are allowed if clinical and radiographic evidence of healing is present	Because intramedullary devices are load sharing, upper extremity strengthening activities are encouraged
12-24	Unrestricted	Unrestricted	If implant is removed, no contact sports for 4 wk after removal	Can consider implant removal during or after this period if radiographs show complete healing

should be draped with the arm free, with exposure continued to the sternoclavicular joint on the affected side. Care should be taken to identify and protect the middle branch of the supraclavicular nerve. Periosteal stripping of the medial and lateral fragments must be avoided, and the soft-tissue attachments and blood supply of comminuted fracture fragments must be preserved. The medial fragment canal should be prepared as deeply as possible, continuing at least 50 mm past the fracture site when using hybrid fixation. If it is not possible to achieve that depth, the surgeon should consider reversing the orientation of the device or switch to a different type of fixation such as a titanium flexible nail or a plate-and-screw construct. The exit point in the lateral fragment should be halfway between the conoid tubercle of the clavicle and the acromioclavicular joint and at the equator or midpoint of the lateral fragment. If the medullary canal cannot accommodate the 4.2-mm hybrid device, a titanium flexible nail with a smaller diameter or plate fixation should be considered. If a rigid intramedullary fixation device is used, it is important not to lose the normal curvature of the clavicle; if a titanium flexible nail device is used, the surgeon should consider prebending it before implantation. Using the longest possible intramedullary nail helps achieve the highest level of stability and reduce the chance of device failure. The soft-tissue attachments should be left on the comminuted fragments and secured back onto the main fragments with absorbable cerclage sutures. Patients should be cautioned to avoid repeated overhead use of their injured extremity to prevent excessive torque on the clavicle and avoid lifting more than 5 to 10 lb with the affected side until bridging callus is seen.

Bibliography

Abo El Nor T: Displaced mid-shaft clavicular fractures: Surgical treatment with intramedullary screw fixation. *Arch Orthop Trauma Surg* 2013;133(10):1395-1399.

Assobhi JE: Reconstruction plate versus minimal invasive retrograde titanium elastic nail fixation for displaced midclavicular fractures. *J Orthop Traumatol* 2011;12(4):185-192.

Bachoura A, Deane AS, Kamineni S: Clavicle anatomy and the applicability of intramedullary midshaft fracture fixation. *J Shoulder Elbow Surg* 2012;21(10):1384-1390.

Bain GI, Eng K, Zumstein MA: Fatal air embolus during internal fixation of the clavicle: A case report. *JBJS Case Connect* 2013;3(1):e24.

Barlow T, Beazley J, Barlow D: A systematic review of plate versus intramedullary fixation in the treatment of midshaft clavicle fractures. *Scott Med J* 2013;58(3):163-167.

Böhme J, Bonk A, Bacher GO, Wilharm A, Hoffmann R, Josten C: Current treatment concepts for mid-shaft fractures of the clavicle: Results of a prospective multicentre study [German]. *Z Orthop Unfall* 2011;149(1):68-76.

Canadian Orthopaedic Trauma Society: Nonoperative treatment compared with plate fixation of displaced midshaft clavicular fractures: A multicenter, randomized clinical trial. *J Bone Joint Surg Am* 2007;89(1):1-10.

Chen YF, Wei HF, Zhang C, et al: Retrospective comparison of titanium elastic nail (TEN) and reconstruction plate repair of displaced midshaft clavicular fractures. *J Shoulder Elbow Surg* 2012;21(4):495-501.

Duan X, Zhong G, Cen S, Huang F, Xiang Z: Plating versus intramedullary pin or conservative treatment for midshaft fracture of clavicle: A meta-analysis of randomized controlled trials. *J Shoulder Elbow Surg* 2011;20(6):1008-1015.

Ferran NA, Hodgson P, Vannet N, Williams R, Evans RO: Locked intramedullary fixation vs plating for displaced and shortened mid-shaft clavicle fractures: A randomized clinical trial. *J Shoulder Elbow Surg* 2010;19(6):783-789.

Frigg A, Rillmann P, Perren T, Gerber M, Ryf C: Intramedullary nailing of clavicular midshaft fractures with the titanium elastic nail: Problems and complications. *Am J Sports Med* 2009;37(2):352-359.

Fu TH, Tan BL, Liu HC, Wang JW: Anatomical reduction for treatment of displaced midshaft clavicular fractures: Knowles pinning vs. reconstruction plating. *Orthopedics* 2012;35(1):e23-e30.

Harnroongroj T, Jeerathanyasakun Y: Intramedullary pin fixation in clavicular fractures: A study comparing the use of small and large pins. *J Orthop Surg (Hong Kong)* 2000;8(2):7-11.

Houwert RM, Wijdicks FJ, Steins Bisschop C, Verleisdonk EJ, Kruyt M: Plate fixation versus intramedullary fixation for displaced mid-shaft clavicle fractures: A systematic review. *Int Orthop* 2012;36(3):579-585.

Jubel A, Andemahr J, Bergmann H, Prokop A, Rehm KE: Elastic stable intramedullary nailing of midclavicular fractures in athletes. *Br J Sports Med* 2003;37(6):480-483, discussion 484.

Jubel A, Andermahr J, Schiffer G, Tsironis K, Rehm KE: Elastic stable intramedullary nailing of midclavicular fractures with a titanium nail. *Clin Orthop Relat Res* 2003;408:279-285.

Kettler M, Schieker M, Braunstein V, König M, Mutschler W: Flexible intramedullary nailing for stabilization of displaced midshaft clavicle fractures: Technique and results in 87 patients. *Acta Orthop* 2007;78(3):424-429.

Khalil A: Intramedullary screw fixation for midshaft fractures of the clavicle. *Int Orthop* 2009;33(5):1421-1424.

King PR, Ikram A, Lamberts RP: The treatment of clavicular shaft fractures with an innovative locked intramedullary device. *J Shoulder Elbow Surg* 2015;24(1):e1-e6.

Kleweno CP, Jawa A, Wells JH, et al: Midshaft clavicular fractures: Comparison of intramedullary pin and plate fixation. *J Shoulder Elbow Surg* 2011;20(7):1114-1117.

Lee YS, Huang HL, Lo TY, Hsieh YF, Huang CR: Surgical treatment of midclavicular fractures: A prospective comparison of Knowles pinning and plate fixation. *Int Orthop* 2008;32(4):541-545.

Liu HH, Chang CH, Chia WT, Chen CH, Tarng YW, Wong CY: Comparison of plates versus intramedullary nails for fixation of displaced midshaft clavicular fractures. *J Trauma* 2010;69(6):E82-E87.

Millett PJ, Hurst JM, Horan MP, Hawkins RJ: Complications of clavicle fractures treated with intramedullary fixation. *J Shoulder Elbow Surg* 2011;20(1):86-91.

Ngarmukos C, Parkpian V, Patradul A: Fixation of fractures of the midshaft of the clavicle with Kirschner wires: Results in 108 patients. *J Bone Joint Surg Br* 1998;80(1):106-108.

Perren SM: Evolution of the internal fixation of long bone fractures: The scientific basis of biological internal fixation. Choosing a new balance between stability and biology. *J Bone Joint Surg Br* 2002;84(8):1093-1110.

Richardson M, Asadollahi S, Richardson L: Management of acute displaced midshaft clavicular fractures using Herbert cannulated screw: Technique and results in 114 patients. *Int J Shoulder Surg* 2013;7(2):52-58.

Saha P, Datta P, Ayan S, Garg AK, Bandyopadhyay U, Kundu S: Plate versus titanium elastic nail in treatment of displaced midshaft clavicle fractures: A comparative study. *Indian J Orthop* 2014;48(6):587-593.

Smekal V, Irenberger A, Struve P, Wambacher M, Krappinger D, Kralinger FS: Elastic stable intramedullary nailing versus nonoperative treatment of displaced midshaft clavicular fractures: a randomized, controlled, clinical trial. *J Orthop Trauma* 2009;23(2):106-112.

Smith SD, Wijdicks CA, Jansson KS, et al: Stability of mid-shaft clavicle fractures after plate fixation versus intramedullary repair and after hardware removal. *Knee Surg Sports Traumatol Arthrosc* 2014;22(2):448-455.

Thyagarajan DS, Day M, Dent C, Williams R, Evans R: Treatment of mid-shaft clavicle fractures: A comparative study. *Int J Shoulder Surg* 2009;3(2):23-27.

Wang K, Dowrick A, Choi J, Rahim R, Edwards E: Post-operative numbness and patient satisfaction following plate fixation of clavicular fractures. *Injury* 2010;41(10):1002-1005.

Wenninger JJ Jr, Dannenbaum JH, Branstetter JG, Arrington ED: Comparison of complication rates of intramedullary pin fixation versus plating of midshaft clavicle fractures in an active duty military population. *J Surg Orthop Adv* 2013;22(1):77-81.

Wijdicks FJ, Houwert M, Dijkgraaf M, et al: Complications after plate fixation and elastic stable intramedullary nailing of dislocated midshaft clavicle fractures: A retrospective comparison. *Int Orthop* 2012;36(10):2139-2145.

Wijdicks FJ, Houwert RM, Millett PJ, Verleisdonk EJ, Van der Meijden OA: Systematic review of complications after intramedullary fixation for displaced midshaft clavicle fractures. *Can J Surg* 2013;56(1):58-64.

Wijdicks FJ, Van der Meijden OA, Millett PJ, Verleisdonk EJ, Houwert RM: Systematic review of the complications of plate fixation of clavicle fractures. *Arch Orthop Trauma Surg* 2012;132(5):617-625.

Zehir S, Zehir R, Şahin E, Çalbıyık M: Comparison of novel intramedullary nailing with mini-invasive plating in surgical fixation of displaced midshaft clavicle fractures. *Arch Orthop Trauma Surg* 2015;135(3):339-344.

Chapter 53

Options for Management of Distal Clavicle Fractures and Acromioclavicular Joint Separation

Randa Berdusco, MD, MSc, FRCS

Peter B. MacDonald, MD, FRCS

Distal Clavicle Fractures

Distal clavicle fractures are classified on the basis of their relationship to the coracoclavicular (CC) ligaments in the Neer classification and the Craig subclassification (**Figure 1**). Type I fractures occur lateral to the CC ligaments and typically have minimal displacement because the trapezoid and conoid ligaments remain intact. Type II fractures are characterized by detachment of the CC ligaments from the medial segment. These fractures are subdivided into type IIA fractures, which occur medial to the intact CC ligaments, and type IIB fractures, which occur between a disrupted conoid ligament and an intact trapezoid ligament. The trapezoid ligament remains attached to the lateral clavicular fragment. Type II fractures are often characterized by substantial clavicular displacement (>100% of the width of the clavicle) and instability because the medial fragment is pulled superiorly and posteriorly by the trapezius muscle while the lateral fragment is drawn distally by the weight of the arm and medially via scapular rotation and the pull of the pectoral and latissimus dorsi muscles. Type III fractures extend into the acromioclavicular (AC) joint and typically have minimal displacement because the CC ligaments remain intact.

Type I and III lateral clavicle fractures are typically managed nonsurgically with sling immobilization. Type III fractures may lead to eventual AC arthrosis or osteolysis requiring distal clavicle excision. Type II fractures are often managed surgically because of their displacement and inherent instability and the increased risk of nonunion with nonsurgical management. Advanced patient age (65 years or older), smoking, and the amount of fracture displacement have been shown to be independent risk factors for nonunion. The clinical relevance of nonunion after distal clavicle fracture has been called into question because nonunion does not appear to affect functional outcomes, and nonsurgical management is associated with fewer complications. However, surgical management of displaced type II distal clavicle fractures remains the most common treatment, although no consensus exists as to the optimal method of surgical fixation. A multitude of surgical procedures, each with advantages and disadvantages, are described in the literature with high rates of fracture union, good functional outcomes, and acceptable complication rates.

Case Presentation

A 36-year-old man is seen in the clinic after sustaining a direct lateral blow to his right shoulder while playing hockey. Clinical examination reveals a moderate bump deformity and point tenderness over the distal clavicle. Preoperative radiographs demonstrate a displaced type IIA distal clavicle fracture. After discussion of the options, surgical treatment with distal clavicle locking plate fixation is chosen. This treatment was chosen because of the presence of good bone stock and fixation potential as well as the high risk of nonunion associated with nonsurgical treatment of this fracture type.

Indications

Indications for surgical management of distal clavicle fractures include open fractures, compromised overlying skin, and associated neurovascular injury requiring surgical management. Nonsurgical management may be considered, especially in elderly patients or those with contraindications to surgical treatment; however, the authors of this chapter prefer to manage displaced

Dr. MacDonald or an immediate family member has received research or institutional support from Arthrex, ConMed Linvatec, and Össur, and serves as a board member, owner, officer, or committee member of American Shoulder and Elbow Surgeons. Neither Dr. Berdusco nor any immediate family member has received anything of value from or has stock or stock options held in a commercial company or institution related directly or indirectly to the subject of this chapter.

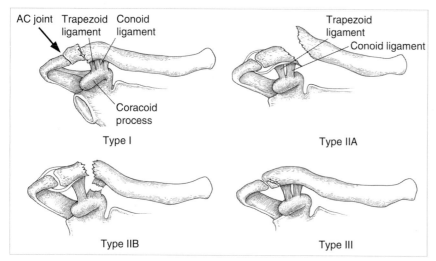

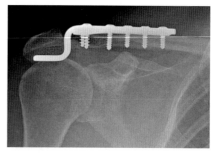

Figure 2 AP radiograph of a right shoulder demonstrates a type II distal clavicle fracture with a small distal fracture fragment that is insufficient to hold adequate screw fixation. A hook plate was used rather than a distal clavicle locking plate.

Figure 1 Illustration shows types I, IIA, IIB, and III in the Craig subclassification of the Neer classification of distal clavicle fractures. Type I fractures occur lateral to the intact coracoclavicular (CC) ligaments. Type IIA fractures occur medially to the intact CC ligaments. Type IIB fractures occur between the CC ligaments, disrupting the conoid and leaving the trapezoid intact. Type III fractures occur laterally to the intact CC ligaments, extending into the acromioclavicular (AC) joint. (Reproduced from Banerjee R, Waterman B, Padalecki J, Robertson W: Management of distal clavicle fractures. *J Am Acad Orthop Surg* 2011;19[7]:392-401.)

type II distal clavicle fractures with early surgical fixation using a low-profile pre-contoured distal clavicle locking plate. Achieving early fracture reduction and stability helps avoid the increased risk of nonunion associated with nonsurgical management and the greater complication rate associated with delayed fixation. Indications for later surgical management include symptomatic malunion, nonunion, and AC joint arthrosis.

A displaced type II distal clavicle fracture with CC ligamentous injury disrupts the superior shoulder suspensory complex. Fracture fixation and bony union typically are adequate to restore the stability of the complex; however, biomechanical evidence suggests that the combination of a distal clavicle locking plate and CC stabilization results in increased stiffness, maximum resistance to compression, and decreased displacement of type II distal clavicle fractures. If reinforcement of vertical clavicular stability is desired, heavy nonabsorbable sutures can be passed and secured under the base of the coracoid and around

or through the medial clavicular segment. As an alternative, a CC fixation device that keys into a custom distal clavicle plate can be used to augment the distal clavicle fixation.

If it becomes clear on open intraoperative assessment that distal fixation cannot be achieved with locking screw purchase because the lateral fragment is too small, comminuted, or of poor bone quality, a clavicular hook plate can be inserted through a lateral extension of the incision (**Figure 2**).

Controversies and Alternative Approaches

Because nonsurgical management of displaced type II clavicle fractures demonstrates functional outcomes equivalent to those of surgical management despite higher rates of nonunion in retrospective case series, some authors have questioned the necessity of surgical stabilization. Nonsurgical management avoids the risk of surgical complications and remains a viable option for minimally displaced type II clavicle fractures

if the patient is willing to accept the associated cosmetic deformity and increased risk of nonunion.

In addition to open internal fixation using distal clavicular locking or hook plates, numerous other surgical procedures have been described for the management of type II distal clavicle fractures. Primary or supplementary fixation methods include plate fixation (T-plates, distal radius plates, double plating), interfragmentary sutures, tension-band or cerclage wiring, transacromial or intramedullary fixation (Kirschner wires or Knowles pin), CC screw fixation, a modified Weaver-Dunn procedure, CC ligament repair or reconstruction, suture or sling techniques, and, most recently, arthroscopic CC stabilization using a double-button suture construct.

Results

Numerous retrospective case series have demonstrated high union rates, good functional outcomes, and acceptable rates of complications after the surgical management of type II distal clavicle fractures. Because of the heterogeneity and evolution of the techniques, together with the retrospective nature of the studies, the small size of the case series, and differing definitions of complications, no consensus has been reached.

The literature on nonsurgical and surgical management options (not including arthroscopic stabilization) is summarized in **Table 1**.

Technical Keys to Success: Distal Clavicle Locking Plate Fixation

SETUP/EXPOSURE

- The patient is positioned supine in a modified beach-chair position with the head of the bed elevated 30°.
- A 1-L intravenous bag is placed under the patient between the scapulae, and the patient's head is rotated to the contralateral side.
- Preoperative fluoroscopic images are obtained to ensure that adequate views of the distal clavicle can be obtained.
- The arm is draped free, with adequate exposure of the clavicle and AC joint.
- An anterior horizontal incision using a standard anterosuperior approach to the clavicle is made.
- Dissection is carried down to the distal clavicle, and the fracture site is delineated after the removal of any interfragmentary debris or hematoma. Care must be taken to avoid stripping any comminuted fragments and to preserve the superior AC joint ligaments.

INSTRUMENTS/EQUIPMENT/ IMPLANTS REQUIRED

- The authors of this chapter recommend preparing a supplemental CC stabilization technique (such as heavy nonabsorbable sutures, suture anchors, or a double-button construct) for use in situations in which increased vertical stability may be helpful, such as in patients with proximal segment instability or severe displacement that makes fracture reduction difficult to achieve or maintain and in patients with increased physical demands or higher expectations of postoperative results.

PROCEDURE

- The fracture is anatomically reduced and held in place with the use of a small reduction clamp. Kirschner wires may be used to aid in fracture reduction.
- If the fracture pattern allows for placement of an interfragmentary lag screw, a 3.5-mm small-fragment countersunk screw is placed to avoid interference with the plate.
- A precontoured low-profile distal clavicle locking plate is sized and positioned on the superior clavicle. Handheld plate benders are used if needed for additional contouring.
- The plate is placed on the reduced clavicle and held by a reduction clamp.
- The plate is secured with multiple divergent locking screws placed in the lateral fragment and with nonlocking and locking screws placed in the medical clavicle shaft.
- Anatomic fracture reduction and adequate hardware position may be confirmed with the use of intraoperative fluoroscopy; however, the technical difficulty of obtaining adequate intraoperative images often makes direct visualization of the fracture preferable.

WOUND CLOSURE

- The deltotrapezial fascia is approximated over the plate and meticulously closed to cover the superior clavicle.
- Subcuticular closure is performed.

Rehabilitation

Postoperatively, the patient uses a sling for 6 weeks. Radiographs are obtained in the recovery room and at 6 weeks postoperatively to evaluate alignment and evidence of healing. A gentle pendulum shoulder exercise program and active elbow, wrist, and hand range of motion are begun immediately; however, complete immobilization is recommended if patient compliance is a concern. The rehabilitation protocol is summarized in **Table 2**.

Avoiding Pitfalls

To optimize patient selection, preoperative discussion with the patient regarding expectations and physical demands as well as nonsurgical treatment options and the possible need for a secondary procedure for hardware removal is recommended. If surgical fixation is chosen, the authors of this chapter prefer early intervention (<3 weeks from the date of injury) to avoid the increased complication rate and poorer functional outcomes observed with delayed surgical management.

The authors of this chapter do not recommend nonlocked plating (**Figure 3**), Kirschner wires, or CC screw fixation because serious complications, such as fixation failure, wire migration, and hardware breakage or pullout, have been reported with these techniques. If a hook plate is used, the authors of this chapter recommend routine plate removal at 3 to 6 months postoperatively, after bony union of the distal clavicle fracture is achieved. This time frame for plate removal helps prevent acromial osteolysis, hook migration, rotator cuff impingement or damage, and the poorer functional outcomes that have been reported in the literature if hook plates are left in place for more than 6 months postoperatively.

AC Joint Separation

The AC joint is stabilized in the horizontal plane by the AC ligaments, especially the posterior and superior portions. The trapezoid and conoid CC ligaments provide vertical stability. The Rockwood modification of the Tossy classification includes six types of AC joint injury (**Table 3**).

Superior displacement is defined radiographically by an increase in the CC interspace compared with the

Table 1 Results of Treatment of Type II Distal Clavicle Fractures

Authors	Journal (Year)	Technique (No. of Fractures)	Outcomes	Failure Rate (%)	Comments
Robinson and Cairns	*J Bone Joint Surg Am* (2004)	Nonsurgical management (101)	No difference in functional outcome scores between patients with nonunion and those with union or between surgical and nonsurgical management	14 (delayed surgery to manage persistent symptoms) 24 (nonunion)[a]	Mean follow-up, 6.2 yr (range, 2-10 yr)
Oh et al	*Arch Orthop Trauma Surg* (2011)	Nonsurgical management (60) Hook plate (162) Coracoclavicular stabilization (105) Intramedullary fixation (42) Interfragmentary fixation (16) Kirschner wire plus tension-band wiring (40)	All functional outcome scores were satisfactory No significant difference in functional outcome scores between nonsurgical and surgical treatment 98% union across all types of fixation	33 (nonunion after nonsurgical management)	Systematic review of 21 studies Complication rates higher with surgical management (22.2%) compared with nonsurgical management (6.7%) Higher rates of complications associated with hook plate (40.7%) and Kirschner wire plus tension-band wiring (20.0%) fixation compared with coracoclavicular stabilization (4.8%), intramedullary fixation (2.4%), and interfragmentary fixation (6.3%)
Stegeman et al	*Acta Orthop* (2013)	Hook plate (143) Other plates: distal radius locking (20), double (9) Intramedullary fixation: Knowles pins (68), coracoclavicular screws (30), malleolar screws (10) Suture anchoring/tension bands: Kirschner wires with suture anchors (10), tension-band suturing (43), synthetic absorbable tape (6) Synthetic polyester fiber arterial graft (11)	Similar functional outcomes across all types of fixation (all good to excellent) 98% union across all types of fixation	2 (nonunion)	Meta-analysis of 21 studies Longer time to union with hook plate fixation compared with pin fixation (avg 10 wk longer) Higher complication rates associated with hook plate fixation (11 times higher compared with intramedullary fixation and 24 times higher compared with suture anchoring)
Zhang et al	*Int Orthop* (2014)	Hook plate (322) Distal locking plate (186)	Similar excellent functional outcome scores across both groups 98% union rate for both groups	2 (nonunion)	Systematic review of 21 studies Higher complication rate with hook plate (30.4%) compared with locking plate (7.5%)

[a] Percentage based on the 87 patients who did not have delayed surgery.

contralateral side. The posterior displacement of type IV AC joint separations is best visualized on axillary radiographs. Type V injuries involve complete tearing of the AC and CC ligaments with a more than 100% increase of the CC interspace and associated rupture of the deltotrapezial fascia, resulting in a subcutaneous distal clavicle.

Table 2 Rehabilitation Protocol After Fixation of Distal Clavicle Fracture

Postoperative Week	ROM	Strengthening	Return to Play	Comments/ Emphasis
0-2	Gentle pendulum exercise program	None	Not allowed	Sling immobilization
2-6	Gentle pendulum exercise program	None	Not allowed	Sling immobilization
6-12	Supine passive and active-assisted ROM; progressive active ROM is begun at 8 wk	Permitted at 10 wk if clinical and radiographic signs of healing are evident	Not allowed	Physical therapy initiated
12-24	Unrestricted	Allowed after clinical and radiographic signs of healing	Permitted at 4-6 mo if clinical and radiographic signs of healing are evident	—

ROM = range of motion.

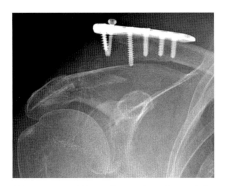

Figure 3 AP radiograph of a right shoulder demonstrates lateral failure of a nonlocking plate 5 weeks after fixation of a distal clavicle fracture.

The extremely rare type VI AC joint dislocation is characterized by inferior subcoracoid or subacromial displacement of the distal clavicle.

Type I and II AC joint separations typically are managed nonsurgically, with a brief period of sling immobilization and return to physical activity after pain has subsided and symmetric shoulder range of motion and strength are restored. The management of type III AC joint separations remains controversial. Historically, these injuries were managed surgically until numerous case series reported good to excellent functional outcomes with nonsurgical management. Reports of persistent pain

and symptoms on long-term follow-up after nonsurgical management have led to renewed enthusiasm for surgical management of acute type III AC joint separations in an attempt to improve functional outcomes, particularly in young overhead athletes, patients who work as laborers, and patients with higher functional demands. The literature, however, is limited by the use of outdated and heterogeneous surgical techniques, retrospective study designs, and variable outcome measures. The current consensus regarding the management of type III AC joint separations is that nonsurgical and surgical management typically result in similar functional outcomes, but surgical management is associated with a higher complication rate and longer time required to return to work or previous activities. A trial of 3 to 6 months of nonsurgical management for type III AC joint separations is therefore recommended, although surgical treatment should be considered in patients with higher demands, skin compromise, or failure of initial nonsurgical treatment.

Surgical management of type V injuries is widely accepted to address the associated cosmetic deformity and maximize patient function; however, no consensus exists as to the optimal

surgical technique. The rare type IV and VI AC joint separations also are managed surgically.

Case Presentation

A 21-year-old man is seen in the clinic after falling onto the lateral aspect of his left shoulder with the arm in an adducted position. Clinical examination is performed with the patient in the sitting and standing positions, and a subcutaneous prominence of the distal clavicle is noted. Preoperative radiographs, including a bilateral Zanca view (AP view of the AC joint with 10° to 15° cephalic tilt), indicate a type V separation of the left AC joint (**Figure 4**). After discussion of the surgical and nonsurgical options, the patient chooses surgical treatment.

Indications

Surgical management of AC joint separation is indicated in patients with type IV, V, and VI injuries; open fractures; compromised skin; or previous failed nonsurgical treatment. Surgical management also can be considered in high-demand patients with acute type III separation. Numerous techniques have been described, all of which have the goals of eliminating the possibility of hardware or soft-tissue failure, eliminating the possibility of late degenerative

Table 3 Summary of the Rockwood Acromioclavicular Joint Injury Classification

Injury Type	Acromioclavicular Ligament	CC Ligaments	Deltotrapezial Fascia	Displacement
I	Sprained/partially torn	Intact	Intact	Nondisplaced
II	Disrupted	Sprained	Intact	<25% increase in CC distance
III	Disrupted	Disrupted	Injured	25%-100% increase in CC distance
IV	Disrupted	Disrupted	Detached	Posterior through trapezius
V	Disrupted	Disrupted	Detached	>100% increase in CC distance
VI	Disrupted	Disrupted	Detached	Subcoracoid or subacromial

CC = coracoclavicular.

disease of the AC joint, and producing a cosmetically and functionally acceptable result.

The authors of this chapter prefer to manage high-grade AC joint separations with open distal clavicle resection and anatomic CC stabilization using a free semitendinosus muscle allograft or autograft. Autograft is preferred to reduce the risk of infection and accelerate graft incorporation. Because of the minimal soft-tissue coverage in this region, infection is more than a theoretical risk, particularly in persons who smoke or have diabetes and other patients at risk for wound healing complications. The reconstruction is combined with heavy suture augmentation passed under the coracoid and around the clavicle, in addition to reinforcement of the AC joint with the excess graft limbs.

Regardless of the technique or modifications used, attention to detail at every step is important to ensure a stable, lasting construct. The following principles are imperative: accurate reduction of the AC joint to correct vertical and horizontal instability, repair or reconstruction of the CC ligaments with supplemental augmentation (tape, sutures, rigid implant) to maintain stability during initial healing, distal clavicle excision (only in patients with chronic separation and underlying AC joint arthritis), and careful repair of the deltotrapezial fascia.

Preoperative templating to ascertain the appropriate distances of the CC

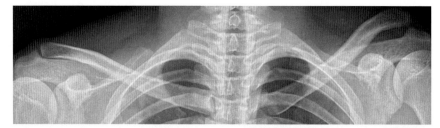

Figure 4 Bilateral AP radiograph of the acromioclavicular joints demonstrates a type V separation of the left acromioclavicular joint.

stabilization tunnels from the lateral clavicle may be helpful because medial tunnel placement is a risk factor for early loss of reduction. Trapezoid and conoid tunnel placement at 17% and 24% of the clavicular length (or 25 and 45 mm medial to the AC joint) has been shown to be effective in preventing loss of reduction.

Concomitant intra-articular shoulder pathology is not uncommon with high-grade AC separations, with a reported incidence of up to 30%. Preoperative MRI evaluation and subsequent arthroscopy have been increasingly used to identify and treat associated injuries, such as superior labrum anterior to posterior lesions, labral tears, and rotator cuff pathology, at the time of surgical management.

Controversies and Alternative Approaches

Nonsurgical treatment remains an option in patients with type V injuries who are poor candidates for surgery or who

are willing to accept the cosmetic and functional results of nonsurgical treatment. The multitude of surgical techniques can be divided into soft-tissue and bony repairs. In soft-tissue repair techniques, the focus is on repair or reconstruction of the AC and/or CC ligaments. The classic technique involves a distal clavicle resection and transfer of the coracoacromial ligament from the acromion to the clavicle. Subsequent modifications of this technique and numerous alternative approaches have been reported.

Arthroscopic or arthroscopically assisted techniques that include reconstruction of the CC ligaments using graft or synthetic material also have gained in popularity. Advantages of these techniques include the ability to address concomitant intra-articular shoulder pathology, limited soft-tissue dissection resulting in a decreased risk of wound complications, and facilitation of rehabilitation to promote earlier return to activities. The primary disadvantages of arthroscopic reconstructive techniques are their technical difficulty and increased surgical costs.

Bony repair involves the use of internal rigid fixation to reestablish the AC joint and to obtain secondary soft-tissue healing. This fixation may consist of CC screw fixation and pins or plates (commonly the hook plate) that transfix the AC joint. Disadvantages of rigid fixation include the need for a secondary procedure for hardware removal and the possibility of hardware pullout, migration, infection, and damage to the AC joint that may result in late arthritis.

Results

Numerous heterogeneous retrospective case series have examined the surgical management of type III and type V AC joint separations. A recent systematic review identified 120 studies describing 162 techniques for surgical reconstruction of the AC joint. No consensus exists regarding a superior technique; however, several biomechanical studies support anatomic reconstruction of the AC joint because these techniques re-create the native stability more closely compared with other techniques. Recent studies of anatomic reconstruction techniques are summarized in **Table 4**. Although loss of reduction over time is commonly observed and complication rates are substantial, the outcomes of AC joint reconstruction are largely satisfactory.

Technical Keys to Success: Semitendinosus Autograft Anatomic Reconstruction

SETUP/EXPOSURE
- The patient is positioned supine in a modified beach-chair position with the head of the bed elevated 30°.
- A 1-L intravenous bag is placed under the affected scapula, and the patient's head is rotated to the contralateral side.
- The arm is draped free, with adequate exposure of the AC joint.

- The contralateral leg is draped free to expose the hamstring harvest site at the knee.

PROCEDURE
- An incision is made in the Langer lines from the posterior extent of the distal clavicle anteriorly to the level of the coracoid.
- Dissection is carried down to the distal clavicle, which is typically herniated through the trapezial fascia in patients with type V AC joint dislocation.
- Soft-tissue release is performed to achieve reduction of the AC joint.
- The distal 5 mm of the clavicle is resected perpendicular to the shaft of the clavicle with a small oscillating saw.
- Dissection is carried down to the coracoid via splitting of the overlying anterior deltoid fibers.
- Subperiosteal dissection is performed around the coracoid base (approximately 3 cm from its tip).
- A hemostat, curved forceps, and a curved suture-passing device are passed around the coracoid base.
- A single No. 1 monofilament suture is passed around the coracoid to be used later for graft shuttling.
- The semitendinosus autograft is harvested from the contralateral knee through an oblique incision at the pes anserinus with the use of a tendon stripper. Care must be taken to release all fibrous bands to the gastrocnemius muscle.
- The graft is prepared on the back table with the use of No. 2 nonabsorbable sutures whipstitched along both graft limbs.
- Careful exposure of the coracoid through a deltoid-splitting incision and medial and lateral release of the coracoid fascial attachments are performed, after which the No. 1 suture is used to shuttle the graft around the coracoid.
- Two No. 5 high-strength

nonabsorbable sutures are used for augmentation.
- The use of a curved suture passer facilitates subcoracoid suture passage.
- The distal clavicle is prepared with two drill holes at the insertion points of the trapezoid and conoid ligaments (**Figure 5**). These drill holes are created by passing a guidewire and then reaming the appropriate diameter determined via measurement of the ends of the semitendinosus graft (typically 5 to 6 mm).
- The graft limbs are passed through their respective holes in the clavicle to anatomically reconstruct the CC ligament. The graft limbs should remain uncrossed.
- The clavicle is reduced, and the No. 5 FiberTape augmentation sutures (Arthrex) are securely tied, with the knots located inferiorly between the clavicle and the coracoid. These sutures act as an internal splint until tendon-graft incorporation occurs biologically.
- With the clavicular reduction manually maintained, the passed graft ends are equally tensioned superiorly, and two bicortical, bioabsorbable polyetheretherketone interference screws are placed into the reamed holes to secure the graft to the clavicle (**Figure 6, A**).
- The excess free ends of the tendon graft are folded over, and the limb of the trapezoid ligament is sutured laterally toward the acromion or passed through a 5-mm drill hole in the acromion.
- The conoid limb is sutured laterally to the limb of the trapezoid ligament to further supplement the AC joint reconstruction (**Figure 6, B**).

WOUND CLOSURE
- The deltoid muscle and the deltotrapezial fascia are meticulously closed to cover the graft and

Table 4 Results of Anatomic Acromioclavicular Joint Reconstruction

Authors	Journal (Year)	Technique (No. and Type of Injuries)	Outcomes[a]	Failure Rate (%)	Comments
Tauber et al	*Am J Sports Med* (2009)	Semitendinosus autograft (12, chronic)	Excellent patient satisfaction and functional outcomes ASES score, 96 ± 5 Constant-Murley score, 93 ± 7	8.3	Use of semitendinosus autograft resulted in better clinical and radiographic outcomes compared with use of a modified Weaver-Dunn procedure ($P < 0.001$) The 1 failure involved loss of reduction after a traumatic fall
Carofino and Mazzocca	*J Shoulder Elbow Surg* (2010)	Semitendinosus allograft (17, 6-12 wk after injury)	Good-to-excellent functional outcomes ASES score, 92 ± 5 Constant-Murley score, 94.7 ± 5 SST score, 11.8 ± 0.4	17.6	Persistent pain accounted for 1 failure, 1 chronic infection, 1 loss of reduction
Salzmann et al	*Am J Sports Med* (2010)	Arthroscopically assisted with 2 double flip buttons (23, acute)	Good-to-excellent functional outcomes	34.8 (radiographic)	3 clinical failures excluded from the study required revision surgery The radiographic failures consisted of undercorrection, posterior displacement, or both Immediate arthroscopic anatomic reduction of an acute acromioclavicular separation provides satisfactory clinical outcome at intermediate follow-up Arthroscopic expertise required
Lädermann et al	*J Shoulder Elbow Surg* (2011)	Acromioclavicular and coracoclavicular nonabsorbable sutures (37, acute)	Excellent patient satisfaction and functional outcomes Constant-Murley score, 96 ± 7.7 DASH score, 7 ± 10.8	5.4	4 nonresorbable Ethibond No. 6 sutures (Ethicon) were used 1 failure required revision
Glanzmann et al	*Arch Orthop Trauma Surg* (2013)	Arthroscopically assisted double flip button (21, acute)	High patient satisfaction and functional outcomes Constant-Murley score, 90.2 ± 6.5 SST score, 11.5 (range, 8-12)	19	High patient satisfaction despite loss of radiographic reduction in 6 patients 2 of the 4 failures required revision
Martetschläger et al	*Am J Sports Med* (2013)	Cortical fixation buttons (13) or tendon grafts (46) with or without arthroscopic assistance (31 acute, 26 chronic)	Excellent patient satisfaction and functional outcome scores reported for the 43 patients without complication ASES score, 91 (range, 63-100)	23.1 (button group) 28.2 (tendon graft group)	No significant functional difference between patients with or without complications

ASES = American Shoulder and Elbow Surgeons shoulder outcome; DASH = Disabilities of the Arm, Shoulder and Hand; SST = Simple Shoulder Test.

[a] All results are mean or mean ± standard deviation values unless otherwise noted.

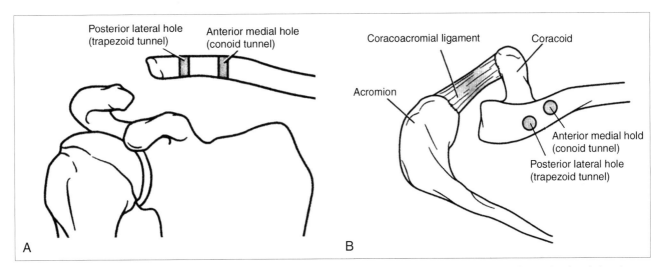

Figure 5 Illustrations of the frontal (**A**) and overhead (**B**) views of the shoulder show the two drill holes in the distal clavicle corresponding to the insertions of the trapezoid and conoid ligaments. The drill holes are placed thus in the semitendinosus autograft anatomic reconstruction technique.

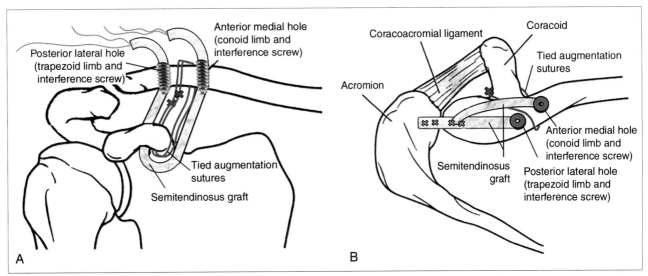

Figure 6 Illustrations show the method of graft passage in the semitendinosus autograft anatomic reconstruction technique. **A,** Frontal view of a shoulder shows the tied augmentation sutures passed under the coracoid and over the clavicle (purple), the passed semitendinosus graft fixed with two bicortical interference screws, and the excess graft ends that have been previously whipstitched (blue). **B,** Overhead view of a shoulder shows the excess semitendinosus graft ends folded laterally and fixed (with suture or through an acromion drill hole) for reinforcement of the acromioclavicular joint.

the superior clavicle.

- Wound closure is completed with a subcuticular suture.

Rehabilitation

Postoperatively, the patient uses a sling for 6 weeks, with only gentle range of motion of the elbow, wrist, and hand permitted. Pendulum shoulder exercises are delayed until 6 weeks postoperatively to avoid graft loosening or failure. Postoperative radiographs are obtained at 6 weeks (**Figure 7**). The rehabilitation protocol is summarized in **Table 5**. Rehabilitation begins with passive range of motion and progresses to active range of motion at postoperative week 8 and strengthening at postoperative week 10. Sport-specific exercises are begun at postoperative week 16, with return to noncontact sports at postoperative week 20 and contact sports 6 months postoperatively.

Avoiding Pitfalls

The complication rate associated with AC joint stabilization techniques is estimated to be 25% to 30%. Complications include superficial or deep wound infection, neurovascular injury, loss of reduction, residual cosmetic deformity, fracture of the clavicle or coracoid, implant failure, implant migration or irritation, persistent pain or dysfunction, adhesive capsulitis, development of late AC joint arthritis, and distal clavicle osteolysis. The complication most commonly observed by the authors of this chapter is an early partial loss of reduction; however, most patients do not experience symptoms and do not require additional surgical treatment.

Careful exposure and dissection around the coracoid is important to avoid injury to the major neurovascular bundle. Practice on a cadaver specimen is advised for surgeons who are not familiar with the local anatomy. Exposure and drilling of the clavicle must be done carefully, with adequate distance between drill holes to avoid fracture. To achieve an anatomic repair, the drill holes should be 25 and 45 mm medial from the distal end of the clavicle. After the graft is passed, reduction of the AC joint must be ensured before the graft is secured. Fracture of the clavicle between the two reamed holes can occur during the process of securing the graft or the bioabsorbable suture. This complication is a concern in contact athletes and patients with poor bone quality. If a fracture occurs, the graft and the augmentation sutures can be secured around the entire distal clavicle. The prominent semitendinosus tendon must be carefully covered during closure to avoid prominence or wound healing complications.

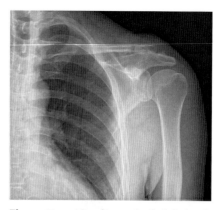

Figure 7 AP radiograph of a left shoulder obtained 6 weeks postoperatively demonstrates a type V acromioclavicular joint separation reconstructed with the use of a semitendinosus autograft. The excess trapezoid graft limb was used to reinforce the acromioclavicular joint laterally through an acromion drill hole. In this patient, the coracoclavicular ligament tunnels were placed too distally on the clavicle, which may increase the risk for clavicular fracture.

Table 5 Rehabilitation Protocol After Acromioclavicular Stabilization

Postoperative Week	ROM	Strengthening	Return to Play	Comments/Emphasis
0-2	Gentle ROM of elbow, wrist, and hand only	None	Not allowed	Sling immobilization
2-6	Gentle ROM of elbow, wrist, and hand only	None	Not allowed	Sling immobilization
6-10	Pendulum and full passive-assisted ROM is begun at 6 wk Progressive active ROM is begun at 8 wk	None	Not allowed	Physical therapy initiated
10-24	Full active and passive ROM allowed	Permitted at 10 wk	Permitted at 6 mo	Sport-specific exercises are begun at wk 16 Return to noncontact sports is allowed at 20 wk

ROM = range of motion.

Bibliography

Arrigoni P, Brady PC, Zottarelli L, et al: Associated lesions requiring additional surgical treatment in grade 3 acromioclavicular joint dislocations. *Arthroscopy* 2014;30(1):6-10.

Banerjee R, Waterman B, Padalecki J, Robertson W: Management of distal clavicle fractures. *J Am Acad Orthop Surg* 2011;19(7):392-401.

Beitzel K, Cote MP, Apostolakos J, et al: Current concepts in the treatment of acromioclavicular joint dislocations. *Arthroscopy* 2013;29(2):387-397.

Carofino BC, Mazzocca AD: The anatomic coracoclavicular ligament reconstruction: Surgical technique and indications. *J Shoulder Elbow Surg* 2010;19(2 suppl):37-46.

Checchia SL, Doneux PS, Miyazaki AN, Fregoneze M, Silva LA: Treatment of distal clavicle fractures using an arthroscopic technique. *J Shoulder Elbow Surg* 2008;17(3):395-398.

Cook JB, Shaha JS, Rowles DJ, Bottoni CR, Shaha SH, Tokish JM: Clavicular bone tunnel malposition leads to early failures in coracoclavicular ligament reconstructions. *Am J Sports Med* 2013;41(1):142-148.

Craig EV: Fractures of the clavicle, in Rockwood CA, Green DP, Bucholz RW, Heckman JD, eds: *Rockwood and Green's Fractures in Adults,* ed 4. Philadelphia, PA, Lippincott-Raven, 1996, pp 1109-1193.

Fukuda K, Craig EV, An KN, Cofield RH, Chao EY: Biomechanical study of the ligamentous system of the acromioclavicular joint. *J Bone Joint Surg Am* 1986;68(3):434-440.

Glanzmann MC, Buchmann S, Audigé L, Kolling C, Flury M: Clinical and radiographical results after double flip button stabilization of acute grade III and IV acromioclavicular joint separations. *Arch Orthop Trauma Surg* 2013;133(12):1699-1707.

Good DW, Lui DF, Leonard M, Morris S, McElwain JP: Clavicle hook plate fixation for displaced lateral-third clavicle fractures (Neer type II): A functional outcome study. *J Shoulder Elbow Surg* 2012;21(8):1045-1048.

Goss TP: Double disruptions of the superior shoulder suspensory complex. *J Orthop Trauma* 1993;7(2):99-106.

Grutter PW, Petersen SA: Anatomical acromioclavicular ligament reconstruction: A biomechanical comparison of reconstructive techniques of the acromioclavicular joint. *Am J Sports Med* 2005;33(11):1723-1728.

Johansen JA, Grutter PW, McFarland EG, Petersen SA: Acromioclavicular joint injuries: Indications for treatment and treatment options. *J Shoulder Elbow Surg* 2011;20(2 suppl):S70-S82.

Khan LA, Bradnock TJ, Scott C, Robinson CM: Fractures of the clavicle. *J Bone Joint Surg Am* 2009;91(2):447-460.

Klein SM, Badman BL, Keating CJ, Devinney DS, Frankle MA, Mighell MA: Results of surgical treatment for unstable distal clavicular fractures. *J Shoulder Elbow Surg* 2010;19(7):1049-1055.

Korsten K, Gunning AC, Leenen LP: Operative or conservative treatment in patients with Rockwood type III acromioclavicular dislocation: A systematic review and update of current literature. *Int Orthop* 2014;38(4):831-838.

Lädermann A, Grosclaude M, Lübbeke A, et al: Acromioclavicular and coracoclavicular cerclage reconstruction for acute acromioclavicular joint dislocations. *J Shoulder Elbow Surg* 2011;20(3):401-408.

Li X, Ma R, Bedi A, Dines DM, Altchek DW, Dines JS: Management of acromioclavicular joint injuries. *J Bone Joint Surg Am* 2014;96(1):73-84.

Loriaut P, Moreau PE, Dallaudiere B, et al: Outcome of arthroscopic treatment for displaced lateral clavicle fractures using a double button device. *Knee Surg Sports Traumatol Arthrosc* 2015;23(5):1429-1433.

MacDonald PB, Alexander MJ, Frejuk J, Johnson GE: Comprehensive functional analysis of shoulders following complete acromioclavicular separation. *Am J Sports Med* 1988;16(5):475-480.

Madsen W, Yaseen Z, LaFrance R, et al: Addition of a suture anchor for coracoclavicular fixation to a superior locking plate improves stability of type IIB distal clavicle fractures. *Arthroscopy* 2013;29(6):998-1004.

Martetschläger F, Horan MP, Warth RJ, Millett PJ: Complications after anatomic fixation and reconstruction of the coracoclavicular ligaments. *Am J Sports Med* 2013;41(12):2896-2903.

Milewski MD, Tompkins M, Giugale JM, Carson EW, Miller MD, Diduch DR: Complications related to anatomic reconstruction of the coracoclavicular ligaments. *Am J Sports Med* 2012;40(7):1628-1634.

Neer CS II: Fracture of the distal clavicle with detachment of the coracoclavicular ligaments in adults. *J Trauma* 1963;3:99-110.

Neer CS II: Fractures of the distal third of the clavicle. *Clin Orthop Relat Res* 1968;(58):43-50.

Oh JH, Kim SH, Lee JH, Shin SH, Gong HS: Treatment of distal clavicle fracture: A systematic review of treatment modalities in 425 fractures. *Arch Orthop Trauma Surg* 2011;131(4):525-533.

Rieser GR, Edwards K, Gould GC, Markert RJ, Goswami T, Rubino LJ: Distal-third clavicle fracture fixation: A biomechanical evaluation of fixation. *J Shoulder Elbow Surg* 2013;22(6):848-855.

Rios CG, Arciero RA, Mazzocca AD: Anatomy of the clavicle and coracoid process for reconstruction of the coraco-clavicular ligaments. *Am J Sports Med* 2007;35(5):811-817.

Robinson CM, Cairns DA: Primary nonoperative treatment of displaced lateral fractures of the clavicle. *J Bone Joint Surg Am* 2004;86(4):778-782.

Robinson CM, Court-Brown CM, McQueen MM, Wakefield AE: Estimating the risk of nonunion following nonoperative treatment of a clavicular fracture. *J Bone Joint Surg Am* 2004;86(7):1359-1365.

Rockwood CA Jr: Injuries to the acromioclavicular joint, in Rockwood CA Jr, Green DP, eds: *Rockwood and Green's Fractures in Adults,* ed 2. Philadelphia, PA, JB Lippincott, 1984, pp 860-910.

Rokito AS, Zuckerman JD, Shaari JM, Eisenberg DP, Cuomo F, Gallagher MA: A comparison of nonoperative and operative treatment of type II distal clavicle fractures. *Bull Hosp Jt Dis* 2002-2003;61(1-2):32-39.

Salzmann GM, Walz L, Buchmann S, Glabgly P, Venjakob A, Imhoff AB: Arthroscopically assisted 2-bundle anatomical reduction of acute acromioclavicular joint separations. *Am J Sports Med* 2010;38(6):1179-1187.

Smith TO, Chester R, Pearse EO, Hing CB: Operative versus non-operative management following Rockwood grade III acromioclavicular separation: A meta-analysis of the current evidence base. *J Orthop Traumatol* 2011;12(1):19-27.

Stegeman SA, Nacak H, Huvenaars KH, Stijnen T, Krijnen P, Schipper IB: Surgical treatment of Neer type-II fractures of the distal clavicle: A meta-analysis. *Acta Orthop* 2013;84(2):184-190.

Takase K, Kono R, Yamamoto K: Arthroscopic stabilization for Neer type 2 fracture of the distal clavicle fracture. *Arch Orthop Trauma Surg* 2012;132(3):399-403.

Tauber M, Gordon K, Koller H, Fox M, Resch H: Semitendinosus tendon graft versus a modified Weaver-Dunn procedure for acromioclavicular joint reconstruction in chronic cases: A prospective comparative study. *Am J Sports Med* 2009;37(1):181-190.

Thomas K, Litsky A, Jones G, Bishop JY: Biomechanical comparison of coracoclavicular reconstructive techniques. *Am J Sports Med* 2011;39(4):804-810.

Tischer T, Salzmann GM, El-Azab H, Vogt S, Imhoff AB: Incidence of associated injuries with acute acromioclavicular joint dislocations types III through V. *Am J Sports Med* 2009;37(1):136-139.

Tossy JD, Mead NC, Sigmond HM: Acromioclavicular separations: Useful and practical classification for treatment. *Clin Orthop Relat Res* 1963;(28):111-119.

van der Meijden OA, Gaskill TR, Millett PJ: Treatment of clavicle fractures: Current concepts review. *J Shoulder Elbow Surg* 2012;21(3):423-429.

Weaver JK, Dunn HK: Treatment of acromioclavicular injuries, especially complete acromioclavicular separation. *J Bone Joint Surg Am* 1972;54(6):1187-1194.

Zhang C, Huang J, Luo Y, Sun H: Comparison of the efficacy of a distal clavicular locking plate versus a clavicular hook plate in the treatment of unstable distal clavicle fractures and a systematic literature review. *Int Orthop* 2014;38(7):1461-1468.

Chapter 54

Open Surgical Management of Glenoid Rim Fractures

Michael Knesek, MD

Matthew D. Saltzman, MD

Guido Marra, MD

Introduction

Glenoid fractures are less common than other upper extremity fractures. However, they are important to address because of the role that the glenohumeral joint plays in shoulder stability and mobility. Classification systems have been described for fractures of the glenoid fossa and glenoid rim, although no correlation between fracture pattern and functional outcomes of subsequent surgical management has been identified. Surgical and nonsurgical management options are available, and treatment selection depends on the type of glenoid fracture. A thorough understanding of the anatomy and fracture morphology is necessary to facilitate management of fractures requiring surgical intervention.

Case Presentation

A 57-year-old, right-hand–dominant man slips on a wet surface and falls onto his right upper extremity while walking near a drinking fountain and sustains a fracture-dislocation of his right

shoulder. He is evaluated in the emergency department, where the shoulder is relocated. The patient is referred for surgical intervention. Radiographs and a CT scan are obtained (**Figure 1**). During further evaluation in the orthopaedic clinic, the patient reports subluxation of the shoulder and a sense of instability. The patient has no neurovascular injury and no notable medical comorbidities.

After discussion of the risks and benefits of surgical and nonsurgical management, the patient elects to proceed with surgical intervention that includes open reduction and internal fixation with cannulated screws through a deltopectoral approach. In this particular patient, the subscapularis split approach was used for exposure of the fracture. Kirschner wires (K-wires) were used as joysticks to manipulate the fracture fragment and provide preliminary reduction and stabilization. Final fixation was achieved using cannulated screws. At the most recent 6-month follow-up, the patient was doing well, with forward elevation to 180°, external rotation to 60°, and radiographic maintenance of alignment with no signs of

osteoarthritis and no further instability or redislocation.

Indications

Fractures of the scapula account for approximately 0.4% to 1% of all fractures, with fractures of the glenoid making up approximately 10% of scapular fractures. Most glenoid fractures are not substantially displaced; therefore, surgical management typically is not required. The most common type of glenoid fracture is an anterior avulsion or rim fracture, which accounts for approximately 75% to 85% of all glenoid fossa fractures.

Glenoid rim fractures are the result of a direct impact of the humeral head into the glenoid rim during a subluxation or dislocation event and can involve one-third of the articular surface. Most commonly, these fractures occur as a result of sports injuries in younger patients; however, they also can occur as a result of motor vehicle accidents or as pathologic fractures resulting from minor trauma in older individuals. Glenoid fossa fractures that extend into the scapular neck and body can result from high-energy trauma. Several classifications of glenoid fractures and glenoid rim fractures have been developed (**Figure 2**). The Ideberg classification is the most widely accepted system; Goss

Dr. Saltzman or an immediate family member has received royalties from Tornier and serves as a paid consultant to Medacta and Tornier. Dr. Marra or an immediate family member has received royalties from and serves as a paid consultant to Zimmer and serves as a board member, owner, officer, or committee member of the American Shoulder and Elbow Surgeons, the American Academy of Orthopaedic Surgeons, and the Association of Bone and Joint Surgeons. Neither Dr. Knesek nor any immediate family member has received anything of value from or has stock or stock options held in a commercial company or institution related directly or indirectly to the subject of this chapter.

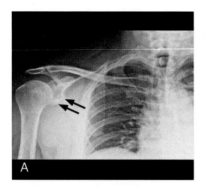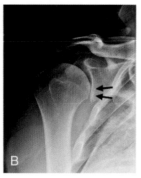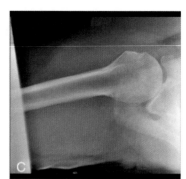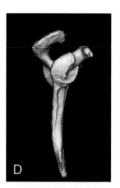

Figure 1 Images of a right shoulder. AP (**A**) and Grashey (**B**) radiographs demonstrate fracture of the anteroinferior glenoid rim (arrows). **C,** Axillary radiograph demonstrates concentric reduction of the glenohumeral joint. **D,** Three-dimensional CT reconstruction demonstrates fracture of the anteroinferior glenoid rim involving approximately one-third of the glenoid diameter.

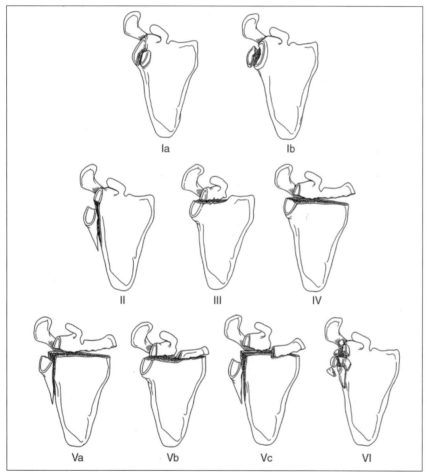

Figure 2 Illustration depicts classification of glenoid fractures of the scapula. Type Ia, anterior rim fracture. Type Ib, posterior rim fracture. Type II, fracture line through the glenoid fossa exiting at the lateral border of the scapula. Type III, fracture line through the glenoid fossa exiting at the superior border of the scapula. Type IV, fracture line through the glenoid fossa exiting at the medial border of the scapula. Type Va, combination of types II and IV. Type Vb, combination of types III and IV. Type Vc, combination of types II, III, and IV. Type VI, comminuted fracture. (Reproduced from Goss TP: Scapular fractures and dislocations: Diagnosis and treatment. *J Am Acad Orthop Surg* 1995;3[1]:22-33.)

subsequently modified it. The Bigliani classification of bony Bankart glenoid rim fractures includes type I, consisting of a displaced avulsion with attached capsule; type II, involving a medially displaced fragment malunited to the glenoid rim; and type III, involving erosion of the glenoid rim with less than 25% deficiency (type IIIA) or greater than 25% deficiency (type IIIB).

Regardless of the mechanism of injury, the size of a glenoid fracture typically determines the approach. The authors of this chapter typically manage fractures that involve more than 21% to 25% of the glenoid with open reduction and internal screw fixation, whereas smaller fracture patterns are typically managed arthroscopically.

Controversies and Alternative Approaches

Glenoid rim fractures can be managed through open or arthroscopic surgical approaches. Treatment recommendations depend on the size of a fracture and the experience of the surgeon. Similarly, fixation techniques depend on the size and quality of the bone fragment. Fractures that involve less than 25% of the glenoid surface (Bigliani types I, II, and IIIA) can be managed with suture anchor repair, whereas larger fragments (type IIIB) require screw fixation. After open surgical reduction is performed, cannulated screws are often used to achieve definitive fixation. Larger glenoid rim fractures with bone loss can be managed with the use of bone grafting or coracoid process transfer procedures.

Each treatment method has advantages and disadvantages. Arthroscopy decreases the risk of surgical morbidity and is often less painful compared with open surgical dissection. The arthroscopic approach typically spares either the split or tenotomy of the subscapularis tendon, which speeds functional recovery. Some surgeons argue that visualization and reduction of the fracture are best achieved arthroscopically. Others suggest that an open approach allows for better anatomic visualization and reduction. This typically is a matter of surgeon preference.

Complications inherent to suture anchor fixation include anchor pullout, chondral damage resulting from inappropriate placement of anchors superficial to subchondral bone, and suture failure. However, these complications are reported less commonly than those resulting from cannulated screw fixation. The authors of this chapter prefer nonabsorbable plastic suture anchors because of the complications associated with metal suture anchor fixation. In patients with smaller fractures, reduction and internal fixation through an arthroscopic approach can be achieved with suture anchor fixation. In patients with larger fractures or more complex fracture patterns, an open approach is used to obtain fixation with cannulated screws. Complications related to metal or titanium screw impingement or loosening have been reported in the literature.

Nonunion or malunion is generally managed on a case-by-case basis. Management is based on the amount of fragment resorption and bone loss of the anterior glenoid. When substantial bone loss of the anterior glenoid is present, anatomic (such as iliac crest bone graft or osteoarticular allograft) or nonanatomic (such as Latarjet or Bristow) reconstruction of the anterior glenoid is indicated.

 Results

Published results of open reduction and internal fixation of glenoid rim fractures are summarized in **Table 1**. Although larger glenoid rim fractures typically are managed with open reduction and internal fixation, evidence indicates that nonsurgical management can be successful in certain patients. In a study of 14 patients with larger (>5 mm) anteroinferior glenoid rim fractures with greater than 2 mm of displacement and concentric reduction of the glenohumeral joint on AP radiographs, the mean Constant score was 98 and all fragments had healed with a small step-off (0.5 to 11 mm) at 5.6-year follow-up. No recurrent dislocation or subluxation and no symptomatic osteoarthritis were reported.

Several studies have reported outcomes after surgical management of glenoid rim fractures with a deltopectoral approach and internal fixation. In a study of 10 patients with glenoid rim fractures that involved more than 25% of the glenoid surface and were managed with cannulated screw fixation, a mean Constant score of 81.9 and a mean Rowe score of 90 were reported at mean 30-month follow-up. Radiographic evidence of anatomic union was identified in nine patients. Reported complications included screw loosening in one patient and screw impingement in three patients. The mean patient age was 46.6 years.

A similar study performed in the Netherlands reported outcomes for 14 patients who underwent open reduction and internal fixation for Ideberg (Goss modification) type 1a or 2 fractures. Excellent results were reported in 11 patients and good results in 3 patients. The median Rowe score was 90, and the median Quick Disabilities of the Arm, Shoulder and Hand score was 4.6. Despite these outcome measures, the authors of the study reported disappointing functional outcomes in 21% of the patients at median 4-year follow-up.

In a longer term retrospective review of 29 patients with mean follow-up of 6.5 years, all patients sustained a traumatic anterior shoulder dislocation in combination with a larger (>25%) glenoid rim fracture that was treated with open reduction and internal screw fixation. Mean patient age was 41.6 years. The mean Constant score was 93.3, and the mean Disabilities of the Arm, Shoulder and Hand score was 10.1. Eight patients required hardware removal, and six patients had radiographic evidence of osteoarthritis at follow-up. Isokinetic muscular strength measurements showed statistically significant differences in external rotation and muscular endurance compared with the unaffected side. Twenty-seven patients reported overall satisfaction after surgical treatment.

 Technical Keys to Success

Setup/Exposure

- The patient is placed in the semi–beach-chair position on a radiolucent table with the torso and head of the bed elevated 30° to 45° (**Figure 3**).
- A rolled support is placed behind the medial border of the scapula to stabilize and protract the scapula on the chest wall.
- A C-arm is positioned so that the beam is perpendicular to the plane of the shoulder and the C-arm can be rotated to obtain intraoperative imaging. The ability to obtain an AP image in the scapular plane and an axillary view is confirmed.

Table 1 Results of Open Reduction and Internal Fixation of Glenoid Rim Fracture

Authors	Journal (Year)	Technique (No. of Patients)	Outcomes	Failure Rate (%)	Comments
Scheibel et al	*Knee Surg Sports Traumatol Arthrosc* (2004)	Suture anchor fixation of glenoid rim fractures involving <25% of the articular surface (15) Cannulated screw fixation of glenoid rim fractures involving >25% of the articular surface (10)	Suture anchor fixation: avg Constant score, 85.5; avg Rowe score, 94 Cannulated screw fixation: avg Constant score, 81.9; avg Rowe score, 90	0	Suture anchor fixation: avg follow-up, 22 mo Cannulated screw fixation: avg follow-up, 30 mo Anatomic healing was achieved in 20% after suture anchor fixation and in 90% after cannulated screw fixation 3 patients treated with cannulated screw fixation had screw impingement, and 1 patient had screw loosening No recurrent subluxation or redislocation in either group
Maquieira et al	*J Bone Joint Surg Br* (2007)	Nonsurgical management in patients with concentrically reduced glenohumeral joint (14)	Avg Constant score, 98 Subjective shoulder value, 97	0	Avg follow-up, 67.2 mo Avg intra-articular step-off of 3 mm noted on CT No patient had symptomatic glenohumeral osteoarthritis No redislocation or recurrent subluxation Apprehension test results were negative in all patients
Tauber et al	*Knee Surg Sports Traumatol Arthrosc* (2008)	Arthroscopic cannulated screw fixation (10)	Mean Rowe score, 94 Good-to-excellent results in 90%	10 (redislocation)	Avg follow-up, 24 mo Avg fragment size was 26% of glenoid articular surface 1 patient had traumatic redislocation, and 1 patient required removal of symptomatic hardware
Raiss et al	*Knee Surg Sports Traumatol Arthrosc* (2009)	Open screw fixation (29)	Mean Constant score, 93.3 Mean DASH score, 10.1	0	Avg follow-up, 78 mo 6 patients had radiographic signs of osteoarthritis at follow-up 8 patients required revision surgery to remove symptomatic screws No redislocation or subluxation reported
Van Dijkman et al	*Acta Orthop Belg* (2010)	3.5-mm cannulated screw fixation (14)	Median Rowe score, 90 Median QuickDASH score, 4.6 Results were excellent in 11 patients and good in 3	0	Avg follow-up, 48 mo 3 patients had a disappointing functional outcome No redislocation or subluxation reported

DASH = Disabilities of the Arm, Shoulder and Hand.

- The patient is prepped and draped per the surgeon's usual protocol.
- A deltopectoral approach is used. The skin is mobilized from the deltoid and pectoralis major tendon, and the interval is dissected from the deltoid origin on the clavicle to the humeral insertion. This dissection facilitates deeper exposure.

Instruments/Equipment/Implants Required

- A C-arm is necessary for patient setup and exposure.
- Glenoid rim, Hohmann, and/or

ribbon retractors are needed for medial retraction on the scapula.

- A deep Gelpi retractor is most helpful for the subscapularis split approach.
- A Fukuda retractor is necessary for humeral head retraction.
- Suture anchors and suture-passing devices as well as a cannulated screw set are used.
- Latarjet instrumentation may be required. Different sets are available for salvage if open reduction and internal fixation cannot be performed.
- A small-fragment set is needed. For example, 2.7-mm screws are helpful for smaller comminuted fractures.

Procedure

- The clavipectoral fascia is identified and opened lateral to the muscular portion of the conjoined tendon.
- The subscapularis bursa is identified and resected, exposing the subscapularis.
- Tenotomy of the subscapularis tendon is done medial to the tendon insertion on the lesser tuberosity. The tendon is dissected from the underlying capsule to the scapular neck and reflected medially.
- The capsule is incised longitudinally from the humeral insertion, leaving some attachment to allow for repair.
- The capsule is divided to the glenoid rim between the anterior band of the inferior glenohumeral ligament and the middle glenohumeral ligament.
- A ribbon retractor is placed along the scapular neck between the subscapularis tendon and the capsule.
- A Fukuda retractor or a sharp Hohmann retractor is used to retract the humeral head posteriorly (**Figure 4**).
- An elevator is used to dissect the subscapularis from the anterior glenoid neck.

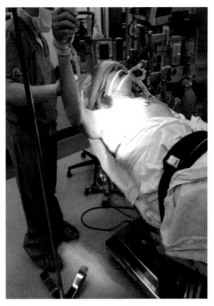

Figure 3   Photograph shows a patient placed in the beach-chair position on a radiolucent table with the torso elevated approximately 30° to 45°.

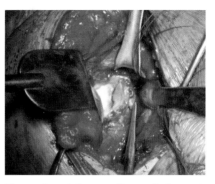

Figure 4   Intraoperative photograph of a shoulder obtained after subscapularis split and capsulotomy shows the use of a Fukuda retractor to retract the humeral head and the use of an anterior glenoid neck retractor on the anterior glenoid. The large glenoid rim fragment is clearly visible.

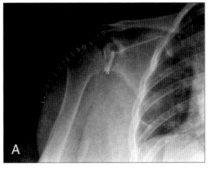

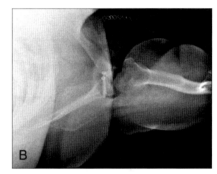

Figure 5   Postoperative Grashey (**A**) and axillary (**B**) radiographs of a shoulder demonstrate extra-articular placement of two cannulated screws with appropriate reduction and compression of the glenoid rim fragment.

- The axillary nerve, which runs along the ventral surface of the subscapularis muscle, is identified and protected.
- A thin, flexible ribbon retractor is placed on the anterior scapular neck to expose the entire anterior glenoid, including the glenoid rim and fossa.
- Clear visualization of the cranial and caudal extent of the fracture line is confirmed.
- An assessment of associated labral pathology is performed.

- The fracture site is cleaned, and an anatomic reduction is performed under direct visualization.
- Provisional fixation is achieved with K-wires.
- Reduction is confirmed with fluoroscopic imaging.
- Guidewires and cannulated screws are placed, with care taken to ensure that the screws are placed extra-articularly. Placement is confirmed visually and radiographically.

Table 2 Rehabilitation Protocol After Open Reduction and Internal Fixation of Glenoid Rim Fracture

Postoperative Week	ROM	Strengthening	Return to Play	Comments/Emphasis
0-2	None	None	None	—
2-6	Pendulums, passive ROM of glenohumeral joint	Isometric periscapular strengthening	None	Radiography at 6 wk
6-12	Active-assisted, progressing to active as tolerated	Light weight training	None	—
12-24	Unlimited passive and active	Unrestricted weight training	Return to play as tolerated with sport-specific therapy	No lifting in which the patient cannot see the back of his or her hands

ROM = range of motion.

Wound Closure

- The subscapularis tenotomy is repaired with nonabsorbable sutures, and the wound is closed in a layered fashion.
- If the subscapularis tendon split technique, in which the superior two-thirds and inferior one-third of the musculotendinous junction were separated was used, the tendon is repaired with absorbable sutures to reapproximate the split at the end of the procedure.
- Postoperative radiography or fluoroscopy, including AP, Grashey, and axillary views, is used to confirm hardware placement and concentric reduction of the joint (**Figure 5**).

Rehabilitation

Rehabilitation includes stages of immobilization, range of motion (ROM), and strengthening (**Table 2**). Strict immobilization is required for the first 2 weeks postoperatively, after which repeat radiographs are obtained to monitor healing. Pendulum exercises are begun approximately 3 weeks postoperatively, and passive ROM exercises are begun approximately 4 to 6 weeks postoperatively. For the second stage of rehabilitation, postoperative weeks 6 to 12, more active-assisted ROM is allowed, and early weight training with light resistance is begun. Three months postoperatively, unrestricted ROM is allowed, and more aggressive weight training is begun. For the first year postoperatively, overhead lifting is restricted to activities in which patients can see the back of their hands.

Avoiding Pitfalls

Adequate preoperative imaging is necessary to define the size and location of a fracture. The use of CT with three-dimensional reconstruction and humeral subtraction provides a clear image of fracture morphology. During the surgical procedure, the surgeon should have bone grafting instrumentation available so that augmentation or a Latarjet procedure can be performed if needed. A K-wire can be used as a joystick to manipulate the fracture fragment before reduction. After preliminary reduction and stabilization is achieved, cannulated screws are used for definitive anatomic reduction and fixation. Two screws should be used to ensure adequate fixation and minimize further rotation of the rim fragment. Imaging studies, including AP, Grashey, and axillary views, should be obtained to confirm fracture reduction and hardware placement.

For more comminuted fractures involving the glenoid rim, the authors of this chapter consider removal of the smaller fragments followed by fixation with small-fragment screws and incorporation of as much bone stock as is feasible. For patients with fracture lines that are more horizontal, the treating surgeon should consider using the posterior Judet approach and anatomic fixation using a scapular plating system. Alternatively, in patients who have substantial involvement of the scapular body along with a horizontal fracture line, fixation can be achieved by placing a Steinmann pin from the supraglenoid tubercle, starting posterior to the clavicle, through a limited posterior approach.

Bibliography

Bahk MS, Kuhn JE, Galatz LM, Connor PM, Williams GR Jr: Acromioclavicular and sternoclavicular injuries and clavicular, glenoid, and scapular fractures. *J Bone Joint Surg Am* 2009;91(10):2492-2510.

Bigliani LU, Newton PM, Steinmann SP, Connor PM, Mcllveen SJ: Glenoid rim lesions associated with recurrent anterior dislocation of the shoulder. *Am J Sports Med* 1998;26(1):41-45.

Goss TP: Fractures of the glenoid cavity. *J Bone Joint Surg Am* 1992;74(2):299-305.

Itoi E, Lee SB, Berglund LJ, Berge LL, An KN: The effect of a glenoid defect on anteroinferior stability of the shoulder after Bankart repair: A cadaveric study. *J Bone Joint Surg Am* 2000;82(1):35-46.

Kim YS, Lee BG, Rhee YG, Lee CH: Arthroscopic reduction and internal fixation for displaced anterior glenoid rim and greater tuberosity fractures. *J Orthop Sci* 2014;19(3):497-501.

Leung KS, Lam TP, Poon KM: Operative treatment of displaced intra-articular glenoid fractures. *Injury* 1993;24(5):324-328.

Maquieira GJ, Espinosa N, Gerber C, Eid K: Non-operative treatment of large anterior glenoid rim fractures after traumatic anterior dislocation of the shoulder. *J Bone Joint Surg Br* 2007;89(10):1347-1351.

Raiss P, Baumann F, Akbar M, Rickert M, Loew M: Open screw fixation of large anterior glenoid rim fractures: Mid- and long-term results in 29 patients. *Knee Surg Sports Traumatol Arthrosc* 2009;17(2):195-203.

Schandelmaier P, Blauth M, Schneider C, Krettek C: Fractures of the glenoid treated by operation: A 5- to 23-year follow-up of 22 cases. *J Bone Joint Surg Br* 2002;84(2):173-177.

Scheibel M, Magosch P, Lichtenberg S, Habermeyer P: Open reconstruction of anterior glenoid rim fractures. *Knee Surg Sports Traumatol Arthrosc* 2004;12(6):568-573.

Tauber M, Moursy M, Eppel M, Koller H, Resch H: Arthroscopic screw fixation of large anterior glenoid fractures. *Knee Surg Sports Traumatol Arthrosc* 2008;16(3):326-332.

Theivendran K, McBryde CW, Massoud SN: Scapula fractures: A review. *Trauma* 2008;10(1):25-33.

Van Dijkman BA, Schep NW, Luitse JS, Ponsen KJ, Kloen P, Goslings JC: Patient related functional outcome of glenoid rim fractures treated with open reduction and internal fixation. *Acta Orthop Belg* 2010;76(6):730-734.

Wiedemann E: Fractures of the scapula [German]. *Unfallchirurg* 2004;107(12):1124-1133.

Chapter 55

Open Reduction and Internal Fixation of Glenoid Fractures: Posterior Approach

William D. Regan, MD, FRCSC

Cameron M. Anley, MD

Introduction

Fractures of the scapula are uncommon, accounting for 0.4% to 1% of all fractures. Of these, only 10% involve the glenoid cavity. Approximately 90% of glenoid fractures are minimally displaced or nondisplaced, leaving only 10% that require surgical intervention. However, a recent study reported that up to 80% of glenoid fractures were managed surgically.

The Ideberg classification of glenoid fractures was initially proposed in 1984, and the Goss modification subdivided type V of this classification (**Figure 1**). This widely used classification system presents management options and approaches for each type of fracture. In this system, glenoid fractures are classified as either glenoid rim (type I) or glenoid fossa (types II to VI) fractures. Several other classification systems, including the most recent AO/Orthopaedic Trauma Association glenoid fracture classification, which requires further validation, have been proposed.

Glenoid rim fractures differ from small body avulsions that occur as a result of impaction of the dislocating humeral head and the anterior aspect of the glenoid. A glenoid rim fracture results from a lateral force that drives the humeral head onto the anterior or posterior rim, producing a larger fracture. Type II to IV glenoid fossa fractures occur when a more substantial lateral force drives the proximal humerus into the glenoid cavity, resulting in a transverse fracture that may extend in one or more directions depending on the direction of the force.

Glenoid and scapular fractures are generally the result of high-energy blunt trauma; therefore, concomitant injuries are common. Concomitant injuries can be local, such as vascular or brachial plexus injuries, or generalized, such as thoracic injuries (fractured ribs, pulmonary contusion, and pneumothorax), abdominal injuries (splenic or liver lacerations), head injuries, and spinal injuries. Because these life-threatening injuries take priority in the acute phase, scapular fractures are often overlooked or neglected. The surgeon should be aware of these associations, should ask pertinent questions, and, if possible, examine for swelling, crepitus, or ecchymosis around the shoulder as well as scrutinize chest radiographs for evidence of a fracture. When a glenoid fracture is suspected, further imaging, including true AP and axillary radiographs, should be obtained. If a normal axillary view cannot be obtained because of pain, a Velpeau axillary lateral view should be requested. Occasionally, an AP radiograph of the shoulder with the humerus in external rotation and neutral abduction can be helpful. This position helps to place the glenoid "in plane," thereby improving visualization of the fracture. Because of the complexity of glenoid fractures and the difficulty of visualization, CT may be required to further assess the fracture pattern and displacement.

Although a variety of approaches have been described to address glenoid fossa fractures, this procedure remains technically challenging. The posterior approach is used in the surgical treatment of approximately 80% of patients with glenoid fractures and is used for Ideberg type Ib, II, III, IV, and V fractures. The Judet posterior approach was initially described in 1964; however, in an attempt to limit the dissection required, a variety of modifications, including the limited posterior approach and the two-portal approach, have been reported on with favorable results. Knowledge of the internervous planes is essential to prevent nerve damage, specifically to the accessory, axillary, and suprascapular nerves.

As with any surgical intervention, good preoperative planning is essential. All appropriate imaging, as

---

Neither of the following authors nor any immediate family member has received anything of value from or has stock or stock options held in a commercial company or institution related directly or indirectly to the subject of this chapter: Dr. Regan and Dr. Anley.

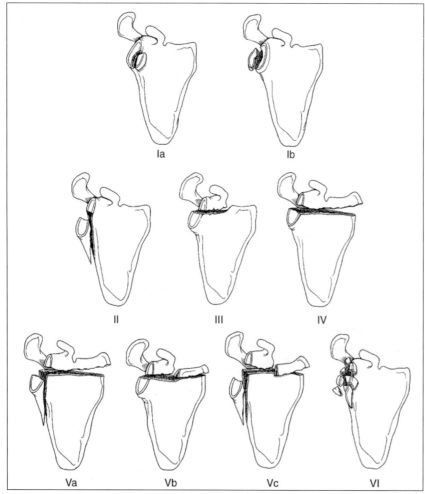

Figure 1 Illustration shows the classification system for fractures of the glenoid cavity. Type Ia, anterior rim fracture. Type Ib, posterior rim fracture. Type II, fracture line through the glenoid fossa exiting at the lateral border of the scapula. Type III, fracture line through the glenoid fossa exiting at the superior border of the scapula. Type IV, fracture line through the glenoid fossa exiting at the medial border of the scapula. Type Va, combination of types II and IV. Type Vb, combination of types III and IV. Type Vc, combination of types II, III, and IV. Type VI, comminuted fracture. (Reproduced from Goss TP: Scapular fractures and dislocations: Diagnosis and treatment. *J Am Acad Orthop Surg* 1995;3[1]:22-33.)

previously discussed, should be reviewed. Three-dimensional CT reconstruction may help the surgeon visualize the fracture pattern and the required reduction.

 Case Presentation

A 30-year-old man is injured in a motor vehicle accident. A right glenoid fracture and cervical fracture are noted on the initial chest radiograph, and further radiographs of the right shoulder (AP, axillary, transscapular lateral, and external AP views) are obtained to confirm the diagnosis (**Figure 2**). A CT scan is obtained to further define the fracture pattern and assist in preoperative planning.

An Ideberg type Va fracture is diagnosed. After appropriate medical stabilization, the patient undergoes open reduction and internal fixation (ORIF)

of the glenoid and scapula through a Judet posterior approach. Adequate reduction is confirmed on postoperative radiographs (**Figure 3**). The patient undergoes rehabilitation, starting with passive range of motion and progressing to active-assisted range of motion and, finally, resistive exercise combined with aggressive activity.

 Indications

Given the paucity of reported outcomes after ORIF of glenoid fractures, nonsurgical management should always be considered in patients with these fractures. However, in certain patients, surgical management may be required. The principal goal of surgical management is the reduction of fracture fragments to prevent instability and degenerative joint disease. General indications for surgical intervention in patients with open fractures and vascular injuries apply. Additional indications for glenoid fossa and neck fractures are based on the degree of incongruity, the presence of instability, and the risk of nonunion.

In patients with incongruity, ORIF is indicated in those with a loss of joint concentricity and a step-off of 5 to 10 mm. The exact amount of step-off that should be accepted ranges from 2 mm to 10 mm in the literature. Many authors have suggested that surgical treatment should be considered in patients with displacement of 5 mm, which is the average thickness of the articular cartilage, although 10 mm is accepted as a definite indication for surgical treatment. In patients with instability, subluxation of the humeral head (most commonly inferior or anterior-posterior) and larger fracture fragments (>25% for anterior fragments or >33% for posterior fragments) are indications for ORIF. The risk of nonunion depends on the size of the fracture gap. In patients with a gap greater than 10 mm despite joint concentricity and secondary congruence

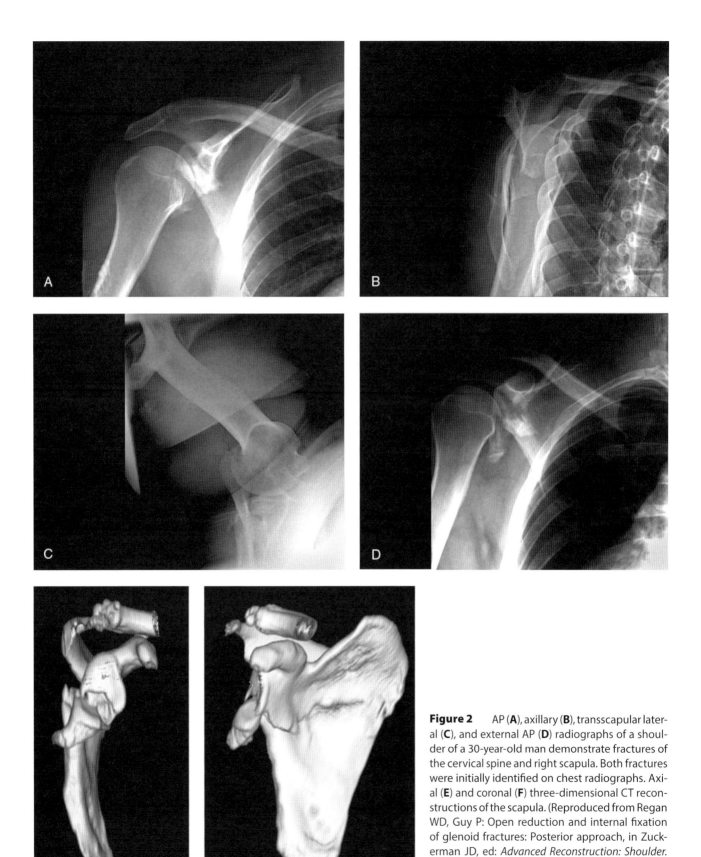

Figure 2 AP (**A**), axillary (**B**), transscapular lateral (**C**), and external AP (**D**) radiographs of a shoulder of a 30-year-old man demonstrate fractures of the cervical spine and right scapula. Both fractures were initially identified on chest radiographs. Axial (**E**) and coronal (**F**) three-dimensional CT reconstructions of the scapula. (Reproduced from Regan WD, Guy P: Open reduction and internal fixation of glenoid fractures: Posterior approach, in Zuckerman JD, ed: *Advanced Reconstruction: Shoulder*. Rosemont, IL, American Academy of Orthopaedic Surgeons, 2007, pp 405-415.)

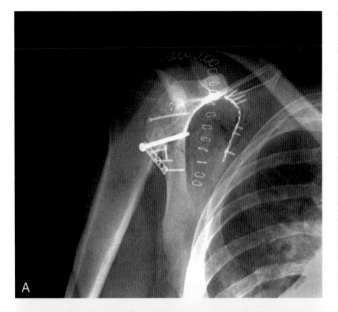

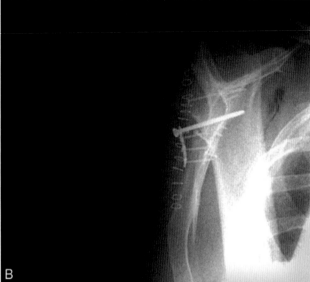

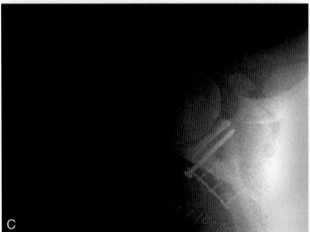

Figure 3   Postoperative AP (**A**), transscapular lateral (**B**), and axillary (**C**) radiographs of the shoulder of the patient whose imaging studies are shown in Figure 2 demonstrate fracture reduction. (Reproduced from Regan WD, Guy P: Open reduction and internal fixation of glenoid fractures: Posterior approach, in Zuckerman JD, ed: *Advanced Reconstruction: Shoulder.* Rosemont, IL, American Academy of Orthopaedic Surgeons, 2007, pp 405-415.)

(no subluxation), ORIF should be considered to reduce the risk of nonunion.

Indications for surgical management of fractures of the scapular neck remain controversial. Most of these fractures can be managed nonsurgically without substantial morbidity. However, these recommendations are based on small series with differing surgical indications. Surgical treatment should be considered in patients with more than 40° of scapular angulation and 1 to 2 cm of medial or anterior-posterior translation. Indications are summarized in **Table 1**.

Contraindications to ORIF include associated injuries that are life threatening (chest or head injuries) or that may preclude acceptable patient positioning (unstable cervical fractures) and active or suspected infection. In addition, ORIF should not be performed in patients with preexisting glenohumeral osteoarthritis. In this situation, total shoulder arthroplasty can be considered after union has occurred.

 Controversies and Alternative Approaches

The indications for surgical management of glenoid fractures in patients with double disruption of the superior shoulder suspensory complex remain controversial. Because of the rarity of these injuries, only a few small studies have been published, with conflicting results. The most common fracture pattern is a glenoid fracture with an ipsilateral clavicle fracture, referred to as a floating shoulder. Options include nonsurgical management of both fractures, ORIF of the clavicle alone, or ORIF of both fractures. Although initial studies suggested better results in patients treated with ORIF, later studies refuted these findings. A comparative study showed slightly better forward elevation and external rotation in patients who underwent ORIF but no

Table 1 Indications for Surgical Management of Glenoid Fractures

Fracture Site	Indication	Type of Displacement	Amount of Displacement	Recommended Imaging	Comment
Glenoid fossa	Incongruity	Articular step	≥5 mm (possible indication) ≥10 mm (definitive indication)	True AP radiograph of glenoid AP radiograph with passive external rotation CT with or without coronal scapular plane reconstruction	Most step displacements occur in patients with a transverse fracture
		Concentricity	Loss of congruency (absence of secondary congruence)	AP axillary radiographs CT axial and coronal scapular plane reconstruction	None
	Instability	Subluxation	Humeral head does not lie in middle of glenoid	AP, transscapular lateral, and axial radiographs Axial CT	Indication applies to both glenoid fossa and glenoid rim fractures
		Articular involvement	>25% of the anterior wall or >33% of the posterior wall	Axillary radiograph Axial CT	Indication applies to both glenoid fossa and glenoid rim fractures
	Nonunion risk	Gap and/or space between fragments	≥10 mm	All radiographic views Axial CT	Concern that a large gap may prevent callus formation and union
Glenoid neck	Angulation (instability)	Transverse or coronal angulation	40°	All radiographic views CT in all planes	Severe angulation may cause impingement, subluxation, or dislocation
	Translation	Medial or anterior-posterior	>1 cm (relative indication) >2 cm (surgical management considered)	AP radiograph and CT in patients with medial displacement Axillary radiographs and CT in patients with AP displacement	Severe translation may cause impingement and abductor weakness
Adjacent structures	Instability and/ or risk of nonunion	Associated clavicle fracture	Not yet determined	AP radiograph	Controversial indication with conflicting reports Comparative studies show better forward elevation and external rotation with surgical management
	Instability and/ or risk of nonunion	Associated suspensory ligament injury	Not yet determined	AP radiograph	Associated injuries (at least two) to the glenoid process, the coracoid process, the coracoclavicular ligament, the distal clavicle, the acromioclavicular joint, or the acromion process may be an indication for repair

Adapted from Regan WD, Guy P: Open reduction and internal fixation of glenoid fractures: Posterior approach, in Zuckerman JD, ed: *Advanced Reconstruction: Shoulder.* Rosemont, IL, American Academy of Orthopaedic Surgeons, 2007, pp 405-415.

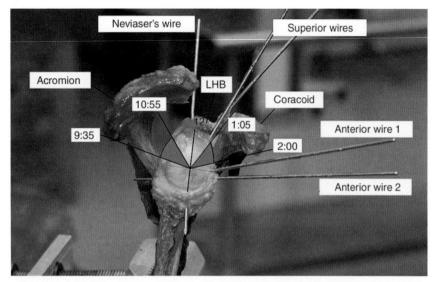

Figure 4 Photograph of a cadaver specimen shows the positions of the coracoid and acromion relative to the glenoid. Shaded areas indicate clock-face positions on the glenoid. The posterior wire has been removed in this photograph. LHB = long head of the biceps. (Reproduced with permission from Marsland D, Ahmed HA: Arthroscopically assisted fixation of glenoid fractures: A cadaver study to show potential applications of percutaneous screw insertion and anatomic risks. *J Shoulder Elbow Surg* 2011;20[3]:481-490.)

overall significant difference between the groups. It is generally accepted that these injuries can be managed nonsurgically if the fracture is minimally displaced or nondisplaced. However, the exact amount of acceptable displacement remains debated.

Arthroscopically assisted fracture reduction and percutaneous fixation of glenoid fractures has received increased interest in the past few years. An obvious advantage of arthroscopy is the accurate reduction of the fracture without the need for major soft-tissue dissection. However, it poses a risk to surrounding neurovascular structures, limiting its usefulness to specific fracture configurations that allow cannulated screws to be passed perpendicular to the fracture line. The authors of a recent cadaver study inserted wires into the glenoid from five different positions and measured the distance to the neurovascular structures. Using 15 mm as the criterion for a safe distance, the authors established the safe zone for percutaneous screw insertion (**Figure 4**) as being

between the 7:40 and 2:50 clock-face positions posteriorly and superiorly, whereas the anterior approach places the cephalic vein, the musculocutaneous nerve, and the inferior branch of the suprascapular nerve in danger. The positions of the acromion and coracoid, which may physically limit screw insertion, should be taken into consideration. The published results of arthroscopically assisted reduction and fixation are limited to case series and small studies of type II and III fractures, with the largest published study having 18 patients. After 2-year follow-up, the authors of that largest study concluded that arthroscopically assisted reduction and percutaneous cannulated screw fixation is a safe and effective method for the treatment of Ideberg type III glenoid fractures.

In patients with severely comminuted fractures that preclude fixation, and in patients with an unsuccessful outcome after nonsurgical or surgical intervention, delayed arthroplasty may be considered after union has occurred.

In certain patients in whom arthroplasty is not possible, arthrodesis of the glenohumeral joint may be considered.

Results

Because displaced glenoid fractures requiring surgical intervention are uncommon, the results of surgical management are limited to a few studies with limited patient numbers. In addition, the variety of fracture patterns, treatment indications, and outcome scoring systems further complicate the interpretation of these studies. With these limitations taken into account, the published studies generally demonstrate favorable results of ORIF, with mostly good and excellent outcomes. The published studies are summarized in **Table 2**.

Technical Keys to Success

Setup/Exposure

- After careful consideration of associated injuries (head, thoracic, abdominal, and spinal) and appropriate consultation, the patient is placed in the prone or lateral decubitus position.
- A beanbag may be useful for stabilization of the torso, especially in patients with multiple injuries.
- A well-padded Mayo stand is used as an adjustable arm rest to allow the affected limb to be draped free and mobilized during the procedure.
- Bony landmarks are outlined with a marking pen.
- The incision is marked along the scapular spine, beginning laterally at the posterior acromion, progressing to the superomedial corner of the scapula, and extending distally along the medial border of the scapula.

Table 2 Results of Surgical Management of Glenoid Fossa Fractures

Author(s)	Journal (Year)	Technique (No. of Patients)	Outcomes	Comments
Kavanagh et al	*J Bone Joint Surg Am* (1993)	ORIF (10 [9 with posterior approach, 1 with anterior approach])	8 patients had little or no pain 8 patients had mildly limited ROM No OA	9 patients available for follow-up Mean follow-up, 48 mo 1 patient had HO
Leung et al	*Injury* (1993)	ORIF (11 with posterior approach, 3 with anterior approach)	All rates good (Rowe score)	Mean follow-up, 30.5 mo Pneumothorax developed in 2 patients during surgery, likely related to initial chest injuries
Mayo et al	*Clin Orthop Relat Res* (1998)	ORIF (27)	24 patients had anatomic reduction 3 patients had <2 mm nonunion Functional ratings: 6 excellent, 16 good, 3 fair, 2 poor No OA	Mean follow-up, 43 mo Complications included superficial wound dehiscence 2 patients had infraspinatus palsy (resolved spontaneously)
Adam	*Int Orthop* (2002)	ORIF (10 [7 with posterior approach])	No rating scale used 9 patients had occasional or no pain 8 patients had excellent or good results 2 patients had severe to moderately limited motion	Mean follow-up, 59.2 mo 9 patients had multiple injuries 1 patient had infection with loss of fixation 1 patient had hematoma 1 patient developed OA
Schandelmaier et al	*J Bone Joint Surg Br* (2002)	ORIF (16 with posterior approach, 6 with anterior approach)	19 patients had excellent ROM 19 patients had little to no pain Mean Constant score, 79 (median was 94; 4 patients scored <50)	Mean follow-up, 120 mo 2 patients had failure of fixation 2 patients had complete brachial plexus palsy 2 patients had deep infection 1 patient required revision surgery
Anavian et al	*J Bone Joint Surg Am* (2012)	ORIF (21 with posterior approach, 7 with anterior approach, 5 with combined approach)	Mean DASH score, 10.8 Mean SF-36 subscores comparable with those of the general population Mean ROM: forward flexion, 151°; abduction, 105°; external rotation, 52°; internal rotation to T5	Mean follow-up, 27 mo 1 intra-articular screw 1 patient had postoperative stiffness 1 patient had HO
Lewis et al	*J Orthop* (2013)	ORIF (7 with posterior approach, 4 with anterior approach, 4 with combined approach)	Mean DASH score, 10 (range, 0.83-29.17) Mean ASES score, 90 (range, 41.7-100)	Mean follow-up, 49 mo No hardware failure or infections
Sen et al	*Indian J Orthop* (2014)	ORIF (all 8 with posterior approach)	Constant score, 87.24 4 excellent, 2 good, 1 fair, 1 poor	Mean follow-up, 87.6 mo 2 patients had superficial wound infection

ASES = American Shoulder and Elbow Surgeons shoulder outcome; DASH = Disabilities of the Arm, Shoulder and Hand; HO = heterotopic ossification; OA = osteoarthritis; ORIF = open reduction and internal fixation; ROM = range of motion; SF-36 = Medical Outcomes Study 36-Item Short Form.

Adapted from Regan WD, Guy P: Open reduction and internal fixation of glenoid fractures: Posterior approach, in Zuckerman JD, ed: *Advanced Reconstruction: Shoulder*. Rosemont, IL, American Academy of Orthopaedic Surgeons, 2007, pp 405-415.

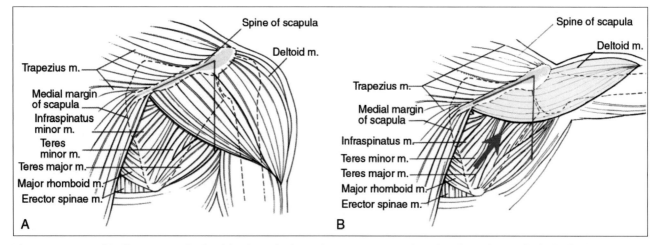

Figure 5   **A** and **B,** Illustrations of a shoulder show the limited posterior approach to the glenoid. Note the lack of deltoid detachment required on abducting the arm to 90° in panel B. The arrow indicates the deltoid-infraspinatus muscle interval inferior to the scapular spine. (Reproduced from Regan WD, Guy P: Open reduction and internal fixation of glenoid fractures: Posterior approach, in Zuckerman JD, ed: *Advanced Reconstruction: Shoulder.* Rosemont, IL, American Academy of Orthopaedic Surgeons, 2007, pp 405-415.)

- The limited posterior approach or the classic extensile exposure may be used.

LIMITED POSTERIOR APPROACH

- In the limited posterior approach, an incision is made from the lateral third of the scapular spine to the posterior aspect of the acromion at its lateral tip and extended caudally or distally approximately 3 to 4 cm in a midlateral plane (**Figure 5, A**).
- In the original description of the Judet approach, the posterior deltoid is dissected sharply off the scapular spine and acromion, beginning at the lateral tip of the acromion, and retracted laterally. The deltoid-infraspinatus muscle interval inferior to the scapular spine is then identified. In the limited posterior approach, detachment of the deltoid is avoided by abducting the arm to 90° (**Figure 5, B**). The inferior border of the deltoid is then elevated, facilitating retraction.
- A minimal release of the medial attachment of the deltoid from the scapular spine is performed to expose the glenohumeral joint deep to the infraspinatus tendon.

- The limited posterior approach places the axillary nerve at a slightly increased risk of injury because it is retracted during the exposure. Therefore, if this approach is used, particular care must be taken to avoid excessive tension on the axillary nerve.
- The internervous plane between the infraspinatus (suprascapular nerve) and teres minor (axillary nerve) is developed, exposing the lateral border of the scapula to the inferior aspect of the glenoid. The posterior glenohumeral joint capsule is incised in the same horizontal fashion and elevated subperiosteally from the posterior glenoid process. A retractor is inserted into the joint to retract the humeral head anteriorly.

EXTENSILE EXPOSURE

- In the extensile exposure, a so-called safe interval is developed by detaching the teres minor inferiorly from the inferior aspect of the glenohumeral joint capsule.
- Additional dissection from the posteroinferior aspect of the joint is performed to expose the more posteroinferior fracture fragments.

- The triceps may be detached from the inferior glenoid to improve exposure if needed.
- If additional access to the medial aspect of the scapular spine and scapular body is necessary, the infraspinatus is further elevated off of the scapular body to improve fracture visualization and avoid potential neurovascular injury. To accomplish this elevation, the skin incision over the scapular spine is extended medially to the superomedial corner of the scapula (**Figure 6, A**). The incision then curves distally along the medial edge of the scapula. The infraspinatus is elevated from the lateral border of the scapula, with its neurovascular pedicle arising from the suprascapular nerve (**Figure 6, B and C**).
- Complete extensile exposure involves detaching the posterior deltoid from the scapular spine to provide additional exposure and relieve tension in the neurovascular bundle (**Figure 7**).

SUPERIOR EXPOSURE

- Superior access may be necessary in combination with the posterior

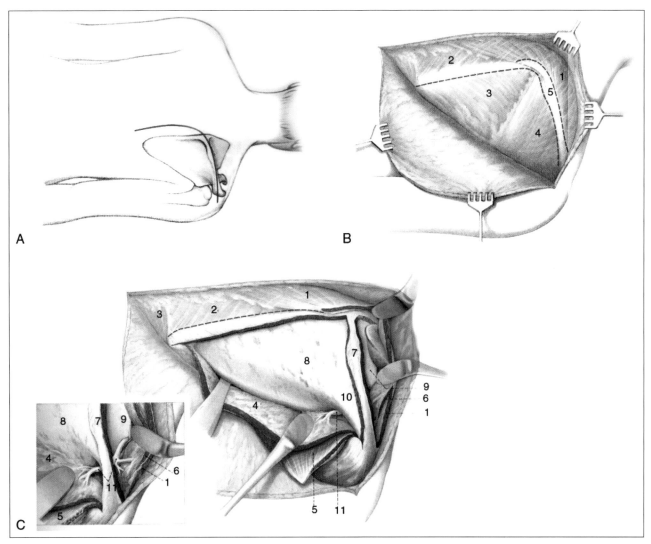

Figure 6 Illustrations of a shoulder show the Judet approach. **A,** The skin incision is indicated by the red arc. **B,** Detachment of the scapular musculature (dashed line). 1 = trapezius muscle, 2 = greater rhomboid muscle, 3 = infraspinatus muscle, 4 = deltoid muscle, 5 = scapular spine. **C,** Exposure of the posterior aspect of the scapula after subperiosteal detachment of the musculature. Inset, Exposure of the course and muscular branches of the suprascapular nerve after detachment of the supraspinatus and infraspinatus muscles. 1 = trapezius muscle, 2 = greater rhomboid muscle, 3 = latissimus dorsi muscle, 4 = infraspinatus muscle, 5 = deltoid muscle, 6 = supraspinatus muscle, 7 = scapular spine, 8 = infraspinatus fossa, 9 = supraspinatus fossa, 10 = scapular neck, 11 = suprascapular nerve. (Reproduced from Regan WD, Guy P: Open reduction and internal fixation of glenoid fractures: Posterior approach, in Zuckerman JD, ed: *Advanced Reconstruction: Shoulder.* Rosemont, IL, American Academy of Orthopaedic Surgeons, 2007, pp 405-415.)

approach when the fracture plane is transverse and involves a larger superior fragment.

- To improve fixation, a superior-to-inferior screw can be placed through a superior (often percutaneous) approach.
- The excision is extended over the superior aspect of the

shoulder posterior to the acromioclavicular joint in the interval between the clavicle and the acromion.

- The trapezius muscle and underlying supraspinatus muscle are split in line with their fibers to expose the superior aspect of the glenoid process.

Instruments/Equipment/Implants Required

- A variety of fixation devices are available. A 2.7- or 3.5-mm reconstruction plate and screws and/or 3.5- or 4.0-mm cannulated screws are most commonly used.
- Locking plates can be helpful in patients with thin bone.

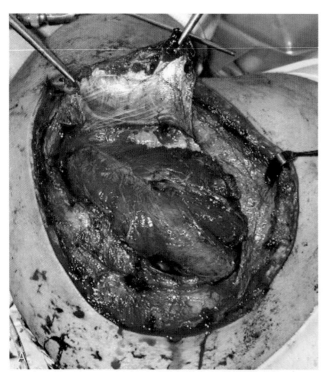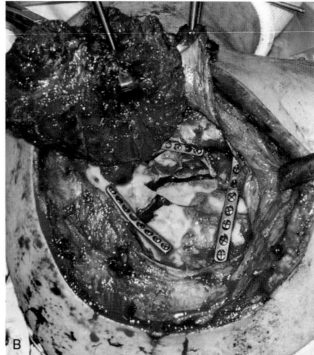

Figure 7 Intraoperative photographs of the shoulder of the patient described in Figure 2 show the extensile approach (**A**) and detachment of the posterior deltoid (**B**). (Reproduced from Regan WD, Guy P: Open reduction and internal fixation of glenoid fractures: Posterior approach, in Zuckerman JD, ed: *Advanced Reconstruction: Shoulder*. Rosemont, IL, American Academy of Orthopaedic Surgeons, 2007, pp 405-415.)

- Kirschner wires should be available for temporary fixation.

Procedure

- After the posterior glenoid has been exposed, reduction of the articular fragments can be attempted. Reduction of the scapular body with Kirschner wires may be necessary before the articular surface can be reconstructed.
- Realignment of the medial portion of the scapular body may facilitate reduction.
- Fixation devices are applied as needed to maintain the reduction, with care taken to avoid intra-articular penetration.
- After fixation has been achieved, the shoulder is moved through a range of motion to assess the rigidity of the fixation.

Wound Closure

- The wound is thoroughly irrigated, and hemostasis is obtained.
- Wound closure is performed in layers.
- The infraspinatus is reattached to the medial border of the scapula and adjacent fascia with 1-0 bioabsorbable suture.
- If necessary, the deltoid is reattached to the scapular spine with 1-0 bioabsorbable suture.
- The subcutaneous layer and skin are closed, and a dressing is applied.
- The patient is moved off the surgical table with careful consideration of associated injuries.
- A simple sling is applied for comfort, and analgesia is provided as required.

Rehabilitation

A variety of postoperative regimes are presented in the literature, many of which are based on the personal experience of the authors and follow the basic principles of rehabilitation after surgical management of shoulder fractures. Rehabilitation should be tailored to the patient according to the surgical approach used and the rigidity of the fixation. The basic rehabilitation protocol is summarized in **Table 3**.

Avoiding Pitfalls

Minimization of complications is key to a successful outcome after ORIF of a displaced glenoid fracture. The overall complication rate after ORIF of displaced glenoid fractures is low. The most

Table 3 Rehabilitation Protocol After Open Reduction and Internal Fixation of Glenoid Fractures

Postoperative Week	ROM	Strengthening	Return to Play	Comments/Emphasis
0-4	Passive Goals: forward elevation of 90°, external rotation of 30°, internal rotation to thoracolumbar junction	No	No	Radiographs at 4 wk to confirm reduction and fixation Consider extending this phase of rehabilitation to 6 wk if fracture was highly comminuted or fixation is questionable
4-12	Active assisted Goals: Progressing to full ROM	No	No	Repeat examination and radiographs at 12 wk If fracture has united, proceed to next phase of rehabilitation
12-24	Resistive exercise combined with aggressive activity Goal: full ROM	Yes	After 4-6 mo	Rehabilitation continues until ROM and strength have been maximized, normally 4-6 mo

ROM = range of motion.

common complications are infection (4.2%); rotator cuff pathology (0.9%); hematoma (1.9%); hardware-related complications, such as implant failure (3.8%) or the need for hardware removal (7.1%); nerve injury (2.4%); heterotopic ossification (1.4%); instability (0.5%); and, in the long term, posttraumatic arthritis (1.9%). Many of these complications can be avoided with meticulous preoperative planning and surgical technique. Although uncommon, infection is one of the most feared complications and should always be considered in patients with a loss of fixation. The risk of infection can be reduced with the use of preoperative prophylactic antibiotics in

accordance with local guidelines, careful soft-tissue management and dissection, removal of devitalized tissue, and meticulous hemostasis. If infection develops, it should be managed aggressively with isolation and antibiotic sensitivity analysis of the organism(s), thorough débridement of the area, maintenance of bony stability, and adequate antibiotic treatment, taking into account the duration of the treatment and sensitivity of the organism(s), in consultation with infectious disease specialists.

Heterotopic ossification and stiffness may develop after management of glenoid fractures. Prophylactic regimes are available to reduce the risk

of heterotopic ossification, although no specific guidelines related to glenoid fractures have been developed. Early mobilization is important to prevent postoperative stiffness. To reduce the risk of nerve palsy, attention to detail and knowledge of the surgical approach are essential. Axillary or suprascapular nerve palsy may result in weakness and compromise the outcome of the surgical procedure. Careful dissection of internervous planes and conversion to a more extensile approach when needed to avoid nerve tension are important. To limit joint wear and the progression of arthritis, all potential loose fragments in comminuted fractures must be removed.

Bibliography

Adam FF: Surgical treatment of displaced fractures of the glenoid cavity. *Int Orthop* 2002;26(3):150-153.

Anavian J, Gauger EM, Schroder LK, Wijdicks CA, Cole PA: Surgical and functional outcomes after operative management of complex and displaced intra-articular glenoid fractures. *J Bone Joint Surg Am* 2012;94(7):645-653.

Cole PA, Gauger EM, Schroder LK: Management of scapular fractures. *J Am Acad Orthop Surg* 2012;20(3):130-141.

Goss TP: Fractures of the glenoid cavity. *J Bone Joint Surg Am* 1992;74(2):299-305.

Ideberg R, Grevsten S, Larsson S: Epidemiology of scapular fractures: Incidence and classification of 338 fractures. *Acta Orthop Scand* 1995;66(5):395-397.

Jaeger M, Lambert S, Südkamp NP, et al: The AO Foundation and Orthopaedic Trauma Association (AO/OTA) scapula fracture classification system: Focus on glenoid fossa involvement. *J Shoulder Elbow Surg* 2013;22(4):512-520.

Kavanagh BF, Bradway JK, Cofield RH: Open reduction and internal fixation of displaced intra-articular fractures of the glenoid fossa. *J Bone Joint Surg Am* 1993;75(4):479-484.

Lantry JM, Roberts CS, Giannoudis PV: Operative treatment of scapular fractures: A systematic review. *Injury* 2008;39(3):271-283.

Leung KS, Lam TP, Poon KM: Operative treatment of displaced intra-articular glenoid fractures. *Injury* 1993;24(5):324-328.

Lewis S, Argintar E, Jahn R, Zusmanovich M, Itamura J, Rick Hatch GF: Intra-articular scapular fractures: Outcomes after internal fixation. *J Orthop* 2013;10(4):188-192.

Marsland D, Ahmed HA: Arthroscopically assisted fixation of glenoid fractures: A cadaver study to show potential applications of percutaneous screw insertion and anatomic risks. *J Shoulder Elbow Surg* 2011;20(3):481-490.

Mayo KA, Benirschke SK, Mast JW: Displaced fractures of the glenoid fossa: Results of open reduction and internal fixation. *Clin Orthop Relat Res* 1998;(347):122-130.

Nork SE, Barei DP, Gardner MJ, Schildhauer TA, Mayo KA, Benirschke SK: Surgical exposure and fixation of displaced type IV, V, and VI glenoid fractures. *J Orthop Trauma* 2008;22(7):487-493.

Pizanis A, Tosounidis G, Braun C, Pohlemann T, Wirbel RJ: The posterior two-portal approach for reconstruction of scapula fractures: Results of 39 patients. *Injury* 2013;44(11):1630-1635.

Salassa TE, Hill BW, Cole PA: Quantitative comparison of exposure for the posterior Judet approach to the scapula with and without deltoid takedown. *J Shoulder Elbow Surg* 2014;23(11):1747-1752.

Schandelmaier P, Blauth M, Schneider C, Krettek C: Fractures of the glenoid treated by operation: A 5- to 23-year follow-up of 22 cases. *J Bone Joint Surg Br* 2002;84(2):173-177.

Sen RK, Sud S, Saini G, Rangdal S, Sament R, Bachhal V: Glenoid fossa fractures: Outcome of operative and nonoperative treatment. *Indian J Orthop* 2014;48(1):14-19.

Soslowsky LJ, Flatow EL, Bigliani LU, Mow VC: Articular geometry of the glenohumeral joint. *Clin Orthop Relat Res* 1992;(285):181-190.

van Noort A, van Loon CJ, Rijnberg WJ: Limited posterior approach for internal fixation of a glenoid fracture. *Arch Orthop Trauma Surg* 2004;124(2):140-144.

van Oostveen DP, Temmerman OP, Burger BJ, van Noort A, Robinson M: Glenoid fractures: A review of pathology, classification, treatment and results. *Acta Orthop Belg* 2014;80(1):88-98.

Yang HB, Wang D, He XJ: Arthroscopic-assisted reduction and percutaneous cannulated screw fixation for Ideberg type III glenoid fractures: A minimum 2-year follow-up of 18 cases. *Am J Sports Med* 2011;39(9):1923-1928.

Zlowodzki M, Bhandari M, Zelle BA, Kregor PJ, Cole PA: Treatment of scapula fractures: Systematic review of 520 fractures in 22 case series. *J Orthop Trauma* 2006;20(3):230-233.

Chapter 56

Surgical Management of Scapular Body Fractures

Frank R. Avilucea, MD

William T. Obremskey, MD, MPH, MMHC

Introduction

Scapular fractures account for fewer than 1% of all fractures and are often the result of high-energy trauma. Most of these are extra-articular injuries involving the scapular neck or body; thus, extra-articular injuries constitute the most common scapular fracture pattern. Historically, observation was the predominant treatment of patients with scapular fractures because these injuries are often identified late or are missed in the presence of associated injuries of higher acuity. A systematic review published in 2006 identified that although 80% of intra-articular glenoid fractures were managed surgically, 99% of extra-articular injuries were managed nonsurgically. Several subsequent reports have questioned the nonsurgical management of extra-articular scapula fractures. A long-term follow-up study of patients treated with immobilization and early motion identified that 50% of patients with scapular deformity had shoulder symptoms including pain. In addition, a study published in 2011 showed significant improvement in shoulder strength and motion after surgical correction of extra-articular malunions.

Surgical management is done to restore length, rotation, and alignment with minimal soft-tissue injury. Fixation should provide stability, allowing early physical therapy. The surgical approach should provide adequate exposure of the fracture, minimize soft-tissue injury, and enable fracture reduction. The use of three-dimensional (3D) CT reconstruction will help determine the surgical approach. Acute fractures are more easily reduced during initial hospitalization but may be mobilized and reduced up to 3 weeks after the date of the injury. Fractures managed after delayed presentation may require greater dissection to release callus formation.

Case Presentation

A 22-year-old male football player is seen in the emergency department with left shoulder pain after a motorcycle crash. Physical examination reveals the arm held at the side. The patient is unable to initiate abduction or forward flexion. Sensation and motor function are found to be intact for all peripheral nerves. Radiographs reveal an extra-articular scapular fracture with the lateral border displaced 3 cm and angulated 20° (**Figure 1, A** and **B**). To facilitate preoperative planning, 3D CT reconstructions of the injury are obtained (**Figure 1, C** and **D**). The patient has no associated injuries. After surgical management, radiographic assessment demonstrates fracture reduction and fixation (**Figure 1, E** and **F**). At 6-month follow-up, the patient has full range of motion (ROM) symmetric to the contralateral side (**Figure 1, G, H**, and **I**).

Indications

Some surgeons do not think that extra-articular scapula fractures should be managed surgically. However, recent studies support internal fixation in patients with substantial displacement of the scapular neck leading to compromised shoulder function. The authors of a 1991 study recommended open reduction and internal fixation (ORIF) of scapular neck fractures in patients in whom the lateral border of the neck is laterally displaced 9 mm relative to the glenoid or in whom angular displacement exceeds 40°. Although ORIF has been recommended for descriptive indications, including grossly displaced fractures of the acromion or coracoid process, displaced fractures of the anatomic neck, and unstable fractures of the surgical neck, several recent studies suggest measurable indications for

Dr. Obremskey or an immediate family member serves as a board member, owner, officer, or committee member of the Orthopaedic Trauma Association and the Southeastern Fracture Consortium. Neither Dr. Avilucea nor any immediate family member has received anything of value from or has stock or stock options held in a commercial company or institution related directly or indirectly to the subject of this chapter.

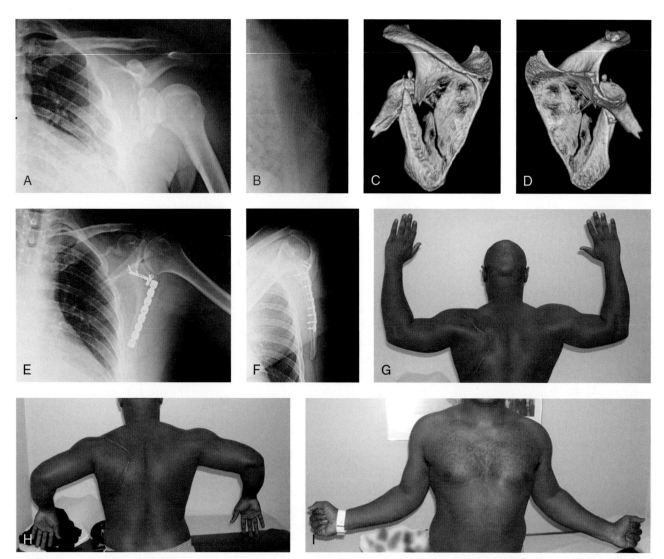

Figure 1 AP (**A**) and scapular Y (**B**) radiographs of an extra-articular scapular fracture demonstrate substantial multiplanar fracture displacement. **C** and **D,** Three-dimensional CT reconstructions obtained for topographic fracture characterization in preoperative planning. Postoperative AP (**E**) and scapular Y (**F**) radiographs demonstrate restoration of the lateral scapular border, glenopolar angle, and anteroposterior and mediolateral osseous relationships. **G** through **I,** Clinical photographs obtained at 6-month follow-up show symmetric scapulothoracic and shoulder motion with no subjective deficit.

surgical management, including at least 4 mm step-off of an articular glenoid fracture, at least 20 to 25 mm displacement of the glenohumeral articulation, at least 25° to 45° of angular deformity in the semicoronal plane visualized on the scapular Y radiograph, shortening of at least 25 mm, and a glenopolar angle of less than or equal to 20° to 22°. In patients with scapular deformities that warrant consideration of surgical management, 3D CT reconstructions should

be obtained to improve assessment of the deformity and facilitate preoperative planning.

The decision to proceed with surgical or nonsurgical treatment takes into account several factors, including radiographic findings, demographic characteristics, clinical deficits, and patient history. Demographic characteristics that favor surgical treatment include younger patient age, injury of the dominant extremity, and overhead vocational

(such as carpentry) or avocational (such as tennis, throwing sport, swimming) use of the arm. Clinical examination findings that support surgical treatment include a so-called droopy shoulder, an inability to actively abduct or forward flex the arm or tolerate passive arm motion, and the presence of neurologic injury. Patients reporting instability and/or shoulder dysfunction may benefit from surgical stabilization. Finally, a patient's overall clinical scenario is a critical determinant of both the timing of fixation and whether surgical treatment is pursued. A patient with severe lung injury would likely undergo delayed fixation, whereas a patient who holds strong religious preferences against blood transfusion or is in favor of only lifesaving surgical intervention may prefer nonsurgical treatment despite radiographic or clinical findings.

Controversies and Alternative Approaches

The primary controversy surrounds the indications for surgical management. In many trauma centers, displaced extra-articular scapula fractures are never managed surgically. Most studies report union achieved with nonsurgical management, likely because the scapula is encompassed by a robust muscular envelope and rich vascular supply enabling callus formation. In addition, the shoulder has a tremendous capability for compensatory motion. It remains unclear, however, whether compensatory motion results in dysfunction. Although no published studies have compared surgical and nonsurgical management, a few series demonstrate a positive correlation between decreased glenopolar angle and negative clinical outcome.

Results

As a result of greater understanding of the anatomy, injury, and surgical approaches and new recognition of dysfunction related to malunion, the management of scapular fractures has gradually changed. Results are summarized in **Table 1**.

In a systematic review analyzing 22 studies that included 520 surgically and nonsurgically treated patients, 99% of scapular body fractures were managed nonsurgically and 14% of those

had fair to poor outcomes. Similarly, of the 83% of scapular neck fractures managed nonsurgically, 20% had fair to poor outcomes. In a 1991 study of 113 patients with 116 scapular fractures managed nonsurgically, 2 patients with displaced scapular body fractures reported no pain or loss of motion; however, crepitus with active ROM was subjectively noted. In the same study, 40% of patients with displaced scapular neck fractures reported weakness with exertion involving abduction. In a study of 129 patients treated with sling immobilization followed by active motion activities, 25% reported persistent shoulder symptoms; fair or poor outcomes were reported by 32% of patients with a scapular neck fracture compared with 22% of patients with a scapular body fracture.

In a systematic review of 17 studies including 243 patients with scapular fractures managed surgically, good to excellent results were reported in 83.4% of patients, and the complication rate was low. In a more recent study of 84 patients with scapular neck and body fractures managed surgically, radiographic assessment demonstrated union in all patients, and no infections were reported. In a study of clinical outcomes after surgical management, researchers reported a mean Disabilities of the Arm, Shoulder and Hand score of 14 at 26-month follow-up in addition to symmetric motion and near-complete recovery of strength. These studies suggest that displaced unstable fractures of the scapular neck or body are effectively and successfully addressed with open surgical management.

Limited data are available on clinical outcomes after surgical management of displaced extra-articular scapula fractures. In a small series of patients with malunion and concomitant shoulder dysfunction who underwent surgical osteotomy, reorientation, and fixation of the scapula, preoperative and postoperative functional measures were obtained.

Mean follow-up was 39 months. All fractures united radiographically, and a statistically significant improvement in the mean Disabilities of the Arm, Shoulder and Hand score was observed. The marked improvement in this cohort suggests that a subset of patients with acute extra-articular scapula fractures would benefit from surgical treatment.

Technical Keys to Success

Setup/Exposure
- General anesthesia is administered.
- The patient may be placed in the lateral decubitus position such that the affected shoulder is tilted forward, enabling access to the posterior aspect of the shoulder girdle (**Figure 2, A**). This position provides appropriate access to the injury and allows the surgeon to obtain a scapular Y fluoroscopic image (**Figure 2, B**) for assessing sagittal plane correction and fixation.
- Alternatively, the patient may be positioned prone with the ipsilateral arm draped free and a small bump placed beneath the anterior chest.
- If the patient has an ipsilateral displaced clavicle, then the displaced clavicle is typically reduced and stabilized before the scapular fracture is addressed. The lateral position allows access to the clavicle and the scapula without repositioning.
- The entire forequarter is widely prepped and draped, enabling unrestricted motion of the shoulder.
- Bony landmarks are palpated in the posterior shoulder and marked with a sterile pen (**Figure 3, A**). In muscular patients, grasping the scapula and attempting to protract and retract the shoulder allows the surgeon to better identify the bony landmarks.
- In patients with an anterior scapula

Table 1 Results of Management of Scapular Fractures

Authors	Journal (Year)	Technique (No. of Patients)	Outcomes and Comments
Hardegger et al	*J Bone Joint Surg Br* (1984)	Judet (37)	To prevent late disability, anatomic repositioning of glenoid fracture-dislocations, scapular neck fractures, and displaced apophyseal fractures is needed Mean follow-up, 78 mo
Ada and Miller	*Clin Orthop Relat Res* (1991)	Nonsurgical (113)	24 patients available for follow-up Patients with displaced scapular neck and spine fractures should undergo surgical treatment Minimum follow-up, 15 mo
Bozkurt et al	*Injury* (2005)	Nonsurgical (18)	A glenopolar angle ≤20° is predictive of shoulder dysfunction Mean follow-up, 25 mo
van Noort and van Kampen	*Arch Orthop Trauma Surg* (2005)	Nonsurgical (24)	Good clinical results and no neurologic disability Mean follow-up, 66 mo
Gosens et al	*J Shoulder Elbow Surg* (2009)	Nonsurgical (26)	Worse functional outcome with nonsurgical treatment in patients with concomitant injuries than in patients with isolated scapular fracture Mean follow-up, 22 mo
Herrera et al	*J Bone Joint Surg Br* (2009)	Posterior Judet (19) Anterior Judet (2) Combined anterior and posterior Judet (1)	Surgical treatment prevents malunion in patients with delayed presentation Mean follow-up, 26.4 mo
Jones et al	*J Orthop Trauma* (2009)	Modified Judet (37)	This approach enables excellent visualization of the scapula or glenoid while minimizing iatrogenic injury of the posterior rotator cuff Mean follow-up, 12 mo
Schofer et al	*Arch Orthop Trauma Surg* (2009)	Nonsurgical (137)	Nonsurgical management of scapular fracture results in decreased range of motion Mean follow-up, 65 mo
Bartoníček and Frič	*Int Orthop* (2011)	Posterior Judet (22)	Stable fixation of the lateral border is necessary to restore anatomic reduction of the scapula, and it improves clinical outcome Mean follow-up, 26 mo
Cole et al	*J Orthop Trauma* (2011)	Posterior Judet (5)	Surgical reconstruction of scapular malunion results in improved shoulder function Mean follow-up, 39 mo
Dimitroulias et al	*Clin Orthop Relat Res* (2011)	Nonsurgical (49)	Increased Injury Severity Score and presence of rib fractures are associated with worse clinical outcome Mean follow-up, 15 mo

fracture requiring access to the coracoid or anterior glenoid, the patient is positioned in the beach-chair position with an arm board attached to the extremity; the affected extremity may also be secured with the use of a shoulder positioner.

JUDET APPROACH

- The extensile Judet incision is the classic approach for scapular neck and body fractures. This posterior approach allows visualization of the infraspinatus fossa and the scapular borders and neck by elevating the infraspinatus muscle out of its fossa from lateral to medial, maintaining the neurovascular pedicle, and placing it inverted superolaterally out of the surgical field. This enables access to medial, lateral, and superior bone stock for fixation.

- This incision is the standard approach for managing severely comminuted fractures with multiple exit points through the borders requiring extensive visualization and in cases of substantial callus formation or late malunion.

- The incision parallels the palpable scapular spine beginning at the base of the acromion and extends medially toward the medial angle (**Figure 3, A**). The incision then courses toward the inferior angle of the scapula.

- A large skin flap with the underlying subcutaneous tissue is elevated off the underlying fascia to expose the posterior deltoid, infraspinatus, teres minor, and teres major muscles (**Figure 3, B**).

- Dissection proceeds with release of the infraspinatus muscle. The medial scapular border is sharply reflected and carefully elevated off the infraspinatus fossa with the use of a Cobb elevator in a subperiosteal fashion (**Figure 3, C** and **D**).

- The suprascapular nerve enters the surgical field laterally as it descends from the spinoglenoid notch. The ascending branch of the circumflex scapular artery is encountered on the lateral border of the scapula body inferior to the glenoid neck (on average, 4 cm inferior to the articular surface). The branch is often clotted; however, if it bleeds it should be ligated because it will bleed quickly if injured. Vascular clips are often useful to achieve hemostasis.

- Although the Judet approach exposes the entire posterior surface of the scapular body, the subscapularis is preserved on the anterior surface, maintaining blood supply to the scapular body.

- Exposure of all fragments allows fixation with minifragment or small-fragment plating systems (**Figure 3, E**). All essential scapular attachments of the infraspinatus muscle are released.

- Care must be taken to identify and protect the nerve and artery

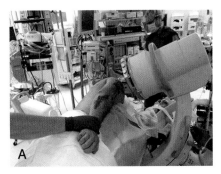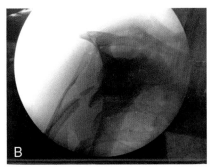

Figure 2   **A,** Intraoperative photograph shows a patient placed on a radiolucent table in the lateral decubitus position with the shoulder girdle leaning slightly forward to enable intraoperative imaging. **B,** Scapular Y fluoroscopic image obtained intraoperatively to assess anteroposterior reduction and fixation. (Courtesy of Chad Corrigan, MD, Wichita, KS.)

branches extending to the infraspinatus muscle as they exit the spinoglenoid notch to avoid denervation and devascularization.

MODIFIED JUDET APPROACH

- As with the standard Judet approach, the initial incision courses along the scapular spine to the superomedial angle of the scapula and is directed toward the inferior angle (**Figure 3, A**).

- A large skin flap with the underlying subcutaneous tissue is developed as described previously, enabling exposure of the posterior shoulder girdle musculature (**Figure 3, B**). This dissection is developed in the areolar plane between the muscle and subcutaneous tissue.

- Spreading with heavy scissors often helps identify the correct plane.

- The perforating vessels can be controlled with electrocautery; however, dissection with electrocautery often makes it difficult to maintain the correct plane.

- The plane between the deltoid and infraspinatus muscles is developed with blunt or sharp dissection to identify the interval between the posterior deltoid and the infraspinatus muscles.

- Sharp dissection or Bovie electrocautery is used to release the fascial

origin of the posterior deltoid off the scapular spine. The fascial cuff is tagged for reattachment at the conclusion of the procedure.

- The deltoid is reflected anterolaterally to allow visualization of the infraspinatus, teres minor, and teres major muscles (**Figure 4, A**).

- Alternatively, if the deltoid is not too large it can be left attached, instead mobilizing the plane between the deltoid and infraspinatus and elevating the deltoid with a deep retractor.

- The plane between the teres minor and infraspinatus muscles is lateral and distal on the scapula and may be developed with blunt dissection (**Figure 4, B**). In the modified Judet approach, the infraspinatus remains in the scapular fossa; the infraspinatus is minimally dissected and left attached to the scapula. The muscle is mobilized only on the periphery of the scapula to expose sufficient bone to facilitate internal fixation.

- After the plane is developed, the ascending branch of the circumflex scapular artery is exposed and ligated if it was not torn and clotted as a result of the fracture. The artery is often located at the fracture site.

- This area of the fracture on the lateral border is exposed on the

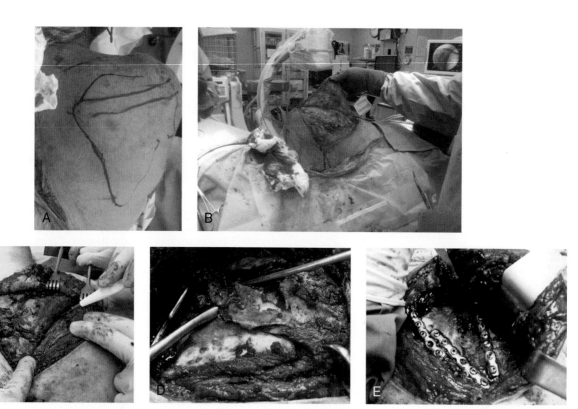

Figure 3 Intraoperative photographs show the Judet approach. **A,** The scapular borders are marked to identify essential bony landmarks to guide the skin incision. **B,** A large skin flap is elevated, exposing the underlying fascia. The infraspinatus is elevated off the medial border and carefully elevated off the fossa (**C**), enabling exposure of the fracture (**D**) for reduction and stabilization (**E**).

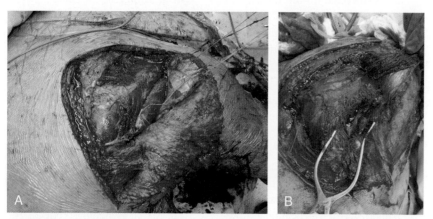

Figure 4 Intraoperative photographs of the modified Judet approach. **A,** Appearance of the shoulder after release and reflection of the posterior deltoid muscle off the scapular spine. **B,** The interval between the infraspinatus and teres minor muscles is bluntly separated, exposing the scapula.

respectively, permits visualization of the lateral border of the scapula.

- The use of nonstatic retractors may decrease the risk of muscle ischemia and necrosis of the infraspinatus and teres minor muscles. Although the interval lies between the teres minor and the infraspinatus, the teres major is also retracted.

- The medial border of the scapula or the scapular spine is exposed at the fracture site, and the periosteum is cleared to allow reduction and plate placement (**Figure 5, I** and **J**).

DELTOPECTORAL APPROACH
- A classic deltopectoral incision is made.
- The cephalic vein is identified and retracted laterally.
- The interval between the deltoid and pectoralis major muscles is identified and bluntly developed down the level of the clavipectoral

dorsal side of the scapula so that if the artery is lacerated, it does not retract anteriorly and bleed excessively.
- Vascular clips should be readily available for use in case the vessel

is inadvertently transected before ligation.
- Gentle caudal and cranial retraction of the superior border of the teres minor muscle and the inferior border of the infraspinatus muscle,

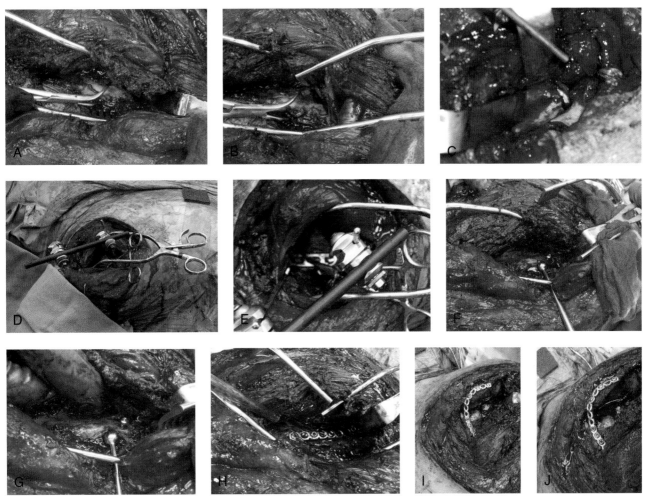

Figure 5 Intraoperative photographs show the modified Judet approach. Fracture reduction is achieved with small-pointed reduction clamps (**A** and **B**) and a 4.0-mm Schanz pin (**C**). External fixator clamps and a bar are used to maintain fracture reduction (**D**) during fixation (**E**). **F** and **G,** A ball-spiked pusher is used to correct deformity and achieve bony reduction. **H** through **J,** Note the fairly broad exposure for placement of fixation with this approach. (Courtesy of Chad Corrigan, MD, Wichita, KS.)

fascia, which is opened to expose the coracobrachialis and subscapularis muscles.

- An uncommon scapular fracture that may be encountered is the superior glenoid fracture that extends to the coracoid process, resulting in displacement of the coracoid process. This fragment is difficult to reduce and stabilize. A percutaneous portal at the junction of the clavicle may be used. This fragment is often minimally displaced and can be left with some displacement because it is not essential for joint stability and is non–weight-bearing. If reduction

is required, the surgeon can access the coracoid and the coracoclavicular ligaments by extending the deltopectoral interval proximally to the level of the clavicle.

- An unstable anterior glenoid fragment can be accessed by taking down or splitting the subscapularis tendon, and the coracoid process can be stabilized with a long 3.5-mm screw.

LATERAL BORDER APPROACH

- The lateral border approach is oriented over the glenoid neck or lateral border of the scapula, with the

skin incision over the bony landmarks. Visualization of the fracture for reduction and fixation is challenging with this approach in muscular patients and in obese patients. The lateral border approach can be used if only a lateral baseplate is needed for fixation.

- A straight incision of approximately 6 cm is made, and dissection is extended to the deltoid fascia, which is divided in line with its fibers at the inferior edge.
- The deltoid muscle is retracted cephalad, enabling exposure of the external rotators.

- The fascia overlying the infraspinatus and teres minor muscles is divided in line with its fibers to expose the interval between these two muscle bellies.
- Blunt dissection in this interval exposes the fracture site.
- Care must be taken with cephalad retraction of the infraspinatus muscle to avoid tethering or injuring the suprascapular nerve that exits at the base of the acromion in the spinoglenoid notch.
- The ascending branch of the circumflex scapular artery may be encountered at the lateral border of the scapula approximately 4 cm distal to the glenoid rim. The vessel may be cauterized or clipped if necessary.

SUPERIOR APPROACH

- The superior approach to the scapula involves an incision extending along the prominent posterior border of the lateral acromion and acromial spine.
- The incision is taken down to the posterior border of the acromion between the fascia of the deltoid and trapezius muscles.
- The deltoid muscle is elevated off the posterior aspect of the acromial spine and reflected with the infraspinatus muscle to expose the bone at the fracture site.
- The neck and base of the acromion, including the entire acromial spine, may be exposed to the vertebral border for visualization if necessary.
- A lamina spreader is used to distract the fragments to débride callus and hematoma while the fracture edges are cleared of interposed periosteum.

Instruments/Equipment/Implants Required

- A radiolucent table is used, with the patient placed in a prone or lateral

position. With lateral positioning, a beanbag is placed.
- 3.5- or 2.7-mm plates and screws (locking or nonlocking) are used. The authors of this chapter routinely use nonlocking 2.7-mm implants.
- A small external fixator should be made available in case of malunions or late fixation.
- A ball-spiked reduction tool is used.
- Small and medium reduction clamps are used.
- Nonabsorbable 2.0 suture is used.
- Two drains are placed during wound closure.

Procedure

- Because surgical management of scapular fractures is often delayed, the reduction of the lateral border and the neck of the scapula may be particularly difficult in the patient with a highly displaced and angulated glenoid.
- The lateral scapular border can be reduced with the use of small-pointed reduction clamps (**Figure 5, A** and **B**).
- Alternatively, 4.0-mm Schanz pins (**Figure 5, C**) may be placed into the glenoid neck and lateral scapula to facilitate fragment manipulation and fracture reduction. After fracture reduction is obtained, these pins may be secured with bars to maintain reduction during fixation (**Figure 5, D** and **E**).
- A 2.0- or 2.5-mm drill bit may also be used to place a hole into the distal lateral border of the scapula, enabling the use of a ball-spiked pusher (**Figure 5, F** and **G**) to control lateral-to-medial deviation of the distal lateral fragment; one or two Kirschner wires are then placed to maintain fracture reduction.
- When the modified Judet approach is used, mobilization, reduction, and fixation can be particularly difficult in patients treated more

than 10 days after the injury.
- In patients with acute injuries, reduction can be accomplished with the use of Kirschner wires or 4-mm Schanz pins placed into the lateral border, glenoid neck, or spine of the scapula. The wires or pins can be mobilized to manipulate the fracture and achieve improved reduction.
- Small-pointed reduction clamps may be used to maintain the reduction.
- A small external fixator may also be applied.
- If it is necessary to medialize the scapular body in a controlled fashion, a hole can be drilled at the lateral wall; a ball-spiked pusher can then be used to enable gentle pushing of the scapular body in the medial direction until reduction of the lateral border is achieved.
- Buttress plating of the lateral border with 2.7- or 3.5-mm reconstruction plates is done through the Judet or modified Judet approach (**Figure 5, H, I,** and **J**).
- The authors of this chapter prefer to use 2.7-mm nonlocking plates, which are easier to contour, offer more points of fixation, and have a lower profile than 3.5-mm plates. On the lateral border of the scapula, 2.7-mm dynamic compression or reconstruction plates are used, whereas 2.7-mm reconstruction plates are used on the scapular body or spine.
- Reduction and fixation is complete when all fracture fragments have been reduced and stabilized to allow early motion.

Wound Closure

- Repair of the deltoid to the scapular spine through drill tunnels is completed with nonabsorbable suture.
- In a similar fashion, the fascia between the infraspinatus and rhomboid muscles is reapproximated at

Table 2 Rehabilitation Protocol After Management of Fractures of the Scapular Body and Neck

Postoperative Week	ROM	Strengthening	Return to Play
0-2	Full active and passive ROM is begun 1 or 2 d postoperatively; passive and active-assisted ROM are advanced as pain subsides After hospital discharge, physical therapy is continued and home therapy using pulleys and supine-assisted motion is commenced	Ipsilateral elbow, wrist, and hand exercise program using 3- to 5-lb weights	None
2-6	—	At 5 wk postoperatively, shoulder strengthening and resistance with 3- to 5-lb weights is begun	None
6-12	—	Strength and endurance training is begun at approximately 9 wk	None
12-24	—	—	Normal activity is resumed at 3 mo

ROM = range of motion.

the medial scapular border through drill holes.

- Because a large subcutaneous flap is present, drains are placed to exit superiorly and laterally to minimize the potential for seroma formation. Drains are kept in place until minimal output is present.

- Layered closure of the skin flap is completed. The authors of this chapter prefer to use subcuticular monofilament closure because it offers good cosmetic results and may help avoid infection by sealing the wound.

Rehabilitation

Postoperative rehabilitation is directed at maintaining motion because the shoulder tends to become stiff with immobility. Therefore, full active-assisted and passive ROM are emphasized beginning 1 or 2 days postoperatively. Under the direction of a physical therapist, passive ROM and active-assisted motion are advanced as the patient's pain subsides. After patients are discharged from the hospital, they commence a home therapy program using pulleys and supine-assisted motion with push-pull sticks. An ipsilateral elbow, wrist, and hand exercise program using 3- to 5-lb weights is encouraged to promote edema reduction and prevent muscular atrophy. At 5 weeks postoperatively, a program of shoulder strengthening and resistance with 3- to 5-lb weights is commenced, followed by strength and endurance training beginning at approximately 9 weeks postoperatively. At 3 months, restrictions are removed and the patient resumes normal activity. The rehabilitation protocol is summarized in **Table 2**.

Avoiding Pitfalls

Preoperative review of all imaging, particularly the 3D CT reconstruction of the fracture, is necessary to plan the surgical approach and understand the maneuvers required to achieve reduction. In the setting of scapular fracture that extends from the superior glenoid to the base of the coracoid, the superior glenoid fragment is difficult to reduce and stabilize. Surgeons should consider accepting some displacement of this

fragment because it is not critical to shoulder stability or function. Attempted reduction may be more harmful than residual displacement.

The modified Judet approach limits muscle dissection by following muscular planes. When using this approach, the surgeon should take care to develop the plane between the posterior deltoid and the underlying infraspinatus muscles before sharply dissecting the fascia of the posterior deltoid origin to enable anterolateral reflection of the deltoid. This step should be accomplished without entering the lateral deltoid, and the surgeon must ensure that a cuff of fascia remains for fixation at the conclusion of the procedure. In a muscular patient, it is possible to dissect between the teres minor and teres major muscles, resulting in limited exposure of the scapular neck and lateral border.

The classic Judet approach allows for excellent exposure of the scapular fossa to the lateral border. The infraspinatus muscle should be carefully elevated off its fossa, particularly toward the lateral half, where the suprascapular neurovascular bundle resides at the level of the spinoglenoid notch. In addition, in patients with a fractured scapular body, the surgeon should take care to avoid entrapment of the suprascapular nerve within the fracture.

Identification of the ascending branch of the circumflex scapular artery is important because it is typically located at the glenoid fracture location and can bleed profusely. The artery should be identified and cauterized or clipped before transection because it can retract anteriorly and become difficult to control.

The complication rates after ORIF of scapular fractures are low. Because of the proximity of the suprascapular, axillary, and musculocutaneous nerves to the surgical site, the potential for nerve injury exists. Stiffness is common after any shoulder surgical procedure, particularly in patients who have had a substantial period of immobilization preoperatively or postoperatively. Aggressive physical therapy targeted at obtaining full ROM should begin immediately postoperatively.

■ Bibliography

Ada JR, Miller ME: Scapular fractures: Analysis of 113 cases. *Clin Orthop Relat Res* 1991;(269):174-180.

Anavian J, Conflitti JM, Khanna G, Guthrie ST, Cole PA: A reliable radiographic measurement technique for extra-articular scapular fractures. *Clin Orthop Relat Res* 2011;469(12):3371-3378.

Anavian J, Wijdicks CA, Schroder LK, Vang S, Cole PA: Surgery for scapula process fractures: Good outcome in 26 patients. *Acta Orthop* 2009;80(3):344-350.

Armstrong CP, Van der Spuy J: The fractured scapula: Importance and management based on a series of 62 patients. *Injury* 1984;15(5):324-329.

Bartoníček J, Frič V: Scapular body fractures: Results of operative treatment. *Int Orthop* 2011;35(5):747-753.

Bozkurt M, Can F, Kirdemir V, Erden Z, Demirkale I, Başbozkurt M: Conservative treatment of scapular neck fracture: The effect of stability and glenopolar angle on clinical outcome. *Injury* 2005;36(10):1176-1181.

Cole PA, Gauger EM, Herrera DA, Anavian J, Tarkin IS: Radiographic follow-up of 84 operatively treated scapula neck and body fractures. *Injury* 2012;43(3):327-333.

Cole PA, Talbot M, Schroder LK, Anavian J: Extra-articular malunions of the scapula: A comparison of functional outcome before and after reconstruction. *J Orthop Trauma* 2011;25(11):649-656.

Dimitroulias A, Molinero KG, Krenk DE, Muffly MT, Altman DT, Altman GT: Outcomes of nonoperatively treated displaced scapular body fractures. *Clin Orthop Relat Res* 2011;469(5):1459-1465.

Gosens T, Speigner B, Minekus J: Fracture of the scapular body: Functional outcome after conservative treatment. *J Shoulder Elbow Surg* 2009;18(3):443-448.

Hardegger FH, Simpson LA, Weber BG: The operative treatment of scapular fractures. *J Bone Joint Surg Br* 1984;66(5):725-731.

Herrera DA, Anavian J, Tarkin IS, Armitage BA, Schroder LK, Cole PA: Delayed operative management of fractures of the scapula. *J Bone Joint Surg Br* 2009;91(5):619-626.

Imatani RJ: Fractures of the scapula: A review of 53 fractures. *J Trauma* 1975;15(6):473-478.

Jones CB, Cornelius JP, Sietsema DL, Ringler JR, Endres TJ: Modified Judet approach and minifragment fixation of scapular body and glenoid neck fractures. *J Orthop Trauma* 2009;23(8):558-564.

Khallaf F, Mikami A, Al-Akkad M: The use of surgery in displaced scapular neck fractures. *Med Princ Pract* 2006;15(6):443-448.

Kim KC, Rhee KJ, Shin HD, Yang JY: Can the glenopolar angle be used to predict outcome and treatment of the floating shoulder? *J Trauma* 2008;64(1):174-178.

Lantry JM, Roberts CS, Giannoudis PV: Operative treatment of scapular fractures: A systematic review. *Injury* 2008;39(3):271-283.

McGahan JP, Rab GT, Dublin A: Fractures of the scapula. *J Trauma* 1980;20(10):880-883.

McGinnis M, Denton JR: Fractures of the scapula: A retrospective study of 40 fractured scapulae. *J Trauma* 1989;29(11):1488-1493.

Nordqvist A, Petersson C: Fracture of the body, neck, or spine of the scapula: A long-term follow-up study. *Clin Orthop Relat Res* 1992;(283):139-144.

Obremskey WT, Lyman JR: A modified Judet approach to the scapula. *J Orthop Trauma* 2004;18(10):696-699.

Pace AM, Stuart R, Brownlow H: Outcome of glenoid neck fractures. *J Shoulder Elbow Surg* 2005;14(6):585-590.

Romero J, Schai P, Imhoff AB: Scapular neck fracture: The influence of permanent malalignment of the glenoid neck on clinical outcome. *Arch Orthop Trauma Surg* 2001;121(6):313-316.

Schofer MD, Sehrt AC, Timmesfeld N, Störmer S, Kortmann HR: Fractures of the scapula: Long-term results after conservative treatment. *Arch Orthop Trauma Surg* 2009;129(11):1511-1519.

van Noort A, van Kampen A: Fractures of the scapula surgical neck: Outcome after conservative treatment in 13 cases. *Arch Orthop Trauma Surg* 2005;125(10):696-700.

Wijdicks CA, Armitage BM, Anavian J, Schroder LK, Cole PA: Vulnerable neurovasculature with a posterior approach to the scapula. *Clin Orthop Relat Res* 2009;467(8):2011-2017.

Wilson P: *Experience of the Management of Fractures and Dislocations (Based on Analysis of 4,390 Cases) by Staff of the Fracture Service MGH, Boston.* Philadelphia, PA, JB Lippincott, 1938.

Zlowodzki M, Bhandari M, Zelle BA, Kregor PJ, Cole PA: Treatment of scapula fractures: Systematic review of 520 fractures in 22 case series. *J Orthop Trauma* 2006;20(3):230-233.

Chapter 57
Surgical Management of the Floating Shoulder

Mark A. Schrumpf, MD

Samuel Harmsen, MD

Danielle Casagrande, MD

Introduction

The superior shoulder suspensory complex (SSSC) consists of the glenoid, coracoid process, coracoclavicular ligaments, distal clavicle, acromioclavicular joint, and acromion process. This ring of osseous and soft-tissue structures supports the shoulder and provides stability between the axial skeleton and the upper extremity (**Figure 1**). This complex ring is supported by an anterior strut (clavicle) and posterior struts (scapular body and spine). Any double disruption of this complex results in an unstable relationship between the axial skeleton and the upper extremity, resulting in a rare injury often referred to as the floating shoulder. Ipsilateral clavicle and scapular neck fractures represent the most common double disruption, and the optimal management of these rare, often high-energy injuries remains controversial. However, floating shoulder injuries can also consist of soft-tissue disruptions of the acromioclavicular and sternoclavicular joints.

Although floating shoulder injuries may be visible on the initial chest radiographs of trauma patients, the presence of concomitant injuries may delay the

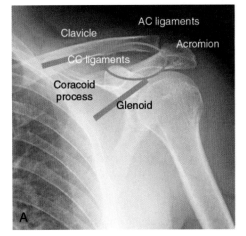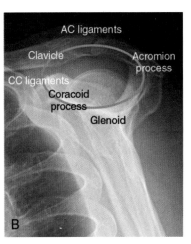

Figure 1   AP (**A**) and scapular Y (**B**) radiographs demonstrate the anatomic structures that comprise an intact superior shoulder suspensory complex. AC = acromioclavicular, CC = coracoclavicular.

identification of a floating shoulder injury. When a floating shoulder is identified, a standard three-view shoulder series consisting of Grashey, scapular Y, and axillary views is the initial imaging of choice. Although these radiographs are often sufficient for evaluation of the clavicular fracture, the scapular fracture can be difficult to evaluate with radiographs alone. Therefore, a CT scan of the shoulder including the entirety of the scapula is recommended. Three-dimensional CT reconstructions can

be particularly helpful in evaluating the involvement of the scapular spine, scapular body, and glenoid neck.

The timing of surgical intervention is critical. Although fixation of the clavicle can often be accomplished quickly, it usually requires general anesthesia because regional anesthesia frequently does not cover the whole field. Additionally, surgical fixation of the scapula is often an involved and lengthy procedure. Therefore, surgical management should be delayed until the patient is well resuscitated and any head, neck, and chest injuries have been stabilized. Fixation of most floating shoulder injuries can be done within the first 1 to 2 weeks after fracture. However, if the

Dr. Schrumpf or an immediate family member serves as a paid consultant to Tornier. Neither of the following authors nor any immediate family member has received anything of value from or has stock or stock options held in a commercial company or institution related directly or indirectly to the subject of this chapter: Dr. Harmsen and Dr. Casagrande.

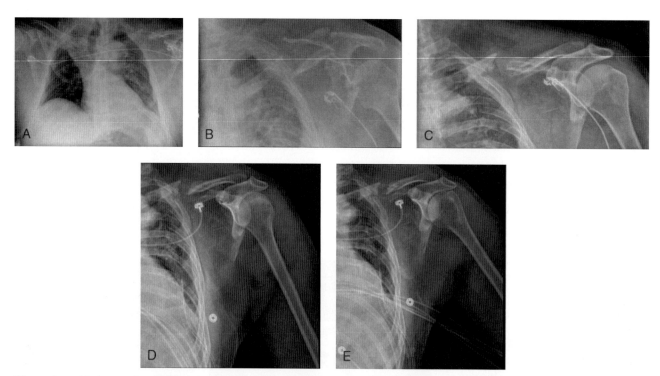

Figure 2 AP chest radiograph (**A**), AP (**B**) and sunrise (**C**) radiographs of the clavicle, and internal rotation AP (**D**) and external rotation AP (**E**) radiographs of the shoulder demonstrate a floating shoulder with a comminuted, widely displaced fracture of the clavicle and a fracture of the glenoid neck. Multiple rib fractures, bilateral pneumothoraces, and a left-side scapulothoracic disassociation are also seen.

surgeon plans to rely on fixation of the clavicular fracture alone for reduction of a displaced scapular fracture, earlier intervention may be preferable. As additional time passes, the likelihood of successful indirect reduction decreases.

The first step in surgical intervention is deciding on fixation of both the clavicle and the scapula or fixation of the clavicle alone. The authors of this chapter recommend evaluation of intraoperative fluoroscopic images to guide this decision. Standard indications for scapular fixation include a glenopolar angle of less than 20°, angulation greater than 40°, and/or displacement greater than 1 cm.

Case Presentation

A 38-year-old man is transported to the emergency department via ambulance following an automobile-pedestrian collision. The patient has a closed head injury as well as a floating left shoulder. The patient also has bilateral hemopneumothoraces, multiple rib fractures, and scapulothoracic dissociation on the left side (**Figure 2**). As in many patients with floating shoulder injuries, the fractures of the shoulder girdle occurred as a result of high-energy trauma that resulted in severe and devastating injuries.

Surgical management consisting of clavicular fixation with a superior plate successfully restored the length and stability of the SSSC (**Figure 3**). Nonsurgical management was chosen for the scapular neck injury because the glenopolar angle was approximately 40° and no intra-articular extension of the fracture was observed. In addition, the prone patient positioning and surgical dissection that would have been required for a Judet approach for scapular fixation were considered too dangerous to attempt in this patient because of the severe injuries to the chest wall and lungs. The patient achieved uneventful union of the clavicular and scapular neck fractures; however, the closed head injury sustained at the time of the initial injury limited his ability to make a full functional recovery. The neurologic status of the limb is an important consideration in deciding whether surgical management is necessary or appropriate for any given patient. Nevertheless, it is difficult to know at the time of injury to what extent a neurologic injury may recover. Therefore, it should be assumed that at least a partial neurologic recovery will be achieved.

Indications

Individual fractures of the clavicle and scapular neck can be managed nonsurgically with good to excellent results. However, if these fractures are displaced or unstable, they are best managed with open reduction and internal fixation (ORIF). Current recommendations for fixation of clavicular fractures include comminution, greater than 2 cm of shortening, or greater than 100% displacement of the fracture fragments. In patients with these indications, surgical treatment has been reported to result in improved union rates, improved time to union, increased patient satisfaction, increased shoulder strength and endurance, and decreased pain. Indications for surgical fixation of scapular fractures include 1 cm of displacement, angulation in the coronal or sagittal plane greater than 40°, associated intra-articular glenoid fractures with displacement of greater than 2 to 5 mm, and/or a glenopolar angle less than 20° to 30° (**Figure 4**). Surgical management in these patients has shown good to excellent results and improvements in range of motion. The authors of this chapter use these indications independently for both the clavicle and the scapular neck in the treatment of floating shoulder injuries.

In patients with a floating shoulder, a scapular neck fracture can lead to increased displacement of the clavicular fracture, and clavicle fracture can lead to increased displacement of the scapular fracture. This disruption results in altered muscular forces across these structures and can result in increased instability of the SSSC. Surgical management of the floating shoulder is recommended in these instances. Restoration of the anterior strut with reduction and fixation of the clavicle restores the anatomic alignment of the shoulder and often leads to indirect reduction and stabilization of the glenoid neck fracture. This indirect reduction results in restoration of the posterior strut as well. Therefore, restoration of the stability of the SSSC can frequently be accomplished by ORIF of the clavicular fracture alone, as in the case presented in this chapter.

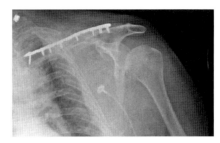

Figure 3 Postoperative AP radiograph of the shoulder described in Figure 2 after open reduction and internal fixation of the clavicle. The scapular fracture was acceptably reduced by means of the clavicular fixation; thus, no further intervention was necessary.

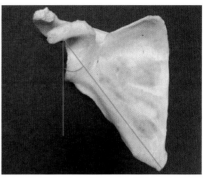

Figure 4 Photograph of a cadaver specimen shows determination of the glenopolar angle, which is calculated by measuring the angle subtended by a line drawn parallel to the glenoid and a line drawn from the inferior angle of the scapula to the superior margin of the glenoid on a Grashey radiograph.

Surgical management of the clavicular fracture is relatively easy from a technical standpoint and has a low complication profile. Both plate osteosynthesis and intramedullary nail fixation have shown good results in the management of floating shoulder injuries. Occasionally, however, indirect reduction does not occur and the scapular neck displacement persists. The authors of this chapter recommend using intraoperative fluoroscopy to assess the displacement and stability of the scapular neck after fixation of the clavicle. If substantial displacement remains, ORIF of the scapular neck should be performed.

Other factors that should be considered when choosing between surgical and nonsurgical treatment include the patient's preinjury level of function, age, hand dominance, and concomitant injuries. Floating shoulder injuries are often the result of high-energy trauma and can be associated with severe injuries to the chest, head, spine, abdominal cavity, and extremities. Early stabilization of the floating shoulder in polytrauma patients can be beneficial in patient care, transfers, early mobilization, occupational therapy, and respiratory therapy. However, some patients may not be stable enough to undergo a prolonged surgical procedure. In these patients, surgical stabilization of the clavicle alone is preferred, regardless of scapular

displacement. If the patient's condition is too unstable to allow surgical intervention, nonsurgical management is acceptable.

Controversies and Results

Because the floating shoulder is rare, great controversy exists regarding whether this injury should be managed surgically or nonsurgically. Furthermore, when surgical fixation is chosen, the question of whether fixation of the clavicle alone or fixation of both the clavicle and the scapula should be performed has not been clearly resolved. Although several published series have addressed these questions, consensus has not been reached (**Table 1**). One reason for this lack of clarity is variation in the definition of a floating shoulder. Whereas the original definition includes any combined fractures of the clavicle and scapula, some authors have proposed that the stability of coracoacromial and acromioclavicular ligaments should be considered. Although the Goss definition of the SSSC is comprehensive, the definitions used in the published literature are not uniform. Nonetheless,

Table 1 Results of Surgical Treatment of Floating Shoulder Injury[a]

Authors	Journal (Year)	Technique (No. of Patients)	Outcomes	Comments
Edwards et al	*J Bone Joint Surg Am* (2000)	Sling immobilization (20)	19 patients had uneventful healing 17 patients had excellent and 3 patients had good results by Herscovici rating Avg Constant score, 96	Nonsurgical management of floating shoulder injuries, especially those with <5 mm of displacement, can result in patient satisfaction
Egol et al	*J Bone Joint Surg Am* (2001)	Nonsurgical treatment (12) or ORIF (7)	No significant difference in SF-36, DASH, or ASES scores Forward flexion statistically greater in the surgical group	Surgical group weaker in both external and internal rotation The authors of the study concluded that patient satisfaction can be achieved with either surgical or nonsurgical treatment
van Noort et al	*J Bone Joint Surg Br* (2001)	Nonsurgical treatment (28) or surgical (clavicle only) treatment (7)	Better avg Constant score in the nonsurgical group compared with the surgical group (76 and 71, respectively) Lower avg Constant score in patients with caudal dislocation in both groups (nonsurgical, 42; surgical, 62)	The authors of the study recommended nonsurgical treatment of patients with nondisplaced ipsilateral fractures and surgical treatment of patients with fracture of the clavicle and caudally displaced fracture of the scapular neck
Izadpanah et al	*J Trauma Acute Care Surg* (2012)	Plate fixation (9) or titanium elastic nail fixation (7)	No significant differences in ASES scores, Constant score, or glenopolar angle	Titanium elastic nail fixation resulted in shortening of the clavicle in patients with Orthopaedic Trauma Association type B and C clavicular fractures
Pailhes et al	*Int J Shoulder Surg* (2013)	Nonsurgical treatment with sling immobilization (24) or surgical treatment (16)	No significant differences in avg Constant, SST, Oxford shoulder, SANE, SF-12, or DASH scores	Of the 16 surgically treated patients, the clavicle only was treated in 10, the scapula only was treated in 3, and both the clavicle and the scapula were treated in 3 Consecutive series Loss of lateral offset influenced the results negatively Osteoarthritis occurred in 5 patients (12.5%) without correlation to fracture patterns and type of treatment
Yadav et al	*Bone Joint J* (2013)	Surgical fixation of clavicle alone (12) or nonsurgical treatment with figure-of-8 brace (13)	Clinical outcomes for pain, quality of life, strength, and ROM better in the surgical group at 3 mo Only ROM remained significantly different 2 yr postoperatively	The authors of this study did not compare fixation of the clavicle alone with fixation of both the clavicle and the scapular neck No correlation was noted between glenopolar angle and outcome 2 yr postoperatively

ASES = American Shoulder and Elbow Surgeons shoulder outcome; DASH = Disabilities of the Arm, Shoulder and Hand; NR = not reported; ORIF = open reduction and internal fixation; ROM = range of motion; SANE = Single Assessment Numeric Evaluation; SF-12 = Medical Outcomes Study 12-Item Short Form; SF-36 = Medical Outcomes Study 36-Item Short Form; SST = simple shoulder test.

[a] Failure rate was not reported in any of these studies.

several retrospective studies can help guide management of this rare injury. In a study of nine patients with ipsilateral fractures of the clavicle and the scapular neck, the seven patients treated with clavicle fixation alone had excellent results, whereas the two patients treated nonsurgically had decreased range of motion and a drooping shoulder. The authors of the study therefore strongly recommended ORIF of the clavicle in patients with these injuries.

However, a review of 13 patients treated nonsurgically used the same criteria as the previously mentioned study and found that all but one patient had good or excellent functional results. In a study of 20 patients with floating shoulder injuries that were managed nonsurgically, all patients had excellent or good results and regained strength equal to that of the uninjured extremity. A study of 15 patients who underwent surgical fixation of both the clavicle and the scapula found that 14 patients experienced healing with good or excellent functional results. Although those studies did not compare surgical and nonsurgical treatment, several studies that did were no more revealing. One study comparing surgical and nonsurgical treatment showed no significant difference between groups with regard to functional outcome measures. However, forward flexion was greater and external and internal rotation were weaker in surgically treated patients compared with those treated nonsurgically. In a review of eight patients treated nonsurgically and nine treated surgically, five patients in each group had excellent or good results. The authors of the study suggested that associated injuries heavily influenced the outcomes and that substantially displaced fractures should therefore be managed surgically if associated injuries allow. Other studies have attempted to use qualitative measures to guide treatment. A review of 24 patients treated nonsurgically and 16 treated surgically revealed no significant differences between groups. However, the authors of the study noted that the loss of lateral offset influenced the functional results negatively. The authors of a multicenter study concluded that a floating shoulder injury is not inherently unstable and can be managed nonsurgically in the absence of caudal dislocation of the glenoid, which the authors described as inferior angulation of the glenoid greater than 20°. A prospective study comparing nonsurgical treatment with surgical treatment consisting of clavicle fixation alone indicated a significant improvement in the glenopolar angle in the surgical group. Despite this finding, no significant correlation between the change in glenopolar angle and the Herscovici score was found at 2-year follow-up. Although the literature is informative, it does not provide clear guidelines for management of the floating shoulder. Future research may provide a consensus, although a randomized prospective study of such a rare injury is unlikely.

 Technical Keys to Success

Setup/Exposure

- For ORIF of the clavicle, the patient may be positioned either in the beach-chair position or supine on a radiolucent table. The authors of this chapter prefer the beach-chair position when its use is not precluded by other injuries.
- The ipsilateral arm is prepped and draped free to facilitate the surgical procedure.
- Although the lateral position allows both the clavicular and scapular fractures to be addressed without repositioning the patient, the authors of this chapter think that this position results in poor exposure of both fractures. Any time saved by not repositioning the patient is lost as a result of the increased difficulty of reduction and the poor surgical exposure.

Procedure
CLAVICULAR FRACTURE FIXATION

- The clavicle is approached through an anterior incision made in line with the clavicle. The incision is placed slightly inferior to the anteroinferior border of the clavicle to reduce wound healing complications and prominence of the scar.
- The platysma muscle is encountered below the skin and should be divided longitudinally so that it can be repaired over the plate at the conclusion of the procedure.
- Many supraclavicular nerves often run perpendicular to the incision. The surgeon should preserve as many of these nerves as possible to help prevent numbness and painful neuromas.
- The clavicle is approached with sharp dissection, and an elevator is used to expose the bone for plate fixation. Care should be taken not to be overzealous in stripping the fracture and devascularizing small fragments and comminution.
- After the fracture is exposed, it is reduced anatomically. Repositioning of the affected arm, the use of reduction forceps, and the use of Kirschner wires as joysticks can be helpful in achieving reduction.
- Lag screws can be used for stabilization and compression of larger fragments.
- For the reduction of long, oblique fractures, racking hitch sutures often can be used instead of bulky reduction forceps.
- Plates can be placed in the anteroinferior position, the superior position, or an orthogonal 90-90 position.
- Because of the complex shape of the clavicle, a 3.5-mm reconstruction plate or a precontoured plate is recommended. The authors of this chapter prefer to use a precontoured plate and typically place the plate over the apex of the fracture rather than use the same plate position for all clavicular fractures.
- After the fracture has been reduced and fixed, a fluoroscopic image of the shoulder should be obtained to check for reduction of the scapular fracture. In the patient with more than 1 cm of displacement of the scapular fracture, angulation in the coronal or sagittal plane greater than 40°, and/or a glenopolar angle less than 20° to 30°, the surgeon

should strongly consider proceeding with fixation of the scapular fracture.

SCAPULAR FRACTURE FIXATION

- The first step in addressing the scapular fracture is to reposition the patient. The authors of this chapter recommend a prone position unless the patient's pulmonary status precludes this position.

- Some fractures can be addressed with the patient in the lateral decubitus position; however, the weight of the arm often causes persistent medialization of the glenoid neck fragment, making reduction difficult.

- Regardless of the selected position, the arm is prepped and draped free to allow for indirect manipulation of the fracture fragments.

- The Judet approach is typically used for scapular fracture fixation. This approach allows excellent exposure to the medial and lateral borders of the scapula, the scapular spine, and the glenoid neck. The incision is a hockey stick–shaped approach beginning on the posterolateral border of the acromion, extending medially to the medial border of the scapula, and angling sharply toward the inferior pole of the scapula. However, when addressing a simple glenoid neck fracture, a more limited posterior glenohumeral approach or a modified Judet approach can be used as an alternative.

- Regardless of the approach, full-thickness flaps including skin and subcutaneous tissues are elevated off the fascia, exposing the posterior deltoid, infraspinatus, and teres minor muscles.

- The interval between the posterior deltoid and the underlying rotator cuff is dissected bluntly.

- In the standard Judet approach, the origins of the posterior deltoid and the infraspinatus are sequentially elevated off their bony insertions. A cuff of tissue, especially of the deltoid, should be left along the acromion for later repair.

- The entire infraspinatus can be lifted out of the infraspinatus fossa on its neurovascular pedicle because the innervation of the infraspinatus comes from the suprascapular nerve as it exits from the spinoglenoid notch. In patients with simpler fractures for whom a modified Judet approach is appropriate, elevation of either the lateral deltoid or the infraspinatus can be avoided without substantial loss of exposure. When possible, leaving the infraspinatus attached to the scapula and simply working through the interval between the infraspinatus and the teres minor can improve postoperative function of the rotator cuff.

- With some fracture patterns, the addition of a deltopectoral approach can be helpful. This approach is essential when addressing anterior glenoid rim fractures or coracoid fractures. An oblique skin incision is placed between the acromioclavicular joint and the coracoid and is extended to the inferomedial insertion of the deltoid on the humerus. The standard interval between the deltoid and the pectoralis major is opened, exposing the clavipectoral fascia and the underlying conjoint tendon and rotator cuff. In many patients, the interval between the deltoid and the pectoralis major is indicated by the presence of the cephalic vein and a fat stripe. To gain access to the glenoid, the rotator interval can be opened and the subscapularis can be taken down from the lesser tuberosity with sharp dissection or a lesser tuberosity osteotomy. Care should be taken to protect the axillary nerve that lies on the anterior muscle belly of the subscapularis.

- Before the reduction is attempted, all fracture lines should be mobilized and débrided.

- Reduction maneuvers are performed with Kirschner wires, reduction forceps, and manipulation of the free arm.

- Fixation of the scapula is performed with 2.7- or 3.5-mm reconstruction plates. Because much of the membranous portion of the scapula cannot accommodate plate-and-screw fixation, plates are positioned along the more substantial areas of the scapula (the medial and lateral borders, the scapular spine, and/or the glenoid neck).

- If intra-articular extension of the fracture lines is observed, posterior arthrotomy should be considered. In most patients, the intra-articular fragments are amenable to lag screw fixation.

- After fixation has been completed, the arm should be assessed fluoroscopically to ensure stability of the shoulder and the absence of intra-articular screws.

Wound Closure

- The infraspinatus and the deltoid are reattached to their origins to facilitate good postoperative function of the shoulder. Strong No. 2 nonabsorbable sutures with a polyethylene core are used.

- Wound closure is performed in a layered fashion. No. 0, 2-0, and 3-0 absorbable synthetic sutures are used to close fascial layers, deep subcutaneous tissues, and deep dermal layers, respectively. A 0.25-inch, round, closed-wound drain is used subfascially when a moderate amount of oozing occurs from the traumatized tissues. The skin is closed with an interrupted 3-0 nylon suture.

Table 2 Rehabilitation Protocol After Surgical Management of Floating Shoulder Injury[a]

Postoperative Week	ROM	Strengthening	Return to Play/Work	Comments/Emphasis
0-2	Pendulum exercises are started immediately or when associated injuries allow	None	None	A sling is used for comfort Hand, wrist, and elbow ROM exercises are encouraged immediately
2-6	Passive and active-assisted ROM is initiated, followed by progression of active motion as pain allows	None	None	Sling use is discontinued when no longer required for comfort
6-12	Active ROM is progressed	Resistive training and strengthening initiated	May return to light-duty work (lifting <10 lb) and conditioning	Radiographs are obtained at 6 wk and assessed for healing
≥12	Active ROM with no limits	No restrictions	Return to normal activity level, full work duties, and full-contact sports is allowed	Recommendations are based on the assumption that bony union of the fractures has occurred and the patient is pain free Patients can expect improvement in functional level for up to 1 yr

ROM = range of motion.

[a] Recommendations depend on the severity of injury, comorbidities, type of work or sport, and preinjury level of function.

Rehabilitation

Physical therapy is critical to successful outcomes after surgical fixation of floating shoulder injuries. Pain, weakness, and stiffness are common. Stable anatomic reduction and aggressive early motion, including pendulum exercises and hand, wrist, and elbow range-of-motion exercises, can help reduce the risk of these complications (**Table 2**). Two weeks postoperatively, sling use may be discontinued if no longer needed for comfort. Passive and active-assisted range of motion are initiated, followed by progression of active motion as tolerated. At 6 weeks, radiographs are obtained and assessed for healing, active range of motion is progressed, and resistive training and strengthening are initiated. The patient may return to light-duty work (lifting <10 lb) and conditioning. At 12 weeks, the patient may return to normal activities if bony union of the fractures has occurred and the patient is pain free, although improvement in functional level may continue up to 1 year postoperatively. The rehabilitation protocol is individualized based on the severity of injury, comorbidities, type of work or sport, and preinjury level of function.

Avoiding Pitfalls

To successfully manage floating shoulder injuries, the surgeon must be comfortable with the posterior approach and have experience working with complex fractures. Early recognition of a floating shoulder injury is often the first step in successful management. Because severe injuries are often sustained contemporaneously, the diagnosis may be delayed.

During clavicular fracture fixation as well as scapular fracture fixation, open communication between the orthopaedic surgeon and the anesthesiologist is essential. Rapid changes in the patient's respiratory status may signal an iatrogenic pneumothorax. Injury to the subclavian vessels, which are close to the surgical field, is a rare complication. Plunging of the drill must be avoided, especially if superior plate fixation is selected for the clavicle.

Anteroinferior plating has been reported to be safer than superior plating because of the anterior-to-posterior direction of the screws, which places more distance between instruments and major neurovascular structures as well as the apex of the lung. Additionally, longer screws can be used with the anterior plate position because of the geometry of the clavicle. Finally, plate prominence tends to be less of an issue with anterior positioning. However, the anterior plate position is more technically demanding. Superior plating places the plate on the tension side of the bone, which facilitates fracture reduction but increases the risk of pullout resulting from the weight of the arm. In patients with extremely comminuted fractures, orthogonal 90-90 plate configurations can allow for easy bridging of the fracture fragments and increased rigidity of the construct.

Reattachment of the deltoid and infraspinatus to their origins is essential for good shoulder function postoperatively. This step is best accomplished with the use of drill holes or suture anchors to ensure adequacy of the repair. In the management of an intra-articular fracture of the glenoid, additional elevation of a portion of the infraspinatus off the greater tuberosity can greatly improve posterior exposure of the glenoid fracture. The infraspinatus can be repaired with the use of suture anchors or transosseous repair techniques.

Because the primary goal in the surgical management of clavicular fractures in a floating shoulder is restoration of length and improvement of the medialization of the glenoid, nonrigid forms of fixation such as elastic nails should not be used. Nonrigid fixation methods are less likely to maintain the length of the fracture and restore the strut to the SSSC.

Bibliography

Edwards SG, Whittle AP, Wood GW II: Nonoperative treatment of ipsilateral fractures of the scapula and clavicle. *J Bone Joint Surg Am* 2000;82(6):774-780.

Egol KA, Connor PM, Karunakar MA, Sims SH, Bosse MJ, Kellam JF: The floating shoulder: Clinical and functional results. *J Bone Joint Surg Am* 2001;83(8):1188-1194.

Ganz R, Noesberger B: Treatment of scapular fractures [German]. *Hefte Unfallheilkd* 1975;126:59-62.

Goss TP: Double disruptions of the superior shoulder suspensory complex. *J Orthop Trauma* 1993;7(2):99-106.

Herscovici D Jr, Fiennes AG, Allgöwer M, Rüedi TP: The floating shoulder: Ipsilateral clavicle and scapular neck fractures. *J Bone Joint Surg Br* 1992;74(3):362-364.

Izadpanah K, Jaeger M, Maier D, Kubosch D, Hammer TO, Südkamp NP: The floating shoulder: Clinical and radiological results after intramedullary stabilization of the clavicle in cases with minor displacement of the scapular neck fracture. *J Trauma Acute Care Surg* 2012;72(2):E8-E13.

Kloen P, Sorkin AT, Rubel IF, Helfet DL: Anteroinferior plating of midshaft clavicular nonunions. *J Orthop Trauma* 2002;16(6):425-430.

Labler L, Platz A, Weishaupt D, Trentz O: Clinical and functional results after floating shoulder injuries. *J Trauma* 2004;57(3):595-602.

Leung KS, Lam TP: Open reduction and internal fixation of ipsilateral fractures of the scapular neck and clavicle. *J Bone Joint Surg Am* 1993;75(7):1015-1018.

McKee MD, Pedersen EM, Jones C, et al: Deficits following nonoperative treatment of displaced midshaft clavicular fractures. *J Bone Joint Surg Am* 2006;88(1):35-40.

Pailhes RG, Bonnevialle N, Laffosse J, Tricoire J, Cavaignac E, Chiron P: Floating shoulders: Clinical and radiographic analysis at a mean follow-up of 11 years. *Int J Shoulder Surg* 2013;7(2):59-64.

Ramos L, Mencía R, Alonso A, Ferrández L: Conservative treatment of ipsilateral fractures of the scapula and clavicle. *J Trauma* 1997;42(2):239-242.

van Noort A, te Slaa RL, Marti RK, van der Werken C: The floating shoulder: A multicentre study. *J Bone Joint Surg Br* 2001;83(6):795-798.

Williams GR Jr, Naranja J, Klimkiewicz J, Karduna A, Iannotti JP, Ramsey M: The floating shoulder: A biomechanical basis for classification and management. *J Bone Joint Surg Am* 2001;83(8):1182-1187.

Yadav V, Khare GN, Singh S, et al: A prospective study comparing conservative with operative treatment in patients with a 'floating shoulder' including assessment of the prognostic value of the glenopolar angle. *Bone Joint J* 2013;95(6):815-819.

Chapter 58

Pectoralis Major Tendon Transfer for Management of Medial Scapular Winging

Jon J.P. Warner, MD

Stephen A. Parada, MD

Amit Sood, MD

Introduction

Scapular winging is an uncommon condition that results in abnormal motion of the scapula, causing pain and decreased function of the upper extremity. The diagnosis can be made with a thorough physical examination and proper diagnostic studies. The most common type of scapular winging is medial winging resulting from a palsy of the long thoracic nerve that leads to dysfunction of the serratus anterior muscle. This dysfunction causes the scapula to displace from the ribs when forward flexion is attempted. If nonsurgical management is unsuccessful, surgical management should be considered. Surgical management of medial winging of the scapula can consist of transfer of the entire pectoralis major tendon, which is referred to as the direct procedure, or transfer of the sternal portion only, which is referred to

as the indirect procedure. Allograft or autograft tissue can be used to augment the tendon transfer.

The authors of this chapter prefer to transfer the sternal head of the pectoralis major tendon (indirect procedure) and augment the graft with autograft consisting of the gracilis and semitendinosus tendons. Augmentation of the graft with autograft provides a robust fixation to the inferior scapula and makes it easier to set the desired tension. In the experience of the authors of this chapter, transfer of the entire pectoralis major tendon is not necessary for functional reconstruction; therefore, the clavicular head is left intact. The authors of this chapter use an incision over the pectoralis major tendon for the tendon harvest and a separate incision over the inferior border of the scapula for insertion of the graft into the inferior angle.

Case Presentation

A 32-year-old man reports shoulder pain and loss of shoulder motion that has persisted for more than 1 year. He reports difficulty with overhead activities and posterior shoulder pain when sitting with his back against a hard surface. He does not report any trauma, but he had a viral illness more than 1 year earlier. Extensive physical therapy and a subacromial injection performed by a previous healthcare provider resulted in no improvement. Physical examination reveals an inability to reach full forward flexion, and posterior scapular winging is evident with resisted flexion of the affected arm (**Figure 1, A**). The scapular compression test, in which the clinician applies an anteriorly directed force on the posterior aspect of the scapula with one hand while stabilizing the anterior chest wall with the other hand and having the patient attempt forward flexion, results in improved motion (**Figure 1, B**). Electromyography demonstrates chronic injury of the long thoracic nerve with no other involvement. Because the patient's symptoms have been present for more than 1 year, long thoracic nerve palsy has been documented electromyographically, and nonsurgical management has failed,

Dr. Warner or an immediate family member has received royalties from and serves as a paid consultant to Tornier; has stock or stock options held in IMASCAP and OrthoSpace; has received nonincome support (such as equipment or services), commercially derived honoraria, or other non–research-related funding (such as paid travel) from Arthrex, Breg, DJO, Mitek Sports Medicine, Smith & Nephew, and Tornier; and serves as a board member, owner, officer, or committee member of the American Shoulder and Elbow Surgeons, the San Diego Shoulder Institute, and the Steadman Philippon Research Institute. Neither of the following authors nor any immediate family member has received anything of value from or has stock or stock options held in a commercial company or institution related directly or indirectly to the subject of this chapter: Dr. Parada and Dr. Sood.

the patient is offered a pectoralis major tendon transfer with autograft hamstring augmentation. The procedure is performed without complication, and at 1-year follow-up, the patient has full forward flexion with no evidence of scapular winging (**Figure 2**).

 Indications

Pectoralis major tendon transfer is indicated after failure of nonsurgical management of scapular winging.

Controversies and Alternative Approaches

Many surgeons think that the additional benefits of augmenting the transfer are not worth the added morbidity of harvesting autograft tendons or using allograft tissue. Some shoulder surgeons lack sufficient expertise in harvesting lower extremity autograft tissue or do not readily have access to allograft tissue. Tensor fascia lata autograft is the most common reported

tissue augmentation and usually entails harvesting a large rectangular section (5 × 20 cm) and twisting the harvested section into a tubular graft. Complications such as seroma or hematoma formation at the graft harvest site can necessitate subsequent surgical procedures. A cadaver anatomic study performed to determine the length of the pectoralis major tendon needed to transfer to the inferior pole of the scapula demonstrated that, with the patient's arm in 45° of abduction, the length of a direct transfer would easily reach the inferior pole, and the authors of the study suggested that added graft was not needed for length. Despite this result, the authors of this chapter think that the added bulk of the graft results in a more sturdy transfer. However, good results have been reported with transfer of the sternal head of the pectoralis major tendon and no added graft.

Some authors have described harvesting the entire tendon with a cortical flake of bone and then transferring the sternal head to the scapula and reattaching the clavicular head to its insertion. The authors of this chapter have not found this technique necessary and prefer to avoid the added morbidity of detaching and reinserting the clavicular head. If transfer of the entire tendon is

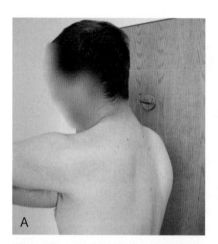

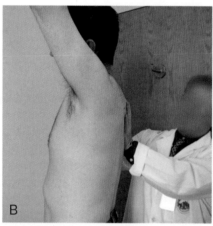

Figure 1 **A,** Clinical photograph of a patient with long thoracic nerve palsy that results in medial scapular winging with attempted forward flexion. **B,** Clinical photograph shows an examiner performing the scapular compression test, with increased forward flexion as the result.

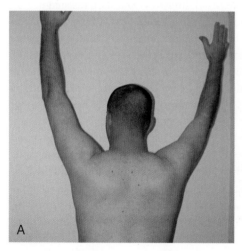

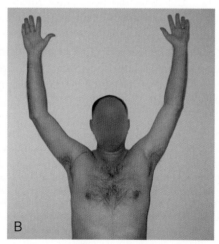

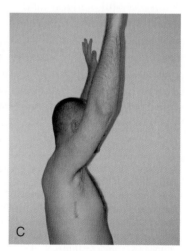

Figure 2 Clinical photographs of the same patient shown in Figure 1 taken 1 year after pectoralis major tendon transfer show the patient performing forward flexion with no scapular winging (**A**), the location of the surgical incisions (**B**), and the position of the lateral incision (**C**).

planned, harvesting the tendon with a cortical flake of bone may result in a faster healing time because of bone-to-bone healing. However, in a multicenter retrospective review, no differences were found between patients who had an indirect transfer and those who had a direct transfer.

Transfer of the pectoralis major tendon has been performed through one long incision; however, the authors of this chapter think that tunneling the graft through soft tissue is easy and that connecting the two incision sites offers no benefit. The use of an incision over the pectoralis major tendon harvest site and an additional incision at the inferior pole of the scapula offers a more cosmetic alternative to a longer incision covering both areas.

Some surgeons perform pectoralis major tendon transfer with the patient placed in the lateral decubitus position to facilitate access to the tensor fascia lata for harvest as well as anterior and posterior access to the shoulder girdle. Because the authors of this chapter use autograft hamstrings, the lateral decubitus position is not feasible. The patient positioning described in this chapter facilitates exposure of the pectoralis major tendon from an anterior incision and allows access to the inferior pole of the scapula. The use of a pneumatic arm holder can further aid this exposure.

Results

Good results can be attained in the management of scapular winging, but prompt diagnosis is key. Often, patients have undergone previous surgical treatment based on incorrect diagnoses. One literature review found that patients with scapular winging were most commonly misdiagnosed as having rotator cuff disorders; other misdiagnoses included glenohumeral instability, peripheral nerve disorders, cervical spine disease, acromioclavicular disorders, and thoracic outlet syndrome.

With the appropriate diagnosis, nonsurgical management of scapular winging may be successful, with recovery often requiring up to 24 months. However, as many as 25% of patients may have persistent serratus anterior palsy. If nonsurgical management of medial scapular winging is unsuccessful, pectoralis major tendon transfer with or without autograft tissue augmentation can lead to substantial improvement in pain and functional results. Success rates range from 74% to 100%, with resolution of winging and improvement in pain with normal scapulothoracic kinematics. Previous studies have reported improvement in range of motion (ROM), with postoperative forward flexion ranging from 144° to 175°. Many studies also have shown marked improvement in pain scores. In a recent large multicenter study consisting of 26 patients with average 21.8-month follow-up and with most patients treated using an indirect pectoralis major tendon transfer with autograft hamstring augmentation, the researchers found statistically significant improvements in ROM (forward flexion and external rotation), American Shoulder and Elbow Surgeons scores, pain scores, and visual analog scale scores. The authors of a 1998 study using the method described in this chapter reported satisfactory results in seven of eight patients. Results of the studies are summarized in **Table 1**.

One complication of the indirect procedure is stretching of the allograft tissue, which may result in recurrent scapular winging. Previously published studies have reported rates ranging from zero to 26% for this complication. Although cadaver studies have demonstrated that the sternal head of the pectoralis major tendon is adequate for direct repair of the scapula, the authors of this chapter suggest that this technique may cause iatrogenic traction injury to the medial and lateral pectoral nerves and result in scapular winging, which has been a reported complication. Other complications include infection, adhesive capsulitis, hematoma, seroma, and pain. Despite these complications, most patients have good outcomes, with an overall low complication rate. Patient compliance with postoperative physical therapy, especially with the use of a biofeedback device, is critical in achieving optimal outcomes.

Technical Keys to Success

Setup/Exposure

- The setup for this procedure depends on the planned incisions and the need to harvest autograft. The preferred method of the authors of this chapter is described.
- The patient is placed in a supine position for the initiation of general anesthesia. Placement of an endotracheal tube is necessary because complete paralysis is required for this procedure.
- After induction of anesthesia, the patient is positioned with slight flexion at the waist and lateral tilt to the contralateral side to allow access to the anterior and posterior aspects of the shoulder (**Figure 3**).
- The entire scapula is exposed, with the shoulder girdle freely mobile.
- A pneumatic arm holder can be placed on the ipsilateral side and oriented to facilitate positioning of the arm for harvesting and transfer of the tendon.
- The entire arm and hemithorax on the surgical side, as well as the ipsilateral leg, are prepped and draped in the usual sterile fashion.
- The authors of this chapter use an occlusive, antibiotic-impregnated adhesive covering to ensure that no skin is exposed in the surgical field.

Table 1 Results of Pectoralis Major Transfer to Manage Scapular Winging Caused by Long Thoracic Nerve Palsy

Author(s)	Journal (Year)	Technique (No. of Patients)	Outcomes	Failure Rate (%)	Comments
Post	*J Shoulder Elbow Surg* (1995)	Indirect transfer with fascia lata autograft (8)	All excellent	0	Mean follow-up, 27 mo 1 hematoma, 1 seroma All patients returned to work
Connor et al	*Clin Orthop Relat Res* (1997)	Indirect transfer with fascia lata autograft (11)	7 excellent, 3 satisfactory, 1 unsatisfactory	9	Mean follow-up, 41 mo 1 recurrence of scapular winging as a result of noncompliance with physical therapy
Warner and Navarro	*Clin Orthop Relat Res* (1998)	Indirect transfer with autograft hamstring (8)	7 satisfactory, 1 postoperative infection	12.5	Mean follow-up, 32 mo
Perlmutter and Leffert	*J Bone Joint Surg Am* (1999)	Indirect transfer with fascia lata autograft (16)	8 excellent, 5 good, 1 fair	12.5	Mean follow-up, 51 mo 2 failures revised to scapulothoracic fusion Both failures were attributed to the use of individual strips of fascia lata
Noerdlinger et al	*J Shoulder Elbow Surg* (2002)	Indirect transfer with fascia lata autograft (15)	2 excellent, 5 good, 4 fair, 4 poor	26.7	Mean follow-up, 64 mo 2 adhesive capsulitis, 1 lateral thigh muscle bulge No patients were pain free with all activities 12 patients indicated that they would undergo the procedure again 13 patients returned to work
Steinmann and Wood	*J Shoulder Elbow Surg* (2003)	Indirect transfer with fascia lata autograft (9)	4 excellent, 2 good, 3 poor	33.3	Mean follow-up, 70 mo 2 adhesive capsulitis, 1 thigh seroma
Galano et al	*Clin Orthop Relat Res* (2008)	Direct transfer (10)	All patients were satisfied and had improvements in forward flexion as well as ASES and VAS scores	10	Mean follow-up, 44 mo 2 superficial infections 1 tendon loosening converted to scapulothoracic fusion
Tauber et al	*J Shoulder Elbow Surg* (2008)	Direct transfer (12)	10 excellent, 2 good	8.3	Mean follow-up, 92.5 mo 1 tendon rupture resulting from a fall required revision
Streit et al	*J Shoulder Elbow Surg* (2012)	Direct transfer (4) Indirect transfer with hamstring autograft (22)	Statistically significant improvements in forward flexion and external rotation as well as ASES and VAS scores	No failures or poor results noted	Mean follow-up, 21.8 mo 5 patients had recurrent scapular winging

ASES = American Shoulder and Elbow Surgeons, VAS = visual analog scale.

Procedure

HAMSTRING TENDON HARVEST

- A sterile tourniquet is routinely used during tendon harvest.
- The hamstring tendons are harvested according to standard technique with the use of a tendon stripper.
- The harvested tendon is prepared on the back table while the tourniquet is deflated, hemostasis is achieved, and the wound is closed and a compressive dressing applied.

TENDON GRAFT PREPARATION

- The tendon is freed of soft tissue using Metzenbaum scissors.
- A running whipstitch of No. 2 nonabsorbable sutures is sewn from the midpoint of the tendon to each end.
- The smaller end of the tendon,

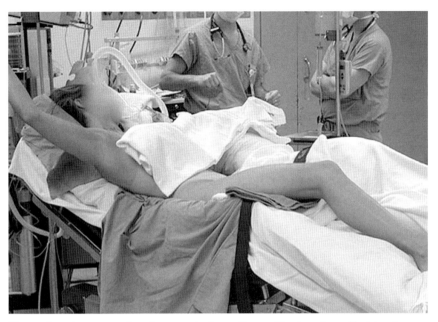

Figure 3 Intraoperative photograph shows the positioning of a patient to allow access to the shoulder as well as the ipsilateral leg for hamstring harvest during pectoralis major tendon transfer.

which is the proximal part, is tubularized with a wrapping technique using No. 2 nonabsorbable sutures.

- The tendon is placed in a moistened sponge for safekeeping until it is needed.

PECTORALIS MAJOR TENDON HARVEST

- An 8-cm incision is made from the coracoid process distally in the skin crease lines of the anterior axillary fold.
- Sharp dissection is performed down to the fascia overlying the deltoid and the pectoralis major muscles.
- The upper and lower borders of the pectoralis major tendon are exposed, and the deltopectoral interval is dissected.
- The interval between the sternal and clavicular heads of the pectoralis major tendon is identified. A Penrose drain is passed around the sternal portion of the muscle using a tonsil clamp.
- The patient's arm is internally rotated, and the sternal head is dissected free from the clavicular head from

medial to lateral, defining the tendon insertion onto the lateral lip of the bicipital groove.

- The short and long heads of the biceps are protected while a No. 15 blade is used to transect the tendon at the attachment of the sternal head to the humerus. The tendon is taken directly off the bone; however, no actual bone is elevated with the tendon. The clavicular attachment is preserved.
- No. 2 nonabsorbable sutures are placed in a modified Mason-Allen configuration to the end of the tendon.
- The previously harvested graft is woven through the pectoralis major tendon in a Pulvertaft fashion so that the tendon end is lengthened by approximately 8 cm. This weaving is done with one short limb of the graft at the level of the pectoralis major tendon and the longer limb projecting forward.
- No. 2 nonabsorbable sutures are used to sew the graft into the pectoralis major tendon so that a funnel shape is created, tubularizing the

end of the tendon so that it can slide through the soft-tissue tunnel when transferred (**Figure 4**).

- After the tubularization is completed, the tendon is placed back into the incision with a moistened sponge placed over it.

SCAPULAR EXPOSURE AND TENDON TRANSFER

- The arm is placed in flexion and abduction to bring the inferior angle of the scapula forward.
- A 5-cm incision is made in the skin crease lines over the inferior border of the scapula. The subcutaneous tissues are sharply dissected down to the latissimus dorsi muscle.
- The latissimus dorsi muscle is split in line with its fibers, first with electrocautery and then with a Cobb elevator, until the inferior border of the scapula and the teres major muscle are clearly identified.
- Electrocautery is used to divide the soft tissue off the inferolateral border of the scapula. This plane is developed with a Cobb elevator and electrocautery medially on the external and deep surfaces of the scapula, clearing away the soft tissue.
- The thickened lateral ridge of the scapula should be visible, with the thinner scapular body more medial to it.
- Cobra retractors are placed behind the scapula, and an oval burr is used to create a hole through the inferomedial border of the scapula just medial to the lateral thickened ridge. The diameter of this hole must be large enough to allow passage of the graft.
- A right-angle clamp is used to pass a suture loop through the hole that was created in the scapula.
- A soft-tissue tunnel along the chest wall is created, first from inferior to superior and then from superior to inferior, and fully dilated; the

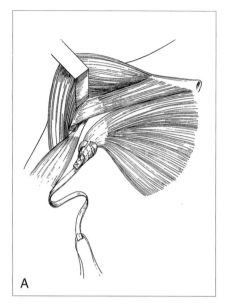

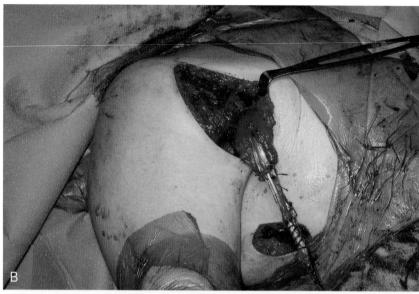

Figure 4 **A,** Illustration depicts the autograft hamstring secured in a Pulvertaft fashion to the pectoralis major tendon. **B,** Intraoperative photograph shows the autograft hamstring secured in a Pulvertaft fashion to the pectoralis major tendon and demonstrates the resulting length. (Panel A reproduced with permission from Warner JJ, Navarro RA: Serratus anterior dysfunction: Recognition and treatment. *Clin Orthop Relat Res* 1998;[349]:139-148.)

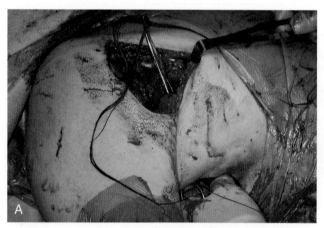

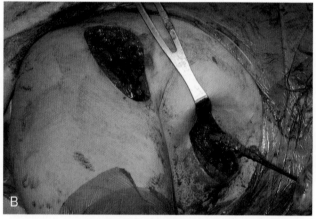

Figure 5 Intraoperative photographs show the passage of sutures with the use of a Kelly clamp that is placed from the distal incision to the proximal incision through a soft-tissue tunnel (**A**) and the appearance of the graft after passage through the soft-tissue tunnel (**B**).

tendon will be transferred through this tunnel. The tunnel is created bluntly with the use of a Schnidt tonsil clamp and finger dissection, with no sharp dissection needed (**Figure 5**). In large patients, a tunnel dilating system from the vascular surgery set can be used; however, the authors of this chapter rarely find it necessary.

- A clamp placed inferiorly is used to

retrieve the sutures in the end of the hamstring tendons and pull them distally to the incision made over the inferior border of the scapula.
- The tendon should be able to freely slide along the chest wall and to have full excursion without being tethered.
- The suture loop previously placed through the hole in the scapula is used to transfer the hamstring

tendons through that same hole (**Figure 6**). The scapula is pushed forward along the chest wall while this step is done.

- The pectoralis major tendon is advanced until the native pectoralis major tendon touches the deep surface of the scapula.
- The tendon is fixed in place by sewing the sutures that were previously passed through the tendon back to

the tendon itself with a free needle. An additional No. 2 nonabsorbable suture is then used to reinforce the previous stitch. Usually, eight simple stiches of the No. 2 nonabsorbable suture are used to secure the graft.

- At this point, the surgeon verifies that the graft is securely fixed and the scapula is held forward in its proper position with excellent tension in the pectoralis major tendon.

Wound Closure

- The wound is irrigated, and the split in the latissimus dorsi muscle is closed with interrupted No. 2 nonabsorbable sutures.
- The incision is closed in layers in a routine fashion (**Figure 7**).
- A drain is not routinely used.
- The patient is placed in a shoulder immobilizer.

 Rehabilitation

The rehabilitation protocol for pectoralis major tendon transfer is summarized in **Table 2**. Postoperative care consists of sling immobilization for the first 4 weeks to allow for healing. Early passive ROM is allowed to permit passage of the tendon in the soft-tissue tunnel. This passive ROM consists of pendulum motion that is begun 1 week postoperatively and physical therapy that is begun after the first postoperative visit (approximately 10 days postoperatively), with flexion limited to 90° and abduction limited to 45°. At 4 weeks postoperatively, the sling is removed and gentle active ROM is begun. Biofeedback training may begin as early as 2 months postoperatively depending on the patient's functional recovery. Biofeedback training is performed by placing electrodes over the pectoralis major muscle and allowing the biofeedback device to give visual and audible feedback in response to electromyographic

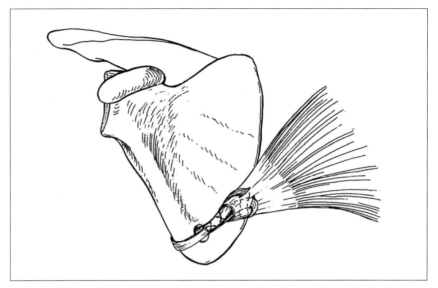

Figure 6 Illustration depicts the final construct of the autograft hamstring secured to itself after having been passed through the hole in the scapula. (Reproduced with permission from Warner JJ, Navarro RA: Serratus anterior dysfunction: Recognition and treatment. *Clin Orthop Relat Res* 1998;[349]:139-148.)

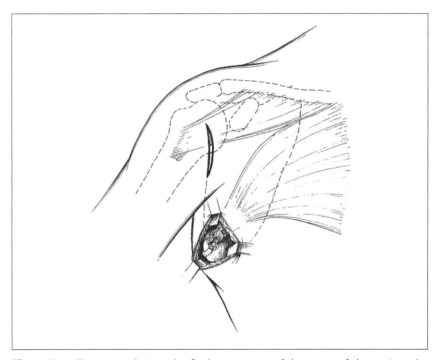

Figure 7 Illustration depicts the final appearance of the autograft hamstring, the transferred tendon, and the two surgical incisions. (Reproduced with permission from Warner JJ, Navarro RA: Serratus anterior dysfunction: Recognition and treatment. *Clin Orthop Relat Res* 1998;[349]:139-148.)

activity in the muscle. The patient starts in the lateral decubitus position to eliminate the effects of gravity and adducts the flexed arm against resistance to promote contraction of the pectoralis major muscle. Resistance is maintained for 5 seconds in multiple repetitions. The next step is to have the patient

Table 2 Rehabilitation Protocol After Pectoralis Major Transfer to Manage Scapular Winging

Postoperative Week	ROM	Strengthening	Return to Play	Comments
0-4	Pendulums are permitted after 1 wk Passive ROM is begun after the first postoperative visit at 10 d, with flexion limited to 90° and abduction limited to 45°	None	None	Remain in shoulder immobilizer for first 4 wk Lifting >20 lb prohibited
4-12	Gentle active ROM is begun at 4 wk	None	None	Sling removed at 4 wk Biofeedback training is initiated 2 mo postoperatively if functional recovery permits
12-52	No limits on ROM	Begin strengthening with physical therapy	None	—
≥52	No limits on ROM	Continue strengthening	May return to contact/collision sports	—

ROM = range of motion.

attempt flexion of the shoulder anterior to the plane of the scapula while maintaining contraction of the pectoralis major muscle, which is verified through audible and visible signals from the biofeedback device. Mild resistance may be applied to adduction during the flexion maneuver if the patient has difficulty maintaining contraction of the pectoralis major muscle during shoulder flexion. After the patient is able to perform these movements in the lateral decubitus position, the patient is transitioned to the upright position, and similar training is performed. Usually at least two to four sessions of physical therapy are necessary to achieve the desired ROM. At 3 months postoperatively, the limitations on ROM are lifted, and a strengthening exercise program may be initiated. Lifting of more than 20 lb with the affected arm and participating in contact and collision sports are prohibited for 1 year postoperatively.

 Avoiding Pitfalls

Patient positioning is of paramount importance, and initial draping must allow for access to the entire scapula. Positioning the patient with a slight amount of lateral tilt to the contralateral side will accomplish this goal. Positioning must also allow for ease of access to any site for harvest of autograft to augment the transfer. The authors of this chapter prefer to irrigate and close the hamstring incision site and place a compressive dressing over it for the remainder of the procedure to lessen the risk of symptomatic hematoma or seroma.

The incision to harvest the pectoralis major tendon should be made more medial or more extensile than a standard deltopectoral incision to allow for clear identification of the pectoralis major muscle. If only the sternal head of the pectoralis major tendon is used for the transfer, care must be taken to identify the raphe between the two heads of the pectoralis major tendon. The authors of this chapter use a Penrose drain passed on a tonsil clamp so that traction can be placed on the inferior aspect of the muscle-tendon junction. When traction is placed with the Penrose drain, the increased visualization may demonstrate that the drain is not in the correct plane. In that instance, the position of the drain should be adjusted before the tenotomy of the sternal head is performed. Both the conjoined tendon and the long head of the biceps tendon must be identified and protected throughout the pectoralis major tendon release or they can be inadvertently tenotomized.

Regardless whether graft augmentation is chosen, it is necessary to tubularize the tendon of the pectoralis major tendon before attempting to pass it through the soft tissue to the inferior pole of the scapula. Creating the scapular tunnel too inferiorly could fracture the inferior cortex of the scapula and make it impossible for the tendon to be pulled through and secured. The tunnel is easily created with a burr and should be positioned so that the inferior aspect of the tunnel remains proximal to the thicker cortical bone of the inferior pole of the scapula. After the tendon is passed through the inferior pole of the scapula, the surgeon must be sure to reduce the scapula anteriorly against the chest wall before securing the tendon to itself. Failure to do so will allow residual winging.

Bibliography

Connor PM, Yamaguchi K, Manifold SG, Pollock RG, Flatow EL, Bigliani LU: Split pectoralis major transfer for serratus anterior palsy. *Clin Orthop Relat Res* 1997;(341):134-142

Galano GJ, Bigliani LU, Ahmad CS, Levine WN: Surgical treatment of winged scapula. *Clin Orthop Relat Res* 2008;466(3):652-660.

Gozna ER, Harris WR: Traumatic winging of the scapula. *J Bone Joint Surg Am* 1979;61(8):1230-1233.

Iceton J, Harris WR: Treatment of winged scapula by pectoralis major transfer. *J Bone Joint Surg Br* 1987;69(1):108-110.

Litts CS, Hennigan SP, Williams GR: Medial and lateral pectoral nerve injury resulting in recurrent scapular winging after pectoralis major transfer: A case report. *J Shoulder Elbow Surg* 2000;9(4):347-349.

Noerdlinger MA, Cole BJ, Stewart M, Post M: Results of pectoralis major transfer with fascia lata autograft augmentation for scapula winging. *J Shoulder Elbow Surg* 2002;11(4):345-350.

Perlmutter GS, Leffert RD: Results of transfer of the pectoralis major tendon to treat paralysis of the serratus anterior muscle. *J Bone Joint Surg Am* 1999;81(3):377-384.

Post M: Pectoralis major transfer for winging of the scapula. *J Shoulder Elbow Surg* 1995;4(1 pt 1):1-9.

Povacz P, Resch H: Dynamic stabilization of winging scapula by direct split pectoralis major transfer: A technical note. *J Shoulder Elbow Surg* 2000;9(1):76-78.

Srikumaran U, Wells JH, Freehill MT, Tan EW, Higgins LD, Warner JJ: Scapular winging: A great masquerader of shoulder disorders. *J Bone Joint Surg Am* 2014;96(14):e122.

Steinmann SP, Wood MB: Pectoralis major transfer for serratus anterior paralysis. *J Shoulder Elbow Surg* 2003;12(6):555-560.

Streit JJ, Lenarz CJ, Shishani Y, et al: Pectoralis major tendon transfer for the treatment of scapular winging due to long thoracic nerve palsy. *J Shoulder Elbow Surg* 2012;21(5):685-690.

Tauber M, Moursy M, Koller H, Schwartz M, Resch H: Direct pectoralis major muscle transfer for dynamic stabilization of scapular winging. *J Shoulder Elbow Surg* 2008;17(1 suppl):29S-34S.

Warner JJ, Navarro RA: Serratus anterior dysfunction: Recognition and treatment. *Clin Orthop Relat Res* 1998;(349):139-148.

Chapter 59

Combined Transfer of the Rhomboid and Levator Scapulae Muscles for Management of Trapezius Palsy (Eden-Lange Procedure)

Adam D. Hall, MD

William J. Mallon, MD

Joseph B. Wilson, MD

Introduction

Scapular dyskinesis secondary to spinal accessory nerve damage and resultant trapezius palsy can be a disabling injury. Initial management is usually nonsurgical, consisting of aggressive physical therapy, with the goal of strengthening the scapular rotators. If symptoms are not relieved with nonsurgical management, muscle and tendon transfer procedures are often indicated to restore scapular stability. The Eden-Lange procedure, which consists of transferring the rhomboid muscles and the levator scapulae muscle laterally to increase their moment arm, is a well-described procedure with reasonably good results.

Case Presentation

A 28-year-old, right-hand–dominant man presents, upon referral, with complete denervation of the trapezius muscle as diagnosed by electromyelography (EMG). The patient sustained traumatic injuries after a fall from a height of 18 feet (5.5 m) onto his head, neck, and right shoulder; the fall occurred a few months before he presented to the institution of the authors of this chapter. The patient was initially diagnosed as having possible scapular fracture and rotator cuff disease, and he underwent extensive nonsurgical treatment that included long courses of physical therapy (6 months' duration). On an EMG study done to investigate persistent shoulder dysfunction and pain, along with vague neuropathic symptoms (nondermatomal hand paresthesia), denervation of the trapezius muscle was noted. The patient was subsequently referred for treatment.

On physical examination, the patient has considerable atrophy of the trapezius muscle with an asymmetric neckline. Active examination reveals Medical Research Council grade 4+ lateral winging with active forward elevation of 100°, which improves to 170° with lifting and stabilization of the scapula. Active external rotation of 70° is noted, along with internal rotation to the ninth thoracic vertebra (T9). Normal function is noted on examination of the patient's rhomboid muscles, levator scapulae muscle, and serratus anterior muscle, and the patient's cervical range of motion is painless and full.

No evidence of fracture or additional pathology is noted on standard radiographs. No marked abnormalities are demonstrated on MRI of the cervical spine.

Based on the clinical findings and the patient's diagnostic workup, combined transfer of the rhomboid and levator scapulae muscles is identified as the best treatment option and is subsequently performed. At final follow-up (1 year postoperatively), the patient notes substantial improvement, with no pain, markedly improved function in the affected shoulder, full range of shoulder motion, and minimal scapular winging.

Indications

Trapezius palsy occurs as a result of pathology affecting the spinal accessory nerve (cranial nerve XI). The etiology of spinal accessory nerve dysfunction and subsequent trapezius palsy may be idiopathic, traumatic, viral, or iatrogenic. Iatrogenic causes are most common,

Dr. Mallon or an immediate family member serves as a board member, owner, officer, or committee member of the American Shoulder and Elbow Surgeons. Neither of the following authors nor any immediate family member has received anything of value from or has stock or stock options held in a commercial company or institution related directly or indirectly to the subject of this chapter: Dr. Hall and Dr. Wilson.

Table 1 Results of Combined Transfer of the Rhomboid and Levator Scapulae Muscles

Authors	Journal (Year)	Technique	Mean Follow-up (yr)	Outcomes
Bigliani et al	*J Bone Joint Surg Am* (1996)	Modified Eden-Lange	7.5	ASES scores were excellent in 13 of 22 patients, satisfactory in 6, and unsatisfactory in 3
Romero and Gerber	*J Bone Joint Surg Br* (2003)	Eden-Lange	32	Mean Constant score was excellent in 9 of 12 patients, fair in 2, and poor in 1
Teboul et al	*J Bone Joint Surg Am* (2004)	Eden-Lange	2.9	Based on clinical assessment and subjective satisfaction, outcomes were excellent in 3 of 7 patients, good in 1, and poor in 3

ASES = American Shoulder and Elbow Surgeons shoulder outcome.

primarily resulting from surgical procedures on the posterior cervical triangle (such as lymph node biopsy).

Diagnosis of trapezius palsy is often delayed or missed. Vague shoulder pain is a frequent complaint and may override the patient's concern for functional loss. Signs of trapezius palsy include lateral winging, trapezius atrophy, asymmetric neckline, weakness of abduction and forward elevation, and decreased range of shoulder motion. These signs may be subtle in the acute period, and a high index of suspicion should be maintained in patients with known iatrogenic risk factors.

Differential diagnosis for spinal accessory nerve palsy includes nerve root avulsion, serratus anterior palsy (medial winging), herniated cervical disk, neuromuscular disease (including Parsonage-Turner syndrome), and cerebrovascular accident (stroke). Evaluation with EMG should be considered to confirm the diagnosis. In patients for whom muscle transfers are being considered, EMG is especially useful to assess the function of the muscles to be transferred.

Management of trapezius palsy may be surgical or nonsurgical, depending on the severity of the symptoms and the physical demands of the patient. For patients in whom palsy resulted from blunt trauma, some physicians proceed with observation and symptomatic treatment for up to 6 weeks, emphasizing physical therapy. In other patients, especially in

those with suspected iatrogenic etiology, nerve exploration may be indicated for up to 12 months after injury. Treatment options at this early stage (that is, the first 12 months) may include neurolysis, nerve repair, nerve grafting, and nerve transfer. Shoulder bracing, physiotherapy, and electrical stimulation also have been suggested with varied symptomatic and functional results.

Combined transfer of the rhomboid and levator scapulae muscles for the management of trapezius palsy is generally indicated for patients in whom nonsurgical treatment and/or nerve procedures have been unsuccessful. The optimal timing of transfer is controversial, but the authors of this chapter generally suggest muscle transfers after 12 months of unrelieved symptoms and/or symptoms that interfere with activities of daily living. Muscle transfer may be considered earlier in patients with poor prognostic factors for nerve procedures, such as spontaneous spinal accessory nerve palsy.

Alternative Approaches

Alternative options are most viable in the first 3 months after injury, particularly in patients with a known etiologic event. Nerve procedures should be considered as a potential primary treatment in patients with a known etiologic event. Scapulothoracic fusion as an alternative

to dynamic muscle transfer is best reserved for patients with global shoulder girdle weakness, such as facioscapulohumeral muscular dystrophy, or for patients with symptoms and difficulties that persist even after muscle transfers. Other static procedures to stabilize the scapula to the spine tend to fail with time; thus, they have fallen out of favor in the management of trapezius palsy.

Results

In the experience of the authors of this chapter, improved scapular stability and decreased periscapular pain are typically achieved with the Eden-Lange and modified Eden-Lange procedures. However, some minor residual winging is common, and although the scapular stabilizing muscles are made stronger by the Eden-Lange procedure, they are not usually as strong and stable as a native scapula.

Results of the Eden-Lange and modified Eden-Lange procedures are summarized in **Table 1**. To the knowledge of the authors of this chapter, few studies have evaluated outcomes of combined transfers of the rhomboid and levator scapulae for trapezius palsy. Substantial variation between the studies summarized in **Table 1** should be noted. The authors of the studies published in 2003 and 2004 used the original transfers as described by Eden, whereas the authors of the study published

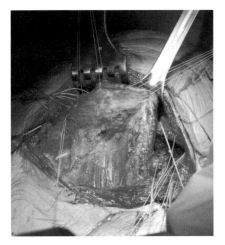

Figure 1 Intraoperative photograph of a shoulder shows the incision with the rhomboid muscles and the levator scapulae muscle taken off the medial scapular border and tagged for future transfer. (Courtesy of Louis U. Bigliani, MD, New York, NY.)

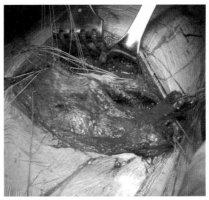

Figure 2 Intraoperative photograph of a shoulder shows drill holes placed in the medial scapular border with sutures from the rhomboid muscles passed through the holes. (Courtesy of Louis U. Bigliani, MD, New York, NY.)

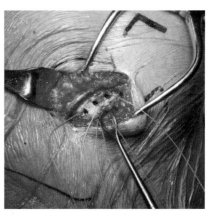

Figure 3 Intraoperative photograph of a shoulder shows drill holes placed through the scapular spine through a second lateral incision. (Courtesy of Louis U. Bigliani, MD, New York, NY.)

in 1996 used a modified procedure in which the rhomboid minor was transferred separately. In two studies, patients were immobilized in an abduction splint postoperatively, whereas in the third study the patients' arms were secured to the chest with a bandage for 6 weeks postoperatively. In one study, early passive motion was begun on the first postoperative day, but in the other two studies, passive and active motion were begun 6 weeks postoperatively.

 Technical Keys to Success

- The patient is placed in either the lateral decubitus or prone position to facilitate exposure. The upper back and surgical extremity are prepped, and the arm is draped free.
- The authors of this chapter prefer a single, continuous incision with a horizontal limb along the scapular spine and a vertical limb centered between the medial scapular border and the adjacent spinous processes.

Some surgeons use two incisions, with a medial incision to dissect out the rhomboid muscles and the levator scapulae muscle and a second incision along the scapular spine for reattachment of the transferred muscles.

- The trapezius muscle is split near its insertion on the scapular spine.
- The rhomboid muscles and the levator scapulae muscle are then identified and raised from their insertions with a small piece of bone to facilitate incorporation at the muscle transfer site.
- The rhomboid muscles may be separated for transfer, consistent with the modification described by Bigliani, by transferring the rhomboid minor to the supraspinous fossa and the rhomboid major to the infraspinous fossa. The decision to use the modified Eden-Lange procedure is based on surgeon preference (**Figure 1**).
- After the rhomboid muscles are separated, each muscle is mobilized to allow adequate excursion to the transfer sites (**Figure 2**). The dorsal scapular nerve must be protected during this portion of the procedure.

- The supraspinatus and infraspinatus muscles are elevated from their respective fossae in a medial-to-lateral direction to allow transfer of the rhomboid muscles 4 cm from the medial border. Drill holes are made 1.5 cm apart (**Figure 3**), with two in the superior fossa and four in the inferior fossa.
- Next, attention is turned to the transfer of the levator scapulae muscle (**Figure 4**).
- A No. 2 nonabsorbable braided suture is used to attach each of the rhomboid muscles to the desired site using a horizontal mattress technique (**Figures 5** and **6**). A towel clip can be placed on the scapular spine to control the scapula. The towel clip can be pulled medially to allow the repair to be done more easily.
- The trapezius, deltoid, and supraspinatus muscles are elevated from the scapular spine, 5 to 7 cm from the posterolateral border of the acromion. This step must be done carefully to avoid injury to the suprascapular nerve.
- Three drill holes are then placed in the scapular spine, 1.5 cm apart, to allow attachment of the levator

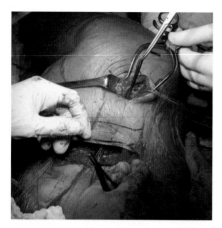

Figure 4 Intraoperative photograph of a shoulder shows passage of the sutures used to tag the levator scapulae muscle from the medial to the lateral incision via a soft-tissue tunnel. (Courtesy of Louis U. Bigliani, MD, New York, NY.)

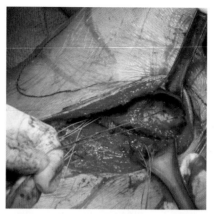

Figure 5 Intraoperative photograph of a shoulder shows the appearance of the surgical site in preparation for tying down the rhomboid muscles to the scapular blade via the sutures passed through the drill holes. (Courtesy of Louis U. Bigliani, MD, New York, NY.)

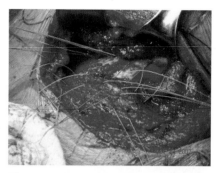

Figure 6 Intraoperative photograph of a shoulder shows the appearance of the surgical site after all the sutures have been passed and in preparation to finish transferring the rhomboid muscles to the midscapular blade on the infraspinatus fossa. (Courtesy of Louis U. Bigliani, MD, New York, NY.)

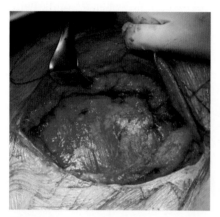

Figure 7 Intraoperative photograph of a shoulder shows the appearance of the rhomboid muscles after they have been transferred to the infraspinatus fossa. (Courtesy of Louis U. Bigliani, MD, New York, NY.)

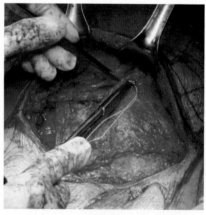

Figure 8 Intraoperative photograph of a shoulder shows side-to-side repair of the trapezius muscle. (Courtesy of Louis U. Bigliani, MD, New York, NY.)

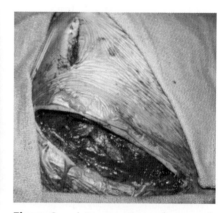

Figure 9 Intraoperative photograph of a shoulder shows the appearance of the incisions after trapezial muscle repair and before skin closure. (Courtesy of Evan L. Flatow, MD, New York, NY.)

scapulae muscle to the transfer site using two horizontal mattress sutures.
- After the muscle transfers are completed, the infraspinatus and supraspinatus muscles are closed over the transferred rhomboid muscles and the levator scapulae muscle (**Figure 7**).
- The wound is closed in layers, taking care to securely close the trapezial split (**Figures 8** and **9**), and a

drain is placed at the discretion of the surgeon.
- Postoperatively, the patient's shoulder is immobilized using a padded shoulder immobilizer or a shoulder abduction brace.

Rehabilitation

The rehabilitation protocol is summarized in **Table 2**. For the first 4 weeks

postoperatively, the patient wears the sling and can perform gentle range of motion of the hand, wrist, and elbow. After the first 4 weeks postoperatively, active range of motion is begun, and gentle strengthening is added as the patient progresses. Twelve weeks from the date of surgery, the patient is cleared for all activities without restriction.

Table 2 Rehabilitation Protocol After Combined Transfer of the Rhomboid and Levator Scapulae Muscles (Eden-Lange Procedure)

Postoperative Week	ROM	Strengthening	Comments/Emphasis
0-4	None; abduction brace is worn	None	Healing of transfers
5-12	Active ROM is begun	Gentle strengthening	Conditioning of transfer muscles, achievement of dynamic scapular stability
≥13	Unrestricted	Unrestricted	Maintenance of dynamic scapular stability Return to play is prohibited until approximately 6 mo postoperatively

ROM = range of motion.

Avoiding Pitfalls

When dividing the atrophied trapezius muscle, care must be taken to avoid iatrogenic injury to the underlying muscles. With medial division of the muscles, the rhomboid muscles and the levator scapulae muscle are at risk for injury, whereas with lateral division of the muscles, the rotator cuff muscles are at risk for injury.

Elevation, separation, and mobilization of the rhomboid muscles and the levator scapulae muscle should be done carefully by staying directly on the scapula to avoid damaging the dorsal scapular nerve and its insertions into the transfer muscles. Damage to the dorsal scapular nerve may cause permanent impairment of the transfer muscles, thus leading to failure of the procedure.

When transferring the levator scapulae muscle laterally, care must be taken to avoid injury to the suprascapular nerve. Injury to the suprascapular nerve will adversely affect the outcome of any shoulder procedure.

Draping the entire extremity free allows for manipulation during the procedure. This is helpful in the early phases of the procedure to assist with identification and dissection of the involved structures. It also is important in the latter portions of the procedure when the transfer is being completed to assist with obtaining adequate tension and scapular reduction.

Bibliography

Bigliani LU, Compito CA, Duralde XA, Wolfe IN: Transfer of the levator scapulae, rhomboid major, and rhomboid minor for paralysis of the trapezius. *J Bone Joint Surg Am* 1996;78(10):1534-1540.

Bigliani LU, Perez-Sanz JR, Wolfe IN: Treatment of trapezius paralysis. *J Bone Joint Surg Am* 1985;67(6):871-877.

Duralde XA, Bigliani LU: Neurologic disorders, in Hawkins RJ, Misamore GW, eds: *Shoulder Injuries in the Athlete.* New York, NY, Churchill Livingstone, 1996, pp 259-262.

Eden R: Zur Behandlung der Trapeziuslahmung mittelst Muskelplastik. *Deutsche Zeitschrift für Chirurgie* 1924;184:387-397.

Galano GJ, Bigliani LU, Ahmad CS, Levine WN: Surgical treatment of winged scapula. *Clin Orthop Relat Res* 2008;466(3):652-660.

Lange M: Treatment of paralysis of the trapezius [Article in undetermined language]. *Langenbecks Arch Klin Chir Ver Dtsch Z Chir* 1951;270:437-439.

Lee JH, Levine WN: Eden-Lange procedure for trapezius palsy, in Wiesel SW, ed: *Operative Techniques in Orthopaedic Surgery*. Philadelphia, PA, Wolters Kluwer, 2011, pp 3301-3307.

Meininger AK, Figuerres BF, Goldberg BA: Scapular winging: An update. *J Am Acad Orthop Surg* 2011;19(8):453-462.

Romero J, Gerber C: Levator scapulae and rhomboid transfer for paralysis of trapezius: The Eden-Lange procedure. *J Bone Joint Surg Br* 2003;85(8):1141-1145.

Steinmann SP, Spinner RJ: Nerve problems about the shoulder, in Rockwood CA, Matsen FA, Wirth MA, Lippitt SB, eds: *The Shoulder,* ed 4. Philadelphia, PA, Saunders Elsevier, 2009, pp 1366-1369.

Teboul F, Bizot P, Kakkar R, Sedel L: Surgical management of trapezius palsy. *J Bone Joint Surg Am* 2004;86(9):1884-1890.

Wiater JM, Bigliani LU: Spinal accessory nerve injury. *Clin Orthop Relat Res* 1999;(368):5-16.

Chapter 60
Scapulothoracic Fusion to Manage Facioscapulohumeral Muscular Dystrophy

Anthony A. Romeo, MD

Chris R. Mellano, MD

Mandeep S. Virk, MD

Peter N. Chalmers, MD

 ## Introduction

The functional role of the shoulder is twofold. First, the shoulder creates a sphere about which the hand is placed in space. Second, the shoulder provides a stable fulcrum enabling the arm and hand to work. The glenohumeral joint and scapulothoracic articulation work in concert to achieve these two shoulder functions.

Scapulothoracic motion accounts for approximately one-third of shoulder range of motion. Disorders affecting the muscles that attach to the scapula and coordinate scapulothoracic motion or injury to the nerves that innervate these muscles can result in scapulothoracic winging and dysfunction. Scapulothoracic dysfunction can manifest as periscapular pain;

cosmetic asymmetry; and diminished shoulder motion, strength, and endurance. Surgery may be warranted in patients with diminished shoulder function resulting from periscapular muscle dysfunction. If the periscapular muscle dysfunction is the result of an isolated muscle dysfunction, such as a long thoracic nerve palsy resulting in a dysfunctional serratus anterior and medial scapular winging, a tendon transfer may be beneficial to restore proper scapulothoracic function. However, if scapulothoracic dysfunction is caused by multiple periscapular muscle dysfunctions or function is not restored with tendon transfer, a scapulothoracic fusion (STF) should be considered to improve shoulder function, reduce periscapular pain, and enhance cosmesis (**Figure 1**).

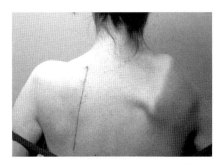

Figure 1 Clinical posterior photograph of a patient who initially presented with bilateral scapular winging resulting from facioscapulohumeral dystrophy and who then underwent scapulothoracic fusion of the left scapula. Note the improved appearance of the treated left shoulder compared with the untreated right shoulder. (Reproduced with permission from Diab M, Darras BT, Shapiro F: Scapulothoracic fusion for facioscapulohumeral muscular dystrophy. *J Bone Joint Surg Am* 2005;87[10]:2267-2275.)

 ## Case Presentation

A 23-year-old man has left shoulder pain and weakness with attempted overhead activity that has progressively worsened for many years. Physical examination demonstrates wasting of the facial muscle and periscapular muscles. Scapular medial winging is evident with attempted motion, and active forward elevation is limited to 80°. The patient

Dr. Romeo or an immediate family member has received royalties from, is a member of a speakers' bureau or has made paid presentations on behalf of, and serves as a paid consultant to Arthrex; has received research or institutional support from Arthrex, DJO Surgical, Smith & Nephew, and Össur; has received nonincome support (such as equipment or services), commercially derived honoraria, or other non–research-related funding (such as paid travel) from Arthrex; and serves as a board member, owner, officer, or committee member of the American Orthopaedic Society for Sports Medicine and the American Shoulder and Elbow Surgeons. None of the following authors or any immediate family member has received anything of value from or has stock or stock options held in a commercial company or institution related directly or indirectly to the subject of this chapter: Dr. Mellano, Dr. Virk, and Dr. Chalmers.

reports that his grandfather had similar shoulder weakness and deformity. The diagnosis of facioscapulohumeral dystrophy (FSHD) was made after muscle biopsy confirmed the clinical suspicion. Scapulothoracic fusion was performed using posterior iliac crest autograft. At 6-month follow-up, the patient demonstrates painless active forward elevation of 120°, and radiographs demonstrate successful scapulothoracic fusion.

 Indications

The types of scapulothoracic dysfunction that may benefit from STF can be described as dystrophic or nondystrophic. The most common form of muscular dystrophy that may benefit from STF is FSHD. FSHD is the third most common muscular dystrophy after the Duchenne and Becker types. Most commonly, FSHD results from a 4q35 deletion, and it is an autosomal dominant progressive muscle dystrophy that uniquely affects the facial, shoulder girdle, and arm muscles (and may extend to abdominal, hip, and foot musculature). Phenotypically, wasting of the facial muscles is seen first, followed by weakness and atrophy of muscles about the shoulder girdle and arm. Within the shoulder girdle and arm, FSHD commonly affects the serratus anterior, rhomboids, trapezius, and teres major and minor muscles; less commonly, FSHD affects the pectoralis, biceps, and triceps muscles. The deltoid and rotator cuff are often unaffected. Although FSHD is inherited in an autosomal dominant pattern, there is often variable penetrance without a clear familial history, and the appearance can often be asymmetric from one shoulder to the other. FSHD is a relatively slow progressive dystrophy and usually is not diagnosed until the second decade of life. Patients may report severe periscapular pain with attempted shoulder activity as well as weakness or inability

to raise the arm above shoulder level. The shoulder at rest is typically asymptomatic, and scapular winging is seen only with attempted activity. Diagnosis begins with clinical suspicion and may be confirmed with muscle biopsy, electromyography, and genetic testing.

Nondystrophic causes of painful scapulothoracic dysfunction include failed tendon transfer procedures, brachial plexus injuries, cerebrovascular injury, cleidocranial dysostosis, Sprengel deformity, and medial clavicle insufficiency.

 Contraindications

Candidates for STF should be counseled about the surgical goals and limitations. Periscapular pain will most predictably improve after STF. Shoulder and arm function after STF, however, is reliant on well-functioning deltoid, rotator cuff, and arm musculature. Caution is required with the use of STF to manage any dystrophic or nondystrophic condition that includes impairment of shoulder abduction and arm strength. Although FSHD is an autosomal-dominant inherited disorder, persons with FSHD can experience various degrees of muscle dysfunction. Some patients with FSHD have well-preserved deltoid, biceps, and triceps function, whereas others have severe weakness of all muscle groups. Preoperative deltoid, biceps, and triceps strength may be retained after STF, but such strength does not typically improve after surgery. Thus, the severity of the dysfunction of the shoulder abductors and arm musculature preoperatively predicts shoulder and arm function after STF. Patients with FSHD who are candidates for STF should be preoperatively evaluated for shoulder abduction and arm muscle function and counseled accordingly. Similarly, patients with nondystrophic presentation and with axillary or suprascapular nerve dysfunction will have a poor functional result after STF.

Patients with pulmonary dysfunction should also be counseled about the surgical risks. On average, the STF procedure reduces vital lung capacity by 20% or more. Routine pulmonary function tests should be performed, particularly in an individual who is considering bilateral staged procedures.

 Controversies and Alternative Approaches

Nonsurgical treatment options of severe scapulothoracic dysfunction, including FSHD, are limited. Orthoses are not well tolerated and are difficult to use by patients who have severe weakness. Alternative surgical options for scapular dysfunction include tendon transfers or scapulopexy. Scapulopexy is a procedure in which a soft-tissue checkrein is created between the scapula and the rib cage to prevent abnormal scapular movement and provide a stable base for scapulohumeral motion while allowing a small amount of scapulothoracic motion.

Tendon transfers about the shoulder can be an effective treatment of isolated periscapular muscle dysfunction. A long thoracic nerve palsy resulting in dysfunction of the serratus anterior muscle can benefit from transfer of the pectoralis major muscle to the lateral border of the scapula. Similarly, paralysis of the trapezius, which is usually associated with spinal accessory nerve palsy during cervical lymph node surgical dissection, can benefit from transfer of the rhomboid and levator muscles (Eden-Lange procedure). Both forms of periscapular tendon transfers rely on the normal function of the remaining periscapular musculature. Patients with FSHD typically do not have isolated periscapular muscle dysfunction and thus, are not appropriate candidates for tendon transfers.

Scapulopexy is also an alternative

to STF. Several variations of the scapulopexy procedure exist; however, the common goal is to create a soft-tissue checkrein against scapular winging and weakness. Long-term concerns of scapulopexy include possible deterioration of the soft-tissue scapular restraints over time.

 Results

STF is an uncommon procedure and, thus, only level IV evidence is available. The most contemporary case series reported are summarized in **Table 1**. The most commonly reported indication for STF is treatment of FSHD and, less commonly, nondystrophic causes (such as periscapular neurologic injury). Case reports exist for rare indications (such as clavicle insufficiency). Regardless of surgical indication, the patient can be counseled to expect good relief of the periscapular pain with attempted arm elevation. Furthermore, modest improvements in range of motion and strength can be expected. Most patients can achieve active elevation of the arm above 100°, and an average 30° improvement in arm elevation is gained. However, in some patients with FSHD, deltoid strength may diminish as the disease progresses and, thus, an initially good functional result after surgery may deteriorate over time. Cosmetic improvement can also be expected for the drooping shoulder appearance, although some patients dislike the square shoulder contour.

Reported fixation techniques include cerclage wiring with or without plate application, rush rods, and even screws alone. The rate of symptomatic hardware is high in some reports (range, 50% to 100%, depending on the fixation method). Most authors report the use of autogenous iliac crest bone graft; however, in a recent report on the use of femoral head allograft, nonunion rates were similar to those for posterior iliac crest autograft.

Overall, although these procedures are effective, patients must be informed that high complication rates have been reported (>50%). Serious complications may include brachial plexus injury, pneumothorax, nonunion, rib fractures (wire cutout), and deep infection. Minor complications may include adhesive capsulitis of the glenohumeral joint, symptomatic hardware, prominent inferior scapular border, and disappointment with cosmetic appearance. With the exception of revision surgery for nonunion or brachial plexus injury, most complications are not associated with negative long-term sequelae.

 Technical Keys to Success

The goals of STF are to prepare the posterior ribs and anteromedial scapula surfaces for fusion and to create immediate rigid internal fixation of the scapula to the posterior ribs until fusion is achieved. To accomplish these two goals, the surgeon must have a thorough understanding of the relevant osseous and soft-tissue anatomy.

The medial border of the scapula has sufficient bone stock (typically, 4 ± 1 SD mm) to support fixation; however, the middle of the scapula is often paper-thin. The scapular spine is the most prominent osseous landmark of the scapula, and the prominent C7 spinous process is the most identifiable spinal landmark. The scapular spine separates the supraspinatus fossa (which contains the supraspinatus muscle) superiorly and the infraspinatus fossa (which contains the infraspinatus and teres minor) inferiorly. The osseous landmarks of the scapular spine and T4 spinous process are used as references for properly positioning the scapula in space relative to the thorax.

Knowledge of the soft-tissue anatomy around the scapula is equally important both for dissection and for proper preparation of the fusion site. The

muscle layers within this dissection can be compartmentalized into three distinct layers: superficial, intermediate, and deep. The superficial layer includes the trapezius and the latissimus dorsi muscles. The muscle fibers of the trapezius are oriented in three distinct divisions—upper, middle, and lower—and converge to insert over the scapular spine and surrounding fascia. The trapezial bursa lies between the trapezius tendon and the superomedial border of the scapula. The intermediate layer includes tendinous attachments to the medial border of the scapula, including the rhomboid major and minor and levator scapula superiorly, as well as the spinal accessory nerve. The deep layer includes muscle attachments to the anteromedial border of the scapula, including the serratus anterior and the subscapularis. Deep to the subscapularis, the subscapularis bursa overlies the ribs and intercostal muscles. The erector spinae can also be a useful longitudinal landmark for medial exposure of the ribs.

Preoperative Considerations

Pulmonary function tests are performed routinely to evaluate for baseline vital lung capacity, especially in a patient who is considering staged bilateral procedures. Somatosensory-evoked potential neuromonitoring is routinely used to alert the clinician to brachial plexus traction throughout the procedure, especially during scapular reduction. Intraoperative consultation with a thoracic surgeon may be required for insertion of a chest tube if a pneumothorax is created. Discussion with an anesthesiologist preoperatively regarding the use of paralytic agents (such as succinylcholine chloride) is encouraged. Typically, paralytic agents are contraindicated for patients with Duchenne or Becker muscular dystrophy because of increased risk of malignant hyperthermia, rhabdomyolysis, and life-threatening hyperkalemia. Patients with FSHD

Table 1 Results of Scapulothoracic Fusion

Author(s)	Journal (Year)	Technique	Outcomes	Failure Rate	Comments
Letournel et al	*J Bone Joint Surg Am* (1990)	Fourth rib taken through a window in the scapula and fixed with a 6-hole plate and cerclage wires; no bone graft used	3 pneumothoraces, 1 pleural effusion requiring drainage, 2 rib stress fractures (asymptomatic), 1 pseudarthrosis (asymptomatic) Avg active FE improved from 75° to 108°	11% nonunion (asymptomatic)	9 patients with FSHD (16 shoulders) Age range, 17-36 yr Mean follow-up, 69 mo (range, 24-133 mo)
Twyman et al	*J Shoulder Elbow Surg* (1996)	18-gauge cerclage wires, autograft ICBG	3 pneumothoraces, 1 brachial plexus injury, 1 nonunion, 2 rib fracture Avg active FE improved from 56° to 96°	8% nonunion (revision arthrodesis required)	6 patients with FSHD (12 shoulders) Mean age, 30 yr (range, 17-44 yr) Mean follow-up, 48.5 mo (range, 12-80 mo) Patients underwent early postoperative active ROM
Bizot et al	*J Shoulder Elbow Surg* (2003)	Cerclage wires, autograft ICBG	2 pneumothoraces requiring chest tube insertion, 1 frozen shoulder, 1 nonunion Avg active FE improved from 83° to 101°	10% nonunion	10 patients with chronic serratus anterior dysfunction resulting from long thoracic nerve palsy Mean age, 39 yr (range, 22-57 yr) Mean follow-up, 74.4 mo (range, 12-180 mo)
Diab et al	*J Bone Joint Surg Am* (2005)	Cerclage wires around 5 ribs, autograft ICBG	6 excellent, 3 good, 2 fair Avg FE improved from 75° to 145°	0	11 patients with FSHD Mean age, 17 yr (range, 11-22 yr) Mean follow-up, 75.6 mo (range, 24-120 mo) Study authors noted deterioration of ROM as the disease process progressed to involve the deltoid muscle
Jeon et al	*J Shoulder Elbow Surg* (2005)	Cerclage wires around 4 ribs, rush rod, autograft ICBG	1 asymptomatic nonunion, removal of prominent hardware in 6 Avg active FE improved from 80° to 98°	17% nonunion (asymptomatic)	6 patients with brachial plexus palsy Mean age, 30 yr (range, 22-39 yr) Mean follow-up, 49 mo (range, 28-89 mo)
Rhee and Ha	*J Shoulder Elbow Surg* (2006)	Cerclage wires, plate, autograft ICBG	1 pleural effusion requiring aspiration Avg FE improved from 71° to 109°	0	6 patients with FSHD (9 shoulders) Mean age, 25 yr (range, 15-27 yr) Mean follow-up, 102 mo (range, 56-118 mo)
Sewell et al	*J Bone Joint Surg Br* (2012)	Cerclage wires, plate, autograft ICBG	3 pneumothoraces, 2 rib fractures, 3 pleural effusions, 6 nonunions Avg FE improved from 59° to 97°	26% nonunion (revision arthrodesis required)	34 patients with various presentations (42 shoulders) Mean age, 30 yr (range, 15-75 yr) Mean follow-up, 60 mo (range 24-127 mo)
Van Tongel et al	*J Bone Joint Surg Am* (2013)	Screw fixation, autograft ICBG	1 pneumothorax, 4 early failures due to noncompliance, 2 fractures through arthrodesis site Avg active FE improved from 65° to 119°	18% nonunion (revision arthrodesis required)	21 patients with FSHD (32 shoulders) Mean age, 26 yr (range 16-62 yr) Mean follow-up, 88 mo (24-174 mo)

FE = forward elevation, FSHD = facioscapulohumeral dystrophy, ICBG = iliac crest bone graft, ROM = range of motion.

Table 1 Results of Scapulothoracic Fusion (*continued*)

Author(s)	Journal (Year)	Technique	Outcomes	Failure Rate	Comments
Cooney et al	*J Shoulder Elbow Surg* (2014)	Cerclage wires, femoral head allograft, 2 plates	1 nonunion, 1 brachial plexus injury resolved, 1 pleural effusion, 1 chest infection Avg active FE improved from 70° to 115°	7% nonunion (revision arthrodesis with auto-graft ICBG required)	11 patients with FSHD (14 shoulders) Mean age, 33 yr (range, 18-50 yr) Mean follow-up, 29 mo (range, 6-50 mo)
Goel et al	*J Shoulder Elbow Surg* (2014)	Cerclage wires, plate, autograft ICBG	3 pleural effusions, 1 hemo-pneumothorax, 1 pulmonary embolus, 1 infection, 6 hardware removals Avg active FE improved from 90° to 117°	17% nonunion (revision arthrodesis required)	10 patients with various presentations (12 shoulders) Mean age, 43 yr (range, 19-67 yr) Mean follow-up, 41 mo (range, 8-72 mo)

FE = forward elevation, FSHD = facioscapulohumeral dystrophy, ICBG = iliac crest bone graft, ROM = range of motion.

are not at increased risk of malignant hyperthermia, and paralytic anesthesia can be safely provided.

Video 60.1 Scapulothoracic Fusion for Facioscapulohumeral Muscular Dystrophy. Anthony A. Romeo, MD (39 min)

Surgical Equipment

- Two curved Adson elevators, a curved gouge, and a high-speed burr are needed.
- Eight 18-gauge Luque wires, a five-hole pelvic reconstruction plate, plate benders, jet twisters, and heavy wire cutters are also used.
- Synthetic bone graft is used.

Setup/Exposure

- The patient is intubated, given general anesthetic, and placed in a prone position.
- The contralateral arm is placed on an arm holder with the elbow slightly forward, so that the humerus is in the plane of the scapula and the elbow is positioned in 90° of flexion and 90° of abduction.
- The ipsilateral arm can be placed in a similar position on an arm holder or, alternatively, the arm can be prepped into the surgical field and

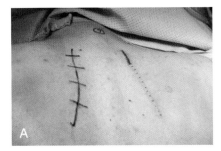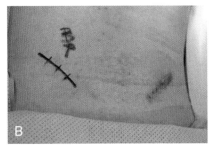

Figure 2 Intraoperative photographs show bony landmarks and planned surgical incision marked on a patient undergoing scapulothoracic fusion. **A,** The vertebra prominens (C7) is marked. The surgeon then counted down the T1-T4 processes and marked the incision equidistant from the medial border of the scapula and the spinous processes. The incision curves slightly distal and lies parallel to the medial border of the scapula. The previous contralateral incision can be seen. **B,** The posterior superior iliac spine bone graft harvest site is seen on the left. The lateral iliac crest was palpated and the line for the longitudinal incision drawn just distal to the posterior iliac crest. Outer table iliac crest harvest was planned for this patient, and the surgeon planned to avoid violating the crest to decrease postsurgical discomfort. The contralateral incision is seen.

held to the side of the body, where it can be manipulated in the so-called chicken wing position to enhance anteromedial scapular exposure.
- The surgical field to be prepped and draped should include the contralateral scapula and the entire back (including the vertebra prominens [C7]) distally to just above the buttock (for posterior iliac crest bone graft harvest).
- Bony landmarks are marked, including the vertebra prominens (C7), the T1-T4 spinous processes

(counted down from C7), the scapular spine, and the medial border of the scapula.
- The longitudinal incision is marked equidistant between the medial scapular border and the vertebral spinous processes; typically, this incision curves distally parallel to the medial border of the scapula (**Figure 2, A**).
- The location of the incision for the posterior iliac crest bone graft is slightly distal to the posterior iliac crest, beginning at the posterior

superior iliac spine and extending laterally toward the lateral iliac crest.

- Bone graft is harvested from the outer table of the posterior ilium (**Figure 2, B**).

Procedure

STEP 1: EXPOSE THE TRAPEZIUS AND LOCATE THE SCAPULAR SPINE

- The skin is injected with local anesthetic (0.5% bupivacaine hydrochloride with epinephrine).
- The skin is incised by means of sharp knife dissection.
- Bovie electrocautery is used for hemostasis, and the superficial fascia of the trapezius is divided longitudinally along the incision line.
- The skin flap is raised laterally to expose the trapezius attachment to the scapular spine as well as the fascia. The orientation of the muscle fibers of the trapezius aids in visualizing the division between the upper, middle, and lower trapezius.
- The lateral spine of the scapula is palpated.

STEP 2: DIVIDE THE TRAPEZIUS AND EXPOSE THE MEDIAL BORDER OF THE SCAPULA

- The trapezius muscle is incised directly along the inferior border of the scapular spine, curving distally to follow the medial border of the scapula.
- The supraspinatus and infraspinatus are elevated subperiosteally off the superior and inferior borders, respectively, of the scapular spine.
- The origins of the infraspinatus and teres minor are elevated off the medial border of the scapula.
- Partial release of the tendon of the trapezius insertion onto the scapular spine is performed to enhance exposure of the supraspinatus fossa and superomedial border of the scapula. At this point in the surgical dissection, the rhomboids are

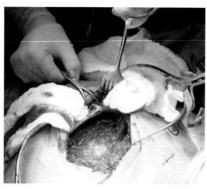

Figure 3 Intraoperative photograph shows periosteal dissection of the rhomboid attachments to the medial border of the scapula performed to expose the medial scapular border. Lap pads are placed in the supraspinatus fossa (right) and infraspinatus fossa (left) for hemostasis. A towel clip was placed through the scapular spine and used to lift the scapula away from the thorax.

seen medial to the medial scapular border, and the supraspinatus and infraspinatus and teres minor are elevated to expose the suprascapular fossa and infrascapular fossa with the skeletonized scapular spine in between.

STEP 3: SKELETONIZE THE VENTROMEDIAL BORDER OF THE SCAPULA

- A towel clip is placed into the scapular spine and used to elevate the scapula to enhance exposure of the medial border of the scapula.
- The rhomboid attachments are dissected off the medial border of the scapula (**Figure 3**).
- The dissection is carried to the ventral surface of the scapula to release the origin of the serratus anterior and the subscapularis off the subscapularis fossa (**Figure 4**).

STEP 4: EXPOSE THE DEEP SUBSCAPULARIS BURSAL LAYER

- The dissection is taken down to the deep layer of the subscapularis bursa, located between the

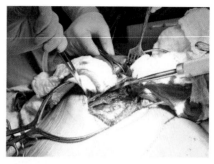

Figure 4 Intraoperative photograph of the medial border of the scapula. A Cobb elevator is used to elevate the muscular origins of the serratus anterior and subscapularis off the ventromedial surface of the scapula to expose the subscapularis fossa.

subscapularis and the thoracic cage. To enter the subscapularis bursa, the rhomboid muscles are elevated medially and the serratus and subscapularis muscles laterally along a relatively avascular longitudinal raphe that can be divided longitudinally. The subscapularis bursa is highly vascular, with traversing branches from the intercostal vessels, and patience is required to achieve meticulous hemostasis.

STEP 5: EXPOSE RIBS 3 THROUGH 6

- The vertebra prominens is palpated through the incision, and the ribs are counted from 1 through 6. Ribs 3 through 6 are identified and the subscapularis bursa is divided directly over each of those ribs.
- A periosteal elevator is used to perform periosteal dissection to expose the dorsal surface.
- A curved blunt Adson elevator is used subperiosteally to dissect the parietal pleura off the ventral surface of each rib (**Figure 5**).
- The intercostal neurovascular bundles, which lie within a groove on the inferior aspect of each rib, should be elevated with the musculature.
- To create an adequate surface area for fusion, each rib is dissected from

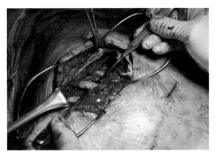

Figure 5 Intraoperative photograph shows blunt curved Adson elevators used to elevate the intercostal muscles, intercostal neurovascular bundles, and parietal pleura off the ventral surface of ribs 3 through 6 to allow for safe wire passage.

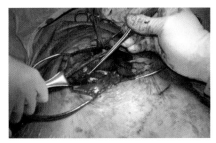

Figure 6 Intraoperative photograph shows ribs 3 through 6 exposed from the lateral border of the erector spinae muscle to 6 cm laterally. The Cobb elevator is used to indicate interposition of the intercostal muscles over the dorsal aspect of the ribs. This interposition must be resected to avoid interference with fusion.

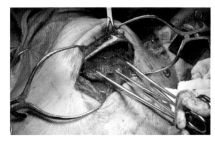

Figure 7 Intraoperative photograph shows the use of clamps to pull the serratus anterior and a portion of the subscapularis into the surgical field. Approximately 6 cm of muscle must be excised to prevent interposition in the fusion site.

the lateral border of the erector spinae musculature to approximately 6 cm laterally. This is performed for each rib.

- The intercostal muscles are excised to avoid muscular interposition in the fusion site (**Figure 6**).

STEP 6: CREATE ADEQUATE SCAPULAR FUSION SURFACE AREA

- The serratus anterior muscle and part of the subscapularis are excised to achieve adequate bone surface area for STF (**Figure 7**).
- Beginning from the anteromedial border of the scapula and extending approximately 6 cm laterally, the muscle of the serratus anterior and subscapularis is excised to prevent any muscle interposition in the fusion site (**Figure 8**).

STEP 7: PREPARE THE FUSION SURFACES WITH A HIGH-SPEED BURR

- A high-speed burr is used to prepare the dorsal surface of the ribs for fusion. Light burring of the dorsal rib cortex is performed until punctate bleeding is seen (**Figure 9**).
- Care should be taken to avoid complete decortication of the rib to avoid wire cutout and loss of rigid fixation as well as to achieve fusion.
- The medial portion of the scapula is

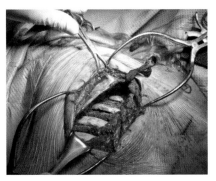

Figure 8 Intraoperative photograph shows dissection of ribs 3 through 6 and excision of the intercostal muscles as well as the serratus anterior and subscapularis muscles to achieve the proper fusion surface area.

prepared with the high-speed burr in a similar fashion.

STEP 8: HARVEST POSTERIOR ILIAC CREST BONE GRAFT

- As previously noted, the incision is begun at the posterior superior iliac spine and extended laterally just inferior to the iliac crest.
- Subcutaneous dissection is taken down to the fascial layer overlying the posterior iliac crest. Rather than release the fascia insertion onto the superior aspect of the posterior iliac crest, the dissection is made just distal to the

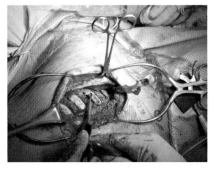

Figure 9 Intraoperative photograph shows use of a high-speed burr to prepare the dorsal surface of the ribs and the ventral surface of the medial scapula.

superior crest down through the origin of the gluteus maximus. The senior author of this chapter (A.A.R.) thinks that patients tolerate this dissection better and experience less pain at the iliac crest.

- Using a curved 0.75-in osteotome inserted through a small cortical window, the outer table is opened and a curved gouge is used to harvest the corticocancellous bone (**Figure 10**).
- Approximately 20 to 30 mL of autograft is harvested, and this can be supplemented with additional synthetic bone graft to ensure adequate bone mass for STF.

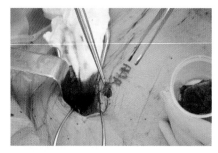

Figure 10 Intraoperative photograph shows posterior iliac crest bone graft harvest. The fascial attachment to the superior crest is untouched; instead, the gluteus maximus origin is elevated off the posterior crest and a cortical window is made. A curved gouge is used to harvest approximately 20 to 30 mL of corticocancellous bone graft. In this case, use of synthetic bone graft was planned in addition to the autograft.

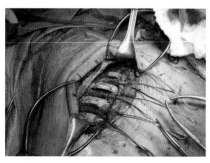

Figure 11 Intraoperative photograph shows 18-gauge Luque wire doubled in half and curved at the end and passed under each rib (3 through 6). A blunt elevator was used to create a path ventral to the rib for safe passage of the Luque wire.

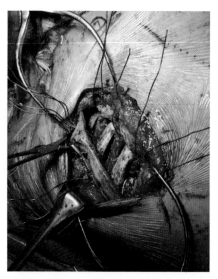

Figure 12 Intraoperative photograph shows placement of a five-hole reconstruction plate that was contoured to match the posteromedial scapular border. One limb of each wire has been passed through the adjacent scapular holes and through the plate. The scapular spine is provisionally positioned over the T4 rib with the towel clip.

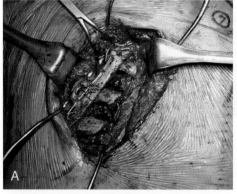
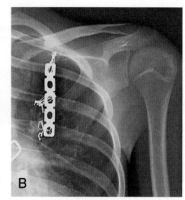

Figure 13 **A,** Intraoperative photograph shows the final reduction and fixation of the scapulothoracic fusion. The bone graft has been packed under the scapula before final fixation of the wires, and the additional bone graft and synthetic graft will be added before closure. **B,** Postoperative radiograph demonstrates appropriate reduction and fixation. Depending on patient size, only three ribs may be available for fusion.

STEP 9: CREATE HOLES IN THE SCAPULA AND PASS WIRES AROUND THE RIBS

- A high-speed burr is used to create holes in the scapula to accept the wires. Four holes are created in the scapula, one for each corresponding rib.
- The most proximal hole is made in the supraspinatus fossa in preparation to receive wire to be passed around the T3 rib.
- The hole for the T4 rib is made below the scapular spine, and the T5 and T6 holes are created distal to this. These holes are placed approximately 1 cm lateral to the medial border of the scapula.
- The 18-gauge Luque wires are passed under each rib. To pass the wires without injury to the underlying parietal pleura, the wires are bent in half and curved at the tip so that the rounded end is passed under the rib. An elevator is used to depress the soft tissue down and away from the rib to create a path for wire passage (**Figure 11**).
- After each doubled Luque wire is passed under each of the four ribs (T3-T6), the wires are cut in half to create two separate wires under each rib, for a total of eight wires.
- A five-hole pelvic reconstruction plate is contoured to match the posteromedial border of the infraspinatus fossa. The function of the plate is to act as a washer to distribute the forces of the wires evenly and thus to avoid wire cutout through the scapula or ribs.
- One limb of each wire is passed through the previously created holes in the scapula and through holes one, three, and five in the plate. The wires are passed so as to create an X-shaped configuration on the ribs (**Figure 12**). Alignment of the scapular spine with the T4 rib is confirmed.
- The autograft bone is placed over the ribs at the site of anticipated

Table 2 Rehabilitation Protocol After Scapulothoracic Fusion

Postoperative Week	Range of Motion	Strengthening	Return to Activities	Comments/Emphasis
0-6	Exercises of the hand and wrist	None	None	Gunslinger brace is used
6-12	Active forward elevation	None	Sedentary work is permitted	Gunslinger brace is discontinued
12-24	Active	Strengthening is begun	Sedentary work is permitted	—
≥24	Active	Strengthening exercises are continued	Return to sports and work is allowed	—

fusion. Additional synthetic bone graft is added between the ribs to enhance the fusion surface area.

- The scapula is reduced to the final desired position, which consists of slight abduction of the inferomedial border of the scapula in relation to the long axis of the spine. This position of slight abduction may help prevent subacromial impingement with glenohumeral motion.
- A jet wire twister is used to twist the wires down over the plate to secure the fixation. Heavy wire cutters are used to clip the free ends of wire, and the wire ends are rotated to avoid complications resulting from symptomatic hardware (**Figure 13**).
- Additional bone graft can be placed under the medial border as needed.
- Prior to closure, the wound is filled with saline, and a Valsalva maneuver is performed to evaluate for the presence of a pneumothorax. A small pneumothorax may be monitored clinically; however, a larger pneumothorax should be treated with a chest tube insertion by a thoracic surgeon.

Wound Closure

- To decrease dead space, the rhomboid is sutured to the supraspinatus as well as the infraspinatus and teres minor with No. 2 braided, nonabsorbable suture while the needle is passed through the medial border of the scapula.
- The lateral trapezius insertion onto the scapular spinal is repaired with size 0 absorbable suture.
- The deep dermal layer and skin are closed in standard fashion.
- A bulky dressing is applied to the wound.

Rehabilitation

A postoperative rehabilitation regimen is presented in **Table 2**. A gunslinger brace is applied immediately postoperatively, and hand, wrist, and elbow exercises are begun. Two to 3 weeks postoperatively, pendulum exercises are allowed. Six weeks postoperatively, bracing is discontinued. Physical therapy that includes active range of motion and strengthening exercises is begun 3 months postoperatively. Return

to sedentary work is allowed 6 weeks postoperatively, and return to sports and heavy labor is allowed 6 months postoperatively.

Avoiding Pitfalls and Complications

Potential intraoperative complications include pneumothorax during wire passage around ribs and brachial plexus palsy during scapular reduction. The use of curved blunt Adson elevators to dissect around each rib can decrease the risk of pneumothorax. Similarly, the use of somatosensory-evoked potential monitoring will alert the surgeon to brachial plexus traction.

The lack of fusion formation is typically the result of a technical failure: either inadequate fixation or inadequate preparation of the fusion site. To avoid wire cutout and loss of fixation, the surgeon should use 18-gauge Luque wires rather than cables and tighten them with jet wire twisters. All soft tissue between the ribs should be removed to avoid soft-tissue interposition in the fusion site.

Bibliography

Bizot P, Teboul F, Nizard R, Sedel L: Scapulothoracic fusion for serratus anterior paralysis. *J Shoulder Elbow Surg* 2003;12(6):561-565.

Cooney AD, Gill I, Stuart PR: The outcome of scapulothoracic arthrodesis using cerclage wires, plates, and allograft for facioscapulohumeral dystrophy. *J Shoulder Elbow Surg* 2014;23(1):e8-e13.

DeFranco MJ, Nho S, Romeo AA: Scapulothoracic fusion. *J Am Acad Orthop Surg* 2010;18(4):236-242.

Demirhan M, Uysal O, Atalar AC, Kilicoglu O, Serdaroglu P: Scapulothoracic arthrodesis in facioscapulohumeral dystrophy with multifilament cable. *Clin Orthop Relat Res* 2009;467(8):2090-2097.

Diab M, Darras BT, Shapiro F: Scapulothoracic fusion for facioscapulohumeral muscular dystrophy. *J Bone Joint Surg Am* 2005;87(10):2267-2275.

Elhassan B, Chung ST, Ozbaydar M, Diller D, Warner JJ: Scapulothoracic fusion for clavicular insufficiency: A report of two cases. *J Bone Joint Surg Am* 2008;90(4):875-880.

Goel DP, Romanowski JR, Shi LL, Warner JJ: Scapulothoracic fusion: Outcomes and complications. *J Shoulder Elbow Surg* 2014;23(4):542-547.

Jeon IH, Neumann L, Wallace WA: Scapulothoracic fusion for painful winging of the scapula in nondystrophic patients. *J Shoulder Elbow Surg* 2005;14(4):400-406.

Letournel E, Fardeau M, Lytle JO, Serrault M, Gosselin RA: Scapulothoracic arthrodesis for patients who have fascioscapulohumeral muscular dystrophy. *J Bone Joint Surg Am* 1990;72(1):78-84.

Rhee YG, Ha JH: Long-term results of scapulothoracic arthrodesis of facioscapulohumeral muscular dystrophy. *J Shoulder Elbow Surg* 2006;15(4):445-450.

Sewell MD, Higgs DS, Al-Hadithy N, Falworth M, Bayley I, Lambert SM: The outcome of scapulothoracic fusion for painful winging of the scapula in dystrophic and non-dystrophic conditions. *J Bone Joint Surg Br* 2012;94(9):1253-1259.

Twyman RS, Harper GD, Edgar MA: Thoracoscapular fusion in facioscapulohumeral dystrophy: Clinical review of a new surgical method. *J Shoulder Elbow Surg* 1996;5(3):201-205.

Van Tongel A, Atoun E, Narvani A, Sforza G, Copeland S, Levy O: Medium to long-term outcome of thoracoscapular arthrodesis with screw fixation for facioscapulohumeral muscular dystrophy. *J Bone Joint Surg Am* 2013;95(15):1404-1408.

 Video Reference

Romeo AA: Video. *Scapulothoracic Fusion for Facioscapulohumeral Muscular Dystrophy.* Chicago, IL, 2015.

Chapter 61
Glenohumeral Arthrodesis

Joaquin Sanchez-Sotelo, MD, PhD

Introduction

Glenohumeral arthrodesis was commonly performed before the development of shoulder arthroplasty. Currently, arthrodesis is considered a salvage procedure that is appropriate for select patients. Current indications include neuromuscular conditions (for example, sequels of brachial plexus palsy), severe destruction of the glenohumeral joint that cannot be reconstructed (especially in patients in whom the deltoid or axillary nerve is compromised), and recurrent instability after multiple failed procedures in the young, active patient. Keys to success include bone preparation, position of fusion, internal fixation, and postoperative management.

Case Presentation

A 32-year-old right-hand–dominant man sustained a penetrating gunshot injury to his right shoulder region, which resulted in an open fracture of the right proximal humerus, an axillary nerve injury, and an associated fracture of the coracoid. He underwent open reduction and internal fixation of the proximal humerus fracture with a long humeral locking compression plate and fixation of the coracoid with a mini-plate.

Two years after the initial procedure, the man had pain in and reduced use of his right shoulder. On physical examination, his anterior incision was well healed with some scarring of the skin in the axillary region. His range of motion included active elevation to 20°, passive elevation to 60°, active external rotation to -10°, passive external rotation to 10°, and active internal rotation to the level of L1. He had decreased sensation in the area of the axillary nerve with active but weak deltoid contraction.

Plain radiographs and CT revealed a proximal humerus malunion (marked superior displacement of the greater tuberosity) with osteonecrosis, a long humeral locking compression plate, and a small fragment plate in the coracoid (**Figure 1**). Intra-articular fluid cultures were negative. The man's electromyography showed evidence of upper trunk brachial plexopathy and superimposed injuries to the subscapularis and axillary nerves, with evidence of incomplete re-innervation.

The man underwent hardware removal and glenohumeral arthrodesis with the use of two interfragmentary screws and a neutralization plate (**Figure 2**). The man's shoulder was immobilized in a long-arm spica cast for 2 months postoperatively. At 1 year postoperatively, the patient had active elevation to 120°, active external rotation to 30°, and active internal rotation to the back pocket (**Figure 3**) and reported no pain.

Indications

The patient discussed in the case presentation is a good example of a candidate for glenohumeral arthrodesis. The combination of arthritis, rotator cuff dysfunction secondary to malunion, severe stiffness, deltoid insufficiency, and associated persistent dysfunction of the brachial plexus and axillary nerve are unlikely to be managed with other procedures in a younger patient who plans to remain physically active.

The indications for glenohumeral osteoarthritis have evolved over time. **Table 1** summarizes the current indications for glenohumeral arthrodesis. Traditionally, glenohumeral arthrodesis has been indicated for patients who have lack of motor function (paralysis), tuberculosis, or other refractory deep infections. It also is indicated for patients who undergo tumor resection and those who experience the sequela of shoulder trauma with deltoid insufficiency, such as primary muscular damage, axillary nerve injury, or brachial plexus injuries.

Dr. Sanchez-Sotelo or an immediate family member has received royalties from Stryker; has received research or institutional support from Biomet, DePuy Synthes, Stryker, and Zimmer; and serves as a board member, owner, officer, or committee member of the American Academy of Orthopaedic Surgeons and the American Shoulder and Elbow Surgeons.

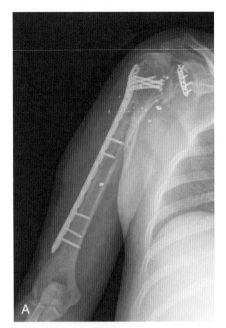
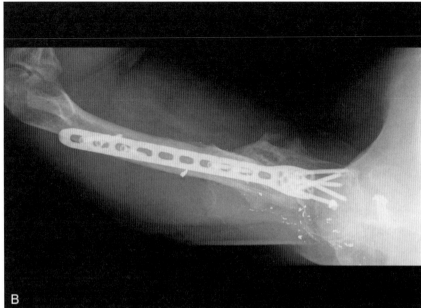

Figure 1   AP (**A**) and axillary (**B**) shoulder radiographs demonstrate a proximal humerus malunion with posttraumatic osteonecrosis and osteoarthritis after failed internal fixation of an open proximal humerus fracture with shaft extension.

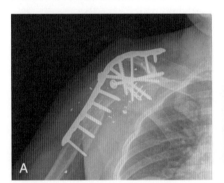
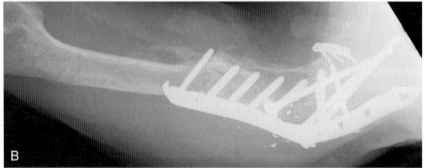

Figure 2   AP (**A**) and axillary (**B**) shoulder radiographs obtained after hardware removal and glenohumeral arthrodesis demonstrate a solid union.

Currently, reverse shoulder arthroplasty is considered for patients who have conditions for which arthrodesis was commonly indicated. Reverse shoulder arthroplasty is considered in patients who undergo tumor resection if the function of the deltoid can be preserved. Although reverse shoulder arthroplasty has become the procedure of choice for patients who have massive irreparable rotator cuff tears or pseudoparalysis, arthrodesis is still considered for ultra-young patients who have massive irreparable rotator cuff tears or pseudoparalysis because of concerns

for implant longevity. The relative indications for reverse arthroplasty and fusion must be individualized to each patient. Age is considered in the decision-making process, but there is no absolute age limit for either procedure. Complete absence of deltoid function may be managed with transfer of the pectoralis major combined with reverse arthroplasty in patients who are willing to accept the potential for mechanical failure of the implant. Pectoralis major transfer and reverse arthroplasty also could be attempted as a reconstructive alternative later in life for patients who

have symptomatic fusion; however, most patients who have longstanding glenohumeral arthrodesis are satisfied with their outcome and do not seek additional surgery.

Persistent instability after multiple failed stabilization procedures is currently a relatively common indication for glenohumeral arthrodesis. Patients who have persistent instability after multiple failed stabilization procedures typically are young and have substantial soft-tissue and bone deficiencies, sometimes with an underlying collagen disorder, such as Ehlers-Danlos syndrome. Some

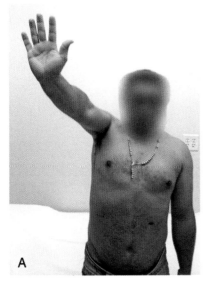
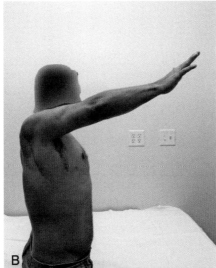
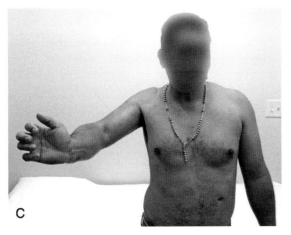
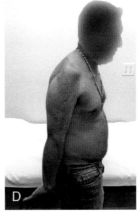

Figure 3 Photographs of a man taken 1 year after he underwent glenohumeral arthrodesis show active shoulder motion in elevation (**A**), flexion (**B**), external rotation (**C**), and internal rotation (**D**).

Table 1 Current Indications for Glenohumeral Arthrodesis

Paralysis (ie, brachial plexus injuries, poliomyelitis)

Glenohumeral osteoarthritis in the presence of deltoid dysfunction (most commonly after trauma)

Refractory deep infection (eg, tuberculosis, refractory osteomyelitis)

Resection of a tumor

Recurrent instability after multiple failed procedures in younger patients who have marked soft-tissue or bony deficiencies

Massive irreparable rotator cuff tear with pseudoparalysis if reverse arthroplasty is contraindicated

Failed shoulder arthroplasty not amenable to revision arthroplasty

patients may have cartilage damage secondary to dislocation arthropathy or chondrolysis.

Failed shoulder arthroplasty can often be salvaged with implant revision. However, patients who have catastrophic bone loss or severe deltoid dysfunction may be better candidates for arthrodesis rather than revision arthroplasty. One challenge of arthrodesis after failed arthroplasty is the magnitude of bone loss. The author of this chapter prefers to use structural iliac crest bone graft in these patients. Failure rates are no higher with the use of such bone graft.

 Controversies and Alternative Approaches

Shoulder hemiarthroplasty, reverse total shoulder arthroplasty, and resection arthroplasty are alternatives to glenohumeral arthrodesis. Shoulder hemiarthroplasty may help improve arthritic pain and motion; however, in patients without a functioning deltoid, active use of the shoulder will likely be more limited with hemiarthroplasty compared with arthrodesis. In addition, rotator cuff insufficiency may lead to instability with either subluxation or frank dislocation after hemiarthroplasty. Pain on the glenoid side of the joint may continue and progressive glenoid erosion may develop after hemiarthroplasty.

Some surgeons consider reverse total shoulder arthroplasty to salvage shoulders that are similar to the shoulder described in the case presentation, even in the absence of a completely intact deltoid. Surgeons should understand that the range of motion typically reported after reverse total shoulder arthroplasty for rotator cuff-tear arthropathy does not reflect that of patients who undergo reverse total shoulder arthroplasty for posttraumatic conditions. The complication rate after reverse total shoulder arthroplasty in patients who have posttraumatic conditions is high. In addition, although younger patients who undergo reverse total shoulder arthroplasty are expected to experience a substantial rate of mechanical failure, this outcome has not been confirmed in the literature.

Permanent resection arthroplasty of the glenohumeral joint has been reported to provide some pain relief; however, it is clearly associated with less function and is seldom considered, except after

Table 2 Results of Glenohumeral Arthrodesis

Authors	Journal (Year)	Technique (No. of Patients)	Outcomes	Comments
Cofield and Briggs	J Bone Joint Surg Am (1979)	Glenohumeral arthrodesis with internal fixation (70)	Union achieved in 96% 75% had no or mild pain Function: trunk level (75%), head level (50%), overhead (25%)	Indications: paralysis, rotator cuff tear, osteoarthritis, infection, instability, and rheumatoid arthritis Mean follow-up: 9.6 yr Subjective satisfaction: 82% Results did not deteriorate over time Complications: postoperative fracture (14%), infection (1.5%), and hardware removal (24%)
Rybka et al	J Bone Joint Surg Am (1979)	Glenohumeral arthrodesis with internal fixation and external splits (39)	Union achieved in 90% 90% had no or mild pain Good or excellent results in 68%	Indication: rheumatoid arthritis Mean follow-up: 6 yr Subjective satisfaction: 95% Complications: postoperative fracture (2.5%) and hardware removal (10%)
Richards et al	Clin Orthop Relat Res (1985)	Glenohumeral arthrodesis with internal fixation (14)	Union achieved in 100% 78% had no or mild pain Minimum abduction, 60°	Indication: brachial plexus injury Mean follow-up: 2.6 yr All patients believed function improved Complications: hardware removal (50%)
Diaz et al	J Shoulder Elbow Surg (2003)	Glenohumeral arthrodesis (8)	Union achieved in 100% Mean VAS pain score, 3.1 Mean VAS function score, 4.7	Indication: instability Mean follow-up: 2.9 yr Subjective satisfaction: 100% Complications: hardware removal (62%) and acromioclavicular joint resection (25%)
Fuchs et al	Clin Orthop Relat Res (2005)	Primary glenohumeral arthrodesis (8) Salvage glenohumeral arthrodesis (13)	Toronto Extremity Salvage Score, 81%	Indication: tumor resection Mean follow-up: 11 yr Complications: 43%
Scalise and Iannotti	J Bone Joint Surg Am (2008)	Glenohumeral arthrodesis (7)	Union achieved in 42%; union achieved in 71% after secondary bone grafting Mean Penn pain score, 26 Mean Penn function score, 26	Indication: failed arthroplasty Mean follow-up: 4 yr 4 patients required vascularized fibular autograft Complications: secondary bone grafting (57%) and hardware removal (28%)
Atlan et al	J Hand Surg Am (2012)	Glenohumeral arthrodesis with massive subacromial corticocancellous bone autograft (26) Glenohumeral arthrodesis with cancellous bone graft (28)	Union achieved in 76%; union achieved in 94% after additional surgery Abduction >45° in 75%, rotation >45° in 65%	Indication: brachial plexus injury Mean follow-up: 3 yr Graft used between acromion and humeral head Only 12% of patients were immobilized Complications: secondary bone grafting (24%) and infection (3.7%)

Penn = Penn Shoulder Score, SPADI = shoulder pain and disability index, SSV = subjective shoulder value, VAS = visual analog scale.

catastrophic failure of shoulder arthroplasty in elderly patients who are not candidates for further reconstructive efforts. Uncontrolled osteomyelitis also is an indication for resection arthroplasty. Modern mobile cement spacers allow some motion and pain relief. Some patients in whom a temporary spacer is placed for the management of infection

Table 2 Results of Glenohumeral Arthrodesis (*continued*)

Authors	Journal (Year)	Technique (No. of Patients)	Outcomes	Comments
Porcellini et al	*Arthroscopy* (2014)	Arthroscopic-assisted glenohumeral arthrodesis (12)	Union achieved in 83%; union achieved in 100% after additional bone grafting Mean SPADI score improved 60 points	Indications: instability, deep infection, rotator cuff deficiency, brachial plexus palsy Mean follow-up: 2 yr Complications: secondary bone grafting (17%)
Thangarajah et al	*Bone Joint J* (2014)	Glenohumeral arthrodesis (6)	Union achieved in 100% Mean SSV score, 42 Mean Oxford Shoulder Instability score, 24	Indications: epileptic-associated instability Mean follow-up: 3 yr Cast immobilization for 3 mo Complications: hardware removal (16%) and postoperative fracture (16%)

Penn = Penn Shoulder Score, SPADI = shoulder pain and disability index, SSV = subjective shoulder value, VAS = visual analog scale.

function reasonably well with the spacer in place and elect not to undergo further surgery.

 Results

Results of glenohumeral arthrodesis are presented in **Table 2**. Union rates have ranged from 75% to 100%, with higher nonunion rates in one study on arthrodesis after failed arthroplasty. Most patients achieve a functional range of elevation but experience considerable rotation restriction. Reported complication rates range from 5% to 50%, which, in part, reflects the need for hardware removal in some patients.

 Technical Keys to Success

Exposure

- The author of this chapter performs glenohumeral arthrodesis via the anteromedial approach (**Figure 4**).
- The neutralization plate must be placed across the acromion and proximal humerus underneath the deltoid.
- The soft tissue between the humeral head and acromion is excised, including any residual rotator cuff that could become interposed.

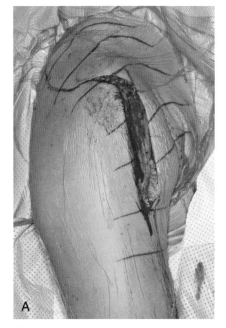
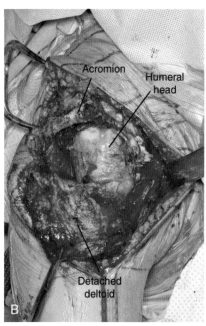

Figure 4 Intraoperative photographs of a shoulder show the anteromedial approach for glenohumeral arthrodesis. **A,** The skin incision courses along the spine of the scapula and curves in a lazy S fashion over the deltopectoral interval. **B,** The anteromedial approach combines a deltopectoral approach with detachment of the deltoid origin from the clavicle, acromion, and spine of the scapula.

Bone Preparation

- The humeral head, glenoid, and acromion are prepared to bleeding bone to promote healing and preserve the strength of the subchondral bone.
- The humeral head must be adequately contoured to maximize contact between the acromion and

the glenoid at the desired arthrodesis site (**Figure 5**).

Selective Bone Grafting

- In some patients who undergo tumor resection or salvage of a failed shoulder arthroplasty, marked bone loss of the proximal humerus makes adequate contact at the

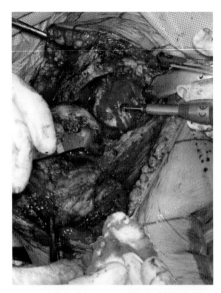

Figure 5 Intraoperative photograph of a shoulder shows contouring and preparation of the humeral head, glenoid, and inferior surface of the acromion to bleeding bone, which facilitates contact and promotes union.

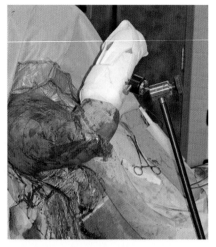

Figure 6 Intraoperative photograph shows the most commonly recommended position of a patient's arm for glenohumeral arthrodesis, which combines 40° to 45° of internal rotation, 20° of flexion, and 20° of abduction. A higher degree of abduction may result in a higher active elevation but may cause increased periscapular pain.

arthrodesis site extremely difficult.
- Allograft, nonvascularized iliac crest bone graft, and vascularized fibular autograft may be considered depending on the amount of bone loss.

Patient Positioning
- Various studies have proposed small variations in the position of a patient's arm for glenohumeral arthrodesis. Most surgeons agree that 40° to 45° of internal rotation and 20° of flexion allows the patient's hand to easily reach his or her face (**Figure 6**).
- The amount of abduction will influence how much active elevation will be achieved. The author of this chapter tends to select between 20° and 40° of abduction. More abduction may lead to worse periscapular pain and make it difficult for the patient to rest his or her arm at his or her side.
- Higher abduction angles are typically selected for patients who are

overweight to facilitate hygiene in the axillary region.
- The desired position of the patient's arm can be maintained during surgery by a surgical assistant or with the use of a mechanical arm holder.

Adequate Internal Fixation
- The author of this chapter prefers to combine interfragmentary screw fixation with plate neutralization. Another option is to osteotomize the acromion to ensure apposition to the greater tuberosity.
- Adequate proximal screw fixation may be difficult to achieve because of the skeletal morphology of the scapula.
- Provisional fixation of the humeral head to the glenoid may be achieved with two Steinmann pins.
- The plate is carefully contoured to the spine of the scapula, acromion, humeral head, and humeral shaft.
- Fixation is achieved by replacing the two Steinmann pins with partially-threaded cancellous screws

for compression and plate fixation for neutralization (**Figure 7**).

Soft-Tissue Coverage Over the Plate
- Prominence of the plate on the posterosuperior aspect of the scapula may be uncomfortable, especially for slender patients.
- The deltoid should be advanced over the plate at the time of wound closure to provide the best possible soft-tissue coverage of the plate under the skin (**Figure 8**).

Rehabilitation

Glenohumeral arthrodesis requires protection of the shoulder until the fusion mass is solid. Rehabilitation programs concentrate on isometric exercises with the arm immobilized in a cast or brace for the first few weeks postoperatively, after which exercises to strengthen the scapular stabilizing musculature and the elbow are begun (**Table 3**).

Avoiding Pitfalls

Several pitfalls, including suboptimal positioning, inadequate bone contact and compression, inaccurate plate contouring and screw fixation along the scapula, poor soft-tissue coverage of the plate, inadequate postoperative protection, adverse biologic aspects of healing, poor rehabilitation, and postoperative fracture, may compromise the outcome of glenohumeral arthrodesis. The position of a patient's arm at the time of arthrodesis, especially with regard to abduction, may be difficult to estimate accurately in the operating room. A large, hand-held, sterile goniometer may be helpful. After the optimal position of a patient's arm is established, it is important to maintain it with a combination of external assistance and temporary fixation.

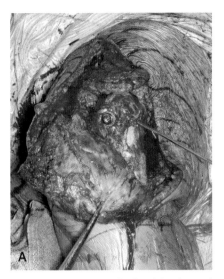
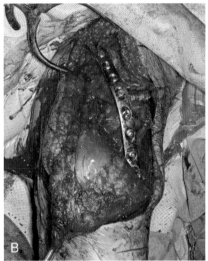
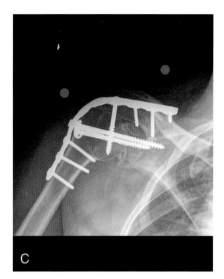

Figure 7 Images of a shoulder show glenohumeral arthrodesis with the use of interfragmentary screws and a neutralization plate. **A,** Intraoperative photograph shows provisional fixation with Steinmann pins, which are later replaced by large-fragment, partially-threaded, cancellous compression screws. **B,** Intraoperative photograph shows plate neutralization across the spine of the scapula, acromion, and humeral shaft, which requires adequate plate contouring. **C,** AP radiograph demonstrates solid arthrodesis, which was achieved with the use of compression screws and a neutralization plate. Note the fusion of the humeral head to both the glenoid and the acromion as well as adequate plate fixation proximally, distally, and across the humeral head.

The humeral head must be compressed to the glenoid and the acromion to achieve the best possible contact. As previously mentioned, bone graft may be necessary in patients who have substantial bone loss.

The author of this chapter prefers to use a malleable template to understand the plate contour necessary for each patient. If the plate is not contoured accurately, it may displace the arthrodesis to an undesirable position, make screw fixation difficult to achieve, and/or irritate soft tissue postoperatively as a result of prominent hardware. Screw fixation in the scapula may be difficult. The most proximal screw holes will be very close to a patient's head and neck, which complicates drilling at the desired angle. The bone stock of the scapula is somewhat limited in most patients. In most patients, the author of this chapter attempts to direct the screws to the spine of the scapula and use cancellous screws proximally.

The plate used for neutralization may be uncomfortable after postoperative swelling subsides. The author of

this chapter makes a conscious effort to cover the plate with as much muscle as possible. Patients should be counseled preoperatively on the possibility of postoperative plate discomfort.

Plate neutralization may allow for less postoperative shoulder protection; however, nonunion and hardware failure may still occur. The author of this chapter prefers to use a postoperative long-arm spica cast for postoperative protection after glenohumeral arthrodesis (**Figure 9**). Although a long-arm spica cast guarantees patient compliance, it may not be well tolerated in some patients. A shoulder brace or immobilizer may be used instead of a long-arm spica cast in compliant patients who have good bone quality.

Successful union also requires attention to adverse biologic conditions. Many patients who undergo glenohumeral arthrodesis have a history of previous surgery. Therefore, observation for and the treatment of deep infection are essential. The author of this chapter delays glenohumeral arthrodesis in patients who are smokers until the use

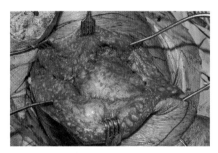

Figure 8 Intraoperative photograph of a shoulder shows meticulous deltoid repair and complete coverage of the plate with soft tissue, which helps minimize hardware-related irritation.

of tobacco products has ceased. Patients are advised to avoid smoking 3 months before the procedure and 6 months after the procedure, or until union is confirmed.

A common misconception after glenohumeral arthrodesis is that rehabilitation is not beneficial postoperatively because the glenohumeral joint is fused. Glenohumeral arthrodesis shifts the use of the upper extremity from the glenohumeral joint muscles to the periscapular muscles. Therefore, core

Table 3 Rehabilitation Protocol After Glenohumeral Arthrodesis

Postoperative Week	ROM	Strengthening	Return to Play	Comments/Emphasis
1-8	Wrist and hand active ROM	Isometric exercises in the cast for deltoid, elbow flexion and extension, scapular retraction, shoulder shrugs	N/A	Cast or brace immobilization
8-12	Elbow passive and AAROM Shoulder AAROM	Scapular stabilizing exercises	N/A	Emphasis on restoration of elevation and external rotation
12-20	Active ROM	Plyometrics Open chain (free weights) Core strengthening	N/A	Emphasis on deltoid and periscapular muscle strengthening

AAROM = active-assisted range of motion, N/A = not applicable, ROM = range of motion.

strengthening and scapular stabilizing exercises are necessary after glenohumeral arthrodesis to help patients achieve the best possible outcomes.

One of the main complications after glenohumeral arthrodesis is fracture of the humeral shaft below the plate. Fracture of the humeral shaft below the plate typically occurs as a result of the large lever arm of the upper extremity over the fusion site or because of a patient's inability to protect the upper extremity as a result of the lack of glenohumeral motion. Patients should be counseled preoperatively on the possibility of postoperative fracture.

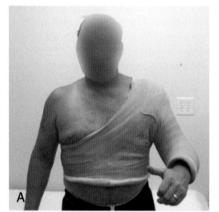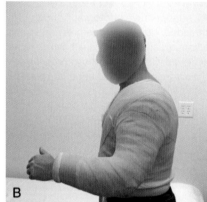

Figure 9 Forward-facing (**A**) and side-facing (**B**) photographs of a man who underwent glenohumeral arthrodesis show postoperative protection of the shoulder with a long-arm spica cast.

Bibliography

Atlan F, Durand S, Fox M, Levy P, Belkheyar Z, Oberlin C: Functional outcome of glenohumeral fusion in brachial plexus palsy: A report of 54 cases. *J Hand Surg Am* 2012;37(4):683-688.

Cofield RH, Briggs BT: Glenohumeral arthrodesis: Operative and long-term functional results. *J Bone Joint Surg Am* 1979;61(5):668-677.

Diaz JA, Cohen SB, Warren RF, Craig EV, Allen AA: Arthrodesis as a salvage procedure for recurrent instability of the shoulder. *J Shoulder Elbow Surg* 2003;12(3):237-241.

Fuchs B, O'Connor MI, Padgett DJ, Kaufman KR, Sim FH: Arthrodesis of the shoulder after tumor resection. *Clin Orthop Relat Res* 2005;(436):202-207.

Porcellini G, Savoie FH III, Campi F, Merolla G, Paladini P: Arthroscopically assisted shoulder arthrodesis: Is it an effective technique? *Arthroscopy* 2014;30(12):1550-1556.

Richards RR, Waddell JP, Hudson AR: Shoulder arthrodesis for the treatment of brachial plexus palsy. *Clin Orthop Relat Res* 1985;(198):250-258.

Rybka V, Raunio P, Vainio K: Arthrodesis of the shoulder in rheumatoid arthritis: A review of forty-one cases. *J Bone Joint Surg Br* 1979;61(2):155-158.

Scalise JJ, Iannotti JP: Glenohumeral arthrodesis after failed prosthetic shoulder arthroplasty. *J Bone Joint Surg Am* 2008;90(1):70-77.

Thangarajah T, Alexander S, Bayley I, Lambert SM: Glenohumeral arthrodesis for the treatment of recurrent shoulder instability in epileptic patients. *Bone Joint J* 2014;96(11):1525-1529.

Chapter 62

The Next Edition: The Future of Shoulder Reconstruction

Jeffrey S. Abrams, MD

Robert H. Bell, MD

John M. Tokish, MD

Introduction

The purpose of the second edition of *Advanced Reconstruction Shoulder: Arthroscopy, Arthroplasty, and Fracture Management*, is to present a comprehensive, state-of-the-art approach to shoulder reconstruction. Readers who are familiar with the first edition will note considerable changes and innovations in the field. With advances in communication and information technology, the rate of progress in shoulder reconstruction continues to accelerate, and the next edition of this text will undoubtedly require substantial revision to keep pace. Furthermore, the number and scope of adjunctive technologies that can enhance anatomic restoration of the shoulder continues to increase. New applications in orthobiologics, nanotechnology, and computer-assisted navigation are moving from innovative to mainstream. The application of some of the following innovative advances may well be featured in the next edition of this publication.

Orthobiologics

With increased understanding of the complex process of musculoskeletal healing, orthobiologic techniques have evolved to allow for the manipulation of this process to enhance tissue healing. Platelet-rich plasma (PRP) is perhaps the best studied orthobiologic product. It is well understood that platelets contain super-concentrations of the growth factors required for tissue healing and regeneration. More controversial is which combination of growth factors is best suited for various pathologic conditions, how best to deliver and activate those factors, and whether the demonstrated in vitro effects of PRP translate into clinical success.

For example, in injured skeletal muscle, fibrosis is part of the healing process, but it is detrimental to muscle regeneration and retained function. After muscle injury, growth factors such as transforming growth factor-β1 (TGF-β1) act as potent inducers of extracellular matrix production and fibrosis, and it appears as if abolishing the fibrotic effects of these growth factors enables the full recovery of skeletal muscle function. Recent studies have shown that the injection of PRP into injured muscle results in substantial increases in satellite cell activation and markers of myofiber regeneration.

The regeneration of skeletal muscle would have tremendous application in the management of chronic, retracted rotator cuff tear with fatty infiltration. Several approaches have been studied to preserve rotator cuff function in this setting, and results are mixed. In a sheep model, the use of continuous traction on a chronically torn rotator cuff was shown to partially reverse fatty infiltration and improve muscle architecture. Although the application of this technology in humans is lacking, the concept that muscle atrophy and fatty infiltration could be reversed will undoubtedly stimulate further study on the topic. The

Dr. Abrams or an immediate family member has received royalties from Smith & Nephew; serves as a paid consultant to Smith & Nephew, ConMed Linvatec, Mitek Sports Medicine, and Rotation Medical; serves as an unpaid consultant to Ingen Technology and KFx Medical; has stock or stock options held in Smith & Nephew, Cayenne Medical, Ingen Technology, KFx Medical, and Rotation Medical; and serves as a board member, owner, officer, or committee member of the American Shoulder and Elbow Surgeons and the Arthroscopy Association of North America. Dr. Bell or an immediate family member has received royalties from OrthoHelix and DePuy Synthes; is a member of a speakers' bureau or has made paid presentations on behalf of Smith & Nephew; serves as a paid consultant to Smith & Nephew; serves as an unpaid consultant to Exactech; has stock or stock options held in OrthoHelix and Cayenne Medical; and serves as a board member, owner, officer, or committee member of the American Shoulder and Elbow Surgeons and the Orthopaedic Learning Center. Dr. Tokish or an immediate family member is a member of a speakers' bureau or has made paid presentations on behalf of Arthrex; serves as a paid consultant to Arthrex, DePuy Synthes, and Mitek Sports Medicine; and serves as a board member, owner, officer, or committee member of the Arthroscopy Association of North America.

same authors also investigated chronic fatty atrophy from a pharmacologic standpoint. Using an animal model of rotator cuff tears, they noted that the administration of anabolic steroid could limit fatty infiltration and partially preserve muscle function. A more recent sheep model by the same authors was less promising, however; neither adjuvant therapy with anabolic steroid nor insulin-like growth factor significantly reversed fatty infiltration of muscle in chronic rotator cuff tears. The development and use of novel techniques to stimulate muscle regeneration will undoubtedly become a major focus for innovative technologies in rotator cuff pathology.

 ## Tendon Healing

Research on the use of orthobiologics, including PRP, to enhance tendon healing in the rotator cuff is in its infancy. Currently, at least six level I, II, and III studies exist that compare surgical results after rotator cuff repair with and without PRP augmentation. In one systematic review of five studies, the use of PRP augmentation in the repair of small- to medium-sized rotator cuff tears resulted in lower retear rates compared with repair alone. Large tears were not improved with the use of PRP, however, and no clinical outcome measure demonstrated improvement with PRP augmentation in any breakdown of the data. In a more recent randomized trial, PRP augmentation and repair were compared with standard repair in 48 patients who had large to massive tears. Retear rates were significantly lower with PRP augmentation than with conventional repair alone (56% and 20%, respectively; $P = 0.023$). In addition, the overall function score was significantly higher with the use of PRP ($P = 0.043$).

Thus, it appears as if there are conditions for which certain growth factor combinations result in improved healing after rotator cuff repair. It remains to be seen how individual PRP preparations may be altered or applied in the clinical setting to improve healing and clinical outcomes.

 ## Cartilage Damage and Osteoarthritis

Chondral damage and degeneration are among the most difficult conditions to manage in a patient with shoulder pain. Although basic science research on the orthobiologic treatment of these conditions is promising, clinical validation is lacking. One strategy involves the use orthobiologics in cartilage restoration as an adjunct to established techniques. Evidence is growing that the orthobiologic augmentation of microfracture, for example, may improve the quality of the repair tissue and the clinical outcomes of patients with chondral defects. An additional emerging orthobiologic application is the augmentation of cartilage transplantation with mesenchymal stem cells derived from bone marrow, synovium, or other sources to regenerate hyaline and hyaline-like cartilage.

The manipulation of pluripotent stem cells to differentiate down a chondrogenic pathway is becoming increasingly understood. The exposure of the cells to growth factors such as the TGF-β superfamily is one of the most studied and effective chondrogenic influences, and the delivery of these factors from marrow-derived stem cells has shown increased chondrogenesis in a rat model. In a rabbit model, constructs seeded with stem cells regenerated hyaline tissue and restored a smooth cartilage surface better compared with constructs seeded with chondrocytes, which produced fibrocartilage-like tissue with a discontinuous superficial cartilage contour.

Obtaining enough chondrocytes to effect a clinical change is challenging, and, eventually, the use of amniotic stem cells may offer a solution. Amnion has been shown to contain large numbers of cells that are able to be manipulated to differentiate into chondrocytes with the addition of bone morphogenetic proteins (BMPs), such as BMP-2. BMPs are widely available and are immunologically privileged, which should minimize host rejection response in their use as allografts.

More experienced orthopaedic surgeons will appreciate the tremendous decline in the surgical treatment of patients with rheumatoid arthritis as the result of monumental advances in disease-modifying antirheumatic drugs (DMARDs). The search for similar drugs to manage osteoarthritis is accelerating because the medical management of osteoarthritis has moved beyond the use of traditional anti-inflammatory and pain-relieving medications to true disease-modifying technologies. DMARDs are used with the goal of modifying chondrocyte metabolism and thereby affecting matrix degradation. Examples of DMARDs are antiapoptotic agents, poloxamer (P188), caspase inhibitors, doxycycline, and risedronate. Although the clinical application of DMARDs to manage osteoarthritis is not yet a reality, basic science research in this area is promising.

 ## Nanotechnology

The use of polymer nanofibers has tremendous potential in musculoskeletal regenerative medicine. Structural composition at this size allows for fiber orientation and matrix structural properties that mimic the native biologic milieu. For example, one challenge in tendon-to-bone healing is the tremendous mechanical mismatch in the transition zone of the two tissues. Bone has a modulus of approximately 20 GPa, whereas the modulus of tendon is closer to 200 MPa. Nanofiber technology offers a scaffold structure that mimics this transition zone, which may provide a truly anatomic approach for tendon-to-bone healing. Recent studies have shown that the structural properties of these scaffolds can manipulate cells to produce certain types of extracellular matrix. In a study of the effect of fiber size on human tendon fibroblasts, the use of polymer nanofibers resulted in a higher cell number and greater proliferation of total collagen and proteoglycan production compared with the use of microfibers. In addition, tendon fibroblasts have been shown to adhere and proliferate on electrospun nanofiber scaffolds. These scaffolds can add strength, act as growth factor delivery systems to stimulate the tenocyte, and approximate the native tendon/bone anatomic transition zone to improve healing and regenerative properties in vivo. The use of nanotechnology for scaffolding, delivering drugs and growth factors, and structural recreation of biologic structures has the potential to transform shoulder reconstruction into shoulder regeneration.

 ## Computer-Assisted Navigation

Typically, the goal of shoulder reconstruction is to restore a patient's anatomy to a state as close as possible to the native, pre-diseased condition. This can be challenging because native anatomy is variable and difficult to ascertain on standard imaging. The discovery that tuberosity malposition is among the most important risk factors for unsatisfactory outcomes after proximal humerus fracture has led to an increased emphasis on anatomic restoration of the tuberosities after open reduction and internal fixation and after hemiarthroplasty. Subsequently, a computer-assisted technique was designed to optimize reduction of the tuberosities, and more accurate restoration of anatomy was achieved with this technology compared with traditional methods.

In total shoulder arthroplasty, improper positioning of the glenoid component can lead to loosening, instability, and premature wear. Reliable intraoperative anatomic landmarks for the placement of the glenoid component are lacking. Even with modern surgical technique performed by highly trained arthroplasty surgeons, glenoid version malpositioning of 7° to 12° has been reported. Recently, efforts have been directed toward developing a computer-assisted navigation system that can improve accuracy in all phases of glenoid implantation. In one published study, glenoid version was substantially improved with the aid of computer navigation. The authors of a separate study reported that surgeons were highly consistent in their use of this technique, and concluded that preoperative planning using three-dimensional modeling and computer navigation can improve implant positioning.

An improved understanding of anatomy is spurring research in the area of patient-specific instrumentation. In approximately 40% of patients who are treated with reverse shoulder arthroplasty, glenoid morphology is found to be abnormal. The placement of the glenoid along the anatomic center line may not be possible, and it may be necessary to direct the glenoid on an alternative path to achieve adequate fixation. Although computer-assisted navigation can help design this path preoperatively, translation of this technology into the operating room can be time-consuming and technically demanding. With patient-matched instrumentation, the preoperative computer-assisted technology can be used to design drill guides that match individual anatomy based on preoperatively determined anatomic reference points. In a randomized clinical trial evaluating the clinical accuracy of patient-specific instrumentation, the technology was found to be most effective in patients with substantial retroversion. The use of patient-specific instrumentation resulted in 9° greater accuracy compared with the use of traditional surgical techniques. The accuracy of patient-specific instrumentation was recently validated in a reverse shoulder arthroplasty model. The authors of that study demonstrated improved accuracy and a nearly 20% reduction in intraoperative time with patient-specific instrumentation compared with intraoperative computer-assisted navigation. Further study is required to determine the threshold at which improved accuracy in positioning translates into improved clinical outcomes and the cost-effectiveness of these tools.

 ## Conclusion

The field of shoulder reconstruction continues to evolve at an accelerated pace. In the future, shoulder surgeons will be able to incorporate the translational sciences that combine biologic augmentation with reconstructive approaches. Such a combination may allow the evolution from reconstructive to regenerative approaches to the shoulder. The authors of this chapter look forward to reports of new and innovative techniques and technologies in the next edition of this publication.

Bibliography

Barber FA, Hrnack SA, Snyder SJ, Hapa O: Rotator cuff repair healing influenced by platelet-rich plasma construct augmentation. *Arthroscopy* 2011;27(8):1029-1035.

Bergeson AG, Tashjian RZ, Greis PE, Crim J, Stoddard GJ, Burks RT: Effects of platelet-rich fibrin matrix on repair integrity of at-risk rotator cuff tears. *Am J Sports Med* 2012;40(2):286-293.

Bicknell RT, DeLude JA, Kedgley AE, et al: Early experience with computer-assisted shoulder hemiarthroplasty for fractures of the proximal humerus: Development of a novel technique and an in vitro comparison with traditional methods. *J Shoulder Elbow Surg* 2007;16(3 suppl):S117-S125.

Boileau P, Krishnan SG, Tinsi L, Walch G, Coste JS, Molé D: Tuberosity malposition and migration: Reasons for poor outcomes after hemiarthroplasty for displaced fractures of the proximal humerus. *J Shoulder Elbow Surg* 2002;11(5):401-412.

Boileau P, Walch G: The three-dimensional geometry of the proximal humerus: Implications for surgical technique and prosthetic design. *J Bone Joint Surg Br* 1997;79(5):857-865.

Bokor DJ, O'Sullivan MD, Hazan GJ: Variability of measurement of glenoid version on computed tomography scan. *J Shoulder Elbow Surg* 1999;8(6):595-598.

Castricini R, Longo UG, De Benedetto M, et al: Platelet-rich plasma augmentation for arthroscopic rotator cuff repair: A randomized controlled trial. *Am J Sports Med* 2011;39(2):258-265.

Chahal J, Van Thiel GS, Mall N, et al: The role of platelet-rich plasma in arthroscopic rotator cuff repair: A systematic review with quantitative synthesis. *Arthroscopy* 2012;28(11):1718-1727.

Chen H, Sun J, Hoemann CD, et al: Drilling and microfracture lead to different bone structure and necrosis during bone-marrow stimulation for cartilage repair. *J Orthop Res* 2009;27(11):1432-1438.

Cyprien JM, Vasey HM, Burdet A, Bonvin JC, Kritsikis N, Vuagnat P: Humeral retrotorsion and glenohumeral relationship in the normal shoulder and in recurrent anterior dislocation (scapulometry). *Clin Orthop Relat Res* 1983;(175):8-17.

Erisken C, Zhang X, Moffat KL, Levine WN, Lu HH: Scaffold fiber diameter regulates human tendon fibroblast growth and differentiation. *Tissue Eng Part A* 2013;19(3-4):519-528.

Farr J, Cole B, Dhawan A, Kercher J, Sherman S: Clinical cartilage restoration: Evolution and overview. *Clin Orthop Relat Res* 2011;469(10):2696-2705.

Frankle MA, Teramoto A, Luo ZP, Levy JC, Pupello D: Glenoid morphology in reverse shoulder arthroplasty: Classification and surgical implications. *J Shoulder Elbow Surg* 2009;18(6):874-885.

Gerber C, Meyer DC, Frey E, et al: Neer Award 2007: Reversion of structural muscle changes caused by chronic rotator cuff tears using continuous musculotendinous traction: An experimental study in sheep. *J Shoulder Elbow Surg* 2009;18(2):163-171.

Gerber C, Meyer DC, Nuss KM, Farshad M: Anabolic steroids reduce muscle damage caused by rotator cuff tendon release in an experimental study in rabbits. *J Bone Joint Surg Am* 2011;93(23):2189-2195.

Gerber C, Meyer DC, Von Rechenberg B, Hoppeler H, Frigg R, Farshad M: Rotator cuff muscles lose responsiveness to anabolic steroids after tendon tear and musculotendinous retraction: An experimental study in sheep. *Am J Sports Med* 2012;40(11):2454-2461.

Hendel MD, Bryan JA, Barsoum WK, et al: Comparison of patient-specific instruments with standard surgical instruments in determining glenoid component position: A randomized prospective clinical trial. *J Bone Joint Surg Am* 2012;94(23):2167-2175.

Jo CH, Kim JE, Yoon KS, et al: Does platelet-rich plasma accelerate recovery after rotator cuff repair? A prospective cohort study. *Am J Sports Med* 2011;39(10):2082-2090.

Jo CH, Shin JS, Lee YG, et al: Platelet-rich plasma for arthroscopic repair of large to massive rotator cuff tears: A randomized, single-blind, parallel-group trial. *Am J Sports Med* 2013;41(10):2240-2248.

Kähäri VM, Larjava H, Uitto J: Differential regulation of extracellular matrix proteoglycan (PG) gene expression: Transforming growth factor-beta 1 up-regulates biglycan (PGI), and versican (large fibroblast PG) but down-regulates decorin (PGII) mRNA levels in human fibroblasts in culture. *J Biol Chem* 1991;266(16):10608-10615.

Karduna AR, Williams GR, Iannotti JP, Williams JL: Total shoulder arthroplasty biomechanics: A study of the forces and strains at the glenoid component. *J Biomech Eng* 1998;120(1):92-99.

Levy JC, Everding NG, Frankle MA, Keppler LJ: Accuracy of patient-specific guided glenoid baseplate positioning for reverse shoulder arthroplasty. *J Shoulder Elbow Surg* 2014;23(10):1563-1567.

Ma B, Xie J, Jiang J, Shuler FD, Bartlett DE: Rational design of nanofiber scaffolds for orthopedic tissue repair and regeneration. *Nanomedicine (Lond)* 2013;8(9):1459-1481.

Mazor M, Lespessailles E, Coursier R, Daniellou R, Best TM, Toumi H: Mesenchymal stem-cell potential in cartilage repair: An update. *J Cell Mol Med* 2014;18(12):2340-2350.

Menetrey J, Kasemkijwattana C, Day CS, et al: Growth factors improve muscle healing in vivo. *J Bone Joint Surg Br* 2000;82(1):131-137.

Moran CJ, Pascual-Garrido C, Chubinskaya S, et al: Restoration of articular cartilage. *J Bone Joint Surg Am* 2014;96(4):336-344.

Nguyen D, Ferreira LM, Brownhill JR, et al: Improved accuracy of computer assisted glenoid implantation in total shoulder arthroplasty: An in-vitro randomized controlled trial. *J Shoulder Elbow Surg* 2009;18(6):907-914.

Nguyen D, Ferreira LM, Brownhill JR, Faber KJ, Johnson JA: Design and development of a computer assisted glenoid implantation technique for shoulder replacement surgery. *Comput Aided Surg* 2007;12(3):152-159.

Randelli P, Arrigoni P, Ragone V, Aliprandi A, Cabitza P: Platelet rich plasma in arthroscopic rotator cuff repair: A prospective RCT study, 2-year follow-up. *J Shoulder Elbow Surg* 2011;20(4):518-528.

Smith L, Xia Y, Galatz LM, Genin GM, Thomopoulos S: Tissue-engineering strategies for the tendon/ligament-to-bone insertion. *Connect Tissue Res* 2012;53(2):95-105.

Tay LX, Ahmad RE, Dashtdar H, et al: Treatment outcomes of alginate-embedded allogenic mesenchymal stem cells versus autologous chondrocytes for the repair of focal articular cartilage defects in a rabbit model. *Am J Sports Med* 2012;40(1):83-90.

Thomopoulos S, Genin GM, Galatz LM: The development and morphogenesis of the tendon-to-bone insertion: What development can teach us about healing. *J Musculoskelet Neuronal Interact* 2010;10(1):35-45.

Verborgt O, De Smedt T, Vanhees M, Clockaerts S, Parizel PM, Van Glabbeek F: Accuracy of placement of the glenoid component in reversed shoulder arthroplasty with and without navigation. *J Shoulder Elbow Surg* 2011;20(1):21-26.

Warren RF, Coleman SH, Dines JS: Instability after arthroplasty: The shoulder. *J Arthroplasty* 2002;17(4 suppl 1):28-31.

Wei JP, Nawata M, Wakitani S, et al: Human amniotic mesenchymal cells differentiate into chondrocytes. *Cloning Stem Cells* 2009;11(1):19-26.

Williams GR Jr, Wong KL, Pepe MD, et al: The effect of articular malposition after total shoulder arthroplasty on glenohumeral translations, range of motion, and subacromial impingement. *J Shoulder Elbow Surg* 2001;10(5):399-409.

Wright-Carpenter T, Opolon P, Appell HJ, Meijer H, Wehling P, Mir LM: Treatment of muscle injuries by local administration of autologous conditioned serum: Animal experiments using a muscle contusion model. *Int J Sports Med* 2004;25(8):582-587.

Xie J, Li X, Lipner J, et al: "Aligned-to-random" nanofiber scaffolds for mimicking the structure of the tendon-to-bone insertion site. *Nanoscale* 2010;2(6):923-926.

Index

Page numbers with *f* indicate figures;
page numbers with *t* indicate tables

A

Achilles tendon allograft
    for anterior capsule and subscapularis reconstruction,
        133–134, 134*f*, 135*f*
    for massive irreparable RCTs, 277, 277*f*
    MDI and, 162, 164, 167, 168*f*
    for prosthetic instability after shoulder arthroplasty, 499
    reconstruction, 133, 135*f*
AC joint. *See* Acromioclavicular joint
Acromial arch, Bigliani type 2, 187
Acromial fracture, 451, 493
Acromioclavicular (AC) joint, 321*f*, 322*f*
    arthropathy in, 335
    arthrosis, 631–632
    capsule, 41
    OA, 322*f*
    procedures of, arthroscopic portals for, 16
    repair and reconstruction of
        rehabilitation, 351, 352*t*
        surgical methods, 347
        surgical procedure for, 348–350, 348*f*, 349*f*, 350*f*,
            351*f*, 352*f*
        types of injury, 345, 346*f*
    separation of
        injury classification, 633–635, 636*t*
        management results of, 637, 638*t*
        rehabilitation for, 639, 640*f*, 640*t*
        semitendinosus autograft anatomic reconstruction
            for, 637–639, 639*f*
        subperiosteal dissection for, 637
        treatment options, 636–637
    subacromial space and, 378
Acromiohumeral interval, 254
Acromion, ossification of, 333
Acromioplasty, 10
    for articular-sided tear, in overhead throwing athlete,
        229*t*
    avoidance of, 15
    for bursal-sided tear, 229*t*
        with acromial spurring, 233
    concomitant, 233
    for glenohumeral OA, 378, 381*t*, 384
    for os acromiale, 337, 338*t*, 341*t*
    with TSA, 426
Adhesive capsulitis
    arthroscopic capsular release for
        procedure for, 369–370, 369*f*, 370*f*, 371*f*

rehabilitation for, 370–371, 371*t*
    results of, 368, 368*t*
  with comma sign, 304
  as complication of
    pectoralis major tendon transfer, 693
    STF, 709
  diagnostic arthroscopy for, 369
  lateral release and, 305
Allografts
  Achilles tendon
    for anterior capsule and subscapularis, 133–134,
        134*f*, 135*f*
    for massive irreparable RCTs, 277, 277*f*
    MDI and, 162, 164, 167, 168*f*
    for prosthetic instability after shoulder arthroplasty,
        499
    reconstruction, 133, 135*f*
  for anterior instability resulting from severe humeral
    bone loss, 112–118, 116*t*, 117*f*
  bulk, for failed shoulder arthroplasty, 511
  deltopectoral approach for, 176
  distal tibia, 83, 84*t*
    for anterior instability, 85–87
    for GBL, 85–86
  femoral head, 709, 711*t*
    bulk, 510–512
    for glenoid defects, 475*f*
    impacted, 467*f*
  human dermal, for open capsular repair, 92, 92*f*
  of humeral head, 112*f*
  for MDI, in patients with Ehlers-Danlos syndrome, 167
  meniscal
    glenoid resurfacing and, 394
    lateral, 392
  for prosthetic instability after shoulder arthroplasty,
    498–499, 502*t*
Anterior capsular plication, 153
Anterior capsule and subscapularis reconstruction,
  Achilles tendon allograft for, 133–134, 134*f*, 135*f*
Anterior dislocations, closed reduction for, 131
Anterior glenohumeral stabilization, 11*t*
Anterior glenoid rim fractures, 684. *See also* Glenoid rim
  fractures
Anterior shoulder instability, 58*f*
  arthroscopic Bankart repair for
    equipment, 60
    exposure, 60, 61*f*
    procedure, 60–63, 61*f*, 62*f*, 63*f*
    rehabilitation, 63, 64*t*
    results of, 59–60, 59–60*t*
  with moderate GBL, 70*f*, 71*f*, 72*f*, 73*f*
    procedure for, 73–77, 74*f*, 75*f*, 76*f*

for frozen shoulder, 384
of glenohumeral OA, 384, 384*f*
Capsular repair, 69
open with human dermal allograft, 92, 92*f*
posterior, 441, 443
Capsular shift
anterior, rehabilitation for, 169*t*
anteroinferior, 62, 231
arthroscopic, 160
for MDI, 162–163
Bankart repair and, 112
open, 91
humerally based, 35*t*, 164
inferior, 100, 149, 162, 165*f*, 166*f*, 167*f*
Neer and Foster, 167
open, 123, 160
open inferior, 147, 162
plication and, 152
posterior, rehabilitation for, 169*t*
posterior-inferior, 34
for posterior labral repair, 177
reduction of capsular volume with, 166
Capsular stretching
posterior, 123, 238
tendon pull-off and, 167
Capsulorrhaphy
posterior, 34, 35*t*, 36, 37*f*, 38, 153*f*, 500
open, 35, 147–154, 149*f*, 152*f*, 153*f*, 154*f*
thermal, 39, 71, 160
C-arm fluoroscope, 382*f*, 544, 558*f*
Cartilage
damage to, 728
transplantation of, 728
Catheter, scalene, 371
Cavitation, 567
CC ligament. *See* Coracoclavicular ligament
Cephalic vein, 13*t*
Cerebral oxygenation, 6
during beach-chair position, 5
Cerebrovascular accident, 702
Cervical disk, herniated, 702
Cervical spine, 3
Chondrolysis, 718
drug-induced, 369
glenohumeral, 160
for glenohumeral joint, 160
Chronic glenohumeral dislocation, shoulder
arthroplasty for
anatomic, 136*f*, 140–142, 142*f*
patient evaluation, 131–132, 133*f*, 134*f*, 135*f*, 136*f*
physical examination for, 132
rehabilitation for, 143, 143*t*
results, 138–140, 139–140*t*
reverse, 137–138, 138*f*, 142–143

Clavicle, distal
excision of, 11*t*
osteolysis, 321, 323, 324*t*, 640
Clavicle fractures, 604*f*
distal. *See* Distal clavicle fractures
fixation of, 683–684
medial intramedullary fixation of, 627
middle third, intramedullary fixation of, 614*f*, 615–616, 616*f*
flexible, 616
implant removal for, 627
procedure for, 619–627, 622*f*, 623*f*, 624*f*, 626*f*
rehabilitation for, 627, 628*t*
results of, 617–619, 618–619*t*
rigid, 616–617
types of, 616, 617*f*
middle third, plate-and-screw fixation of, 614–615
ORIF of
anterior *versus* superior plating, 604–605
exposure, 605–606, 606*f*
hardware failure, 609
infection and, 609
intramedullary nailing *versus* plating, 604
intraoperative vascular injury, 609
nonunion and, 608
procedure for, 606–607, 606*f*
rehabilitation for, 607–608, 607*t*
results of, 605, 605*t*
setup for, 605, 606*f*
technique, 604*f*, 606*f*, 608
traumatic, 415
Clavipectoral fascia, 26, 29*f*, 115, 164
dense, 13
division of, 181
identification of, 427
incision of, 140
release of, 545
Closed reduction
for anterior dislocations, 131
failure of, 497
intramedullary nailing and, 534
with percutaneous pin fixation, 540, 557
Cobb elevator, 457
Collagen disorders, open surgical revision in MDI and, 159
allograft procedure in patients with Ehlers-Danlos syndrome, 167
anterior approach, 167–168, 169*t*
diagnosis after failed surgical management of, 161–162
nonsurgical treatment for, 162
posterior approach, 168, 169*t*
reasons for failed surgical repair of, 159–161
rehabilitation for, 168–169, 170*t*
results of, 163–164, 164*t*
surgical treatment for, 162–163, 164–165, 165–167, 165*f*, 166*f*, 167*f*

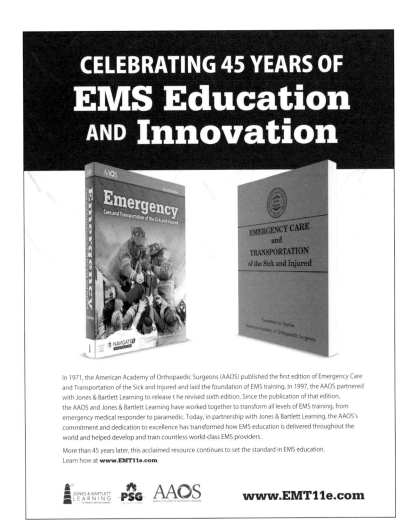
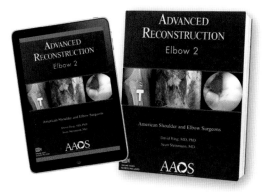
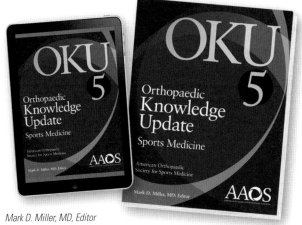

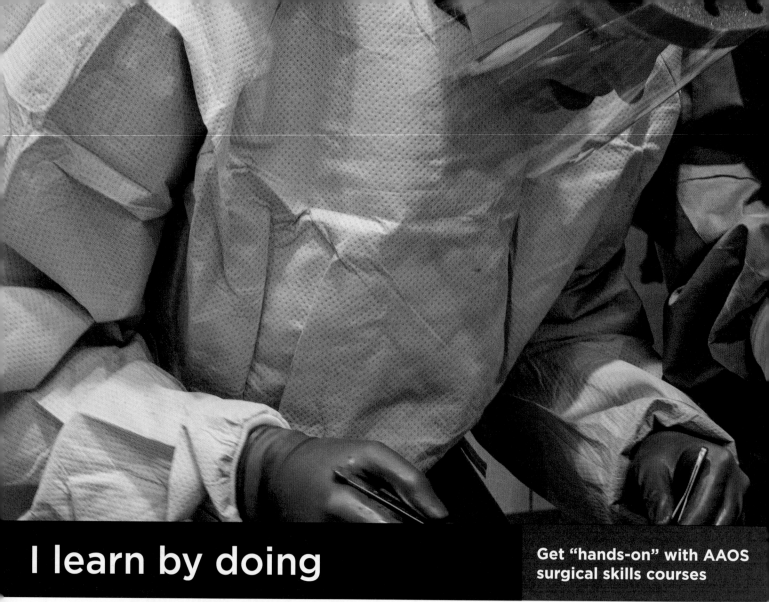

I learn by doing

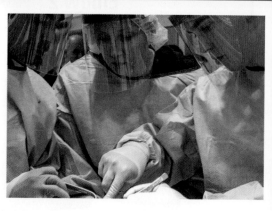
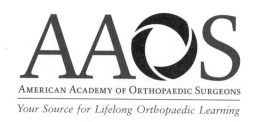